J. B. Lippincott Company
Philadelphia
London Mexico City New York
St. Louis São Paulo Sydney

Breast Disea

Breast Diseases

Edited by

Jay R. Harris, M.D.

Associate Professor
Department of Radiation Therapy
Harvard Medical School
Clinical Director
Joint Center for Radiation Therapy
Boston, Massachusetts

Samuel Hellman, M.D.

Physician-in-Chief
Incumbent of the Benno C. Schmidt
Chair in Clinical Oncology
Memorial Sloan-Kettering Cancer Center
New York, New York

I. Craig Henderson, M.D.

Associate Professor of Medicine
Harvard Medical School
Medical Coordinator
Breast Evaluation Center
Division of Medical Oncology
Dana-Farber Cancer Institute
Boston, Massachusetts

David W. Kinne, M.D.

Attending Surgeon
Chief, Breast Service
Memorial Sloan-Kettering
Cancer Center
Associate Professor of Surgery
Cornell University Medical College
New York, New York

51 Contributors

Developmental Editor: Richard Winters
Manuscript Editor: Patrick O'Kane
Indexer: Sandra King
Art Director: Tracy Baldwin
Production Coordinator: Charlene Catlett Squibb
Compositor: Ruttle, Shaw & Wetherill
Printer/Binder: Halliday Lithograph

6 5 4 3 2 1

Library of Congress Cataloging-in-Publication Data

Breast diseases

Includes bibliographies and index.
1. Breast—Diseases. I. Harris, Jay R. [DNLM:
1. Breast Diseases. WP 840 B8283]
RG491.B742 1987 618.1′9 86-15328
ISBN 0-397-50760-7

The authors and publisher have exerted every effort to ensure that drug selection and dosage set forth in this text are in accord with current recommendations and practice at the time of publication. However, in view of ongoing research, changes in government regulations, and the constant flow of information relating to drug therapy and drug reactions, the reader is urged to check the package insert for each drug for any change in indications and dosage and for added warnings and precautions. This is particularly important when the recommended agent is a new or infrequently employed drug.

Contributors

Laurie J. Bauman, Ph.D
Research Associate
Department of Social Work
Memorial Sloan-Kettering Cancer Center
New York, New York

John Bostwick III, M.D.
Professor of Surgery
Division of Plastic Surgery
Department of Surgery
Emory University School of Medicine
Atlanta, Georgia

Mary Ellen Bowles, M.S.W.
Social Worker and Research Associate
Breast Service
Memorial Sloan-Kettering Cancer Center
New York, New York

Blake Cady, M.D.
Associate Professor of Surgery
Harvard Medical School
Chief, Surgical Oncology
New England Deaconess Hospital
Boston, Massachusetts

George P. Canellos, M.D.
Professor of Medicine
Harvard Medical School
Chief, Division of Medical Oncology
Dana-Farber Cancer Institute
Physician, Brigham & Women's Hospital
Boston, Massachusetts

Grace H. Christ, M.S.W.
Director of Social Work
Memorial Sloan-Kettering Cancer Center
New York, New York

Steven E. Come, M.D.
Director, Hematology-Oncology Ambulatory Unit
Beth Israel Hospital
Assistant Professor of Medicine
Harvard Medical School
Boston, Massachusetts

James L. Connolly, M.D.
Associate Pathologist
Beth Israel Hospital
Assistant Professor of Pathology
Harvard Medical School
Consultant in Pathology
Dana-Farber Cancer Institute
Boston, Massachusetts

Charles N. Cornell, M.D.
Associate Professor of Orthopedic Surgery
Cornell University Medical Center
Associate Attending Orthopedic Surgeon
The Hospital for Special Surgery
New York, New York

Stephen P. Ethier, Ph.D.
Assistant Member
Michigan Cancer Foundation
Detroit, Michigan

Edward L. Feldman, M.D.
Director, Retina Unit
Beth Israel Hospital
Associate Staff
Massachusetts Eye and Ear Infirmary
Clinical Assistant in Ophthalmology
Harvard Medical School
Boston, Massachusetts

Jack Fishman, Ph.D.
Professor, Laboratory of Biochemical Endocrinology
The Rockefeller University
New York, New York

Kathleen M. Foley, M.D.
Associate Professor of Neurology and Pharmacology
Cornell University Medical College
Chief, Pain Service
Associate Attending Neurologist
Department of Neurology
Memorial Sloan-Kettering Cancer Center
New York, New York

Rebecca Gelman, Ph.D.
Associate Professor of Biostatistics
Harvard School of Public Health
Dana-Farber Cancer Institute
Boston, Massachusetts

J. Peter Glass, M.D.
Associate Professor of Clinical Neurology
The University of Texas System Cancer Center
M.D. Anderson Hospital & Tumor Institute
Houston, Texas

Stacey M. Gore, M.D.
Clinical Fellow
Division of Hematology-Oncology
Beth Israel Hospital
Instructor in Medicine
Harvard Medical School
Boston, Massachusetts

Frank E. Gump, M.D.
Professor of Surgery
Columbia University College of Physicians and Surgeons
Chief, Breast Service
Columbia-Presbyterian Medical Center
New York, New York

Jay R. Harris, M.D.
Associate Professor
Department of Radiation Therapy
Harvard Medical School
Clinical Director
Joint Center for Radiation Therapy
Boston, Massachusetts

Daniel F. Hayes, M.D.
Instructor in Medicine
Dana-Farber Cancer Institute
Harvard Medical School
Boston, Massachusetts

Samuel Hellman, M.D.
Physician-in-Chief
Incumbent of the Benno C. Schmidt Chair in Clinical Oncology
Memorial Sloan-Kettering Cancer Center
New York, New York

I. Craig Henderson, M.D.
Associate Professor of Medicine
Harvard Medical School
Medical Coordinator
Breast Evaluation Center
Division of Medical Oncology
Dana-Farber Cancer Institute
Boston, Massachusetts

W. David Henner, M.D., Ph.D.
Assistant Professor of Medicine
Harvard Medical School
Dana-Farber Cancer Institute
Boston, Massachusetts

Gloria H. Heppner, Ph.D.
Senior Vice-President
Michigan Cancer Foundation
Detroit, Michigan

Jimmie C. Holland, M.D.
Chief, Psychiatry Service
Memorial Sloan-Kettering Cancer Center
Professor of Psychiatry
Cornell University Medical Center
New York, New York

Susan McKenney Keohan, R.N., M.S.N.
Coordinator, Breast Evaluation Center
Dana-Farber Cancer Institute
Boston, Massachusetts

David W. Kinne, M.D.
Attending Surgeon
Chief, Breast Service
Memorial Sloan-Kettering Cancer Center
Associate Professor of Surgery
Cornell University Medical College
New York, New York

Daniel B. Kopans, M.D.
Associate Professor of Radiology
Harvard Medical School
Director of Breast Imaging
Assistant Director of Ambulatory Care Radiology
Massachusetts General Hospital
Boston, Massachusetts

Joseph M. Lane, M.D.
Professor of Orthopedic Surgery
Cornell University Medical College
Chief Attending Surgeon, Orthopedic Oncology
Memorial Sloan-Kettering Cancer Center
Chief Associate Attending
Metabolic Bone Disease
Hospital for Special Surgery
New York, New York

Susan M. Love, M.D., F.A.C.S.
Director of Breast Clinic
Beth Israel Hospital
Surgical Oncologist
Dana-Farber Cancer Institute
Clinical Instructor
Harvard Medical School
Boston, Massachusetts

Beryl McCormick, M.D.
Assistant Attending Radiation Oncologist
Memorial Sloan-Kettering Cancer Center
New York, New York

Anthony B. Miller, M.D.
Professor, Department of Preventive Medicine and Biostatistics
University of Toronto
Toronto, Ontario, Canada

C. Kent Osborne, M.D.
Professor of Medicine
University of Texas Health Science Center
Attending Physician
Medical Center Hospital
San Antonio, Texas

Michael P. Osborne, M.D., M.S., F.R.C.S., F.A.C.S.
Assistant Attending Surgeon
Memorial Hospital for Cancer & Allied Diseases
Assistant Member
Department of Surgery
Memorial Sloan-Kettering Cancer Center
Associate Professor of Surgery
Cornell University Medical College
Visiting Associate Physician
The Rockefeller University Hospital
Adjunct Faculty Member
The Rockefeller University
New York, New York

Robert T. Osteen, M.D.
Department of Surgery/Oncology
Brigham & Women's Hospital
Assistant Physician in Surgical Oncology
University Health Services at Harvard Medical School
Boston, Massachusetts

Leroy M. Parker, M.D.
Assistant Professor of Medicine
Harvard Medical School
Assistant Physician in Medicine
Dana-Farber Cancer Institute
Associate Physician
Brigham & Women's Hospital
Boston, Massachusetts
Chief of Medical Oncology
Norwood Hospital
Norwood, Massachusetts
Chief of Medical Oncology
Southwood Community Hospital
Norfolk, Massachusetts

W. Bradford Patterson, M.D.
Visiting Professor of Surgery
Harvard Medical School
Chief, Division of Cancer Control
Dana-Farber Cancer Institute
Boston, Massachusetts

Jeanne A. Petrek, M.D.
Assistant Attending Surgeon
Memorial Sloan-Kettering Cancer Center
Assistant Professor of Surgery
Cornell University Medical College
Visiting Associate Physician
The Rockefeller University Hospital
Adjunct Faculty Member
The Rockefeller University
New York, New York

Abram Recht, M.D.
Assistant Professor of Radiation Therapy
Harvard Medical School
Staff Radiation Therapist
Joint Center for Radiation Therapy
Clinical Associate
Breast Evaluation Clinic
Dana-Farber Cancer Institute
Boston, Massachusetts

Mary Ann Rose, M.D.
Instructor, Harvard Medical School
Staff Radiation Therapist
Joint Center for Radiation Therapy
Clinical Associate
Breast Evaluation Clinic
Dana-Farber Cancer Institute
Boston, Massachusetts

Paul Peter Rosen, M.D.
Attending Pathologist
Department of Pathology
Memorial Sloan-Kettering Cancer Center
New York, New York

Julia H. Rowland, Ph.D.
Clinical Assistant
Psychiatry Service
Memorial Sloan-Kettering Cancer Center
Instructor of Psychology
Department of Psychiatry
Cornell University Medical College
New York, New York

Lowell E. Schnipper, M.D.
Chief, Oncology Division
Beth Israel Hospital
Associate Professor of Medicine
Harvard Medical School
Boston, Massachusetts

Stuart J. Schnitt, M.D.
Instructor in Pathology
Harvard Medical School
Associate in Pathology
Beth Israel Hospital
Consultant in Pathology
Dana-Farber Cancer Institute
Boston, Massachusetts

Thomas A. Sheldon, M.D.
Instructor, Joint Center for Radiation Therapy
Harvard Medical School
Boston, Massachusetts
Staff Radiation Therapist
Elliot Hospital
Manchester, New Hampshire

Robert L. Shirley, M.D.
Assistant Clinical Professor of Obstetrics and Gynecology
Harvard Medical School
Senior Staff Obstetrician and Gynecologist
Brigham & Women's Hospital
Staff Member
Dana-Farber Cancer Institute
Boston, Massachusetts

Sumner A. Slavin, M.D.
Clinical Instructor in Plastic Surgery
Harvard Medical School
Boston, Massachusetts

Ian E. Smith, M.D., F.R.C.P. (Edin)
Honorary Senior Lecturer
Institute of Cancer Research
Consultant Medical Oncologist
Royal Marsden Hospital
London, England

Mark J. Stillman, M.D.
Research Fellow
Department of Neurology
Memorial Sloan-Kettering Cancer Center
Cornell University Medical College
New York, New York

Mark E. Weinstein, M.D.
Instructor in Surgery
Harvard Medical School
Associate Surgeon
Beth Israel Hospital
Boston, Massachusetts

Wick R. Williams, Ph.D.
Associate Epidemiologist
Fox Chase Cancer Center
Philadelphia, Pennsylvania

Marvin Zelen, Ph.D.
Professor and Chairman
Department of Biostatistics
Harvard School of Public Health
Chief of Division of Biostatistics and Epidemiology
Dana-Farber Cancer Institute
Boston, Massachusetts

Foreword

The past twenty years have witnessed a startling revolution in the diagnosis and treatment of diseases of the breast. Mammography has clearly enabled the detection of some lesions at a much earlier stage than was previously possible. Pathologists have participated in this upheaval by sharpening the criteria for the microscopic diagnosis of both premalignant and malignant lesions. Perhaps of greatest importance has been the realization that the classical Halstedian radical mastectomy does not offer more prolonged or more frequent survival than less mutilating alternatives such as local excision combined with radiotherapy. This revelation, ultimately brought to full fruition by the advent of prospective randomized trials in Milan and in the United States, has led also to a full reconsideration of the biology of breast cancer. The concept of orderly progression of cancer from the breast to axillary lymph nodes prior to wider dissemination, a thesis upon which the radical mastectomy was based, has given way to an understanding that invasive breast cancer is very often already a systemic disease at the time of discovery, especially when the axillary lymph nodes are found to be involved. The demonstration of the efficacy of adjuvant chemotherapy offers new hope for improved outcome in treatment, and finally the effectiveness of these chemotherapeutic agents and of tamoxifen in advanced breast cancer has completely eliminated the use of oophorectomy and adrenalectomy.

It is in this setting that *Breast Diseases* has been launched by the many who have played an important role in bringing about this revolution. The book offers its readers a comprehensive and definitive work on all diseases of the breast with particular emphasis on breast cancer. It will provide much to all students of diseases of the breast whether they be surgeons, oncologists, radiotherapists, pathologists, or generalists. I know of no persons better able to describe the current state of the art than the authors of this fine book.

William Silen, M.D.

Preface

Perhaps the diseases and treatment of no other organ have had more manifold significance for our culture than those of the breast. Mammary cancer has been described in many cultures and can even be found recorded in early Egyptian hieroglyphics. Not only is breast cancer important because of its frequency and clinical implications, the breast itself has important cultural significance. In certain contexts it is a symbol of motherhood, nourishment, and security while in others it represents beauty and femininity. The trauma of loss of the breast has been vividly presented in the martyrdom of St. Agatha, who for refusing the sexual advances of a Roman general was punished by bilateral breast amputation. This strong symbolic and emotional context has made the discussion of the management of breast diseases difficult, heated, and sometimes contentious.

Within recent years the physiology of the breast has become better understood. The normal physiologic conditions of the breast, various benign diseases, and breast cancer have been clearly separated. The significance, prognosis, relation to breast cancer, and treatment of these benign diseases and conditions have been elucidated. Epidemiological studies have shown marked differences in the incidence of breast cancer within populations and within a variety of physiological states. These findings have suggested hypotheses as to the etiology and natural history of breast cancer. Increased patient awareness and the development of screening mammography have resulted in earlier diagnosis of the disease.

In this past century, medicine has made important therapeutic advances. Breast cancer treatment has become the paradigm for cancer treatment. The radical en bloc dissection described by Halsted and Meyers was based on the notion of predictable centrifugal spread. Although it resulted in improved results for many, physicians were frustrated by the all-too-frequent appearance of distant metastases despite proper application of this important regional technique. With changes in our understanding of the natural history of breast cancer and the development of effective radiation therapy, breast-preserving surgical procedures combined with radiation have resulted in an acceptable alternative to mastectomy. Adjuvant chemotherapy and hormonal therapy have been applied successfully first in the adult in the management of primary breast cancer. Advanced breast cancer has also been shown to be amenable to hormonal manipulation, chemotherapy, and radiation therapy.

The developments in our understanding of the disease and the variety of treatments available have provided major roles for the surgeon, medical oncologist, radiation oncologist, diagnostic radiologist, and pathologist. The primary care physician and gynecologist have had increasing roles in early diagnosis and in counseling the high-risk patient. These diverse treatment options necessitate a coordinated, cohesive, multidisciplinary approach. This book is an attempt to present our current understanding of breast diseases and treatments in such a multidisciplinary context. We have attempted to provide primary data whenever possible in order to allow the reader the opportunity to judge the conclusions presented. While the contributors to this book are from a number of institutions, the editors and a large majority are from two institutions: Harvard Medical School and the Memorial Sloan-Kettering Cancer Center. This is intended to present both a multidisciplinary and a coherent approach to breast diseases.

Jay R. Harris, M.D.

Samuel Hellman, M.D.

I. Craig Henderson, M.D.

David W. Kinne, M.D.

Contents

The color illustrations are to be found between pages 80 and 81.

Breast Development and Anatomy

1

Michael P. Osborne

The breasts, or mammary glands, of mammals are important for the survival of the newborn and thus of the species. Nursing of the young in the animal kingdom has many physiological advantages for the mother, such as aiding postpartum uterine involution, as well as for the neonate in terms of the transfer of immunity and bonding. In humans, social influences have reduced the prevalence of breastfeeding of neonates, and may have interfered with its physiological role. Recently, it has become increasingly apparent that the advantages of nursing are substantial for both mother and child.

An understanding of the morphology and physiology of the breast and the many endocrine interrelationships of both is essential to the study of the pathophysiology of the breast and the management of benign, preneoplastic, and neoplastic disorders.

EMBRYOLOGY

During the fifth week of human fetal development, the ectodermal primitive milk streak, or "galactic band," develops from axilla to groin on the embryonic trunk.[1] In the region of the thorax, the band develops to form a mammary ridge, whereas the remaining galactic band regresses. Incomplete regression or dispersion of the primitive galactic band leads to accessory mammary tissues, found in 2% to 6% of adult women.

At 7 to 8 weeks of gestation, a thickening occurs in the mammary anlage (milk hill stage), followed by invagination into the chest wall mesenchyme (disc stage) and tridimensional growth (globular stage). Further invasion of the chest wall mesenchyme results in a flattening of the ridge (cone stage) at 10 to 14 weeks of gestation. Between 12 and 16 weeks, mesenchymal cells differentiate into the smooth muscle of the nipple and areola. Epithelial buds develop (budding stage) and then branch to form 15 to 25 strips of epithelium (branching stage) at 16 weeks; these strips represent the future secretory alveoli.[2] The secondary mammary anlage then develops, with differentiation of hair follicle, sebaceous gland, and sweat gland elements, but only the sweat glands develop fully at this time. It is believed that, phylogenetically, the breast parenchyma develops from sweat-gland tissue. In addition, special apocrine glands develop to form Montgomery's glands around the nipple. The developments described thus far are independent of hormonal influences.

During the third trimester of pregnancy, placental sex hormones enter the fetal circulation and induce canalization of the branched epithelial tissues (canalization stage); this process continues from the 20th to the 32nd week of gestation. At about term, 15 to 25 mammary ducts are formed, with coalescence of duct and sebaceous glands near the epidermis. Parenchymal differentiation occurs at 32 to 40 weeks with the development of lobular-alveolar structures that contain colostrum (end-vesicle stage). There is a fourfold increase in mammary gland mass at this time, and the nipple-areolar complex develops and becomes pigmented. In the neonate, the stimulated mammary tissue secretes colostral milk (sometimes called witch's milk), which can be expressed from the nipple for 4 to 7 days postpartum in the majority of neonates of either sex. In the newborn, colostral secretion declines over a 3 to 4 week period owing to involution of the breast following withdrawal of placental hormones. During early childhood, the end-vesicles become further canalized and develop into ductal structures by further growth and branching.

ABNORMAL BREAST DEVELOPMENT

Congenital Abnormalities

The most frequently observed abnormality seen in both sexes is an accessory nipple (polythelia). Ectopic nipple tissue may be mistaken for a pigmented nevus, and may occur at any point along the milk streak from the axilla to the groin. Rarely, accessory true mammary glands develop. These are most often located in the axilla (polymastia). During pregnancy and lactation, an accessory breast may swell; occasionally, if there is an associated nipple, it may function.

Hypoplasia is the underdevelopment of the breast, congenital absence of a breast is termed *amastia*. When breast tissue is lacking but a nipple is present, the condition is termed *amazia*. A wide range of breast abnormalities have been described and may be classified as follows.[3,4]

1. Unilateral hypoplasia, contralateral normal
2. Bilateral hypoplasia with asymmetry
3. Unilateral hyperplasia, contralateral normal
4. Bilateral hyperplasia with asymmetry
5. Unilateral hypoplasia, contralateral hyperplasia
6. Unilateral hypoplasia of breast, thorax, and pectoral muscles (Poland's syndrome)

The majority of these abnormalities are not severe. The severest deformity, amastia or marked breast hypoplasia, is associated with hypoplasia of the pectoral muscle in 90% of cases,[5] but the reverse does not apply. Of those women with pectoral muscle abnormalities, 92% have a normal breast.[6] Congenital abnormalities of the pectoral muscle are usually manifested by the lack of the lower third of the muscle and an associated deformity of the ipsilateral rib cage. The association between absence of the pectoral muscle, chest wall deformity, and breast abnormalities was first recognized by Poland in 1841. The original description, however, did not note the concomitant abnormalities of the hand (synbrachydactyly with hypoplasia of the middle phalanges and central skin webbing),[7] and considerable controversy has evolved concerning the validity of the eponym for this congenital syndrome.[8,9]

Acquired Abnormalities

The most common—and avoidable—cause of amazia is iatrogenic. Injudicious biopsy of a precociously developing breast results in excision of most of the breast bud and subsequent marked deformity during puberty. The use of radiation therapy in prepubertal females to treat either hemangioma of the breast or intrathoracic disease may also result in amazia. Traumatic injury of the developing breast, such as that resulting from a severe cutaneous burn with subsequent contracture, may also result in severe deformity.

NORMAL BREAST DEVELOPMENT DURING PUBERTY

Puberty in girls begins at the age of 10 to 12 years as a result of the influence of hypothalamic gonadotropin-releasing hormones secreted into the hypothalamic-pituitary portal venous system. The basophilic cells of the anterior pituitary release follicle-stimulating hormone (FSH) and luteinizing hormone (LH). Follicle-stimulating hormone causes the primordial ovarian follicles to mature into graafian follicles, which secrete estrogens, primarily in the form of 17-β-estradiol. These hormones induce the growth and maturation of the breasts and genital organs. During the first 1 to 2 years after menarche, there is unbalanced hypothalamic-adenohypophyseal function owing to the fact that the maturation of the primordial ovarian follicles does not result in ovulation or a luteal phase. Therefore, ovarian estrogen synthesis predominates over luteal progesterone synthesis. The physiological effect of estrogens on the maturing breast is to stimulate longitudinal ductal growth of ductal epithelium. Terminal ductules also form buds that precede future breast lobules. Simultaneously, periductal connective tissues increase in volume and elasticity, with enhanced vascularity and fat deposition. These initial changes are induced by estrogens synthesized in immature ovarian follicles, which are anovulatory; subsequently, mature follicles ovulate and the corpus luteum releases progesterone. The relative role of these hormones is not clear. In experimental studies, estrogens alone induce a pronounced ductular increase, whereas progesterone alone does not. The two hormones together produce full ductular-lobular-alveolar development of mammary tissues.[10]

The evolution of the breast from childhood to maturity has been divided into five phases by Tanner.[11]

Phase I (age: puberty): Preadolescent elevation of the nipple with no palpable glandular tissue or areolar pigmentation

Phase II (age: 11.1 ± 1.1 years): Presence of glandular tissue in the subareolar region. The nipple and breast project as a single mound from the chest wall

Phase III (age: 12.1 ± 1.09 years): Increase in the amount of readily palpable glandular tissue with enlargement of the breast and increased diameter and pigmentation of the areola. The contour of the breast and nipple remains in a single plane.

Phase IV (age: 13.1 ± 1.15 years): Enlargement of the areola and increased areolar pigmentation. The nipple and areola form a secondary mound above the level of the breast

Phase V (age: 15.3 ± 1.7 years): Final adolescent development of a smooth contour with no projection of the areola and nipple

MORPHOLOGY

The Adult Breast

The adult breast lies between the second and sixth ribs in the vertical axis, and between the sternal edge and the midaxillary line in the horizontal axis (Fig. 1-1). The average breast measures 10 cm to 12 cm in diameter and its average thickness centrally is 5 cm to 7 cm. Breast tissue also projects into the axilla as the axillary tail of Spence. The contour of the breast varies, but is usually domelike

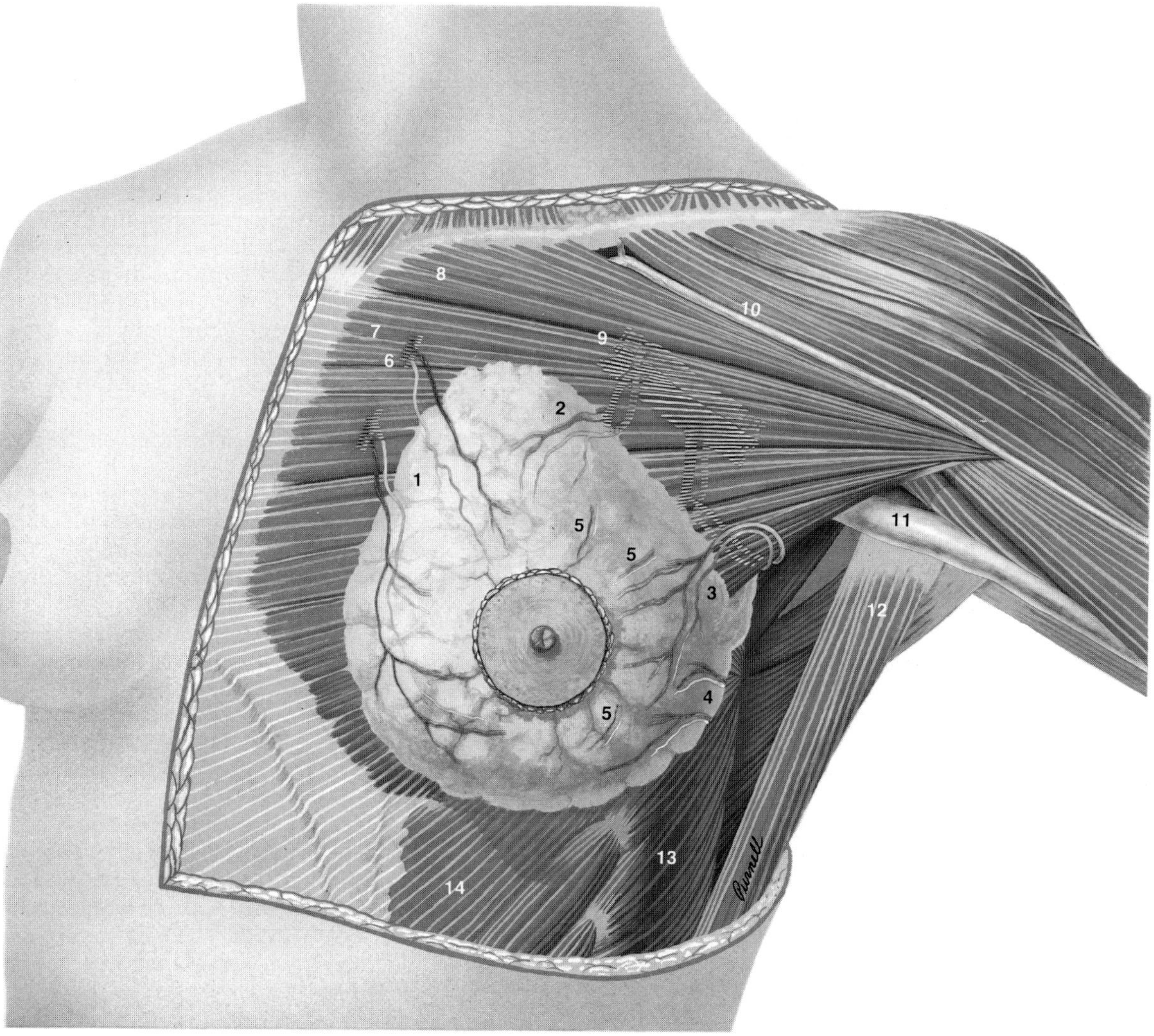

FIGURE 1-1. Normal anatomy of the breast and pectoralis major muscle.

1. *Perforating branches from internal mammary artery and vein*
2. *Pectoral branches from thoracoacromial artery and vein*
3. *External mammary branch from lateral thoracic artery and vein*
4. *Branches from subscapular and thoracodorsal arteries and veins*
5. *Lateral branches of third, fourth and fifth intercostal arteries and veins*
6. *Internal mammary artery and veins*
7. *Sternocostal head of pectoralis major muscle*
8. *Clavicular head of pectoralis major muscle*
9. *Axillary artery and vein*
10. *Cephalic vein*
11. *Axillary sheath*
12. *Latissimus dorsi muscle*
13. *Serratus anterior muscle*
14. *External abdominal oblique muscle*

with a conical configuration in the nulliparous woman and pendulous in the parous woman. The breast comprises three major structures: skin, subcutaneous tissue, and breast tissue, with the last comprising both parenchyma and stroma. The parenchyma is divided into 15 to 20 segments that converge at the nipple in a radial arrangement. The collecting ducts draining each segment are 2 mm in diameter with subareolar lactiferous sinuses 5 mm to 8 mm in diameter. Between 5 and 10 major collecting milk ducts open at the nipple although some contend that the correct number is 15 to 20 major ducts. Sartorius, however, showed that many of the openings seen at the nipple were blind pits.

The nomenclature of the duct system is varied. The branching system may be named in a logical fashion, starting with the collecting ducts in the nipple and extending to the ducts draining each alveolus, as illustrated in Table 1-1.

Each duct drains a lobe made up of 20 to 40 lobules. Each lobule consists of 10 to 100 alveoli or tubulosaccular secretory units. The microanatomy has been described in detail by Parks.[12] The stroma and subcutaneous tissues of the breast contain fat, connective tissue, blood vessels, nerves, and lymphatics.

The skin of the breast is thin and contains hair follicles, sebaceous glands, and eccrine sweat glands. The nipple, which is located over the fourth intercostal space in the nonpendulous breast, contains abundant sensory nerve endings, including Ruffini-like bodies and end-bulbs of Krause. Also, there are sebaceous and apocrine sweat glands, but no hair follicles. The areola is circular and pigmented, measuring 15 mm to 60 mm in diameter. Morgagni's tubercles, located near the periphery of the areola, are elevations formed by the openings of the ducts of Montgomery's glands. Montgomery's glands are large, sebaceous glands capable of secreting milk; they represent an intermediate stage between sweat and mammary glands. Fascial tissues envelop the breast. The superficial pectoral fascia envelops the breast and is continuous with the superficial abdominal fascia of Camper. The undersurface of the breast lies on the deep pectoral fascia, covering the pectoralis major and anterior serratus muscles. Connecting these two fascial layers are fibrous bands (Cooper's suspensory ligaments) that represent the "natural" means of support of the breast.

Blood Supply of the Breast

The principal blood supply to the breast is derived from the internal mammary and lateral thoracic arteries. Approximately 60% of the breast, mainly the medial and central parts, is supplied by the anterior perforating branches of the internal mammary artery. About 30% of the breast, mainly the upper outer quadrant, is supplied by the lateral thoracic artery. The pectoral branch of the thoracoacromial artery; the lateral branches of the third, fourth, and fifth intercostal arteries; and the subscapular and thoracodorsal arteries all make minor contributions to the blood supply.

Table 1-1
Nomenclature of the Breast Epithelial System

Major Ducts	*Terminal Duct-Lobular Unit*
Collecting ducts	Terminal ducts
Lactiferous sinuses	Extralobular
Segmental ducts	Intralobular
Subsegmental ducts	Lobules
	Alveoli

Lymphatic Drainage of the Breast

Lymph Vessels

The subepithelial or papillary plexus of the lymphatics of the breast are confluent with the subepithelial lymphatics over the surface of the body. These valveless lymphatic vessels communicate with subdermal lymphatic vessels and merge with Sappey's subareolar plexus. The subareolar plexus receives lymphatic vessels from the nipple and areola and communicates by way of vertical lymphatic vessels that are equivalent to those connecting the subepithelial and subdermal plexus elsewhere.[13] Lymph flows unidirectionally from the superficial to deep plexus and from the subareolar plexus via the lymphatic vessels of the lactiferous duct to the perilobular and deep subcutaneous plexus. The periductal lymphatic vessels lie just outside the myoepithelial layer of the duct wall.[14]

Flow from the deep subcutaneous and intramammary lymphatic vessels moves centrifugally toward the axillary and internal mammary lymph nodes. Injection studies using radiolabeled colloid[15] have demonstrated the physiology of lymph flow and have countered the old hypothesis of centripetal flow toward Sappey's subareolar plexus. It has been estimated that about 3% of the lymph from the breast flows to the internal mammary chain, whereas 97% flows to the axillary nodes.[16] Drainage of lymph to the internal mammary chain may be observed following injection of any quadrant of the breast.

Axillary Lymph Nodes

The topographical anatomy of the axillary lymph nodes has been studied as the major route of regional spread in primary mammary carcinoma. The anatomical arrangement of the axillary lymph nodes has been subject to many different classifications. The most detailed studies are those of Pickren, which show the pathologic anatomy of tumor spread.[17] Axillary lymph nodes may be grouped as the apical or subclavicular nodes lying medial to the pectoralis minor muscle and the axillary vein lymph nodes grouped along the axillary vein from the pectoralis minor muscle to the lateral limit of the axilla; the interpectoral (Rotter's) nodes lying between the pectoralis major and minor muscles along the lateral pectoral nerve; the scapular group comprising the nodes lying along the subscapular vessels; and the central nodes lying beneath the lateral border of the pectoralis major muscle and below the pectoralis minor muscle (Fig. 1-2). Other groups can be iden-

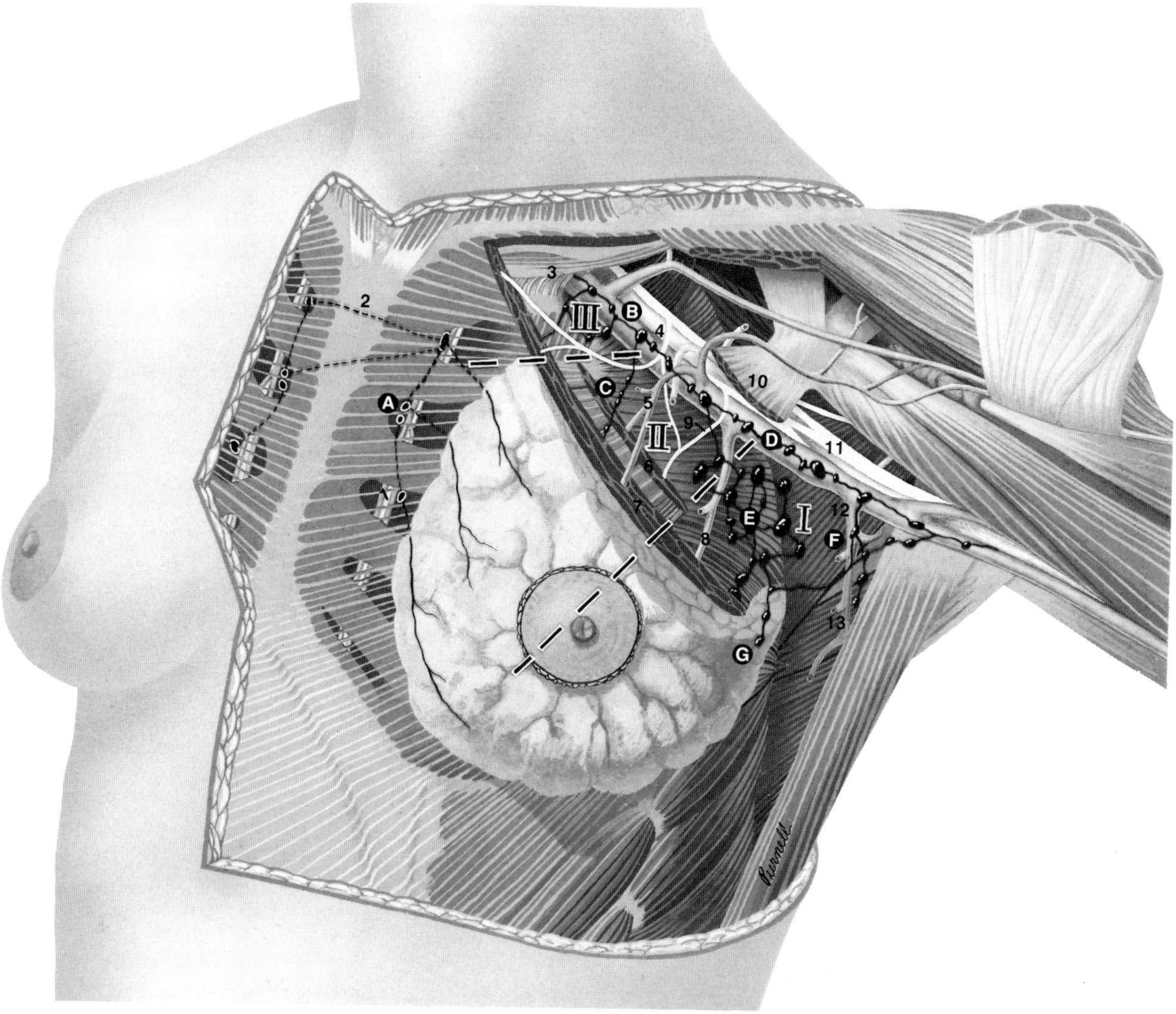

FIGURE 1-2. The lymphatic drainage of the breast showing lymph node groups and levels.

1. *Internal mammary artery and vein*
2. *Substernal cross drainage to contralateral internal mammary lymphatic chain*
3. *Subclavius muscle and Halsted's ligament*
4. *Lateral pectoral nerve (from the lateral cord)*
5. *Pectoral branch from thoracoacromial vein*
6. *Pectoralis minor muscle*
7. *Pectoralis major muscle*
8. *Lateral thoracic vein*
9. *Medial pectoral nerve (from the medial cord)*
10. *Pectoralis minor muscle*
11. *Median nerve*
12. *Subscapular vein*
13. *Thoracodorsal vein*

A. *Internal mammary lymph nodes*
B. *Apical lymph nodes*
C. *Interpectoral (Rotter's) lymph nodes*
D. *Axillary vein lymph nodes*
E. *Central lymph nodes*
F. *Scapular lymph nodes*
G. *External mammary lymph nodes*

Level I lymph nodes: lateral to lateral border of pectoralis minor muscle
Level II lymph nodes: behind pectoralis minor muscle
Level III lymph nodes: medial to medial border of pectoralis minor muscle

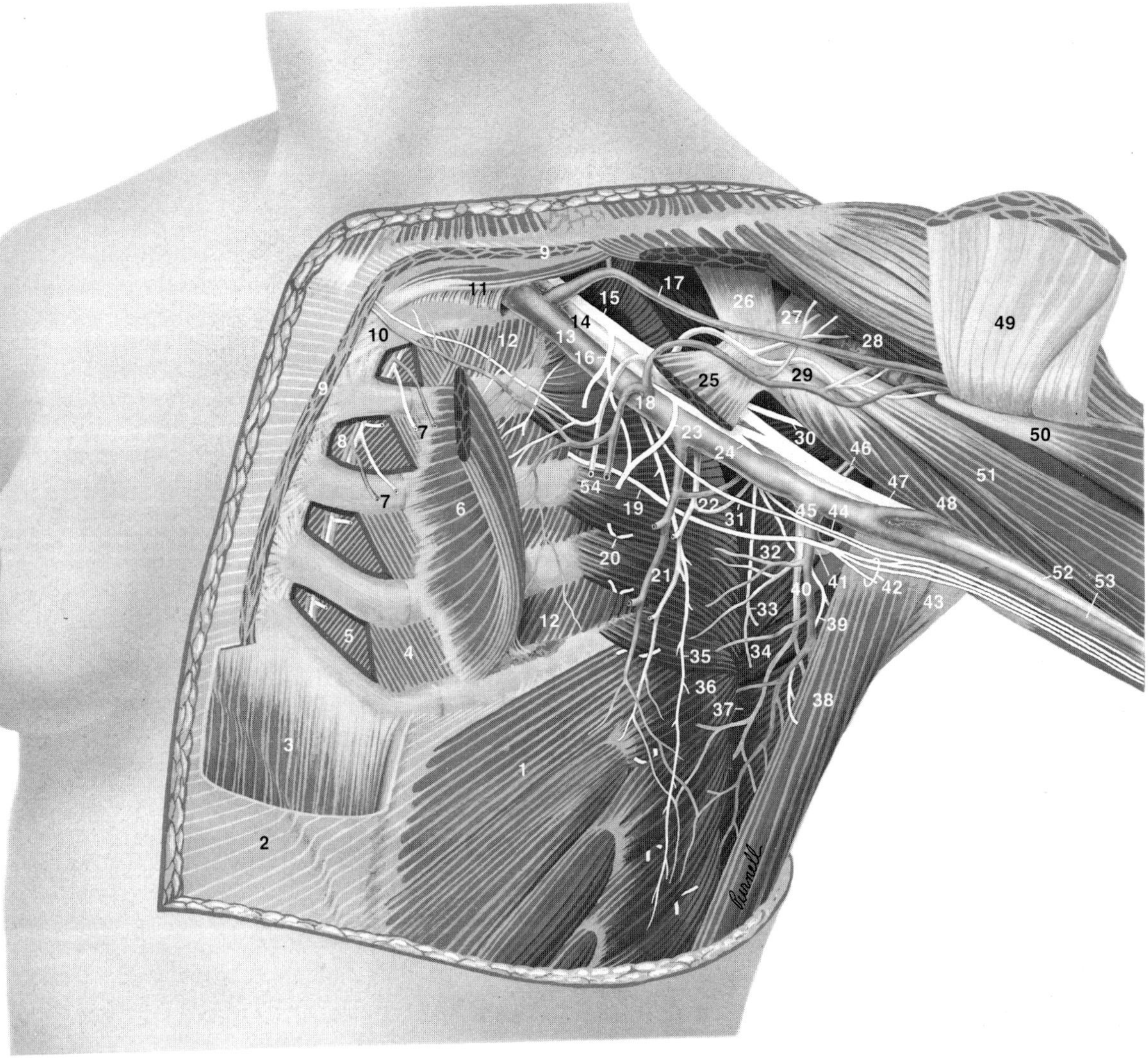

tified, such as the external mammary nodes lying over the axillary tail and the paramammary nodes that are located in the subcutaneous fat over the upper, outer quadrant of the breast.

An alternative method of delineating metastatic spread, for the purposes of determining pathologic anatomy and metastatic progression, is to divide the axillary lymph nodes into arbitrary levels.[18] Level I lymph nodes lie lateral to the lateral border of the pectoralis minor muscle, level II nodes lie behind the pectoralis minor muscle, and level III lymph nodes are located medial to the medial border of the pectoralis minor muscle (Fig. 1-3). These levels can only be determined accurately by marking them at the time of surgery with tags.

Internal Mammary Lymph Nodes

The internal mammary nodes lie in the intercostal spaces in the parasternal region. The nodes lie close to the internal mammary vessels in extrapleural fat and are distributed in the intercostal spaces as shown in Figure 1-2. From the second intercostal space downward, the internal mammary nodes are separated from the pleura by a thin layer of fascia in the same plane as the transverse thoracic muscle. The number of lymph nodes described in the internal mammary chain varies. The nodes lie medial to the internal mammary vessels in the first and second intercostal spaces in 88% and 76% of cases, respectively, whereas they lie lateral to the vessels in the third intercostal space in 79% of cases. The prevalence of nodes in each intercostal space is as follows: first space, 97%; second space, 98%; third space, 82%; fourth space, 9%; fifth space, 12%; and sixth space, 62%.[19] The pathologic anatomy of this route of lymphatic drainage in the spread of breast disease has been described by Handley[20] and Urban.[21]

In the presence of nodal metastases, obstruction of the physiologic routes of lymphatic flow may occur and alternative pathways may then become important. The alternative routes that have been described are deep, sub-

FIGURE 1-3. Chest wall muscles and vascular anatomy.

1. *External abdominal oblique muscle*
2. *Rectus sheath*
3. *Rectus abdominis muscle*
4. *Internal intercostal muscle*
5. *Transverse thoracic muscle*
6. *Pectoralis minor muscle*
7. *Perforating branches from internal mammary artery and vein*
8. *Internal mammary artery and vein*
9. *Cut edge of pectoralis major muscle*
10. *Sternoclavicular branch of thoracoacromial artery and vein*
11. *Subclavius muscle and Halsted's ligament*
12. *External intercostal muscle*
13. *Axillary vein*
14. *Axillary artery*
15. *Lateral cord of brachial plexus*
16. *Lateral pectoral nerve (from the lateral cord)*
17. *Cephalic vein*
18. *Thoracoacromial vein*
19. *Intercostobrachial nerve*
20. *Lateral cutaneous nerves*
21. *Lateral thoracic artery and vein*
22. *Scapular branches of lateral thoracic artery and vein*
23. *Medial pectoral nerve (from medial cord)*
24. *Ulnar nerve*
25. *Pectoralis minor muscle*
26. *Coracoclavicular ligament*
27. *Coracoacromial ligament*
28. *Cut edge of deltoid muscle*
29. *Acromial and humeral branches of thoracoacromial artery and vein*
30. *Musculocutaneous nerve*
31. *Medial cutaneous nerve of arm*
32. *Subscapularis muscle*
33. *Lower subscapular nerve*
34. *Teres major muscle*
35. *Long thoracic nerve*
36. *Serratus anterior muscle*
37. *Latissimus dorsi muscle*
38. *Latissimus dorsi muscle*
39. *Thoracodorsal nerve*
40. *Thoracodorsal artery and vein*
41. *Scapular circumflex artery and vein*
42. *Branching of intercostobrachial nerve*
43. *Teres major muscle*
44. *Medial cutaneous nerve of forearm*
45. *Subscapular artery and vein*
46. *Posterior humeral circumflex artery and vein*
47. *Median nerve*
48. *Coracobrachialis muscle*
49. *Pectoralis major muscle*
50. *Biceps brachii muscle, long head*
51. *Biceps brachii muscle, short head*
52. *Brachial artery*
53. *Basilic vein*
54. *Pectoral branch of thoracoacromial artery and vein*

sternal, cross drainage to the contralateral internal mammary chain,[22,23] superficial presternal crossover, lateral intercostal and mediastinal drainage,[24] and spread via the rectus abdominis muscle sheath to the subdiaphragmatic and subperitoneal plexus (Gerota's pathway). This last route allows the direct spread of tumor to the liver and retroperitoneal lymph nodes. Substernal crossover may be demonstrated using isotope imaging of the lymph nodes, and may be of significance in early breast cancer.[25]

Muscular and Neural Anatomy

The important muscles in the region of the breast are the pectoralis major and minor, serratus anterior, and latissimus dorsi muscles, as well as the aponeurosis of the external oblique and rectus abdominis muscles (see Fig. 1-3).

The pectoralis minor muscle arises from the outer aspect of the third, fourth, and fifth ribs, and is inserted into the medial border of the upper surface of the coracoid process of the scapula. The muscle is usually prefixed rather than postfixed, and is innervated by the medial pectoral nerve which arises mainly from the medial cord of the brachial plexus (C8, T1 segmental origin) and descends posteriorly to the muscle crossing the axillary vein anteriorly. The nerve enters the interpectoral space, passing through the muscle itself in 62% of cases and around the lateral border as a single branch in 38% of cases.[26] Varying numbers of branches passing through the muscle provide motor supply to the lateral part of the pectoralis major muscle. The terms medial and lateral pectoral nerves are confusing; the standard terminology refers to their brachial plexus origin rather than their anatomical positions. Changes in terminology have been proposed, but have not been generally accepted to date. The arrangement of these nerves is of particular importance in performing the modified radical (Patey) mastectomy.

The serratus anterior muscle stabilizes the scapula on the chest wall. The muscle arises by a series of digitations from the upper eight ribs laterally; its origin from the first rib is in the posterior triangle of the neck. At its origin from the fifth, sixth, seventh, and eighth ribs, it interdigitates with the origin of the external oblique muscle. The muscle inserts into the vertebral border of the scapula on its costal surface and is supplied by the long thoracic nerve of Bell (the nerve to the serratus anterior muscle). The origin of this important nerve is the posterior aspect of the C5, C6, and C7 roots of the brachial plexus. It passes posteriorly to the axillary vessels, emerging on the chest wall high in the medial part of the subscapular fossa. The nerve lies superficial to the deep fascia overlying the anterior serratus muscle, and marks the posterior limit of dissection of the deep fascia. Preservation of the nerve to the serratus anterior muscle as it passes downward is essential to avoid "winging" of the scapula and loss of shoulder power.

The latissimus dorsi muscle, the largest muscle in the

body, is characterized by a very wide origin from the spinous processes and supraspinous ligaments of the seventh thoracic vertebra downward, including all the lumbar and sacral vertebrae. The muscle inserts, by a narrow tendon forming the posterior axillary fold, into a 2.5-cm insertion in the bicipital groove of the humerus. As the muscle spirals around the teres major muscle, the surfaces of the muscle become reversed to the point of insertion. The muscle is supplied by the thoracodorsal nerve (the nerve to the latissimus dorsi muscle) which arises from the posterior cord of the brachial plexus with segmental origin from C6, C7, and C8. The nerve passes behind the axillary vessels, approaches the subscapular vessels from the medial side, and then crosses anterior to these vessels to enter the medial surface of the muscle. The nerve passes through the axilla and is intimately involved in the scapular group of lymph nodes. Resection of the nerve does not result in any important cosmetic or functional defect, but it should nevertheless be preserved when possible.

An important landmark in the apex of the axilla is the origin of the subclavius muscle, which arises from the costochondral junction of the first rib. At the tendinous part of the lower border of this muscle, two layers of the clavipectoral fascia fuse together to form a well-developed band, the costocoracoid ligament, which stretches from the coracoid process to the first costochondral junction (Halsted's ligament). At this point, the axillary vessels (the vein being anterior to the artery) enter the thorax, passing over the first rib and beneath the clavicle. There are many unnamed small branches of the axillary vein that pass to its lower border from the axilla. Near the apex, a small artery, the highest thoracic artery, arises from the axillary artery and lies on the first and second ribs.

Muscular Abnormalities

Congenital absence of the sternocostal head of the pectoralis major muscle and its associated abnormalities have been described earlier in this chapter. In 5% of cadavers, a sternalis muscle may be found lying longitudinally between the sternal insertion of the sternocleidomastoid muscle and the rectus abdominis muscle. The pectoralis minor muscle is inserted into the head of the humerus as well as the coracoid process of the scapula in 15% of cases. Part of the tendon then passes between the two parts of the coracoacromial ligament to insert into the coracohumeral ligament. Rarely, the axillopectoral muscle arises as a separate part of the latissimus dorsi muscle and crosses the base of the axilla superficially, then passes deep to the pectoralis major muscle to join its insertion or to continue to the coracoid process (Langer's axillary arch). This anatomical arrangement may cause compression of the axillary vessels[27] and difficulty in orientation during axillary dissection.

Microscopic Anatomy of the Adult Breast

In the immature breast, the ducts and alveoli are lined by a two layer epithelium consisting of a basal cuboidal layer and a flattened surface layer. In the presence of estrogens at puberty and subsequently, this epithelium proliferates, becoming multilayered (Fig. 1-4A). Three alveolar cell types have been observed: superficial (luminal) A-cells, basal B-cells (chief cells), and myoepithelial cells.

Superficial, or luminal, A-cells are dark, basophilic, staining cells that are rich in ribosomes. Superficial cells

FIGURE 1-4. *(A)* One normal, inactive lobule from the breast of a 35-year-old woman. Alveolar cells are small and the lumina are inconspicuous. Much of the lobular space is occupied by capillaries and stroma. (Hematoxylin and eosin stain, original magnification × 40). *(B)* Portions of three adjacent, lactating lobules from the breast of a 25-year-old woman who was three weeks postpartum. Note the cytoplasmic vacuolization of the alveolar cells which have proliferated, leading to marked enlargement of the lobule. (Hematoxylin and eosin stain, original magnification × 40).

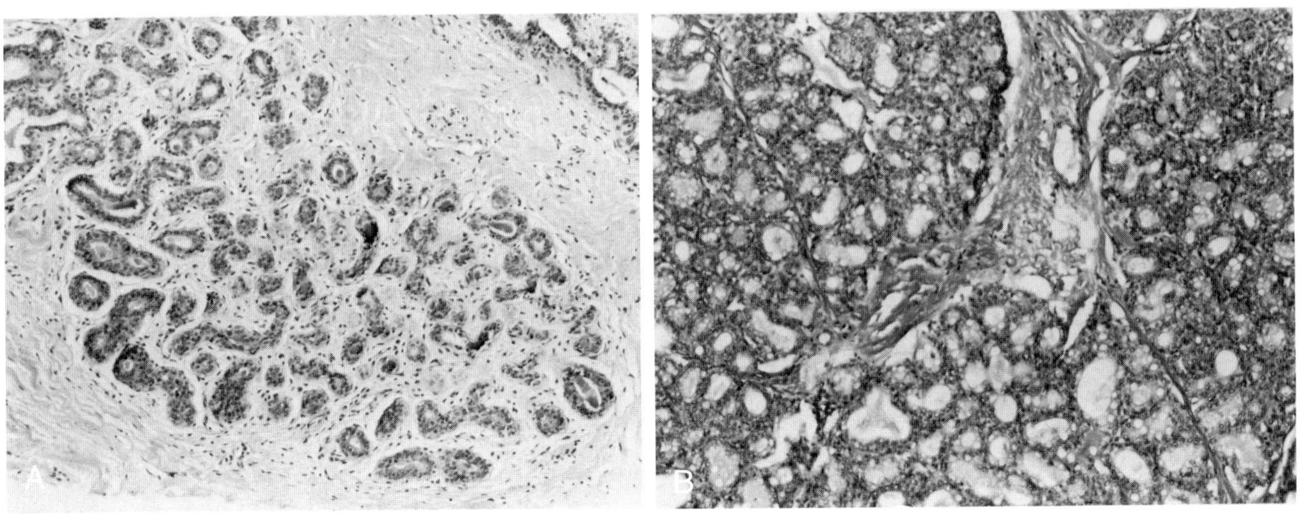

undergo intercellular dehiscence with swelling of the mitochondria and become grouped, forming buds within the lumen.

Basal B-cells, or chief-cells, are the major cell type in mammary epithelium. They are clear, with an ovoid nucleus without nucleoli. Where the basal cells are in contact with the lumen, there are microvilli on the cell membrane. Intracytoplasmic filaments are similar to those in myoepithelial cells, suggesting their differentiation toward that cell type.

Myoepithelial cells are located around alveoli and small excretory milk ducts between the inner aspect of the basement membrane and the tunica propria. Myoepithelial cells are arranged in a branching, starlike fashion. The sarcoplasm contains filaments 50 nm to 80 nm in diameter; these myofilaments are inserted via hemidesmosomes into the basal membrane. These cells are not innervated, but are stimulated by the steroid hormones prolactin and oxytocin.

PHYSIOLOGY

Microscopic Morphology and the Menstrual Cycle

Histologic changes in the normal breast have been identified in relation to the endocrine variations of the menstrual cycle.[28] Normal menstrual-cycle–dependent histologic changes in both stroma and epithelium have been observed and are summarized in Table 1-2.

Cyclic Changes in the Breast During the Menstrual Cycle

Cyclic changes in the sex-steroid hormone levels during the menstrual cycle profoundly influence breast morphology. Under the influence of FSH-LH during the follicular phase of the menstrual cycle, increasing levels of estrogen secreted by the ovarian graafian follicles stimulate breast epithelial proliferation. During this proliferative phase, the epithelium exhibits sprouting with increased cellular mitoses, ribonucleic acid (RNA) synthesis, increased nuclear density, enlargement of the nucleolus, and changes in other intercellular organelles. In particular, the Golgi apparatus, ribosomes, and mitochondria increase in size or number. During the follicular phase, at the time of maximal estrogen synthesis and secretion midcycle, ovulation occurs. A second peak occurs in the midluteal phase, at which time luteal progesterone synthesis is maximal. Similarly, progestogens induce changes in the mammary epithelium during the luteal phase of ovulatory cycles. Mammary ducts dilate and the alveolar epithelial cells differentiate into secretory cells with a partly monolayer arrangement. The combination of these sex-steroid hormones and other hormones results in the formation of lipid droplets in the alveolar cells and some intraluminal

Table 1-2
*Morphologic Criteria for Phase Assignment**

				Epithelium			
Phase	*Days*	*Stroma*	*Lumen*	*Cell Types*	*Orientation of Epithelial Cells*	*Mitoses*	*Active Secretion*
I Proliferative	3–7	Dense, cellular	Tight	Single, predominantly pale eosinophilic cell	No stratification apparent	Present average 4/10 HPF†	None
II Follicular	8–14	Dense, cellular, collagenous	Defined	Luminal columnar basophilic cell; intermediate pale cell; basal clear cell with hyperchromatic nucleus (myoepithelial)	Radial around lumen	Rare	None
III Luteal	15–20	Loose, broken	Open with some secretion	Luminal basophilic cell; intermediate pale cell; prominent vacuolization of basal clear cell (myoepithelial)	Radial around lumen	Absent	None
IV Secretory	21–27	Loose, edematous	Open with secretion	Luminal basophilic cell; intermediate pale cell; prominent vacuolization of basal clear cell (myoepithelium)	Radial around lumen	Absent	Active apocrine secretion from luminal cell
V Menstrual	28–2	Dense, cellular	Distended with secretion	Luminal basophilic cell with scant cytoplasm	Radial around lumen	Absent	Rare

* After Vogel et al: The correlation of histologic changes in the human breast with the menstrual cycle. Am J Pathol 104:24-34, 1981.
† HPF, high-power field.

secretion. The changes in breast epithelium in response to hormones are mediated through either intracellular steroid receptors or membrane-bound peptide receptors. The presence of steroid receptors for estrogen and progestogens in the cytosol of normal mammary epithelium has been demonstrated.[29] It is through the binding of these hormones to specific receptors that the molecular changes, with their observed morphologic effects, are induced as physiologic changes. Similarly, membrane receptors are present to mediate the actions of prolactin. Increases in endogenous estrogen may also exert a histamine-like effect on the mammary microcirculation,[30] resulting in an increased, maximal blood flow 3 to 4 days premenstrually with an average increase in breast volume of 15 cm to 30 cm.[31] Premenstrual breast fullness is attributable to increasing interlobular edema and enhanced ductular-acinar proliferation under the influence of estrogens and progestogens. With the onset of menstruation, following a rapid decline in the circulating levels of sex-steroid hormones, secretory activity of the epithelium regresses. Postmenstrually, tissue edema is reduced and regression of the epithelium ceases as a new cycle begins with concomitant rises in estrogen levels. Minimum breast volume is observed 5 to 7 days after menstruation. However, the breast does not appear to return to its original state each time, but continues to show further development of mammary alveoli.

Breast Changes During Pregnancy

During pregnancy, marked ductular, lobular, and alveolar growth occurs as a result of the influence of luteal and placental sex steroids, placental lactogen, prolactin, and chorionic gonadotropin (Fig. 1-4*B*). In experimental studies, these effects are observed when estrogen and progesterone cause a release of prolactin by reducing the hypothalamic release of prolactin inhibiting factor (PIF).[32] Prolactin in humans is also released progressively during pregnancy and probably stimulates epithelial growth and secretion.[33] Prolactin increases slowly during the first half of pregnancy; during the second and third trimester, blood levels of prolactin are 3 to 5 times greater than normal, and mammary epithelium initiates protein synthesis.

In the first 3 to 4 weeks of pregnancy, marked ductular sprouting occurs with some branching, and lobule formation occurs under estrogenic influence. At 5 to 8 weeks, breast enlargement is significant, with dilatation of the superficial veins, heaviness, and increasing pigmentation of the nipple-areolar complex. In the second trimester, lobule formation exceeds ductular sprouting under progestogenic influence. The alveoli contain colostrum, but no fat, which is secreted under the influence of prolactin. From the second half of pregnancy onward, increasing breast size results not from mammary epithelial proliferation, but from increasing dilatation of the alveoli with colostrum, as well as hypertrophy of myoepithelial cells, connective tissue, and fat. If these processes are interrupted by early delivery, lactation may be adequate from 16 weeks of pregnancy onward.

At the beginning of the second trimester, the mammary alveoli, but not the milk ducts, lose the superficial layer of A-cells. Prior to this, as in the nonpregnant woman, the two-layer structure is maintained. In the second and third trimesters, this monolayer differentiates into a colostrum-cell layer and accumulates eosinophilic cells, plasma cells, and leukocytes around the alveoli. As pregnancy continues, colostrum, composed of desquamated epithelial cells, accumulates. Aggregations of lymphocytes, round cells, and desquamated phagocytic alveolar cells (foam cells) may be found in colostrum; these are termed Donné's corpuscles.

Lactation

Following parturition, an immediate withdrawal of placental lactogen and sex-steroid hormones occurs. During pregnancy, these hormones antagonize the effect of prolactin on mammary epithelium. Concomitant to the abrupt removal of the placental hormones, luteal production of the sex-steroid hormones also ceases. A nadir is reached on the fourth to fifth days postpartum; at this time, the secretion of PIF from the hypothalamus into the hypothalamoadenohypophyseal portal system decreases. This reduction in PIF secretion allows the transmembrane secretion of prolactin by pituitary lactotrophs. Sex-steroid hormones are not necessary for successful lactation, and physiologic increases such as may occur with postpartum ovulatory cycles do not inhibit it.

Prolactin, in the presence of growth hormone, insulin, and cortisol, converts the mammary epithelial cells from a presecretory to a secretory state. During the first four or five days after birth, the breasts enlarge owing to the accumulation of secretions in the alveoli and ducts. The initial secretion is of colostrum, a thin, serous fluid that is, at first, sticky and yellow. Colostrum contains lactoglobulin which is identical to blood immunoglobulins. The importance of these immunoglobulins is unknown; many maternal antibodies cross the placenta, so transferring passive immunity to the fetus *in utero*. Fatty acids, such as decadienoic acid, phospholipids, fat-soluble vitamins, and lactalbumin in colostrum have considerable nutritional value. Following colostrum secretion, transitional milk and then mature milk are elaborated.

Mechanisms of Milk Synthesis and Secretion

The effects of prolactin are mediated through membrane receptors in the mammary epithelial cells. The release of prolactin is maintained and stimulated by suckling, as is the release of adrenocorticotropic hormone (ACTH). The mammary cells are cuboidal or cylindrical, depending on the degree of intracellular accumulation of secretions. The deoxyribonucleic acid (DNA) and RNA of the nuclei increase, and abundant mitochondria, ribosomes, and rough endoplasmic reticulum with a prominent Golgi apparatus are apparent in the epithelial cells. Complex protein, milk fat, and lactose synthetic pathways are activated, as are water-ion transport mechanisms. These processes are initiated by the activation of hormone-specific membrane receptors. Changes in cyclic adenosine monophosphate (AMP) stimulate milk synthesis through the induction of messenger and transfer RNA. Prolactin stimulates cyclic-AMP–induced protein kinase activity, resulting in the phosphorylation of milk proteins. Polymerase activity and cellular transcription are enhanced.[34]

Large fat vacuoles develop and move toward the apex of the cell. At the same time, the nucleus also moves toward the apex. As the water intake of the cell increases, longitudinal cellular striations may be observed. Ultimately, the vacuoles pass from the cell along with part of the cell membrane and cytoplasm; the apical cell membrane reconstitutes as secretion takes place. Enhanced activity occurs during suckling. Fat is secreted chiefly through an apocrine mechanism, lactose is secreted through a merocrine one, and the secretion of proteins occurs as a result of a combination of mechanisms. Ions enter the milk by diffusion and active transport. Relatively little holocrine is thought to be secreted. The end result of secretion and subsequent intraductal dilution by extracellular fluid is milk, comprising a suspension of proteins—casein, α-lactalbumin, and β-lactoglobulin—and fat in a lactose-mineral solution. The white appearance of milk is due to emulsified lipids and calcium caseinate, whereas the yellow color of butterfat is due to the presence of carotenoids.

Mechanisms of Milk Ejection

The removal of milk by suckling is aided by active ejection. Sensory nerve endings in the nipple-areolar complex are activated by tactile stimuli. Impulses pass by way of sensory nerves through the dorsal roots to the spinal cord. In the spinal cord, impulses are relayed through the dorsal, lateral, and ventral spinothalamic tracts to the mesencephalon and lateral hypothalamus. Inhibition of secretion of prolactin inhibiting factor allows the unimpeded secretion of prolactin from the anterior pituitary. Simultaneously, through a different pathway in the paraventricular nucleus, the synthesis of oxytocin occurs. Oxytocin is released from the posterior pituitary neurovesicles by impulses traveling along the neurosecretory fibers of the hypothalamoneurohypophyseal tract. Oxytocin released into the systemic circulation acts on the myoepithelial cells, which contract and eject milk from the alveoli into the lactiferous ducts and sinuses. This phenomenon is specific to oxytocin, and changes in intramammary ductal pressures of 20 mm Hg to 25 mm Hg may be observed in relation to peak blood levels. Oxytocin also acts on the uterus and cervix to promote involution. This effect may be stimulated by cervical dilatation and by vaginal stretching via the ascending afferent neural pathways (Ferguson reflex).

Complex neuroendocrine interactions determine normal lactation. An appreciation of these mechanisms is essential to the understanding of abnormalities and to the treatment of problems of lactation.

THE MALE BREAST

In males, the lack of a sustained pubertal surge of estrogen results in the breast remaining rudimentary. In some males, however, a breast similar to the shape and size of the female breast may develop.

Gynecomastia

The development in a male of a breast configuration that is similar to that of the female breast is termed *gynecomastia.* The palpation of a firm, subareolar mass without the contour of a female breast is indicative of *mammaplasia,* not gynecomastia, but this distinction is rarely made. The incidence of gynecomastia has been evaluated in various groups of normal males:

Boy scouts aged 11 to 14 years[35] 39%
Military reservists[36] 36%
Veterans[37] 32%
Subjects older than 59 years of age undergoing autopsy[38] 40%

This condition affects the left breast more frequently than the right.[39,40]

The etiology of mammaplasia/gynecomastia varies, but may be classified into four major groups:

1. Hormonal causes
2. Drug-related causes
3. Systemic disease
4. Idiopathic causes

The multiplicity of clinical associations and drug-related changes are shown in the accompanying display.

Hormonal Causes

Physiologic hormonal changes in the body that may induce gynecomastia occur during three periods: the neonatal period, puberty, and senescence.[41–49] In neonates, transplacental hormonal stimulation may occur, and a colostrum-like discharge may be secreted. Pubertal gynecomastia may be related to an estradiol-testosterone imbalance.[50] Serum levels of estradiol have been found to be high in relation to serum testosterone.[51] These changes, usually occurring between 11 and 15 years of age, tend to disappear spontaneously within 2 years.[35] Senescent gynecomastia is associated with declining serum testosterone levels and an unchanged level of serum estradiol.[52]

Nonphysiologic (pathologic) causes of estradiol-testosterone imbalance include primary or secondary hypogonadism and Klinefelter's syndrome.

Neoplasms in the testis or adrenal glands may cause

Causes of Gynecomastia

Hormonal Causes

Physiologic

- Changes in the neonatal period
- Changes during puberty
- Changes in senescence

Pathologic

- Primary testicular failure
    - Pubertal testicular failure
    - Postpubertal testicular failure
    - Klinefelter's syndrome
- Secondary testicular failure
    - Radiation
    - Orchitis
    - Cryptorchidism
    - Trauma
    - Hydrocele
    - Varicocele
    - Spermatocele
    - Tuberculosis
    - Leprosy
- Endocrine disorders
    - Hyperthyroidism, hypothyroidism
- Neoplastic hormone production
    - Nonectopic
        - Testicular
            - Seminoma, teratoma
            - Choriocarcinoma
            - Interstitial (Leydig) cell
            - Androblastoma
            - Embryonal cell carcinoma
    - Adrenal
        - Hyperplasia, carcinoma
    - Pituitary
        - Adenoma
    - Ectopic
        - Bronchogenic carcinoma
        - Hepatoma

Drugs

- Amiloride
- Amphetamines
- Anabolic steroids
- Busulfan
- Chlorpromazine
- Cimetidine
- Clomiphene
- Diazepam
- Diethylstilbestrol
- Digoxin
- Diphenylhydantoin
- D-penicillamine
- Ergotamine tartrate
- Estramustine
- Estrogen
- Fluphenazine
- Flutamide
- Guanabenz
- Heroin
- Isoniazid
- Ketocanazole
- Leuprolide
- Marijuana
- Methadone
- Methyldopa
- Metronidazole
- Neuroleptic drugs
- Perphenazine
- Phenothiazines
- Procarbazine
- Prochlorperazine
- Propranolol
- Ranitidine
- Reserpine
- Spironolactone
- Sulindac
- Tamoxifen
- Theophylline
- Thiazide
- Thiethylperazine
- Thioridazine
- Trifluoperazine
- Tricyclics
- Vincristine

Systemic Disorders

- Chronic liver disease
- Chronic renal disease
- Malnutrition
- Chronic pulmonary disease
- Chronic neurological disease
- Rheumatic fever
- Lymphoma
- Carcinoma of the colon
- Carcinoma of the prostate
- Ulcerative colitis
- Starvation

Idiopathic

- Cause unknown

gynecomastia due to hormone secretion by the tumor. Other tumors may secrete ectopic hormones that reflect the pluripotent cell origin rather than the normal function of the tissue of origin.

Drug-Related Causes

Many drugs have been found to cause gynecomastia as a side effect.[53–64] Frequently, drug-induced gynecomastia is unilateral and the breast may be tender or painful.

Systemic Disease

Gynecomastia may occur in patients with advanced alcoholic cirrhosis, chronic renal failure, chronic pulmonary disease, and malnutrition.[65–67] Breast development in male patients with these disorders may be mediated by endocrine changes.

Idiopathic Causes

Gynecomastia in apparently healthy young adult men frequently remains unexplained. A familial association has been noted.[68]

REFERENCES

1. Hamilton NJ, Boyd JD, Mossman HW: Human embryology, p 428. Cambridge, Heffer, 1968
2. Hughes ESR: Development of mammary gland. Ann R Coll Surg Engl 6:99, 1950
3. Maliniac JW: Breast deformities and their origin, p 163. New York, Grune & Stratton Inc., 1950.
4. Simon BE, Hoffman S, Kahn S: Treatment of asymmetry of the breasts. Clin Plast Surg 2:375, 1975
5. Trier WC: Complete breast absence. Plast Reconstr Surg 36:430, 1965

6. Pers M: Aplasias of the anterior thoracic wall, the pectoral muscle, and the breast. Scand J Plast Reconstr Surg 2:125, 1968
7. Beals RK, Crawford S: Congenital absence of the pectoral muscles. Clin Orthop 119:166, 1976
8. McDowell F: On the propagation, perpetuation and parroting of erroneous eponyms such as "Poland's syndrome." Plast Reconstr Surg 59:561, 1977
9. Ravitch MM: Poland's syndrome: A study of an eponym. Plast Reconstr Surg 59:508, 1977
10. Vorherr H: The Breast: Morphology, Physiology and Lactation. New York, Academic Press, 1974
11. Tanner JM: Wachstum und Reifung des Menschen. Stuttgart, Georg Thieme Verlag, 1962
12. Parks AG: The micro-anatomy of the breast. Ann R Coll Surg Engl 25:235, 1959
13. Spratt JS, Shieber W, Dillard B: Anatomy and Surgical Technique of Groin Dissection. St Louis, CV Mosby, 1965
14. Bonsor GM, Dossett JA, Jull JW: Human and Experimental Breast Cancer. Springfield, IL, Charles C Thomas, 1961
15. Turner-Warwick RT: The lymphatics of the breast. Br J Surg 46:574, 1959
16. Hultborn KA, Larsen LG, Raghnult I: The lymph drainage from the breast to the axillary and parasternal lymph nodes: Studied with the aid of colloidal AU^{198}. Acta Radiol 43:52, 1955
17. Pickren JW: Lymph node metastases in carcinoma of the female mammary gland. Bull Roswell Park Meml Inst 1:79, 1956
18. Berg JW: The significance of axillary node levels in the study of breast carcinoma. Cancer 8:776, 1955
19. Stibbe EP: The internal mammary lymphatic glands. J Anat 52:257, 1918
20. Handley RS, Thackray AC: Invasion of internal mammary lymph nodes in carcinoma of the breast. Br Med J 1:61, 1954
21. Urban JA, Marjani MA: Significance of internal mammary lymph node metastases in breast cancer. Am J Roentgenol 111:130, 1971
22. Rouviere H: Anatomie des lymphatiques de l'homme. Paris, Masson, 1932
23. Ege GN: Internal mammary lymphoscintigraphy. Radiology 118:101, 1975
24. Thomas JM, Redding WH, Sloane JP: The spread of breast cancer: Importance of the intrathoracic lymphatic route and its relevance to treatment. Br J Cancer 40:540, 1979
25. Osborne MP, Jeyasingh K, Jewkes RF, et al: The preoperative detection of internal mammary lymph node metastases in breast cancer. Br J Surg 66:813, 1979
26. Moosman DA: Anatomy of the pectoral nerves and their preservation in modified mastectomy. Am J Surg 139:883, 1980
27. Boontje AH: Axillary vein entrapment. Br J Surg 66:331, 1979
28. Vogel PM, Georgiade NG, Fetter BF, et al: The correlation of histologic changes in the human breast with the menstrual cycle. Am J Pathol 104:23, 1981
29. Wittliff JL, Lewko WM, Park DC, et al: Hormones, receptors and breast cancer. In McGuire WL (ed): Steroic binding proteins of mammary tissues and their clinical significance in breast cancer, Vol 10, pp 327-330. New York. Raven Press, 1978.
30. Zeppa R: Vascular response of the breast to estrogen. J Clin Endocrinol Metab 29:695, 1969
31. Dabelow A: Die Milchdrüse. In Bargman W (ed): Handbuch der Mikroskopishen Anatomie des Menschen, vol 3, part 3. Berlin, Springer-Verlag, 1957
32. MacLeod RM, Abad A, Eidson LL: *In vivo* effect of sex hormones on the *in vitro* synthesis prolactin and growth hormone in normal and pituitary tumor-bearing rats. Endocrinology 84:1475, 1969
33. Tyson JE, Hwang P, Guyda H, et al: Studies of prolactin secretion in human pregnancy. Am J Obstet Gynecol 113:14, 1972
34. Turkington RW: Multiple hormonal interactions. The mammary gland. In Litwack G (ed): Biochemical Actions of Hormones, pp 55-80. New York, Academic Press, 1972
35. Nydick M, Bustos J, Dale JH: Gynecomastia in adolescent boys. JAMA 178:449, 1961
36. Nuttal FQ: Gynecomastia as a physical finding in normal men. J Clin Endocrinol Metab 48:338, 1979
37. Carlson HE: Current concepts: Gynecomastia. N Engl J Med 303:671, 1980
38. Williams MJ: Gynecomastia: Its incidence, recognition and host characterization in 447 autopsy cases. Am J Med 334:103, 1963
39. Bannayan GA, Hajdu SI: Gynecomastia: Clinicopathologic study of 351 cases. Am J Clin Pathol 57:431, 1972
40. Kapdi CC, Parekh NJ: The male breast. Radiol Clin North Am 21:137, 1983
41. Knorr D, Bidlingmaier F: Gynecomastia in male adolescents. Clin Endocrinol Metab 4:157, 1975
42. Sbar S: Unilateral gynecomastia. N Engl J Med 286:1367, 1972
43. Molina C, Aberkane B: Les gynecomasties des tuberculeux pulmonaires. Sem Hop Paris 36:834, 1960
44. Bercovici JP, Mauvais-Jarvis P: Hyperthyroidism and gynecomastia: Metabolic studies. J Clin Endocrinol Metab 35:671, 1972
45. Greenwood SM, Goodman JR, Schneider G: Choriocarcinoma in man: Relationship of gynecomastia to chronic somatotrophin and estrogens. Am J Med 51:416, 1971
46. Stewart WK, Fleming LW, Wotiz HW: Feminizing syndrome in male subjects with adrenal cortical neoplasms. Am J Med 37:455, 1984
47. McCullagh FP, Alivisatos JG, Schaffenburg CA: Pituitary tumor of gynecomastia lactation. J Clin Endocrinol Metab 16:397, 1956
48. Hardy JD: Gynecomastia associated with lung cancer. JAMA 173:1462-1465, 1960
49. Summerskill WH, Adson MA: Gynecomastia as sign of hepatoma. Am J Dig Dis 7:250, 1962
50. Lee PA: The relationship of concentrations of serum hormones to pubertal gynecomastia. Z Kinderheilkd 115:89, 1973
51. Large DM, Anderson DC: Twenty-four-hour profiles of circulating androgens and oestrogens in male puberty with and without gynecomastia. Clin Endocrinol (Oxf) 8:277, 1978
52. Rubens R, Dhont M, Vermuelen A: Further studies on Leydig cell function in old age. J Clin Endocrinol Metab 39:40, 1974
53. Clarke E: Spironolactone therapy and gynecomastia. JAMA 193:163, 1965
54. Dardick KR: Gynecomastia associated with theophylline. J Fam Pract 18:141, 1984
55. Delle Fave GF, Tamburrano F, De Magistris L: Gynecomastia with cimetidine. Lancet 1:1319, 1977
56. Edidin DV, Levitsky LL: Prepubertal gynecomastia associated with estrogen-containing hair cream. Am J Dis Child 136:587, 1982
57. Harmon J, Aliapoulios MA: Gynecomastia in marijuana users. N Engl J Med 287:936, 1972
58. Lardinois CK, Mazzaferri EL: Cimetidine blocks testosterone synthesis. Arch Intern Med 145:920, 1985
59. Spence RW, Celestin LR: Gynecomastia associated with cimetidine. Gut 20:154, 1979
60. Mendelson JH, Mendelson JE, Patch VA: Plasma testosterone levels in heroin addiction and during methadone maintenance. J Pharmacol Exp Ther 192:211, 1975
61. Reid DM, Martynoga AK, Muki G: Reversible gynecomastia

associated with D-penicillamine in a man with rheumatoid arthritis. Br Med J 285:1083, 1982

62. Rodstein M: Gynecomastia: Unusual manifestation of digitalis toxicity. GP 26:95, 1962
63. DeFelice R, Johnson DG, Galgiani J: Gynecomastia with ketoconazole. Antimicrob Agents Chemother 19:1073, 1981
64. Fagan TC, Johnson DG, Grosso DS: Metronidazole-induced gynecomastia. JAMA 254:3217, 1985
65. Jacobs EC: Gynecomastia following severe starvation. Ann Intern Med 28:792, 1948
66. Lloyd CW, Williams RH: Endocrine changes associated with Laennec's cirrhosis of liver. Am J Med 4:315, 1948
67. Nagel TC, Freinkel N, Bell RH: Gynecomastia, prolactin and other peptide hormones in patients undergoing chronic hemodialysis. J Clin Endocrinol Metab 36:428, 1973
68. Edwards JA, Bannerman RN: Familial gynecomastia. Birth Defects 7:193, 1971

Benign Breast Disorders

2

Susan M. Love Stuart J. Schnitt
James L. Connolly Robert L. Shirley

HISTORICAL DESCRIPTIONS

The confusion that runs rampant on the subject of benign breast disease is not new. Patey stated in 1949, "I would like to support the plea of Cheatle for the abolition of the term chronic mastitis which has lost almost all precision and value; its sole remaining virtue is that no one can agree on a term to replace it."[1] He further noted that Deaver and McFarland, in 1918, were able to collect 23 different terms for this entity. Thirty years ago, Lewison and Lyon stated that, "Benign breast disease enfolds in its indiscriminate embrace a galaxy of 'synonyms,' all of which are in common use and many of which describe what may actually be the same lesion."[2] Pathologically, this term is ubiquitous and nonspecific, and is often applied to any biopsy of benign breast tissue. This fact moved Foote and Stewart in 1945 to state that, "The term 'chronic cystic mastitis' is so ingrained in the minds of some pathologists that this diagnosis of a locally excised portion of breast almost amounts to a surgicopathological reflex."[3] Even radiographic studies have not yielded a strict definition of this phrase, which is used generally to describe dense breast tissue.

Historically, Brodie is thought to have provided the first clear description of cystic disease in 1846.[4] Shortly thereafter, Birkett[5] (1850), Velpeau[6] (1856), and Bryant[7] (1887) published descriptions of benign breast disease and clearly distinguished between cystic disease (gross cysts) and what they described as the pain syndrome. Reclus[8] (1883) and then Schimmelbusch[9] (1892) carefully described the histologic features of the disease and, by emphasizing the pathologic component, contributed to the tendency to consider the clinical pain syndrome and gross cystic disease as the same phenomenon. Cheatle and Cutler (1931) not only restressed the distinct nature of these clinical entities, but also were the first to acknowledge that nodularity of the breasts was not necessarily pathologic, but occurred regularly under physiologic conditions, such as menstruation.[10] Geschickter[11] (1943) and Patey[1] (1949) continued to differentiate among the clinical syndromes, including mastodynia or pain, adenosis or nodularity, and cystic disease or gross cysts. Haagensen (1956), in his classic book on the breast, maintained a distinction between pain, physiologic nodularity, and gross cystic disease, although he emphasized the last of these.[12]

Although the European literature continues to make these distinctions, there has been a tendency in the United States to ignore them and to include all benign breast syndromes and pathology under the label of "fibrocystic disease." This practice confuses normal physiologic phenomena with a disease process and is based on the assumption that all nonmalignant breast symptoms spring from the same pathophysiology.[13] Rather than having a unifying effect, this approach tends to cause increased confusion and has prevented the systematic study of benign breast disease in all of its manifestations.[14]

An attempt will be made in this chapter to review previous studies regarding epidemiology, etiology, and treatment of benign breast conditions, acknowledging the fact that they are far from clear. Clinically, the subject will be organized according to common symptom complexes. Finally, all noncancerous pathologic entities will be discussed separately at the end of the chapter.

EPIDEMIOLOGIC VIEW

It is virtually impossible to estimate the incidence of benign breast disorders. The subjectiveness in any one woman's evaluation of her own breasts, as well as the variation in the physician observer's designation of disease, invalidates any clinical estimates. In order to gain some degree of reproducibility, most studies rely on data from women who have undergone biopsies for benign conditions. This approach, too, is subject to considerable bias, since not every woman with lumpy breasts will undergo a biopsy, and since the decision to biopsy is influenced strongly by the presence of other risk factors for malignant disease.

For example, biopsies are done more frequently in women in their 40s than in those in their 20s, not necessarily because of a greater incidence of benign disease, but because of a greater risk that a lump could actually be cancerous. This phenomenon would lead one to believe that benign breast conditions requiring biopsy are more common in older women, which is not necessarily a valid conclusion. Moreover, the practice of labeling all noncancerous biopsy results as indicative of "fibrocystic disease" tends to overestimate the actual incidence of pathology. These difficulties notwithstanding, it is useful to review the published data regarding the epidemiology and risk factors for benign breast problems.

Clinically defined, benign breast symptoms are very common and have been estimated to occur in 50% of women at some point in their lifetime. In a case control study conducted by Cole in Boston from 1968 to 1969, the age-standardized incidence rate for histologically diagnosed fibrocystic disease and fibroadenoma was 89.4 and 32.8 per 100,000 woman years, respectively.[15] Cole found that the incidence rises in women 45 years of age or younger, and then declines sharply. This study suffers from the bias inherent in using biopsies, however, possibly underestimating the incidence in younger women. Hislop and Elwood conducted a 30-year cohort study of nurses in British Columbia and found that, by the age of 50 years, the subjects' cumulative risk for benign breast disorders (determined by questionnaire) was 17% for those undergoing biopsy and 31% for those with symptomatic disease.[16] In autopsy studies, the incidence of histologic fibrocystic disease may be determined with only slightly greater accuracy. Davis summarized eight autopsy studies conducted prior to 1964 and found evidence of cystic disease in 58.5% of a total of 725 breasts in women who had had no symptoms of breast disease while living.[17] Cystic disease was bilateral in 43% of these women. The average incidence of gross cysts was 21%, whereas the average incidence of coexisting gross and microscopic cysts and of cystic disease with epithelial hyperplasia was 58.3% and 30.6%, respectively. Kramer and co-workers studied the breasts of women older than 70 years of age and found histologic evidence of fibrocystic disease in 67%.[18] Thus, although the incidence of clinical features may decrease in the postmenopausal period, the histologic features persist.

Natural History and Risk Factors

Generally, the clinical and epidemiologic literature are in agreement with regard to the age incidence of various patterns of benign breast conditions.[19] These reports show that benign breast symptoms occur predominantly in women of menstruating age, with a mean age of 39 years and a range of 18 to 67 years. Fibroadenomas tend to occur in younger women, whereas gross cysts are more common in perimenopausal women ranging in age from 35 to 60 years (with a mean age of 43 years). Only 15% of gross cysts occur in the postmenopausal period. The incidence rates for patients undergoing biopsy and those with symptomatic disease show an early peak at the age of 20 to 24 years, followed by a brief decline and then a steady increase that is sustained until, but not beyond, menopause.[16,19,20]

The risk factors for benign breast disorders appear to be distinct from those for breast cancer.[21] Breast disease warranting biopsy has been associated with a history of premenstrual breast discomfort, irregular menses, and spontaneous abortions; a family history of both benign and malignant breast disease; lack of use of oral contraceptives; a low incidence of obesity; small breasts; and late natural menopause.[15,16,22]

Few analyses of the comparative incidences of benign breast disorders in various races have been conducted. The general clinical impression has always been that the incidence is decreased in rural Africans, first-generation Chinese immigrants, and American Indians.[23] This premise, however, may reflect these groups' access to medical care rather than an actual absence of breast disorders. Fibrocystic or hyperplastic lesions were diagnosed in a greater number of white women than black women, whereas a greater number of blacks than whites were reported to have fibroadenoma.[24] Schuerch and colleagues compared benign biopsy results from the National Cancer Center Hospital in Tokyo and 263 biopsy results from Memorial Hospital in New York. They found that hyperplastic lesions were twice as common in the American women, whereas solitary papillomas with prominent epithelial proliferation and sclerosis were more common in the Japanese women.[25]

Exogenous Hormone Use and Benign Breast Disorders

Many studies and much confusion exist regarding the relationship of benign breast disorders to oral contraceptive use. Early studies showed a reduced incidence of "fibrocystic disease" evaluated by biopsy with the use of any oral contraceptive.[26–28] Many studies have shown no difference in benign breast disease with "ever" use, but a reduced risk with "long-term" use.[29–33] Although most studies show the effect to be limited to current use only,[20,27,30,34] some have demonstrated that it may persist for several years after the drug is discontinued.[30,33,35] A recent study by Berkowitz showed no evidence of a reduction in risk correlating with duration of use among either current or past users of oral contraceptives who were premenopausal, and an increased incidence of "fibrocystic disease" in postmenopausal women who had taken oral contraceptives premenopausally.[37]

One of the limitations of these studies is that they are restricted to patients with breast lumps who have undergone biopsy. Janerich suggested that the reduced risk observed in many of these studies may be related to a reluctance of physicians to prescribe oral contraceptives to women with preexisting breast conditions.[32] Hislop tried to correct for this and for the biopsy bias by performing a cohort study and by limiting his observations on oral contraceptive use to the period preceding the first diagnosis of benign breast disease.[16] He found that long-term contraceptive use reduced the risk of developing signs of benign breast disease, as well as the risk of undergoing biopsy for these signs. The results of Hislop's research were confirmed in a study by Brinton.[20] Paradoxically, oral contraceptives appear to protect against benign problems, yet have no effect on the risk of developing breast cancer. LiVolsi attempted to explain this phenomenon by analyzing her data according to the degree of epithelial proliferation in biopsy specimens of oral contraceptive users.[38] She concluded that long-term use of oral contraceptives protects against the forms of histologic fibrocystic disease that are not strongly associated with an increased risk of breast cancer, but not against the premalignant forms. Recent studies, however, have failed to confirm a linear relationship between the use of oral contraceptives and the degree of atypical hyperplasia in biopsies.[39–41] In a case control and intracase comparison, Berkowitz found that oral contraceptive use might be associated with an increased incidence of sclerosing adenosis in premenopausal women and of gross cysts in postmenopausal women.[39]

In evaluating these studies, the fact that the formulation of the contraceptive pill has changed since its introduction in the 1960s must be considered. The initial pills had more estrogen and progesterone than do current types. It is interesting to note that the first group of studies of the relationship between oral contraceptives and benign breast disorders, conducted in the mid 1970s, all showed a reduction in incidence of breast disorders, in both current and "ever" users.[23] However, recent studies have shown that only current users of contraceptives derive any protective effect.[20,33] Most recently, the study of Berkowitz revealed no evidence that long-term use of oral contraceptives in premenopausal women was associated with a decreased frequency of benign breast symptoms among either current or past users.[39] A reduction in the dose of estrogen, progesterone, or both has been postulated to explain this shift. Brinton, who studied various formulations, found a relationship between the dose of progesterone and the incidence of benign breast problems,[20] as did the Royal College of General Practitioners.[30]

Other exogenous hormones have been less well studied. Fechner examined breast tissue from 43 women who had been receiving postmenopausal estrogen replacement and found a slightly higher, but not statistically significant, incidence of epithelial hyperplasia.[42] Other researchers, however, have noted that prior use of estrogen replacement therapy among postmenopausal women was associated with an increased risk of fibrocystic breast disease, fibroadenoma, and gross cysts.[39,43] This risk increased with duration of use and was higher in women who had undergone bilateral oophorectomy than in other postmenopausal women.

ETIOLOGY

Although there is general agreement that the breast is hormonally controlled, few data exist regarding the mechanisms of action and interaction of these hormones and the response of breast tissue. Recent evidence suggests that a neuroendocrine imbalance is a likely cause of benign breast disorders, but the data are far from conclusive. An impediment to evaluating much of the research is the lack of a clear definition of which women are being studied. Nevertheless, hormones seem to have an etiologic role in mastalgia, if not in breast nodularity, and a difference in hormonal patterns may serve to further distinguish between these two clinical entities.

In 1941, Geschickter postulated that a relative hyperestrinism was a mechanism responsible for mastodynia and breast nodularity.[11] He felt that this hormonal imbalance could reflect either high estrogen or low progesterone levels in the luteal phase, basing this theory on animal experiments showing the induction of adenosis in rats receiving large doses of estrone. His observations were supported by Kier and co-workers.[44]

Estrogen is the hormone responsible for development of the ductal epithelium, whereas progesterone is associated with lobular-alveolar proliferation. Progesterone may also act as an antiestrogen, antagonizing the action of estradiol on duct cells[45] by decreasing the concentration of estrogen receptors.[46] Bassler showed that large doses of estrogen, administered to castrated rats, induced proliferation and dilation of lobules with formation of cysts and epithelial proliferation, as well as an increase in circumcanalicular and intralobular connective tissue.[47] In contrast, when estradiol was administered to castrated female rats in combination with progesterone, normal mammary development occurred. Similarly, Cowie found that administering a combination of hexoestriol and progesterone to castrated goats resulted in normal mammary development, whereas increasing the estrogen dose produced cysts and epithelial proliferation.[48] Bassler also found that nongonadal hormones, especially the pituitary lactotropic hormones, may induce stromal fibrosis and epithelial hyperplasia in the rat model.[47]

Recently, England postulated that an increase in estrogen levels in the luteal phase was a factor in mastodynia and nodularity.[49] However, this theory has not been borne out in clinical studies, which invariably have demonstrated normal estradiol levels in affected patients.[50–52] An alternative theory suggests that a deficiency of progesterone occurs in the luteal phase. Such a deficiency was demonstrated by Sitruk-Ware,[50] but not confirmed by Walsh.[53,54] It has been proposed that the ratio of estrogen to progesterone, and not the absolute value of each, is the important factor.[55] This theory is difficult to evaluate, however, since the estrogen-progesterone ratio varies throughout the cycle. Estradiol values may even vary diurnally.[56] In addition, recent studies have shown that progesterone concentrations in the midluteal and late luteal phases rapidly fluctuate within large ranges (2.3–40 ng/ml), often within minutes.[57] Therefore, a single estimation of plasma progesterone in the midluteal or late luteal phase cannot be expected to reflect accurately the adequacy of the corpus luteum or the actual estrogen-progesterone ratio.[57]

Other investigators have focused their attention on the role of prolactin in the development of mastodynia and nodularity in women. Although prolactin has been demonstrated to be in the high-normal range in patients with breast symptoms,[58,59] patients with prolactinomas do not have a higher incidence of benign breast disease,[60] and medically induced hyperprolactinemia using metoclopromide does not usually cause breast pain.[61] Several studies have shown an exaggerated response of prolactin to the thyrotropin releasing hormone (TRH) test in patients with mastodynia, suggesting a hyperresponsiveness and possible functional hyperprolactinemia.[59,62,63] This premise is supported by the fact that bromocriptine, a prolactin inhibitor and dopamine agonist, is efficacious in alleviating symptoms of mastodynia, regardless of an initial normal level of prolactin.[64,65] Kumar and colleagues demonstrated an increased responsiveness to TRH and domperidone, a dopamine receptor blocking drug, in patients with cyclic mastalgia and breast nodularity, but not in those with noncyclic mastalgia.[62] They attributed this response to an increased dopaminergic inhibition of prolactin release which is specific for prolactin since stores of thyroid stimulating hormone (TSH) and the dopaminergic inhibition of TSH were unaltered. In contrast, Watt-Boolsen showed that the prolactin and TSH response to submaximal doses of metoclopromide were identical.[63] These studies are not completely comparable since they employed different dopamine antagonists and different subsets of patients. Watt-Boolsen did confirm that basal serum levels of prolactin were significantly higher in patients with cyclic mastalgia than in those without mastalgia, and that the TRH-induced rise in prolactin was highest in the group of patients with cyclic mastalgia.[63]

A hormonal distinction between nodularity and mastalgia has recently been supported by studies combining sonographic evaluation of the breast with midluteal phase endocrine profiles in 25 women with significant mastalgia and 15 asymptomatic fertile women. Not surprisingly, a 50% incidence of fibrocystic disease (nodularity) confirmed by sonography was observed both in the group with mastalgia and in the normal patients. Sonographic evidence of fibrocystic disease did not correlate with clinical symptoms or luteal phase abnormalities. Patients with mastalgia, however, demonstrated normal midluteal levels of estradiol with significantly lower midluteal progesterone levels, as well as prolactin hyperresponsiveness to TRH.[66]

The most consistent hypothesis regarding the role of hormonal dysfunction in benign breast disease is that of Mauvais-Jarvis and co-workers.[67] Their hypothesis implicates dysovulation, or an inadequate corpus luteum, and the consequent decreased ratio of progesterone to estrogen, which is related to an abnormality in gonadotropin secretion.[67] They cite as clinical support the observation that physiologic anovulatory cycles occur most commonly in women who are at either end of the reproductive life span—that is, at menarche or menopause—both of which are periods characterized by a high incidence of benign breast problems.[68] Ovulation may also be disturbed at any time by external stress which, in turn, may alter cyclic hypothalamic regulation, setting the stage for subsequent hormonal imbalance leading to mastalgia.

High normal levels of prolactin may reflect the altered estrogenic status in these women since it is known that estrogen has a direct stimulatory effect on lactotrophic cells. In turn, an excess of prolactin suppresses progesterone production by the luteinized granulosa cell, leading to luteal insufficiency and relative estrogen excess, producing a vicious cycle. Although stress does not act directly on pituitary prolactin, it increases β-endorphin secretion, which increases dopamine turnover and thus, prolactin stimulation. Such an intermittent, stress-related hypersecretion of prolactin could accentuate or induce an inadequate corpus luteum. In addition, the prolactin hyperresponsiveness to TRH testing seen in patients with mastalgia has been found to increase in the presence of dysovulation with unopposed estrogen.[69] The inability to prove this hypothesis is partly attributable to a limited understanding of the underlying neuroendocrinologic mechanisms. Recent studies have elegantly demonstrated the complexity of pulsatile gonadotropin releasing hormone, luteinizing hormone, and progesterone secretion, and have underscored the inaccuracy of isolated blood samples in diagnosing abnormalities.[57,70]

Clinically, there are several appealing aspects to this theory, including an explanation for the element of stress in mastodynia; the common clinical finding of cyclic mastodynia that persists for a period of a few months, subsequently resolving spontaneously; and the clinical observation of a relationship between breast pain and infertility and premenstrual syndrome symptoms. How these hormonal variations actually cause pain, however, is still unknown. There must be an element of end-organ responsiveness, as well as hormonal variation, involved since the breasts often have different levels of sensitivity. One explanation may be found in the hormone receptors for prolactin, as well as for estrogen and progesterone.[71] Although the latter have been better studied in patients with fibroadenoma, there is evidence that patients with lesions characterized by marked cellularity and little fibrosis have more receptors than those with lesions that are mostly fibrous. Certainly, hormone receptors help to explain the breast tissue's response to variations; whether they also are involved in the complex phenomenon of mastalgia has yet to be studied.

A variety of other hormonal alterations have been described in women with benign breast disorders.[19] These include an increase in luteinizing hormone,[72] an increased urinary testosterone level in women with epithelial hyperplasia,[73] and elevation of peripheral androgens and sex-hormone-binding globulin.[74]

CLINICAL FEATURES

Clinically, the most useful classification system for benign breast disease is based on symptoms and physical findings (see the section on pathology, later in this chapter). Six general categories have been identified:

1. Physiologic, cyclic swelling and tenderness
2. Nodularity: significant lumpiness, both cyclic and noncyclic

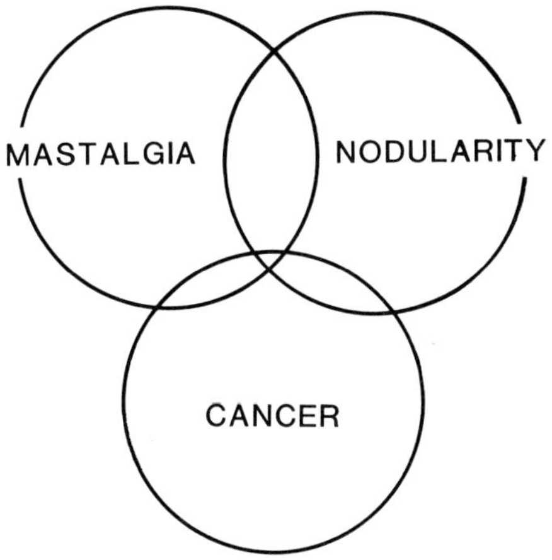

FIGURE 2-1. The relationship between mastalgia, nodularity, and breast cancer.

3. Mastalgia: severe pain, both cyclic and noncyclic
4. Dominant lumps, including gross cysts and fibroadenomas
5. Nipple discharge, including intraductal papilloma and duct ectasia
6. Infections and inflammations, including subareolar abscess, lactational mastitis, breast abscess, and Mondor's disease

This schema indicates the variety of benign breast disorders, many of which do not have a pathologic counterpart, that are seen by clinicians. It acknowledges the fact that many women have premenstrual swelling and tenderness that is mild and probably physiologic, and that should not be termed a disease or even a symptom requiring treatment. In addition, it emphasizes the fact that a woman may have pain and no lumps, lumps and no pain, or both (Fig. 2-1). It should be noted that pain, lumpiness, or both may occur unilaterally or bilaterally; most commonly, one breast predominates. Some French investigators believe that there may be a progression from mastodynia to increased nodularity and then to "chronic fibrocystic disease."[67] However, they and others have delineated distinct hormonal, sonographic, and mammographic findings for each of the categories.[66]

Physiologic, Cyclic Swelling and Tenderness

Physiologic, cyclic swelling and tenderness represent the normal variations in size, shape, and tenderness that occur in a menstruating woman's breasts. Since these sensations are limited to the reproductive years, they are obviously hormonally controlled. Robinson and Short showed that sensitivity to pain and touch in the breast and areola varies with the menstrual cycle, with maximal sensitivity occurring midcycle and during menstruation.[75] Histologic studies of the breast throughout the menstrual cycle show a sequence of changes in epithelial cells, from nonsecretory to potentially secretory, with distinct morphological correlates of hormone responsiveness in different phases.[76,77] At some time in their lives, most women will have some form of mild, premenstrual tenderness or sensitivity. The distinction between normal sensitivity and swelling and mastalgia or nodularity is one of degree and persistence.

Nodularity

A general pattern of persistent lumpiness or nodularity differs from the clinical manifestation of a dominant lump. In the former, the general texture may be finely granular, nodular, or even grossly lumpy, and the abnormality is diffuse. In contrast, a single lump is distinct, persistent, and unchanging. Physiologic nodularity may vary with the menstrual cycle or it may be stable. It may involve either the whole breast or a particular area, such as the axillary tail or superior aspect. Nodularity is often bilateral, but may be more exaggerated in one breast than the other. Although this condition may be associated with tenderness, it is not necessarily painful.

In some patients, an area that feels like a distinct lump on palpation may be found at surgery to merge indistinctly with the rest of the breast tissue. These areas, termed by Patey in 1949 as pseudolumps,[1] probably represent most of what is often described as "fibrocystic disease." Autopsy studies of asymptomatic women have shown "fibrocystic disease" in 90%; therefore, a biopsy of a pseudolump or questionable area may, and often will, be diagnosed as "fibrocystic disease."[13] However, since most of the histologic entities included under this umbrella term do not form gross lumps or have a mechanism for causing pain, they are probably incidental findings. Since this connection between clinical nodularity and pathologic fibrocystic disease is tenuous, or at least controversial, pathologic entities will be discussed separately.

Breast Pain (Mastalgia)

The prevalence of severe mastalgia is unknown, but has been estimated to be as high as 50%. The term does not refer to pain that is associated with dominant lumps, such as gross cysts or cancer. A recent German study of 700 women in whom mammograms were performed for various indications found that more than half of the women complained of mastalgia.[78] A quarter mentioned experiencing frequent, diffuse breast pain, one-third had had pain for years, and one-third complained of localized pain. That mastalgia is a symptom of importance to those who experience it is evidenced by the large number of patients who present to special breast pain clinics.[79–81] Many women with mild forms of mastalgia or mastodynia who seek medical advice because they are concerned that they may have cancer may be reassured following a careful examination. These women are different from those who present with severe pain requesting relief. Watt-Boolsen estimates the risk of developing severe breast pain to be approximately 5%, based on the frequency of breast pain in series of patients with mammary tumors or "fibrocystic disease."[82] Wisbey and colleagues, in their study of the natural history of mastalgia, found that 70% of patients with severe pain (5% of all patients with mastalgia) thought, in retrospect, that their pain should have been treated.[83] The lack of research on mastalgia and the resulting lack of treatment options reflect a historical clinical bias that breast pain is primarily a psychoneurotic symptom. This general impression has gained support as a result of the lack of a histologic or radiographic correlate of breast pain in most studies.[78,82] American researchers have tended to lump breast pain in the overall category of "fibrocystic disease," considering pain and nodular breasts to be the same entity, and perpetuating the myth that all pain is caused by cysts.[81] The lack of a precise definition has invalidated most studies of both pain and other forms of "fibrocystic disease." European researchers have considered mastalgia a separate entity, however, and have, in some instances, demonstrated a hormonal basis for this phenomenon (see the section on etiology, above).

Preece and his group studied mastalgia, not only demonstrating that women with breast pain are no more neurotic than women with varicose veins,[84] but also classifying the different types of breast pain[80] and studying their natural history.[83] They were able to describe six specific groups of patients based on clinical, radiologic, and pathologic findings. Their six categories of breast pain included cyclic mastalgia (thought to be hormonal), duct ectasia or periductal mastitis, Tietze syndrome or costochondritis, trauma, sclerosing adenosis, and cancer. Bishop and Blamey used a similar system, but included the categories of "trigger spot," continuous breast pain, and cyclic breast pain.[85]

The category of cyclic mastalgia, the most common type of breast pain (40%–60%) in both studies[83,85] (Table 2-1), included all patients with pain that in some way varied in intensity with the menstrual cycle. Breast pain was significantly worse in degree or duration than the usual premenstrual discomfort, and could persist for most of the cycle. In most patients, it began in their third decade and, in many, persisted until menopause. About 60% of this group had complete or substantial relief of symptoms during follow-up. In most patients, this remission was related to some hormonal event, such as pregnancy, menopause, or oral contraceptive use. Thus, it is not surprising that this type of breast pain is the one most responsive to hormonal manipulation (see section on treatment, below). Blichert-Toft and Watt-Boolsen described cyclic pain as affecting the whole mammary gland, sometimes most severely in the upper, outer quadrant.[82] This type of breast pain occurs bilaterally in more than 50% of affected patients, but it may also be unilateral. Especially in unilateral cases, the pain may radiate to the ipsilateral axilla and down the arm. It may or may not be accompanied by nodularity on physical examination.

Preece's category of duct ectasia (25%)[80] probably corresponds to Bishop's trigger spot group,[85] including pain that has no discernible pattern in time but is precisely localized, consistent, and of short duration. If this trigger spot is excised, the pathologic examination is usually unremarkable, and the pain may or may not disappear. The Welsh study also described a second group of patients with continuous pain that was diffuse, persistent, and of long duration.[83] This type of pain is usually characterized by a continuous burning or aching that is unrelated to the cyclic changes accompanying menstruation. Sclerosing adenosis has been thought to be one source of pain in this group because of the occasional finding, on histologic examination, of perineural involvement in patients with this condition.[80] Perineural involvement is quite rare, however, and is almost certainly incidental. Continuous, nonlocalized pain has sometimes been thought to be the end stage of severe, cyclic mastalgia.[67] Symptoms improved spontaneously in less than 50% of the noncyclical group; in general, noncyclical breast pain does not seem to be hormonally sensitive.[67]

Other causes of breast pain, although less common, are more precisely characterized. Trauma can be a cause of pain, which is usually strictly localized to the site of a previous injury or surgical scar. This type of pain may occur at any time up to 30 years after the trauma, and is often related to fat necrosis or hematoma. Pregnancy causes an increase in breast sensitivity[75] and breast pain may be its first sign. Another common cause of breast pain, Tietze syndrome or costochondritis,[80,85] affected 11% of the patients in Preece's series and 4% of those in Bish-

Table 2-1
Differential Diagnosis of Mastalgia

Diagnosis	*Wisbey*[83] (No. patients / %)	*Bishop*[85] (No. patients / %)	*Preece*[80] (No. patients / %)
Cyclic mastalgia	174/67%	44/53%	93/40%
Noncylic mastalgia	67/25%	8/9%	81/35%
Trigger spot		6/7%	
Continuous		2/2%	
Nonbreast origin		22/26%	27/12%
Tietze syndrome	17/6%	3/4%	25/12%
Cervical root radiculopathy		17/20%	
Unclassified		8/10%	

op's. It is an inflammation of the costochondral junction that can occur spontaneously or following radiation therapy and that is characterized by tenderness on deep palpation. It usually resolves spontaneously, but it may be treated with anti-inflammatory agents.[86] Radiculopathy of the cervical root may also be interpreted as breast pain. This pain is usually not confined to the breast, but extends into the neck and along the outer border of the arm.[85] It often affects the C6 or C7 roots as a result of narrowing of the disc space. It may be detected by careful motor, sensory, and reflex testing, and confirmed by radiographic studies. Mechanical approaches to treatment have been most successful, including physiotherapy, application of a cervical collar, or, in some cases, traction.[87] Finally, cancer may cause localized pain, so any clinical work-up should include a careful physical examination, mammogram, and biopsy, if indicated.

Dominant Lumps

Dominant lumps are clinically benign breast lesions that are distinct, persistent, and relatively unchanging. Their main importance lies in the fact that they must be distinguished from carcinoma. The most common lesions that form dominant lumps are gross cysts, galactoceles, and fibroadenomas. Sometimes, however, less common pathologic entities may present as dominant lumps (see the section on pathology, below). Most of the time, the first step in diagnosing a dominant lump will involve a needle aspiration to determine if the mass is cystic or solid. This may be done easily on an outpatient basis with a 22-gauge needle and syringe. If the lesion is cystic, the fluid is removed and the cyst is collapsed (Fig. 2-2). If, however, the lesion is solid, it must be removed to rule out cancer definitively. Dominant lumps do not usually respond to the hormonal or other therapeutic maneuvers that are sometimes effective in treating mastalgia or nodularity.

FIGURE 2-2. Aspiration of a gross cyst.

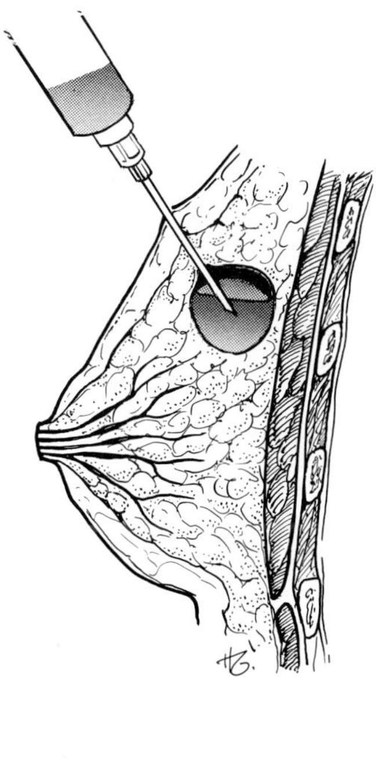

Gross Cysts

Gross cysts, or macrocysts, are the most common dominant lump found in the breast. A gross cyst, as described by Haagensen, is a distinct entity consisting of a palpable, fluid-filled sac within the breast tissue.[12] These cysts may occur in patients as young as 25 years of age, but are most common in those between the ages of 35 and 50 years. Most commonly, the development of gross cysts ceases with menopause, although occasionally, a postmenopausal woman will develop a gross cyst, particularly if she has been receiving estrogen replacement therapy.[88]

Clinically, gross cysts may be silent or painful, and may cause palpable lumps or be seen only on ultrasonography. The consistency of these cysts depends on the pressure of the fluid within them and the amount of normal breast tissue surrounding them. With a low amount of pressure, they will appear soft and fluctuant; however, when the cyst is tense or deep, it may feel like a solid tumor. These cysts are often solitary, but may also be multiple, feeling somewhat like a cluster of grapes upon palpation. They may develop almost overnight or more gradually, and may resolve as rapidly. The presenting symptom of a rapidly developing cyst is often localized pain, thought to result from the distention of the surrounding tissue or possibly, from escape of cystic fluid into the surrounding breast tissue, invoking a sterile inflammatory reaction. Discharge from the nipple is only occasionally associated with gross cysts.

Gross cysts are often demonstrated by mammography or ultrasonography in a palpably normal breast. These asymptomatic radiographic lesions probably do not require treatment. The main significance of gross cysts is that they often form dominant lumps and, therefore, must be differentiated from cancerous masses. Aspiration is both diagnostic and therapeutic. Although ultrasonography is a valuable tool in distinguishing between cystic and solid lesions, it is usually not necessary. Initial fear that aspiration would deposit cancer cells along the needle tract has not been borne out in careful clinical follow-up studies,[88,89] and most surgeons agree that aspiration is the treatment of choice.[90,91] The procedure is done with a 20- or 22-gauge needle and syringe. Local anesthesia may be used, but the procedure is not usually painful. A cyst may contain as little as 0.5 ml of fluid, or as much as 50 ml to 60 ml. The fluid in a cyst will vary from straw-colored to brown, green, or black, but it is not usually grossly bloody. There is some controversy over the value of having the cystic fluid analyzed for cytology.[92] However, most surgeons agree that this is not cost-effective. If a cyst recurs, it may be reaspirated. The indications for open surgical excision include a mass that does not completely disappear with aspiration (other than the rim of compressed breast tissue which resolves spontaneously over one to two weeks); fluid in the cyst that is grossly bloody (except in the case of a bloody tap, which yields fresh blood); and a gross cyst that recurs more than twice.[93] These situations may represent an intracystic papilloma or papillary carcinoma. Some clinicians will inject a cyst with air or contrast material after aspiration to demonstrate the absence of these lesions. Although this practice produces elegant radiographs, it is usually not cost-effective.

Since cystic fluid is readily obtainable, many investigators have analyzed it for electrolytes,[94] proteins,[19,95,96] and hormones.[19,97–101] Perhaps the most useful of these investigations has led to the analysis of gross cystic disease protein as a marker in advanced breast cancer.[102] Other clinical applications of these basic studies are lacking at this time.

The relationship of gross cysts to cancer has been controversial. Haagensen reported a fourfold increase in the incidence of subsequent cancer after 40 years of follow-up of his 2017 sequential patients.[103] Harrington and Lesnick demonstrated an incidence of subsequent cancer that was 3.5 times greater than normal over a period of 13 years in women with gross cysts.[88] The average interval from the aspiration of a breast cyst to the development of cancer was 7.9 years. Other authors have disputed this relationship.[104] Some explanation for this discrepancy may be forthcoming from Dupont's and Page's most recent work, which shows that the incidence of breast cancer in patients with gross cysts and a family history of breast cancer (in mother, sister, or daughter) was increased threefold, whereas gross cysts alone did not confer any significant increased risk (1.5).[105] It may actually be this confounding influence of family history on the risk attributed to the presence of gross cysts that is reflected in the previous studies rather than the gross cysts alone.

A few patients will develop multiple cysts that cause anxiety and discomfort. These can usually be managed by periodic aspirations until menopause brings relief. Rarely, bilateral mastectomies have been performed in such patients.

Galactoceles

A galactocele is a simple, milk-filled cyst, probably formed by overdistention of a lactiferous duct. Usually, it presents as a firm, nontender mass in the breast tissue, commonly in the upper quadrants beyond the areolar border. Diagnostic aspiration is often curative. Ice packs are usually applied to the peripheral adjacent breast tissue. On rare occasions, reaspiration, as many as four times, has been necessary, but surgical resection is rarely needed. Interestingly, there is not a clear association between galactoceles and either preexisting or subsequent gross cysts.

Fibroadenomas

Fibroadenomas are the most common benign solid tumors of the female breast. They may be seen at any time after puberty, but occur most frequently in women in their third decade and represent the most common breast tumors in women younger than 25 years of age. These tumors may also be seen in postmenopausal women, but it is most likely that the fibroadenomas in these patients develop prior to menopause and become clinically apparent with involution of the surrounding breast tissue. Fibroadenomas are said to occur more frequently in blacks. In addition, although Haagensen has the impression that the incidence of multiple tumors is greater in blacks than in Caucasians, the incidence of multiplicity in his own series of 123 cases of multiple fibroadenomas was about 20% for each group.[12] Fibroadenomas are hormonally responsive and may increase in size toward the end of each menstrual cycle. Recent studies have demonstrated the presence of estrogen receptors in fibroadenomas, which may explain this occurrence. Pregnancy may induce considerable enlargement of these tumors. Interestingly, the incidence of fibroadenomas appears to be decreased in oral contraceptive users.[20]

Clinically, fibroadenomas are painless, well-circumscribed, freely movable tumors with a rounded, lobulated, or discoid configuration. They are usually rubbery-firm but, when calcified, may be stony hard. Differentiation from a solitary cyst may, at times, be difficult.[12] Although these tumors may become quite large, they are usually 2 cm to 4 cm in diameter when excised.

Simple gross excision is the treatment of choice for these tumors because they will not regress spontaneously, and tend to enlarge over time. Very small fibroadenomas and those detected only on mammography may sometimes be watched, rather than excised, depending on the clinical situation (see the section on pathology, below, for information on special types of fibroadenomas).

Nipple Discharge

The secretion of fluid from the nipple of a newborn baby or any mature woman is not unusual, nor is it a sign of breast pathology. In the presence of growth hormone, insulin, and adrenal hormones, and with the stimulation of estrogen, progesterone, and prolactin, the breast secretes. At the breast clinic of the Free Hospital for Women, using a special suction device, we were able to demonstrate nipple secretion in 83% of the consecutive breasts examined. Hot compresses, or a warm, soapy examination prior to suction was used in each case. These women were unselected, nonpregnant, and many were in their seventh, eighth, and ninth decades. The normal color of these secretions may be clear, brown, green, blue, milky, yellow, or a mixture of these.

Galactorrhea

Most endocrinologists define galactorrhea as the spontaneous secretion of a milky discharge. This discharge is usually due to stimulation of the breast by elevated prolactin secretion from the pituitary. Because hyperprolactinemia inhibits the pulsatile secretion of gonadatropin releasing hormone, menstrual irregularities (most commonly, oligomenorrhea or amenorrhea) are also often

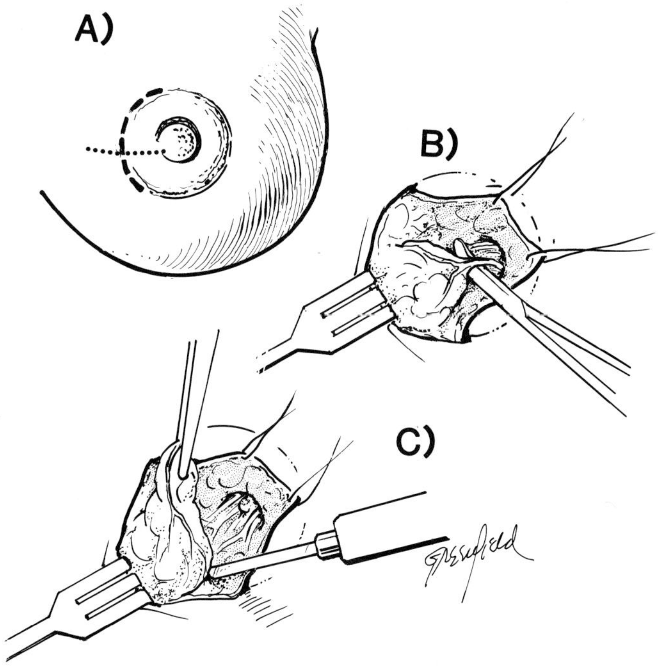

FIGURE 2-3. Excision of a single duct or a chronic subareolar abscess. *(A)* Incision can be circumareolar or radial. *(B)* Identifying entire duct. *(C)* Removing entire involved duct with core of breast tissue (note that remaining ducts are intact).

present. However, hyperprolactinemia may be manifested either as menstrual disorders or as galactorrhea alone. Since the clinical measurement of human prolactin became possible, hyperprolactinemia has been found to be fairly common. Prolactin secretion may be elevated in thyroid disorders, or as a result of breast or chest stimulation, surgical scars, use of oral contraceptives or many of the drugs that are used for central nervous system sedation and tranquilization, brain tumors or craniopharyngiomas, or commonly, benign pituitary adenomas and prolactinomas.

The appropriate evaluation of a woman with galactorrhea includes thyroid function tests and measurement of prolactin levels. A repeat prolactin level measurement is often wise in unclear cases. When significant hyperprolactinemia is demonstrated (*i.e.,* $> 50\mu/ml$), and in other special cases, a computed tomography (CT) scan of the pituitary fossa and visual field measurements by an ophthalmologist are indicated. Initial management of small prolactinomas should be conservative, with annual prolactin and CT scan measurements. Bromocriptine therapy will restore normal ovulatory function to many women, and may be responsible for apparent shrinkage of the adenomas. Transsphenoidal resection is quite successful for symptomatic or enlarging tumors.

Abnormal Nipple Discharge

When nipple discharge is grossly bloody or persistently guaiac-positive, or when the secretion has a sticky, clear character, further evaluation is indicated. Cytologic studies obtained with frosted or albumin-coated glass slides may help to distinguish between benign and malignant causes of abnormal secretion. The presence of erythrocytes and papillary clusters of 30 ductal cells or more suggests a malignant process.[106] Contrast ductographic mammography is available and, in some cases, might help localize the area from which the discharge originates. The tumor may often be localized by palpation of the circumareolar region. Pressure over the area of the breast harboring the papilloma (the pressure point) results in discharge from the nipple.[12] Less frequently, the lesion may be discovered because of a small, palpable tumor beneath the areola. Rarely, papillomas may cause nipple retraction.

Occasionally, duct resection may be performed over a probe placed in the bleeding duct if the mass can be localized, but usually, nipple-flap duct resection is more accurate in determining the source of discharge. With this technique (Fig. 2-3), a circumareolar incision is made and the areola is undermined to the nipple base, where a teasing dissection then reveals the lactiferous duct sinuses. Gentle occlusion of the suspect duct allows its positive identification if the secretion is thereby stopped. The positively identified duct is then divided and its peripheral course followed out through the breast parenchyma; a 1-cm, circumferential cuff of tissue is included with the duct. This dissection is continued, guided by duct traction, to the deep fascia or to the fatty margins of the breast. The resulting specimen is tagged with a marker on the central duct end so that the pathologist can orient the tissue. Some surgeons have recommended removing the major duct system, rather than a single duct, if the lesion is not well localized and the woman is past childbearing age (Fig. 2-4).[12,107–109]

The most common causes of occult blood in nipple discharge are, in order of frequency, intraductal papilloma, duct ectasia, "fibrocystic disease," and carcinoma (Table 2-2). One series showed the incidence of occult cancer to be 5.9% in 270 patients undergoing duct resection.[110] The pathology of these entities will be discussed separately.

Grossly bloody nipple discharge may be smeared for cytology and managed conservatively in two special situations: during pregnancy or lactation and during adjuvant chemotherapy for carcinoma. Spontaneous cessation of bleeding in these instances suggests bloody degeneration of intraductal lesions, such as papillomas.

Breast Infections

Excluding puerperal events, infection of the human breast is rare. Those infections that do occur may be thought of as *intrinsic* (attributable to disorders in breast structure or function), or *extrinsic* (coincidentally involving the breast). Intrinsic infections include puerperal mastitis; lactational breast abscesses; chronic, recurrent, subareolar

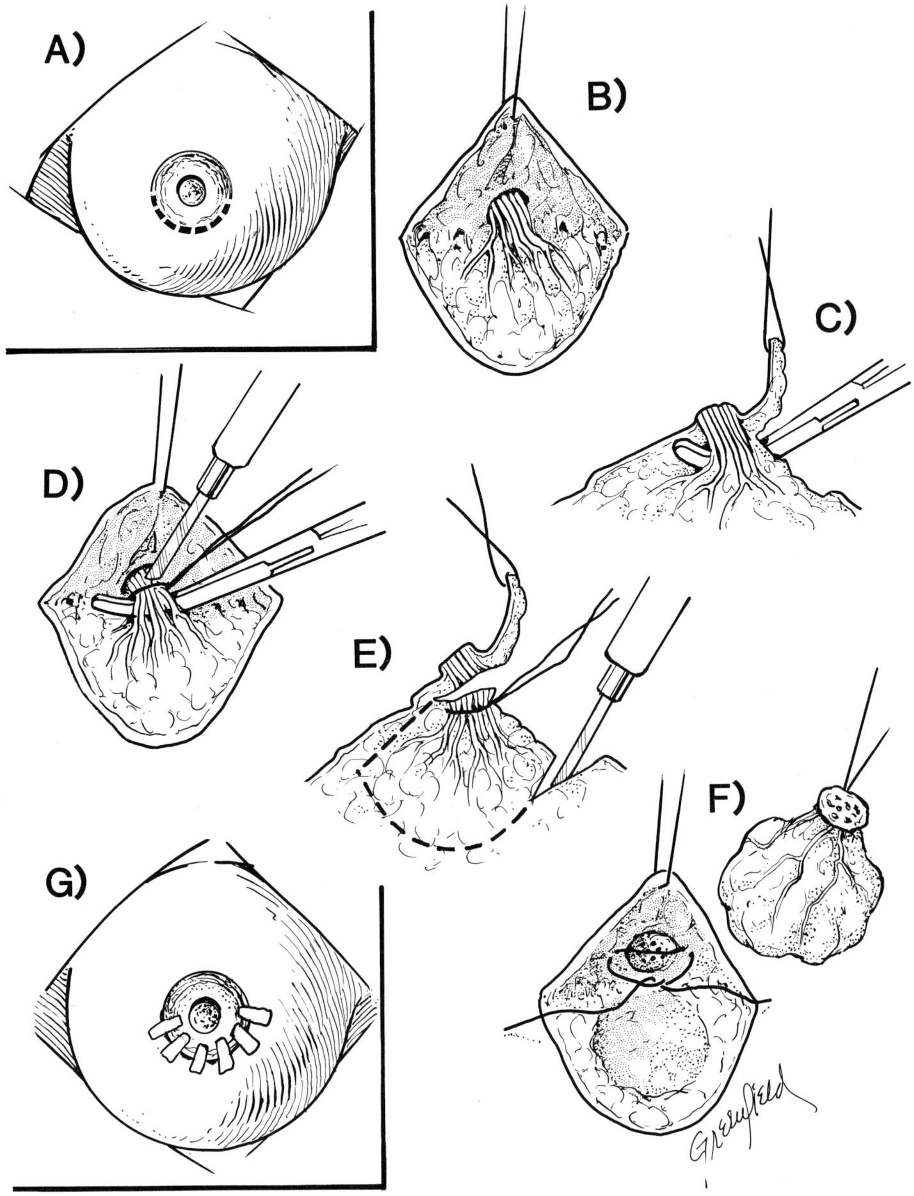

FIGURE 2-4. Excision of the major duct system. *(A)* Circumareolar incision. *(B)* Undermining areola. *(C)* Isolating lactiferous sinuses. *(D)* Transecting end of major duct system. *(E)* Removing core of surrounding breast tissue. *(F)* Specimen has been removed and cavity is being closed. *(G)* Incision closed.

abscesses; and acute mastitis associated with macrocystic breast disease.

Intrinsic Mastitis

POSTPARTUM CHANGES. During the postpartum period, the lactating breasts normally undergo a one- to three-day period of engorgement, marked by swelling, firmness, edema, and discomfort. This usually subsides without incident after a short interval. In bottlefeeding mothers, applications of ice packs and a firm binding are time-honored symptomatic treatments. At least partial abatement or postponement of this engorgement phase may be achieved through the use of hormonal therapy, which blunts the otherwise crescendo outpouring of prolactin at this time. Therapeutic regimens of estrogen, androgen, androgen and estrogen, or bromocriptine are all mostly successful in improving patients' symptoms of engorgement. However, the detrimental effects of sex steroids on the risk of thromboembolic complications, and their theoretical late effects on endocrine organs have lowered enthusiasm for lactation-suppression steroid therapy. In fact, the anxiety-producing details of real or possible side effects provided in the drug package inserts have discouraged most obstetricians and mothers from initiating steroid therapy. Bromocriptine use is also relatively

Table 2-2
Pathology of Nipple Discharges

Pathology	*Urban*[116] (*No. patients / %*)	*Chaudary*[110] (*No. patients / %*)
Intraductal papilloma (papillomatosis)	236/45%	132/45%
Duct ectasia	190/36%	94/32%
Carcinoma	41/8%	16/5%
Infection (chronic subareolar abscess)	42/8%	
Other	13/2.5%	28/10%

rare because of its cost and its frequent side effects, such as hypotension, headaches, dizziness, and nausea.

LACTATIONAL MASTITIS. After the phase of physiologic edema and engorgement, productive lactation should be comfortable, even pleasant. Obstruction to flow of any of the major breast ducts, usually associated with inflammatory areolar skin reactions, causes an obstructive mastopathy. Back pressure from the obstructed duct or lactiferous sinus, combined with forceful milk secretion and ejection, predisposes the patient to bacterial infection, as occurs with obstructions of the urinary, biliary, salivary, or any other high-flow system. This obstructive mastopathy may progress from milk stasis to noninfectious mastitis, and subsequently, to infectious mastitis. Classification into these three stages can be accomplished by laboratory analysis of the secreted milk for leukocyte counts and quantitative cultivation for bacteria.[111] Cases of milk stasis are characterized by leukocyte counts of less than 10^6 and less than 10^3 bacteria per milliliter of milk. Patients with noninfectious mastitis were shown to have leukocyte counts of greater than 10^6, but bacterial counts of less than 10^3 per milliliter of milk. Patients with infectious mastitis had leukocyte counts of greater than 10^6, as well as bacterial counts of greater than 10^3 per milliliter. In practical terms, this differentiation may be made on the basis of the degree of pain, redness, and fever.

Local application of heat is often used in cases of breast soreness during lactation. The heat may help resolve the reaction in the nipple and areolar skin that has caused the obstruction, but the attendant increase in breast metabolism and enhanced milk production and excretion may lead to worsening of the obstructive mastopathy. Efforts to empty the involved segment (including initial nursing on that side, manual expression of milk from that segment, or pumping of that breast); ice packs to reduce the intraluminal pressure via reduced local breast metabolism; and administration of a broad-spectrum antibiotic, such as ampicillin or erythromycin, will usually abort this process quite quickly.[112] The bacteria involved are usually common skin inhabitants, such as *Micrococcus dyogenes,* streptococci, and hemophilus species.

LACTATIONAL BREAST ABSCESS. In less than 10% of patients with infectious mastitis, the infection does not resolve promptly, and breast abscesses develop. A unilocular, superficial abscess may be successfully treated by needle aspiration of the cavity, sensitivity testing, and specific antibiotic therapy. Deep, multilocular, and persistent abscesses, however, require surgical incision and drainage. In order to break down the septae between locules properly, general anesthesia may be necessary. Drains from all cavities must be brought through the skin incisions, which usually can be placed cosmetically within Langer's lines. Lactation suppression may be necessary in cases of breast abscess.

Chronic Recurrent Subareolar Abscess

Chronic, recurrent, subareolar abscesses represent another fairly common infectious process of the breast. In one series of hospitalizations for breast infections, chronic subareolar abscesses were as common as lactational abscesses.[113] Affected patients may experience recurrent abscess formation, spontaneous rupture or drainage of the abscess, and often, chronic formation of areolar fistulas. These abscesses occur in mature women, usually during their reproductive years. Bacterial cultures and antibiotic therapy are essentially useless. Because of the smoldering nature of the clinical problem, and because squamous metaplasia was found in 70% of resected specimens, Crile has coined the term "squamous metaplasia of lactiferous ducts," or SMOLD, to describe this entity.[114] He believes that ruptured hyperkeratotic ducts extrude keratin into the breast stroma, causing a severe inflammatory reaction. It is also possible that this hyperkeratotic squamous metaplasia functionally obstructs the ducts, creating another obstructive mastopathy similar to lactational mastitis. In this case, however, the obstruction occurs slowly because of the low-flow, low-pressure, intraductal flux from secretions in the nonlactating breast.

Cure depends on the removal of the duct by making a flap of the areola and dissecting right under the skin of the nipple, removing about 2 cu cm of tissue (Fig. 2-3). The wound may be sutured primarily or left to heal secondarily according to Smith.[115] Despite apparently adequate surgery, these lesions may be obstinately persistent, recurring in about 50% of patients. Complete excision of the fistulous tract is probably most important, although many authors recommend en bloc excision of the entire major duct system, in addition to excision of the abscess cavity and sinus tract (see Fig. 2-3).[107–109, 116]

Acute Mastitis Associated With Macrocystic Breasts

Occasionally, a patient with known or unrecognized gross cystic disease of the breast will present with localized redness, swelling, pain, and fever. This condition has been observed in teenagers and in patients throughout the menstrual years. Needle aspiration for culture and for cytology should be performed immediately to rule out inflammatory cancer. Slow resolution of this mastitis without remarkable effect by antibiotics is the rule. Any patients in whom the diagnosis is questionable should undergo an open biopsy to further rule out inflammatory carcinoma. This condition probably represents internal rupture of a cyst with inflammatory reaction to the cyst contents.

Extrinsic Infections

Extrinsic infections of the breast occur because the breast represents a significant portion of the integument and is, therefore, subject to any skin disease, and also because of its location on the chest wall with communicating internal mammary vessels from the thoracic cavity. Abscesses of Montgomery's glands and other sebaceous cyst abscesses must be excised if they fail to respond to local heat and antibiotic therapy. Syphilis of the nipple as a primary chancre may be differentiated from Paget's disease by contact cytology and dark-field examination. Secondary syphilis rash and late syphilis gummas are possible in the breast. Antibiotic therapy may be relied upon to reverse luetic changes in the breast. Tuberculosis of the breast, which occurs rarely today, has required simple mastectomy in some cases in the past because of failure of chemotherapy to eradicate its granulomatous foci permanently. Other thoracic diseases, such as metastatic lung cancer and Wegener's granulomatosis, may present in the breast.[117] Basically, all other skin conditions may also affect that skin which has become breast tissue.

TREATMENT OF BENIGN BREAST SYMPTOMS

As in other aspects of benign breast disorders, the literature on treatment is confusing and notably lacks a strictly defined patient population. A number of remedies have been proposed for a variety of benign breast symptoms, and these have produced varying degrees of success. Suggested therapeutic regimens range from the administration of hormones and hormone inhibitors to dietary changes and vitamins, and propose to treat all elements of benign breast conditions from mastalgia to lumpiness and from gross cysts to fibroadenomas. After a review of the pertinent literature on treatment, an overall approach to management will be proposed.

Hormones and Hormone Inhibitors

Progesterone

Current theories on the hormonal basis of mastalgia, if not all benign breast diseases, have led to several modes of treatment with varying efficacy. Since the underlying defect is thought to be a relative insufficiency of progesterone in relation to estrogen in the luteal phase, the most obvious treatment is the administration of progesterone. Geschickter suggested the use of progesterone (corpus luteum therapy) in the 1940s.[11] He described the results of treating 15 patients with mastodynia with intramuscular progesterone (5 mg in oil twice weekly for the last 2 weeks of the menstrual cycle), reporting that all but two patients showed some improvement. Several subsequent, uncontrolled studies have shown an equally favorable response.[118–121] Other progestins, such as norethisterone,[122] norethynodrel,[123] and mastodynon,[127] have all been tried with some success in Europe.[124]

Recent studies on the use of percutaneous progestin alone[126] or in combination with oral progesterone[125] to treat mastalgia and diffuse nodularity have yielded good clinical results. Mammographic results were less clear, but they did not always correlate with symptoms initially.[126] Two randomized controlled studies have confirmed a beneficial effect of oral progesterone on mastalgia [127,128] while one shows it to be worse than placebo.[129]

Experimental support for the use of progesterone for the treatment of pathological precancerous lesions comes from a recent report from Japan showing inhibition of the formation of precancerous, mammary, hyperplastic, alveolar nodules in mice treated with medroxyprogesterone.[130] On the other hand, the use of medroxyprogesterone in beagle dogs has been shown to produce malignant breast nodules.[131] Neither finding has been duplicated in humans.[125]

Bromocriptine

Prolactin is thought to be involved in benign breast disorders only when combined with estrogen excess or progesterone deficiency. Bromocriptine, a prolactin antagonist, may restore normal luteal function in women with luteal insufficiency and moderately elevated prolactin levels and has, therefore, been employed in the treatment of benign breast symptoms.

Dogliotti and co-workers found a marked decrease in pain (89%), mammary tension (80%), nodularity (92%), and tenderness (83%) in 150 patients treated with bromocriptine.[132] Positive results from bromocriptine therapy persisted in 91% of these patients 3 months after discontinuing therapy, and in 70% 1 year later. Several double-blind crossover trials of the use of bromocriptine in the treatment of mastalgia have shown a statistically significant reduction in pain, tenderness, and nodularity.[64,65,133] Durning and Sellwood noted, however, that 30% of their patients had significant side effects, including nausea, headaches, and dizziness, which did not correlate with prolactin levels.[65] They concluded that, although there is a group of patients with severe, cyclic mastalgia who benefit from bromocriptine, in patients with less severe symptoms, the side effects may outweigh the benefits. Marzetti and colleagues[134] noted subjective improvement, as well as improvement in the findings on clinical examination, but no improvement in echography, in their study of bromocriptine and "fibrocystic mastopathy."[134] Their findings support Ayers' hypothesis that mastodynia is hormone-related, but that nodularity, as defined by sonograph, is hormone-independent.[66]

Several authors have used bromocriptine to treat premenstrual syndrome and have noted improvement in the breast symptoms.[135,136]

Danazol

Greenblatt and co-workers were the first to use danazol, a synthetic (2,3 isoxazol) derivative of 17-α-ethinyltestosterone, to treat "fibrocystic disease."[137] The effectiveness of the drug was confirmed in several studies.[138–142] The original studies of its pharmacology confirmed that danazol was a strong antigonadotropin with mild androgenic effects and no other hormonal properties. However, more recent research suggests that it has direct effects on hypothalamic-pituitary function, several classes of steroid receptors, gonadal steroidogenesis, and endogenous steroid metabolism.[143] Mansel performed a double-blind crossover trial of the use of danazol in patients with painful nodular breast disease and found that the danazol-treated patients experienced significant improvement in comparison to the placebo-treated group.[144] They postulated that the mechanism of action is an abolition of the follicle stimulating hormone (FSH)/luteinizing hormone (LH) peak; however, the drug also has mild androgenic effects and possibly progestogenic effects. The androgenic effects may be significant, since androgens have been shown to improve benign breast symptoms.[145] Plasma progesterone levels were shown to be decreased to an anovulatory level, and prolactin levels were not changed. Thus, the exact hormonal mechanism is not clear, and does not easily fit into the luteal insufficiency schema proposed by Mauvais-Jarvis.[67]

The Hjorring project in Sweden also studied danazol in a controlled, double-blind trial and showed that danazol caused a marked and sustained decrease in mastodynia when compared to placebo.[146,147] Changes in palpatory or mammographic findings, or both, were also found more consistently with the use of danazol than with placebo. Side effects included menstrual irregularities, moderate weight gain, and facial hair and voice changes.

Thyroid Hormones

Investigators have attempted to demonstrate a correlation between hypothyroidism and benign breast disorders. Daro demonstrated improvement in cystic mastitis symptoms in 286 patients with clinical or subclinical hypothyroidism.[148] Estes studied 19 women with mastodynia and found that thyroxine produced rapid pain relief in 73% of them, with total relief being reported in 47%.[149] Softening of the breast tissue and decreased nodularity occurred within 3 months. Estes noted that three patients who had high prolactin levels before treatment experienced normalization of their prolactin levels with the administration of thyroxine. He felt that the thyroid hormone had reduced the level of TRH, thus decreasing prolactin levels. More recently, Peters and colleagues studied the ability of thyroxine to normalize the exaggerated prolactin responsiveness to TRH in patients with mastalgia.[150] During an 8-week course of thyroxine, the significantly elevated, TRH-induced, prolactin response in patients was decreased by 50% and reached the level of their control counterparts, whereas the responses of the control subjects were not decreased. Patients exhibited significantly lower levels of progesterone than did the control subjects, although estradiol levels were not different. Peters' group postulated that relative estrogen dominance is the cause of increased prolactin responsiveness to thyroid releasing hormone, and that thyroid hormone may antagonize the effects of estradiol on the lactotroph TRH receptors.[151] The thyroid treatment did not seem to have any effect on the luteal function of patients or control subjects, although clinical mastalgia in those receiving thyroxine was improved when compared to the mastalgia in those receiving placebo.

Tamoxifen

The evidence that benign breast lesions have estrogen receptors and that they respond to hormonal influences has led some investigators to try tamoxifen as a treatment for benign breast disorders.[152] It is known that tamoxifen achieves its effect in hormonally sensitive breast cancers by competing for estrogen receptors in target tissues and possibly by lowering serum prolactin levels. Ricciardi and co-workers found that 71% of patients with severe breast dysplasia who were treated with tamoxifen experienced a complete remission of symptoms and disappearance of lesions as assessed by echography and clinical examination.[152] Although estrogen receptors were assayed in tissue from 10 patients, none were found. In another recent study, Shaaban showed improvements in 30 of 31 patients treated with tamoxifen.[153] A recent randomized controlled study has combined this beneficial effect of tamoxifen in mastalgia. Another estrogen antagonist, ethamoxytriphetol, has also been tested in patients with symptomatic, histologically proven, cystic breast disease, and has been helpful in 22 of 25 patients.[148] Two patients had severe side effects of nausea, anorexia, and epigastric pain.

Other Hormones

Human chorionic gonadotropin hormone effected an improvement in clinical and mammographic findings in

97% of patients in an uncontrolled study, presumably by altering ovarian physiology and improving progestational levels.[156] Use of androgens in some patients has resulted in subjective improvement, but not without side effects, such as hirsutism and virilization.[145] Oral contraceptives and other combinations of estrogen and progesterone have also resulted in some improvement in breast symptoms.[157,158]

Methylxanthine Restriction

The controversy over methylxanthine restriction as a treatment for benign breast disorders is based on studies with poorly defined study groups and indistinct parameters. Minton and colleagues first reported an association between methylxanthine consumption and "fibrocystic disease" in 1979 on the basis of an uncontrolled, subjective, six-month study of 47 women.[159] Sixty-five percent of the women who abstained from methylxanthine experienced relief of symptoms within 6 months. Heyden noted, however, that this condition has a notorious reputation for waxing and waning, and that 87% of the women in his study who were receiving methylxanthine continuously, and who were observed for 6 months, had a change in the number or position of nodules, with 15% showing complete remission.[160]

Two attempts have been made to investigate this association in a more objective manner. Brooks and co-workers used graphic stress telethermometry in an uncontrolled study of 66 patients and found a reduction in both thermal activity and clinical and physical symptoms.[161] Boyle and associates limited their study group to women whose biopsies showed either microcysts or macrocysts. They found a positive association between fibrocystic disease and remembered methylxanthine consumption as compared to the control population,[162] but found no association with caffeine consumption in other forms of histologically benign breast disease or in fibroadenomas. Only the control subjects showed an increase in the likelihood of developing breast symptoms with increasing caffeine use. Thus, although this study may show an increase in actual cysts with methylxanthine use, it does not demonstrate any association of its use with either symptomatology or other histologic categories of benign breast disease.

Several case control studies have examined the association of methylxanthine consumption and benign breast disease. These studies have revealed either slight[163] or no association.[164–166]

The only American randomized, controlled, prospective study conducted was not blinded. Ernster and co-workers randomly assigned 158 women presenting with breast symptoms to either a group told to eliminate methylxanthine consumption or a group given no dietary recommendation.[167] A nonblinded nurse practitioner then serially graded the physical findings relating to nodularity. Although the overall change in palpable breast lumps was significant, the absolute change, quadrant to quadrant, was minor and of questionable clinical significance. There was no change in mammographic findings, nor was there any association between breast caffeine levels and improvement in palpable lumps. The authors felt that the minor decrease in palpable lump scores might well represent observer bias, since the scores of a sizable portion of control subjects were said to worsen, even among those who dramatically reduced caffeine levels on their own. A recent randomized, controlled trial from Milan has confirmed a lack of association between consumption of methylxanthines and fibrocystic disease using physical exam, symptoms and thermography.[168]

Minton's initial contention that methylxanthines increase both fibrocystic disease and, possibly, breast cancer stems from his observation that patients with fibrocystic breast tissue and breast cancer had elevated levels of intracellular cyclic adenosine monophosphate (cAMP) and guanosine monophosphate (GMP).[169,170] He postulated that chronic methylxanthine consumption caused permanently elevated cAMP levels in breast epithelial cells, either as a direct result of inhibition of cyclic nucleotide phosphodiesterase activity, or indirectly, via catecholamine release. He has not, however, demonstrated that systemic levels of caffeine resulting from dietary consumption or any resulting elevation of systemic catecholamine were sufficient to cause increased levels of cAMP. In addition, most cells with an accumulation of cAMP will show a desensitization to the agent, rather than an increase in sensitivity. Barber and associates studied human mammary carcinoma cells and normal mouse mammary epithelial cells to test these hypotheses.[171] They could not demonstrate the ability of methylxanthine at any pharmacologic concentration to increase cAMP levels significantly in mammary epithelial cells. Second, both normal mouse and malignant human mammary epithelial cells showed desensitization, rather than enhancement, to subsequent additions of catecholamines. Although Minton and co-workers claim that both caffeine and a high-fat diet significantly promote dimethylbenzanthracene-induced breast cancer in rats,[172] their statistical analysis has been questioned.[173] In addition, Petrek and colleagues showed caffeine to have an inhibitory effect on diethylstilbestrol (DES)-induced breast cancer in rats.[174]

Thus, the data linking methylxanthines to benign breast disease are far from clear. Minton's initial observations are interesting, but thus far, have not been borne out in controlled studies with clearly defined study populations, nor have the pathophysiological mechanisms been clearly established.

Vitamin E

Abrams was the first to report that vitamin E (α-tocopherol) reduced tenderness and cyst size among patients with chronic cystic mastitis.[175] In small studies, London and co-workers[176] and Sundaram and colleagues[177] demonstrated a clinical response to vitamin E, and postulated that α-tocopherol altered adrenal steroidogenesis.

Most recently, however, in two separate, randomized, double-blind, controlled trials, no significant difference was demonstrated between α-tocopherol and placebo in benign breast disease detected clinically, radiologically, or sonographically. London reported a response in 53% of the patients receiving placebo, and in 55% of those receiving vitamin E.[178] Likewise, no significant difference in sonographic or mammographic findings or hormone levels was found in patients before or after therapy. Ernster and associates confirmed these findings in a similar study.[179] These recent studies again demonstrate the necessity for a double-blind, controlled, randomized trial to evaluate any treatment for such a variable diagnosis as "fibrocystic disease."

Diuretics

Diuretics and salt restriction have been used on a clinical basis to relieve the premenstrual bloated sensation in patients with benign breast disease. This treatment is based on the premise that the swelling is the cause of the pain. However, Preece and colleagues showed quite clearly that there were no changes in total body water premenstrually in patients with breast pain.[180] No controlled studies of diuretics in the treatment of benign breast disease exist.

Prostaglandin Inhibitors

Rolland and co-workers studied prostaglandin levels in patients with benign mastopathy and found significantly higher blood levels of prostaglandin E_2 (PGE_2) compared to the levels in the control subjects.[181] They confirmed the presence of low progesterone levels, but also found somewhat lower estradiol levels. The mammary thermographic responses to prostaglandin inhibitors were determined in both phases of the menstrual cycle and showed fair thermographic evidence of a cooling effect on the breast in the majority of patients.

Surgery

There is no question that any woman who is thought to have a dominant lump should undergo surgical biopsy. The accuracy of needle aspiration cytology in comparison to that of excisional biopsy is still controversial, and is highly dependent upon the skill and experience of the cytopathologist. The purpose of a surgical approach to a perceived dominant lump is, however, diagnostic, and not therapeutic.

In the case of nodular breasts, limited surgery seldom eliminates the problem because it does nothing to change the etiology of the lumpiness. In some types of mastalgia, usually limited to those cases of localized pain associated with a trigger zone, surgery may be useful. Sometimes, surgical excision of this area may relieve the pain. Also, in cases of ductal ectasia or periductal mastitis, as described by Preece,[80] surgical removal of the major ductal system may be curative. (See Fig. 2-4.)

Most authors note that cyclic mastalgia seldom disappears with mastectomy, whether total or subcutaneous. The question then arises as to whether there are breasts so lumpy that they defy accurate follow-up, either clinically or by radiography, and, therefore, should be removed as the only way to ensure against the future development of breast cancer. This is a very controversial proposal since the issue involves the prophylactic removal of a normal body part to prevent the possible development of disease.[182] Only in rare circumstances, and only after multiple opinions and honest discussions with the patient, should this approach even be considered. It should be understood that menopause often brings improvement in the clinical and mammographic findings, so follow-up in these women will not always be so difficult. In addition, cancer risk is actually spread over a lifetime, not just the difficult decade between the ages of 35 and 45 years.[183] Clinicians should be careful not to fall into the trap of thinking or saying, "It would be much easier if you had both your breasts removed." It is often easier for the doctor, who no longer has to take responsibility for detecting cancer, but not for the woman, who must live with her deformed, albeit reconstructed, breasts. Cancerphobia is an overused term that often reflects the fear instilled by a physician, rather than a patient's psychopathology. A realistic explanation of the actual risks is often all that is needed.

In those few cases in which a prophylactic operation is jointly decided upon by the patient and the practitioner, the question arises as to the type of mastectomy that should be performed. It has been documented that a subcutaneous mastectomy does not remove all the breast tissue,[184] and that, at least in rats, removing a portion of breast tissue does not reduce the cancer risk proportionately.[185] Thus, a subcutaneous mastectomy that removes 90% of the breast tissue does not decrease the cancer risk by 90%, but leaves 10% of the breast tissue at full risk. A subcutaneous mastectomy, therefore, is not a good prophylactic operation. In addition, there have been several reports of cancers developing in the flaps after subcutaneous mastectomy.[182,186–188] A standard simple or total mastectomy, with or without reconstruction, is a better prophylactic operation, although the cosmetic results are less satisfactory.[120,182]

Other Modes of Treatment

Many other treatment regimens for benign breast disorders have been suggested anecdotally, including the use of an "adequate supporting brassiere" in mastodynia;[189] the withdrawal of ginseng tea;[190] the injection of steroids directly into the breast;[191] the administration of vitamin A, vitamin B complex, or iodine; and the use of oral evening primrose oil.[129] The Welsh group, in a nonrandomized, uncontrolled study, has shown orally administered evening primrose oil to be superior to placebo in the treatment of severe mastalgia.[129]

OVERALL MANAGEMENT OF BENIGN BREAST DISORDERS

The management of dominant lumps, nipple discharge, infections, and inflammations of the breast has already been reviewed. Most important is the rule that any dominant lump that does not yield fluid on aspiration should be examined by biopsy to rule out cancer.

Most patients who present to the physician with physiologic, cyclic swelling and tenderness, mild mastalgia, or nodularity are seeking reassurance that they do not have cancer. A careful examination and, in patients older than 35 years of age, a mammogram will help rule out this possibility. An explanation of the hormonal nature of the breast symptoms is very helpful in assuaging the patient's anxiety and is usually all the treatment that is necessary.[129] This is often a good time to teach or review with the patient the importance of breast self-examination and regular mammographic screening as early detection methods. If the physician has any question about the results of a physical examination, it is often advisable to see the patient at a different point in her menstrual cycle or to reexamine her in 3 months. Again, if there is a suspicious area, the patient should be referred to a surgeon for biopsy to rule out cancer.

In severe, noncyclic mastalgia, routine measures to rule out cancer must be taken; then, an attempt may be made to better characterize the pain. It may be localized to one area of the breast or chest wall, or it may be diffuse and bilateral. Costochondritis and cervical radiculopathy should be sought and appropriately treated with anti-inflammatory agents, physiotherapy, or a cervical collar. Any questionable area on mammogram or physical examination may be surgically excised. It must be noted, however, that the presence of a trigger zone does not necessarily mean that the pain is treatable surgically. Persistent, idiopathic, noncyclic pain will usually not be relieved by conventional means, and symptomatic analgesia may be all that can be offered.[129] Patients usually respond to a frank discussion of the current lack of research on breast pain and reassurance that the pain is usually not a manifestation of cancer.

Severe, cyclic breast pain is somewhat more amenable to treatment because of its probable hormonal etiology. Affected patients have pain in their breasts that starts at ovulation and persists until menstruation. They may have only one pain-free week per month. They often state that they cannot wear a brassiere or tolerate palpation, and are seeking treatment as well as reassurance. In young women in their 20s, the contraceptive pill may be helpful because it delivers a stable amount of hormones every month. Danazol and bromocriptine will often provide relief for these women; however, these drugs are expensive and have significant side effects. Most women are not willing to take such potent drugs for symptomatic relief. Currently, there is no middle range treatment available that has withstood the test of a randomized, controlled trial. French researchers have found that topical progesterone gel shows some promise,[125] and Welsh investigators have reported uncontrolled studies that provide evidence of benefit from oral evening primrose oil,[129] a remedy currently popular within the holistic health movement.

At this time of limited research and understanding of the etiology of mastalgia, a careful explanation to the patient of the limits of knowledge is often helpful. It is important for the physician to acknowledge that the woman does, in fact, have pain, that they are not alone, and that the perfect remedy is not yet available. Additional reassurance may be derived from the fact that most cyclic mastalgia is completely relieved by menopause.

Severe nodularity usually causes more concern to the physician than to the patient. Unfortunately, there is no known treatment that reliably and permanently resolves these noncystic lumps, short of surgery. It is important not to fall into the trap of recommending a prophylactic mastectomy because it would be easier than trying to follow those lumps. If a physician is uncomfortable following such a patient, the patient should be referred to another physician. Careful breast self-examination, examination by a physician, and yearly mammograms are the best methods currently available for observing these patients. Again, reassurance that menopause brings atrophy of the breast tissue and replacement by fat is encouraging to both the physician and patient. None of the proposed dietary, vitamin, or hormonal treatment regimens have, in fact, been advocated for this group of women with severely lumpy breasts.

Currently, there is no solid evidence to support dietary restriction or vitamin therapy in patients with benign breast symptoms. In addition, no one has been able to demonstrate that symptomatic treatment of benign breast disorders in any way reduces the subsequent risk of breast cancer. Therefore, the question must be asked whether it is fair to encourage women to undertake the expense and hardship of changing their lifestyle for questionable gain. It is important to recognize that a nontoxic therapy is not always justified because of its placebo effect if there is no objective evidence of benefit.[192] Most importantly, a woman needs acknowledgment of the validity of her symptoms, reassurance as to her cancer risk, and an honest discussion of current research and symptomatic modes of treatment. She can then decide which approach to symptom relief is best suited for her.

PATHOLOGIC OVERVIEW: "FIBROCYSTIC DISEASE"

As noted earlier, a wide variety of histologic conditions have been included under the broad heading of "fibrocystic disease" of the breast. It must be emphasized that, from a pathologic viewpoint, there is no such specific entity. Histologically, the term encompasses a broad spectrum of changes, some normal variants and some abnormal conditions. The breast is a very inhomogeneous organ. The nonlactating normal breast is composed primarily of adipose and fibrous tissue that is unevenly distributed. This lack of even distribution leads to physiologic inhomogeneity, irregularity, or lumpiness. Biopsy of a lumpy area may show primarily fibrous tissue and mammary epithelium. Although normal, this finding would, in most institutions, be reported as "fibrocystic disease," fibrocystic change, mammary dysplasia, chronic cystic mastitis, or any one of a number of other entities.

Benign breast disorders may be broadly categorized into two groups: localized specific entities (e.g., fibroadenoma), which will be dealt with in individual sections of this chapter; and "fibrocystic disease," which represents a wide variety of changes seen individually or in combination, and which includes cysts, stromal fibrosis, and epithelial proliferative lesions.

The pathologic significance of benign breast disease is twofold. First, a solitary lesion in the breast must be differentiated from carcinoma. Second, the significance of the observed changes with regard to the subsequent risk of developing carcinoma must be determined. The differentiation of a solitary mass from carcinoma is the province of the surgical pathologist and, for the most part, is straightforward. Determining the clinical significance of a breast biopsy in the absence of invasive carcinoma is a much more difficult problem. A number of authors have addressed this issue and have devised a wide variety of classification systems of benign breast abnormalities in an attempt to determine the significance of these lesions. The system adopted by Page and his co-workers,[104,105,193] more recently supported at a consensus meeting of the College of American Pathologists,[194] provides a pragmatic classification system for benign breast pathology. This system separates the various types of benign breast lesions into three clinically relevant groups, each composed of distinct pathologic entities: nonproliferative lesions, proliferative lesions without atypia, and atypical proliferative lesions. Such a system is of greater practical value than is the useless term "fibrocystic disease," and the use of the latter should be abandoned.

Nonproliferative Lesions

Nonproliferative lesions, as defined by Page and co-workers,[104] include cysts, papillary apocrine changes, mild hyperplasias of the usual type, epithelial-related calcifications, and fibroadenomas.

Cysts in the breast may vary tremendously in size and number, and may be microscopic or macroscopic (Fig. 2-5). They appear to originate from the terminal duct-lobular unit (TDLU), primarily through hormonally regulated dilation and failure to shrink after menstruation. Alternatively, they may arise from an obstructed duct. The epithelium of these cysts is usually two-layered, as seen in normal breast ducts and lobules. Frequently, the epithelium is either reduced to a flattened, attenuated layer or shows metaplasia, usually of the apocrine type. The stroma surrounding these cysts is variably fibrotic and often shows clusters of chronic inflammatory cells.

The breast is a modified apocrine sweat gland; therefore, it is not surprising that a common type of epithelial metaplasia is apocrine in type. Apocrine metaplasia usually occurs in dilated ducts or cysts. It is characterized by a single layer, multiple layers or papillary formations of eosinophilic cells with small, regular, round nuclei.

Mild hyperplasia of the usual type is defined as an increase in the number of epithelial cells to more than two to three layers above the basement membrane without crossing of the lumen. The cells vary in size, are often elliptical, and are not atypical. Mild hyperplasia is a very common finding, especially in biopsies performed in premenopausal women.

Calcifications are common in breast tissue. They may either be seen in blood vessels, free in the stroma, or associated with epithelium. Scattered microcalcifications are commonly seen in lobules. Diffuse microcalcifications are most commonly seen in sclerosing adenosis (see the next section).

Fibroadenomas are discussed in detail elsewhere in this chapter.

Proliferative Disorders Without Atypia

The category of proliferative disorders without atypia includes sclerosing adenosis, ductal involvement with cells characteristic of atypical lobular hyperplasia, moderate or florid hyperplasia of the usual type, and intraductal papillomas, which are discussed later in this chapter.

Sclerosing adenosis most commonly occurs in multiple, microscopic foci. Occasionally, it presents as a palpable mass. It is formed by a proliferation of both stromal and epithelial elements of the TDLU. The hallmark of sclerosing adenosis is a cellular proliferation which, at low-power magnification, is limited to a discrete area and, in fact, is lobular in configuration. Microscopically, at high magnification, these lesions may mimic infiltrating carcinoma (Fig. 2-6). It is often difficult to identify the normal, double-layered epithelium, and solid proliferations of myoid or epithelial cells may occur. The prime significance of sclerosing adenosis is its ability to mimic carcinoma. Adenosis very commonly contains microcalcifications which, on mammography, may raise the suspicion of carcinoma. Since adenosis may occur as a palpable mass, and because of its pseudoinfiltrative appearance, it may create difficulties in differential diagnosis.

Ductal involvement with cells characteristic of atypical lobular hyperplasia is an unusual phenomenon. Microscopically, this condition is characterized by small, regular cells with round nuclei. These cells usually spread beneath the normal ductal epithelium in a pagetoid fashion. In order to be classified in this category of proliferative disorders without atypia, the ductal involvement must not be extensive. Ductal involvement with cells typical of lobular proliferative lesions is not rare, and when extensive, is

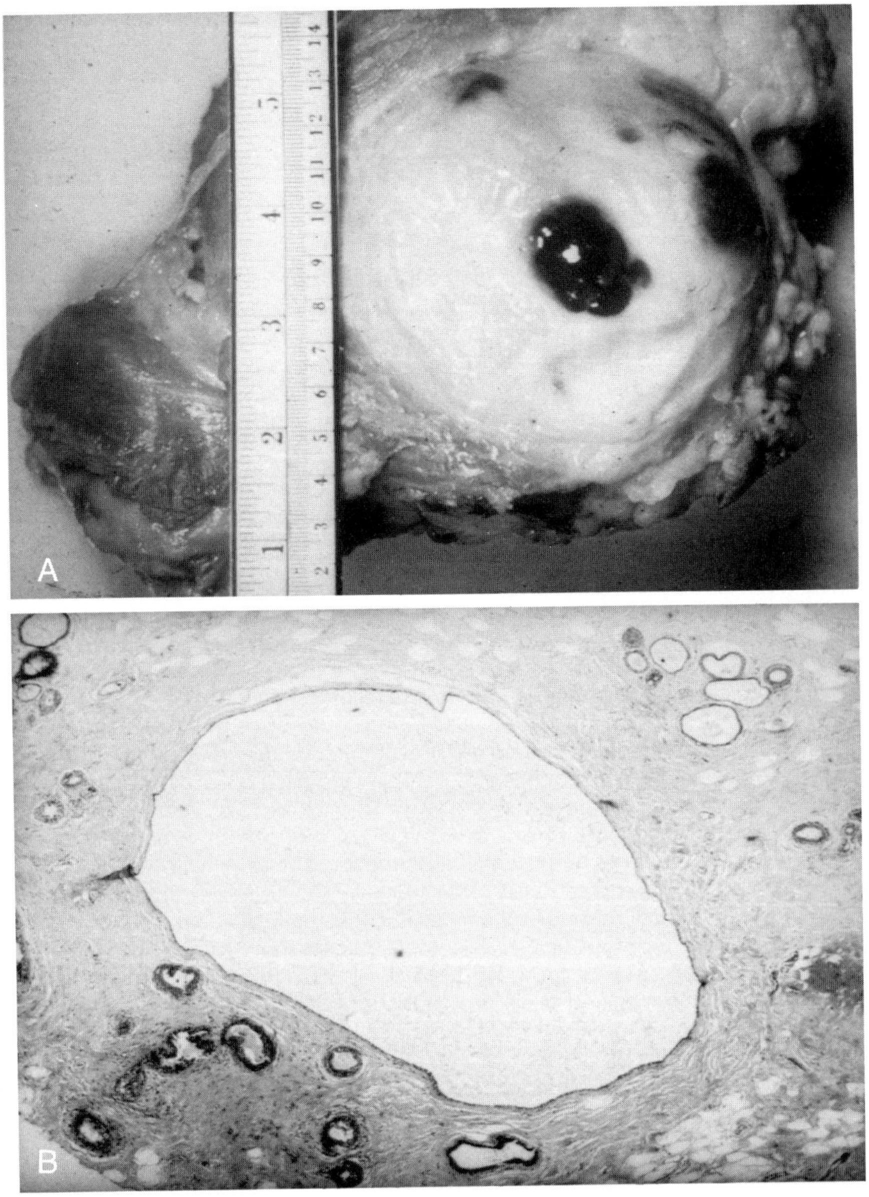

FIGURE 2-5. *(A)* This fibrotic breast tissue contains grossly apparent cysts. The cysts are often blue in color in the fresh state, hence their designation as "blue dome cysts." *(B)* A photomicrograph shows breast tissue containing a cyst that is surrounded by fibrous stroma and lined by a flattened layer of epithelial cells. (x50)

usually seen in conjunction with lobular neoplasia or lobular carcinoma *in situ*.

Moderate and florid hyperplasias of the usual type are the most common types of proliferative lesions of the breast. They are characterized by an increase in cell number within the ducts. Moderate hyperplasia is defined arbitrarily as having more than three cells in height above the basement membrane.[105,193] Florid hyperplasia consists of a proliferation of cells filling at least 70% of the lumen and often distending the involved spaces. Architecturally, the proliferation is either solid or papillary, and contains irregularly spaced openings. The cells are often elongated, as are the nuclei. The nuclei are irregularly placed cell-to-cell, and the chromatin pattern is bland. Two cell populations (epithelial and myoepithelial) are present, although they may be difficult to distinguish in a single area. Fibrovascular stroma may or may not be present. Necrosis is generally lacking or is minimal (Fig. 2-7).

Atypical Proliferative Lesions

The category of atypical proliferative lesions includes both ductal and lobular lesions. These are lesions with some, but not all, of the features of *in situ* carcinomas.[193] The histologic diagnosis of such lesions is, to a large degree, subjective. Even very experienced pathologists may disagree as to whether to classify a given lesion as atypical hyperplasia or carcinoma *in situ*.

Atypical lobular hyperplasia fulfills some, but not all,

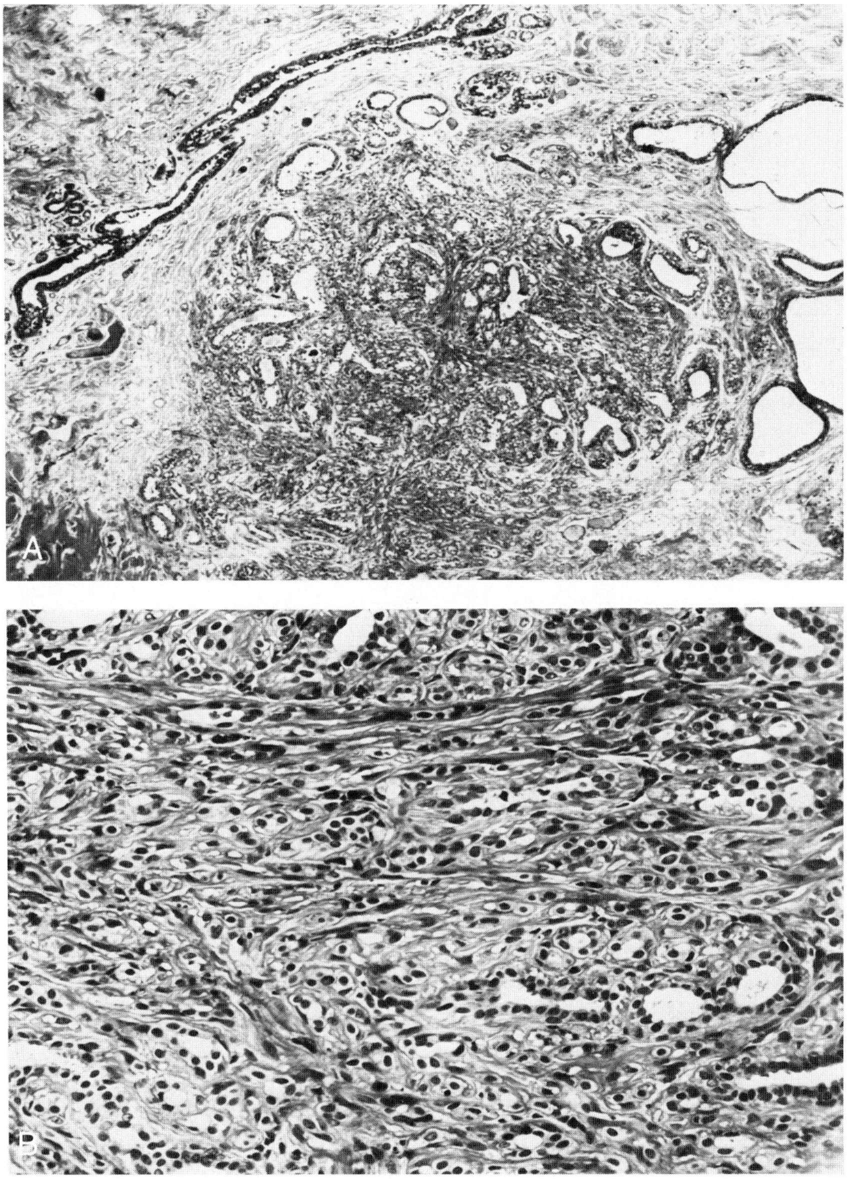

FIGURE 2-6. Sclerosing adenosis. *(A)* A low-power photomicrograph demonstrates a lobulocentric proliferation of stromal and epithelial elements. (x125) *(B)* High-power examination reveals epithelial cells entrapped in a fibrotic stroma. The cells are cytologically benign, but the pattern simulates that of invasive carcinoma. (x300)

of the criteria of lobular carcinoma *in situ* (see Chapter 11 for a detailed discussion of lobular carcinoma *in situ*).[195–198] It is characterized by a proliferation of round to polygonal cells with round, monotonous nuclei. The lobular unit must be less than half-filled with these cells, and no significant distortion of the lobular unit should be present (Fig. 2-8).

Atypical ductal hyperplasia, as defined by Dupont and Page,[104,193] has some, but not all, of the features of ductal carcinoma *in situ*. (See Chapter 11 for a discussion of ductal carcinoma *in situ*.) In general, atypical ductal hyperplasias are similar to florid intraductal hyperplasias, but with focal areas that resemble ductal carcinoma *in situ*. More regular spaces may occur, and the cells may be more spherical than elongated in shape. The nuclei may be more uniform or hyperchromatic than is usually seen in florid intraductal hyperplasia.

"FIBROCYSTIC DISEASE" AND CANCER: EPIDEMIOLOGY AND PATHOLOGY

Many attempts have been made to evaluate the relation between "fibrocystic disease" and cancer. The most common and simplest studies evaluate the coexistence of benign pathology in mastectomy specimens removed because of a malignant condition. These studies show that there is no greater incidence of microscopic "fibrocystic disease" in cancerous breasts than in noncancerous breasts studied at autopsy (Table 2-3). "Fibrocystic dis-

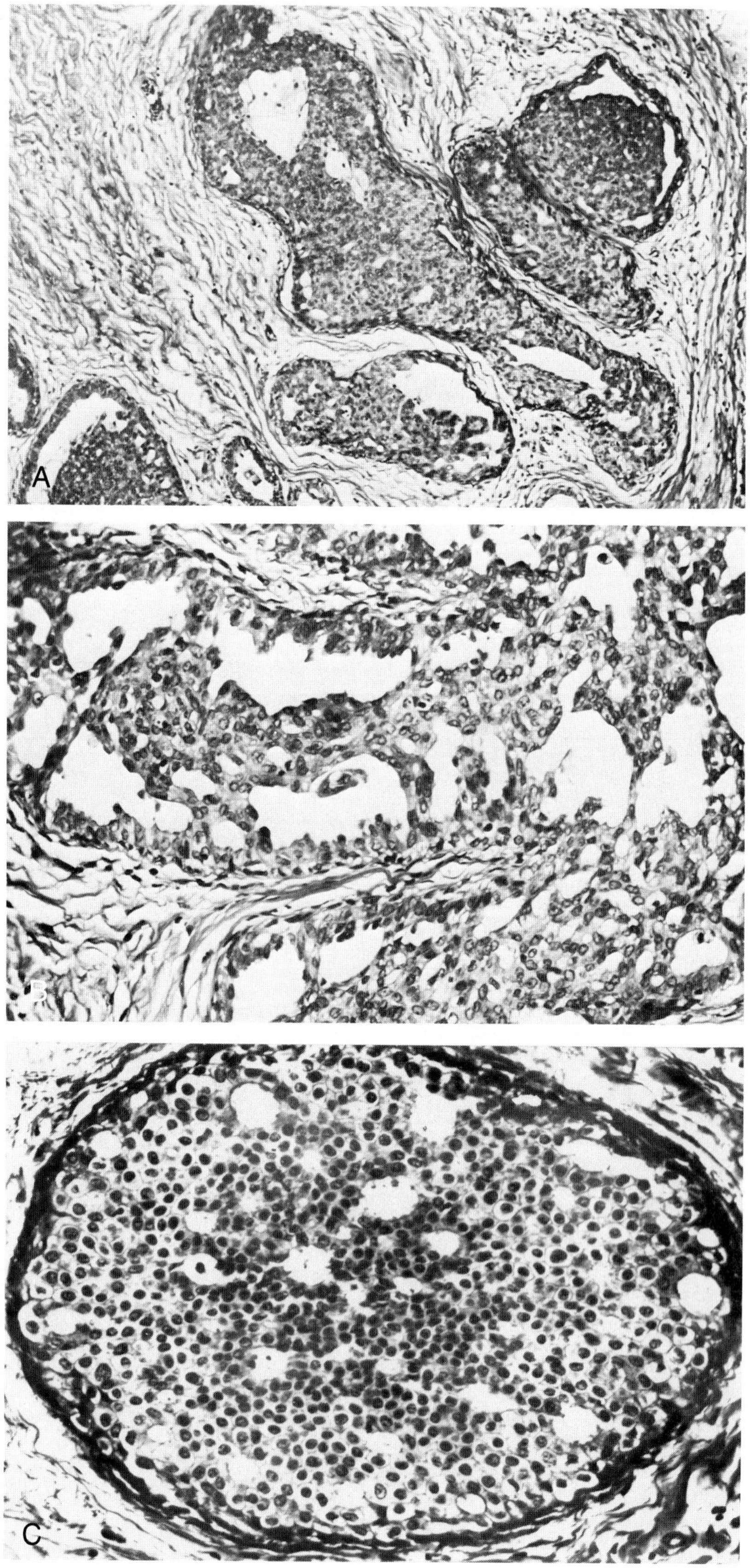

FIGURE 2-7. *(A)* Florid intraductal hyperplasia is characterized by a proliferation of cytologically benign epithelial cells that compromise the lumina of the involved ducts. (x125) *(B)* In intraductal hyperplasia, the proliferating epithelial cells form bridges across the duct lumen, producing spaces that vary in size and configuration. Many of the cells have elliptical nuclei. (x130) (Compare this entity with intraductal carcinoma, depicted in Figure 2-7*C*.) *(C)* In intraductal carcinoma (or ductal carcinima *in situ*), the duct is filled with and distended by a population of cells that are uniform in size and shape and have hyperchromatic nuclei. Lumina in this duct are round and regular (cribriform pattern). (x300) Atypical intraductal hyperplasia displays features that are intermediate between those of hyperplasia (Figs. 2-7*A* and 2-7*B*) and intraductal carcinoma (Fig. 2-7*C*).

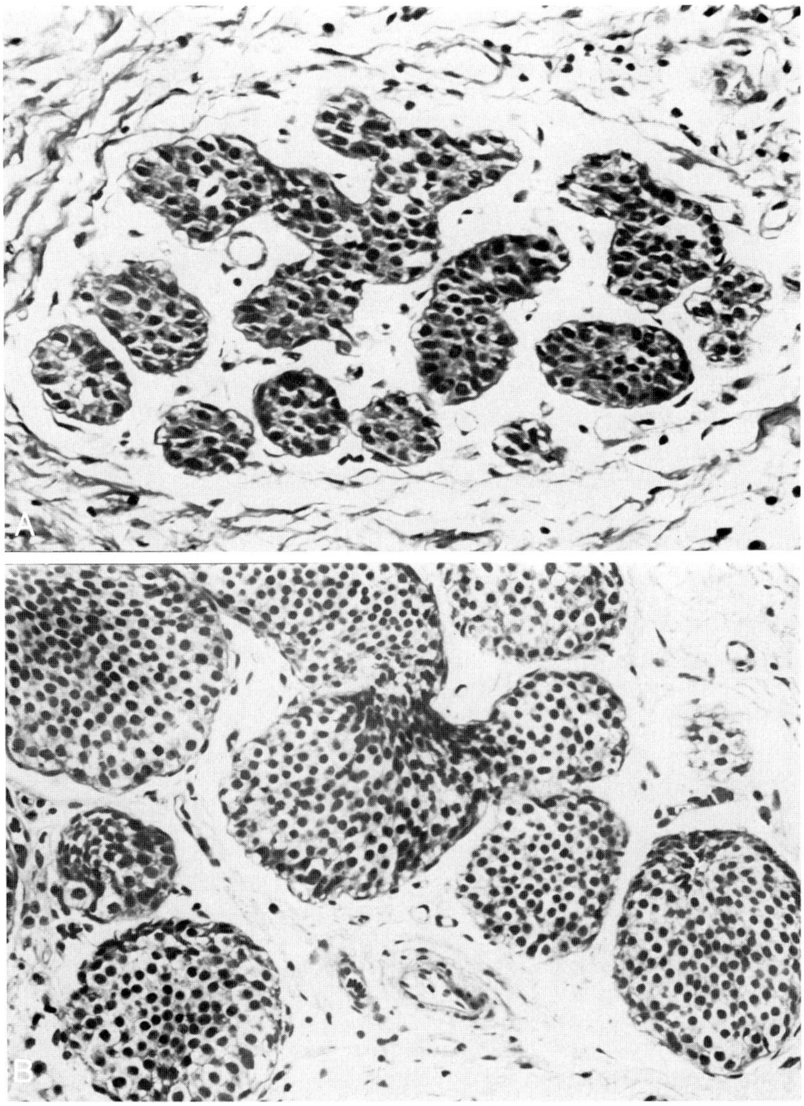

FIGURE 2-8. *(A)* In atypical lobular hyperplasia, terminal ducts and acini contain a proliferation of relatively uniform cells. This proliferation does not distend the involved ductules, and residual ductal lumina are evident. (x350) (Compare this entity with lobular carcinoma *in situ,* depicted in Figure 2-8*B*. *(B)* In lobular carcinoma *in situ,* the terminal ducts and acini are filled with and distended by a solid proliferation of uniform cells with monomorphic nuclei. The ductular lumina have been completely obliterated. (x300)

ease" was found in 58% of autopsied noncancerous breasts, but in only 26% of cancerous breasts. In addition, epithelial hyperplasia, often thought to be a precursor of malignant disease, was at least as common in noncancerous breasts as in cancerous ones (32% and 23%, respectively). Davis and colleagues concluded that the mere finding of coexistent cystic disease was not adequate evidence that cystic change had predisposed a breast to carcinoma.[17]

Two other types of epidemiologic studies have been used to assess the relationship of "fibrocystic disease" to cancer: a retrospective analysis of the number and histology of previous biopsy specimens in patients who subsequently had breast cancer (retrospective case control study), and retrospective cohort studies of patients in whom biopsy specimens showed benign disease and who were then observed to determine the subsequent incidence of cancer.

In the retrospective, case control study, the percentage of previous biopsies in patients with cancer was quite low (about 8%), as compared to the percentage of previous biopsies performed in patients with benign disease (about 14%).[199,200] Thus, once a woman has had a biopsy for benign disease, she is more likely to have a second biopsy, perhaps because of increased surveillance or even anatomic distortion caused by the previous surgery. Roberts and associates recently confirmed this finding in a consecutive series of 791 women who had attended diagnostic breast clinics in Wales.[201] During the period of follow-up, most of the women were found to have no further abnormality, but there was a high level of referral back to the breast clinic, and the biopsy rate was about five times that which was expected. Comparing the number of previous biopsies performed in patients with cancer with the number performed in patients with normal breasts seen in

Table 2-3
Reported Incidence of Microscopic "Fibrocystic Disease" in Breasts Removed for Cancer and in Noncancerous Breasts Studied at Autopsy

Study	No. of Patients	Age Range (yr.)	"Fibrocystic Disease" No.	(%)	Epithelial Hyperplasia No.	(%)	Atypia No.	(%)
Noncancerous Breast Studied at Autopsy								
Frantz[271]*	225	13–85	117	(52)	32	(14)		
Sloss[272]*	100	20–99			33	(33)		
Davis[17]	725	13–99	360	(58)	210	(31)		
Kramer[18]	70	70			48	(69)	7	(10)
Total			360	(58)	258	(32)		
Breasts Removed for Cancer								
Davis[17]	327		128	(40)	38	(12)		
Kern[273]	100	30–90	71	(71)	27	(27)	24	(24)
Karpas[274]	226	20–80+			52	(23)	32	(14)
Fischerman[275]	411	20–80	54	(13)	10	(2)		
Silverberg[276]	398	20–99	157	(40)	30	(8)		
Bonser[277]	220	20–80			123	(56)		
Fisher[278]	1000		206	(21)	349	(35)		
Devitt[199]	594	15–80	133	(22)				
Total			749	(26)	629	(23)		

* These studies were done before 1964, so their totals are included in the totals given for Davis. (Reprinted by permission, Love SM, Gelman RS, Silen WS: Fibrocystic disease of the breast: A non-disease. N Engl J Med 307:1010, 1982).

either a diagnostic or a screening clinic, Chetty and colleagues found no real difference between the two groups.[200]

Evaluation of retrospective cohort studies, in which women with benign biopsy specimens were followed to determine the subsequent incidence of cancer, poses even greater problems. There are statistical difficulties, including unspecified age distributions and periods of follow-up. In addition, only some of the investigators reevaluated the original histology to substantiate the diagnosis; others relied on the pathology reports as adequate evidence of "fibrocystic disease." Finally, each study used a different control to establish the expected risk of cancer. An evaluation of these studies by Love and associates (Table 2-4) showed that there was about a twofold increase in the risk of cancer in patients who had undergone biopsy, no matter what the resulting pathology.[13] Roberts found that this increased risk included not only the patients who had been biopsied, but all women who had attended a special breast clinic.[201] This may reflect a bias resulting from physician or patient referral of high risk patients for increased surveillance. There are several possible epidemiologic explanations for the finding of increased risk secondary to a previous benign biopsy as well. Some of the original benign biopsies might have actually been *in situ* disease, as found by Black in 21% of the cases he reviewed.[202] Also, patients are selected for biopsy on the basis of several subjective criteria, including clinical judgment and relative risk for cancer. Thus, the very process of selection for biopsy could identify a group at higher risk. This premise is supported by Page,[104] who corrected for risk factors and found the lowest increased risk of any of the series.[13] Since having a biopsy makes one more likely to have another, increased surveillance may increase detection without actually increasing the actual incidence of breast cancer. Finally, it should be noted that the majority of these studies were done in the 1950s. It is undoubtedly true that more biopsies are currently done in women with benign conditions who are at lower risk than were done at that time. This trend will increase the denominator (total number of women undergoing biopsy), therefore reducing even further the statistical risk of cancer in women who have had biopsies. Evidence for this is found in a more recent study done from 1972 to 1984 in association with the Breast Cancer Demonstration and Detection Project in Louisville.[203] This study involved the follow-up of a subset of 355 patients with biopsy-proven, chronic, cystic mastitis over a period of 6 to 12 years, and revealed that the incidence of cancer was not significantly different from the expected value.

Although the epidemiologic risk of developing cancer after a previous biopsy has been somewhat discounted, the pathologic precursors have been clarified. A number of studies have demonstrated that the most important pathologic risk factor for the subsequent development of carcinoma is the degree and nature (typical or atypical) of epithelial proliferation.[104,105,193,202,204–209] The relative risks vary from study to study, and depend, to a great extent, on the categorization of the various benign lesions. When biopsy results are categorized as showing nonpro-

Table 2-4
Comparison between Prospective Studies of Patients Who Had Biopsies and Later Had Cancer and the Number of Cancers Predicted by the 1970 and 1976 Surveys of the National Cancer Institute (NCI)

Study	*No. of Patients*	*Average Follow-up (yr)*	*Incidence Reported in Paper*			*Recalculated Incidence**			
						1970 NCI Survey		1976 NCI Survey	
			Observed cancers	*Predicted cancers*	*Increased risk*	*Predicted cancers*	*Increased risk*	*Predicted cancers*	*Increased risk*
Kodlin[206]	2900	7	64	23.8	2.69	20.4	3.13	23.0	2.78
Veronesi[207†]	875	8.75	16	10.1	1.58	10.5	1.52	11.9	1.34
Donnelly[208]	370	17.5	14	8.5	1.64	7	2	8	1.75
Page[104]	925	20	31	22.6	1.37	25.3	1.22	29.1	1.06
Hutchinson [209]	1441	12.9	66	31.5	2.10	26.6	2.48	30.8	2.15
Total	6511		191	96.5	1.98	89.8	2.13	102.8	1.86

* Recalculations were done by assuming that all age groups were followed for the average follow-up period unless follow-up distributions were given, and by using 10-year age groups, as given in papers. The average, age-specific incidence rates of breast cancer were then obtained from the third and fourth NCI surveys.
† The patients treated by mastectomy or androgens were eliminated from the calculations for the purpose of comparison.
(Reprinted by permission, Love SM, Gelman RS, Silen WS: Fibrocystic "disease" of the breast: A non-disease. N Engl J Med 307:1010, 1982).

Table 2-5
Relative Risk of Breast Cancer in Women With Proliferative Disease and in Those Without Proliferative Lesions

	No. of Women	*No. of Cancers*	*Relative Risk†*	*95% Confidence Interval*	*P value*
All patients	3303	134	1.5	1.3–1.8	< 0.0001
Non-proliferative disease	1378	31	0.89	0.62–1.3	0.51
Proliferative disease	1925	103	1.9	1.6–2.3	< 0.0001
Non-proliferative disease without FH *	1243	27	0.86	0.59–1.3	0.43
Non-proliferative disease with FH	135	4	1.2	0.43–3.1	0.78
Proliferative disease without FH	1691	81	1.7	1.4–2.2	< 0.0001
Proliferative disease with FH	234	22	3.2	2.1–4.9	< 0.0001
Cysts without FH	1808	73	1.5	1.2–1.9	0.0008
Cysts with FH	246	21	3	1.9–4.5	< 0.0001

* FH denotes a family history of breast cancer in mother, sister, or daughter.
† As compared with the risk in women from Atlanta (Third National Cancer Survey).
(Reprinted by permission and adapted from Dupont WD, Page DL: Risk factors for breast cancer in women with proliferative breast disease. N Engl J Med 312:146, 1985).

liferative lesions, proliferative lesions without atypia, or atypical proliferative lesions, populations with a low risk of developing breast cancer (versus those with a relatively high risk of developing breast cancer) may be isolated. When additional factors, such as family history and age, are considered, subgroups that are at significantly greater risk of developing breast cancer than the remainder of the population may be identified. Even these data must be viewed with caution, however, since the risk of being diagnosed with a proliferative lesion rests heavily on the degree of medical surveillance.[210]

Nonproliferative Lesions

For patients with nonproliferative lesions, the relative risk of developing breast cancer is low. The relative risk for developing carcinoma for all patients in the study of Dupont and Page[105] was 1.5, as compared with the risk of women from Atlanta (Table 2-5) (Third National Cancer Survey). All patients with nonproliferative lesions had a relative risk of 0.89. Patients with nonproliferative lesions but with no family history of breast cancer in first-degree relatives (mother, sister, or daughter) had a relative risk of 0.86. This risk was only slightly increased (1.2) when there was a family history.

The only group of patients in the nonproliferative category with an increased risk of developing cancer were those with gross cysts plus a family history of breast cancer. The relative risk with gross cysts alone was 1.5, the same as the study population as a whole, but was 3.0 in patients with gross cysts and a family history.

The 15-year absolute risk in the group of patients with nonproliferative disease was only 2%.[102] It can be concluded, therefore, that patients whose biopsy specimens lack proliferative disease, even with a family history of

Table 2-6
Relative Risk of Breast Cancer in Women With Hyperplasia and in Those With Atypical Hyperplasia

	No. of Women	No. of Cancers	Relative Risk†	95% Confidence Interval	P value
Proliferative disease without atypia	1693	73	1.6	1.3–2	0.0001
Atypical hyperplasia	232	30	4.4	3.1–6.3	< 0.0001
Proliferative disease without atypia without FH*	1498	61	1.5	1.2–1.9	0.002
Proliferative disease without atypia but with FH	195	12	2.1	1.2–3.7	0.009
Atypical hyperplasia without FH	193	20	3.5	2.3–5.5	< 0.0001
Atypical hyperplasia with FH	39	10	8.9	4.8–17	< 0.0001

* FH denotes a family history of breast cancer in mother, sister, or daughter.
† As compared with the risk in women from Atlanta (Third National Cancer Survey).
(Reprinted by permission and adapted from Dupont WD, Page DL: Risk factors for breast cancer in women with proliferative breast disease. N Engl J Med 312:146, 1985).

breast cancer, are not at increased risk as long as gross cysts are not present.

Proliferative Disease Without Atypia

The relative risk of the subsequent development of carcinoma in patients with proliferative disease without atypia is low. In comparison to the entire study population, the relative risk is 1.6, and even with a family history, it is only 2.1 (Table 2-6).[102] The 15-year absolute risk was only 4% for these patients. Therefore, even florid hyperplasia, so long as it lacks atypia, does not seem to be a harbinger of carcinoma.

Atypical Proliferative Lesions

The group of patients with atypical hyperplasia has a significant risk of subsequently developing invasive carcinoma. The relative risk of developing carcinoma in this group was 4.4, as compared to the reference population (see Table 2-6). When a positive family history was added, the relative risk rose to 8.9. In comparison to patients who had a negative family history and a biopsy that showed nonproliferative disease, patients with a positive family history and a biopsy showing atypical hyperplasia had a risk 11 times greater than the reference population.[105] This risk approached that of having carcinoma *in situ* demonstrated on biopsy.[201] The therapeutic implications of these findings are complicated by the fact that the risk of invasive carcinoma in these patients was almost equally distributed in both breasts, and a substantial number of cases were bilateral.[193]

BENIGN PATHOLOGIC ENTITIES

There are many pathologic entities that are included in the general category of benign breast disease because they are not malignant. Some of these cause lumps or clinical symptoms, or both, but often, they are found incidentally. Some are true neoplasms or proliferative lesions, whereas others represent reactive, nonneoplastic conditions. These entities will be reviewed to complete the pathologic picture of benign breast problems.

Benign Neoplasms and Proliferative Lesions

Fibroadenomas

The clinical and epidemiologic features of fibroadenomas have been described earlier in this chapter.

On gross examination, fibroadenomas are pseudoencapsulated and are sharply delimited from the surrounding breast tissue. They are usually spherical or ovoid, but may be multilobulated. When cut, the tumor bulges above the level of the surrounding breast tissue. The cut surface is most typically grey-white, and small, punctate, yellow-to-pink, soft areas and slit-like spaces are commonly observed. Occasionally, the tumor has a gelatinous, mucoid consistency.

Microscopically, fibroadenomas have both an epithelial and stromal component (Fig. 2-9). The histologic pattern depends upon which of these components predominates. In general, the epithelial component consists of well-defined, gland-like, and duct-like spaces lined by cuboidal or columnar cells with uniform nuclei. Varying degrees of epithelial hyperplasia are frequently observed. The stromal component consists of connective tissue that has a variable content of acid mucopolysaccharides and collagen. In older lesions and in postmenopausal patients, the stroma may become hyalinized, calcified, or even ossified (ancient fibroadenoma). On rare occasions, mature adipose tissue or smooth muscle may comprise a portion of the stroma.[197,212] The term intracanalicular has been used to describe tumors in which the stromal component compresses the glands into slit-like spaces, whereas pericanalicular tumors are those in which the rounded configuration of the glandular structures is maintained. In fact, these two patterns often coexist in the same lesion, and this distinction has no practical significance.

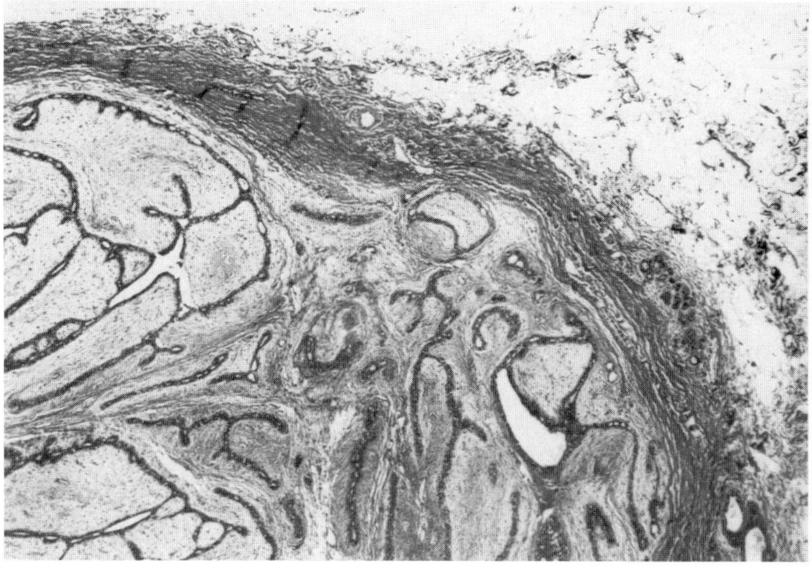

FIGURE 2-9. In this fibroadenoma, the tumor is well circumscribed and separated from the adjacent breast tissue by a rim of dense collagen. Both glandular and stromal elements are apparent. (x50)

JUVENILE FIBROADENOMAS. Most fibroadenomas in adolescents are of the usual type seen in older patients. A minority present a different clinical and pathologic picture and are termed juvenile fibroadenomas. It is important to be aware of these lesions because they may be clinically and microscopically confused with malignant masses. These tumors tend to grow rapidly and may double in size in 3 to 6 months. Venous dilatation may be present in the overlying skin. In some instances, the clinical appearance resembles that of virginal hypertrophy and only surgical exploration will reveal a circumscribed tumor.[213–215] Microscopically, these lesions are more floridly glandular and have greater stromal cellularity than the more common, adult-type fibroadenoma. As for the adult-type fibroadenomas, simple excision is the treatment of choice.

GIANT FIBROADENOMAS. Some tumors that are histologically typical fibroadenomas may attain great size. Unfortunately, several authors have used the terms giant fibroadenoma and benign cystosarcoma phyllodes synonymously, and have created considerable confusion regarding these entities. A lesion that has the microscopic appearance of a conventional fibroadenoma but that is large should still be classified as a fibroadenoma and may be treated adequately by enucleation. The major feature that distinguishes a cystosarcoma phyllodes (preferably called a phyllodes tumor) from a giant fibroadenoma is the cellularity of the stromal component in the former.[197] It must be noted, however, that the distinction between these two entities may be extremely difficult in some cases, as is discussed in Chapter 15. Because juvenile fibroadenomas may attain great sizes, some authors consider them to be variants of giant fibroadenomas.[215]

INFARCTION. Fibroadenomas may undergo partial, subtotal, or total infarction. Pregnancy and lactation are the most common predisposing factors. It has been postulated that a relative vascular insufficiency in the face of increased metabolic activity in the breast underlies this phenomenon.[197]

INVOLVEMENT OF FIBROADENOMAS BY CARCINOMA. This subject has recently been reviewed by Pick and Iossifides[216] and by Azzopardi.[197] Infrequently, carcinoma may occur in association with a fibroadenoma. The most frequent type of carcinoma involving fibroadenomas is lobular carcinoma *in situ,* but intraductal, infiltrating ductal, and infiltrating lobular carcinoma have also been observed. In almost half of the reported cases, the malignant tumor also involves the surrounding breast tissue. The prognosis of carcinoma limited to a fibroadenoma is excellent. Treatment should follow the same principles used in the management of *in situ* or infiltrating carcinomas that occur in breast tissue in the absence of fibroadenomas.

Adenoma

Adenomas of the breast are well-circumscribed tumors composed of benign epithelial elements with sparse, inconspicuous stroma. The last feature differentiates these lesions from fibroadenomas, in which the stroma is an integral part of the tumor. For practical purposes, adenomas may be divided into two major groups: tubular adenomas and lactating adenomas.

TUBULAR ADENOMAS. Tubular adenomas present in young women as well-defined, freely movable nodules that clinically resemble fibroadenomas.[218] Gross examination reveals a well-circumscribed, tan-yellow, firm tumor. On microscopic examination, tubular adenomas are separated from the adjacent breast tissue by a pseudocapsule, and are composed of a proliferation of uniform, small, tubular structures with a scant amount of intervening stroma. The tubules are composed of an inner epithelial layer and an outer myoepithelial layer, and resemble normal breast acini both at the light and ultrastructural level. In some cases, this pattern is admixed with that of a fibroadenoma, suggesting a relationship between the two tumors.

LACTATING ADENOMAS (NODULAR LACTATIONAL HYPERPLASIA). Lactating adenomas present as one or more freely movable masses during pregnancy or the postpartum period.[218] They are grossly well circumscribed and lobulated, and on cut section appear tan and softer than tubular adenomas. On microscopic examination, these lesions have lobulated borders and are composed of glands lined by cuboidal cells with secretory activity, identical to the lactational changes normally observed in breast tissue during pregnancy and the puerperium. Although some authors believe that these lesions are the result of lactational changes superimposed on a preexisting tubular adenoma, others have suggested that they represent *de novo* lesions and are merely nodular foci of hyperplasia in the lactating breast.

O'Hara and Page recently reviewed 42 breast adenomas that demonstrated lactational changes.[219] They observed an overlapping spectrum of morphologic features in fibroadenomas with lactational changes and in lactating and tubular adenomas. These authors suggested that all these lesions may have a common pathogenesis.

Rarely, adenomatous tumors resembling dermal sweat-gland neoplasms are observed as primary lesions in the breast parenchyma (e.g., clear cell hidradenoma and eccrine spiradenoma)[197,218] or nipple (e.g., syringomatous adenoma).[220]

Adenomas of the Nipple

Adenoma of the nipple has been described under a variety of names, including florid papillomatosis of the nipple ducts,[221] subareolar duct papillomatosis,[197] papillary adenoma of the nipple,[222] and erosive adenomatosis of the nipple.[223] It is not, strictly speaking, a true adenoma of the breast, as defined by Hertel and associates,[218] because of its prominent stromal component.

Nipple adenomas are rare lesions that occur most commonly in women in their fourth and fifth decades. They are important tumors to recognize because they may simulate malignant disease, both clinically and pathologically.

Affected patients most often present with a nipple discharge, which is usually bloody but may be serous. This discharge is commonly associated with erythema, soreness, erosion, and scaling of the nipple, thereby closely resembling Paget's disease. On physical examination, the nipple is usually indurated and may be enlarged. A discrete mass may be palpable within the nipple or just deep to it. Gross pathologic examination sometimes reveals a solid, grey-tan, poorly demarcated tumor in the nipple and subareolar region; in other cases, no gross lesion is evident.

Microscopically, the dominant feature is a proliferation of small, gland-like structures. Solid and papillary proliferation of ductal epithelium is also usually evident; however, the papillary pattern may be inconspicuous or totally absent. In advanced lesions, glandular epithelium extends out onto the surface of the nipple. It is this phenomenon that results in the clinically apparent, reddish, granular appearance. Squamous epithelium frequently extends into the superficial regions of the involved ducts, sometimes with the formation of keratinaceous cysts. The lesions usually show considerable stromal fibrosis. This connective tissue may distort and entrap the epithelial elements, resulting in a pattern mimicking invasive carcinoma. The lesion is distinguishable from carcinoma by the preservation of a double layer of epithelium in the proliferating glands (an inner epithelial and outer myoepithelial layer), minimal nuclear atypicality, absence of necrosis, and the overall low-power configuration.

A few cases of carcinoma associated with adenomas of the nipple have been reported.[224,225] However, in the majority of cases, the lesion is entirely benign and is adequately treated by local excision. Reports of recurrence most likely represent cases in which the initial resection failed to remove the lesion completely.

Intraductal Papillomas

SOLITARY INTRADUCTAL PAPILLOMAS. Solitary intraductal papillomas are tumors of the major lactiferous ducts, most frequently observed in women 30 to 50 years of age. In Haagensen's series, the mean age was 48 years.[12] The most frequent presenting symptom of intraductal papilloma is nipple discharge, which may be serous or bloody. Bloody discharge is present in approximately 50% of cases.

Intraductal papillomas are generally less than 1 cm in diameter, usually measuring 3 mm to 4 mm. Occasionally, these lesions may be as large as 4 or 5 cm. On gross examination, papillomas are tan-pink, friable tumors within a dilated duct or cyst. A frankly papillary configuration may or may not be apparent. The tumor is usually attached to the wall of the involved duct by a delicate stalk, but it may be sessile. To identify the papilloma, the involved duct should be opened carefully, using a fine pair of scissors, until the tumor is exposed. Identification of the lesion may be facilitated by the placement of a suture at the end of the involved duct nearest the nipple. Randomly slicing through the excised tissue is not recommended, as a small lesion may be missed.

Microscopically, these tumors are composed of multiple, branching, and interanastomosing papillae, each with a central fibrovascular core and a covering layer of cuboidal to columnar epithelial cells. A myoepithelial cell layer is often discernible between the epithelial cells and the connective tissue stalk (Fig. 2-10). In some areas, the complex growth pattern of the papillae results in the formation of gland-like spaces. Variable amounts of fibrosis may result in the entrapment of epithelial elements, producing a pseudoinfiltrative pattern. In addition, florid epithelial proliferation is sometimes observed. At times, the epithelial cell hyperplasia or fibrosis, or both, and the architectural

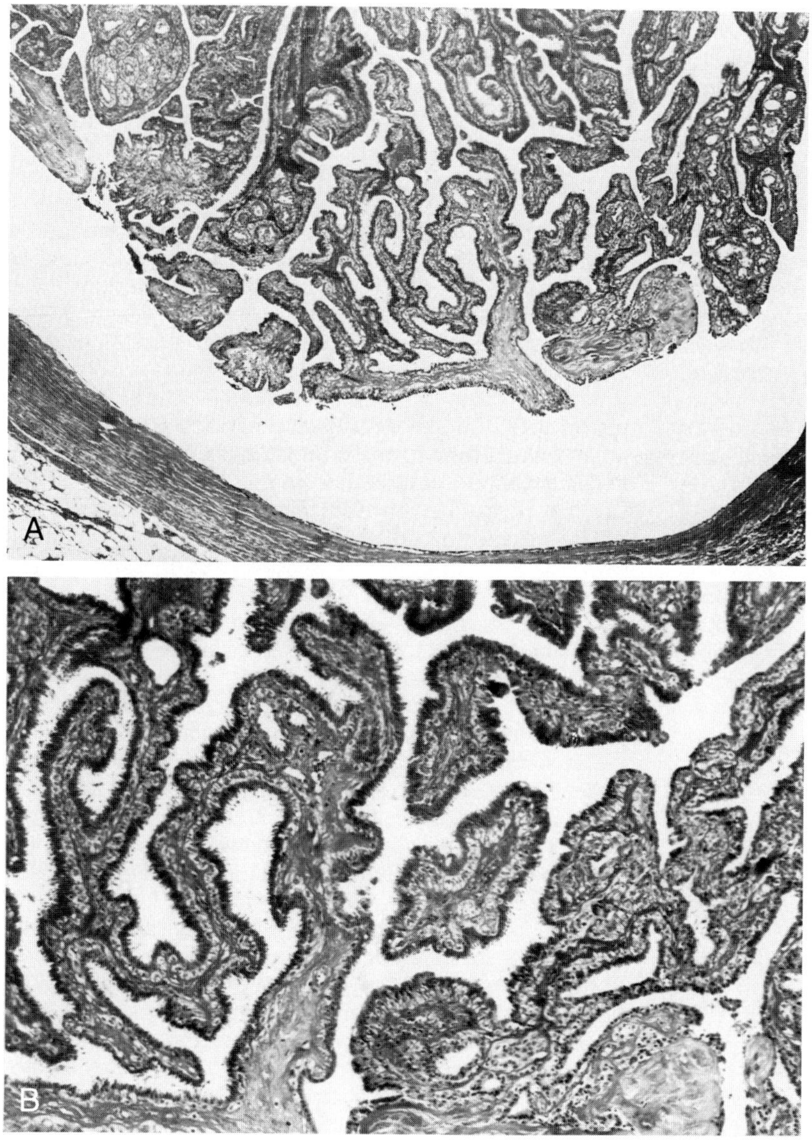

FIGURE 2-10. Intraductal papilloma. *(A)* A low-power photomicrograph demonstrates the papillary lesion within a dilated duct. (x50) *(B)* A higher-power view demonstrates that the papillae are composed of central fibrovascular cores covered by two layers of cells, a myoepithelial layer (lying closer to the cores) and an epithelial layer (lying closer to the duct lumen). (x125)

distortion make it extremely difficult to distinguish between benign papilloma and papillary carcinoma. Features helpful in making this distinction have been elucidated by Kraus and Neubecker[226] and by Azzopardi.[197] In general, benign lesions are characterized by a proliferation composed of two cell types (epithelial and myoepithelial), lack of nuclear hyperchromasia or monomorphism, scant mitotic activity, prominent connective tissue stroma, apocrine metaplasia, lack of necrosis, and the presence of benign proliferative lesions, such as intraductal hyperplasia and sclerosing adenosis, in the adjacent breast tissue. It should be apparent from the foregoing description that careful evaluation of intraductal papillomas can only be accomplished with paraffin-embedded sections. Therefore, we see no place for frozen-section evaluation of papillary lesions of the breast.

Two additional features of intraductal papillomas deserve emphasis because they may create difficulties in histologic interpretation. Papillomas may undergo partial or total infarction, often accompanied by distortion of the adjacent, viable epithelium and production of a pattern that may simulate invasive carcinoma. Squamous metaplasia has been observed in intraductal papillomas. In some cases, it accompanies infarction, but it has also been observed in the absence of infarction. This phenomenon may also result in a disturbing growth pattern that may be confused with carcinoma.[227]

There has been considerable debate in the literature regarding the malignant potential of solitary intraductal papillomas. Available evidence suggests that these lesions rarely undergo malignant transformation. Furthermore, the risk of subsequent carcinoma in a woman who has had an intraductal papilloma appears to be no greater than that in the general population.

MULTIPLE INTRADUCTAL PAPILLOMAS. Compared to solitary intraductal papillomas, multiple intraductal papillomas tend to occur in younger patients, are less often associated with nipple discharge, are more frequently peripheral, and are more often bilateral. Most importantly, these lesions appear to be susceptible to the development of carcinoma. In Haagensen's series of 39 patients with multiple papillomas, simultaneous or subsequent carcinoma of the apocrine papillary and cribriform types was observed in 15 patients (38%).[12] A recent study in which surgically excised specimens from patients with intraductal papillomas were subjected to three-dimensional reconstruction confirms these observations.[228] All 16 cases of multiple papillomas in the series were found to originate in the most peripheral portion of the duct system, the TDLU. Furthermore, carcinoma was found to be associated with these multiple peripheral papillomas in six cases (37.5%). In contrast, no cases of carcinoma were found to be associated with solitary papillomas involving the large ducts. These findings suggest that peripheral papillomas, in contrast to solitary central papillomas, may be highly susceptible to malignant transformation.

Juvenile Papillomatosis (Swiss Cheese Disease)

Juvenile papillomatosis was first recognized as a clinicopathologic entity by Rosen and colleagues in 1980.[229] This lesion occurs most commonly in adolescents and young women (with a mean age of 23 years), but has been seen in women up to 48 years of age. Patients typically present with a painless mass which, on physical examination, is circumscribed, easily movable, and is most often considered to be a fibroadenoma.

On gross pathologic examination, the lesions range in size from 1 cm to 8 cm. Multiple cysts of up to 1 cm in diameter are generally apparent. The microscopic features of juvenile papillomatosis are not unique to this entity, and are all components described as part of "fibrocystic disease." The constellation of histologic features, however, form a characteristic complex. These lesions appear to be well circumscribed but not encapsulated, and are characterized by the following elements: duct papillomatosis, apocrine and nonapocrine cysts, papillary apocrine hyperplasia, sclerosing adenosis, and duct stasis. The epithelial proliferation in these lesions may be quite marked, and the cytologic and architectural features may approach those of intraductal carcinoma.

The majority of patients in whom juvenile papillomatosis has been reported have not reached the age range in which the risk of developing carcinoma is the greatest. Therefore, prolonged follow-up is required to determine the ultimate significance of this entity. Recent reports have suggested that juvenile papillomatosis is associated with an increased risk of breast cancer in the patient's female relatives,[230] and that the patient herself may be at increased risk for developing carcinoma.[231]

Wide excision and careful follow-up appear to be the most prudent approaches to the management of these patients.

Microglandular Adenosis

Microglandular adenosis (MGA) is an uncommon lesion that may be identified as an incidental finding in breast tissue excised for a variety of other lesions, or it may present as a palpable mass. Most women in whom this lesion has been reported are older than 40 years of age, but patients as young as 28 years and as old as 82 years have been reported to have MGA. On gross examination, MGA has generally been described as an ill-defined area of firm, rubbery tissue that is usually 3 cm to 4 cm in diameter. The importance of this lesion resides in the fact that it may be mistaken for a well-differentiated (tubular) carcinoma on histologic examination. Microscopically, the lesion of MGA is characterized by a poorly circumscribed, haphazard proliferation of small, round glands in the breast stroma and adipose tissue. Unlike sclerosing adenosis, MGA does not have a lobulocentric, organoid configuration. The glands are composed of a single layer of cuboidal epithelial cells with clear to slightly eosinophilic cytoplasm and small, regular nuclei. Eosinophilic secretions are frequently present within the glandular lumina. The stroma is typically composed of dense, relatively acellular collagen, which usually demarcates the lesion from the adjacent parenchyma. In some areas, the stroma is minimal and the proliferating glands lie exposed in adipose tissue (Fig. 2-11).

The relationship between MGA and cancer has not been established. Simultaneous or subsequent carcinoma has been reported in 4 of the 13 patients originally reported by Rosen,[232] 1 of the 11 patients described by Tavassoli and Norris,[233] and none of the 6 patients reported by Clement and Azzopardi.[234] More recently, Rosenblum and co-workers described seven cases of MGA associated with carcinoma.[235] In these cases, a spectrum of changes—from typical MGA to atypical glandular proliferations to infiltrating carcinoma—was observed. Thus, in some cases, MGA may be associated with carcinoma. At the present time, the recommended approach to the management of patients with MGA is complete, local excision of the lesion and careful follow-up.

Radial Sclerosing Lesions

Radial sclerosing lesions have been described in the literature by a variety of names, including sclerosing papillary proliferation,[236] nonencapsulated sclerosing lesion,[237] indurative mastopathy,[238] and radial scar.[239] Its importance lies in the fact that it may, on mammographic, gross, and microscopic examinations, simulate carcinoma.

Radial sclerosing lesions are most frequently incidental findings in breast tissue excised because of "fibrocystic

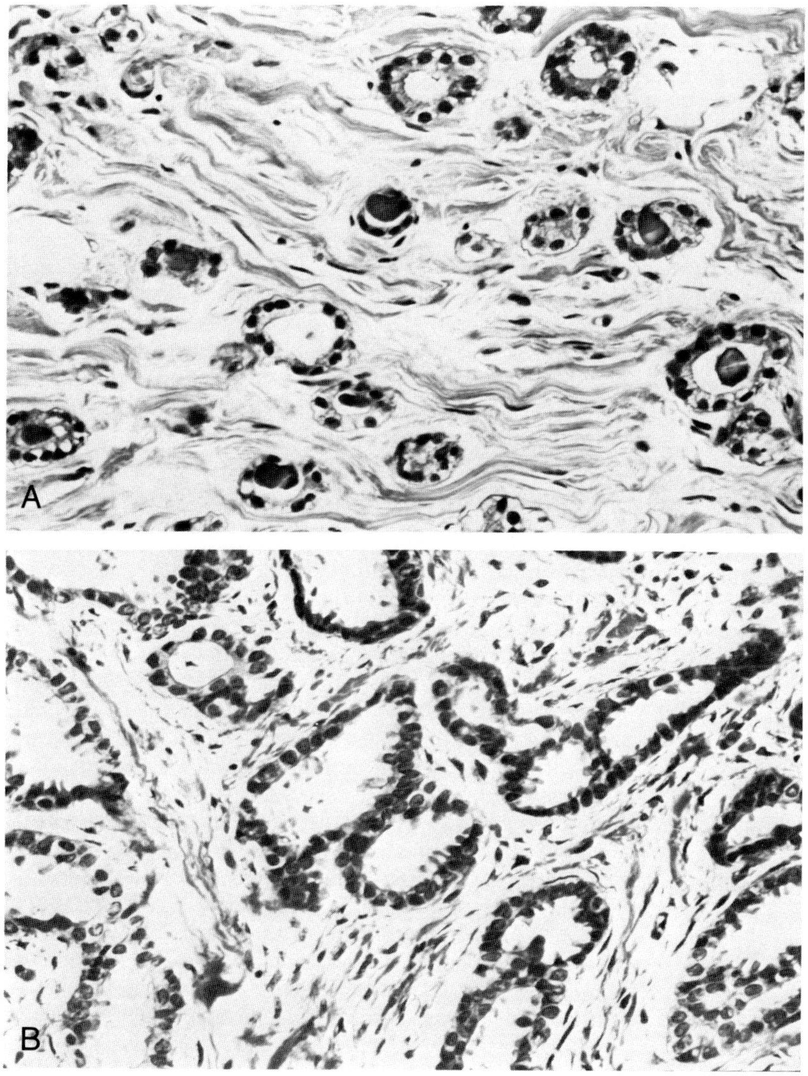

FIGURE 2-11. *(A)* Microglandular adenosis is characterized by a proliferation of small, glandular structures composed of a single layer of epithelial cells. The cells have clear to eosinophilic cytoplasm. The glands are round, and many contain eosinophilic material within their lumina. (x300). (Compare this lesion with that found in cases of tubular carcinoma, depicted in Figure 2-11*B*. *(B)* Well-differentiated, infiltrating, ductal (tubular) carcinoma is composed of well-formed glands, many of which are ovoid and have tapering ends. The epithelial cells that constitute the tubules show minimal nuclear atypicality; apocrine snouts are apparent at the luminal aspect of the cells. (x300)

disease." They are often multiple, with as many as 31 lesions having been observed in a single breast.[240] Occasionally, they are detected by mammography, on which they appear as soft tissue densities with irregular, serrated edges, similar in appearance to carcinomas. These lesions are typically less than 1 cm in diameter and, on gross examination, are irregular, grey-white, and indurated with central retraction, an appearance identical to that of scirrhous carcinoma.

Microscopically, the lesion has a stellate configuration and consists of a central, fibroelastotic core containing entrapped glandular elements. Radiating from this core are ducts with varying degrees of epithelial hyperplasia and papillomatosis. Ducts at the periphery may be dilated cystically. Sclerosing adenosis and apocrine metaplasia frequently accompany the lesion. The surrounding breast tissue typically shows varying degrees of intraductal hyperplasia and adenosis. The entrapped glands in the center of the lesion may be confused with the glands of tubular carcinoma. It is the low-power configuration of the lesion that permits the correct diagnosis.

The significance of radial sclerosing lesions with regard to the subsequent development of carcinoma is controversial. Some authors have argued that these lesions may represent incipient tubular carcinomas[237] or a stage in the development of many invasive breast cancers.[241] A recent autopsy study has demonstrated that these lesions are significantly more common in breasts of cancer patients than in noncancerous breasts;[240] however, this is clearly not sufficient evidence to prove that these lesions are precancerous. Follow-up studies have failed to show an increased incidence of breast cancer in patients who have had a radial sclerosing lesion excised.[236,239] Available evidence suggests that these lesions are best considered to be a part of the fibrocystic complex. It is likely that their premalignant potential is the same as that of their constituent parts.[240] Local excision of these lesions is the treatment of choice.

Lipomas and Adenolipomas

Lipomas consist of encapsulated nodules of mature adipose tissue. Although true lipomas do occur in the breast, the lesion that commonly presents as a lipoma is often merely a fatty area of breast tissue without a true capsule. Adenolipoma is the name applied to a benign fatty tumor of the breast that contains entrapped, lobular, epithelial elements.[197]

Hemangiomas

Benign angiomatous lesions of the breast parenchyma are relatively uncommon.[197] They are usually incidental findings, and generally do not produce palpable masses. In a series of 550 mastectomy specimens from patients with breast carcinoma, the incidence of benign hemangiomas was 1.2%.[242]

Benign vascular lesions of the breast may broadly be divided into four categories: perilobular hemangiomas, angiomatoses, venous hemangiomas, and hemangiomas involving the mammary subcutaneous tissue.[243–246]

The significance of benign angiomatous lesions of the breast is that they must be distinguished from angiosarcomas.[247] Benign angiomas are almost always microscopic in size and lack interanastamosing channels, endothelial proliferation, and atypia.

Chondromatous Lesions

Chondromatous lesions of the breast should be evaluated with caution.[248] Chondromatous change is most often seen in breast carcinomas and sarcomas. Although the carcinomatous or sarcomatous elements are usually obvious, occasionally, a lesion may present with a pure chondromatous picture. In some cases, the chondroid metaplasia seen in malignant breast lesions may be relatively mature.

The most common benign lesion of the breast associated with chondroid metaplasia is the fibroadenoma.

Benign chondromatous metaplasia may occur in the stroma, entrapping adipose tissue or glandular elements. Intraductal papillomas may also contain cartilaginous areas.[197,249]

Leiomyomas

Leiomyomas of the breast are most commonly seen in the areolar region, and rarely occur in the breast parenchyma. The histologic characteristics of leiomyomas of the breast are the same as those found in other tissues.

Neurofibromas and Schwannomas

Neurofibromas and schwannomas are benign tumors of nerve sheath origin. These lesions are most frequently seen in patients with neurofibromatosis, and are most common in the areolar area.[12] The lesions may also occur within the breast parenchyma.

Myoepitheliomas

The myoepithelial cell is a contractile cell located between the basal lamina and ductal or acinar epithelium. Although myoepithelial tumors have been described, they are rare, and many of the reported cases lack adequate documentation. Typically, these lesions are spindle cell tumors, and require electron microscopic examination for definitive diagnosis.[250]

Granular Cell Tumors

Granular cell tumors are uncommonly found in the breast but, when present, simulate carcinoma on clinical, mammographic, and pathologic examination. DeMay and Kay recently reported 12 cases and provided an excellent review of the literature.[251] These tumors occur more commonly in blacks than in whites, and typically appear between puberty and menopause, implicating some hormonal factor in their development. Granular cell tumors of the breast most commonly occur in the upper, inner quadrant in contrast to carcinomas, which occur most frequently in the upper, outer quadrant. Patients present with a palpable mass that may be associated with skin retraction or fixation to skeletal muscles of the chest wall. The similarity of granular cell tumors to carcinoma is also evident on mammographic examination, on which they resemble scirrhous carcinoma. Gross examination of the lesion reveals a grey-white to tan, firm tumor that may be gritty when cut with a knife; these features further support the impression of carcinoma. Microscopically, these lesions are identical to granular cell tumors in other sites, consisting of a poorly circumscribed proliferation of clusters of cells in which the most characteristic feature is prominent granularity of the cytoplasm. On electron microscopic examination, these granules correspond to secondary lysosomes. The nuclei are small and uniform, and lack the features of malignant disease.

Granular cell tumors are almost invariably benign and are adequately treated by wide local excision. Rare cases of malignant granular cell tumors have been reported in both the breast and extramammary sites.

Granular cell tumors were initially considered to be myogenic in origin (hence, their earlier designation as granular cell myoblastomas), but recent ultrastructural and immunohistochemical evidence support a neurogenic origin for these tumors.[252]

Fibromatosis

Approximately 30 cases of fibromatosis of the breast have been reported.[253–256] These lesions are analogous to fibromatoses in other sites (*e.g.,* desmoid tumors of the abdominal wall), and are characterized by a locally invasive, nonencapsulated proliferation of well-differentiated fibroblasts. These tumors have the capacity to recur locally if inadequately excised, but they do not mestastasize. Gump and colleagues have reported the largest series of fibromatosis of the breast (17 cases).[253] In their series, patients ranged in age from 18 to 80 years (with a mean of 48.7 years), and typically presented with a palpable mass that was sometimes associated with skin retraction or fixation to the underlying pectoral muscle. On mammography, these lesions are indistinguishable from carcinomas. Gross pathologic examination reveals an ill-defined, firm, grey-white lesion. Microscopically, fibromatoses consist of interlacing bundles of spindle-shaped cells surrounded by collagen. The cells show minimal to no cytologic atypism, and mitoses are only infrequently encountered. The proliferation tends to surround and entrap preexisting ducts and lobules without destroying them. The edges of the lesion infiltrate irregularly into the adjacent parenchyma. On electron microscopic examination, some tumor cells have the ultrastructural features of fibroblasts, whereas others appear to be myofibroblasts.

The proper treatment for these lesions consists of wide local excision. Although metastases have not been reported, lesions may recur locally. Zayid and Dehmis described an exceptional case in which a patient was treated with mastectomy, subsequently developing multiple tumor recurrences in the chest wall, which ultimately resulted in her death.[257]

Interestingly, two of the reported cases of fibromatosis of the breast have been associated with Gardner syndrome.[255] Another case occurred in a patient with familial multicentric fibromatosis.[257]

Reactive/Inflammatory Lesions

Mammary Duct Ectasia (Periductal Mastitis)

Mammary duct ectasia occurs primarily in perimenopausal and postmenopausal women, and is characterized by dilatation of the subareolar ducts.[12] Considerable controversy exists regarding the most appropriate name for this condition. This controversy has arisen from the fact that some authors consider ductal dilatation to be the primary event, whereas others consider the ectatic ducts to be the consequence of prior periductal inflammation.

Pregnancy and lactation have been implicated in the etiology of this condition. However, a recent study in which parity and breastfeeding were evaluated in patients with duct ectasia and in age-matched control subjects with other breast disorders failed to reveal significant differences between the two groups.[258] In addition, this condition has been reported to occur in men as well as women.[259]

Duct ectasia is a frequent pathologic finding in breast tissue obtained at autopsy and in surgically excised material. It has been observed on microscopic examination in 30% to 40% of women older than 50 years of age. Clinically evident disease, however, occurs much less frequently.[258] This disorder is most often unilateral, but bilateral involvement may be seen in a minority of cases. Patients most frequently present with a mass which may be tender and painful or which may be accompanied by skin retraction. Nipple inversion results from traction on the nipple by ducts that have undergone fibrosis and shortening, and is seen in about 30% to 40% of cases. Nipple discharge, which may be serous, pasty, or bloody, is present in approximately 20% of cases. It should be apparent that the finding of a mass associated with skin and nipple retraction may be mistaken for carcinoma. Indeed, the presumptive diagnosis was carcinoma in 50% of the cases of duct ectasia in Haagensen's series.[12]

A wide spectrum of pathologic changes is observed in this condition. Cut section of the gross specimen often reveals dilated, thick-walled ducts that contain pasty, yellow-brown secretions. The intervening stroma may be fibrotic. On microscopic examination, some cases show prominent inspissation of lipid-rich material within ducts, accompanied by periductal inflammation. Rupture or leakage of these ducts results in release of this material into the adjacent stroma, with subsequent inflammation and fat necrosis. Plasma cells may be a prominent component of the periductal and stromal inflammatory infiltrate. It should be noted that many cases previously designated as plasma cell mastitis probably represent a stage in the evolution of duct ectasia. In other cases, the histologic picture is dominated by periductal fibrosis and ductal dilatation with minimal inflammation.

As alluded to earlier, the pathogenesis of this condition has not been fully established. Available evidence suggests, however, that the primary event is periductal inflammation and that duct ectasia is the ultimate outcome of this disorder. In support of this premise, Dixon and associates have observed that inflammation around nondilated ducts predominates in younger patients with this condition, whereas duct dilatation and nipple retraction are more common in older patients.[258] Thus, the postulated sequence of events in the evolution of this disease is that periductal inflammation leads to periductal fibrosis, which subsequently results in ductal dilatation. It should be noted, however, that the etiology of the initial inflammatory response remains obscure.

Treatment consists of local excision of the involved area of breast tissue.

Fat Necrosis

The importance of fat necrosis lies in the fact that it may closely simulate carcinoma both clinically and on mammographic examination.[12,260] In less than 50% of cases, a prior history of trauma is obtained. This lesion is most common in obese women with pendulous breasts. Areas of fat necrosis are typically situated superficially, and may be fixed to the overlying skin with resultant retraction. Fixation to the chest wall and nipple retraction are rare. The lesion may increase in size for a short period of time after it is discovered. In some patients, the lesion spontaneously regresses, whereas in others, it may persist for years.

The gross appearance of this type of lesion depends on its age. In early lesions, there is hemorrhage and indurated fat. With time, a rounded, firm tumor is formed. The cut surface of the lesion at this stage has a variegated, yellow-grey appearance with focal hemorrhage. Cavitation may subsequently occur owing to liquefactive necrosis. The lesion may eventually be converted to a dense, fibrous scar or may remain a cystic cavity with calcification of its walls.

On microscopic examination, early lesions show cystic spaces surrounded by lipid-laden macrophages and foreign-body–type giant cells with foamy cytoplasm (Fig. 2-12). A variable, acute, inflammatory cell infiltrate may be present, and there may be focal hemorrhage. With time, there is fibroblastic proliferation with deposition of collagen. Scattered, chronic, inflammatory cells are usually present, and focal hemosiderin deposition may be observed. Even in older lesions, scattered, foamy histiocytes and foreign-body giant cells are usually discernible.

A similar pathologic appearance may be seen after surgical trauma to the breast and after radiation therapy for carcinoma (see the section on pathologic changes associated with radiation therapy, below).

Because of its clinical similarity to carcinoma, complete excision of this lesion is required for accurate diagnosis.

Reactions to Foreign Material

Foreign-body–type granulomatous inflammation has been described following injection or implantation of a variety of substances, including paraffin and silicone, within the breast for therapeutic or cosmetic purposes.[216] Clinically, these lesions generally appear as multiple, firm nodules that may be tender.

Mondor's Disease (Phlebitis of the Thoracoepigastric Vein)

Mondor's disease, or phlebitis of the thoracoepigastric vein, has been considered to be rare; however, it is increasingly being recognized.[261–263] It was first mentioned by Flagge in 1869, but was best described by Mondor[264] in 1939 as "a string phlebitis of the chest wall." The disease involves a phlebitis and periphlebitis of the lateral thoracic or thoracoepigastric vein that occurs primarily in women, although men may be affected. Mondor's disease was initially ascribed to local trauma, and is commonly seen following diagnostic, therapeutic, or cosmetic surgery to the breast, or following local radiation therapy. The onset of the disease is often insidious, progressive, and painful. Characteristically, there is a tender fibrous cord fixed to the skin that forms a furrow, or sometimes a dimple. It is usually not erythematous, nor is it associated with hematoma, bruising, or adenopathy. It can appear anywhere along the course of the vein, from the axilla curving laterally around the breast to just below the nipple, where it sometimes arborizes into two or three branches before plunging caudally toward the epigastrium. Elevating the arm, or putting traction on the midinferior breast tissue, will often demonstrate the shallow groove. Haagensen believes that this groove is produced by the fibrosis surrounding the vein, which retracts the surrounding tissue, as well as by the shortening of the vein, which bowstrings the surrounding tissue.[12]

The course of the disease is entirely benign, and most cases will gradually resolve within several weeks to

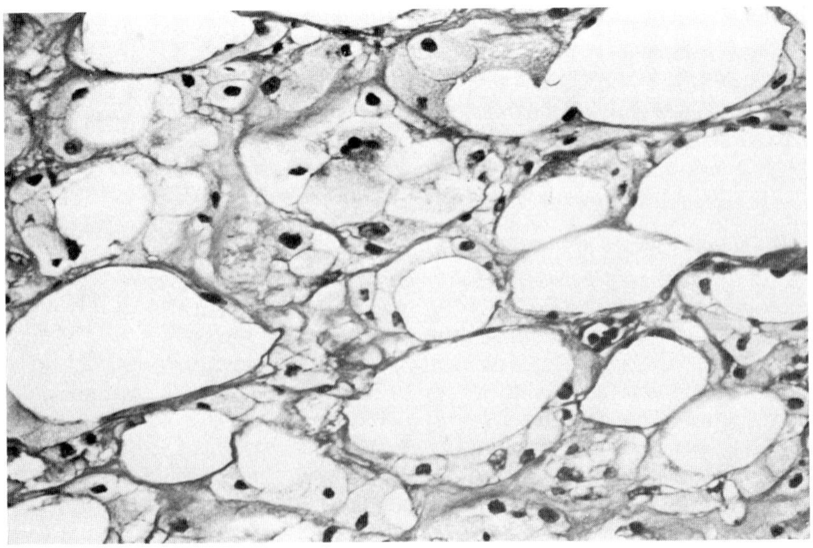

FIGURE 2-12. Fat necrosis. The fatty breast tissue is infiltrated by histiocytes containing foamy cytoplasm. (x300)

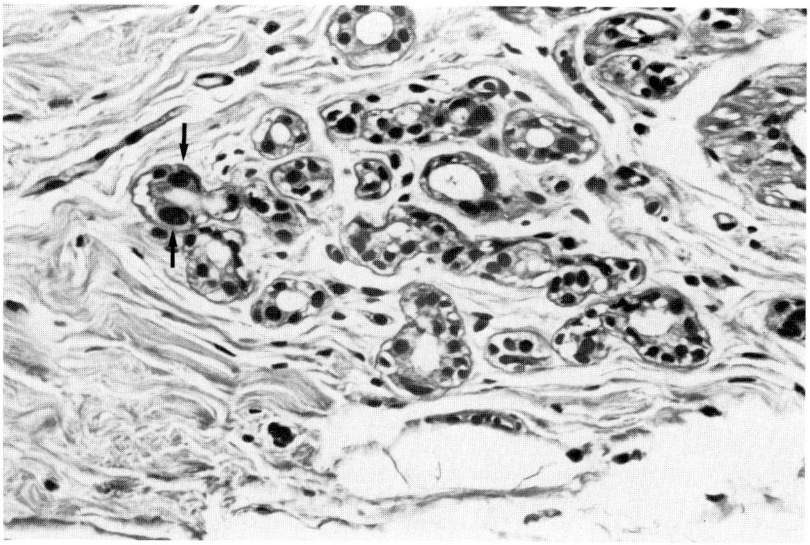

FIGURE 2-13. Radiation effects. This terminal duct-lobular unit contains scattered, enlarged, epithelial cells with large, diffusely hyperchromatic nuclei *(arrows).* Cellular polarity is maintained, and there is no evidence of epithelial cell proliferation. (x300)

months, without active treatment. Pain or discomfort is occasionally treated with anti-inflammatory agents, such as aspirin.

On pathologic examination, the lesion is that of phlebitis and periphlebitis. The obliterative endophlebitis is associated with varying degrees of thrombosis, and the adventitia and media may be completely destroyed in advanced cases.

Mondor's disease is self-limiting and needs no treatment. Its main importance is in recognizing it and differentiating it from the skin retraction or dimpling that may be associated with carcinoma.

Pathologic Changes Associated With Radiation Therapy for Carcinoma

Breast-conserving surgery, followed by radiation therapy, is becoming an increasingly common treatment for patients with early-stage breast cancer. The effects of therapeutic doses of ionizing radiation on the skin of the breast have been well described, and are identical to the radiation-induced alterations occurring in skin from any irradiated site.[265]

Fat necrosis may occur in the breast following local excision and radiation therapy for carcinoma. These lesions may be indistinguishable from carcinoma by clinical and radiographic examination, requiring complete histologic examination for accurate diagnosis.[266]

The most characteristic pathologic finding in breast tissue excised following primary radiation therapy for carcinoma is epithelial cell atypicality in the TDLU, usually associated with varying degrees of lobular sclerosis and atrophy (Fig. 2-13).[267] These changes may be distinguished from carcinoma involving the TDLU by the preservation of polarity and cohesion, and by the absence of cellular proliferation and distention of the involved TDLU in areas of radiation-induced change. Less frequently, epithelial atypia in large (extralobular) ducts, atypical fibroblasts in the stroma, and radiation-related vascular changes may be observed. Interestingly, stromal fibrosis, a characteristic feature of radiation effect in other organs, is so variable among both irradiated patients and nonirradiated control subjects that it is not, by itself, a reliable marker for radiation-induced injury in the breast.

Sarcoidosis

Involvement of the breast by sarcoidosis is rare, but when present, may clinically simulate a neoplasm.[268–270] Histologically, the lesions consist of typical, noncaseating granulomas with varying numbers of giant cells, which are present in the interlobular and intralobular connective tissue. A diagnosis of sarcoidosis should be made only after the exclusion of other causes of granulomatous inflammation, such as mycobacterial, fungal, and parasitic infections or reactions to foreign materials.

REFERENCES

1. Patey DH: Two common non-malignant conditions of the breast. Br Med J 1:96, 1949
2. Lewison EF, Lyons JG: Relationship between benign breast disease and cancer. AMA Arch Surg 66:94, 1953
3. Foote FW, Stewart FW: Comparative studies of cancerous versus noncancerous breasts. Ann Surg 121:a,6; b,197, 1945
4. Brodie B: Lectures on sero-cystic tumors of the breast. London Medical Gazette 25:808, 1840
5. Birkett J: The Diseases of the Breast. London, Longman & Co, 1850
6. Velpeau A: A Treatise on Diseases of the Breast and Mammary Region. Mitchell H (trans): London, Sydenham Society 1856

7. Bryant T: The Diseases of the Breast. London, Cassel & Co, 1887
8. Reclus P: Cystic disease of the breast. Rev Chir 3:761, 1883
9. Schimmelbusch C: Cystadenoma of the mamma. Archiv für klinische Chirurgie 44:117, 1892
10. Cheatle GL, Cutler M: Tumors of the Breast. London, Edward Arnold & Co, 1931
11. Geschickter CF: Diseases of the Breast, 2nd ed. Philadelphia, JB Lippincott, 1945
12. Haagensen CD: Diseases of the Breast. Philadelphia, WB Saunders, 1971
13. Love SM, Gelman RS, Silen WS: Fibrocystic "disease" of the breast: A non-disease. N Engl J Med 307:1010, 1982
14. Hutter RVP: Goodbye to "fibrocystic disease." N Engl J Med 312:179, 1985
15. Cole P, Elwood JM, Kaplan SD: Incidence rates and risk factors of benign breast neoplasms. Am J Epidemiol 108:112, 1978
16. Hislop TG, Elwood JM: Risk factors for benign breast disease: A 30-year cohort study. Can Med Assoc J 124:283, 1981
17. Davis HH, Simons M, Davis JB: Cystic disease of the breast: Relationship to cancer. Cancer 17:957, 1964
18. Kramer WM, Rush BF: Mammary duct proliferation in the elderly. Cancer 31:130, 1973
19. Wang DY, Fentiman IS: Epidemiology and endocrinology of benign breast disease. Breast Cancer Res Treat 6:5, 1985
20. Brinton LA, Vessey MP, Flavel R, et al: Risk factors for benign breast disease. Am J Epidemiol 113:203, 1981
21. Berkowitz GS, Kelsey JL, LiVolsi VA et al: Risk factors for fibrocystic breast disease and its histopathologic components J Natl Cancer Inst 75:43–50, 1985
22. Nomura A, Comstock GW, Tonascia JA: Epidemiologic characteristics of benign breast disease. Am J Epidemiol 105:505, 1977
23. Ernster VL: The epidemiology of benign breast disease. Epidemiol Rev 3:184, 1981
24. Oluwole SF, Freeman HP: Analysis of benign breast lesions in blacks. Am J Surg 137:786, 1979
25. Schuerch C, Rosen PP, Hirota T, et al: A pathological study of benign breast diseases in Tokyo and New York. Cancer 50:1899, 1982
26. Hislop TG, Threlfall WJ: Oral contraceptives and benign breast disease. Am J Epidemiol 120:273, 1984
27. Vessey MP, Doll R, Sutton PM: Oral contraceptives and breast neoplasia: A retrospective study. Br Med J 3:719, 1972
28. Boston Collaborative Drug Surveillance Programme. Oral contraceptives and venous thromboembolic disease, surgically confirmed gall bladder disease, and breast tumours. Lancet 1:1399, 1973
29. Sartwell PE, Arthes FG, Tonascia J: Epidemiology of benign breast lesions: Lack of association with oral contraceptive use. N Engl J Med 288:551, 1973
30. Royal College of General Practitioners: Oral Contraceptives and Health. New York, Pitman, 1974
31. Ory H, Cole P, MacMahon B, et al: Oral contraceptives and reduced risk of benign breast disease. N Engl J Med 294:419, 1976
32. Janerich DT, Glebatis DM, Dugan J: Benign breast disease and oral contraceptive use. JAMA 237:2199, 1977
33. Kelsey JL, Lindfors KK, White C: A case control study of the epidemiology of benign breast diseases with reference to oral contraceptive use. Int J Epidemiol 3:333, 1974
34. Franceschi S, La Vecchia C, Parazzini F, et al: Oral contraceptives and benign breast disease: A case control study. Am J Obstet Gynecol 149:602, 1984
35. Lees AW, Burns PE, Grace M: Oral contraceptives and breast disease in premenopausal Northern Albertan women. Int J Cancer 22:700, 1978
36. Ravnihar B, Seigel DG, Lindtner J: An epidemiologic study of breast cancer and benign breast neoplasia in relation to the oral contraceptive and estrogen use. Eur J Cancer 15:395, 1979
37. Berkowitz GS, Kelsey JL, LiVolsi VA, et al: Oral contraceptive use and fibrocystic breast disease among pre- and postmenopausal women. Am J Epidemiol 120:87, 1984
38. LiVolsi VA, Stadel BV, Kelsey JL, et al: Fibrocystic breast disease in oral-contraceptive users. N Engl J Med 299:381, 1978
39. Berkowitz GS, Kelsey JL, LiVolsi VA et al: Exogenous hormone use and fibrocystic disease by histopathologic component. Int J Cancer 34:443, 1984
40. Pastides H, Kelsey JL, LiVolsi VA, et al: Oral contraceptive use and fibrocystic breast disease with special reference to its histopathology. J Natl Cancer Inst 71:5, 1983
41. Hsieh C, Crosson AW, Walker AM, et al: Oral contraceptive use and fibrocystic breast disease of different histologic classifications. J Natl Cancer Inst 72:285, 1984
42. Fechner RE: Benign breast disease in women on estrogen therapy: A pathological study. Cancer 29:273, 1972
43. Trapido EJ, Brinton LA, Schairer C, et al: Estrogen replacement therapy and benign breast disease. J Natl Cancer Inst 73:1101, 1984
44. Kier LC, Hickey RC, Keettel WC, et al: Endocrine relationships in benign lesions of the breast. Ann Surg 135:782, 1952
45. Vorherr H, Messer RH: Breast cancer: Potentially predisposing and protecting factors. Role of pregnancy, lactation and endocrine status. Am J Obstet Gynecol 130:335, 1978
46. Kuttenn F, Fournier S, Durand JC, et al: Estradiol and progesterone receptors in human breast fibroadenomas. J Clin Endocrinol Metab 52:1225, 1981
47. Bassler, R: The morphology of hormone-induced structural changes in the female breast. Curr Top Pathol 53:1, 1970
48. Cowie AT, Folley SJ, Malprees FH, et al: Studies on the hormonal induction of mammary growth and lactation in the goat. J Endocrinol 8:64, 1952
49. England PC, Skinner LG, Cottrell KM, et al: Sex hormones in breast disease. Br J Surg 62:806, 1975
50. Sitruk-Ware, R, Sterkers N, Mowszowicz I, et al: Inadequate corpus luteal function in women with benign breast diseases. J Clin Endocrinol Metab 44:771, 1977
51. Malarkey WB, Schroeder LL, Stevens VC, et al: Twenty-four-hour preoperative endocrine profiles in women with benign and malignant breast disease. Cancer Res 37:4655, 1977
52. Gorins RC, Cordray JP: Hormonal profile of benign breast disease and premenstrual mastodynia. Eur J Gynaecol Oncol 5:1, 1984
53. Walsh PV, Bulbrook RD, Stell PM, et al: Serum progesterone concentration during the luteal phase in women with benign breast disease. Eur J Cancer Clin Oncol 20:1339, 1984
54. Kumar S, Mansel RE, Wilson DW, et al: Daily salivary progesterone levels in cyclical mastalgia patients and their controls. Br J Surg 73:260, 1986
55. Sitruk-Ware R, Sterkers N, Mauvais-Jarvis P: Benign breast disease. I. Hormonal Investigation. Obstet Gynecol 53:457, 1979
56. Walsh PV, McDicken RD, Bulbrook RD, et al: Serum oestradiol-17β and prolactin concentrations during the luteal phase in women with benign breast disease. Eur J Cancer Clin Oncol 20:1345, 1984
57. Filicori M, Butler JP, Crowley WF Jr: Neuroendocrine regulation of the corpus luteum in the human: Evidence for pulsatile progesterone secretion. J Clin Invest 73:1638, 1984

58. Watt-Boolsen S, Andersen AN, Blichert-Toft M: Serum prolactin and oestradiol levels in women with cyclical mastalgia. Horm Metab Res 13:700, 1981
59. Peters F, Schuth W, Scheurich B, et al: Serum prolactin levels in patients with fibrocystic breast disease. Obstet Gynecol 64:381, 1984
60. Brown RW, Meehan C, Martin FIR, et al: Breast tumors in patients with hyperprolactinemia. Cancer 50:125, 1982
61. Kauppila A, Ylikorkala O: Effects of oral and intravenous TRH and metoclopramide on PRL and TSH secretion in women. Clin Endocrinol 17:617, 1982
62. Kumar S, Mansel RE, Hughes LE, et al: Prolactin response to thyrotropin-releasing hormone stimulation and dopaminergic inhibition in benign breast disease. Cancer 53:1311, 1984
63. Watt-Boolsen S, Eskildsen PC, Blaehr H: Release of prolactin, thyrotropin, and growth hormone in women with cyclical mastalgia and fibrocystic disease of the breast. Cancer 56:500, 1985
64. Mansel RE, Preece PE, Hughes LE: A double blind trial of the prolactin inhibitor bromocriptine in painful benign breast disease. Br J Surg 65:724, 1978
65. Durning P, Sellwood RA: Bromocriptine in severe cyclical breast pain. Br J Surg 69:248, 1982
66. Ayers JW, Gidwani GP: The "luteal breast": Hormonal and sonographic investigations of benign breast disease in patients with cyclic mastalgia. Fertil Steril 40:779, 1983
67. Kuttenn F, Fournier S, Sitruk-Ware R, et al: Progesterone insufficiency in benign breast disease. In Endocrinology of Cystic Breast Disease. New York, Raven Press, 1983
68. Sherman BM, Korenman SG: Inadequate corpus luteum function: A pathophysiological interpretation of human breast cancer epidemiology. Cancer 33:1306, 1974
69. Peillon F, Vincens M, Cesselin F, et al: Exaggerated prolactin response of thyrotropin-releasing hormone in women with anovulatory cycles: Possible role of endogenous estrogens and effect of bromocriptine. Fertil Steril 37:530, 1982
70. Crowley WF Jr, Filicori M, Sprait DI, et al: The physiology of gonadotropin-releasing hormone (GRH) secretion in men and women. Recent Prog Horm Res 41:473, 1985
71. DiCarlo R, Muccioli, DiCarlo F: Hormone receptors in benign breast tumors. In Angeli A, Bradlow HL. Dogliotti L, et al: Endocrinology of Cystic Breast Disease. New York, Raven Press, 1983
72. Golinger RC, Krebs J, Fisher ER, et al: Hormones and the pathophysiology of fibrocystic mastopathy: Elevated luteinizing hormone levels. Surgery 84:212, 1978
73. Secreto G, Recchione C, Fariselli G, et al: High testosterone and low progesterone circulating levels in premenopausal patients with hyperplasia and cancer of the breast. Cancer Res 44:841, 1984
74. Carlstrom K, Doberl A, Gershagen S, et al: Elevated peripheral levels of androgens and of some steroid sensitive plasma proteins in patients with severe fibrocystic breast disease. Acta Obstet Gynecol Scand (Suppl) 123:157, 1984
75. Robinson JE, Short RV: Changes in breast sensitivity at puberty, during the menstrual cycle, and at parturition. Br Med J 1:1188, 1977
76. Fanger H, Ree HJ: Cyclic changes of human mammary gland epithelium in relation to the menstrual cycle—an ultrastructural study. Cancer 34:574, 1974
77. Vogel PM, Georgiade NG, Fetter BS, et al: The correlation of histologic changes in the human breast with the memstrual cycle. Am J Pathol 104:23, 1981
78. Bischoff VJ, Wenderlein JM: Die bedeutung der mastalgie in der mammadiagnostik. Fortschr Geb Rontgenstr 130:706, 1979
79. Atkins HJ: Treatment of chronic mastitis. Lancet 1:707, 1938
80. Preece PE, Hughes LE, Mansel RE, et al: Clinical syndromes of mastalgia. Lancet 2:670, 1976
81. Goodson WH, Mailman R, Jacobson M, et al: What do breast symptoms mean? Am J Surg 150:271, 1985
82. Blichert-Toft M, Watt-Boolsen S: Clinical approach to women with severe mastalgia and the therapeutic possibilities. Acta Obstet Gynecol Scand (Suppl)123:185, 1984
83. Wisbey JR, Kumar S, Mansel RE, et al: Natural history of breast pain. Lancet 2:672, 1983
84. Preece PE, Mansel RE, Hughes LE: Mastalgia: Psychoneurosis or organic disease? Br Med J 1:29, 1978
85. Bishop HM, Blamey RW: A suggested classification of breast pain. Postgrad Med J (Suppl 5)55:59, 1979
86. Peyton FW: Unexpected frequency of idiopathic costochondral pain. Obstet Gynecol 62:605, 1983
87. LeBan MM, Meerschaert JR, Taylor RS: Breast pain: A symptom of cervical radiculopathy. Arch Phys Med Rehabil 60:315, 1979
88. Harrington E, Lesnick G: The association between gross cysts of the breast and breast cancer. Breast 7:13, 1981
89. Herrman JB: Mammary cancer subsequent to aspiration of cysts in the breast. Ann Surg 173:40, 1971
90. Patey DH, Nurck AW: Natural history of cystic disease of breast treated conservatively. Br Med J 1:15, 1953
91. Barnes WC: Management of cystic disease of the breast. Am J Surg 129:324, 1975
92. Greenblatt RB, Vasquez J, Samaras C: Fibrocystic breast disease: Current status of diagnosis and treatment. Postgrad Med 71:159, 1982
93. Murley RS: Treatment of benign breast disease. Ann Coll Surg Engl 58:385, 1976
94. Bradlow HL, Skidmore FD, Schwartz MK, et al: Cations in breast fluid. In Angeli A, et al: Endocrinology of Cystic Breast Disease. New York, Raven Press, 1983
95. Angeli A, Fraira R, Agrimonti F, et al: Steroid binding proteins in breast cyst fluid. In Angeli A, et al: Endocrinology of Cystic Breast Disease. New York, Raven Press, 1983
96. Gairard B, Gros CM, Koehl C, et al: Proteins and ionic components in breast cyst fluids. In Angeli A, et al: Endocrinology of Cystic Breast Disease. New York, Raven Press, 1983
97. Bradlow HL, Schwartz MK, Fleisher M, et al: Accumulation of hormones in breast cyst fluid. J Clin Endocrinol Metab 49:778, 1979
98. Miller WR, Forrest APM: Androgen conjugates in human breast cyst fluid. In Angeli A, et al: Endocrinology of Cystic Breast Disease. New York, Raven Press, 1983
99. Boccuzzi G, Brignardello E, Agrimonti F, et al: Adrenal androgens and prolactin in human breast cyst fluid: A possible correlation. In Angeli A, et al: Endocrinology of Cystic Breast Disease. New York, Raven Press, 1983
100. DeBoever J, Verheugen C, Van Maele G, et al: Steroid concentrations in serum glandular breast tissue and breast cyst fluid of control and progesterone treated patients. In Angeli A, et al: Endocrinology of Cystic Breast Disease. New York, Raven Press, 1983
101. Melis GB, Guarnieri G, Paoletti FD, et al: Clinical significance of hormonal evaluation in peripheral blood and in breast cyst fluid of women with benign breast disease. In Angeli A, et al: Endocrinology of Cystic Breast Disease. New York, Raven Press, 1983
102. Haagensen DE, Mazoujian G: Relationship of glycoproteins

in human breast cystic disease fluid to breast carcinoma. In Angeli A, et al: Endocrinology of Cystic Breast Disease. New York, Raven Press, 1983
103. Haagensen CD: The relationship of gross cystic disease of the breast and carcinoma. Ann Surg 185:375, 1977
104. Page DL, Vanderzwagg R, Rogers LW, et al: Relationship between the component parts of fibrocystic disease complex and breast cancer. J Natl Cancer Inst 61:1055, 1978
105. Dupont WD, Page DL: Risk factors for breast cancer in women with proliferative breast disease. N Engl J Med 312:146, 1985
106. Takeda T, Suzuki M, Sato Y, et al: Cytologic studies of nipple discharges. Acta Cytol 26:35, 1982
107. Urban JA, Egell RA: Excision of the major duct system of the breast. Cancer 16:516, 1963
108. Leis HP Jr, Cammarata A, LaRaja RD: Nipple discharge significance and treatment. Breast 11:6, 1985
109. O'Brien PH, Kreutner A Jr: Another cause of nipple discharge: Mammary duct ectasia with periductal mastitis. Am Surg 48:577, 1982
110. Chaudary MA, Millis RR, Davies GC et al: The diagnostic value of testing for occult blood. Ann Surg 196:651, 1982
111. Thomsen AC, Espersen T, Maigaard S: Course and treatment of milk stasis, noninfectious inflammation of the breast, and infectious mastitis in nursing women. Am J Obstet Gynecol 149:492, 1984
112. Reid DE, Ryan KJ, Benirschke K: Principles and Management of Human Reproduction, pp. 338-390. Philadelphia, WB Saunders, 1972
113. Golinger RC, O'Neal BJ: Mastitis and mammary duct disease. Arch Surg 117:1027, 1982
114. Crile G, Chatty EM: Squamous metaplasia of lactiferous ducts. Arch Surg 102:533, 1971
115. Smith GV, Shirley RL: Management of benign lesions related to the diagnosis of early breast cancer. In Reid DE, Christian CD: Controversy in Obstetrics and Gynecology, Vol II, p 503. Philadelphia, WB Saunders, 1974
116. Urban JA, Egeli RA: Nonlactational nipple discharge. Cancer 28:130, 1978
117. Deninger HK: Wegener's granulomatosis of the breast. Radiology 154:59, 1985
118. Copeland MM: The treatment of mammary dysplasia with special reference to microcystic and macrocystic disease of the breast. Am J Surg 106:382, 1963
119. Hendrick JW: Results of treatment of cystic disease of the breast. Surgery 44:457, 1958
120. Peacock EE: Biological basis for management of benign diseases of the breast. Plast Reconstr Surg 55:14, 1975
121. Vorherr H: Fibrocystic breast disease: Pathophysiology, pathomorphology, clinical picture and management. Am J Obstet Gynecol 154:161, 1986
122. Meyerick RLL, Smith I: Benign breast swelling. Br Med J 2:585, 1972
123. Ruf H, Codoccioni JL, Serment H: Le norethynodrel dans le syndrome premenstrual, et les dysplasies mammaires. Bull Fed Gynecol Obstet Franc 16:587, 1964
124. Roeder D: Treatment of mastodynia and mastopathy using mastodynon. Med Welt 27:591, 1976
125. Lafaye C, Aubert B: Action de la progesterone locale dans les mastopathies benignes. J Gynecol Obstet Biol Reprod 7:1123, 1978
126. Mauvais-Jarvis P, Sterkers N, Kuttenn F, et al: Traitement des mastopathies benignes par la progesterone, et les progestatifs. J Gynecol Obstet Biol Reprod 7:477, 1978
127. Colin C, Gasparou, Lambotte R: Relationship of mastodynia with its endocrine environment and treatment in a double blind trial with lynestrenol. Arch Gynakol 225, No. I:7, 1978
128. Dennerstein L, Spencer–Gardiner C, Gotts G, et al: Progesterone and the premenstrual syndrome; A double blind crossover trial. Br Med J 290:1617, 1985
129. Page JK, Mansel RE, Hughes SE: Clinical experience of drug treatments for mastalgia. Lancet 2:373, 1985
130. Nagasawa H, Fujii M, Hagiwara K: Inhibition by medroxyprogesterone acetate of precancerous mammary hyperplastic alveolar nodule formation in mice. Breast Cancer Res Treat 5:31, 1985
131. Liang AP, Levenson AG, Layde PM, et al: Risk of breast, uterine corpus and ovarian cancer in women receiving medroxyprogesterone injections. JAMA 249:2909, 1983
132. Dogliotti L, Mussa A, Sandrucci S: Prolactin and benign breast disease with special emphasis on bromocriptine therapy. In Angeli A, et al: Endocrinology of Cystic Breast Disease. New York, Raven Press, 1983
133. Blichert-Toft M, Anderson AN, Henriksen OB, et al: Treatment of mastalgia with bromocriptine: A double-blind crossover study. Br Med J 1:237, 1979
134. Marzetti L, Framarino dei Malatesta ML, Aaragona C: Prolactin and benign breast diseases. In Angeli A, et al: Endocrinology of Cystic Breast Disease. New York, Raven Press, 1983
135. Ylostalo P: Cycle of continuous treatment of the premenstrual syndrome (PMS) with bromocriptine. Eur J Obstet Gynecol Reprod Biol 17:337, 1984
136. Andersen AN, Larsen JF, Steenstrup OR, et al: Effect of bromocriptine on the premenstrual syndrome. A double blind clinical trial. Br J Obstet Gynaecol 84:370, 1977
137. Greenblatt RB, Dmowsky WP, Mahesh VB, et al: Clinical studies with an antigonadotropin-danazol. Fertil Steril 22:102, 1971
138. Lauersen NH, Wilson KH: The effect of danazol in the treatment of chronic cystic mastitis. Obstet Gynecol 48:93, 1976
139. Blackmore WP: Danazol in the treatment of benign breast disease. J Int Med Res 5:101, 1977
140. Montgomery ACV, Palmer BV, Biswas S, et al: Treatment of severe cyclical mastalgia. J R Soc Med 72:489, 1979
141. Asch RH, Greenblatt RB: The use of an impeded androgen—danazol—in the management of benign breast disorders. Am J Obstet Gynecol 127:130, 1977
142. Aksu MF, Tzingounis VA, Greenblatt RB: Treatment of benign breast disease with danazol: A follow-up report. J Reprod Med 21:181, 1978
143. Barbieri RL, Ryan KJ: Danazol: Endocrine pharmacology and therapeutic applications. Am J Obstet Gynecol 141:453, 1981
144. Mansel RE, Hughes LE: The clinical and hormonal effects of treating mastalgia with danazol. In Angeli A, et al: Endocrinology of Cystic Breast Disease. New York, Raven Press, 1983
145. Atkins HJB: The effect of endocrines on fibroadenosis. Br Med J 1:750, 1949
146. Tobiassen T, Rasmussen T, Doberl A, et al: Danazol treatment of severely symptomatic fibrocystic breast disease and long-term follow-up—the Hjorring project. Acta Obstet Gynecol Scand (Suppl)123:159, 1984
147. Doberl A, Tobiassen T, Rasmussen T: Treatment of recurrent cyclical mastodynia in patients with fibrocystic disease. Acta Obstet Gynecol Scand (Suppl)123:177, 1984
148. Daro AF, Gollin HA, Samos FH: The effect of thyroid on cystic mastitis. J Int Coll Surg 41:58, 1964
149. Estes NC: Mastodynia due to fibrocystic disease of the breast controlled with thyroid hormone. Am J Surg 142:764, 1981
150. Peters F, Pickardt R, Breckwoldt M: Thyroid hormones in benign breast disease. Cancer 56:1082, 1985

151. DeLean A, Ferland L, Drouin J, et al: Modulation of pituitary thyrotropin releasing hormone receptor levels by estrogens and thyroid hormones. Endocrinology 100:1496, 1977
152. Ricciardi I, Ianniruberto A: Tamoxifen-induced regression of benign breast lesions. Obstet Gynecol 54:80, 1979
153. Shaaban MM, Morad F, Hassan A: Treatment of fibrocystic mastopathy by an antiestrogen, tamoxifen. Int J Gynaecol Obstet 18:348, 1980
154. Fentiman IS, Caleffi M, Brame K, et al: Double-blind controlled trial of tamoxifen therapy for mastalgia. Lancet i:287, 1986
155. Kistner RW: Observations on the use of a nonsteroidal estrogen antagonist-I. Cystic disease of the breast. Am J Obstet Gynecol 81:233, 1961
156. Morandi G, Marchesoni M, Valdagni C: Chorionic gonadotropins in the therapy of fibrocystic mastosis. Minerva Ginecol 21:1655, 1969
157. Ariel IM: Enovid therapy (norethynodrel with mestranol) for fibrocystic disease. Am J Obstet Gynecol 117:453, 1973
158. Erb H, Kallenberger A: The action of an oral high-dosed oestrogen-progestogen combination on the human breast. Acta Endocrinol 70:143, 1972
159. Minton JP, Foecking MK, Webster DJT, et al: Response of fibrocystic disease to caffeine withdrawal and correlation of cyclic nucleotides with breast disease. Am J Obstet Gynecol 135:157, 1979
160. Heyden S, Muhlbaier LH: Prospective study of "fibrocystic breast disease" and caffeine consumption. Surgery 96:479, 1984
161. Brooks PG, Gart S, Heldfond AJ, et al: Measuring the effect of caffeine restriction on fibrocystic breast disease. J Repro Med 26:279, 1981
162. Boyle CA, Berkowitz GS, LiVolsi VA, et al: Caffeine consumption and fibrocystic breast disease: A case-control epidemiologic study. J Natl Cancer Inst 72:1015, 1984
163. Lawson DH, Jick H, Rothman KJ: Coffee and tea consumption and breast disease. Surgery 90:801, 1981
164. Minton JP, Abou-Issa H, Reiches N, et al: Clinical and biochemical studies on methylxanthine-related fibrocystic disease. Surgery 90:299, 1981
165. Marshall J, Graham S, Swanson M: Caffeine consumption and benign breast disease: A case-control comparison. Am J Public Health 72:610, 1982
166. Lubin F, Ron E, Wax Y, et al: A case-control study of caffeine and methylxanthine in benign breast disease. JAMA 253:2388, 1985
167. Ernster VL, Mason L, Goodson WH, et al: Effects of caffeine-free diet on benign breast disease: A randomized trial. Surgery 91:263, 1982
168. Parazzini F, La Vecchia C, Riundi R, et al: Methylxanthine, alcohol-free diet and fibrocystic breast disease. A factorial clinical trial. Surgery 99:576, 1986
169. Minton JP, Foecking MK, Webster DJT, et al: Caffeine, cyclic nucleotides and breast disease. Surgery 86:105, 1979
170. Elliot JB, Abou-Issa HM, Foecking MK, et al: Cyclic nucleotides as predictors of benign to malignant progression of breast disease. Breast 7:6, 1981
171. Barber R, Goka TJ, Butcher RW: Hormone and methylxanthine action on breast epithelial cells. Life Sci 34:2467, 1984
172. Minton JP, Abou-Issa H, Foecking MK et al: Caffeine and unsaturated fat diet significantly promotes DMBA-induced breast cancer in rats. Cancer 51:1249, 1983
173. Pike MC, Bernstein L: Statistical errors invalidate conclusions in "Caffeine and unsaturated diet significantly promotes DMBA-induced breast cancer in rats." Cancer 55:1855, 1985
174. Petrek JA, Sandberg WA, Cole MN, et al: The inhibitory effect of caffeine on hormone-induced rat breast cancer. Cancer 56:1977, 1985
175. Abrams AA: Use of vitamin E in chronic cystic mastitis. N Engl J Med 272:1080, 1965
176. London RS, Solomon DM, London ED, et al: Mammary dysplasia: clinical response and urinary excretion of 11-deoxy-17-ketosteroids and pregnanediol following α-tocopherol therapy. Breast 4:19, 1978
177. Sundaram GS, London R, Manimekalai S, et al: Alpha-tocopherol and serum lipoproteins. Lipids 16:223, 1981
178. London RS, Sundaram GS, Murphy L, et al: The effect of vitamin E on mammary dysplasia: A double-blind study. Obstet Gynecol 65:104, 1985
179. Ernster VL, Goodson WH, Hunt TK, et al: Vitamin E and benign breast "disease": A double-blind, randomized clinical trial. Surgery 97:490, 1985
180. Preece PE, Richards AR, Owen GM, et al: Mastalgia and total body water. Br Med J 4:498, 1975
181. Rolland PH, Martin PM, Rolland AM, et al: Benign breast disease: Studies of prostaglandin E_2, steroids, and thermographic effects of inhibitors of prostaglandin biosynthesis. Obstet Gynecol 54:715, 1979
182. Humphrey LJ: Subcutaneous mastectomy is not a prophylaxis against carcinoma of the breast: Opinion or knowledge? Am J Surg 145:311, 1983
183. Anderson DE, Badzioch MD: Risks of familial breast cancer. Cancer 56:383, 1985
184. Goldman LD, Goldwyn RM: Some anatomical considerations of subcutaneous mastectomy. Plast Reconstr Surg 51:501, 1973
185. Jackson CF, Palmquist M, Swanson J, et al: The effectiveness of prophylactic subcutaneous mastectomy in Sprague-Dawley rats induced with 7,12-dimethylbenzanthracene. Plast Reconstr Surg 73:249, 1984
186. Eldar S, Meguid MM, Beatty JD: Cancer of the breast after prophylactic subcutaneous mastectomy. Am J Surg 148:692, 1984
187. Pennisi VR: Subcutaneous mastectomy and fibrocystic disease of the breast. Clin Plast Surg 3:205, 1976
188. Goodnight JE, Quagliana JM, Morton DL: Failure of subcutaneous mastectomy to prevent the development of breast cancer. J Surg Oncol 26:198, 1984
189. Wilson MC, Sellwood RA: Therapeutic value of a supporting brassiere in mastodynia. Br Med J 2:90, 1976
190. Palmer BV, Montgomery ACV, Monteiro JCM: Ginseng and mastalgia. Br Med J 1:1284, 1978
191. Crile G: Injection of steroids in painful breasts. Am J Surg 133:705, 1977
192. Henderson IC: Adjuvant chemotherapy of breast cancer: A promising experiment or standard practice? J Clin Oncol 3:140, 1985
193. Page DL, Dupont WD, Rogers LW, et al: Atypical hyperplastic lesions of the female breast: A long-term follow-up study. Cancer 55:2698, 1985
194. Consensus Meeting: Is "fibrocystic disease" of the breast precancerous? Arch Pathol Lab Med 110:171, 1986
195. Haagensen CD, Lane N, Lattes R, et al: Lobular neoplasia (so-called lobular carcinoma *in situ*) of the breast. Cancer 42:737, 1978
196. McDivitt RW, Stewart FW, Berg JW: Tumors of the breast. In Firminger HI (ed): Atlas of Tumor Pathology, 2nd series, Part 2. Washington, DC: Armed Forces Institute of Pathology, 1968
197. Azzopardi JG: Problems in Breast Pathology. Philadelphia, WB Saunders, 1979

198. Rosen PP, Lieberman PH, Braum DWJ, et al: Lobular carcinoma *in situ* of the breast: Detailed analysis of 99 patients with average follow-up of 24 years. Am J Surg Pathol 2:225, 1978
199. Devitt JE: Fibrocystic disease of the breast is not premalignant. Surg Gynecol Obstet 134:803, 1972
200. Chetty U, Wang CC, Forrest APM, et al: Benign breast disease and cancer. Br J Surg 67:789, 1980
201. Roberts MM, Jones V, Elton RA, et al: Risk of breast cancer in women with history of benign disease of the breast. Br Med J 288:275, 1984
202. Black MM, Barclay THC, Cutler SJ, et al: Association of atypical characteristics of benign breast lesions with subsequent risk of breast cancer. Cancer 29:338, 1972
203. Spratt JS, Alagia DP, Greenberg RA, et al: Association of chronic cystic mastopathy, xeromammographic patterns and cancer. Cancer 55:1372, 1985
204. Azzopardi JG: Benign and malignant proliferative epithelial lesions of the breast: A review. Eur J Cancer Clin Oncol 19:1717, 1983
205. Ashikari R, Huvos AG, Snyder RE, et al: A clinicopathological study of atypical lesions of the breast. Cancer 33:310, 1974
206. Kodlin D, Winger EE, Morgenstern NL, et al: Chronic cystic mastopathy and breast cancer: A follow-up study. Cancer 39:2603, 1977
207. Veronesi U, Pizzocaro G: Breast cancer in women subsequent to cystic disease of the breast. Surg Gynecol Obstet 126:529, 1968
208. Donnelly PK, Baker KW, Carney JA, et al: Benign breast lesions and subsequent breast carcinoma in Rochester, Minnesota. Mayo Clinic Proc 50:650, 1975
209. Hutchinson WB, Thomas DB, Hamlin WB, et al: Risk of breast cancer in women with benign breast disease. J Natl Cancer Inst 65:13, 1980
210. Pastides H, Kelsey JL, Holford TR, et al: An epidemiologic study of fibrocystic breast disease with reference to diet epitheliol atypia. Am J Epidemiol 121:440, 1985
211. Page DL, Dupont WD, Rogers LW, et al: Intraductal carcinoma of the breast: Follow-up after biopsy only. Cancer 49:751, 1982
212. Goodman ZD, Taxy JB: Fibroadenomas of the breast with prominent smooth muscle. Am J Surg Pathol 5:99, 1981
213. Oberman, HA: Breast lesions in the adolescent female. In Sommers SC, Rosen PP: Pathology Annual 1979, Part I. Norwalk, CT, Appleton-Century-Crofts, 1979
214. Nambiar R, Kutty K: Giant fibroadenoma (cytosarcoma phyllodes) in adolescent females—a clinicopathologic study. Br J Surg 61:113, 1974
215. Ashikari R, Farrow JH, O'Hara J: Fibroadenomas in the breast of juveniles. Surg Gynecol Obstet 132:259, 1971
216. Symmers W: The breasts. In Symmers W: Systemic Pathology. Edinburgh, Churchill Livingstone, 1978
217. Pick PW, Iossifides IA: Occurrence of breast carcinoma within a fibroadenoma. A review. Arch Pathol Lab Med 108:590, 1984
218. Hertel BF, Zaloudek C, Kempson RL: Breast adenomas. Cancer 37:2891, 1976
219. O'Hara MF, Page DL: Adenomas of the breast and ectopic breast under lactational influences. Hum Pathol 16:707, 1985
220. Rosen PP: Syringomatous adenoma of the nipple. Am J Surg Pathol 7:739, 1983
221. Jones DB: Florid papillomatosis of the nipple ducts. Cancer 8:315, 1955
222. Perzin KH, Lattes R: Papillary adenoma of the nipple (florid papillomatosis, adenoma, adenomatosis). A clinicopathologic study. Cancer 29:996, 1972
223. Smith EJ, Kron SD, Gross PR: Erosive adenomatosis of the nipple. Arch Dermatol 102:330, 1970
224. Gudjonsdottir A, Hagerstrand I, Ostberg G: Adenoma of the nipple with carcinomatous development. Acta Pathol Microbiol Scand [A] 79:676, 1971
225. Bhagavan BS, Patchevsky AS, Koss LG: Florid subareolar duct papillomatosis (nipple adenoma) and mammary carcinoma: Report of three cases. Hum Pathol 4:289, 1973
226. Kraus FT, Neubecker RD: The differential diagnosis of papillary tumors of the breast. Cancer 15:444, 1962
227. Flint A, Oberman HA: Infarction and squamous metaplasia of intraductal papilloma. A benign breast lesion that may simulate carcinoma. Hum Pathol 15:764, 1984
228. Ohuchi N, Abe R, Kasai M: Possible cancerous change of intraductal papillomas of the breast. A 3-D reconstruction study of 25 cases. Cancer 54:605, 1984
229. Rosen PP, Cantrell B, Mullen DL, et al: Juvenile papillomatosis (Swiss cheese disease) of the breast. Am J Surg Pathol 4:3, 1980
230. Rosen PP, Lyngholm B, Kinne DW, et al: Juvenile papillomatosis and family history of breast carcinoma. Cancer 49:2591, 1982
231. Rosen PP, Holmes G, Lesser ML, et al: Juvenile papillomatosis and breast carcinoma. Cancer 55:1345, 1985
232. Rosen PP: Microglandular adenosis. A benign lesion simulating invasive mammary carcinoma. Am J Surg Pathol 7:137, 1983
233. Tavassoli FA, Norris HJ: Microglandular adenosis of the breast. A clinicopathologic study of 11 cases with ultrastructural observations. Am J Surg Pathol 7:731, 1983
234. Clement PB, Azzopardi JG: Microglandular adenosis of the breast—a lesion simulating tubular carcinoma. Histopathology 7:169, 1983
235. Rosenblum MK, Purrazzella R, Rosen PP: Is microglandular adenosis a precancerous disease? A study of carcinoma arising in microglandular adenosis. Lab Invest 52:57A, 1985
236. Fenoglio C, Lattes R: Sclerosing papillary proliferations in the female breast. A benign lesion often mistaken for carcinoma. Cancer 33:691, 1974
237. Fisher ER, Palekar AS, Kotwal N, et al: A nonencapsulated sclerosing lesion of the breast. Am J Clin Pathol 71:240, 1979
238. Rickert RR, Kalisher L, Hutter RVP: Indurative mastopathy: A benign sclerosing lesion of breast with elastosis which may simulate carcinoma. Cancer 47:561, 1981
239. Andersen JA, Gram JB: Radial scar in the female breast. A long-term follow-up study of 32 cases. Cancer 53:2557, 1984
240. Wellings SR, Alpers CE: Subgross pathologic features and incidence of radial scars in the breast. Hum Pathol 15:475, 1984
241. Linell F, Ljungberg O, Andersson I: Breast carcinoma: Aspects of early stages, progression and related problems. Acta Pathol Microbiol Scand [A] (Suppl) 272:14, 1980
242. Rosen PP, Ridolfi RL: The perilobular hemangioma. A benign microscopic vascular lesion of the breast. Am J Clin Path 68:21, 1977
243. Jozefczyk MA, Rosen PP: Vascular tumors of the breast II. Perilobular hemangiomas and hemangiomas. Am J Surg Pathol 9:491, 1985
244. Rosen PP: Vascular tumors of the breast III. Angiomatosis. Am J Surg Pathol 9:652, 1985
245. Rosen PP: Iozefczyk MA, Boram LH: Vascular tumors of the breast IV. The venous hemangioma. Am J Surg Pathol 9:659, 1985
246. Rosen PP: Vascular tumors of the breast V. Nonparenchymal hemangiomas of mammary subcutaneous tissues. Am J Surg Pathol 9:723, 1985

247. Donnell RM, Rosen PP, Lieberman PH, et al: Angiosarcoma and other vascular tumors of the breast: Pathologic analysis as a guide to prognosis. Am J Surg Pathol 5:629, 1981
248. Kaplan L, Walts A: Benign chondrolipomatous tumor of the human female breast. Arch Pathol Lab Med 101:149, 1977
249. Smith BG, Taylor HB: The occurrence of bone and cartilage in mammary tumors. Am J Clin Pathol 51:610, 1969
250. Erlandson RA, Rosen PP: Infiltrating myoepithelioma of the breast. Am J Surg Pathol 6:785, 1982
251. DeMay RM, Kay S: Granular cell tumors of the breast. In Sommers SC, Rosen PP: Pathology Annual 1984, Part 2, pp. 121–148. Norwalk, CT, Appleton-Century-Crofts, 1984
252. Ingram DL, Mossler JA, Snowhite J, et al: Granular cell tumors of the breast. Steroid receptor analysis and localization of carcinoembryonic antigen, myoglobin and S100 protein. Arch Pathol Lab Med 108:897, 1984
253. Gump FE, Sternschein MJ, Wolff M: Fibromatosis of the breast. Surg Gynecol Obstet 153:57, 1981
254. Ali M, Fayemi AO, Braun EV, et al: Fibromatosis of the breast. Am J Surg Pathol 3:501, 1979
255. Rosen Y, Sozos CP, Gardner B: Fibromatosis of the breast. Cancer 41:1409, 1978
256. Hanna WM, Jambrosic J, Fish E: Aggressive fibromatosis of the breast. Arch Pathol Lab Med 109:260, 1985
257. Zayid I, Dehmis C: Familial multicentric fibromatosis-desmoids. Cancer 24:786, 1969
258. Dixon JM, Anderson TJ, Lumsden AB, et al: Mammary duct ectasia. Br J Surg 70:601, 1983
259. Mansel RE, Morgan WP: Duct ectasia in the male. Br J Surg 66:660, 1979
260. Adair FE, Munger JT: Fat necrosis of the female breast: Report of 110 cases. Am J Surg 74:117, 1947
261. Honig C, Rado R: Mondor's disease—superficial phlebitis of the chest wall: A review of seven cases. Ann Surg 153:589, 1961
262. Fischl RA, Kahn S, Simon BE: Mondor's disease. Plast Reconstr Surg 56:319, 1975
263. Tabar L, Dean PB: Mondor's disease: Clinical, mammographic and pathologic features. Breast 7:18, 1981
264. Mondor H: Tonculite sous-cutanee subaigue de la paroi thoracique antero-laterale. Mem Acad de Chir 65:1271, 1939
265. Fajardo, LJ: Pathology of Radiation Injury. New York, Masson Publishing, 1982
266. Clarke D, Curtin JL, Martinez A, et al: Fat necrosis of the breast simulating recurrent carcinoma after primary radiotherapy in the management of early stage breast carcinoma. Cancer 52:442, 1983
267. Schnitt SJ, Connolly JL, Harris JR, et al: Radiation-induced changes in the breast. Hum Pathol 15:545, 1984
268. Gansler TS, Wheeler JE: Mammary sarcoidosis. Two cases and literature review. Arch Pathol Lab Med 108:673, 1984
269. Ross MJ, Merino MJ: Sarcoidosis of the breast. Hum Pathol 16:185, 1985
270. Fitzgibbons PL, Smiley DF, Kern WH: Sarcoidosis presenting initially as breast mass: Report of two cases. Hum Pathol 16:851, 1985
271. Frantz VK, Pickren JW, Melcher GW, et al: Incidence of chronic cystic disease in so-called "normal breasts". A study based on 225 postmortem exams. Cancer 4:762, 1951
272. Sloss PT, Bennett WA, Clagett OT: Incidence in normal breasts of features associated with chronic cystic mastitis. Am J Pathol 33:1181, 1957
273. Kern WH, Brooks RN: Atypical epithelial hyperplasia associated with breast cancer and fibrocystic disease. Cancer 24:668, 1969
274. Karpas CM, Leis HP, Oppenheim A, et al: Relationship of fibrocystic disease to carcinoma of the breast. Ann Surg 162:1, 1965
275. Fischerman K, Bech I, Foged P, et al: Relationship between fibrocystic disease and cancer of the breast. Acta Chir Scand 135:671, 1969
276. Silverberg SG, Chitale AR, Levitt SH: Prognostic implications of fibrocystic dysplasia in breasts removed for mammary carcinoma. Cancer 29:574, 1972
277. Bonser GM, Dosset J, Jull J, et al: Human and Experimental Breast Cancer. London, Pitman Medical, 1961
278. Fisher ER, Gregorio RM, Fisher B, et al: The pathology of invasive breast cancer: A syllabus derived from findings of the national surgical adjuvant breast project (protocol no. 4). Cancer 36:1, 1975

3 Physical Examination and Mammography in the Diagnosis of Breast Disease

David W. Kinne Daniel B. Kopans

SYMPTOMS OF BREAST DISEASE

In several large series of patients with breast cancer, presenting symptoms have been recorded. As summarized by Haagensen, about 75% to 80% of women with breast carcinoma become aware of their disease because of a breast lump.[1] In the majority of cases, the lump is painless, and is often described by patients as a thickening or "something different that was not there before," rather than as a three-dimensional mass. Physicians should be alerted to pursue such vague descriptions.

Pain is an uncommon symptom of breast cancer. Haagensen noted it as the first reported symptom in only 6.2% of 1433 patients, whereas others have reported it as the first symptom noted in 24%[2] and 53%[3] of patients with breast cancer. A common misconception of some physicians and patients is that if a mass is painful or tender on examination, it is benign. A true mass should be explored, even when painful, because carcinoma as an underlying cause is possible.

Nipple discharge (the spontaneous type, not produced only with examination), whether watery, serous, or bloody, occurs in patients with breast carcinoma in 1% to 7.5% of reported cases.[1] The higher figure may include patients whose discharge is due to nipple erosion with Paget's disease. Of greater clinical importance is the percentage of patients with nipple discharge who prove to have breast carcinoma. The benign lesions that cause nipple discharge are papillary in nature, and are frequently difficult to distinguish from malignant tumors. Perhaps this factor accounts for the reports of earlier series of "malignant" tumors in almost 50% of patients with nipple discharge. More recent series, with careful pathologic examinations, report a 10% to 12% incidence of carcinoma in patients with nipple discharge.[1] Whereas most of these patients have a bloody discharge, some have a serous discharge. Spontaneous, bloody nipple discharge in females has been shown by Adair[4] and Haagensen and associates[5] to be caused mostly by benign intraductal papillomas, but all types of discharge have been associated with all types of breast lesions, including carcinoma. Benign lesions, such as fibrocystic disease and periductal mastitis, may be the underlying cause. However, serosanguinous nipple discharge in males is an ominous symptom associated with carcinoma in the majority of cases.[6]

In the absence of a suspicious mass or mammographic abnormality that would indicate the need for biopsy, breast examination in female patients should attempt to determine from which quadrant of the breast the discharge is being produced. With the patient in the supine position, gentle pressure is exerted from beyond the areolar margin toward the nipple in each quadrant until discharge is produced. Hemoccult testing is not routinely done because serous, nonbloody discharge is also of concern. Cytologic analysis of this discharge may be done; reports by Strawbridge and co-workers[7] indicate that 4 of 40 patients tested had carcinoma detected by smears. However, if this discharge is reproducible on physical examination, and if it originates in the same quadrant each time, the generally recommended procedure is a major duct excision of that quadrant through a circumareolar incision, as described in Chapter 2.

Other symptoms occur less frequently and are not often reported by patients. Skin or nipple retraction, nipple erosion, redness of the skin of the breast, or an axillary mass should alert examining physicians to possible underlying carcinoma. Rarely, patients with no breast symptoms will present with symptoms attributable to metastases, such as bone pain.

TECHNIQUES OF BREAST EXAMINATION

Although the techniques and importance of breast examination are taught in medical schools, the current trends of clinical specialization and subspecialization may cause practitioners to lose expertise in or, even worse, to forget to include adequate breast examination as part of the work-up of their patients. To omit breast evaluation from routine examinations or to neglect to advise appropriate patients to undergo mammography may result in a missed opportunity for early detection that is tantamount to omitting a gynecologic examination with a Papanicolaou's smear, or to neglecting to perform a Hemoccult examination of a stool specimen. In diseases in which early detection is so clearly related to improved survival (after appropriate treatment), the value of these relatively simple techniques cannot be overemphasized.

Examination with the Patient in the Sitting Position

Physical examination of the breasts begins with the patient in the sitting position. In this position, obvious asymmetry, bulging of the skin, skin or nipple retraction, or nipple ulceration should be apparent (Fig. 3-1). With the patients' arms raised upward (Fig. 3-2), skin changes in the lower half of the breast, or in the inframammary fold, will become accentuated. Contraction of the pectoralis major muscle, effected by the patient pushing her hands against her hips (Fig. 3-3), may demonstrate an otherwise undetected skin retraction. Next, palpation of the breast with the patient still sitting upright may allow detection of subtle lesions that would be more difficult to palpate if she were supine (Fig. 3-4). The use of talc on the fingers of the examiner's hand reduces the friction between the skin of the hand and the skin of the breast, facilitating deeper palpation of the breast parenchyma. (For the same reason, patients are advised to begin breast self-examination in the shower, using soap on their fingers.) This is particularly true for masses high in the breast or in the axillary tail region, which are more apparent when the surrounding breast tissue is displaced inferiorly while the patient is in the sitting position than when the patient is in the supine position. Examination of the supraclavicular areas and both sides of the neck for the purpose of detecting suspicious lymphadenopathy is best carried out in the upright position also.

FIGURE 3-1. Examination of the patient in the upright position.

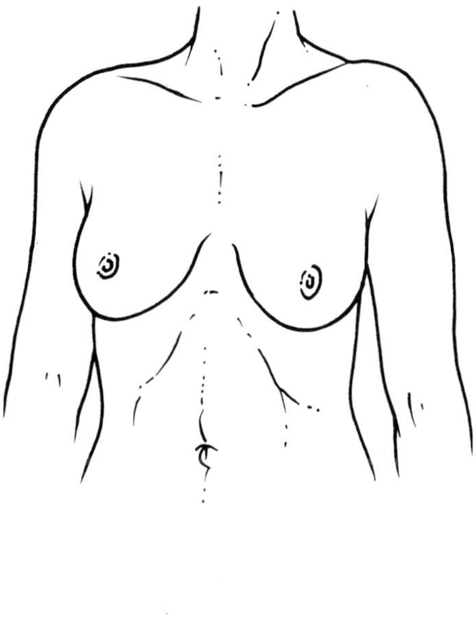

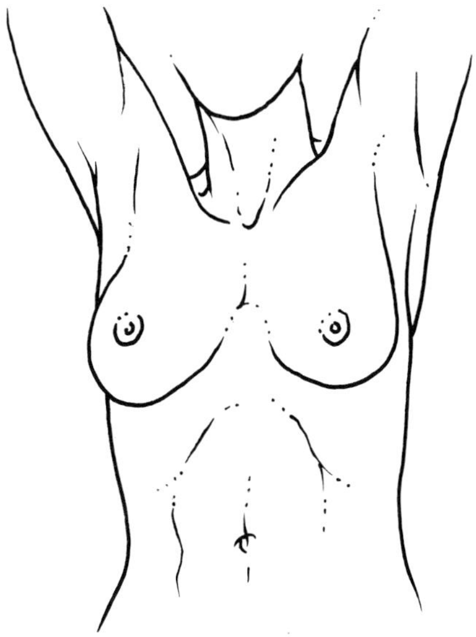

FIGURE 3-2. With the patients' arms raised upward, skin changes in the lower half of the breast and retraction may be detected.

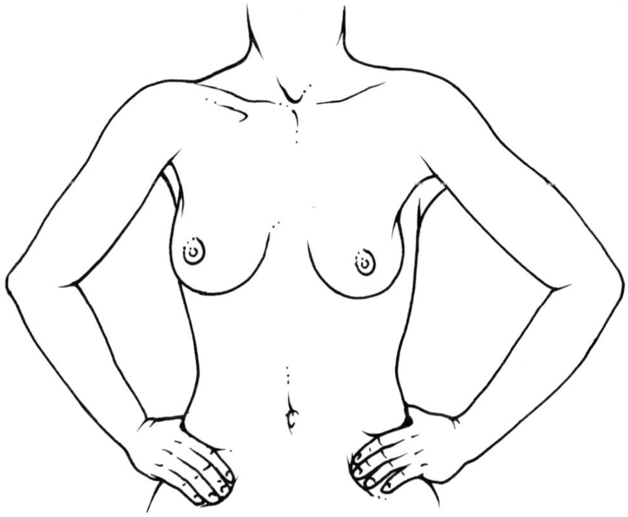

FIGURE 3-3. Contraction of the pectoralis major muscles to reveal or accentuate any skin retraction.

The axilla is examined with the patient's right arm flexed at the elbow and held there by the physician's right hand, a position that allows relaxation of the chest wall musculature (Fig. 3-5). Palpation with the left hand permits assessment of the lower axilla, and with extension higher toward the clavicle, the mid and upper portions of the axilla may be assessed. The left axilla is examined with the

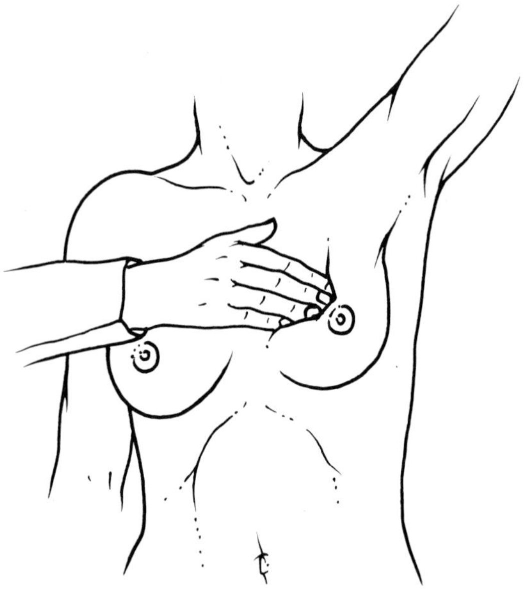

FIGURE 3-4. Initial breast palpation with the patient in an upright position.

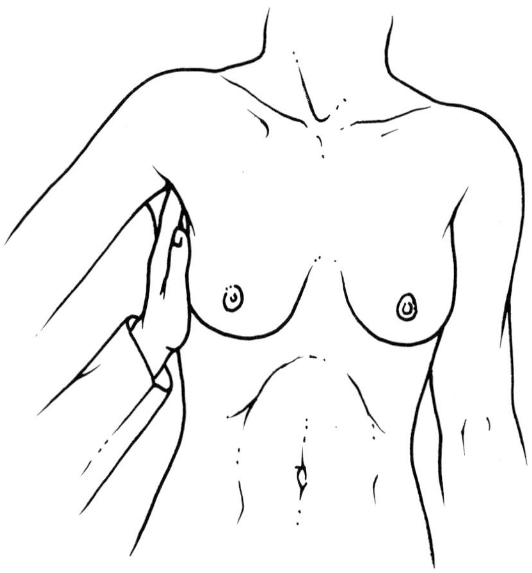

FIGURE 3-5. Examination of the axilla.

right hand, after relaxation of the patient's left arm in the physician's left hand. In heavy or muscular patients, accessibility to the upper levels of the axilla is restricted, but this position allows the most accurate examination. If lymph nodes are palpable, the clinician must assess their level and size, as well as whether they are single or multiple (or matted together), mobile or fixed to underlying structures, soft or firm. Most importantly, the physician must determine whether they are clinically involved or uninvolved (nonsuspicious). Nodes that are considered suspicious for metastases are large in diameter (≥1 cm), firm, irregular, possibly fixed to the underlying chest wall, and multiple or matted together. Many women, especially those subject to low-grade inflammatory processes of the hands or arms (from paper cuts, hangnails, minor abrasions or burns, for example), will have small, soft, mobile, and palpable axillary lymph nodes secondary to lymphadenitis. These nodes are generally less than 1 cm in diameter, and are recorded as being palpable but clinically uninvolved. This latter assessment is recorded in most staging systems. Palpation of the axilla with the patient in the prone position is inaccurate. The proper maneuvers for breast examination have been outlined by Haagensen, who also demonstrated the possible advantage of having patients bend forward in order to exaggerate retraction of subareolar lesions.[8]

Close inspection of the skin and nipple of the breast may reveal abnormalities suggesting an underlying malignant process. Edema of the skin of the breast (appropriately named *peau d'orange*) is occasionally subtle, but is more often rather extensive (Fig. 3-6). This condition is frequently more prominent in the lower half of the breast than in any other region, and is more noticeable when the patient's arms are raised. Although this edema is often attributable to lymphatic obstruction from a deep-seated carcinoma in the breast, it may also be caused by extensive axillary lymph node involvement with metastatic (or occasionally, benign) disease. Thus, it may be present in the breasts of patients who have undergone axillary lymph node dissection for another disease, such as malignant melanoma.

The technique for retraction of the skin and nipple, which may be accentuated by contraction of the pectoralis

FIGURE 3-6. Edema (peau d'orange) of periareolar skin of the breast. A recent incisional biopsy site is noted in the lower outer quadrant.

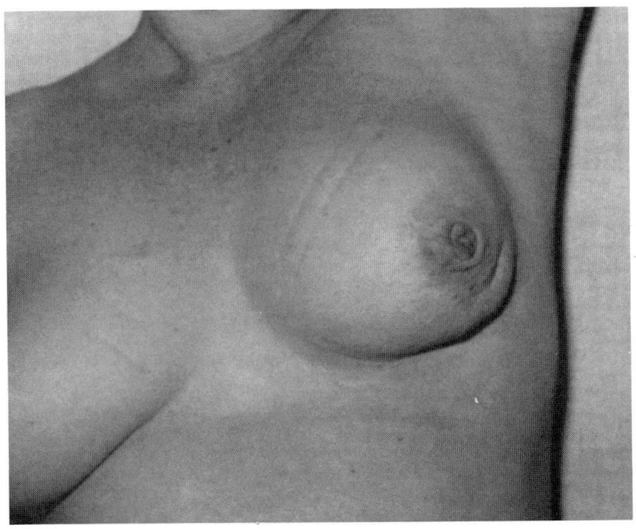

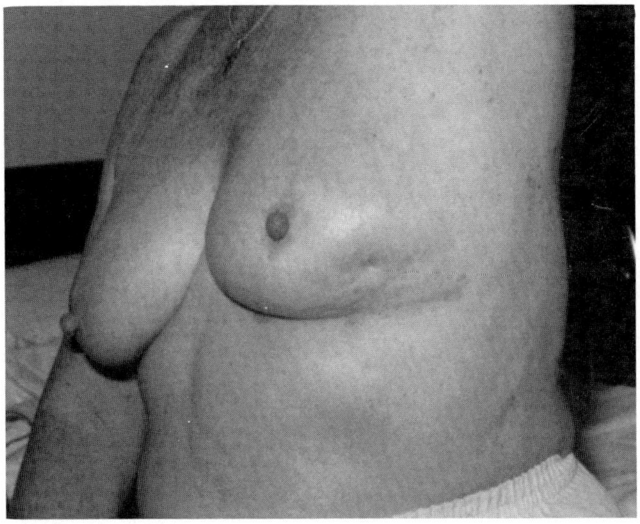

FIGURE 3-7. Skin retraction of the lateral aspect of the breast with the arm raised.

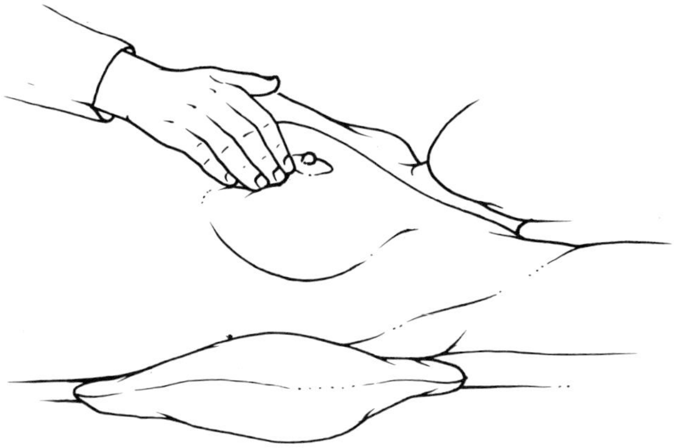

FIGURE 3-8. The breast examination with the patient lying supine with ipsilateral shoulder elevated by a folded sheet or a small pillow.

major muscle, is shown in Figure 3-7. Although some benign conditions, such as fat necrosis, may cause this retraction, a high index of suspicion of an underlying carcinoma should be raised.

Erythema of the skin of the breast is an ominous sign. Although it may be caused by an inflammation, such as periductal mastitis or even abscess formation, inflammatory carcinoma should be considered a possibility. As discussed in Chapter 15, this very aggressive form of breast cancer presents with reddened skin, which is usually warm, and with a raised erysipeloid edge. Color Plate 1 shows a patient who recently underwent biopsy of the left breast accomplished through a circumareolar incision that included overlying skin, to check for subdermal lymphatic invasion of carcinoma.

Inspection of the nipple for either retraction or ulceration is important. The latter, which may begin as a minimal process involving a portion of the nipple, raises the suspicion of Paget's disease. This early form of breast carcinoma, which originates in and extends along the major ducts, and which expresses itself as a nipple abnormality, is discussed in detail in Chapter 15. In a more advanced state, the entire nipple may become ulcerated or involved with an exophytic tumor mass, as shown in Color Plate 2.

Examination with the Patient Lying Supine

The patient is subsequently asked to assume a supine position. The breast is best examined when it is positioned on top of and splayed out over the chest wall. This position is best accomplished with a small pillow (or folded sheet) placed beneath the ipsilateral shoulder to elevate the breast, and with the ipsilateral arm raised above the patient's head (Fig. 3-8). Breast examination is most accurate when the least possible amount of breast tissue is present between the skin and chest wall; it is least accurate when the converse is true. (An example of the latter is when patients who report breast lumps have examined their breasts with the ipsilateral hand, thus violating the two important principles described above.) The examiner must assess the entire breast, with the examination extending from the sternum to the midaxillary line, and superiorly from the clavicle to the lower rib cage. Usually, examination with the hand as a unit, exerting gentle pressure using the pulps of the fingers rather than the fingertips, will most accurately assess the breast parenchyma.

This is the most important part of the examination, and small lesions must be sought. Carcinomas of less than 1 cm in diameter are palpable in some women; in others, very large lesions may be hidden. The examiner must assess the background consistency of the breasts; in premenopausal patients who are examined premenstrually, clumps of engorged glandular tissue may seem impossible to assess. A repeat examination 1 to 2 weeks after a menstrual period may reveal a marked improvement, with decreased glandular elements. Postmenopausal patients have a higher ratio of fat to glandular elements, making palpation (and mammographic examination) more accurate. No cyclic changes occur in these patients, so indiscrete thickenings may be more significant in them than they are in premenopausal patients.

The examiner is searching for three-dimensional masses or significant thickenings. On palpation, firm masses or areas that are three-dimensional (measurable), irregular, and fixed to the skin or underlying fascia are characteristic of carcinoma. Benign lesions tend to be softer, smoother with more regular borders, and not fixed. Fibroadenoma, the most common benign disease of the breast occurring in younger women, is the easiest condition to appreciate. These lesions are clearly demarcated, and feel like marbles despite the dense, glandular, parenchymal tissue present in these young women. Gross cysts are soft and circumscribed, and the fluid may be ballottable occasionally. Sclerosing adenoses tend to be firm, small (<1 cm in diameter), peripherally-located nodules that frequently appear close to the skin. Other benign lesions have been described in Chapter 2.

The clinician must assess each patient individually, assigning each to one of three categories, based on the results of the examination: suspicious, questionable, or nonsuspicious. Of course, mammography (and other tests, such as sonography) may be helpful in making this decision.

Examination in Selected Patients

Two major differences between premenopausal/perimenopausal and postmenopausal patients make examination in the latter group easier. The increased ratio of glandular to fat elements, together with the fibrocystic (and cyclic hormonal) changes in breast tissue in the younger patients contributes to an increased "lumpiness" or decreased homogeneity on palpation in this age group.

PREMENOPAUSAL/PERIMENOPAUSAL PATIENTS. The following is the recommended sequence of appraisal in a premenopausal or perimenopausal patient with a suspicious, but not obviously malignant, mass. As has been described in Chapter 2, aspiration of the dominant lesion (usually with a 20-gauge needle, small syringe, and no local anesthesia) will establish whether the lesion is cystic or solid. Typical cysts yield nonbloody fluid that is frequently clear, yellow, greenish, or brown, and that may occasionally be turbid. Complete disappearance of the mass should occur following aspiration. Biopsy would be indicated if the mass did not completely disappear, or if the fluid were bloody. Adjacent carcinomas, or intracystic carcinomas, have been found in such instances. Although we have not found cytologic analysis of typical cystic fluid (after complete disappearance of the mass) to be helpful, it is indicated if the fluid is bloody or if the mass is not a cyst. A cytologic report of breast cancer facilitates subsequent discussions with patients regarding their treatment options, although preliminary excision is advisable for accurate histologic classification, estrogen receptor protein (ERP) determination, and assessment of margins. A diagnosis of malignant disease established by cytologic examination serves a two-stage purpose in many respects, allowing both a preliminary diagnosis and a discussion of treatment options with patients prior to definitive therapy. For patients in whom complete disappearance of a mass occurs following aspiration of nonbloody fluid, mammography is advised. If mammographic results are negative, a repeat examination (1 to 2 weeks postmenstruation) within 2 to 3 months is advised. If the same cyst recurs after a second aspiration, excision to rule out intracystic papillary carcinoma is advised. However, if no further cysts recur, follow-up at close intervals (every 4 to 6 months) is recommended. This approach to patient management is represented in Figures 3-9 and 3-10.

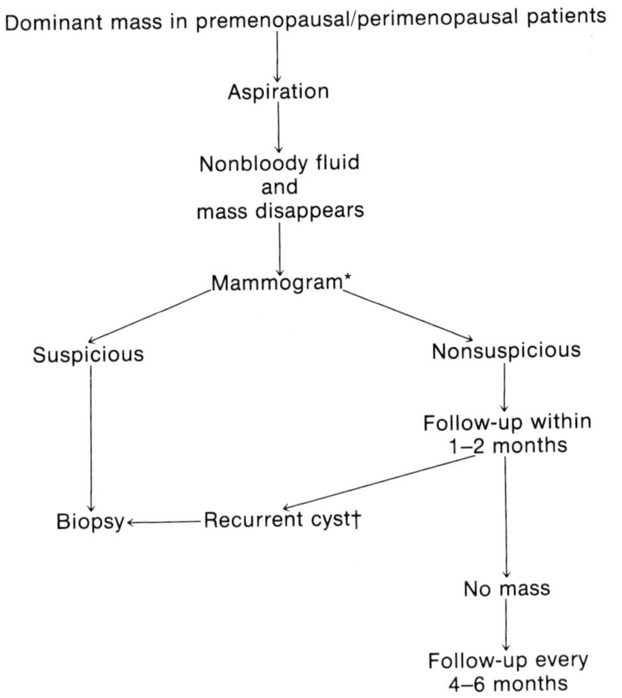

* Mammography is recommended for appropriate age groups if it has not been done recently.

† Excisional biopsy is indicated if the same cyst recurs after two aspirations.

FIGURE 3-9. Flow diagram indicating management of premenopausal patients whose dominant masses disappear with aspiration of nonbloody fluid.

Some patients may belong in a third category: those patients in whom a few drops of cystic fluid are removed with aspiration and mammography is nonsuspicious, but thickening remains. Although these patients usually have benign disease, a biopsy is generally advised.

It should be emphasized that the vast majority of patients with this presentation will never require biopsy. However, clinicians, with the help of mammographic studies, must be satisfied that no area of suspicion is overlooked in the evaluation of their patients.

POSTMENOPAUSAL PATIENTS. Postmenopausal patients are usually easier to evaluate owing to a decrease in the ratio of glandular tissue to fat in the breast and a decline in fibrocystic and cyclic activity in glandular tissue. However, microscopic evidence of fibrocystic disease persists in postmenopausal patients, and hormonal replacement may induce a degree of otherwise unexpected nodularity. Aspiration in this group is not undertaken to rule out cysts (or to obviate the need for biopsy by withdrawal of cystic fluid with disappearance of the mass), but is utilized solely for aspiration cytology. Patients in whom dominant masses or significant, asymmetrical thickenings are found should undergo biopsy, following mammography, for the purpose of assessing other areas. Short-term

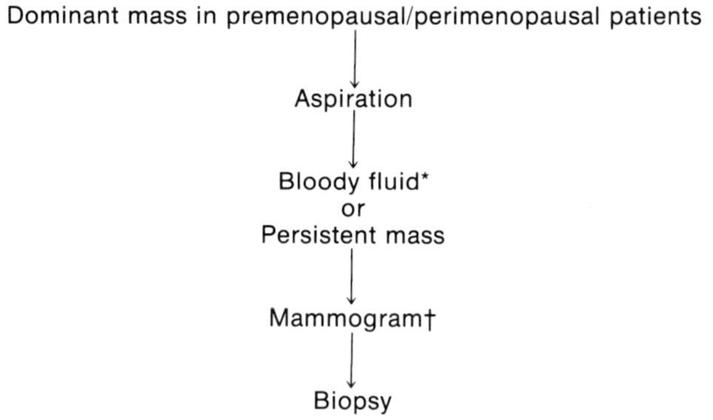

* Cytologic studies may be useful, but a benign diagnosis does not eliminate the need for biopsy.

† A biopsy will be done in any event; other areas of suspicion, as suggested by mammography, are also targeted for biopsy.

FIGURE 3-10. Management of premenopausal patients whose dominant masses do not disappear after aspiration.

follow-up, owing to the lack of hormonal cycles, is unnecessary in postmenopausal patients. Evaluation of nondominant nodularity, referred to as postmenopausal thickening, is more difficult. As outlined in Figure 3-11, mammography is of greater importance in the early assessment of such areas than is cytologic analysis, which is not relied upon as often owing to the sampling difficulties inherent in such indiscrete, often diffuse lesions. Figure 3-12 indicates the appropriate sequence for management of postmenopausal patients with discrete masses.

POSTMASTECTOMY PATIENTS. Examination of the chest wall, axilla, supraclavicular area, and ipsilateral arm is important in postmastectomy patients. A locally recurrent mass usually presents as a nodule in the epidermis or dermis, or less often, in the muscle. Although these nodules are frequently small and are often attributable to scar tissue or suture granuloma, biopsy is indicated to ensure that they do not represent carcinoma. Examination of the parasternal area may reveal a subtle prominence or bulging suggestive of internal mammary lymph node metastases. Such changes are often difficult to detect, and routine radiographic studies of the chest, rib, or sternum are often not helpful, although they should be done initially in an attempt to demonstrate any mediastinal or bony involvement. When these studies are normal, further investigation with a computed tomography (CT) scan or lymphoscintigraphy of the internal mammary lymph node, or both, may help to establish the diagnosis. Frequently, incisional biopsy of an interspace is required for accurate diagnosis.

Certain types of extensive skin involvement in advanced breast cancer or recurrent masses postmastectomy are termed *en cuirasse* carcinomas. As originally described by Velpeau, this type of carcinoma occurs in patients with advanced breast cancer and is characterized by involvement of the skin and subcutaneous tissues of the upper trunk. Fortunately, it is rarely seen today. This type of recurrence may arise after mastectomy for advanced disease, and the process extends across the chest wall and to the supraclavicular areas, where a recent incisional biopsy has been done. This type of recurrence, which is refractory to most types of treatment, will be discussed further in Chapter 14. (See Color Plate 6).

Inspection of the ipsilateral arm in postmastectomy patients with lymphedema will, on rare occasions, reveal the presence of reddish-purple nodules, as illustrated in Color Plate 3. A recent biopsy scar is evident in this photograph. Biopsy confirmed the presence of lymphangiosarcoma (Stewart-Treves syndrome), a high-grade, aggressive sarcoma that may present as a few nodules or that may coalesce, spreading to involve the entire extremity. A further description and discussion of the management of lymphangiosarcoma appears in Chapter 15.

BREAST SELF-EXAMINATION

The benefits of this examination for patients, or the lack thereof, will be discussed in Chapter 5. Most clinicians dealing with patients having breast disease encourage this practice, realizing it is carried out with difficulty, and is sometimes infrequently performed in many patients. Most would question how it could not benefit their patients. However, scientific evidence that breast cancers are detected earlier by patients as a result of this examination is lacking. Assertions of potential harm, especially in younger patients (owing to increased anxiety and to the performance of increased numbers of benign biopsies), are difficult to envision. Considering that breast disease is so common in Western societies, we would be remiss in not informing patients of these risks and of their role in early detection.

Thorough descriptions of breast self-examination (BSE) have been published in medical textbooks,[1] and handouts, published by several concerned organizations, including the National Institutes of Health,[9] are available for patients. Physicians dealing with female patients in age groups that are at risk for breast cancer (as well as women 25 to 30 years of age) should instruct them in BSE techniques and should provide pamphlets describing these techniques. Premenopausal patients are advised to do this examination monthly, 1 to 2 weeks after their menstrual period. They should be warned that premenstrual examination is inaccurate and may reveal many "lumps" that will subside after the period. As patients become comfortable with BSE, examination throughout the monthly cycle is most instructive. Many patients with multiple areas of dense, glandular breast tissue are able to report accurately on improvement in these areas, or on the development of new nodules that should concern them and their examining physician. Clinicians are soon able to identify those patients in their practice who carry out BSE regularly and those who do not, as well as those in the former group who are inaccurate and those who are reliable examiners. The reports of patients who prove to be

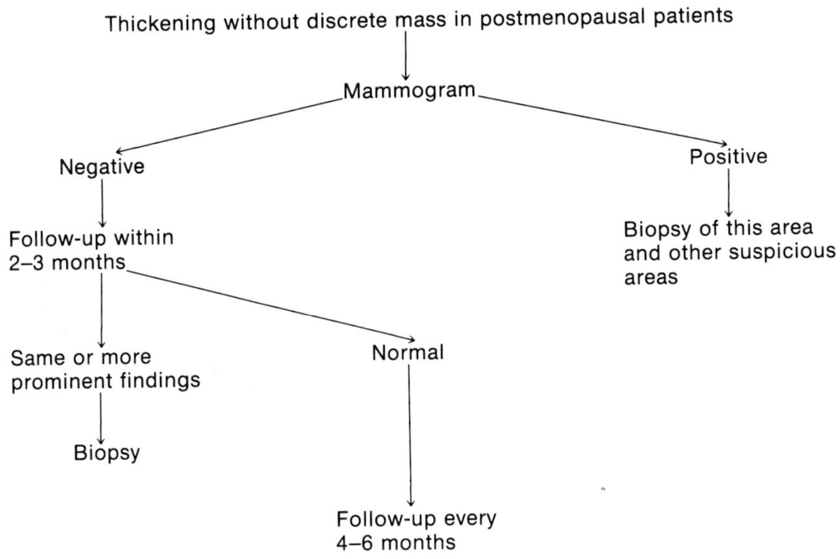

FIGURE 3-11. Management of postmenopausal patients with indiscrete nodularity (thickening).

* Aspiration cytology may be done at these times; a benign diagnosis with persistence of thickening or mammographic abnormalities, or both, does not eliminate the need for biopsy.

reliable examiners, especially, should be carefully heeded, particularly when a change for the worse has been noted.

Physicians must recognize that many patients are anxious about this examination. The dense areas of glandular tissue that are so commonly present may be frightening to many patients. If reassurance and instruction in BSE are not successful, a subgroup who cannot or will not perform this procedure regularly is created. Apart from questions about the efficacy of BSE in early detection of breast cancer, most reports document that BSE is practiced regularly by a minority of women,[10–12] and that the quality of the examination is inadequate in most.[13–15] These problems are difficult to assess, and are, perhaps, rooted in the fear of discovery of breast cancer, the treatment entailed, and the uncertainty of the outcome.

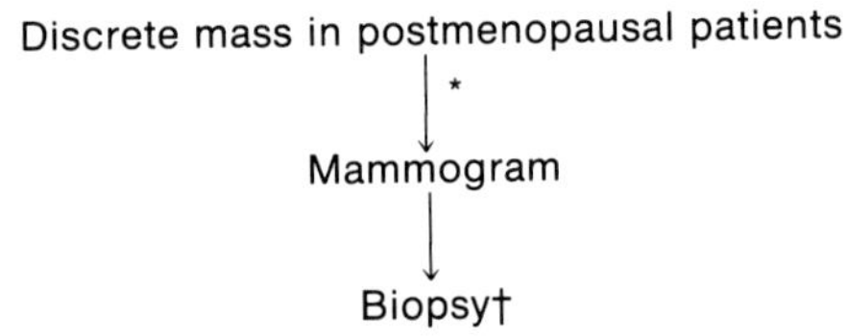

* Aspiration cytology may be done at this time; however, a benign diagnosis does not eliminate the need for biopsy.

† A biopsy of the mass and any other areas that appear suspicious on mammography is performed.

FIGURE 3-12. Management of postmenopausal patients with dominant masses

MAMMOGRAPHY

The first x-ray studies of the breast were performed on mastectomy specimens by Salomon in 1913. The technique became clinically relevant following the work of Gros and similar advances made by Gershon-Cohen.[16] Leborgne helped to advance the morphologic principles, many of which remain relevant today.[17] Egan developed techniques to standardize the study and helped make mammography a clinically significant technique.[18] The first significant screening study was undertaken in the 1960s by the Health Insurance Plan of New York (HIP)[19] This was followed by a large-scale project in the 1970s, undertaken by the American Cancer Society and the National Cancer Institute, that involved the screening of more than 275,000 women by physical examination and mammography in 27 centers across the nation. This Breast Cancer Detection Demonstration Project (BCDDP) paralleled the increased use of xeromammography, which permitted x-ray imaging of the breast with lower doses than plain film and improved image quality.[20] Mammography came under fire following concerns raised by Bailar in 1976 that the doses used in the 1960s might pose a risk of x-ray carcinogenesis that might offset any gains derived from screening.[21] This assessment halted much of the routine mammography and was a setback for screening in this country. It did serve to stimulate the development of improved equipment to permit low-dose studies and led to more detailed assessment of mammographic risk.[22] Modern mammographic equipment using high-resolution film/screen combinations delivers less than 0.3 cGy to the midplane of the breast for a two-view study.[23] Based on studies of women exposed to high doses from other sources in the past, this dose carries

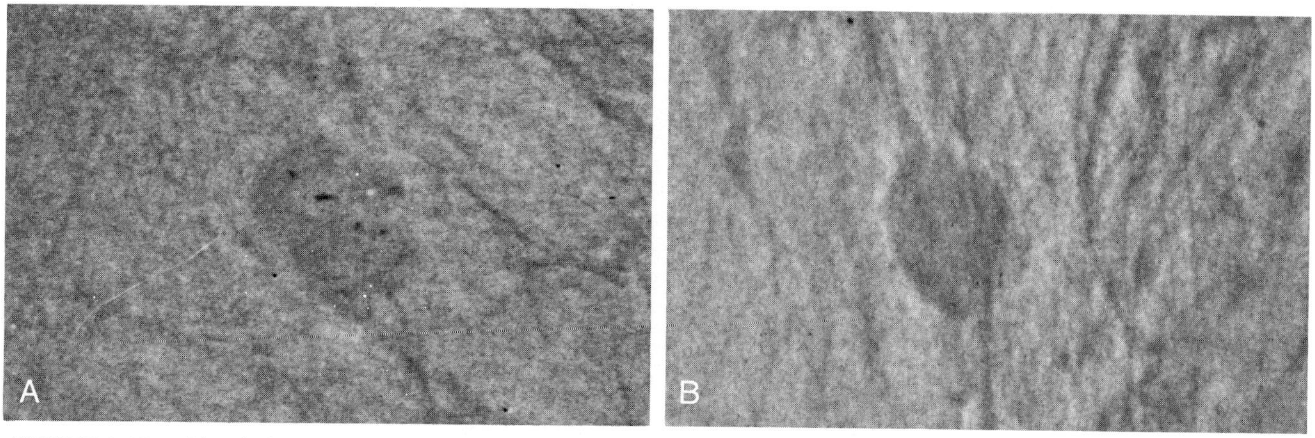

FIGURE 3-13. *(A)* Lobulated mass with associated microcalcifications proven at biopsy to be a benign fibroadenoma. *(B)* Similar lobulated mass proven at biopsy to be an infiltrating ductal carcinoma.

a theoretical risk of one cancer per one million women studied.[24] Not only is this effect too small to prove or disprove (since approximately 800 cancers occur naturally in a population this size each year), but it is a lower risk than is associated with many normal daily activities, such as driving a car.

Although breast cancer spreads both hematogenously and by the lymphatics, prognosis is directly related to the size of the lesion[25] and to axillary involvement at the time of diagnosis. Data from the BCDDP demonstrated that mammographic scanning can help reduce the number of women with positive nodes by 50%.[26] Evidence for the efficacy of screening for breast cancer comes from the two available randomized controlled studies: the HIP study in the 1960s[27] and the ongoing Swedish study reported in 1985.[28] These two studies demonstrated a reduction in mortality from breast cancer in the screened population. The efficacy of screening will be discussed in greater detail in Chapter 5.

It has been clearly established that x-ray mammography has the ability to detect clinically occult, nonpalpable breast cancers that are frequently at an earlier stage than larger, palpable lesions. Nevertheless, it must be repeatedly emphasized that mammography does not demonstrate all breast cancers, and that the findings on physical examination and mammography are complementary. The information derived from one should rarely negate concerns raised by the other. A negative mammogram does not preclude the possibility of palpable breast cancer and should never result in delaying the biopsy of a clinically suspicious mass. Similarly, a negative physical examination should not delay the biopsy of a suspicious lesion detected on mammography.

The distinction between detection and diagnosis must be clearly understood. The goal of screening asymptomatic women is to detect occult lesions at an earlier stage than that at which they might otherwise be detected. A fairly high false-positive rate may be tolerated as long as there is a low false-negative rate. Positive predictive value may be low as long as sensitivity is high. This holds true for x-ray mammography. Small lesions may be detected, but there is a significant overlap in the appearance of benign and malignant processes in the breast (Figs. 3-13 and 3-14). This factor increases the importance of accurate preoperative localization of such lesions for surgical excision to avoid the loss of an unnecessarily large amount of breast tissue. Since the positive predictive value of a palpable mass that is examined by biopsy is between 20% and 30%,[29] it is reasonable for the same parameters to be accepted for an imaging technique used as a screening test if a significant number of cancers may be detected at an earlier stage. Mammography fulfills this expectation.[30] An even lower predictive value might be reasonable if a significant number of cancers could be discovered at an even earlier stage.

The term *diagnosis,* within the context of breast disease, is frequently loosely employed. Diagnosis is the characterization of a lesion whose presence has already been detected, as a result of either palpation or mammography. Mammography is sensitive and can detect many early cancers, but frequently, it cannot be relied upon to distinguish these lesions from other benign lesions that it reveals. The radiographic characteristics of benign lesions often overlap with those of malignant processes. Nevertheless, mammography may be diagnostic in lesions that have spiculated, ill-defined margins (Fig. 3-15). This particular characteristic is rarely seen with benign processes, although uncommon lesions, such as indurative mastopathy, granular cell myoblastoma, extra-abdominal desmoids, and fat necrosis, may mimic this classic malignant change. For all practical purposes, a lesion with spiculated, ill-defined margins can be said, with a 99% degree of certainty, to indicate breast cancer. With the exception of calcified fibroadenomas (Fig. 3-16) and radiolucent lesions, such as lipomas, galactoceles, fat necrosis (Fig. 3-17) and the typical intramammary lymph node, (Fig. 3-18)

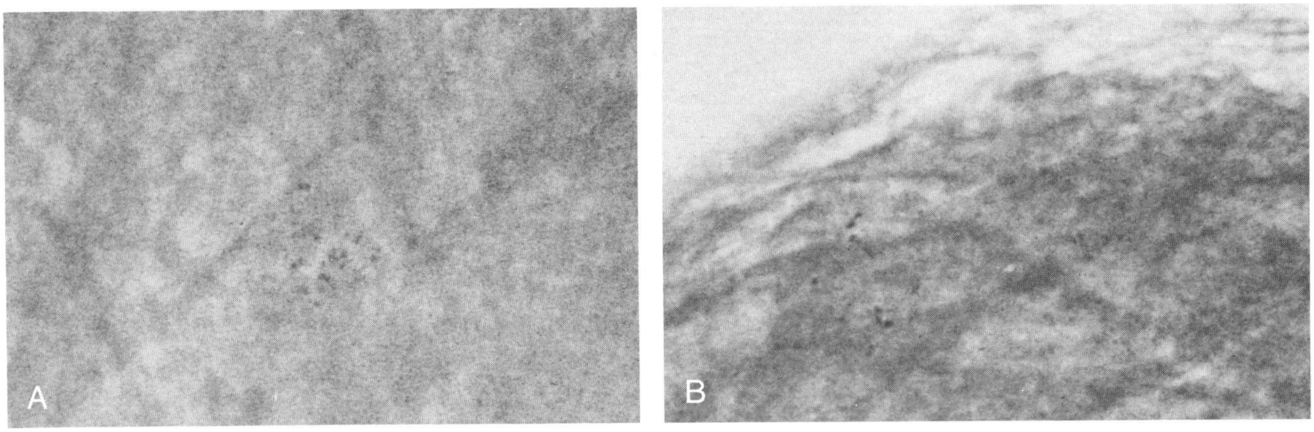

FIGURE 3-14. *(A)* Clustered microcalcifications proven at biopsy to be benign adenosis. *(B)* Similar clustered microcalcifications proven at biopsy to be intraductal carcinoma.

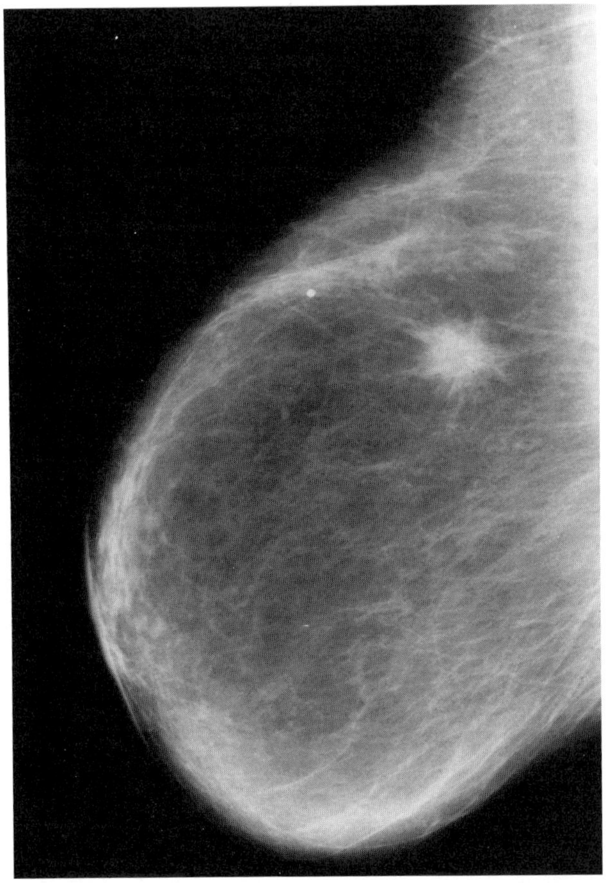

FIGURE 3-15. Typical spiculated appearance of infiltrating ductal carcinoma. This is a diagnostic appearance by mammography.

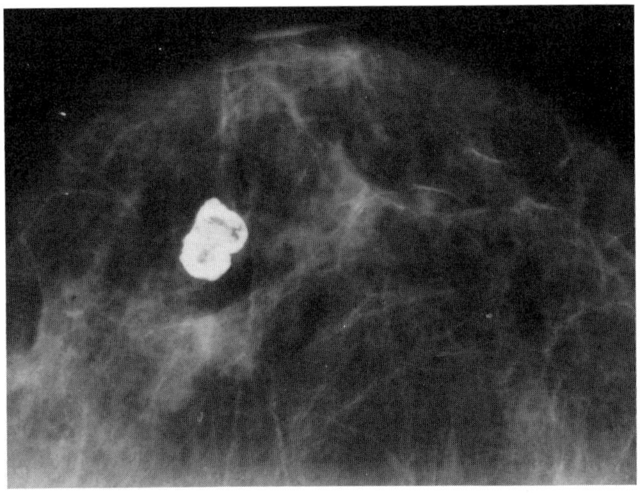

FIGURE 3-16. The pathognomonic appearance of a calcified, involuting fibroadenoma.

mammography cannot, in most instances, be used to determine that a lesion is benign, at least not with sufficient certainty to obviate the need for a biopsy.

Although mammography is not a truly diagnostic procedure and cannot rule out the presence of an intramammary malignant process, it is, nevertheless, an important study to perform in symptomatic patients. This is true despite the fact that a biopsy will be performed regardless of the mammographic findings. Mammography should be considered to be a screening technique in all women, and should be used in the preoperative setting to confirm the presence of a malignant process so that it is not missed at surgery,[31] to detect occult, multicentric, malignant disease by screening the ipsilateral breast (Fig. 3-19), and to detect occult contralateral malignant processes (Fig. 3-20).[32] Fur-

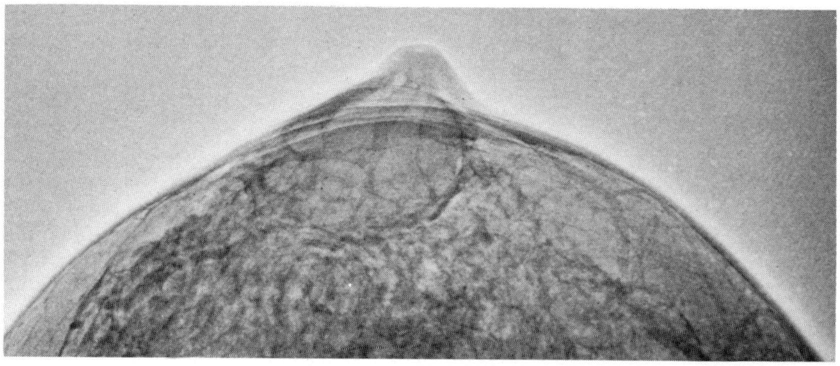

FIGURE 3-17. This subareolar, lucent lesion represents a galactocele containing a fluid of high fat content.

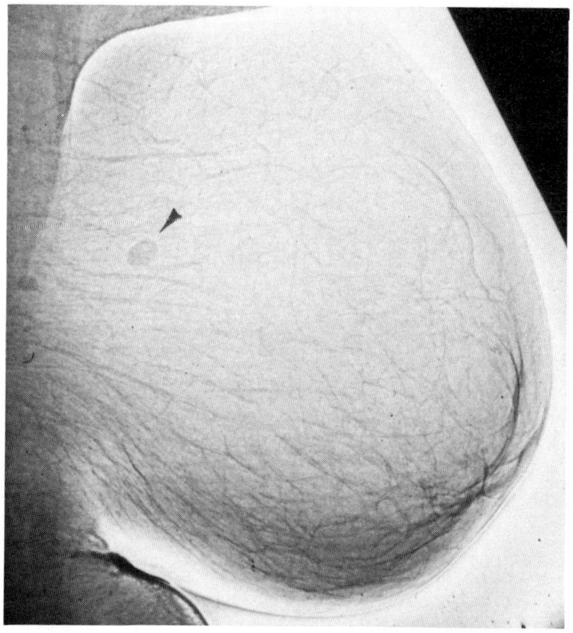

FIGURE 3-18. Typical benign, intramammary lymph node. Note the radiolucent notch that is present (*arrow*).

thermore, a lesion that is palpable may indeed prove to be benign, but an occult cancer elsewhere in either breast may be present. Thus, a woman who has a palpable mass can derive the same benefit from screening as an asymptomatic woman.

X-Ray Mammography

X-ray mammography is a two-dimensional projection of three-dimensional structures. It produces an image through the absorption and scattering characteristics of structures based on their water content or, in the case of calcifications, on the absorption characteristics of the metals involved. Two principal forms of x-ray mammography are currently available. The basic differences between xeromammography and film/screen techniques lie in their detector systems and in the kilovoltage of the radiation employed.

Xeromammography

Xeroradiography is an electrostatic detector system. It consists of an aluminum plate coated with selenium to produce a semi-conductor. Approximately 2000 volts of charge are distributed uniformly across the surface of the detector plate in a conditioner unit. The plate is inserted

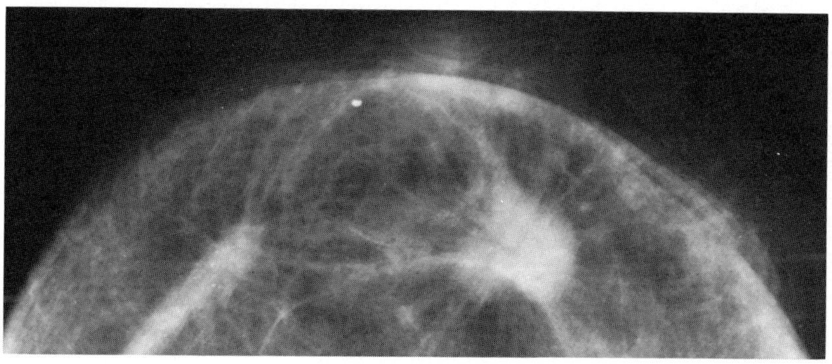

FIGURE 3-19. Mammography in a woman with a palpable mass in the medial subareolar region shows clustered microcalcifications and an ill-defined density. These findings indicate a second, nonpalpable cancerous lesion located laterally in the same breast.

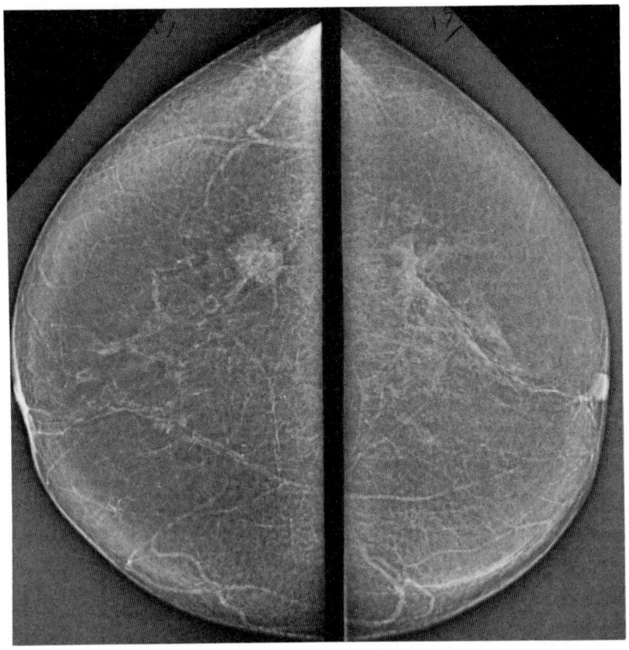

FIGURE 3-20. Palpable lobulated carcinoma in the left breast. A contralateral, nonpalpable, clinically occult cancer was found by mammography in the right breast.

automatically into a cassette that acts as an insulator to avoid discharge on the plate surface and to prevent exposure to light, which would also cause a shift of charges on the plate surface. The breast is placed on the cassette and then an exposure is made utilizing kilovoltages ranging from 35 kvp to 60 kvp. Beam filtration with up to 2 mm of aluminum filtration will significantly reduce the skin entrance dose and somewhat reduce the absorbed dose to the breast.[33] As in all x-ray techniques, the amount of radiation exiting the breast is relative to the absorption and scattering properties of the tissue through which the beam has passed. X-ray interactions in the Xerox plate cause a dissipation of charge on the plate surface that is proportionate to the amount of radiation reaching it, producing a latent charge on the plate surface.[34] The plate is then mechanically removed from the insulating cassette and travels through a processor. A powder is blown on to the surface of the plate and the particles of toner adhere to the plate in proportion to the charge distribution on its surface. The plate is then brought into contact with a plastic-coated paper and the powder image is transferred to the paper. The final step in the process melts the toner into the paper, and the Xerox image is completed. Xeroradiography has the advantage of carrying a lower dose than did the industrial plain film techniques used in the 1960s. There is an additional advantage in the wide exposure latitude of the technique, which permits a uniform image of an organ, such as the breast, whose thickness varies from front to back. The wide exposure latitude diminishes the broad area contrast, but this is compensated for by the property of edge enhancement inherent in the xeroradiographic technique. There is a buildup of charge at transition zones between two areas of differing density, producing an amplification of the edge by an increase of toner particles on one side of the edge and a relative diminution immediately adjacent to the edge. Xeroradiography has the high resolution necessary for imaging the fine structures of the breast and, in particular, for demonstrating the presence of an early malignant lesion.[35] Because of the wide exposure latitude, rigid compression of the breast is not required with xeroradiographic systems, and the chest wall may be imaged as part of the mammographic study. This permits the demonstration of lesions in close proximity to the chest wall. A common misconception is that imaging of the chest wall results in the entire breast being imaged. This assumption is incorrect because the image produced is only tangential to the chest wall, and breast tissue curves behind the ribs, both laterally and medially.

The xeroradiographic technique does produce some technical artifacts. In particular, the degradation of the selenium surface of the plate severely compromises the images. Furthermore, in areas of abrupt change in tissue contrast, the properties that permit edge enhancement can lead to a failure to deposit toner over fairly broad bands. This so-called "toner rob" results in areas that are not imaged satisfactorily, and may be a source of false-negative mammographic results. The problem of toner rob may be ameliorated by using the negative-mode option. This also serves to reduce the dose to the breast by approximately 30%. Xeromammography may be performed with a conventional tungsten anode x-ray tube as long as the lack of geometric sharpness can be reduced to a minimum with a small focal spot or a long source-to-image distance. The Xerox conditioner and processor are specialized equipment.

Film/Screen Mammography

Recent advances in x-ray film and intensifying screen technology have permitted a further reduction in the x-ray dose to the breast.[36] These developments permit the high resolution necessary for mammography, and dose is conserved by utilizing the amplification of the light output of the screen phosphors to expose the x-ray film. Film/screen mammography has the advantage of broad area contrast, which aids in the visualization of mass lesions in the breast. There are fewer technical failures with film/screen imaging, and the standard x-ray film processor may be utilized for film development. Because of the narrow exposure latitude of the film/screen combination, the breast must be firmly compressed between rigid plates in an effort to reduce the thickness variations from front to back. In order to obtain sufficient soft-tissue contrast, a low-kvp spectrum is required. Although this may be accomplished with specially designed tungsten anode systems with special filtration, a molybdenum target is preferred because the radiation produced as a result of the K edge of molybdenum produces a soft tissue differentiation of higher contrast. Compression of the breast is also important in diminishing the overall thickness of the breast and reducing the dose necessary for optimal imaging. Since the relationship of the breast and the thoracic wall is complex, areas of tissue may be difficult to image. To avoid the overlap of the breast with chest structures, and to permit the high level of detail required, the breast must be held away from the chest by rigid plates. This permits the projection of the breast onto the film surface. Resolution of structures as small as 200 μ is required, and a higher resolution is preferable. Rigid compression also reduces the lack of sharpness that results from motion and improves geometric sharpness by pushing the structures of the breast closer to the detector system. Although only a few studies are available, the data that have been collected suggest that there is no significant difference between film/screen and xeroradiography in the detection of breast cancer.[37,38] Based on these findings and the fact that film/screen imaging requires approximately one-third to one-fifth the dose of xeroradiography, film/screen imaging should be preferred for screening the breast, provided it is performed using a dedicated system with a scatter-reducing grid and phototiming to reduce the need for retaking of images. Xerox is helpful in the dense breast or the large breast where scatter becomes a significant problem, and in situations where the ability to angle the tube can aid in breast evaluation.

Normal Mammographic Anatomy

The anatomy of the breast, as seen on mammography, is complex owing to the overlapping nature of the three-dimensional organ projected in two dimensions. One reason for the inability of mammography to demonstrate some breast lesions[39] is the difficulty in projecting all of the mammary parenchyma onto the detector system.[40] This limitation has led to modifications in the standard lateral view. By rotating the tube compression system, the breast is compressed along a 45- to 60-degree axis extending from the axilla to the lower, inner quadrant of the breast. Because of the relationship of the breast to the pectoralis musculature, this oblique projection frequently permits a large volume of breast tissue to be imaged.[41]

Radiographic Anatomy

The skin is easily seen where the x-ray beam is tangential to the breast (Fig. 3-21A). It is virtually always separated from the mammary parenchyma by a layer of radiolucent, subcutaneous fat. The ductal elements converge on the nipple, and the parenchymal cone of the breast is usually delineated by the subcutaneous and retromammary fat. Curvilinear structures are seen coursing through the breast, comprising the planes of Cooper's ligaments (Fig. 3-21B). Although individual ducts are difficult to delineate on most routine two-dimensional mammograms, they frequently appear as serpiginous radiodensities coursing in and out of the plane of projection, producing a nodular appearance. Tortuous blood vessels may be seen. Although one breast may be larger than the other, mammary parenchyma is remarkably symmetrical in most women. Mammography should be performed with attention to producing symmetrically positioned and exposed images so that any variation in symmetry may be appreciated.

Although simplified systems have been devised to categorize the distribution of radiographic densities produced by the various fibrous, adipose, and ductal elements of the breast, there is a marked variation in the distribution and appearance of these structures. The determinants of the distribution of the various elements, as manifested by their shadows projected on the x-ray detector, likely represent a complex relationship between genetics, body habitus, parity, hormonal status, and age. Just as the term fibrocystic disease should probably be eliminated from the clinical evaluation of the breast, terms such as mammary dysplasia, should be eliminated from the radiographic description of the breast. It is unclear what actually constitutes a "normal" breast. Once again, the marked variation in the x-ray appearance of the breast structures in women who do not develop breast cancer makes it difficult to define normal. Furthermore, although horizontal studies suggest a different distribution of parenchymal patterns at a given age, there is little information from longitudinal follow-up of a cohort of women to demonstrate changes over time. Wolfe has published a limited longitudinal study, but his analysis may be affected by comparisons between film images in the 1960s and Xerox images in the early 1970s.[42]

Parenchymal Patterns

Attempts have been made to categorize the breast by evaluating the distribution of structures, as demonstrated by the projection of their shadows onto mammograms. The most generally accepted classification scheme was devised by Wolfe.[43] The mammographic appearance of the breast was grouped into four major categories. A breast that appeared to contain almost all fat with little radiographic density was considered to have an N-1 pattern. Unfortunately, Wolfe suggested that this was the "normal" pattern, implying that other appearances were abnormal. There are no data to prove this contention because most available information is based on the biased results of biopsies and mastectomies. Based on Wolfe's own data, fewer than 50% of women would be classified as "normal." Three other patterns were described. A P-1 pattern indicated mostly fat in the breast, with visible ducts occupying up to 25% of the breast volume. If more than 25% of the breast volume was occupied by visible ducts, the breast was classified as P-2. If the breast contained structures producing diffuse areas of radiographic density, it was considered to have a DY pattern. This, too, was an unfortunate choice of terms since Wolfe decided that this level of density meant mammary dysplasia. There is little justification for this except for a subsequent study of biopsy specimens read by Wellings which lends this classification

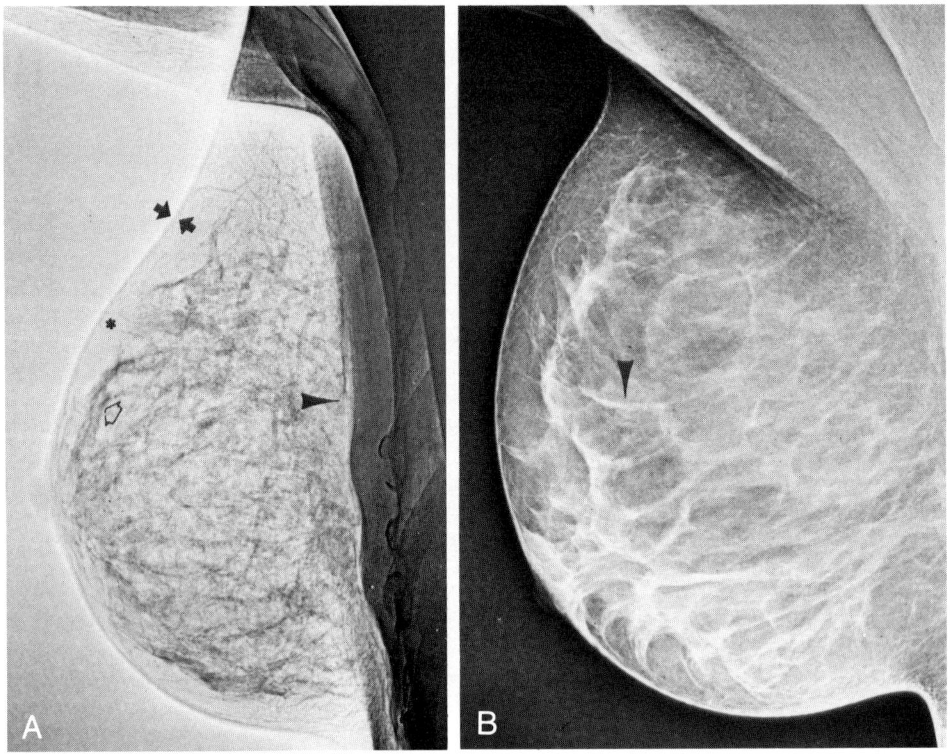

FIGURE 3-21. *(A)* Mediolateral view of a normal breast demonstrated by xerography. The skin (*opposing arrows*), subcutaneous fat (*asterisk*), ducts (*open arrow*), and pectoralis muscle (*single arrow*) are visible. *(B)* The curvilinear density (*arrow*) of Cooper's ligaments is demonstrated.

some support.[44] Wellings' study, however, attempted to explain the overall parenchymal pattern from biopsy tissue removed. This extrapolation is questionable since the tissue removed was, by definition, abnormal. Although the classification system permits gross comparison of breasts, the available data do not justify extrapolating mammographic patterns to predict histologic findings.

Nothing has prompted as many recent studies or as much controversy as the observations by Wolfe in 1976 that women with dense mammary parenchyma, demonstrated by mammography, had a risk of developing breast cancer that was 37 times greater than that of women with mostly fat in their breasts. If true, this would represent the strongest risk indicator yet discovered. Since publication of the original article, numerous studies have refuted Wolfe's original observations, and still others have defended it. Several studies have suggested that it is not the DY pattern, but rather the prominent duct pattern, that is the pattern of greatest risk. None of the supporting studies have suggested the marked increased risk first suggested by Wolfe, but researchers have agreed that some relationship between parenchymal patterns and risk of breast cancer may exist. In reviewing the conflicting studies on increased risk, Boyd and associates criticized the methodology of those contradicting an increased risk.[45] Nevertheless, the magnitude and significance of parenchymal patterns as risk factors remain in question. Compounding the difficulty in assessing parenchymal patterns is the fact that very little data exist to establish what normal parenchymal patterns are. The observations suggesting an increased risk in women with certain radiographic parenchymal patterns warrant further evaluation, but the practical significance of such a risk is uncertain. It is clear that breast cancer may occur in significant numbers of women with any of the parenchymal patterns. Thus, all women are at risk for developing breast cancer, regardless of the parenchymal pattern of their breasts. Given the degree of uncertainty concerning parenchymal patterns, there is certainly insufficient support for extreme actions based on these patterns. Prophylactic mastectomy based on pattern assessment is not warranted, and since there is, as yet, no way of predicting who will develop breast cancer and certainly no way of guaranteeing that a woman is at no risk for developing cancer, parenchymal patterns cannot be used to exclude women from screening programs.

Mammographic Positioning

By convention, a marker should be placed along the cephalic aspect of the breast in the lateral views and along the lateral side of the breast in craniocaudal views (see Fig. 3-10). Although there are those who advocate a single view of each breast for mammographic screening to reduce the cost, time, and radiation exposure, 4% to 6% of

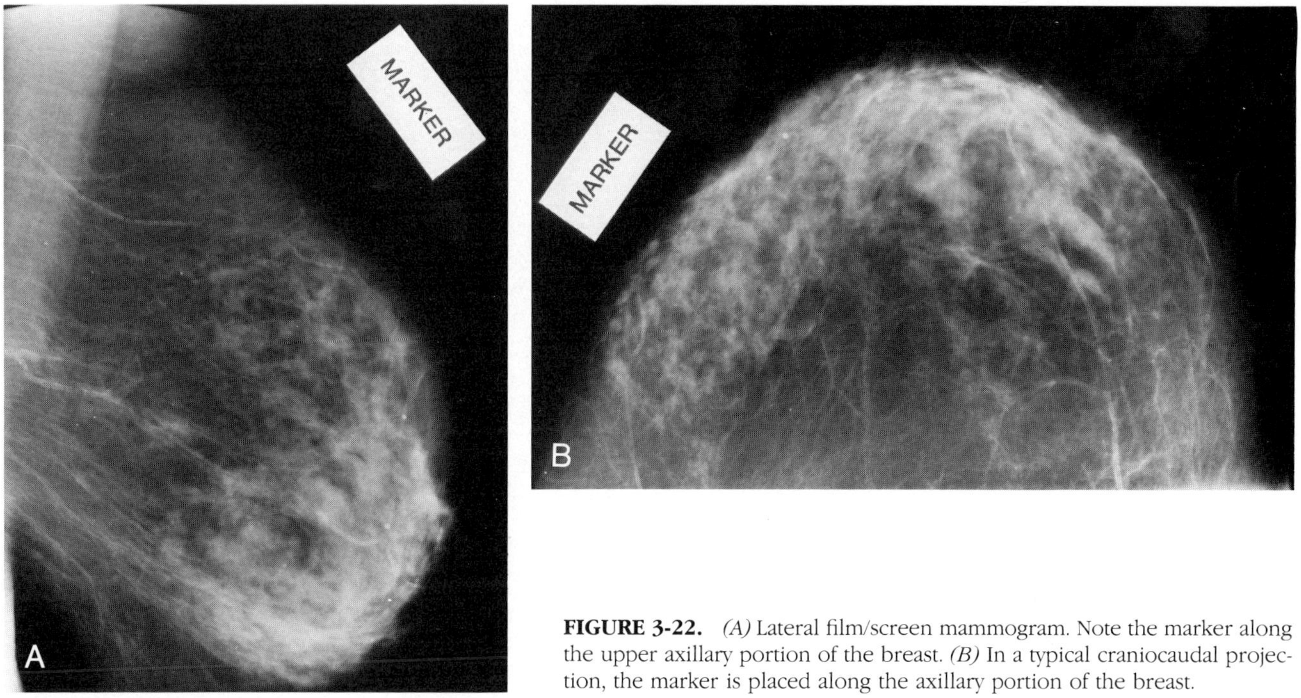

FIGURE 3-22. *(A)* Lateral film/screen mammogram. Note the marker along the upper axillary portion of the breast. *(B)* In a typical craniocaudal projection, the marker is placed along the axillary portion of the breast.

cancers may be missed by a single-view study.[46] At least two views of both breasts are recommended, regardless of the indication for the study. These should be obtained at approximately right angles to one another to permit an understanding, based on two-dimensional images, of the three-dimensional relationship of one structure to another. Because a majority of cancers occur in the lateral half of the breast and positioning is facilitated, a lateromedial side view of the breast is the most common projection. In this projection, the beam enters the breast from the medial side, exposing the film positioned along the lateral surface of the breast (Fig. 3-22A). In an effort to project as much breast tissue as possible onto the detector using dedicated, rigid-compression, mammographic systems, advantage is taken of the muscular anatomy of the chest wall underlying the breast. A rotated compression, or so-called oblique view, compresses the breast along the 45- to 60-degree axis extending from the axilla to the lower inner quadrant. Frequently, it is easier to project more tissue into the field of view of the system when the oblique projection is used than when a straight lateral view is used.

The second view that is usually obtained is the craniocaudal view (Fig. 22B), in which the breast is positioned with the nipple perpendicular to the edge of the recording system. The beam enters from the top of the breast and exits to the detector beneath the breast. In the standard views, the breasts should always be positioned symmetrically. Since the nipple is the only reference point for this heterogeneous organ, and since it may be confused with a mass if its shadow projects over the breast tissue, it should be imaged tangentially to the beam.

Additional views are obtained to best evaluate a palpable abnormality or an abnormality detected on mammography. Physical examination is valuable in tailoring the additional views to ensure that the area in question is optimally imaged[47] and to aid in the decision to employ ultrasonography (see the section on ultrasonography, below) for further evaluation. Exaggerated views are used to place the detector beneath the area in question (Fig. 3-23). This is frequently done in the outer half of the breast, but exaggerating medially is also common. In order to improve the sharpness of the image of some lesions, particularly those that are located in the medial portion of the breast, the detector should be positioned as close to the lesion as possible. For a lateral contact view of an inner-quadrant lesion, the detector is placed against the medial aspect of the breast, with the beam entering from the lateral surface (lateromedial positioning). In order to differentiate overlapping structures from true masses, it is useful to rotate the breast and recompress. This practice separates the projection of structures on opposite sides of the breast which, on the initial views, may have been superimposed, suggesting a lesion. There is no limit to the creativity of novel positioning if a significant problem must be resolved. For example, tangential views of the skin may be used to establish the benign nature of calci-

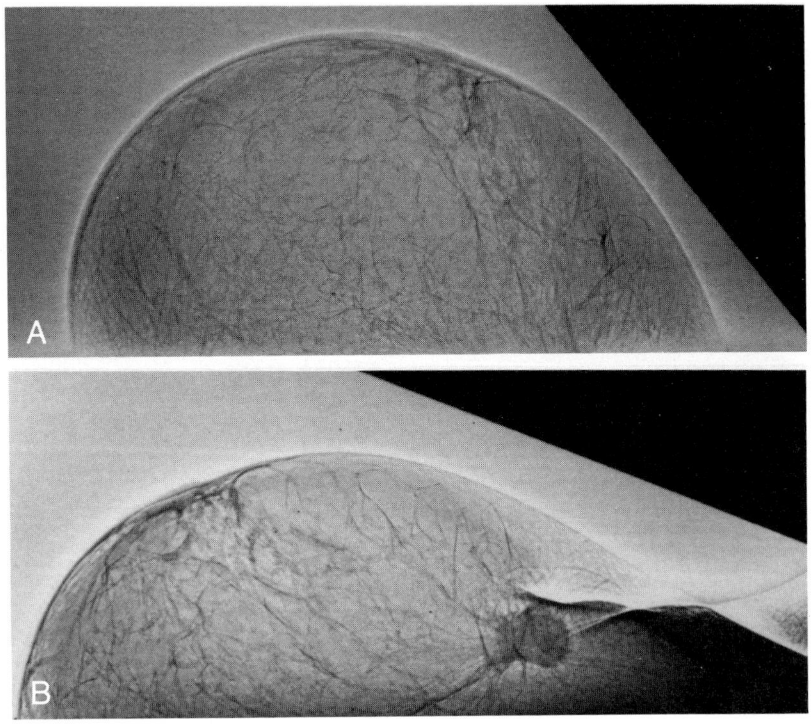

FIGURE 3-23. *(A)* Carcinoma in the lateral left breast is not visible in the standard craniocaudal view. *(B)* Carcinoma is, however, apparent in the exaggerated view toward the axilla.

fications that may appear to be in the breast on initial imaging (see the section on preoperative localization, below).

When visualization of the chest wall is desired, it can only be achieved satisfactorily using xerographic systems. The xerographic plate is placed beneath the ribs. This requires separation of the breast from the detector and results in a decrease in geometric sharpness. If the mammographic system is appropriately designed and has a suitably small focal spot, moving a structure away from the film may be an advantage when obtaining a magnification view. Sickles has repeatedly shown the advantage of magnification to improve the resolution of a system.[48] However, magnification leads to an increased dose and should be reserved for specific purposes, such as confirmation of the presence of microcalcifications; further delineation of benign calcifications, such as vascular deposits; and differentiation between calcifications that are true clusters and those that indicate developing, large, benign calcifications.

The Mammographic Appearance of Breast Cancer

Mammography is an excellent technique for finding lesions in the breast. Its sensitivity has been documented repeatedly. Less widespread is the understanding that mammography is a fairly nonspecific test. Although mammography may detect cancers before they become palpable, it is frequently unable to differentiate such lesions from benign breast changes with similar appearances. Breast cancer may have various manifestations which may be divided into primary and secondary characteristics. A lesion demonstrating primary characteristics has an extremely high probability of being malignant. In fact, benign tumors exhibiting primary malignant characteristics are so rare that one must be certain the lesion has, in fact, been removed and accurately evaluated pathologically before accepting a benign histologic diagnosis.

Secondary signs of malignant disease and the characteristics of many benign lesions may overlap significantly. The probability of a lesion with only secondary signs being malignant is reduced to 20% to 30%.

Primary Mammographic Signs of Malignant Disease

A lesion with spiculated, ill-defined margins (see Fig. 3-15) can be diagnosed as breast cancer with virtually a 99% degree of certainty. Spiculations are radiations of cancer cells and fibrous tissue strands that develop in response to tumor. Scarring from prior surgery (Fig. 3-24) may occasionally produce a similar desmoplastic response, but the breast usually heals without scars that are visible on mammography, and the location of the previous surgery can usually be corroborated in patients with questionable lesions. Frequently, the margins of the lesion are obscured by surrounding tissue, in which case this finding must be distinguished from the ill-defined margins secondary to tumor invasion.

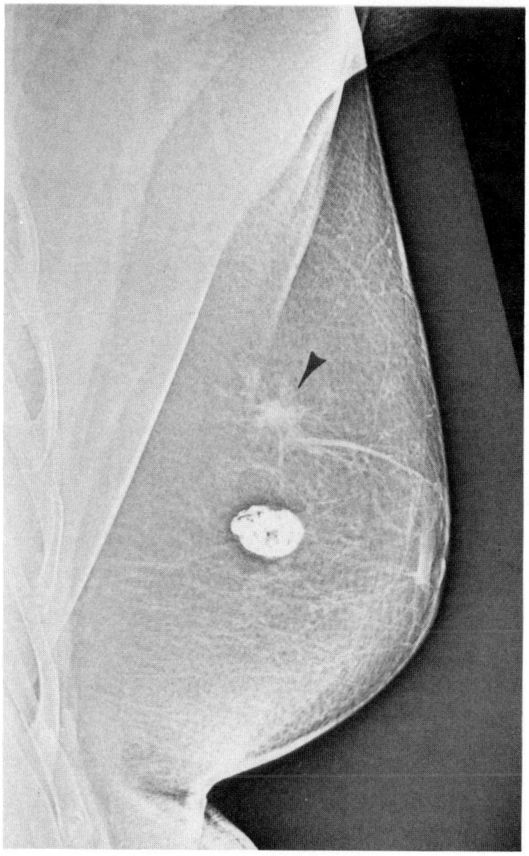

FIGURE 3-24. A postsurgical scar (*arrow*) may be similar in appearance to a malignant process. The large calcification represents a benign, involuting fibroadenoma.

Secondary Mammographic Signs of Malignant Disease

Perhaps the most significant secondary sign of malignant disease is the grouped or clustered microcalcifications that frequently augur the presence of an occult cancer and that may be the earliest findings indicating an intraductal malignant process (Fig. 3-25). Many cancers do not have calcifications that are detectable by mammography. Furthermore, benign processes can cause calcium deposition. However, the presence of five or more calcifications, each of which is under 1 mm in diameter, with the whole group contained within 1 cc of tissue, should be looked upon with suspicion,[49] and in most cases, biopsy is indicated. Despite the fact that up to 80% of such grouped calcifications relate to benign disease, studies have thus far been unable to distinguish accurately between benign and malignant calcifications, and in most instances, biopsy is required. The probability of malignant disease increases with the degree of irregularity in the shapes of the calcifications, as well as their variations in size. Of particular concern are very fine, branching, irregularly shaped calcifications. However, as demonstrated by Sickles,[50] a large number of cancers do not conform to the classic descriptions. An overlap also exists between benign and malignant lesions that have lobulated contours (Fig. 3-26). Breast cancers of all types may appear to be smoothly marginated on mammography (Fig. 3-27), although there is usually at least one area where the margin is poorly defined. Nevertheless, solitary, lobulated densities that are detected on mammography and that do not represent such entities as benign intramammary lymph nodes warrant excision.

Asymmetry of two breasts should be evaluated carefully. Asymmetrical tissue density without specific margins delineating a mass may be seen in many normal women. This is particularly evident in the upper, outer quadrants of the breasts. However, asymmetrical tissue density, when associated with an asymmetrical palpable abnormality, should increase the physician's level of concern (Fig. 3-28).

Asymmetrical ductal structures are frequently described as a secondary sign of malignant disease (Fig. 3-29). Once again, this finding may be seen in normal women, but should be examined by biopsy if a large area of palpable, asymmetrical ducts is noted. The pathologist should be alerted that the malignant process may represent a small area within the overall volume. A solitary, isolated, enlarged duct is unusual, and warrants careful evaluation. Intuitively, one would expect a dilated duct from an obstructive process at the nipple end of the duct. In fact, some cases of isolated dilated ducts have represented a malignant process of the distal portion of the dilated segment.

Asymmetrical enlarged vascular structures have also been included as a secondary sign of malignant disease. If there is no other mammographic abnormality, careful clinical assessment of the involved breast is suggested. However, asymmetrically enlarged vascular structures may be seen in normal breasts. They may also indicate other diagnoses, such as occlusion or collateral flow, as occurs in obstruction of the superior vena cava.

A new density in the breast, when visible on two views (indicating a three-dimensional structure), should be viewed with suspicion. If a cyst is suspected, ultrasonography or aspiration is indicated. If a solid lesion is detected, excision following appropriate localization techniques is indicated.

Architectural distortion is an important secondary sign of malignant disease. In particular, an apparent "pulling-in" of structures toward a point that is eccentric to the nipple should be viewed with a high degree of suspicion (see Fig. 3-29). Benign conditions, such as indurative mastopathy, which produce elastosis and have a spiculated appearance resembling a malignant process may be seen.[51] There is no way to distinguish a benign cause of retraction within the mammary parenchyma from a malignant process, and biopsy is indicated. Similarly, an increase in density or thickening at the edge of the mammary parenchyma which causes an apparent cicatrization of the tissue should be considered suspicious.

Finally, other secondary signs of malignant disease

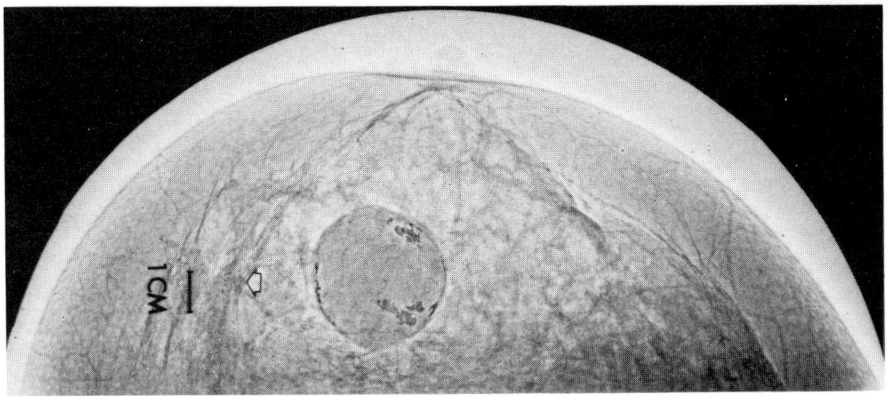

FIGURE 3-25. Clustered microcalcifications (*open arrow*) of a nonpalpable, intraductal carcinoma. The large, spherical, calcified mass is a benign cyst.

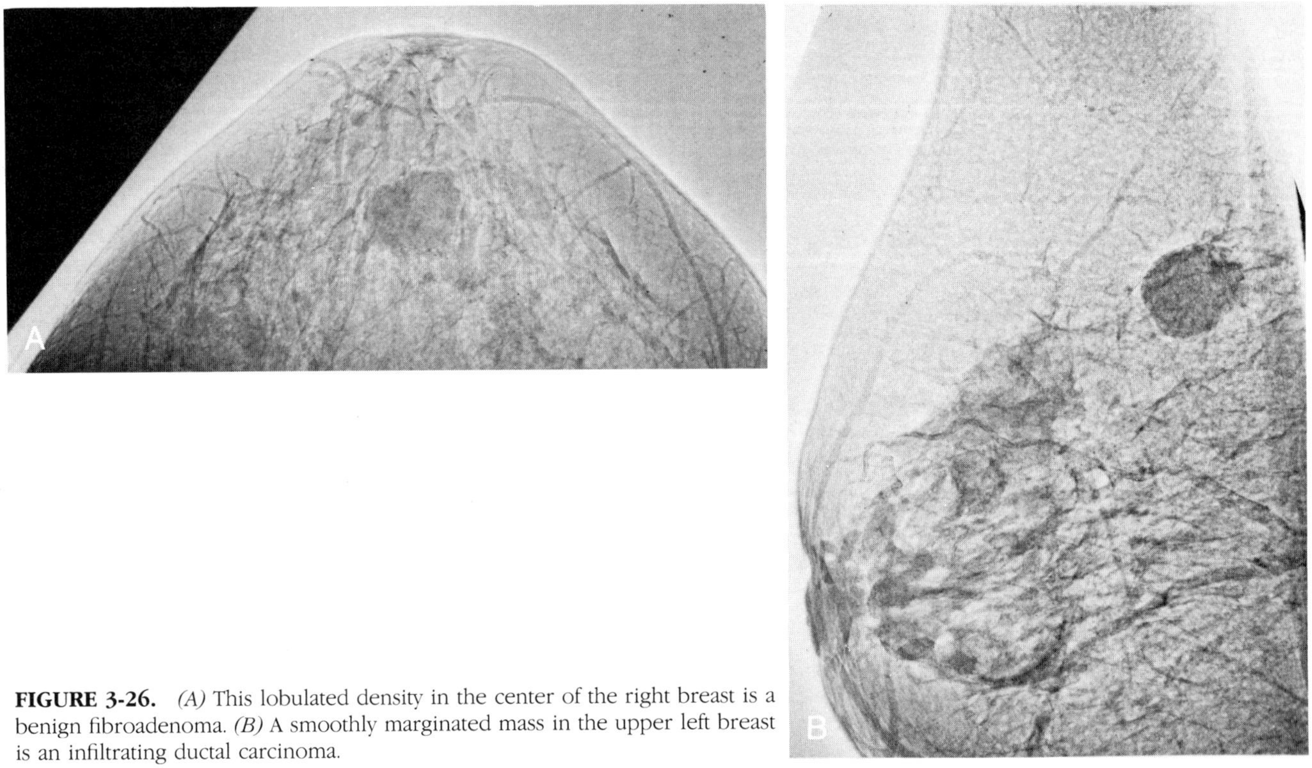

FIGURE 3-26. *(A)* This lobulated density in the center of the right breast is a benign fibroadenoma. *(B)* A smoothly marginated mass in the upper left breast is an infiltrating ductal carcinoma.

may be detected on mammography, but these are usually late changes. They include skin and nipple retraction, skin thickening, an overall increase in density throughout the breast (usually associated with a diffuse malignant process), and enlarged axillary lymph nodes. Once again, it is usually impossible to distinguish between these late malignant changes and benign processes. Benign inflammatory changes in the breast may cause all of these signs, which are visible on mammography and which are indistinguishable from malignant processes. Breast abscesses are frequently not detectable on mammography, or may be indistinguishable from a malignant process. In selected cases, breast ultrasonography and aspiration may be helpful in determining whether a breast abscess is present.

Benign Lesions

There are numerous benign lesions that occur in the breast and that are visible on radiography. Their significance lies in the frequent overlap between benign and malignant characteristics. Fibroadenomas and cysts are the most common masses visible on mammography, and if noncalcified, are indistinguishable from each other. Ultrasonography is useful in differentiating between cystic and solid masses. Intraductal papillomas frequently enlarge sufficiently to be visible as lobulated densities on mammography, but they, too, are indistinguishable from other, fairly well-circumscribed masses. Papillomas and papillomatosis, along with hyperplasia, are relatively common

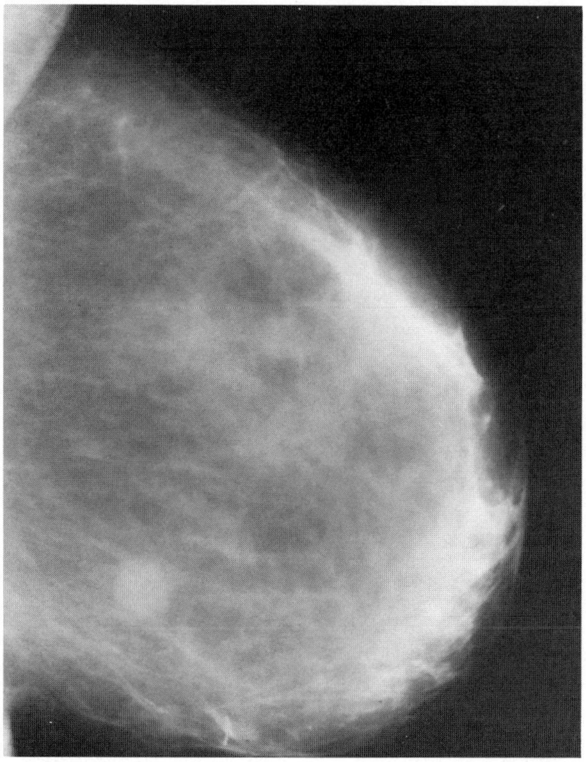

FIGURE 3-27. A round mass with smooth margins was determined to be an infiltrating ductal carcinoma of the right breast.

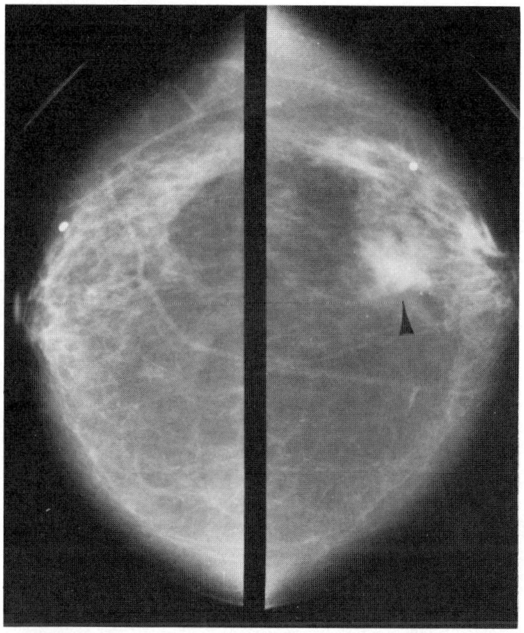

FIGURE 3-28. An asymmetrical density in the right breast (*arrow*) was found to be an infiltrating ductal carcinoma.

causes of microcalcifications that are indistinguishable from those associated with a malignant process.

Several lesions that are visible on mammography may be diagnosed as benign and do not require biopsy. Lesions with a high lipid content usually appear as radiographically lucent lesions on mammography. Lipomas, galactoceles, and a posttraumatic form of fat necrosis known as a traumatic oil cyst[52] present as sharply marginated, encapsulated lesions, with the capsule defined by the fat within the lesion (Fig. 3-30). A relatively uncommon presumed hamartoma of the breast, often called a fibroadenolipoma, has a characteristic heterogeneous appearance with fat, fibrous, and adenomatous elements encapsulated in a lesion that is frequently palpable.

Calcified structures may have characteristic appearances. Fibroadenomas undergoing involution frequently produce large, centrally located calcifications (see Fig. 3-16). When these calcifications are smaller than 1 mm in diameter, multiple, and irregular, the certainty of a benign process is diminished, and biopsy is frequently indicated. It is also important to be aware of the fact that malignant lesions may arise adjacent to benign processes, and that the presence of large calcifications does not exclude the possibility of malignant disease if multiple, fine, irregular calcifications are present immediately adjacent to the fibroadenoma.

Vascular calcifications are rarely difficult to differentiate from malignant calcifications. Vascular deposits form the characteristic parallel appearance seen in arterial deposits elsewhere in the body.

Benign skin calcifications may be confused with intramammary deposits owing to the hemispherical nature of the breast and the potential for projecting skin structures as if they were within the breast structure itself. Techniques have been devised to avoid unnecessary biopsy of these benign deposits, which frequently have characteristic lucent centers and usually do not present a problem in interpretation.

Other large calcifications are commonly found in the breast. The exact etiology of a specific, spherical calcification in the breast is frequently indeterminable. Inflammatory processes involving sloughed ductal material may result in spherical calcifications or large, rod-shaped, "secretory" calcifications that are aligned within the ducts. Fat necrosis is another common cause of large, spherical, benign calcifications.

Isolated lobulated densities in the breast should be regarded with suspicion unless they have the characteristic appearance and location of benign intramammary lymph nodes. These lesions are usually less than 1 cm in diameter and are smoothly defined (see Fig. 3-18). Histologically, they may occur in all parts of the breast, but they have been detected radiographically only in the upper, outer quadrant. Benign intramammary lymph nodes have been seen to extend three-quarters of the way to the nipple, but have not been described in the subareolar region. Frequently, they are fat-infiltrated, which gives them a characteristic hilar notch or central lucency. Extensive fatty replacement may result in the appearance of three or

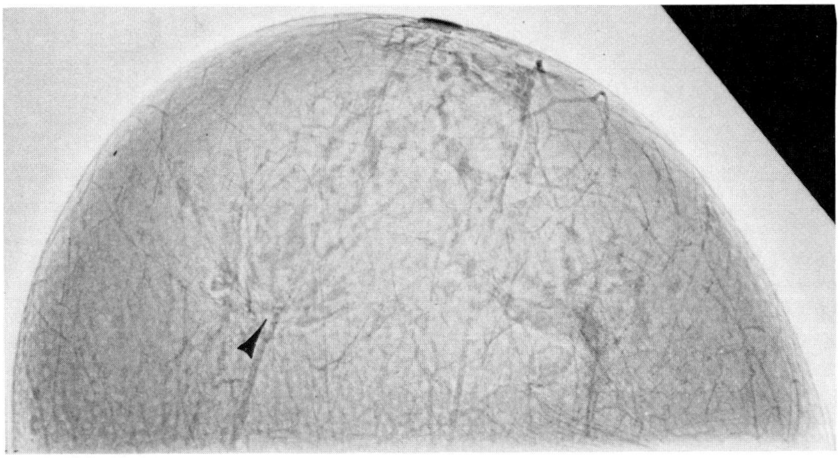

FIGURE 3-29. Architectural distortion (*arrow*) reveals a nonpalpable, infiltrating, ductal carcinoma in the medial left breast.

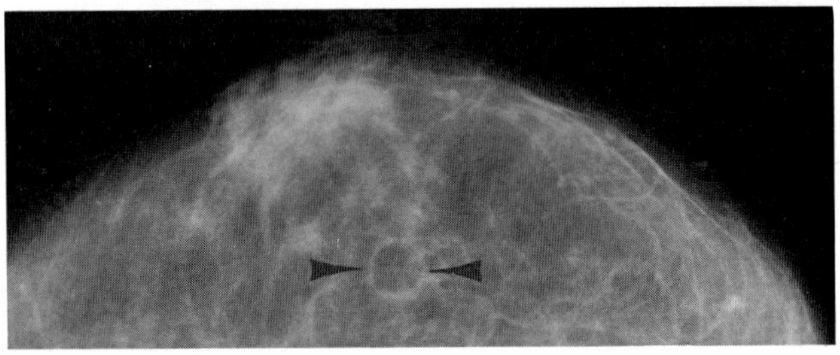

FIGURE 3-30. This lucent lesion, demonstrated in the breast of a patient who had undergone postreduction mammoplasty, is typical of benign, post-traumatic, oil cysts.

more rounded densities immediately adjacent to one another.[50]

If a lesion does not display the characteristics described above, there is no test available, other than biopsy, that can definitively confirm a benign process. Although cancerous lesions of the breast may be smoothly marginated on mammography, such densities, particularly those that are located in several areas of the breast, present a dilemma. A follow-up period of 4 to 6 months has arbitrarily been suggested, and is the most common term of follow-up. If a lesion has primary mammographic signs of malignant disease, its stability over many years does not guarantee a benign process.[54]

Mammographic Interpretation

The ability to interpret a mammogram satisfactorily originates with the performance of the study itself. High-quality x-ray imaging of the breast must be demanded. Dedicated mammographic systems are required. Technologists should be highly trained, and reproducible positioning and exposure values should be sought. The radiologist interpreting the mammograms should be well-trained, and should have an understanding of the technical requirements of the study, as well as an ability to interpret the images produced. As has been emphasized, mammography is sensitive in detecting small breast cancers, but is nonspecific, and certainly is not able to detect all breast cancers. Mammography is able to detect early-stage, nonpalpable breast cancers, but a significant number of benign lesions will be examined by biopsy in the process. Since it may be more difficult to detect cancers in certain types of breast tissue, the mammographic report should indicate the type of breast tissue being evaluated. Since, at this time, the significance of parenchymal patterns is unclear, an assessment of the parenchyma should be done to indicate the sensitivity of the test, not the degree of risk. Mammography relies on the delineation of water-density tumors from surrounding, low-attentuation fat. If the surrounding breast tissue has the same x-ray attentuation as a breast cancer, a sizable lesion may be invisible on a mammogram. Cancers may, nevertheless, be detected in dense, fibroglandular breast tissue if they cause architectural distortion or calcium deposition. Consequently, although the level of sensitivity may be diminished, benefit may be derived from mammographic evaluation, even in women with dense mammary parenchyma. It should be noted that there is frequently no correlation between the mammographic appearance of the breast parenchyma and the clinical assessment. Hard, firm, breast tissue detected on physical examination may merely represent tightly packed fat, as shown by mammography. Similarly, when palpation reveals extremely nodular breast tissue, this condition may merely represent the lobes of the breast containing fat. Conversely, smooth, soft breast tissue detected on clinical examination may appear dense on radiographic examination. Given some of these limitations, it is clear that mammography and physical examination are complementary, not competing, procedures. Physical examination is less sensitive for small cancers than is mammography, but it can detect some small cancers that are invisible on mammography. Furthermore, the architecture of the breast may not permit certain areas of the breast to be imaged satisfactorily by mammography, and these "blind spots" may represent undetected lesions.

The mammographic report should also indicate the

presence or absence of suspicious abnormalities in the breast. The radiologist's degree of concern regarding these abnormalities should also be indicated. Findings can usually be summarized according to one of six degrees of certainty.[16] A spiculated, ill-defined mass should be considered a definite malignant mass.[17] Lesions with multiple secondary signs of malignant disease rate a high probability (greater than 50%) of being malignant,[18] whereas lesions with a single secondary sign of malignant disease have a probability of approximately 20% to 30% of being cancerous.[19] Findings such as numerous calcifications throughout both breasts; multiple, rounded densities; or multiple, vague densities, are most likely benign, but follow-up of an average duration of 4 to 6 months may be suggested.[20] Intramammary lymph nodes, calcified fibroadenomas, and lucent lesions, as well as the calcifications described in the section on benign lesions, do not require follow-up, but should be mentioned in the report.[21] A report of totally negative findings should indicate that the breasts are symmetrical in appearance, without evidence of masses, microcalcifications, or other findings of concern.

The presence of asymmetrical tissue should be noted in the report. Once again, this is of significance primarily in women with palpable abnormalities in the area of symmetry. Mammographic asymmetry should increase the suspicion of a marginally suspicious, palpable asymmetry. When lesions detectable by mammography warrant a biopsy, the report should indicate that a guide may be placed accurately preoperatively to ensure the safe removal of the area in question.

OTHER IMAGING TECHNIQUES

Despite the development of numerous other methods to image the breast, none has approached x-ray mammography's capability of detecting early-stage, nonpalpable cancer. Ultrasonography has a limited role in differentiating between cystic and solid masses. Ultrasonography and computed body tomography (CBT) may be used in selected situations to guide the preoperative localization of occult lesions. All other techniques should be considered experimental, with no demonstrated clinical efficacy for breast evaluation. As new techniques evolve, studies should be conducted to test the detector capability of a system for lesions less than 1 cm in diameter.[55] To replace mammography for screening, any new technique must be at least as capable as x-ray imaging in finding nonpalpable breast cancers.

Thermography

Thermography encompasses a general category of techniques that essentially measure the surface temperature of the skin. These include telethermography, contact plate thermography, and cholesteric crystal and graphic stress telethermography. Theoretically, these represent ideal screening techniques because they are totally passive, recording only the heat given off from the breast and requiring no incident energy on the breast tissue. Unfortunately, the high rates of false-positive and false-negative results from thermographic techniques have made thermography unsuitable for breast cancer detection at this time.[56]

In 1956, Lawson suggested that breast cancers produce an increase in thermal emissions.[57] Subsequent studies have confirmed the fact that some breast cancers do, in fact, increase the temperature of the surrounding tissue, and that if this heat is not dissipated and reaches the skin surface, breast cancer may be detected. Not all breast cancers, however, generate a detectable increase in thermal emission relative to that of benign tissue. Furthermore, normal breast tissue, especially adipose tissue located between a cancerous lesion and the skin surface, acts as an insulating barrier, preventing conduction of heat to the skin. Heat may also be conducted by way of the vascular system, but this also appears to be a variable phenomenon that does not occur with all breast cancers. Some data suggest that the thermal emission generated by a malignant process relates to its differentiation and virulence.[58] This premise suggests the possibility of utilizing thermography, along with other staging criteria, as a prognostic indicator.

Based on published reports, European researchers seem to have had greater success with thermography than have their American counterparts. This observation may relate to the European researchers' more rigorous approach to the technique and their development of a more objective grading system. Results, however, seem to worsen consistently when they are analyzed relative to the stage of the lesion. Clinically occult lesions that are detectable by mammography are frequently undetected by thermography.[59] Proponents of thermography suggest that cancers with little thermal activity are less aggressive and, therefore, need not be detected. This is an unproven and dangerous supposition. Lesions of intermediate virulence, may, in fact, be able to be cured through aggressive screening. Very aggressive tumors may, in fact, be systemic before they break any presently available threshold of detectability. Based on his extensive experience, Gautherie has suggested that thermography may represent one of the strongest risk indicators yet discovered.[60] This theory has not been corroborated but warrants further investigation. It appears that the cancers in Gautherie's series were at a more advanced stage, suggesting that the initial borderline patterns thought to be indicators of risk were, in fact, indicators of a malignant disease that was already present.

Another area that bears further investigation is the prognostic capability of thermography. A relationship between survival and the thermal productivity of a lesion has been suggested.[61] Presumably, this relationship also relates to the aggressiveness of the tumor involved.

At the present time, the data suggest that thermography does not have the ability to detect early-stage lesions that are detectable by mammographic screening. As a consequence, the American College of Radiology has published a policy statement that thermography should not be used to screen asymptomatic women.[62] Certain observations bear further investigation, but thermography should not be used clinically.

Ultrasonography

Ultrasonography utilizes high-frequency sound waves generated by piezoelectric crystals that produce frequencies in diagnostic imaging of 1 MHz to 10 MHz. These crystals are stimulated by electronic pulses that produce vibrations in the piezoelectric material, creating the sound pulses. The resolving capability of ultrasonography depends on a complex interrelationship between frequency, shape of the beam, and tissue interactions. Ultrasonography has been used in breast evaluation for more than 2 decades. It is only within the last 10 years that high-resolution imaging has been available. The technique has never developed a resolution capability that approximates the detail obtained with x-ray imaging of the breast.

Nevertheless, concern over the possible induction of malignant lesions of the breast by ionizing radiation from mammographic studies prompted attempts in the mid-1970s to develop ultrasonographic breast screening techniques. Initial enthusiasm was generated by the ability of ultrasonography to demonstrate large, 3-cm and 4-cm cancers of the breast. Ultrasonographic devices with the capability of evaluating the entire breast were built. Contact systems used in most other parts of the body run the risk of displacing breast tissue from beneath the sound beam from the pressure of the transducer. Consequently, whole-breast ultrasonographic systems relied on either the immersion of the breast in a container of water, which permitted the transducer to scan the breast without placing pressure on the tissues, or scanning of the patient in a supine position using a fluid path contained in a sonolucent membrane placed on the breast.

Although ultrasonography clearly has the ability to differentiate between cystic and solid masses (Fig. 3-31) in the breast, carefully designed and executed studies have failed to demonstrate sufficient sensitivity of the technique in detecting early-stage cancers. In a blind comparison between physical examination, x-ray mammography, and whole-breast ultrasonography, Kopans and colleagues demonstrated a failure of ultrasonography to detect almost 50% of lesions that were less than 2 cm in diameter.[63] Sickles and co-workers had a similar experience.[64] In fact, in most published series, although the overall sensitivity of ultrasonography appears to be quite high, critical review of the data, particularly as they pertain to the detection of early-stage lesions, shows that ultrasonography has a diminished capability in revealing small, cancerous lesions.[65,66] No researchers have published any large series of lesions that were examined by biopsy solely as a result of abnormal ultrasonographic findings. In the series published by Kopans and associates, a follow-up study of abnormalities that were suggested only on ultrasonography failed to demonstrate any clinically evident cancers 3 to 4 years after the study.

There are several reasons why ultrasonography fails to detect small, cancerous lesions, many of which are not only detectable by mammography, but may also be detected on physical examination. The breast is an inhomogeneous organ with numerous scattering and reflecting surfaces. Furthermore, breast cancer is almost universally hypoechoic, and may be similar in echo texture to the hypoechoic fat of the breast. It is difficult to detect a hypoechoic, irregular structure in the presence of a background of normally hypoechoic, irregular tissue. Marked attenuation and scattering of sound, which caused posterior acoustic shadowing, was described in the early literature as a classic sign of malignant disease.[67] Unfortunately, many breast cancers do not produce posterior

FIGURE 3-31. *(A)* A hypoechoic, fairly well circumscribed mass appears as a solid lesion on ultrasonography. *(B)* An anechoic mass is determined to be a cyst on ultrasonography.

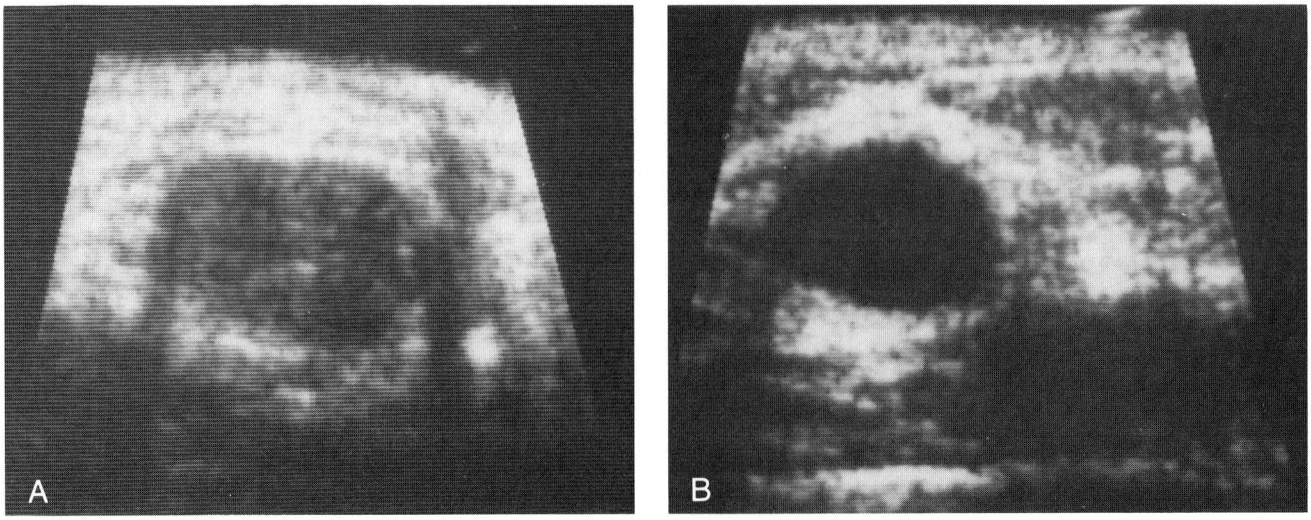

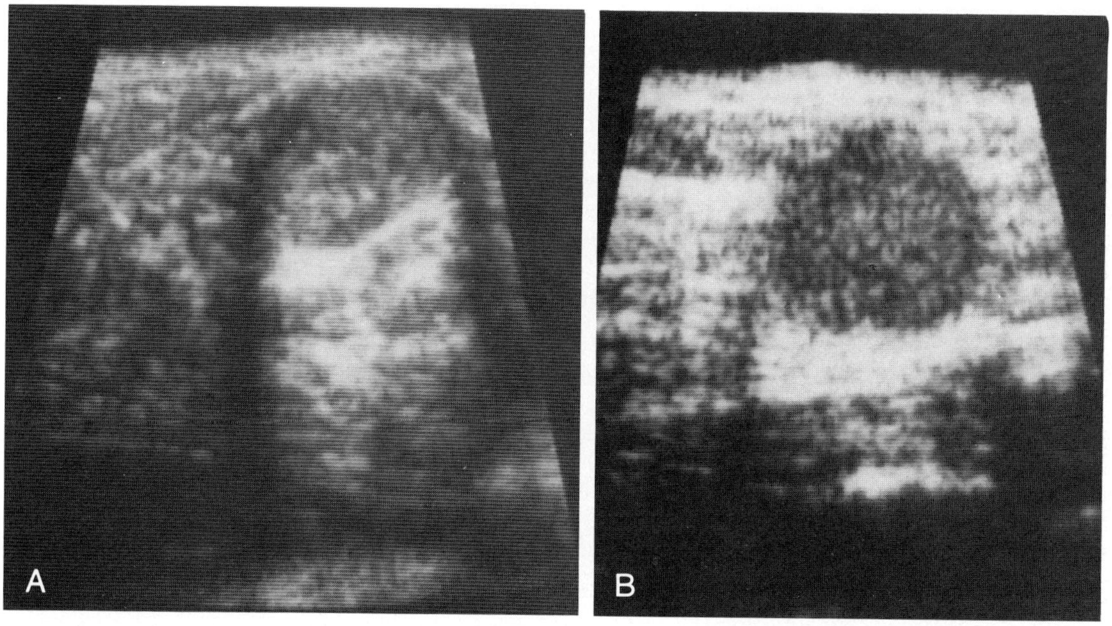

FIGURE 3-32. *(A)* This mass, which showed internal echoes and posterior acoustic enhancement on ultrasonography, proved to be a fibroadenoma at biopsy. *(B)* A similar lesion was found to be an infiltrating ductal carcinoma.

acoustic shadowing,[68,69] and many normal structures of the breast, including the fibrous septations formed by Cooper's ligaments and other benign fibrotic changes in the breast, may produce similar shadowing.

Finally, ultrasonography is also unable to detect the microcalcifications that can only be detected by x-ray mammography and that have proved to be a significant indicator of early-stage breast cancer.

Although ultrasonography has no efficacy for screening asymptomatic women for early signs of breast cancer, it does have a limited role in the evaluation of selected breast lesions. Clinically guided aspiration of a palpable mass is the most cost-effective and efficient way of determining whether a palpable lesion is cystic or solid. A small subset of palpable lesions may defy clinically guided aspiration and still represent benign cysts. These apparently solid masses, when detected preoperatively by mammography, may suggest a cystic process that may be confirmed by ultrasonography. In these situations ultrasonography may be used to guide the successful aspiration of cysts, thus avoiding surgical excision.[70]

Ultrasonography is also useful in the evaluation of a selected group of lesions that are larger than 1 cm in diameter, but that are evident only on mammography. When solitary, a lesion of this type should be examined by biopsy unless it can be demonstrated that it represents a benign cyst. The delineation of a cyst by ultrasonography is quite accurate,[71] and once again, using ultrasonographic guidance, aspiration can be done to confirm this if necessary. In a very limited setting, ultrasonography may also be used to guide the localization of clinically occult, mammographically detected masses that appear to be solid (see the section on localization procedures, below).

Ultrasonography cannot reliably distinguish between benign and malignant solid breast lesions. There is a significant overlap in the appearance of noncystic benign processes in the breast and malignant lesions. Although most benign solid masses are fairly round and well-circumscribed with a homogenous internal echo texture, these characteristics may also be seen in breast cancer (Fig. 3-32). Consequently, ultrasonography should noι be used to differentiate between benign and malignant solid processes. It may be useful in prompting early intervention in some clinically evident lesions that are not of sufficient concern to warrant biopsy. If ultrasonographic examination of a palpable, asymmetrical area demonstrates a hypoechoic mass or an area of isolated hypoechoic tissue with posterior acoustic shadowing, a biopsy should be undertaken (Fig. 3-33).

In summary, there is no role for ultrasonography in the screening of asymptomatic women for early breast cancer. As a consequence, whole-breast ultrasonographic systems are unnecessary. High-resolution contact systems are of value in examining a small subset of clinical cases (described above) to facilitate appropriate care.

Transillumination

The ability to shine visible light through the breast was first described in 1929.[72] The technique has undergone a reevaluation, utilizing wavelengths in the far red and near

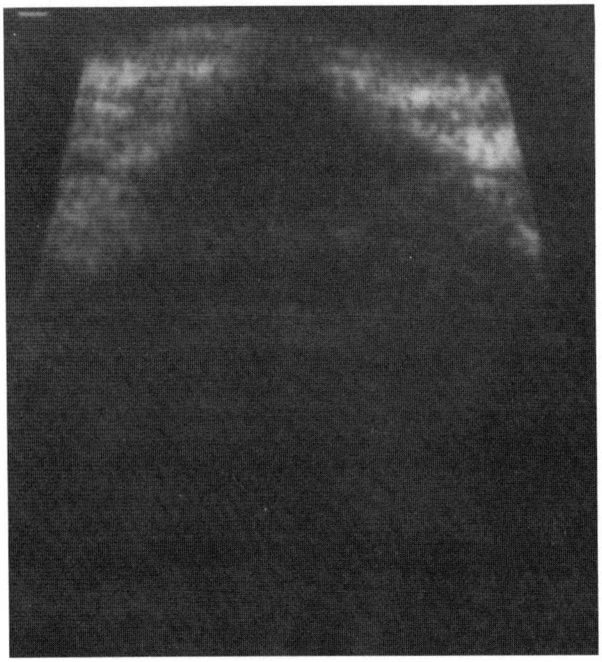

FIGURE 3-33. Palpable asymmetry in this patient was not of sufficient concern to warrant biopsy. A shadowing lesion detected on ultrasonography led to biopsy of an infiltrating ductal carcinoma.

infrared spectrum that appear to be more readily transmitted through the breast. The most widely available system uses filtering of an incandescent light and microprocessing to indicate overall light transmission, producing a ratio of red to infrared signals. It is postulated that the increased blood supply to a tumor produces a greater light absorption, casting a shadow on the skin. In studies of transillumination published in critically reviewed journals, no measure of efficacy in detecting breast cancer has been demonstrated.[69] Optimistic assessment of limited studies has led to a large-scale, triple-blind study that is currently underway to determine what, if any, role light scanning will have in breast evaluation. The major support for light scanning has been anecdotal in nature. Despite relatively poor results in an early study involving a blind evaluation of light scanning,[73] Bartrum and associates were encouraged by the nonblind second reading of the scan that suggested that observer error may have accounted for the initial poor results.

Sickles obtained uniformly poor results using transillumination techniques for the detection of early-stage lesions. However, these data have been criticized because of the older equipment utilized.[74] Marshall used more modern equipment.[75] Based on the fact that his group was able to detect some cases of cancer with the technique, he urged further research but did not support its routine clinical use since all cancers detected by transillumination were also detected by mammography.[75] To further compound the problem, the cancers in his series were usually seen in only one view, and three-dimensional localization was not possible. A recent study by Gesslein and co-workers, in which state-of-the-art equipment with a television detector sensitive to far red and near infrared wavelengths and computer enhancement of the images was used, revealed poor results despite the availability of clinical and mammographic data. This series demonstrated a detector capability that was inferior to that of mammography and diagnostic data that were less specific than those derived from ultrasonography.[76]

The present configuration of transillumination devices involves the use of a broad light source. The breast causes significant scattering of light in these wavelengths, and in fact, it is entirely possible that no light is directly transmitted through the breast. Consequently, resolution is extremely poor. These devices rely on silhouetting cancers on the skin surface opposite to the light source. The technique is extremely operator-dependent and the deeper the lesion within the breast, the more its shadow is obscured by the light scattering around it.[77]

At the present time, there is no proven efficacy for the utilization of light scanning in the detection of or diagnostic differentiation between cystic and solid lesions. Further investigation is warranted, however, and several investigators are exploring the possibility of low-energy laser transillumination, which may permit the use of any light that is directly transmitted. There is no role at this time for transillumination in a clinical setting, except on an experimental basis.

CT Scanning

The great advantage of cross-sectional imaging utilizing computed body tomography may be applied to the breast in a limited fashion. Although Chang and co-workers have reported significant success in detecting small cancerous lesions using precontrast and postcontrast enhanced CT scans,[78] their findings have not been corroborated. The techniques defined by Chang require a radiation exposure that is higher than that of state-of-the-art, two-dimensional mammography, as well as a longer period spent within the scanner. In addition, the intravenous administration of iodinated contrast material is required in CT scanning, and the potential for reactions is well documented. From a practical point of view, CT is useful in a limited number of women in whom a lesion that is detected on mammography, but that can be seen only in a single mammographic projection, is found to warrant biopsy. The inability to triangulate such a lesion with conventional methods precludes an accurate localization. If the lesion cannot be delineated by ultrasonography, CT may be employed to aid in the preoperative positioning of a guide for surgical excision[79] (see the section on localization techniques, below).

Magnetic Resonance Imaging

Magnetic resonance (MR) imaging takes advantage of the electromagnetic properties of hydrogen nuclei in the cells

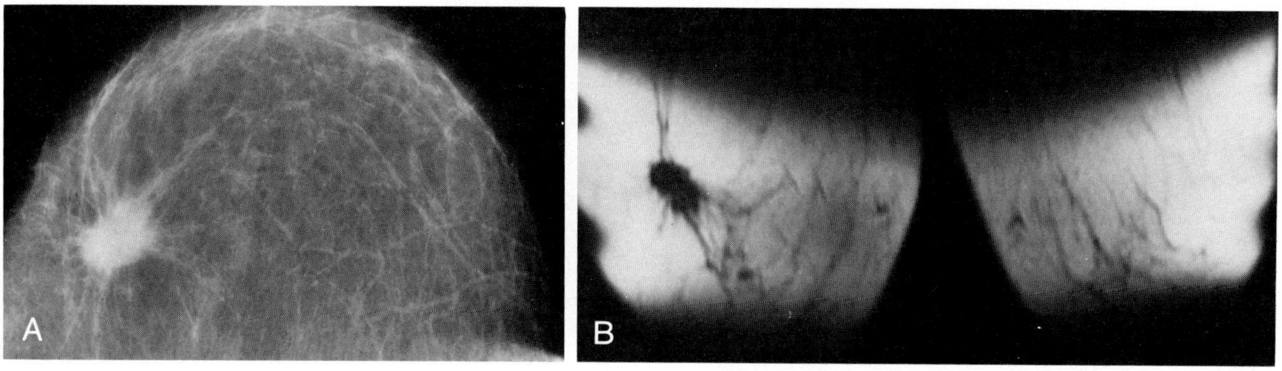

FIGURE 3-34. *(A)* Mammogram of an infiltrating, ductal carcinoma. *(B)* Magnetic resonance imaging demonstrated the same lesion on a TI-weighted image.

of the body. Many of these nuclei act as magnetic dipoles and, when placed in a strong magnetic field, align themselves within the field. Magnetic resonance imaging uses radio-frequency pulses to jolt these dipoles out of line. As they precess within the magnetic field during realignment, the interactions of these dipoles with one another and with the magnetic field produces signals that can be converted into cross-sectional images.

MR imaging of the breast is in the early stages of evaluation. Thus far, the success of MR imaging in delineating breast lesions seems to parallel that of x-ray mammography except that MR imaging is, at this time, unable to detect the microcalcifications that are frequently associated with early-stage cancer. The visibility of a lesion is most closely related to the contrast produced by the fat surrounding it. Lesions that arise within fibroglandular breast tissue are much more difficult to delineate, and many cannot be differentiated from the surrounding normal tissue without prior knowledge of their location.

It is clear that advances in surface coil technology are necessary to improve the signal-to-noise ratio and to gain the resolution required in breast imaging. As presently configured, MR systems cannot replace mammography for the detection of breast cancer because of their lower spatial resolution, the cross-sectional nature of the technique, and the attendant volume-averaging problems created by slice thickness.

The optimistic goal of using MR imaging to differentiate between benign and malignant tissue has yet to be realized. At the present time, morphologic criteria represent the most useful method of differentiation[80] (Fig. 3-34). However, just as with x-ray imaging and ultrasonographic studies of the breast, the morphologic criteria of malignant disease overlap with the characteristics of some benign processes. Malignant lesions may be fairly sharply defined, and many benign lesions have ill-defined margins and irregular shapes that are similar to those that are supposedly characteristic of malignant disease. It is possible that a combination of pulse sequences may result in an algorithmic method of differentiating between benign and malignant masses, but this premise remains to be proven in a large clinical trial.

At this time, MR imaging should be considered an experimental technique with no definite clinical efficacy.

Biopsy

The potential for false-positive and false-negative results from different biopsy techniques must be clearly understood by physicians advising patients in such circumstances. If areas that are suspicious on mammographic or clinical examination, or both, do not resolve (as per the schema in Figures 3-9 through 3-12), a degree of concern regarding the possibility of malignant disease should persist, and such lesions should be removed.

Needle Biopsy

Fine needle biopsy produces a cytologic smear on slides that includes the surrounding tissue or blood, or both. Pathologic interpretation depends on the cytologic features of isolated cells. Aspiration is done with a syringe and a 20-gauge needle. This is similar to the technique used for aspirating cysts (discussed in Chapter 2), and was originally described by Martin and Ellis.[81]

Core needle biopsy by needle aspiration produces a core of tissue that may be difficult to interpret pathologically. This technique requires histologic, not cytologic, interpretation. The possibility that a florid benign process, such as sclerosing adenosis, may be interpreted as malignant is greater with this core specimen than with the specimen obtained by fine needle aspiration. Nevertheless, it is a reliable test in experienced hands. Another type of core technique, the drill biopsy, was described by Ellis to be more useful in scirrhous, fibrotic, or bony lesions.[82]

Incisional Biopsy

With incisional biopsy, a portion of the mass is excised, usually after administration of local anesthesia (although general anesthesia is used if the mass is large and suspicious and if the patient understands the potential

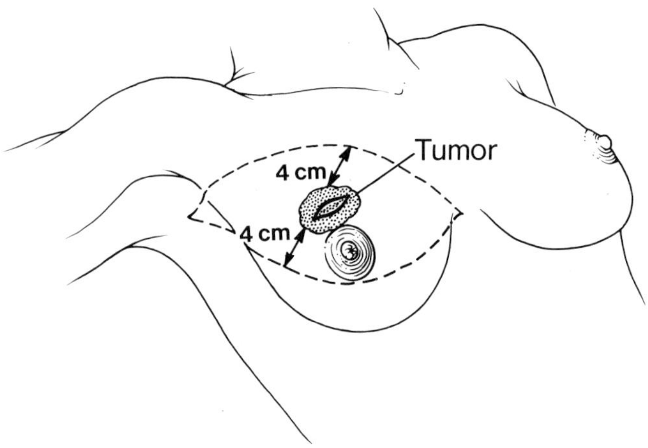

FIGURE 3-35. Incisional biopsy (incomplete removal) of a dominant mass.

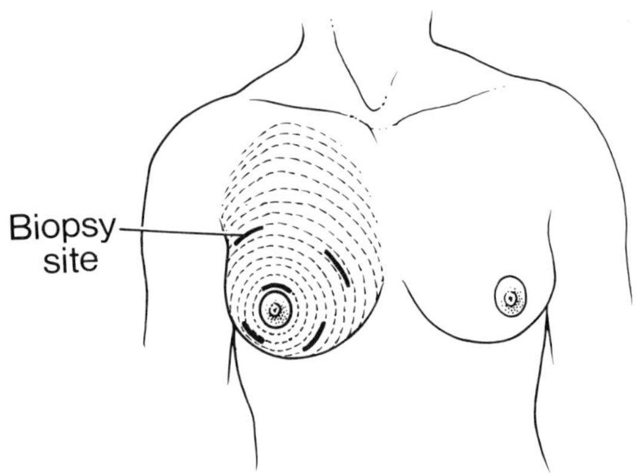

FIGURE 3-36. Curvilinear (Langer's) lines showing ideal incision placement for optimal cosmetic result

benefits of this approach). This procedure is undertaken when the mass is too large for complete excision, the result of which would compromise definitive therapy (usually, mastectomy) (Fig. 3-35); or when a portion of tumor is removed in clearly inoperable circumstances in order to establish the diagnosis and to determine hormone assays.

Excisional Biopsy

Excisional biopsy is the preferred approach for small, potentially curable lesions, and entails complete removal of the suspicious area. It is also indicated in patients with masses that are thought to be benign, to ensure complete removal and histologic evaluation. In patients with suspected malignant masses, this procedure may include the removal of a margin of grossly normal breast tissue. The intact specimen is then delivered to the Pathology Department so that the margins can be inked and assessed by permanent histology for possible margin involvement by cancer. The ideal approach to excisional biopsy is curvilinear, directly over the lesions if they are thought to be malignant, and within skin lines (Langer's lines), as shown in Fig. 3-36. Radial incisions are discouraged except in the cases noted below. Curvilinear incisions are more cosmetic than radial ones, and their placement directly over a malignant tumor facilitates the planning of definitive treatment, whether it involves mastectomy or breast preservation.

Young patients in whom the preoperative diagnosis is clearly benign (especially in those with fibroadenoma) are the exceptions to this rule. In such cases, circumareolar incision, with tunneling through breast tissue to excise the tumor, will result in an optimally cosmetic scar at the areolar margin (Fig. 3-37). However, removal of a malignant lesion by this approach makes subsequent treatment more difficult.

Certain peripheral tumors are difficult to approach, particularly in terms of planning subsequent management.

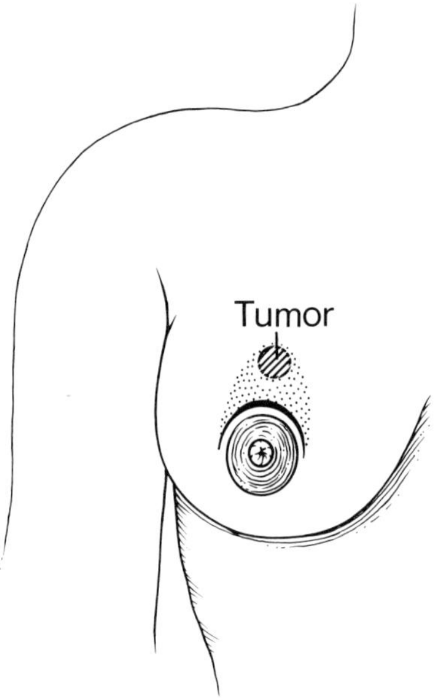

FIGURE 3-37. Circumareolar incision with dissection through the breast for excision of benign lesions in young patients.

Patients commonly present to our center with poorly placed biopsy incisions (where surgeons expected to encounter benign disease, no doubt), and subsequent management, whether by mastectomy or breast preservation approaches, is more complicated simply because of incisional placement. Examples of both optimal and poorly situated incisions are illustrated in Fig. 3-38. Some may disagree with our favored approaches to these unusual situations, but we believe that these recommended incisions are best planned to allow either mastectomy or breast-sparing treatment.

(Fig. 3-38, A). In patients with suspicious axillary lymphadenopathy and no palpable or mammographic abnormality requiring biopsy, a leading possibility is that

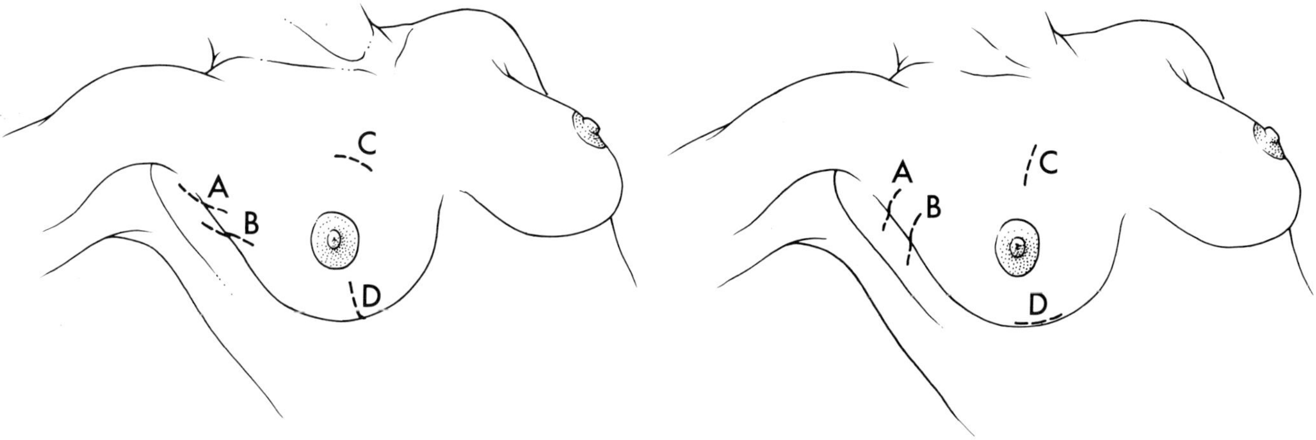

FIGURE 3-38. Examples of incisions for peripheral malignant lesions. (*Left*) Recommended. (*Right*) poor. See text for details.

metastatic breast carcinoma is present in axillary node(s) from an occult primary. Once the diagnosis is established, and in the absence of evidence of distant disease, the appropriate local-regional therapy would be mastectomy (usually, a modified radical approach) or full axillary dissection followed by radiation therapy. In this case, a radial incision, which would allow either surgical approach, is preferable to a curvilinear incision which, although within skin lines, would make subsequent mastectomy difficult.

(Fig. 3-38, B). Lesions of the axillary tail of Spence are quite similar to those just mentioned. Although curvilinear incisions are usually favored in such cases, they make subsequent mastectomy more difficult. Breast preservation through one incision, encompassing the axillary tail primary and the axillary nodes, may be done using a radial approach carried out in a transverse fashion posteriorly into the axilla.

(Fig. 3-38, C). Tumors involving the high, upper-inner quadrant of the breast are difficult to excise. A radial or vertical incision makes subsequent mastectomy difficult and is not cosmetically acceptable for breast-sparing treatment. Curvilinear incisions are, therefore, favored.

(Fig. 3-38, D). Lesions of the inframammary fold, excised by a radial approach, allow either mastectomy or breast preservation. Although the latter may be possible through curvilinear incisions, there is a possibility that the nipple could be pulled inferiorly on closure. Also, mastectomy is more difficult with a curvilinear scar than with a radial scar.

Incisional or excisional biopsy should not be carried out with electrocautery because thermal injury may make histologic interpretation difficult, and estrogen receptor activity may be reduced by heat. However, frozen section is indicated so that hormone receptor determinations may be obtained from fresh tissue.

Although these biopsies may be done in an outpatient setting using local anesthesia, for many patients, excisional biopsies using light general anesthesia are preferred. Patients with deep-seated, indiscrete, or large lesions, or those in whom clear tumor margins are being sought, would benefit from the latter approach.

Fine needle aspiration has increased in usage owing to the cost-effectiveness of this simple outpatient procedure.[83] The incidence of false-negative cytology reports in lesions subsequently determined to be cancerous ranges from 5% to 20%. False-positive rates are very low, often zero, indicating the high specificity of this procedure. If the cytologic examination of a suspicious mass is negative, excisional biopsy is indicated to rule out malignant disease.[84–87] However, some researchers do not remove nonsuspicious masses if the cytologic results are negative; they report no carcinomas developing in these patients.[88,89] This is not a common practice in our hands, however, and excisional biopsy is advised in such cases. Recommended approaches are summarized in Figure 3-39.

A greater number of biopsies are done in outpatients, either by needle aspiration or open biopsy, than in inpatients. Either local anesthesia or general anesthesia (in a same-day surgical setting) is employed. This approach is cost-effective, eliminating the need for hospitalization of patients with benign disease. For patients with malignant disease who understand their treatment options and desire one-step procedures (biopsy and definitive treatment during the same general anesthesia), no cost benefit can be claimed for outpatient biopsy. However, many patients prefer two-step procedures, the first step being the biopsy, which is followed by a discussion of treatment options, the second step being definitive treatment. In the past, two-step procedures were thought to increase the risk of spreading cancer systemically, but recent experience indicates no difference in survival between patients treated by one-step procedures and those undergoing two-step procedures. It has been suggested that certain subsets of patients, especially those with positive axillary nodes or those who undergo incisional biopsies, delaying definitive therapy for more than 2 weeks after biopsy, have a decreased survival rate compared with similarly staged patients treated in one step.[90] These data are inconclusive,

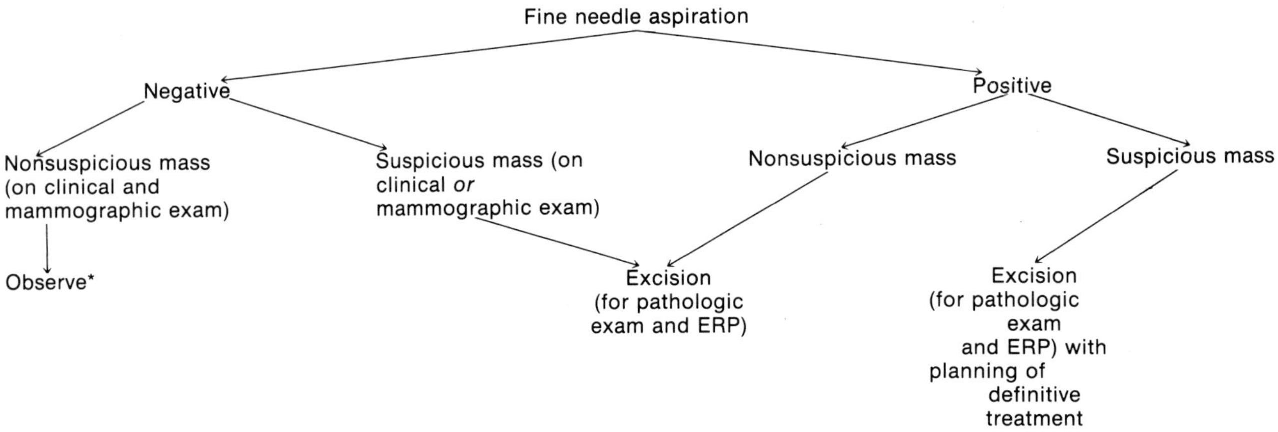

* This policy is advised only if the lesion is vague and indiscrete. Excision to rule out malignant disease is considered safest.

FIGURE 3-39. Recommended sequence of management after fine needle aspiration of a mass.

and no fixed, maximum period of delay between the first and second procedure can be shown to jeopardize long-term results. Most patients, for psychological reasons, will elect to proceed with definitive treatment as soon as they decide what it will be.

PREOPERATIVE LOCALIZATION AND EXCISION OF CLINICALLY OCCULT LESIONS

The primary objective of breast imaging techniques is the early detection of breast cancer at a stage when intervention may substantially alter the course of the disease. Since it is uncertain when metastatic spread occurs, it is desirable to intervene at the earliest possible moment. X-ray mammography has the demonstrated capability of detecting very small abnormalities within the breast, but the technique is usually unable to differentiate between benign and malignant processes, particularly when the lesions are small. In a published review of 500 patients in whom lesions were detected on mammography and biopsy was performed, 23% proved to have malignant disease.[91] This predictive value is similar to that which has appeared in multiple series of lesions requiring biopsy based on clinical findings.[28] Women with cancers detected by mammography are less likely, however, to have involvement of axillary nodes at the time of diagnosis. Nevertheless, because a significant number of biopsies will be undertaken in patients with benign disease, and because of the increased desire for breast conservation in the treatment of women with small cancers, accurate guidance techniques are necessary to permit surgical removal of the lesion in question with sacrifice of the least amount of surrounding tissue. Given this requirement, the technique should offer the least amount of trauma to the patient and should be able to be performed on an outpatient basis.

Numerous methods of localization are presently in use. Quadrant resection and the use of skin markers are unacceptable methods of localizing nonpalpable lesions detected on mammography. Because of the mobility of the breast and the lack of rigid association between surface markers and deeper tissue elements, these methods are extremely inaccurate and lead to the removal of unnecessarily large amounts of normal breast tissue.

All accurate localization techniques require the introduction of a needle in close proximity to the lesion in question. Although surgeons frequently prefer that the needle be advanced toward the lesion from the anterior periareolar region of the breast in a direction similar to that which will be used in surgery, directing needles back toward the chest wall is not only inaccurate, but also unsafe. An increasing number of incidents have occurred in which needles and wire guides have been placed into the pectoralis muscle, the thorax, and the mediastinum. Chest tubes have been required in some instances, and thoracotomies have been undertaken in some patients to retrieve such devices. Furthermore, because of the imaging requirements of mammography, the advancement of needles toward lesions in a direction back toward the chest wall is based on skin measurements that do not correlate well with the position of the lesions seen on mammographic studies.

Safe, accurate positioning is achieved by passing needles parallel to the chest wall, either from the top of the breast, from either side, or occasionally, from beneath the breast.[92] Not only does this approach avoid the possibility of transgressing the thoracic wall, but it also eliminates the theoretical possibility that tumor cells may be seeded deeper into the breast, close to the chest wall. None of the needle localization techniques available is optimal for all situations. Once a needle tip has been positioned close to or in a suspicious lesion, a vital dye

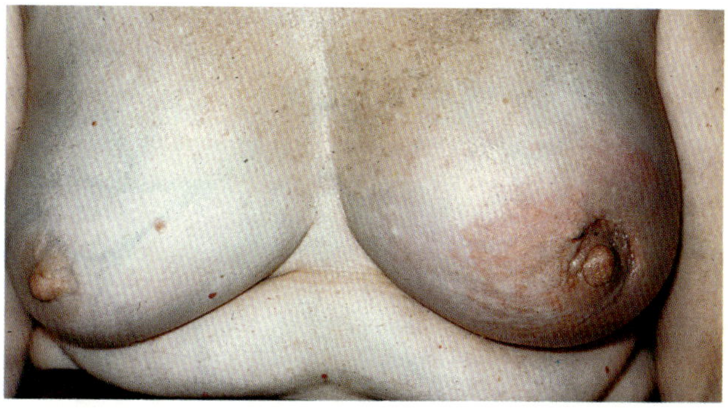

COLOR PLATE 1. Inflammatory breast carcinoma with erythema and erysipeloid edges.

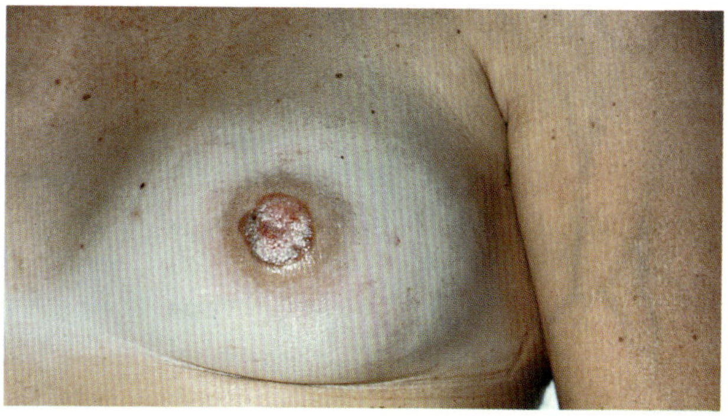

COLOR PLATE 2. Paget's disease of the nipple.

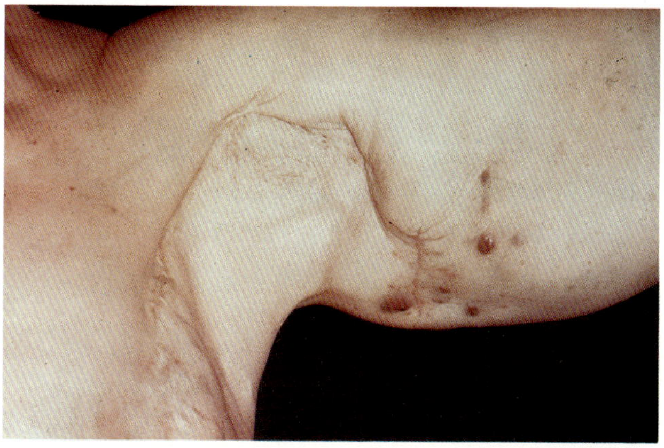

COLOR PLATE 3. Upper, inner aspect of the lymphedematous arm of a postmastectomy patient with lymphangiosarcoma.

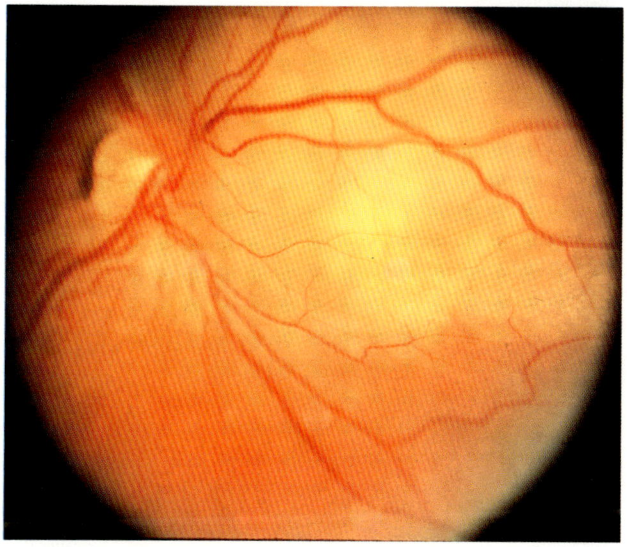

COLOR PLATE 4. Funduscopic photograph of choroidal metastases showing slightly elevated pale yellow lesions with retinal pigment epithelium on the surface.

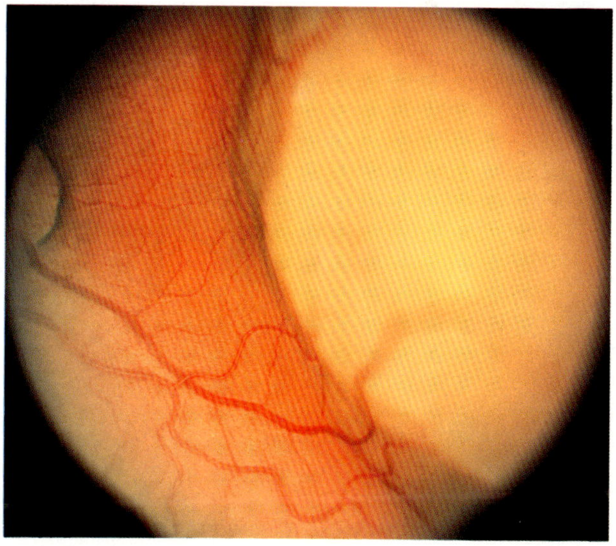

COLOR PLATE 5. Serous retinal detachment characteristic of choroidal metastasis.

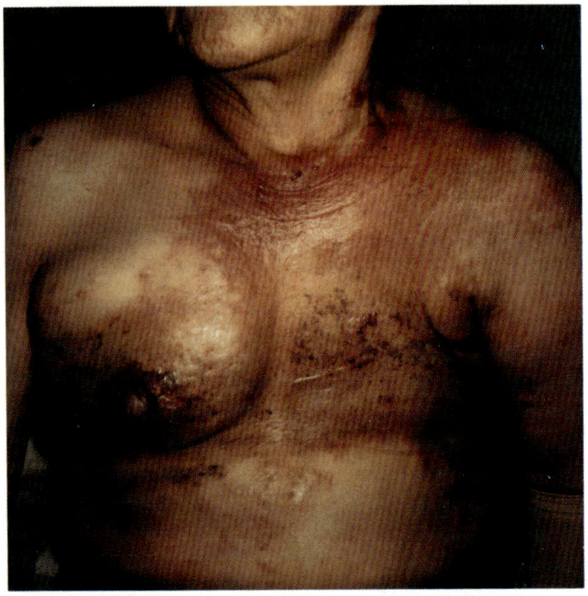

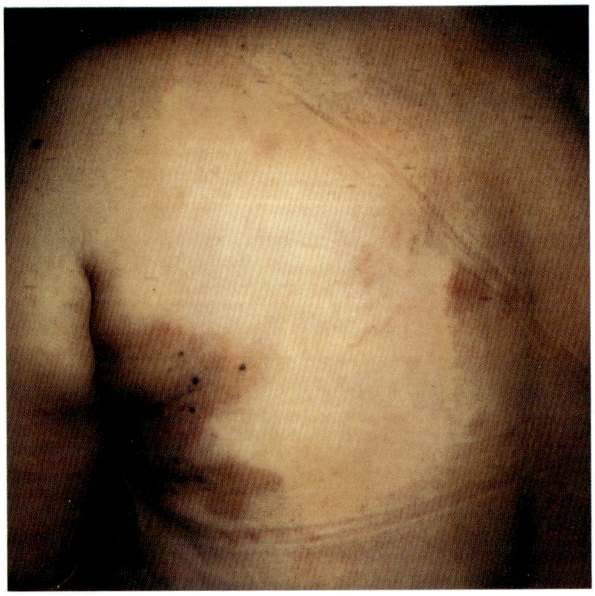

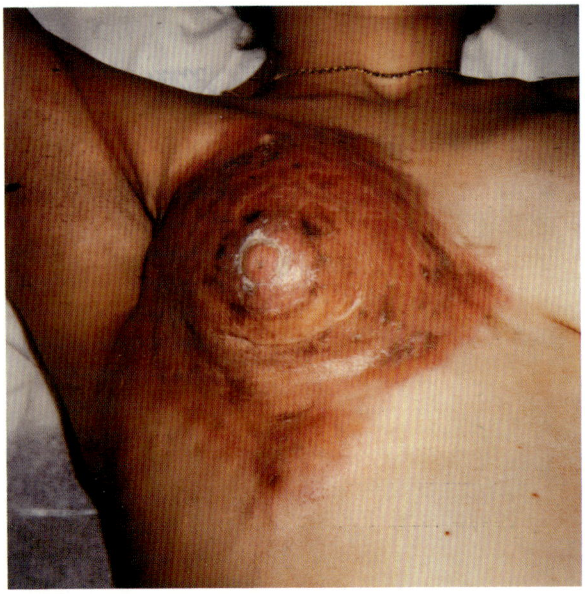

COLOR PLATE 6. *(A, B)* Carcinoma en cuirasse occurring postmastectomy, extending to the posterior thorax, contralateral breast, and neck. *(C)* Carcinoma en cuirasse occurring following primary radiation therapy. Primary was located inferiorly, and initial lesions occurred in the upper quadrant.

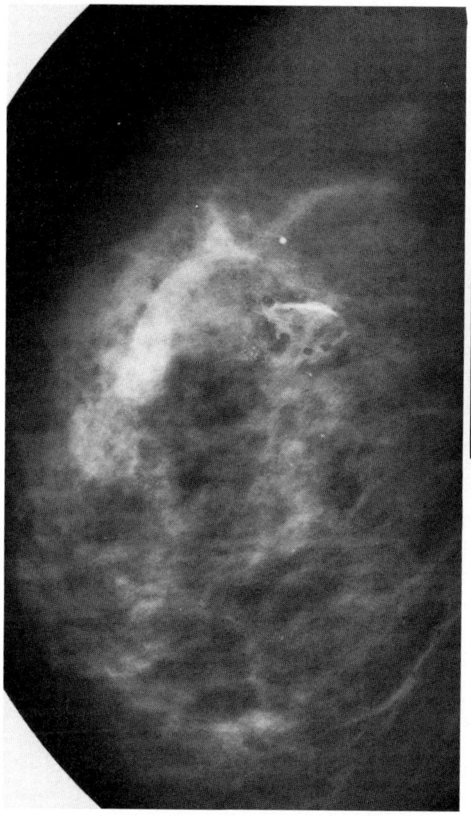

FIGURE 3-40. Lateral view showing dye deep to the calcifications.

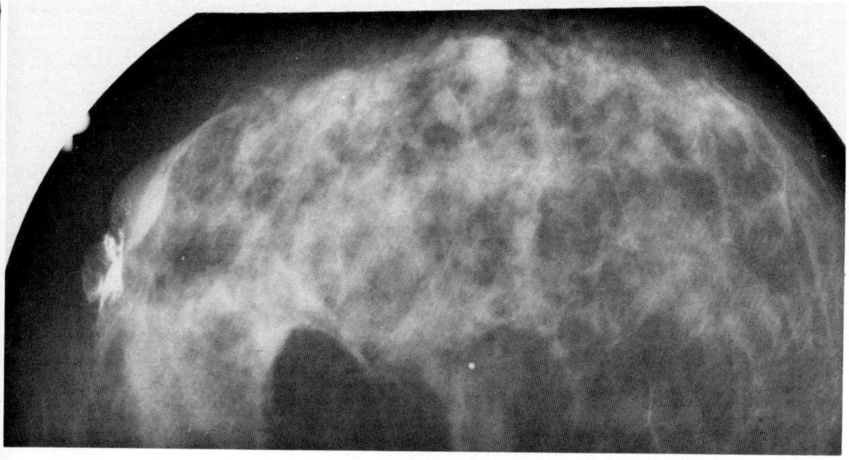

FIGURE 3-41. Cranial-caudal view showing dye adjacent to calcifications.

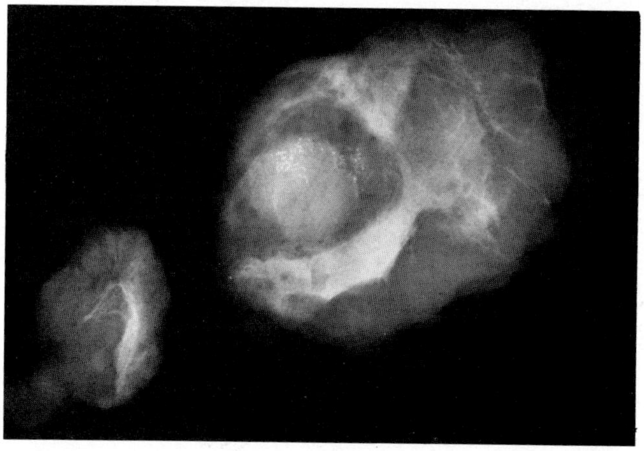

FIGURE 3-42. An X-ray study of the specimen removed from the breast shown in Figures 3-40 and 3-41, showing calcifications. Pathologic studies revealed multifocal, intraductal carcinoma.

may be injected. If mixed with iodinated contrast material, the position of the dye relative to the lesion may be confirmed radiographically. If the biopsy is then performed promptly, the stained tissue containing the lesion can be excised.[93] As shown in two views in Figures 3-40 and 3-41, the relationship between the dye and the suspicious calcifications can be determined. The contrast material is rapidly absorbed, but the surgeon knows that the vital dye is in the same location (and thus has the same spatial relationship to the abnormal area). Specimen radiography (Fig. 3-42) confirms the presence of the lesion in the excised tissue. Pathologic studies of these calcifications indicated multifocal, intraductal carcinoma.

Some surgeons prefer to place the needle within or in close proximity to the lesion to be excised (Figs. 3-43 and 3-44). This permits a thick target, and the stiffness of the needle may be used to facilitate reaching the tissue volume in question. The disadvantage of this technique lies in the possibility that the needle tip will be displaced from the lesion by movement of the breast. In some instances, the needle may back completely out of the breast,

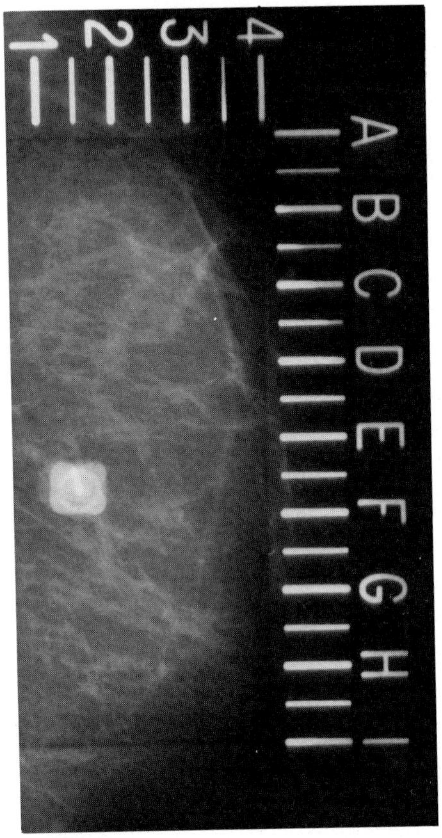

FIGURE 3-43. Using mammographic guidance, a needle is placed directly through or beside the lesion in question. In this figure, a small density is obscured by the hub of the needle that is superimposed on the shaft in the direction of the x-ray beam.

eliminating the necessary guidance. A spring hookwire system has been devised that can be placed accurately in the tumor. This provides a relatively stable, anchored guide for the surgeon[94] (Fig. 3-45).

The method of positioning the needle is similar for all of the guides available.[95] The shortest distance to the lesion is defined by mammography. Utilizing specially designed fenestrated compression plates, the X and Y coordinates of the lesion are directly visible with the breast in the mammographic device (Fig. 3-46). The needle is passed in the direction of the beam in an effort to pierce the lesion or to pass as close as possible to the tissue to be removed. Using this technique, the shaft of the needle should always be within 5 mm of the lesion. If a straight needle technique is employed, the needle should be longer than the depth of the lesion from the skin puncture site with the breast in a relaxed position. This avoids the possibility of the lesion slipping from the needle. If the hookwire system is employed, the needle may be withdrawn to the desired depth and the hookwire engaged. The surgeon then has the option of following wire or needle from the skin entrance site to the lesion or dissecting back from a circumareolar approach. However, when a malignant mass is suspected, an incision over the lesion facilitates complete removal and subsequent definitive therapy, whether it be by breast preservation or mastectomy.

Excision of lesions detected on mammography requires only the removal of a small volume of tissue surrounding the lesion. If the abnormality proves to be benign, there should be virtually no cosmetic defect apparent.

Once the lesion has been removed, it should immediately be radiographed, using mammographic compression, to confirm the presence of the abnormality within the tissue sample. This is especially true when the radiographic abnormality involves clustered microcalcifications. The surgeon should then submit the intact specimen for

FIGURE 3-44. Placement of the needle is assessed with the x-ray beam perpendicular to the shaft of the needle, demonstrating that the lesion has been "skewered" by the needle shaft. Note that the needle should be longer than the depth of the lesion to ensure that the lesion does not slip off the shaft. (Reprinted with permission from Kopans DB, et al: Springhook wire breast lesion localizer: Use with rigid compression systems. Radiology 157:537, 1985.)

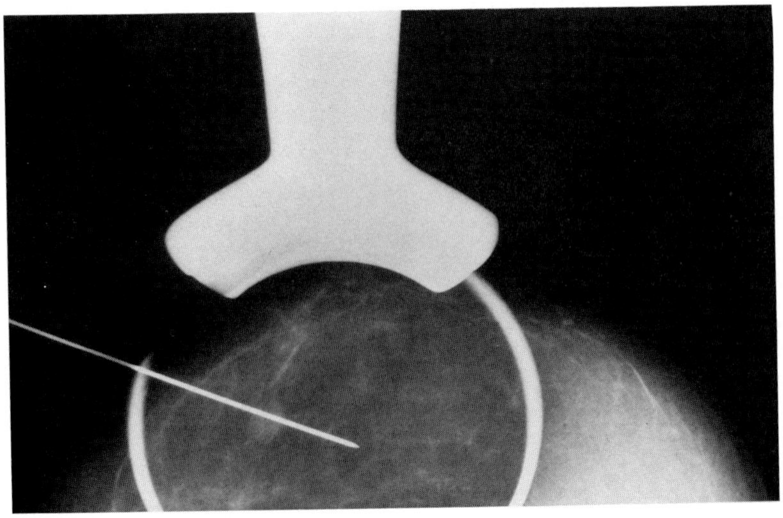

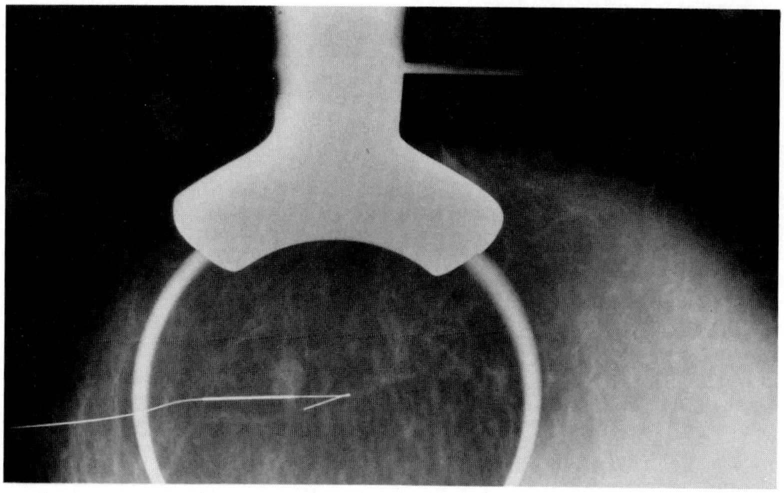

FIGURE 3-45. A springhook wire may be passed through a needle and anchored in the tissue beside the lesion. The needle is then withdrawn, leaving the springhook wire to provide a relatively stable, three-dimensional guide. (Reprinted with permission from Kopans DB, et al: Springhook wire breast lesion localizer: Use with rigid compression systems. Radiology 157:537, 1985.)

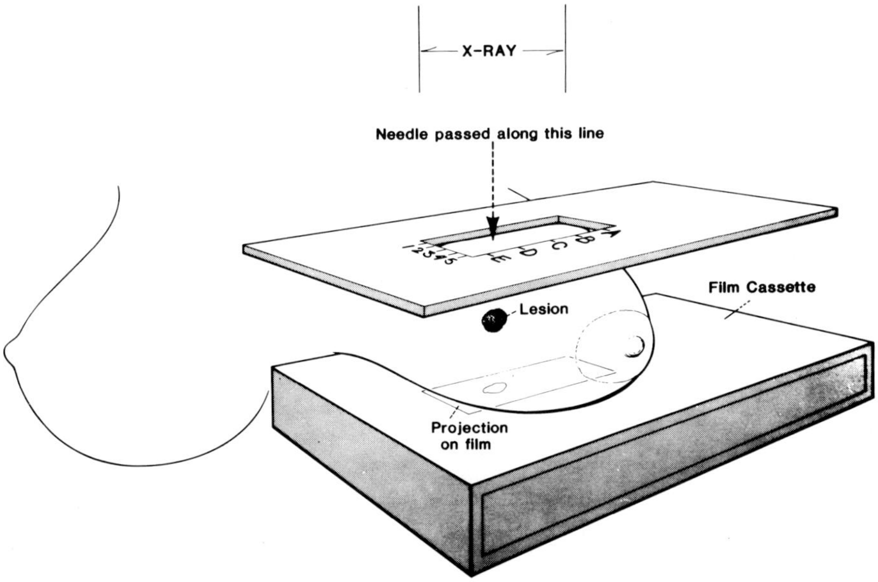

FIGURE 3-46. This is a schematic representation of the direction in which the needle should be passed in an effort to transfix the lesion in question. The compression system is rotated to afford the shortest distance to the lesion.

pathologic study. (The specimen should not be cut into in order to avoid disrupting the pattern of the calcifications.) An x-ray film of the specimen is then compared to the original mammogram to document complete removal of the abnormal area,[96] as shown in Figure 3-42. Close cooperation with the pathologist will help to avoid missing any of the small lesions within the tissue sample. Frozen section analysis may be done. However it is not done routinely, since most lesions detected on mammography are too small for hormone receptor analysis, and the technique of frozen section may miss the lesion completely or, more significantly, may destroy a small cancer, resulting in a missed diagnosis.

In general, needle aspiration biopsy of mammographically detected lesions is not efficacious. Lesions are frequently so small and so mobile within the surrounding tissue that they cannot be pierced by a needle. An aspiration biopsy yielding negative results cannot be trusted, and localization and surgical excision are still required. With positive biopsy results, localization and surgical excision are still required if conservation therapy is to be employed.

Ultrasonography and CT may be used in difficult situations (Fig. 3-47). Ultrasonography may be used to guide the aspiration of cysts that may have defied clinically guided aspiration or that are detected by mammography and cannot be distinguished from malignant processes. Ultrasonography is used to triangulate the lesion; the operator can then utilize this information to aspirate the lesion.[70] Aspiration of such nonpalpable lesions is not necessary if they are clearly demonstrated to be benign cysts on mammography and ultrasonography. If the diag-

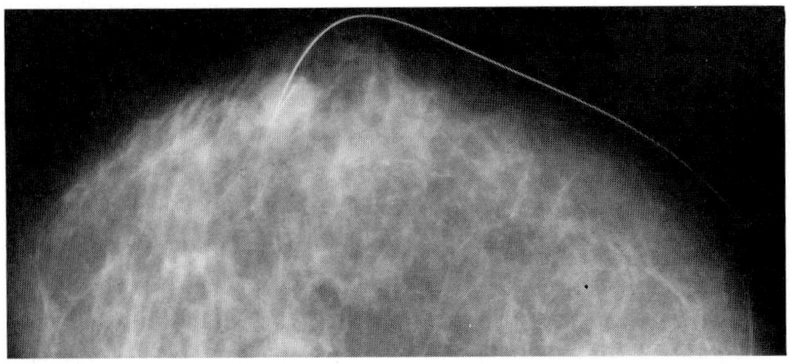

FIGURE 3-47. A wire guide was placed in a nonpalpable mass with the aid of ultrasonographic guidance. This mass was proven at biopsy to be a fibroadenoma.

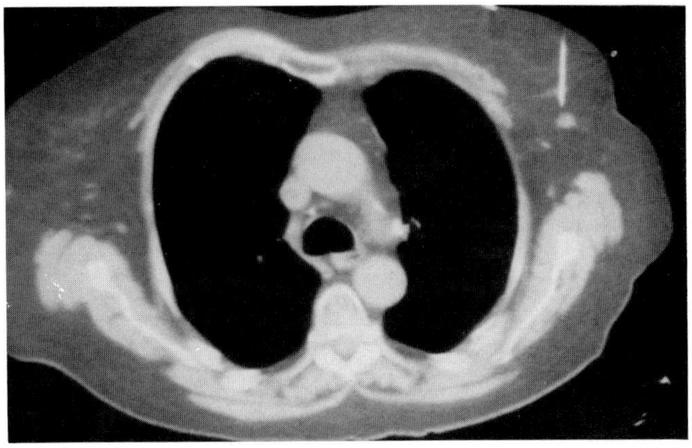

FIGURE 3-48. Computed body tomography was used to localize a nonpalpable, infiltrating ductal carcinoma in the left axilla that could not be localized by any other means.

nosis is questionable and this technique is employed, follow-up mammography within a short period of time is indicated to ensure that a suspicious lesion is not present next to a cyst. Many clinicians would prefer to excise such areas with preoperative needle localization at the outset.

Ultrasonography and CT are useful in the preoperative localization of suspicious lesions that are seen in only one mammographic position.[70,74] Without the information derived from a right-angle view of the tissues in question, the three-dimensional position of a lesion cannot be determined on mammography. Ultrasonography and CT permit evaluation of tissues that are frequently hidden owing to the breast curving around the curving and sloping chest wall (Fig. 3-48).

Accurate localization of clinically occult lesions detected on mammography permits early intervention. Localization and outpatient biopsy are safe techniques that are associated with extremely low morbidity rates. However, careful cooperation between the radiologist, surgeon, and pathologist is mandatory to ensure the success of the technique.

REFERENCES

1. Haagensen CD: Diseases of the Breast. pp 466–477. Philadelphia, WB Saunders, 1971
2. River L, Silverstein J, Grout J, et al: Carcinoma of the breast: The diagnostic significance of pain. Am J Surg 82:733, 1951
3. Corry DC: Pain in carcinoma of the breast. Lancet 1:274, 1952
4. Adair FE: Sanguinous discharge from the nipple and its significance in relation to cancer of the breast. Ann Surg 91:197, 1930
5. Haagensen CD, Stout AP, Phillips JS: Papillary neoplasms of the breast: Benign intraductal papilloma. Ann Surg 133:18, 1951
6. Treves N, Robbins GF, Amoroso WL Jr: Serous and serosanguinous discharge from the male nipple. Arch Surg 73:319, 1956
7. Strawbridge HTG, Bassett AA, Foldes I: Role of cytology in management of lesions of the breast. Surg Gynecol Obstet 152:1, 1981
8. Haagensen CD: Diseases of the Breast, pp 99–148. Philadelphia, WB Saunders, 1971
9. National Institutes of Health: Breast Exams: What You Should Know. NIH Publication No. 84-2000, 1984
10. Foster RS Jr, Lang SP, Costanza MC, et al: Breast self-examination practices and breast cancer stage. N Engl J Med 299:265, 1978
11. Greenwald P, Nasca PC, Lawrence CE, et al: Estimated effect of breast self-examination and routine physician examination on breast cancer mortality. N Engl J Med 299:271, 1978
12. Foster RS Jr, Costanza MC: Breast self-examination practices and breast cancer survival. Cancer 53:999, 1984
13. Huguley CM, Brown RL: The value of breast self-examination. Cancer 47:989, 1981
14. Sheley JF: Inadequate transfer of breast cancer self-detection technology. Am J Public Health 73:1318, 1983
15. Celentano DD, Holtzman D: Breast self-examination competency: An analysis of self-reported practice and associated characteristics. Am J Public Health 73:1321, 1983
16. Gershon-Cohen J: Breast roentgenology. Am J Roentgenol 86:879, 1961
17. Leborgne R: Diagnosis of tumors of the breast by simple roentgenography. Am J Roentgenol 65:1, 1951
18. Egan RL: Experience with mammography in a tumor institution. Radiology 75:894, 1960
19. Shapiro S: Evidence on screening for breast cancer from a randomized trial. Cancer 39:2772, 1977
20. Wolfe J: Mammography. Radiol Clin North Am 12:189, 1974
21. Bailar JC: Mammography: A contrary view. Ann Intern Med 84:77, 1976
22. Feig SA: Hypothetical breast cancer risk from mammography: A reassuring assessment. Breast 5:2, 1980
23. Hammerstein GR, Miller DW, White DR, et al: Absorbed radiation dose in mammography. Radiology 130:485, 1979
24. The effects on populations of exposure to low levels of ionizing radiation, 1980. Washington, DC, National Academy Press, 1980
25. Fisher B, Slack NH, Bross ID: Cancer of the breast: Size of neoplasm and prognosis. Cancer 24:1072, 1980
26. Baker LH: The Breast Cancer Detection Demonstration Projects: Five-year summary report. CA 32, No. 4:194,198, 1982
27. Shapiro S: Ten- to fourteen-year effects of screening on breast cancer mortality. J Natl Cancer Inst 69:349, 1982
28. Tabar L, Gad A, Holmberg LH, et al: Reduction in mortality

from breast cancer after mass screening with mammography. Lancet 1:829, 1985
29. Spivey GH, Perry BW, Clark VA, et al: Predicting the risk of cancer at the time of breast biopsy. Am Surg 48:326, 1982
30. Meyer JE, Kopans DB, Stomper PC, et al: Occult breast abnormalities: Percutaneous preoperative needle localization. Radiology 150:335, 1984
31. Mayer JE, Kopans DB: Analysis of mammographically obvious carcinomas of the breast with benign results upon initial biopsy. Surg Gynecol Obstet 153:570, 1981
32. Kopans DB, Meyer JE, Cohen OM, et al: Palpable breast masses—The importance of preoperative mammography. JAMA 246:2819, 1977
33. Shrivastava PN: Radiation dose in mammography: An energy-balance approach. Radiology 140:483, 1981
34. Feig S, McLelland R (eds): Breast Carcinoma. New York, Masson, 1983
35. Sickles EA: Mammographic detectability of breast microcalcifications. Am J Roentgenol 139:913, 1982
36. Hammerstein GR, Miller DW, White DR, et al: Absorbed radiation dose in mammography. Radiology 130:485, 1979
37. Pagani JJ, Bassett LW, Gold RH: Efficacy of combined film-screen/xeromammography. Am J Roentgenol 135:141, 1980
38. Schmitt EL, Threatt B: Tumor location and detectability in mammographic screening. Am J Roentgenol 139:761, 1982
39. Martin JE, Moskowitz M, Milbrath JR: Breast cancer missed by mammography. Am J Roentgenol 132:737, 1979
40. Bassett LW, Pagani JJ, Gold RH: Pitfalls in mammography. Radiology 136:641, 1980
41. Lundgren B, Jakobsson S: Single view mammography: A simple and efficient approach to breast cancer screening. Cancer 38:1124, 1976
42. Wolfe JN: Breast parenchymal patterns and their changes with age. Radiology 121:545, 1976
43. Wolfe JN: Risk for breast cancer development determined by mammographic parenchymal pattern. Cancer 37:2486, 1976
44. Wellings SR, Wolfe JN: Correlative studies of the histological and radiographic appearance of the breast parenchyma. Radiology 129:299, 1978
45. Boyd NF, O'Sullivan B, Fishell E, et al: Mammographic patterns and breast cancer risk: Methodologic standards and contradictory results. J Natl Cancer Inst 72:1253, 1984
46. Andersson I, Hildell J, Muhlow A, et al: Number of projections in mammography: Influence on detection of breast disease. Am J Roentgenol 130:349, 1978
47. Meyer JE, Kopans DB: Breast physical examination by the mammographer. Appl Radiol 12:103, 1983
48. Sickles EA: Microfocal spot magnification mammography using xeroradiographic and film-screen recording systems. Radiology 131:223, 1979
49. Egan RL, McSweeney MB, Sewell CW, et al: Intramammary calcifications without an associated mass in benign and malignant disease. Radiology 137:1, 1980
50. Sickles EA: Mammographic features of 300 consecutive nonpalpable breast cancers. Presented at the annual meeting American Roentgen Ray Society, Boston, Mass, 1985
51. Cohen MI, Matthies HJ, Mintzer RA, et al: Indurative mastopathy: A cause of false positive mammograms. Radiology 155:69, 1985
52. Hoeffken W, Lanyi M: Mammography. In Rigler LG, Arndt RD, (trans): Rontgenunterschung der Brust mamograph: technique, diagnosis, differential diagnosis, results. Philadelphia, WB Saunders, 1977
53. Meyer JE, Kopans DB, Lawrence WD: Normal intramammary lymph nodes presenting as occult breast masses. Breast 8, No. 1:30, 1982
54. Mayer JE, Kopans DB: Stability of a mammographic mass: A false sense of security. Am J Roentgenol 137:595, 1981
55. Moskowitz M, Feig SA, Cole-Beuglet C: Evaluation of new imaging procedures for breast cancer: Proper process. Am J Roentgenol 140:591, 1984
56. Moskowitz M, Milbrath J, Gartside P, et al: Lack of efficacy of thermography as a screening tool for minimal and Stage 1 breast cancer. N Engl J Med 295:249, 1976
57. Lawson R: Implications of surface temperatures in the diagnosis of breast cancer. Can Med J 75:309, 1956
58. Gautherie M: Thermobiological assessment of benign and malignant breast diseases. Am J Obstet Gynecol 147:861, 1983
59. Feig S, Shaber GS, Schwartz G, et al: Thermography, mammography, and clinical examination in breast cancer screening. Radiology 122:123, 1977
60. Gautherie M, Gros CM: Breast thermography and cancer risk prediction. Cancer 45:51, 1980
61. Jones CH, Greening WD, Davey JB, et al: Thermography of the female breast: A five year study in relation to the detection and prognosis of cancer. Br J Radiol 48:532, 1975
62. American College of Radiology: College policy reviews use of thermography. American College of Radiology Bulletin 40:13, 1984
63. Kopans DB, Meyer JE, Lindfors KK: Whole breast ultrasound imaging—four year follow-up. Radiology 157:505, 1985
64. Sickles EA, Filly RA, Callen PW: Breast cancer detection with sonography and mammography: Comparison using state-of-the-art equipment. Am J Roentgenol 140:843, 1983
65. Cole-Beuglet C, Goldberg BG, Kurtz AB, et al: Ultrasound mammography: A comparison with radiographic mammography. Radiology 139:693, 1981
66. Egan RL, Egan KL: Detection of breast carcinoma: Comparison of automated water-path whole breast sonography, mammography, and physical examination. Am J Roentgenol 143:493, 1984
67. Kobayshi T: Ultrasonic diagnosis of breast cancer. Ultrasound Med Biol 1:383, 1975
68. Cole-Beuglet C, Goldberg BB, Kurtz AB, et al: Clinical experience with a prototype real-time dedicated breast scanner. Am J Roentgenol 139:905, 1982
69. Kopans DB, Meyer JE, Steinbock RT: Breast cancer: The appearance as delineated by whole breast water-path ultrasound scanning. J Clin Ultrasound 10:313, 1982
70. Kopans DB, Meyer JE, Lindfors KK, et al: Breast sonography to guide cyst aspiration and wire localization of occult solid lesions. Am J Roentgenol 143:489, 1984
71. Sickles EA, Filly RA, Callen PW: Benign breast lesions: Ultrasound detection and diagnosis. Radiology 151:467, 1984
72. Cutler M: Transillumination as an aid in the diagnosis of breast lesions: With special reference to its value in cases of bleeding nipple. Surg Gynecol Obstet 48:721, 1929
73. Bartrum RJ, Crow HC: Transillumination light-scanning to diagnose breast cancer: A feasibility study. Am J Roentgenol 142:409, 1984
74. Sickles EA: Breast cancer detection with transillumination and mammography. Am J Roentgenol 142:841, 1984
75. Marshall V, Williams DC, Smith KD: Diaphanography as a means of detecting breast cancer. Radiology 150:339, 1984
76. Geslein GE, Fisher JR, Delaney C: Transillumination in breast

cancer detection: Screening failures and potential. Am J Roentgenol 144:619, 1985
77. Drexler B, Davis JL, Schofield G: Diaphanography in the diagnosis of breast cancer. Radiology 157:41, 1985
78. Chang CHJ, Nesbit DE, Fisher DR, et al: Computed tomography mammography using a conventional body scanner. Am J Roentgenol 138:553, 1981
79. Kopans DB, Meyer JE: Computed tomography guided localization of clinically occult breast carcinoma—The "N" skin guide. Radiology 145:211, 1982
80. El Yousef SJ, Duchesneau RH, Alfidi RJ, et al: Magnetic resonance imaging of breast. Radiology 150:761, 1984
81. Martin HE, Ellis EB: Biopsy by needle puncture and aspiration. Ann Surg 92:169, 1930
82. Ellis F: Needle biopsy in clinical diagnosis of tumors. Br J Surg 34:240, 1947
83. Somers RG, Young GP, Kaplan MJ, et al: Fine needle aspiration biopsy in the management of solid breast tumors. Arch Surg 120:673, 1985
84. Wanebo HJ, Feldman PG, Morton CW, et al: Fine needle aspiration cytology in lieu of open biopsy in management of primary breast cancer. Ann Surg 199:569, 1984
85. Zajdela A, Ghossein NA, Pilleron JP, et al: The value of aspiration cytology in the diagnosis of breast cancer: Experience at the Fondation Curie. Cancer 35:499, 1975
86. Kline TS, Joshi LP, Neal HS: Fine-needle aspiration of the breast—diagnosis and pitfalls: A review of 3545 cases. Cancer 44:1458, 1979
87. Bell DA, Hajdu SI, Urban JA, et al: Role of aspiration cytology in the diagnosis and management of mammary lesions in office practice. Cancer 51:1182, 1983
88. Malberger E, Toledano C, Barzilai A, et al: The decisive role of fine-needle aspiration cytology in the preoperative work-up of breast cancer. Isr J Med Sci 17:899, 1981
89. Kehler M, Ulbrechtsson U: Mammographic fine needle biopsy of non-palpable breast lesions. Acta Radiol (Diagn) (Stockh) 25:273, 1984
90. Kinne DW, Urban JA: The case against outpatient breast biopsy with delayed operative treatment for breast cancer. In Delaney JP, Carlo R: Controversies in Surgery II, pp 385-435. Philadelphia, WB Saunders, 1983
91. Meyer JE, Kopans DB, Stomper PC, et al: Occult breast abnormalities: Percutaneous preoperative needle localization. Radiology 150:335, 1984
92. Kopans DB: Clinically occult breast lesions and interventional procedures in the breast. In Taveras JB: Radiology. Philadelphia, Lippincott (in press)
93. Horns JW, Arndt RD: Percutaneous spot localization of non-palpable breast lesions. Am J Roentgenol 127:253, 1976
94. Kopans DB, Meyer JE: Versatile spring hookwire breast lesion localizer. Am J Roentgenol 138:586, 1982
95. Kopans DB, Meyer JE, Lindfors KK, et al: Use of the spring hookwire breast lesion localizer with rigid compression mammographic systems. Radiology 157:537, 1985
96. Rosen PP, Snyder RE, Urban JA, et al: Correlation of suspicious mammograms and x-rays of breast biopsies done during surgery. Cancer 31:656, 1973

Breast Cancer Epidemiology, Etiology, and Prevention

4

Epidemiology and Prevention

Anthony B. Miller

Breast cancer is the most common malignancy among women in almost all of Europe, in North America, in much of Latin America, and in Australasia.[1] In many of these populations, it is the leading cause of death for women between the ages of 35 and 54 years, and among women younger than 50 it is almost as common as all cancers combined among men. In many Asian countries where the disease was rare, breast cancer is increasing, and second-generation Asian migrants to the United States have rates approaching those encountered in the native white population.[2] In countries where the disease is common, the evidence is convincing that most of the disease is environmental in origin, using the term *environment* to mean all factors external to humans, including life-style.

DESCRIPTIVE EPIDEMIOLOGY OF BREAST CANCER

Data on the incidence of breast cancer for many countries are found in the volumes *Cancer Incidence in Five Continents*, now published by the International Agency for Research on Cancer, but originally by the International Union Against Cancer.[3–6] Breast cancer shows the highest incidence in women in 94 of the 104 sets of incidence data from different registries and racial groups within registries published in Volume 4 of this series.[6] Table 4-1 provides those cancer registries with data in at least two volumes, the age-standardized incidence of breast cancer, and the rate of change in incidence.

The incidence of breast cancer is increasing in almost all the populations considered, on average around 2% per annum. Within the Nordic countries, the rate of increase in Sweden and Finland (6.9% and 3.9%), where rates were lower than in the other countries, was about double that elsewhere. Rates of increase in England and Wales were close to those in Denmark—Oxford excepted (3.2%). The rise in risk in eastern Europe was generally higher than in western Europe. The greatest increase was recorded in Okayama, Japan (11.3%), but that was over a short time period and could have been due to an increase in efficiency of registration. The increase in Miyagi Prefecture, Japan, was low (0.2%) in contrast to that in Hawaiian Japanese (8.0%). In Alameda County, California, the increase in black women (5.7%) was more than twice as great as in white women. The greatest recorded increase in the United States was in Hispanic women in El Paso (9.0%), although this could have been a definitional problem because in the same registry the rates among whites apparently fell. In Bombay, the rate of increase was low (0.4%), although the smallest increases were in Israel in Jews born in Europe, America, or Israel.

There was a general correlation between the incidence of breast cancer and in the rate of change of incidence over time. In the high-risk populations, the upward trend was in general less steep than in those at low risk. This does not mean, however, that the risk is leveling off, as the high-risk Anglo-Saxon and Scandinavian populations still showed a 1% to 2% annual increase. In several of the low-risk populations, the annual percentage increase appears to be accelerating, hence the upward trend was steeper.

The variation in mortality trends was not as great as in incidence rates (Table 4-2). The high-risk Anglo-Saxon in North America and Australasia showed very little change in mortality, the average annual rate of increase ranging from −0.19% to about 0.4%. The rate of increase, however, varied substantially in western and northern European countries, from 0.1% (Denmark) to 3.2% (Portugal). The largest increase was 15%, in Poland. In Japan, the increase was moderate (1.9%). In several other countries

Table 4-1
Incidence of Breast Cancer per 100,000 in Various Countries (Age Standardized to World Population) and Mean Annual Rate of Change

Registry	Midyear	Rate	Midyear	Rate	Rate of Change	
Brazil, Sao Paulo	1969	47.3	1973	56.2	2.22	(4.7%)
Canada						
Alberta	1961	51.2	1975	66.6	1.10	(2.1%)
British Columbia	1970/71	80.0	1975	72.8	−1.60	(−2.0%)
Manitoba	1961	58.5	1975	71.4	0.92	(1.6%)
Maritime provinces	1970/71	58.6	1975	60.3	0.38	(0.6%)
New Brunswick	1963	51.5	1965/66	53.0	0.60	(1.2%)
Newfoundland	1961	37.4	1975	49.6	0.87	(2.3%)
Quebec	1964/65	48.7	1975	63.2	1.38	(2.8%)
Saskatchewan	1961	57.4	1975	62.6	0.37	(0.6%)
Columbia, Cali	1963	31.6	1974	33.2	0.14	(0.4%)
Cuba	1970	28.0	1975	28.5	0.10	(0.4%)
Denmark	1955	43.8	1974/75	58.5	0.77	(1.8%)
Finland	1960	26.3	1973/74	40.1	1.02	(3.9%)
German Dem. Rep.	1965	28.6	1975	37.4	0.88	(3.1%)
Germany, Fed. Rep. Hamburg	1961	37.8	1975	55.7	1.28	(3.4%)
Germany, Fed. Rep. Saarland	1970	50.6	1975	57.2	1.32	(2.6%)
Hawaii						
Hawaiian	1962	52.3	1975	87.5	2.69	(5.1%)
White	1962	62.9	1975	85.6	1.75	(2.8%)
Chinese	1962	44.3	1975	55.3	0.85	(1.9%)
Filipino	1962	19.5	1975	25.7	0.48	(2.5%)
Japanese	1962	23.0	1975	47.1	1.85	(8.0%)
Hungary						
Szabolcs	1964	17.3	1975	20.6	0.30	(1.7%)
Vas	1964	21.4	1975	29.2	0.71	(3.3%)
India, Bombay	1965	20.4	1974	21.2	0.09	(0.4%)
Israel all Jews	1963	44.9	1974	59.9	1.36	(3.0%)
Born Israel	1963	53.6	1974	54.0	0.04	(0.1%)
Born Eur. Am.	1963	60.8	1974	61.7	0.08	(0.1%)
Born Afr. Asia	1963	26.7	1974	34.3	0.69	(2.6%)
Non-Jews	1963	11.0	1974	11.0	0.00	(0.0%)
Jamaica, Kingston	1960/61	31.1	1975	39.0	0.54	(1.7%)
Japan						
Miyagi	1959/60	16.8	1975	17.5	0.04	(0.2%)
Okayama	1966	12.4	1969	16.6	1.40	(11.3%)
Osaka	1970/71	12.1	1975	12.7	0.13	(1.1%)
New Zealand						
Maori	1964	48.2	1974	64.1	1.59	(3.3%)
Non-Maori	1964	50.2	1974	62.6	1.24	(2.5%)
Nigeria, Ibadan	1961	16.8	1964/65	15.3	−0.42	(−2.5%)
Norway	1960	39.0	1975	49.6	0.71	(1.8%)

continued

outside Europe not included in Table 4-2, the increase in mortality has been large. At the upward end of the range, with more than 5% annual increase, were Singapore, Puerto Rico, and Greece, all currently low-risk areas.

Comparison of trends in incidence and mortality may disclose some of the factors responsible for changes in risk. In the United States, Canada, New Zealand, and Scandinavia, a large increase in incidence was associated with a very small increase in mortality. If there was no improvement in the results of treatment, then only about 1 in 10 of the "excess" cancers compared with the beginning of the 1950s was lethal. This would strongly suggest that there was a major change in the diagnosis and definition of breast cancer. Although such changes might be expected in countries that had adopted large-scale screening programs (because of factors such as lead time and overdi-

Registry	*Midyear*	*Rate*	*Midyear*	*Rate*	*Rate of Change*	
Poland						
Cieszyn	1970	18.5	1975	18.9	0.08	(0.4%)
Cracow	1965/66	18.8	1970	19.6	0.18	(1.0%)
Katowice	1965/66	17.0	1973/74	23.8	0.85	(5.0%)
Warsaw city	1965/66	28.4	1975	36.5	0.85	(3.0%)
Warsaw rural	1970	15.3	1975	17.7	0.48	(3.1%)
Puerto Rico	1962/63	16.1	1975	29.5	1.07	(6.6%)
Rhodesia, Bulawayo African	1965	35.5	1970	33.1	−0.48	(−1.4%)
Singapore						
Chinese	1956	10.2	1975	21.9	0.62	(6.1%)
Malay	1970	17.6	1975	14.7	−0.58	(−3.3%)
Indian	1970	25.5	1975	28.2	0.54	(2.1%)
Spain, Zaragoza	1970	30.6	1975	36.5	1.18	(3.9%)
Sweden	1960	29.1	1973	55.2	2.01	(6.9%)
Switzerland, Geneva	1971	70.6	1975	76.1	1.38	(2.0%)
United Kingdom						
Birmingham	1961	46.8	1974/75	56.4	0.71	(1.5%)
Oxford	1964/65	44.0	1975/76	59.3	1.39	(3.2%)
Liverpool	1961	40.4	1970	50.8	1.16	(2.9%)
Southern metropolitan	1961	46.7	1969	48.0	0.16	(0.3%)
Southwestern	1961	44.0	1968	52.1	1.16	(2.6%)
Sheffield	1964/65	46.4	1968/69	49.6	0.80	(1.7%)
United States						
Alameda white	1962	62.4	1975	78.3	1.22	(2.0%)
Alameda black	1962	38.6	1975	67.2	2.20	(5.7%)
Bay area						
White	1971	79.9	1975	83.7	0.95	(1.2%)
Black	1971	57.9	1975	64.1	1.55	(2.7%)
Chinese	1971	44.0	1975	56.8	3.20	(7.3%)
Connecticut	1961	59.3	1975	77.9	1.33	(2.2%)
Detroit						
White	1970	65.7	1975	71.3	1.12	(1.7%)
Black	1970	51.0	1975	62.5	2.30	(4.5%)
Texas, El Paso						
Spanish	1963	34.0	1969	52.3	3.05	(9.0%)
Other white	1963	61.2	1969	53.8	−1.23	(−2.0%)
New Mexico						
Spanish	1970/71	32.4	1975	42.2	2.18	(6.7%)
Other white	1970/71	73.8	1975	78.7	1.09	(1.5%)
Am. Indian	1970/71	26.2	1975	19.3	−1.53	(−5.8%)
New York State	1960	49.1	1975	75.5	1.76	(3.6%)
Utah	1968	56.9	1975	63.8	0.99	(1.7%)
Yugoslavia, Slovenia	1958	21.3	1974/75	34.2	0.78	(3.7%)

agnosis bias, described further in Chapter 5), the increase in incidence in these countries largely preceded the interest that later developed in them in screening for breast cancer. Nevertheless, it seems likely that the changes can be attributed to greater care in the detection and diagnosis of breast abnormalities, with more surgical biopsies performed and more extensive pathologic examination of resected material. However, it would seem that these extra cancers do not have the same biologic potential to cause death.

In countries like the Federal Republic of Germany, Finland, Israel, and Japan, the relative increase in incidence was about two times that in mortality. This implies an average lethality for breast cancer of about 50%. A large increase in mortality compared with incidence was noted in some other countries. This may reflect problems in

Table 4-2
Mortality From Breast Cancer per 100,000 in Various Countries (Age Standardized to World Population) and Mean Annual Rate of Change

Country	*Rate 1950–51*	*Rate 1978–79*	*Rate of Change*
Australia	19.37	18.86	−0.03 (0.1%)
Austria	14.28	18.71	0.25 (1.7%)
Belgium	19.04*	25.49†	0.48 (2.5%)
Canada	22.10	22.77	0.04 (0.2%)
Chile	7.66	11.40	0.21 (2.7%)
Denmark	24.36	24.74	0.02 (0.1%)
Finland	10.73	14.87	0.23 (2.1%)
France	12.73	18.10	0.30 (2.3%)
Germany, Fed. Rep.	14.72	20.52	0.32 (2.2%)
Ireland	17.50	26.54†	0.46 (2.6%)
Israel	16.89	23.20	0.35 (2.1%)
Italy	12.27	18.48†	0.36 (2.9%)
Japan	3.97	5.23	0.07 (1.9%)
Netherlands	23.28	25.79	0.14 (0.6%)
New Zealand	22.80	24.42	0.09 (0.4%)
Norway	17.32	19.05	0.10 (0.6%)
Poland	4.9‡	13.95	0.75 (15%)
Portugal	10.54‡	14.54	0.33 (3.2%)
Sweden	15.83	18.07	0.12 (0.8%)
Switzerland	21.24	23.78	0.14 (0.7%)
United Kingdom			
England and Wales	23.19	27.74	0.25 (1.1%)
Northern Ireland	19.93	25.23	0.29 (1.5%)
Scotland	22.01	27.61	0.31 (1.4%)
United States			
White	21.30	22.19†	0.05 (0.2%)
Nonwhite	18.06	21.17†	0.18 (1.0%)

*1954–1955
†1978 only
‡1956–1957

registration of new cases, improvements in death certification, or lack of comparability between the subpopulation covered by cancer registration and the total population.

Age-Specific Effects

Although in most countries the incidence of breast cancer rises throughout life, the rate of increase in incidence is substantially different before and after the menopause. Figure 4-1 provides two examples of age-specific incidence curves from the United States—Los Angeles whites (non-Hispanic) and blacks (data from 1972–1977), one from Miyagi, Japan (1973–1977), and one from Finland (1971–1976). Rates have in general been rising faster in U.S. blacks than whites (Table 4-1), and Figure 4-1 indicates that the rates in Los Angeles blacks at ages 30 to 39 are now higher than in whites although lower at all other ages, with the greatest gap at the postmenopausal years.

The rates in the Japanese Prefecture of Miyagi are lower at all ages than in Finland or in Los Angeles whites and blacks, and the rates in postmenopausal women do not increase with increasing age, in contrast to Finland and Los Angeles. This difference in the shape of the age-specific curves was originally interpreted by de Waard[7] as evidence for two types of breast cancer, one hormonally induced premenopausally and one nutritionally induced largely postmenopausally. However, examination of temporal trends in breast cancer showed that the differences were largely due to cohort effects, with women contributing to the age-specific rates at younger ages in Japan and to a lesser extent in Finland, having a greater expected lifetime risk of breast cancer than older women from earlier birth cohorts. Thus, contrary to previous interpretations, the effect of age in Japan is very similar to the effect in the West.[8] Analysis of increasing trends of incidence in Iceland during this century also showed that these were interpretable by increases in risk of breast cancer in successive birth cohorts. Thus, the shape of the age-specific incidence curves changed from a "Japanese" to a "western" type of pattern over about 50 years.[9]

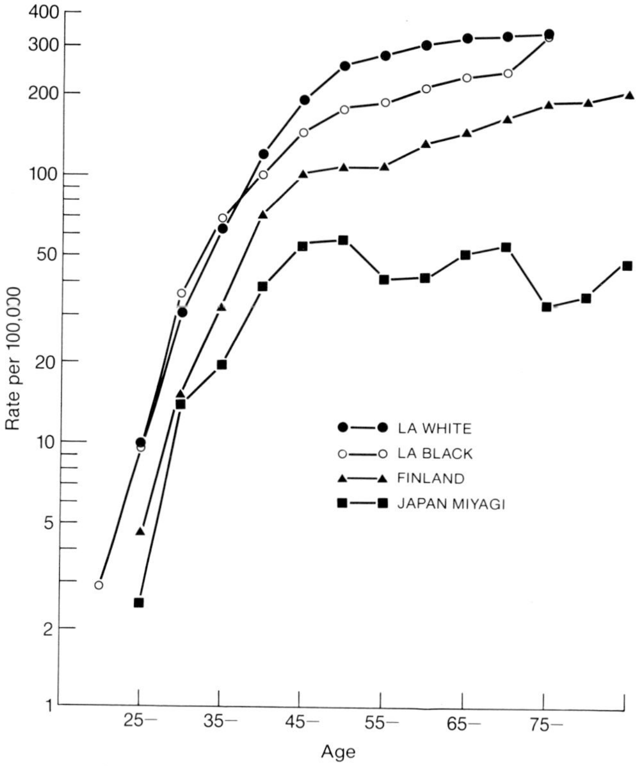

FIGURE 4-1. Examples of age-specific incidence curves for breast cancer.

Projected Incidence and Mortality for Breast Cancer

It is of interest to consider the possible magnitude of the problem of breast cancer in the year 2000, the year chosen by the World Health Organization as a target for "Health for All." The simplest approach is to assume that the latest observed (or estimated) incidence or mortality rates will apply to the world population at the year 2000, using the population projection of the United Nations (1985). Table 4-3 gives the result of these projections for incidence. For many regions, the current observed incidence rates are most likely underestimates and are to be viewed as minimum incidence rates.

The incidence of breast cancer in women is increasing. Assuming a 2% to 3% overall rate of continued increase, the annual number of new cases diagnosed in the year 2000 in the world will probably be between 1.1 and 1.4 million.

HORMONAL RISK FACTORS FOR BREAST CANCER

It has long been recognized that single and nulliparous women are at increased risk of breast cancer.[11–13] However, not until the large international study by MacMahon and colleagues[14] was it recognized that the major factor was the age at which a woman had her first birth. Those with first full-term birth before the age of 20 were at lowest risk, those with first full-term birth after the age of 30 had about a twofold increased risk, and there was a suggestion that those with first birth after the age of 35 had a greater risk than those who had never borne children (Table 4-4). In between, there appeared to be a smooth increase in risk with increasing age at first birth. There seemed to be little additional effect of parity once parity was controlled for age at first birth but a suggestion that second birth before the age of 25 provided some slight additional protection.

These complex relationships have been evaluated in a number of subsequent studies. Some have shown no association between breast cancer risk and age at first birth,[15,16] some have shown associations that vary according to menopausal status,[17] and some appear to have demonstrated some independent effect of parity over and above the effect of age at first birth.[18,19] Nevertheless, it is now generally accepted that age at first birth is possibly the most important aspect of reproductive behavior that influences breast cancer risk,[20] although the proportion of the international differences in incidence that can be explained by differing distributions of age at first birth is small.[21] Additional risk factors that are relevant to the reproductive life of women and that are related to breast cancer risk are age at menarche and age at menopause. Women with an early age at menarche in most but not all studies are at increased risk of breast cancer, the risk ratio being of the order of 1.5.[22] There appears to be a strong correlation among populations between average age at menarche and breast cancer risk.[23] Women with late age at menopause, *i.e.,* beyond the age of 55 years, also appear to be at increased risk of breast cancer, with a risk ratio on the order of 2.0.[24] In contrast, women who have an artificial menopause associated with removal of the ovaries before the age of 45 and particularly if before the age of 40 have a reduced risk of breast cancer.[24,25] This reduced risk appears to be nullified if substitution by estrogens is practiced.[26] A particularly strong effect of reduced risk with irradiation of the ovaries for cancer of the cervix has also been noted. A 65% reduction in risk was observed for women irradiated before age 40, with the reduction increasing from 50% in the first few years to more than 80% more than 15 years after the radiation exposure.[27]

The possibility that reproductive factors vary in their effect according to the age of the woman as well as her menopausal status has been noted in several studies.[15,17,28] However, in one large case-control study designed to evaluate possible differences in risk factors by menopausal status, few differences were found in reproductive risk factors between premenopausal and postmenopausal women.[29] Nevertheless, one study suggested that women younger than 35 years have an increased risk of breast cancer with an early age at first birth,[30] whereas Janerich[31,32] pointed out that there was a higher incidence of breast cancer in married women up to age 35 to 39 than in those who were single, with the reverse later.

Table 4-3
Projected Numbers of New Cases of Cancer of the Breast and of all Sites in Women in the Year 2000 by WHO Region (in Thousands)

		Breast Cancer	
WHO Region	*All Sites*	*No.*	*% of All Sites*
Eastern Africa	111.3	12.1	11
Middle Africa	48.5	5.8	12
Northern Africa	100.9	22.9	23
Southern Africa	31.8	5.5	17
Western Africa	72.0	9.7	14
Caribbean	28.9	5.4	19
Middle America	74.4	10.0	13
Temperate South America	66.7	14.3	21
Tropical South America	303.6	53.0	18
North America	581.0	160.6	28
China	909.7	70.2	8
Japan	163.0	13.7	8
Other East Asia	87.6	8.6	10
Eastern South Asia	288.1	61.6	21
Middle South Asia	645.2	108.0	17
Western South Asia	57.1	12.3	22
Eastern Europe	177.3	33.6	19
Northern Europe	157.7	37.2	24
Southern Europe	244.4	45.0	18
Western Europe	311.0	74.7	24
Australia & New Zealand	29.3	7.4	25
Melanesia	4.1	0.5	12
Micronesia & Polynesia	0.8	0.1	12
USSR	355.0	46.9	13
World Total	4845.6	819.2	17

(International Agency for Research on Cancer: Cancer, Causes and Controls [in press])

Table 4-4
Risk of Breast Cancer Relative to Age at First Birth Less Than 20 Years in an International Study

	Relative Risk For: Age at First Birth (Years)					
Center	*<20*	*20–24*	*25–29*	*30–35*	*35+*	*Nulliparous*
Boston	1.0	1.7	2.4	2.8	3.6	3.1
Glamorgan	1.0	1.3	1.8	1.9	3.3	2.6
Athens	1.0	1.4	1.5	2.1	2.5	1.8
Slovenia	1.0	0.9	1.2	1.4	1.5	1.2
Sao Paulo	1.0	1.3	1.9	1.7	3.6	2.0
Taipei	1.0	0.8	0.7	1.6	2.0	1.9
Tokyo	1.0	1.9	3.0	3.8	5.3	3.8
All centers	1.0	1.2	1.6	1.9	2.4	2.0

(MacMahon B, Cole P, Lin TM, et al: Age at first birth and cancer of the breast. A summary of an international study. Bull WHO 43:209, 1970)

Although undoubtedly associated with hormonal status, the mechanism for these effects is unclear. One hypothesis, modified from that originally proposed by MacMahon and Cole,[33] is that the duration of time between menarche and first completed pregnancy is critical in terms of exposure of breast tissue to exogenous carcinogenic influences. The longer this interval, the greater the probability that exposure to initiating agents will occur. However, delayed pregnancy, with the strong estrogenic stimulus, may encourage promotion of previously transformed cells. Cairns[34] has suggested that stem cells (in which occur the critical mutations that eventually lead to a clone of cells that becomes cancer) in breast tissue increase in number at the time of puberty but reach a final level at the time of first pregnancy. Pike and colleagues[35] have proposed a mathematical model that expresses the effect of hormonal risk factors in terms of breast tissue aging. The implication of these hypotheses is that the events that relate to the probability of breast cancer developing have to affect the age of menarche, the period from then to the first pregnancy, the timing of the first pregnancy, or the age of menopause, largely at the time of adolescence or early adult life. Whatever the mechanism, changes in fertility as a result of conscious choices by women to delay pregnancy are likely to have a critical effect on breast cancer risk in the future. Accordingly, there has to be concern over potential increases in the incidence of breast cancer in the future, with increases being noted in many countries in age at first birth and in the proportion of women who choose to remain nulliparous.

The influence of uncompleted pregnancies is not clear. Some studies suggest that pregnancies that result in an abortion or miscarriage increase the risk of breast cancer.[15,36] However, the effect if present does not seem to be large.[19]

RADIATION INDUCTION OF BREAST CANCER

Breast cancer incidence has been consistently increased following exposure to external low linear energy transfer (LET) radiation in the Japanese atomic bomb survivors, in patients given radiation for postpartum mastitis, and in patients who had multiple fluoroscopy for management of artificial pneumothorax as treatment for pulmonary tuberculosis.[37] In general, the evidence from these studies is consistent, although a recent large Canadian study appears to suggest that the true dose-response relationship may be linear quadratic rather than linear.[38] Increased risk of breast cancer was not noted in patients given radiation for treatment of cancer of the cervix.[39] However, it would be difficult to unravel an effect of radiation in this group known to be at low risk for breast cancer. A suggestion from the followup of female radium dial workers that internally deposited radium increases the risk of breast cancer[40,41] seems not to have been confirmed by a more detailed analysis of the large cohort of U.S. female radium dial workers.[42]

Sensitivity to radiation induction of breast cancer varies by age at first exposure. Sensitivity may be strongest in childhood,[43] slightly less strong in teenage years and the early twenties, but falling off substantially with increasing age at first exposure so that from about the age of 40 years it is difficult to demonstrate an effect.[38,44] Table 4-5 illustrates this from the two largest series. Apart from those first exposed at ages 0 to 9, where in the Canadian series the ratio is based on a comparison involving only three deaths, the parallel between the two series is very close.

Table 4-5
Relationship of Age at First Exposure to Radiation and Breast Cancer Risk

Age at First Exposure	*Atomic Bomb Series**	*Canadian Fluoroscopy Series†*
0–9	2.4	58.0
10–19	2.0	2.5
20–29	1.6	2.8
30–39	1.2	1.2
40–49	1.1	1.0
50+	1.2	0.0

* Ratio of observed to expected cases for those exposed to 10 or more rad. (Tokunaga M, Land CE, Yamamoto T, et al: Breast cancer among atomic bomb survivors. In Boice JD Jr, Fraumeni JF Jr [eds]: Radiation Carcinogenesis Epidemiology and Biological Significance, pp 45–46. New York, Raven Press, 1984)

† Ratio of death rates from breast cancer for those exposed to 100+ rad relative to the unexposed. (Miller AB, Howe GR, Sherman GJ, et al: The Canadian Study of cancer following multiple fluoroscopies. I. Mortality from breast cancer in women. 1950–1980. [in press] 1986)

A "latent period" for cancer induction by radiation has been well recognized. This, for breast cancer, is generally regarded as about 10 to 15 years. However, recent data show no excess risk in irradiated populations until the exposed individuals have reached the age at which breast cancer begins to rise in nonirradiated populations.[38,45] This suggests that other etiologic factors, possibly influencing later stages of carcinogenesis, play an important role in modulating a radiation effect. Radiation itself seems to act as an early stage carcinogen.[46]

The duration of the effect of radiation in increasing the risk of breast cancer is unknown. So far, no irradiated population has been followed for long enough to know whether risk persists throughout life. Nevertheless, the Canadian fluoroscopy series[38] as well as the atomic bomb studies[44] support an effect lasting at least 35 years from first exposure. Indeed, theoretically, if radiation acts on the early stages of carcinogenesis, increased risk should persist throughout life.[46]

DIET AND BREAST CANCER

Several lines of evidence support the importance of nutritional and dietary factors in the etiology of breast cancer. The first derives from animal experimental studies, which have demonstrated that in the presence as well as in the absence of mammary carcinogens, the incidence of mammary tumors in rats increases substantially with high-fat diets, providing that the diet contains at least a small amount of unsaturated fat.[47]

Descriptive Epidemiologic Evidence

The second type of evidence comes from descriptive epidemiology. Changes in incidence and mortality in Iceland[9] and Japan[48] suggest the effects of changing environmental and possibly dietary factors. Studies of migrants[2,49] show the effects of acculturation including dietary change, usually with a slow change in incidence over several generations. In Japanese migrants to California, the incidence of breast cancer in premenopausal women has now almost reached that of the Caucasian population.[2] Similarly, in Israel, substantial changes are occurring in the rates of cancer at ages 35 to 64 years in groups that have migrated there from Africa and Asia, together with a rise in the incidence in those born in Israel, up to the levels experienced by those born in Europe and America.[50] These changes are occurring almost as rapidly for breast cancer as they are for colorectal cancer. Studies of special religious groups[51,52] also suggest the influence of life-style factors on the etiology of breast cancer. However, cohort studies of religious groups who entered orders or changed to a special group in adult life have not shown lower breast cancer rates than expected from the general population. This is true for Adventist women in California,[53] as well as members of strict religious orders in Britain who eschew or eat very little meat.[54] This suggests either that dietary factors in these groups operated before adult life or that the use of high-fat dairy products in substitution for meat maintained a total fat intake similar to normal. Kinlen[54] attempted to make an estimate of dietary fat intake in nuns who eat little or no meat, but found no evidence of an association with breast cancer. Kinlen and colleagues[55] also failed to find to find any indication of lower proportions of breast cancer deaths, or for that matter deaths from cardiovascular disease, among members of a vegetarian society. Nevertheless, the fact that changes in incidence of breast cancer in different populations can be related to changes in successive birth cohorts[8,56] supports the possibility that dietary patterns established relatively early in life are critical for subsequent breast cancer risk.

Correlation Studies

The third line of evidence comes from population studies correlating breast cancer incidence and mortality with total dietary fat and other nutrient intake. Such correlations have been noted internationally,[57–60] within Japan[48] as well as within the United States,[61] for total fat intake. Gaskill and colleagues[62] found a positive correlation in the United States between breast cancer mortality and milk, table fats, beef, calories, protein, and fat, and a negative correlation with egg consumption. The associations with milk and egg consumption remained significant when age of first marriage (as an indicator of age at first birth) was controlled. Hems[63] found that age-standardized breast cancer mortality rates for women of 41 countries during 1970–1971 were positively correlated with total fat, animal protein, and animal calories, independently of other components of diet, for 1964. Differences in childbearing appeared to contribute little to the variation of breast cancer mortality rates between countries. Hems[64] subsequently evaluated changes of breast cancer mortality for women in England and Wales between 1911 and 1975 in relation to changes in the consumption of fat, sugar, and animal protein one to two decades earlier. The association was strongest for fat and sugar intake one decade earlier. The mortality changes were not related to changes in childbearing.

Schrauzer and colleagues[65,66] postulated an inverse relationship between mortality from breast and colon cancer and the consumption of cereals and seafoods. There appeared to be a direct correlation between these cancers and a high intake of fat, sugar, and meat.[67] Schrauzer suggested that food consumption patterns reflected the selenium content of the diets consumed, and he postulated a negative correlation between the selenium intake of population groups and their mortality from cancer.

Nutritionally Associated Risk Factors for Breast Cancer

The fourth, indirect line of evidence comes from the effect of certain risk factors for breast cancer that are themselves probably nutritionally mediated. These are particularly weight, height (and the related indices of body mass dependent on height and weight), and age at menarche.

Obesity and Body Mass

Wynder and colleagues[68] suggested that stocky, and, in particular, somewhat obese women, have a slightly higher chance of developing breast cancer than those of slimmer body build. However, Wynder[69] later pointed out that women in a low socioeconomic class have three to four times more obesity than women in a high socioeconomic class. After matching for socioeconomic factors, he found no clear association between obesity and breast cancer.

Brinkley and colleagues[70] attempted an anthropometric evaluation of the possibility that breast cancer is associated with a particular body type. Weight, sitting height, and biacromial–bi-iliac ratio were among the variables significant in the analysis, which discriminated the cases from the controls, and it was concluded that women with breast cancer tend to be more masculine in type.

In some of the centers in an international collaborative case-control study, an association was found between height, weight, and breast cancer. In Athens,[71] increasing risk was found with increasing height and weight, and with the index weight/height^2. Adjustment for variables associated with height and weight (including schooling as an index of socioeconomic status) failed to abolish this effect. The authors concluded that both height and weight have independent associations with breast cancer risk, the tallest and heaviest deciles of the population having almost twice the risk experienced by the shortest and lightest deciles.

In Sao Paulo,[72] an association of increasing risk with increasing weight was found in women age 50 years or older only, and not in women age 20 to 49. This association was reduced, but not abolished, when the index weight/height^2 was used to control for height.

In a parallel study in Taiwan,[73] there was a significant association of increasing risk with increasing weight, but not for height. Women weighing more than 55 kg (121 lb) had more than twice the breast cancer risk of women weighing less than 45 kg (99 lb). There was a suggestion of a stronger effect of weight in women older than 50 years.

The hypothesis that breast cancer in postmenopausal women was associated with obesity through a hormonal mechanism was proposed by de Waard and colleagues,[74] based on cytologic studies of the vaginal smears of obese postmenopausal women that suggested continuing estrogenic activity. They studied 108 patients with breast cancer and 571 women from the general population. Obesity was defined as a body weight more than 25% above ideal weight. In women age 55 or older, 71% of those with breast cancer were obese compared with 54% of the controls, a significant difference.

de Waard subsequently refined his hypothesis to postulate two types of breast cancer.[75] He suggested that one, occurring largely in premenopausal women, is connected with an endocrine imbalance in which the ovarian hormones are involved; the other, largely occurring in postmenopausal women, has as its major determinant altered hormonal homeostasis related to overnutrition. This hypothesis was supported by a prospective study of 7259 postmenopausal women observed on average for 5.4 years and in whom 70 cases of breast cancer occurred.[76] Increasing risk with both increasing weight and increasing height was found, with women weighing 70 kg (154 lb) or more and 165 cm (5 ft 5 in) or more in height having 3.6 times the risk of women weighing less than 60 kg (132 lb) and less than 160 cm (5 ft 3 in) in height. However, using Quetelet's index (weight [in cm] divided by the square of the height [in kg]) as a measure of degree of overweight as a correction for height removed a large degree of the risk. Therefore, de Waard[77] modified his hypothesis to postulate that body mass rather than overweight (obesity) was the risk factor.

In a further study, de Waard and colleagues[78] evaluated the effect of weight and height on the age-specific incidence of breast cancer using data from the Netherlands and Japan. They computed age-specific curves for different height and weight groups. There was a divergence of the curves in postmenopausal women, with the heavier and taller women showing higher incidence levels. There appeared to be little independent effect for weight if there was an adjustment for its correlation with height. de Waard[77] suggested that lean body mass may be the important variable. However, if height is critical (and it is critical to the calculation of lean body mass), the relevant nutritional factors must begin to operate in adolescence or earlier, rather than in adult life, as was pointed out by MacMahon.[79] de Waard and colleagues[78] suggested that about one-half of the differences in incidence between Holland and Japan could be attributed to differences in body weight and height.

In a case-control study of 400 cases of breast cancer and 400 neighborhood controls in Canada, there was found to be hardly any effect of height, but there was an effect of weight in postmenopausal women when assessed (by questionnaire recall) 12 months before diagnosis and at the time of menopause.[15] The largest difference was in a small group of cases and controls age 70 years or older. There were no differences between premenopausal cases and controls. Later we attempted to replicate these findings in women with breast cancer who were age 65 or older and controls drawn from the population, but we only found a small (and nonsignificant) weight differential, with no greater effect in women age 70 years or older.[80]

Support for the hypothesis of de Waard however, has come from two studies. In a study of 1868 breast cancer patients and 3391 controls in California, lowered risk of breast cancer with higher Quetelet's index was found in premenopausal women.[29] In contrast, in postmenopausal women a markedly higher risk of breast cancer associated with increased Quetelet's index was found. Further, although an estimate of weight gain between age 20 years and interview showed little or no influence on breast cancer risk in the premenopausal women, it was strongly related to risk in postmenopausal women. In a study of 1065 breast cancer patients, 964 surgical and 981 neighborhood controls in Israel, increasing risk of breast cancer was associated with increasing body mass index, especially in women age 60 years or older. Overweight was not a risk factor for premenopausal or younger postmenopausal women. Weight loss during adult life appeared to be protective against breast cancer.[81]

Further, in the long-term prospective study conducted by the American Cancer Society, a significant trend of increasing mortality from breast cancer with increasing weight index was found.[82] For those with a weight index of 140+, there was a mortality ratio of 1.53 in relation to those 90% to 109% of average weight, in contrast to a mortality ratio of 0.82 for those with a weight index of less than 80 (the severely underweight). In addition, in U.S. breast cancer screening program participants, 405 patients with breast cancer identified in the first 2 years were compared with 1156 normal participants.[83] There was increasing risk with increasing weight but little effect of height when adjusted for weight.

Although negative findings have been reported for height and weight and indices of body mass, these tended either to be small studies,[84] used potentially inappropriate controls,[85,86] or were seeking an effect of nutrition using indirect indicators at the population level,[87] an insensitive approach. These studies therefore cannot be regarded as refuting the hypothesis. It may thus be concluded that the bulk of evidence supports the importance of overweight and possibly body mass as a risk factor in postmenopausal women. The evidence is less strong for height, although some studies suggest this as a risk factor, with potential implications for the importance of nutrition in early life.

Age at Menarche

Age at menarche is a risk factor for breast cancer, although the effect is relatively weak.[21,22] Women with an early age at menarche, especially prior to the age of 12, have the highest risk. There is evidence that body weight and food intake are related to early estrus in rats,[88] which supports the hypothesis that a critical body composition of fatness is essential for estrus in the rat, as it appears to be for age at menarche in the human female.[89] Hence the effect of diet and nutrition on breast cancer could be at least partly through age at menarche.[20] Among different populations internationally, the strong correlation between average age at menarche and breast cancer risk supports this possibility.[23]

Other Indirect Indicators of Nutritional Status

Petrakis and colleagues[90] investigated nipple aspirates of breast fluid from nonpregnant healthy women. Cholesterol levels were found to be elevated above plasma levels and to increase with advancing age. Cholesterol epoxide, a carcinogen in animals, was detected in 7 of 17 women, most of whom had high levels of breast fluid cholesterol. Petrakis hypothesized that high dietary fat may increase the level of cholesterol in breast fluid, with local derivation of carcinogenic substances such as cholesterol epoxide.

Direct Assessment of Dietary Factors in Analytic Studies

The final, and presumably most conclusive evidence, should come from studies of diet and nutrition at the individual level, either of the case-control or cohort type. Difficulties with dietary methods have tended to inhibit investigations of this type, but increasing evidence is accumulating.

One case-control study involved 77 breast cancer cases and controls.[91] The cases were discharged from two Adventist-operated hospitals, and the controls, when possible, consisted of two for each case selected from hospitalized cases of hernia and osteoarthritis and a third from the general population of Seventh-Day Adventists. The food questions in the interview were designed to test the hypothesis that high intake of fat, low intake of fiber, or both is associated with risk for breast cancer. Five foods were associated with breast cancer—fried foods in general, fried potatoes, foods fried in hard fats, dairy products except milk, and white bread—with relative risks ranging from 1.6 to 2.6. That for fried potatoes was highest and highly significant.

A second case-control study conducted in four areas of Canada involved 400 newly diagnosed cases and 400 neighborhood controls.[92] Although three different approaches to assessment of diet were used (a 24-hour recall, a 4-day diary, and a detailed quantitative diet history), the final results were derived from the diet history, as this gave a higher response than the diary from the controls and was directed to a period 6 months prior to the time of interview and thus prior to the point of diagnosis of the cases. The mean nutrient intake as estimated by the dietary history alone for six nutrients (total calories, total fat, saturated fat, oleic acid, linoleic acid, and cholesterol) was greater for the cases as a group than for the controls, although the differences were not statistically significant when the premenopausal and postmenopausal groups were considered separately. In a risk ratio analysis, the strongest association in the premenopausal group was for total fat, with weaker associations for saturated fat and cholesterol. When the effect of each nutrient was controlled for the effect of the others, the association for total fat increased in strength while those for saturated fat and cholesterol diminished. In the postmenopausal group, the only consistent finding was for total fat intake. The risk ratios were low (1.6 for total fat in premenopausal women and 1.5 for postmenopausal women), and there was no evidence of a dose-response relationship.

In a reanalysis of these data, Howe[93] found a significant increasing risk with increasing consumption of saturated fat (Table 4-6). This analysis followed the suggestion of Marshall and Graham[94] that increased precision would follow from calculating means of two or more different relatively imprecise methods. Howe[93] combined the data from the 24-hour recall and diet history (6 months before interview). As indicated in Table 4-6, the relative risks for saturated fat intake increased when the data for saturated fat, oleic and linoleic acids, and cholesterol were included simultaneously, whereas the strength of the association and the significance of the trend seemed greater in premenopausal than in postmenopausal women.

Graham and colleagues[95] reported the analysis of food frequency questionnaires administered to 2024 patients with breast cancer and 1463 hospital controls without cancer at Roswell Park Memorial Institute from 1958 to 1965. No association of breast cancer with estimated consumption of animal fat or other dietary factors was found. However, this was a relatively brief questionnaire in which estimates of fat consumption were based on standard portion sizes, and it was not specifically designed to assess the fat hypothesis.

Lubin and colleagues[96] reported the results of a case-control study in northern Alberta involving 577 women between the ages of 30 and 80 years who had breast cancer and were interviewed in 1976–1977, and 826 disease-free controls interviewed subsequently. The questionnaire included information on the frequency with which eight

Table 4-6
Relative Risk Estimates for Estimated Daily Intake of Saturated Fat Based on Mean Values of 24-Hour Recall and Diet History

	Estimated Daily Intake			
	<23.4 g	*23.4–35.4 g*	*>35.4 g*	*p for Trend (Two-Sided)*
All (797) women	1.00	1.27	1.49†	0.028
All (797) women*	1.00	1.70	2.39	0.01
Premenopausal (259) women*	1.00	3.60‡	5.93‡	0.006
Postmenopausal (511) women*	1.00	1.22	1.52	0.358

* Estimates from a model in which intake of saturated fat, oleic and linoleic acids, and cholesterol were included simultaneously.
† p (two-sided) = 0.026
‡ p (two-sided) = 0.01

food items and milk and butter were usually consumed. The major sources of animal fat and animal protein were represented. Using standard portion sizes, estimates of consumption of animal fat were computed. Significant increasing trends of risk with more frequent consumption of beef, pork, and sweet desserts were found. Elevated risks were also noted for the use of butter at the table and for frying with butter and margarine, as opposed to vegetable oils. Risk also increased significantly with increasing indices of consumption of animal fat and animal protein, but not with cholesterol intake.

In an indirect attempt to assess the diet of women with breast cancer, Nomura and colleagues[97] compared the diet of 86 Japanese men whose wives had developed breast cancer with that of the remaining 6774 men in Hawaii who had had dietary data collected in the Japan-Hawaii Cancer Study. They assumed that there is a similarity between the diet of husbands and wives. They found that the husbands of the women with breast cancer consumed more beef or meat, butter/margarine/cheese, corn, and wieners and less Japanese foods than the control spouses.

Preliminary findings from a case-control study in Hawaii have been reported.[98] A positive association between breast cancer risk and the intake of dietary fat (particularly saturated fat) and animal protein in postmenopausal women, especially the Japanese, was noted.

Results from a third case-control study in Canada of diet and breast cancer are now available.[99] In this study, information on frequency of consumption of a limited number of foods was obtained from 846 breast cancer patients and 862 controls using self-administered questionnaires in British Columbia. So far, analyses have only been possible for individual food items and not for nutrients such as total or saturated fat. In premenopausal women, breast cancer risk was increased with recent consumption of foods high in fat content (gravy, beef, pork, whole milk) and reduced with foods low in fat content (fish). In postmenopausal women, risk was increased with pork consumption only. Increased risk was also found for those who consumed visible fat on meat, both recently and in childhood.

Hirayama has been observing a large cohort of Japanese men and women from whom dietary information was collected in the mid 1960s.[100] Associations are now being seen between increased risk of breast cancer and daily consumption of meat (possibly due to higher fat consumption). This is congruent with the increasing incidence and mortality from breast cancer being noted in Japan, as fat consumption has gone up considerably since World War II.

In the report on the study on obesity in Israel,[81] it was noted that an association with dietary fat intake had also been found. The increased risk of breast cancer appeared among women age 50 and older who consumed diets high in fat and animal protein. No correlation was found between overweight and a diet that was high in fat, high in animal protein.

One possible mechanism for the effect of high-fat diets in increasing the risk of breast cancer would be through changes in serum cholesterol plasma lipids. However, prospective studies of women who have had such measurements have failed to find evidence of an association.[101] Nevertheless, if the relevant mechanism is dependent on the levels of fat in the intestine, differences in cholesterol or blood lipids are not only likely to be minimal but irrelevant. Even so, a study of the incidence and mortality of cancer of the breast among women who had previously had total colectomy and terminal ileostomy, mostly for ulcerative colitis or Crohn's disease, failed to find a lower incidence of breast cancer, although there was a slight deficiency of deaths from this cause.[102] These findings suggest that, at least in adult life, the colon may not be involved in the pathogenesis of fat-induced breast cancer.

PREVENTION OF BREAST CANCER

The extent to which prevention of breast cancer is feasible depends on, first, the proportion of breast cancers attributable to various factors and, second, the extent to which women can be persuaded to modify their exposure to these factors. Many studies provide information on the proportion of breast cancers attributable to certain factors; however, it seems unlikely that exposure could be readily altered for all of these, particularly for some hormonally related risk factors. In the following discussion, therefore, we restrict our attention to nulliparity, age at first birth, menopausal estrogens, diet, obesity, and use of antiestrogens.

Nulliparity and Age at First Birth

Miller and colleagues[103] in a study based on data from cancer registries estimated an attributable risk of 1.9% for nulliparity. Two U.S. studies provide data that permit attributable risks for breast cancer in relation to age at first birth to be calculated. Dichotomizing at age 25 years at first birth, the risks in Boston[14] and California[104] were similar. However, although in California the proportion of the controls age 25 years or older at first birth was lower than in Boston, the proportion of nulliparous women was also lower than in Boston. Once attributable risks are related to all breast cancers, the proportion attributable to age 25 or more at first birth was 17% in both areas.

It seems unlikely that all women who plan to have children could be induced to have their first birth before the age of 25 years. Nevertheless, providing information on degree of risk to permit women to make informed choices seems appropriate.

Menopausal Estrogens

Determining the proportion of breast cancers attributable to the use of menopausal estrogens is difficult. One of the studies showing increased risk was based on a cohort of women who had received menopausal estrogens, with comparison made to the general population and with no data on the proportion of women in the general population exposed.[105] Most of the studies were based on selected populations such as screening program participants,[26] retirement communities,[106] or members of prepaid health plans.[107,108] Hence data on exposure in the controls, when provided, is probably not fully representative of the general population but may relate to groups of higher socioeconomic status. Further, the study by Jick and colleagues[107] is only based on cases and controls age 45 to 64, whereas the study by Hoover and associates[105] suggests that much of the risk can be expected in women 15 or more years past the period when use of estrogens for menopausal symptoms began. Nevertheless, some approximation to a possible upper limit of the population-attributable risk can be obtained from two of the studies.

In the study by Ross and colleagues[106] risk was restricted to women with an estimated accumulated dose of conjugated estrogen of 1500 mg or more and to those with intact ovaries. Dichotomizing the population at this level but ignoring ovarian status results in a relative risk of 1.8, an estimate of the proportion of the population exposed of 0.18, and an attributable risk of 12%. If the population is dichotomized into ever/never users of menopausal estrogens, the relative risk falls to 1.1, the estimated proportion of the population exposed increases to 0.49, and the attributable risk becomes 5%. In the study by Hoover and colleagues,[108] risk increased with increasing numbers of prescriptions for menopausal estrogens. Dichotomizing the population into those who had had prescriptions and those who had not results in a relative risk of 1.3, an estimate of the proportion of the population exposed of 0.29, and an attributable risk of 8%.

Diet

A number of different sources of information now support the association of diet, especially high fat in the diet, with risk of breast cancer. Although further work is desirable to clarify the association, the increasing consistency of the evidence derived from the epidemiologic studies and the similar data derived from experimental studies suggest that the association is causal. Indeed, this evidence, together with similar evidence relating to colorectal and other cancers, led a committee of the U.S. National Academy of Sciences[109] to recommend attempts to achieve population reduction of dietary fat intake from the present level of 40% to 30% of available calories. This reduction seems achievable without a major disturbance in dietary habits, is unlikely to be hazardous, and after a period should result in a reduction in the incidence of breast cancer and other fat-associated cancers. It is important that early action be taken to ensure that the population makes appropriate dietary changes. If, as some of the migrant and other descriptive studies suggest, much of the effect of diet and nutrition in increasing the risk of breast cancer operates early in life, there could be a substantial delay before the full impact of primary prevention is seen in the population.[110]

However, clearly more discriminating data are needed on the level of fat intake that should be regarded as optimal. We need to resolve in humans the relative importance of different types of fat, particularly the possible opposed effects of unsaturated and saturated fats. We also need to determine the dose response for cancer induction for total, unsaturated, and saturated fats. Thus we need to answer the question "At what level does further protection from (breast) cancer from lowering fat intake cease?" Does it cease at 30%, as recommended by the National Academy of Sciences (NAS) committee,[109] or should we aim for 25% or even 20% or less? We also need to be concerned about the possibility that adverse effects on health, either through increased incidence of other cancer sites, unexpected effects on cardiovascular disease, and so on, might offset the benefits derived by reducing the incidence of fat-associated cancers.

The NAS Committee on Diet, Nutrition, and Cancer has made recommendations for further research in this area.[111] Further observational analytic epidemiologic studies are clearly needed, both of the case-control and cohort type. Case-control studies could profitably be performed in different populations with differing diets and breast cancer incidence. Cohort studies in which dietary data are collected well in advance of the diagnosis offer the advantage that the dietary information may well be collected at a more relevant time period to the natural history of the cancer, but they also suffer from the disadvantage of less complete dietary information, expense, and long duration of followup required.

Carefully planned intervention studies of dietary factors that may prevent cancer induction should now be initiated in humans. For breast cancer and fat, this will require detailed instruction in the ways to achieve a low-fat diet. Some groups have already initiated pilot studies in this area. Wynder and Cohen[112] have recommended an intervention study of fat reduction in women with Stage II breast cancer, as there is some experimental evidence that supports such an approach in experimental animals. However, a followup of 300 of the cases in our case-control study of diet and breast cancer has failed to find any influence of fat on prognosis of breast cancer, although weight, and possibly obesity in particular, were associated with prognosis.[113] This supports a suggestion by de Waard[114] that weight reduction should be assessed as a means of improving prognosis in women with breast cancer. If intervention studies of reduction in fat intake in women at high risk for breast cancer do proceed, they will have to be carefully planned. They should involve randomization of subjects to experimental and control groups whenever possible. Care will have to be taken to define high risk in a way relevant to the hypothesis under test. Thus it does not seem sensible to define this by, for example, family history. Rather, some attempt should be made to select women at risk by virtue of a high fat intake. The intervention should also be carefully planned to avoid dilution. Thus care will have to be taken to ensure compliance with the intervention in the study group but lack of intervention in the control group. To do this will not be easy, especially if informed consent of all subjects is insisted on. Further, the intervention will not have to be so complex that it would be impossible to use this as an approach to control of breast cancer in the general population subsequently.

This is a formidable list of problems, but care taken in the design stage of a trial will bring dividends later. Some will object to the idea of any trial, suggesting rather that we should act now to advise the public on the actions they should take and monitor the subsequent impact of changes in diet on the cancer rates in the population. Probably both approaches can be supported, yet as the need now is for firmer evidence to justify major shifts of diet in the population, the intervention trial approach would seem to be the most scientifically justifiable.

However, pending the results of such trials, it is still possible to estimate what the possible effect of dietary change might be. In two studies of diet and breast cancer, data were provided that enable population-attributable risks for dietary factors associated with breast cancer to be calculated. On the basis of a case-control study in Canada,[92] Miller[115] computed an attributable risk of 27% for total fat intake. In another study in Canada,[96] although data are not presented to enable attributable risks for fat intake to be estimated, data are available for intake of beef and pork, both strongly associated with fat intake. Dichotomizing the consumption of beef between the authors' levels 4 and 5 and for pork between their levels 3 and 4 results in estimates of attributable risk of 27% and 26%, respectively. Because of the imprecision of dietary methodology, these estimates are likely to be too low rather than too high.[116]

In the United States, objectives for reducing cancer incidence by the year 2000 have been proposed.[117] The dietary objectives proposed to reduce the incidence of breast cancer by 25% and the incidence of other cancers include reduction in fat consumption to 100 g per day, per capita, and reduction in the prevalence of obesity to 5% of the population. Miller,[110] discussing a similar strategy, pointed out that dietary modification might have to start from the age of 5, which could imply a 20-year lag before an effect is observed, and the maximum impact may not be reached for 80 years.

Obesity

A number of studies have pointed to the potential importance of both height and weight in increasing the risk of postmenopausal breast cancer.[29,76,81,82] On the basis of a comparison of breast cancer incidence between the Netherlands and Japan, and using data on height and weight from those populations, de Waard and colleagues[78] estimated that, between the two countries, differences in body weight might explain 37% of the differences in breast cancer incidence and that differences in height might explain 51% of these differences.

A study in California[29] showed a significant effect of an elevated Quetelet's index (weight/height^2) in increasing risk in postmenopausal but not in premenopausal women. From the data presented, an attributable risk for postmenopausal breast cancer of 18% can be estimated for a Quetelet's index of 21.5 or more. In the Bay area of California, the proportion of breast cancer occurring in women older than 55 years is 0.65.[6] Therefore the proportion of breast cancer that might be prevented in that population by reducing obesity is approximately 12%. This is similar to the estimate of 13% made by Miller[115] from the studies by de Waard et al[78] as applied to Canadian data.

As noted above, reduction in the prevalence of obesity has been included in the U.S. strategy for reducing cancer incidence by the year 2000.[117] Miller,[110] however, suggested that although it might be possible to achieve an impact on breast cancer incidence within 5 years by a weight reduction strategy in women age 45 or older, it might take 40 years to achieve a maximum effect.

Antiestrogens

Cuzick and colleagues[118] have suggested that women at high risk for breast cancer should be included in an intervention trial designed to evaluate whether the antiestrogen tamoxifen will reduce breast cancer incidence. Although this agent in clinical practice is relatively free of side effects, these could prove troublesome in premenopausal women who are free of breast cancer. Furthermore, it is such women, especially those with a very strong family history of breast cancer, who are likely to be included in such a trial. Nevertheless, a recent Union Internationale Contre le Cancer (UICC) workshop concluded that a reduction in risk of breast cancer of the order of 30% might be achieved, justifying the testing of the agent in a carefully designed intervention study.[119]

CONCLUSION

As emphasized by a comparison of age-standardized rates by Waterhouse and colleagues,[6] the potential for primary prevention of breast cancer is substantial in those populations with the highest rates. This is as true for those of Japanese stock as it is for those of European. Thus the highest rate in those of European stock is 87.5 in Hawaii whites, the lowest 16.2 in Poland Cieszyn rural, indicating a potential for prevention in Hawaii whites of at least 82%. Similarly, in Los Angeles Japanese the rate is 57.3, in Japan Osaka rural 8.9, indicating a potential for prevention in Los Angeles Japanese of 84%. The main hope for primary prevention seems to be dietary modification, changes that are compatible with primary prevention of colorectal and stomach cancer,[109] aided by reduction in obesity, reduction in use of estrogens at the time of menopause, and possibly some shift back to earlier ages at first birth. The difficulty is the probable long delay before such potentials can be realized.

REFERENCES

1. Parkin DM, Stjernsward J, Muir CS: Estimates of the worldwide frequency of twelve major cancers. Bull WHO 62:163, 1984
2. Dunn JE: Breast cancer among American Japanese in the San Francisco Bay area. Natl Cancer Inst Monogr 47:157, 1977
3. Doll R, Payne P, and Waterhouse J (eds): Cancer Incidence in Five Continents. Berlin, International Union Against Cancer—Springer-Verlag, 1966
4. Doll R, Muir C, Waterhouse J (eds): Cancer Incidence in Five Continents, Vol. 2. Berlin, International Union Against Cancer—Springer-Verlag, 1970
5. Waterhouse J, Muir C, Correa P, et al (eds): Cancer Incidence in Five Continents, Vol. 3. IARC Scientific Publications No. 15. Lyons, International Agency for Research on Cancer, 1976
6. Waterhouse J, Muir C, Shanmugaratnam K, et al (eds): Cancer Incidence in Five Continents, Vol. 4. IARC Scientific Publication No. 42. Lyons, International Agency for Research on Cancer, 1982
7. de Waard F: Premenopausal and postmenopausal breast cancer: One disease or two? J Natl Cancer Inst 65:559, 1980
8. Stevens RG, Moolgavkar SH, Lee JH: Temporal trends in breast cancer. Am J Epidemiol 115:759, 1982
9. Bjarnson O, Day M, Snaedal G, et al: The effect of year of birth on the breast cancer age incidence curve in Iceland. Int J Cancer 13:689, 1974
10. International Agency for Research on Cancer: Cancer, Causes and Control (in press) 1986
11. Logan WPD: Marriage and childbearing in relation to cancer of the breast and uterus. Lancet 2:1199, 1953
12. Mustacchi P: Ramazzini and Rigoni-Stern on parity and breast cancer. Arch Intern Med 108:195, 1961
13. Stocks P: The epidemiology of cancer of the breast. Practitioner 179:233, 1957
14. MacMahon B, Cole P, Lin TM, et al: Age at first birth and cancer of the breast. A summary of an international study. Bull WHO 43:209, 1970
15. Choi NW, Howe GR, Miller AB, et al: An epidemiologic study of breast cancer. Am J Epidemiol 107:510, 1978
16. Adami HO, Hansen J, Jung B, et al: Age at first birth, parity and risk of breast cancer in a Swedish population. Br J Cancer 42:651, 1980
17. Stavraky K, Emmons S: Breast cancer in premenopausal and postmenopausal women. J Natl Cancer Inst 53:647, 1974
18. Tulinius H, Day NE, Johannesson G, et al: Reproductive factors and risk from breast cancer. Int J Cancer 21:724, 1978
19. Brinton LA, Hoover R, Fraumeni JF Jr: Reproductive factors in the aetiology of breast cancer. Br J Cancer 47:757, 1983
20. Miller AB, Bulbrook RD: Special report: The epidemiology and etiology of breast cancer. N Engl J Med 303:1246, 1980
21. MacMahon B, Cole P, Brown J: Etiology of human breast cancer: A review. J Natl Cancer Inst 50:21, 1973
22. Staszewski J: Age at menarche and breast cancer. J Natl Cancer Inst 47:935, 1971
23. Gray GE, Pike MC, Henderson BE: Breast cancer incidence and mortality rates in different countries in relation to known risk factors and dietary practices. Br J Cancer 39:1, 1979
24. Trichopoulos D, MacMahon B, Cole P: Menopause and breast cancer risk. J Natl Cancer Inst 48:605, 1972
25. Lilienfeld A: The relationship of cancer of the female breast to artificial menopause and marital status. Cancer 9:927, 1956
26. Brinton LA, Hoover RN, Szklo M, et al: Menopausal estrogen use and risk of breast cancer. Cancer 47:2517, 1981
27. The Working Group: In Day NE, Boice JD (eds): Second Cancer in Relation to Radiation Treatment for Cervical Cancer. A Cancer Registry Collaboration, pp 137-181. IARC Scientific Publications No. 52. Lyons, International Agency for Research on Cancer, 1983
28. Wynder EL, MacCornack FA, Stellman SD: The epidemiology

of breast cancer in 785 United States Caucasian women. Cancer 41:2341, 1978
29. Paffenbarger RS, Kampert JB, Chang HG: Characteristics that predict risk of breast cancer before and after the menopause. Am J Epidemiol 112:258, 1980
30. Juret P, Couette JE, Brune D, et al: Age at first birth: An equivocal factor in human mammary carcinogenesis. Eur J Cancer 10:591, 1974
31. Janerich DT: Pregnancy, breast cancer risk and maternal fetal genetics. Lancet 1:327, 1979
32. Janerich DT: Pregnancy, breast cancer risk and maternal fetal genetics. Lancet 1:1240, 1979
33. MacMahon B, Cole P: The ovarian etiology of human breast cancer. Recent Results Cancer Res 39:185, 1972
34. Cairns J: Mutation selection and the natural history of cancer. Nature 255:197, 1975
35. Pike MC, Krailo MD, Henderson BE, et al: "Hormonal" risk factors, "breast tissue age" and the age-incidence of breast cancer. Nature 303:767, 1983
36. Pike MC, Henderson BE, Casagrande JT, et al: Oral contraceptive use and early abortion as risk factors for breast cancer in young women. Br J Cancer 43:72, 1981
37. Land CE, Boice JD Jr, Shore RE, et al: Breast cancer risk from low-dose exposure to ionizing radiation. Results of parallel analysis of three exposed populations of women. J Natl Cancer Inst 65:353, 1980
38. Miller AB, Howe GR, Sherman GJ, et al: The Canadian study of cancer following multiple fluoroscopies. I. Mortality from breast cancer in women. 1950–1980 (in preparation)
39. Boice JD, Day NE, Andersen A, et al: Second cancer following radiation treatment for cervical cancer. An international collaboration among cancer registries. J Natl Cancer Inst 74:955, 1985
40. Adams EE, Brues AM: Breast cancer in female radium dial workers first employed before 1930. J Occup Med 22:583, 1980
41. Baverstock KF, Papworth D, Vennart J: Risks of radiation at low dose rates. Lancet 1:430, 1981
42. Stebbings JH, Lucas HF, Stehney AF: Mortality from cancers of major sites in female radium dial workers. Am J Ind Med 5:434, 1984
43. Hildreth N, Shore RE, Hempelmann LH: Risk of breast cancer among women receiving radiation in infancy for thymic enlargement. Lancet 1:273, 1983
44. Tokunaga M, Land CE, Yamamoto T, et al: Breast cancer among atomic bomb survivors. In Boice JD Jr, Fraumeni JF Jr (eds): Radiation Carcinogenesis Epidemiology and Biological Significance, pp 45–46. New York, Raven Press, 1984
45. National Institutes of Health: Report of the National Institutes of Health ad hoc working group to develop radio epidemiologic tables. NIH Publication No. 85–2748. Washington D.C., U.S. Dept. of Health and Human Services, 1985
46. Day NE, Brown C: Multistage models and primary prevention of cancer. J Natl Cancer Inst 64:977, 1980
47. Carroll KK, Hopkins GJ: Dietary polyunsaturated fat versus saturated fat in relation to mammary carcinogenesis. Lipids 14:155, 1979
48. Hirayama T: Changing patterns of cancer in Japan with special reference to the decrease of stomach cancer mortality. In Hiatt HH, Watson JD, Winsten JA (eds): Origins of Human Cancer, pp 55–75. Cold Spring Harbor, NY, Cold Spring Harbor Laboratory, 1977
49. Buell P: Changing incidence of breast cancer in Japanese-American women. J Natl Cancer Inst 51:1479, 1974
50. Steinitz R: Cancer risks in immigrant populations in Israel. In Aoki K (ed): Proceedings of the first UICC Conference on Cancer Prevention in Developing Countries, pp 363–381. Nagoya, University of Nagoya Press, 1982
51. Lyon JL, Gardner JW, West DW: Cancer risk and life-style: Cancer among Mormons from 1967–1975. In Cairns J, Lyon JL, Skolnick M (eds): Cancer Incidence in Defined Populations, Banbury Report 4, pp 3–27. Cold Spring Harbor, NY, Cold Spring Harbor Laboratory, 1980
52. Phillips RL, Kuzma JW, Lotz TM: Cancer mortality among comparable members versus non members of the Seventh Day Adventist Church. In Cairns J, Lyon JL, Skolnick M. (eds): Cancer Incidence in Defined Populations, Banbury Report 4, pp 93–102. Cold Spring Harbor, NY, Cold Spring Harbor Laboratory, 1980
53. Phillips RL, Garfinkel L, Kuzoma JW, et al: Mortality among California Seventh-Day Adventists for selected cancer sites. J Natl Cancer Inst 65:1097, 1980
54. Kinlen LJ: Meat and fat consumption and cancer mortality: A study of strict religious orders in Britain. Lancet 1:946, 1982
55. Kinlen LJ, Herman C, Smith PG: A proportionate study of cancer mortality among members of a vegetarian society. Br J Cancer 48:355, 1983
56. Moolgavkar SH, Day NE, Stevens RG: Two-stage model for carcinogenesis: Epidemiology of breast cancer in females. J Natl Cancer Inst 65:559, 1980
57. Drasar BS, Irving D: Environmental factors and cancer of the colon and breast. Br J Cancer 27:167, 1973
58. Armstrong B, Doll R: Environmental factors and cancer incidence and mortality in difference countries, with special reference to dietary practices. Int J Cancer 15:617, 1975
59. Carroll KK: Experimental evidence of dietary factors and hormone-dependent cancers. Cancer Res 35:3374, 1975
60. Knox EG: Foods and diseases. Br J Soc Prev Med 31:71, 1977
61. Enig MG, Munn RJ, Keeney M: Dietary fats and cancer trends—a critique. Fed Proc 37:2215, 1978
62. Gaskill SP, McGuire WL, Osborne CK, et al: Breast cancer mortality and diet in the United States. Cancer Res 39:3628, 1979
63. Hems G: The contributions of diet and child bearing to breast cancer rates. Br J Cancer 37:974, 1978
64. Hems G: Associations between breast cancer mortality rates, child-bearing and diet in the United Kingdom. Br J Cancer 41:429, 1980
65. Schrauzer GN: Cancer mortality correlation studies. II. Regional associations of mortalities with the consumption of foods and other commodities. Med Hypotheses 2:39, 1976
66. Schrauzer GN, White DA, Schneider CJ: Cancer mortality correlation studies. III. Statistical associations with dietary selenium intakes. Bioinorg Chem 7:23, 1977
67. Schrauzer GN: Selenium and cancer. A review. Bioinorg Chem 5:275, 1975
68. Wynder EL, Bross IJ, Hirayama T: A study of the epidemiology of cancer of the breast. Cancer 13:559, 1960
69. Wynder EL: Identification of women at high risk for breast cancer. Cancer 24:1235, 1969
70. Brinkley D, Carpenter RG, Haybittle JL: An anthropometric study of women with cancer. Br J Prev Soc Med 25:65, 1971
71. Valoras VG, MacMahon B, Trichopoulos D, et al: Lactation and reproductive histories of breast cancer patients in greater Athens, 1965–67. Int J Cancer 4:350, 1969
72. Mirra AP, Cole P, MacMahon B: Breast cancer in an area of high parity. Cancer Res 31:77, 1971
73. Lin TM, Chen KP, MacMahon B: Epidemiologic characteristics of cancer of the breast in Taiwan. Cancer 27:1497, 1971

74. de Waard F, Laive JWJ, Baanders-van Haliwijn EA: On the bimodal age distribution of mammary carcinoma. Br J Cancer 114:437, 1960
75. de Waard F, Baanders-van Haliwijn EA, Huizinga J: The bimodal age distribution of patients with mammary cancer. Cancer 17:141, 1964
76. de Waard F, Baanders-van Haliwijn EA: A prospective study in general practice on breast cancer risk in postmenopausal women. Int J Cancer 14:153, 1974
77. de Waard F: Breast cancer incidence and nutritional status with particular reference to body weight and height. Cancer Res 35:3351, 1975
78. de Waard F, Cornelis JP, Aoki K, et al: Breast cancer incidence according to weight and height in two cities of the Netherlands and Aichi Prefecture Japan. Cancer 40:1269, 1977
79. MacMahon B: Formal discussion of "Breast cancer incidence and nutritional status with particular reference to body weight and height." Cancer Res 35:3357, 1975
80. Burch JD, Howe GR, Miller AB: Breast cancer in relation to weight in women aged 65 years and over. Can Med Assoc 124:1326, 1981
81. Lubin F, Ruder AM, Wax Y, Modan B: Overweight and changes in weight throughout adult life in breast cancer etiology. Am J Epidemiol 122:579, 1985
82. Lew EA, Garfinkel L: Variations in mortality by weight among 750,000 men and women. J Chron Dis 32:563, 1979
83. Brinton LA, Williams RR, Hoover RN, et al: Breast cancer risk factors among screening program participants. J Natl Cancer Inst 62:37, 1979
84. Adami HO, Rimsten A, Stenkvist B, et al: Influence of height, weight and obesity on risk of breast cancer in an unselected Swedish population. Br J Cancer 36:787, 1977
85. Wynder EL, MacGornach FA, Stellman SD: The epidemiology of breast cancer in 875 United States Caucasian women. Cancer 41:2345, 1978
86. Soini I: Risk factors of breast cancer in Finland. Int J Epidemiol 6:365, 1977
87. Hakama M, Soini I, Kuosma E, et al: Breast cancer incidence: Geographical correlations in Finland. Int J Epidemiol 8:33, 1979
88. Frisch RE, Hegsted DM, Yoshinaga K: Body weight and food intake at early estrus of rats on a high fat diet. Proc Natl Acad Sci USA 72:4172, 1975
89. Frisch RE, McArthur J: Menstrual cycles: Fatness as a determinent of minimum weight for height necessary for their maintenance or onset. Science 185:949, 1974
90. Petrakis NL, Gruenke LD, Craig JC: Cholesterol and cholesterol epoxides in nipple aspirates of human breast fluid. Cancer Res 41:2563, 1981
91. Phillips RL: Role of life-style and dietary habits in risk of cancer among Seventh-Day Adventists. Cancer Res 35:3513, 1975
92. Miller AB, Kelly A, Choi NW, et al: A study of diet and breast cancer. Am J Epidemiol 107:499, 1978
93. Howe GR: The use of polytomous dual response data to increase power in case control studies: An application to the association between dietary fat and breast cancer. J Chron Dis 38:663, 1985
94. Marshall J, Graham S: Use of dual response to increase validity of case control studies. J Chron Dis 37:125, 1984
95. Graham S, Marshall J, Mettlin C, et al: Diet in the epidemiology of breast cancer. Am J Epidemiol 116:68, 1982
96. Lubin JH, Burns PE, Blot WJ, et al: Dietary factors and breast cancer risk. Int J Cancer 28:685, 1981
97. Nomura A, Henderson BE, Lee J: Breast cancer and diet among the Japanese in Hawaii. Am J Clin Nutr 31:2020, 1978
98. Kolonel LN, Nomura AMY, Hinds MW, et al: Role of diet in cancer incidence in Hawaii. Cancer Res 43:2397s, 1983
99. Hislop TG, Coldman AJ, Elwood JM, et al: Childhood and recent eating patterns and risk of breast cancer. Cancer Detect Prev 9:47, 1986
100. Hirayama T: Nutrition and cancer—A large-scale cohort study. In Knudsen I (ed): Genetic Toxicology of the Diet, pp 299-311. New York, Alan R. Liss, Inc., 1986
101. Hiatt RA, Friedman GD, Bawol RD, et al: Breast cancer and serum cholesterol. J Natl Cancer Inst 68:885, 1982
102. Rang EH, Kinlen LJ, Herman-Taylor J: A study of cancer of the breast and other sites in women after total colectomy and ileostomy for non-malignant disorders. Lancet 1:1014, 1983
103. Miller AB, Barclay THC, Choi NW, et al: A study of cancer, parity and age at first pregnancy. J Chron Dis 33:585, 1980
104. Henderson BE, Powell D, Rosario I, et al: An epidemiologic study of breast cancer. J Natl Cancer Inst 53:509, 1974
105. Hoover R, Gray LA, Cole P, et al: Menopausal estrogens and breast cancer. N Engl J Med 295:401, 1976
106. Ross RK, Paganini-Hill A, Gerkins VR, et al: A case-control study of menopausal estrogen therapy and breast cancer. JAMA 243:1635, 1980
107. Jick H, Walker AM, Watkins RN, et al: Replacement estrogens and breast cancer. Am J Epidemiol 112:586, 1980
108. Hoover R, Glass A, Finkle WD, et al: Conjugated estrogens and breast cancer risk in women. J Natl Cancer Inst 67:815, 1981
109. National Academy of Sciences: Diet, nutrition, and cancer. Committee on diet, nutrition, and cancer. Assembly of Life Sciences, National Research Council. Washington, DC, National Academy Press, 1982
110. Miller AB: Approaches to the control of breast cancer. In Rich MA, Hager JC, Furmanski P (eds): Understanding Cancer. Clinical and Laboratory Concepts, pp 3–25. New York, Marcel Dekker, 1983
111. National Academy of Sciences: Diet, nutrition, and cancer: Directions for research. Committee on Diet, Nutrition, and Cancer. Commission on Life Sciences, National Research Council. Washington, DC, National Academy Press, 1983
112. Wynder EL, Cohen L: A rationale for dietary intervention in the treatment of postmenopausal breast cancer patients. Nutr Cancer 3:195, 1982
113. Newman SC, Miller AB, Howe GR: A study of the effect of weight and dietary fat on survival time. Am J Epidemiol 123:767, 1986
114. de Waard F: Nutritional epidemiology of breast cancer: Where are we now, and where are we going? Nutr Cancer 4:85, 1982
115. Miller AB: An overview of hormone associated cancers. Cancer Res 38:3985, 1978
116. Jensen OM, Wahrendorf J, Rosenqiest A, et al: The reliability of questionnaire derived historical dietary information and temporal stability of food habits in individuals. Am J Epidemiol 120:281, 1984
117. Greenwald P, Sondik E: Division of Cancer Prevention and Control: Cancer Control. Objectives For the Nation 1985–2000. NCI, National Cancer Institute Monograph #2, Bethesda, MD, September 1986
118. Cuzick J, Wang DY, Bulbrook RD: The prevention of breast cancer. Lancet 1:83–86, 1986
119. Miller AB, Bulbrook RD: UICC multidisciplinary project on breast cancer: The epidemiology, aetiology and prevention of breast cancer. Int J Cancer 37:173, 1986

Endocrine Participation in the Etiology of Breast Cancer

Jack Fishman

The presence of estrogen receptors in the majority of human breast tumors[1] and the clinical response to hormonal therapy[2,3] leave little doubt about the influence of hormones on the progression of the disease in humans. Although a critical role of hormones in the etiology of mammary tumors is clearly evident in animal models of the disease,[4] a similar role in human breast cancer is supported only by indirect epidemiologic evidence. The reduced risk for the disease induced by an early pregnancy,[5] late puberty,[6] or an early natural or surgical menopause[7] is considered to be mediated by hormonal changes associated with these events. The great predominance of breast cancer in women compared with men[8] is also considered to reflect the differences in the gonadal hormones between the sexes. An intense clinical research effort has been mounted over the past three decades to provide firm evidence for and to define the nature of endocrine participation in human breast tumor formation. This effort focused on detecting an association between exogenous hormone intake and the incidence of breast cancer and on the detection of an endogenous hormonal difference that would be securely linked to the presence of or risk for the disease. It may have been expected that prospective and retrospective studies of this nature, with all of the problems and uncertainties of subject and control selection and requiring the use of difficult and often varying analytic procedures, would produce some conflicting results. Unfortunately, this expectation was not only met but was greatly exceeded. The vast amount of data generated in the many studies is frequently in disagreement, and the conclusions derived from it remain imprecise and controversial. As a result, there exists at this time no consensus on the nature, or even on the existence, of an endocrine factor or factors in the initiation of human breast cancer. The large amount of data accumulated and its frequently conflicting nature requires that this topic be reviewed selectively and that only a fraction of the published material be cited. Furthermore, the selection and interpretation of the available data are necessarily subjective and can reflect personal bias. Nevertheless, an attempt will be made to present the prevailing views and the results on which they are based regarding the role of endocrine factors in the incidence of and risk for breast cancer in the human. Although studies concerning the influence of other endocrine components on breast cancer have been reported,[9–11] this discussion will be limited to the gonadal steroid hormones and to prolactin, agents whose relationship to the disease have had the most experimental support. In the interest of clarity, the impact of exogenous hormonal administration and that of endogenous hormonal changes on the incidence of breast cancer in humans will be considered separately.

EXOGENOUS HORMONES

Two large groups of women who have been exposed to exogenous estrogens provide the basis for much of the epidemiologic work attempting to discern a link between estrogen intake and breast cancer incidence. The two populations are women who have used oral contraceptive agents containing an estrogenic component and postmenopausal women given estrogens as replacement. In connection with the studies relating to exogenous estrogens, it is important to stress a point that is frequently obscured if not totally neglected. The term *estrogen* is often used in these studies indiscriminately without regard to the nature of the estrogen used. The structural differences between the different estrogenic compounds employed make this practice of some concern. Thus, the most frequently used postmenopausal estrogens are of equine origin and consist of the sulfated conjugates of a number of different molecules, including some that are unique to the horse and are thus foreign to the human. The estrogenic components in oral contraceptive preparations are partially synthetic derivatives consisting of 17-ethynylestradiol or its methyl ester. The totally synthetic diethylstilbestrol, whose structure is completely different from the natural hormone, has also been used as an estrogen in humans,[12] although its primary use has been in animal husbandry, where its ultimate transmission to humans has generated much concern. It is clearly inappropriate to consider the different molecules as interchangeable, and it is equally incorrect to think of them as fully equivalent to the natural human hormones. Although all estrogens, natural or synthetic, exhibit a commonality in some physiological end points, they do not do so in others. Their metabolic patterns are quite diverse,[13–15] and indeed it can be expected that their pathophysiology as exemplified in any possible tumorigenesis will also be distinct. For this reason, it is important to identify the nature of the exogenous estrogen employed in any of the epidemiologic studies and to consider the use of each such estrogen separately. Furthermore, effects observed with these agents, which are not natural to humans, should not be extrapolated to the natural hormone estradiol and its metabolites.

Oral Contraceptives

The prevalence of the use of oral contraceptives and the chronic nature of their administration have prompted an intense effort to investigate a possible association between these agents and the incidence of breast cancer. The results of these studies, whether retrospective or prospective, are conflicting—some suggesting an increased risk for the disease in oral contraceptive users[16–18] and others failing to detect such a relationship.[19–21] The most recent results, which have the benefit of a larger exposed population and a longer term of exposure, indicate that the use of oral contraceptives is not linked with an enhanced risk for breast cancer but may in fact diminish that risk.[22,23] This protective effect is thought to be mediated by a diminution in benign breast disease that has been observed in oral contraceptive users.[24,25] Because benign breast disease is thought to be a risk factor for cancer,[26,27] this would translate into a diminished rate of breast cancer incidence. This interpretation, however, may be invalid because there are some doubts about whether benign breast disease represents an increased risk for breast cancer.[28] The results of the retrospective epidemiologic studies with oral contraceptives must also be considered with a note of caution if, as has been suggested, the latency of clinically evident breast cancer is 20 years or more.[29,30] If this is the case, the majority of oral contraceptive users have reached that time limit and epidemiologic surprises could still be forthcoming.

The issue of the effect of estrogens in oral contraceptives is complicated by the simultaneous presence of progestogens in these preparations. That this may be a relevant issue is suggested by a recent report of an increased risk for breast cancer following the use of high-progestogen oral contraceptive preparations,[31] although this finding has since been challenged.[32]

Postmenopausal Estrogen Treatment

Postmenopausal estrogen replacement is associated with an increased incidence of endometrial cancer in a dose- and time-related fashion.[33–35] Although some investigators question the validity of this association,[36] the evidence supporting such a causative relationship is very persuasive. A similar relationship between the postmenopausal estrogens and breast cancer has been proposed, since the uterus and the breast are both target organs for the hormone. The results of numerous epidemiologic studies concerned with this question are conflicting and do not allow any definitive conclusion. Several of the studies reveal an increased risk for breast cancer related to the dose and duration of treatment with estrogens,[37,38] whereas others fail to find any increase in breast cancer incidence associated with estrogen replacement therapy.[39,40] A greater risk for the disease with estrogen treatment has been reported in defined groups, such as oophorectomized women,[41] women with benign breast disease,[42] and women with a family history of breast cancer.[42] An assessment of the data available at this time suggests that estrogen replacement therapy is not associated with any substantial increase in the risk for breast cancer, with the possible exception of specific categories of women who are already at greater risk for other reasons. The absence of an effect of postmenopausal estrogens on breast cancer incidence could reflect the long latency of this disease so that its initiation after the menopause would not become clinically evident during the remaining years. Also, the breast could be less vulnerable to tumor initiation postmenopausally than in the early reproductive years. If either of these is the case, then a greater incidence of breast cancer in very long-term users or in women who have received estrogen replacement early in their lives could be expected. This may possibly account for the increased breast cancer risk reported in women who were given replacement estrogens following surgically induced menopause.[41] Clearly this group was exposed to these agents earlier in their lives and thus also for a longer term than the normal menopausal population. It needs to be emphasized that neither the conjugated equine estrogens nor ethynylestradiol, which are the principal estrogens used in hormonal replacement therapy, are identical to the human ovarian product and that their biologic consequences can be different.

Other studies suggestive of a connection between the use of exogenous estrogens and increased breast cancer risk concern the treatment of prostatic cancer with estrogens, when more than the expected cases of breast cancer were observed,[43] and the use of the hormone to inhibit excessive height in girls, when breast abnormalities were noted in the recipients.[44] The number of subjects in these studies was small, and these results must be considered tentative.

Prolactin

Earlier studies suggested that the clinical use of dopamine antagonists, such as the rauwolfia drugs and the phenothiazines, which lead to an elevation of prolactin secretion, resulted in an increased incidence of breast tumors.[45] Subsequent investigations, however, failed to confirm this relationship,[46,47] and the current consensus is that the pharmacological elevation of prolactin secretion does not cause an increase in the incidence of breast cancer.

ENDOGENOUS HORMONES

A role for endogenous hormones, particularly estrogens, in the initiation of human breast cancer rests on indirect but nevertheless fairly compelling epidemiologic evidence. As already noted, the protective effect of an early first pregnancy, an early menopause, and a late menarche is thought to reflect the associated changes in estrogen secretion. The protective effect of an oophorectomy early in life and the low incidence of the disease in men support a role for endogenous estrogens in the initiation or development of breast malignancies. This apparent relationship motivated many investigators to search for a hormonal difference in the endogenous hormones between women with the disease and matched controls who had no clinical evidence of breast cancer. Extensive measurements of plasma and urinary estrogens, however, failed to identify a consistent and reproducible distinction between cases and controls. Studies that reported the existence of such a difference[48,49] are matched by an equal number of studies that failed to find one.[50,51] Much of the disagreement between the various studies may reside in the different sampling or analytic procedures employed. A further potential defect in these investigations is that they were mostly limited to estradiol, estrone, and estriol, the three earliest identified endogenous estrogens, and that they omitted the consideration of other biotransformation products of the female sex hormone, which often are the major quantitative metabolites.

A recent report of an elevation in breast cancer patients of the amount of the estradiol in plasma that is free and is not complexed with the sex-hormone-binding globulin and albumin[52] has not been confirmed.[53] A series of reports from one group of investigators that plasma and urinary androgens, particularly testosterone and androstanediol, are elevated in pre- and postmenopausal breast cancer patients relative to controls[54,55] needs to be considered in the light of other communications that low plasma and urinary androgens are characteristic of breast cancer patients.[56,57] The elevated androgens in premenopausal breast cancer patients observed in the Italian studies[54,55] is consistent with the hypothesis that anovulatory cycles in which the estrogen secretion is accompanied by an inadequate progesterone formation and is hence "unopposed" increases the risk for breast cancer.[58,59] This hypothesis, which has had considerable acceptance, has recently been questioned by investigators who suggest that the opposite is true and that the number of normal ovulatory cycles correlates better with an increased risk for the disease.[60]

Prolactin levels have also been measured in breast cancer patients and in controls. Some studies reported finding increased levels of the hormones in patients,[61,62] whereas others were not able to confirm this finding.[63,64] Prolactin concentrations have also been reported to be increased in daughters of patients.[65] The inconsistency in these various studies may be due to the small number of cases examined in some of the instances and the difficulties of establishing consistent plasma levels of prolactin, which is subject to episodic secretion and is profoundly influenced by unrelated factors such as diet or stress.

Estradiol Metabolites

Another avenue of investigation of the possible endocrine differences in breast cancer patients was directed to the qualitative aspect of the problem, particularly the metabolism of estradiol. The biotransformation of estradiol in the human is dominated by oxidative processes. The principal pathways are the reversible oxidation to estrone,[66] which is followed by the irreversible 16α-hydroxylation to 16α-hydroxyestrone and estriol,[67] or by hydroxylation at position two leading to the catechol estrogens.[68] The view that an abnormal metabolism of estradiol is the factor linking the estrogens to breast cancer risk has much to commend it and it led to a popular theory called the estriol hypothesis.[69] This concept was based on the perception of estriol, a metabolite of estradiol, as an impeded estrogen that functioned as an estrogen antagonist,[70,71] and a decrement in its formation therefore increased the risk for breast tumorigenesis. The pre-eminence of estriol in the estrogenic profile of human pregnancy[71] was then considered responsible for the protection conferred by a full-term pregnancy in early reproductive life. This hypothesis has, however, recently come under attack on both biologic and epidemiologic grounds. The pharmacology of estriol when it is administered so as to reproduce physiological conditions does not appear to differ greatly from that of estradiol in that it behaves as a full estrogen agonist.[72,73] There has also been little supporting evidence that the urinary or plasma estrogenic profile in breast cancer patients is deficient in estriol relative to controls.[74,75]

PROSPECTIVE STUDIES

The absence of any consistent differences in ovarian hormone secretion or excretion between breast cancer patients and controls is not entirely unexpected when considered retrospectively. Breast cancer is acknowledged to be a disease in which in most cases the initiation and clinical diagnosis are separated by many years.[29,30] Hence a hormonal environment that is present and is responsible for the initiation of the tumor during the woman's reproductive years will not be reflected in the endocrine profiles of her postmenopausal period. Disruption of the hypothalamic-pituitary-ovarian axis by, at the very least, the stress of the disease would suggest that even in the premenopausal patient the hormonal secretion will be altered from its predisease condition. The realization of this inconstancy of the hormonal milieu has led to a rethinking of the validity of retrospective studies and has led to a series of prospective efforts in which the above issues would not play a role. One such prospective study was the massive investigation carried out by Bulbrook and colleagues,[56,57] who obtained urine and plasma specimens from the female population of the island of Guernsey and measured their hormonal contents after a number of cases of breast cancer were diagnosed in the population. Comparison of the results between women who eventually developed the disease and those who did not showed that the adrenal androgens were decreased in the urine of the subjects who went on to develop breast cancer, but no such differences were observed in the case of estrogens—at least at the current stage of this continuously progressive study.[76]

HIGH-RISK POPULATIONS

All-inclusive prospective studies of the above type require an almost prohibitive investment in time and effort, and therefore many investigators took a more restrictive approach and compared populations considered at enhanced risk for the disease with controls in whom the defined risk factor was absent. The selective nature of such protocols reduces the effort required but contains the defect that the results obtained may not provide statistically valid differences because of the inherent scatter in groups in which the risk is moderately increased and in which the disease occurs in only some members. The principal categories that were examined in this way consisted of those in whom the increased risk was conferred by family history, reproductive history, race, or geographic location. The results reported from a series of such investigations were again frequently conflicting, with some studies reporting the existence of hormonal differences associated with increased risk that could not, however, be confirmed in other studies. Nevertheless, these investigations may yet provide valuable insights into the cause of breast cancer, because the measurements are conducted closer to the probable time of tumor initiation and because they are not compromised by the overt presence of the disease. One study of the urinary and plasma estrogen levels in women who were daughters of breast cancer patients, and thus were at increased risk, found elevated concentrations of the female hormone,[77] but this increase was not found in other studies.[78] In one investigation in which young women at risk for familial breast cancer and matched low-risk controls were sampled daily throughout one menstrual cycle, the adrenal, pituitary, and gonadal hormone levels in urine or plasma did not differ between the two groups.[79] The sole exceptions were the estrone and estradiol glucuronide conjugates in urine, which were significantly lower in the high-risk group.[80] This decrease appeared to be compensated for by an increase in the urinary excretion of estrone sulfate, with the differential being maximal during the periovulatory period.[81] These results have not yet been independently replicated, but if they are confirmed, they could provide a valuable clue to the endocrine cause of familial and possibly nonfamilial breast cancer.

Women who were considered to be at decreased risk for breast cancer because they had a first full-term pregnancy before the age of 24 were also studied for the presence of a possible endocrine distinction. Their urinary estrogens were compared with those of women who lacked this protective characteristic. The estrogens of the lower-risk group were observed to exhibit a higher estriol ratio due to an increased excretion of estriol relative to estrone and estradiol.[82] This observation supports the estriol hypothesis that was referred to earlier but that is no longer widely accepted.

Other divergent risk categories that were also studied for possible endocrine differences were Japanese and Caucasian women, since the former exhibit a greatly diminished incidence of breast cancer. The results of such comparative studies by different investigators are again inconsistent with those of some workers reporting the presence of significant endocrine differences between the two populations and others failing to observe such differences.[83,84] An important factor in these studies is that the risk for breast cancer increases in Oriental women on their migration to the United States and becomes almost equal to that of the general population in their daughters,[85] suggesting that the risk factors differentiating between these groups are environmental rather than genetic.

HORMONE-RELATED ENVIRONMENTAL FACTORS

The role of environment, particularly diet, has received wide attention as a factor in the incidence of breast cancer.[86,87] The environmental influences responsible for the increased incidence of the disease may well be mediated via the endocrine system.[88,89] Thus, obesity is associated with increased peripheral estrogen biosynthesis and also with a hyperestrogenic shift in estrogen metabolism, in that less of the nonestrogenic catechol estrogens are formed.[90,91] The greater risk for breast cancer [92,93] and its poorer prognosis in these women who develop the disease are then possibly the result of these hormonal changes related to obesity. Similarly, recent studies have shown that dietary manipulations can profoundly affect estrogen metabolism,[95] presumably by alterations of the cytochrome P-450 complex in the liver responsible for estrogen biotransformation, and this may be the effective mediator by which diet influences breast cancer risk.

Another environmental factor in estrogen-related cancer that has captured recent interest is cigarette smoking. Cigarette smoking decreases estrogen levels in body fluids[96] and has been reported to decrease the risk for endometrial cancer,[97] presumably achieving both effects by influencing estrogen biosynthesis or metabolism. However, an earlier report that smoking exerts a similar beneficial effect on breast cancer risk[98] has been refuted.[99]

ESTRADIOL-TRANSFORMING ENZYMES

Another approach at identifying an endocrine difference that could be associated with breast cancer involved a retrospective examination of the *in vivo* enzymatic activities responsible for the dominant estradiol biotransformations, specifically the 17 β-ol dehydrogenase and the 2- and 16α-hydroxylases. A study employing a radiometric procedure that provides information on the extent of these transformations without the need of isolating the specific metabolites found that the activities of these enzymes did not change with age or reproductive status in normal women,[100] suggesting that a measure of these activities could be used as a time-independent constant. Studies in postmenopausal women with breast cancer and matched controls showed that while 17 β-ol dehydrogenase and 2-hydroxylase activities were the same in both groups, the 16α-hydroxylase in the cancer patients was elevated by 50%.[101] Since these enzymic activities do not change with age,[100] these results suggested that this endocrine difference was present at the time of tumor initiation and could have had a role in this event. The possibility that 16α-hydroxylation of estrogens is a factor in the etiology of breast cancer gains support from two other observations. One is that inbred mouse strains with a high incidence of mammary tumors also show high 16α-hydroxylation but low-incidence strains exhibit low 16α-hydroxylation.[102] The second observation is that one of the products of the enzyme, 16α-hydroxyestrone, forms covalent adducts with biologic macromolecules by a mechanism that is unique to this endogenous estrogen.[103,104] This hypothesis, therefore, allows for a rational progression from a metabolic distortion leading to a greater production of a metabolite that then exhibits abnormal subcellular behavior in estrogen target tissue.

In summary, although there is abundant evidence that various hormones, particularly the estrogens, are relevant in the etiology of breast cancer, the nature of the role that they play has not been clarified. The results of the numerous studies comparing hormonal concentrations in patients and normal subjects have been so conflicting that at this time no clear conclusions can be drawn from them. Nevertheless, some tantalizing and possibly valuable observations regarding distortions in estrogen metabolism and the subcellular effects of its products offer hope of eventually uncovering the endocrine factors involved in the initiation of some categories of breast cancer.

REFERENCES

1. McGuire WL: Estrogen receptors in human breast cancer. J Clin Invest 52:73, 1973
2. McGuire WL: Endocrine therapy of breast cancer. Annu Rev Med 26:353, 1975
3. Legha SS, Davis HL, Muggia FM: Hormonal therapy of breast cancer: new approaches and concepts. Ann Int Med 88:69, 1978
4. Heuson JC, Legros N, Heuson-Stiennon JA, et al: Hormone dependency of rat mammary tumors. In Heuson JC, Mattheiem WH, Rozencweig M (eds): Breast Cancers: Trends in Research and Treatment, New York, Raven Press, 1976
5. MacMahon B, Cole P, Lin T, et al: Age at first birth and breast cancer risk. Bull WHO 43:209, 1970
6. Staszewski J: Age at menarche and breast cancer. J Natl Cancer Inst 47:935, 1971
7. Trichopoulos D, MacMahon B, Cole P: Menopause and breast cancer risk. J Natl Cancer Inst 48:605, 1972
8. Crichlow RW: Breast cancer in men. Semin Oncol 1(2): 145, 1974
9. MacFarlane IA, Robinson EL, Bush H, et al: Thyroid function in patients with benign and malignant breast disease. Br J Cancer 41:478, 1978
10. Malarkey WB, Schroeder LL, Stevens VC, et al: Twenty-four hour preoperative endocrine profiles in women with benign and malignant disease. Cancer Res 37:4657, 1977
11. Welsch CW, Iturri GC, Brennan MJ: DNA synthesis in human, mouse and rat mammary carcinomas *in vitro*. Cancer 38:1272, 1976
12. Noller KL, Fish CR: Diethylstilbestrol usage: Its interesting past, important present, and questionable future. Med Clin North Am 58:793, 1974
13. Valette A, Carasco G, Verine A, et al: Differential effects of oestradiol and ethynyl oestradiol on lipid metabolism in the female rat. J Endocrinol 79:405, 1978
14. Leibl H, Spona J: Differential stimulation by 17β-estradiol and synthetic estrogens of progesterone-receptor and of translocation of estrogen-receptor in rat pituitary and uterus. Endocrinology 110:265, 1982
15. Niemela AO, Elo HA: Effects of oestradiol-17β and diethylstilbestrol on progesterone-induced protein production in chick oviduct: evidence for differences in the actions of steroidal and non-steroidal estrogens. J Endocr 96:465, 1983
16. Paffenbarger RS, Fasal E, Simmons ME, et al: Cancer risk as related to use of oral contraceptives during fertile years. Cancer 39(Suppl):1887, 1977
17. Kelsey JL, Holford TR, White C, et al: Oral contraceptives and breast disease: An epidemiological study. Am J Epidemiol 107:236, 1978
18. Pike MC, Henderson BE, Casagrande JT, et al: Oral contraceptive use and early abortion as risk factors for breast cancer in young women. Br J Cancer 43:72, 1981
19. Ravnihar B, Seigel DG, Lindtner J: An epidemiologic study of breast cancer and benign breast neoplasias in relation to the oral contraceptive and estrogen use. Eur J Cancer 15:395, 1979
20. Harris NV, Weiss NS, Francis AM, et al: Breast cancer in relation to patterns of oral contraceptive use. Am J Epidemiol 116:643, 1982
21. The Centers for Disease Control Cancer and Steroid Hormone Study: Long-term oral contraceptive use and risk of breast cancer. JAMA 249:1591, 1983
22. Rosenberg L, Miller DR, Kaufman DW, et al: Breast cancer and oral contraceptive use. Am J Epidemiol 119:167, 1984
23. Kelsey JL, Fischer DB, Holford TR, et al: Exogenous estrogens and other factors in the epidemiology of breast cancer. J Natl Cancer Inst 67:327, 1981
24. Fasal E, Paffenbarger RS Jr: Oral contraceptives as related to cancer and benign lesions of the breast. J Natl Cancer Inst 55:767, 1975
25. LiVolsi VA, Stadel BV, Kelsey JL, et al: Fibrocystic breast diseases in oral contraceptive users. N Engl J Med 299:381, 1978
26. Haagensen CD, Lane N, Lattes R, et al: Lobular neoplasia (so-called lobular carcinoma *in situ*) of the breast. Cancer 42:737, 1978
27. Coombs LJ, Lilienfeld AM, Bross ID, et al: A prospective study of the relationship between benign breast diseases and breast carcinomas. Prev Med 8:40, 1979
28. Dupont WD, Page DL: Risk factors for breast cancer in women with preoperative breast disease. N Engl J Med 312:146, 1985
29. Collins VP, Loeffler RK, Tivey H: Observation on growth rates of human tumors. Am J Roentgenol 76:988, 1956
30. Tokunaga M, Norman JE, Asano M, et al: Malignant breast tumors among atomic bomb survivors, Hiroshima and Nagasaki. J Natl Cancer Inst 42:1347, 1978
31. Pike MC, Henderson BE, Krailo MD, et al: Breast cancer in young women and use of oral contraceptives: Possible modifying effect of formulation and age at use. Lancet ii:926, 1983
32. Gillmer MG: Breast cancer and oral contraceptives. Lancet ii:1145, 1983
33. Antunes CMF, Stolley PD, Rosenshein NB, et al: Endometrial cancer and estrogen use: Report of a large case-control study. N Engl J Med 309:9, 1979
34. Weiss NS, Szekely DR, English DR, et al: Endometrial cancer in relation to patterns of menopausal estrogen use. JAMA 242:261, 1979
35. Hulka BS, Fowler WC, Kaufman DG, et al: Estrogen and endometrial cancer: Cases and two control groups from North Carolina. Am J Obstet Gynecol 137:92, 1980
36. Gordon GS, Greenberg BG: Exogenous estrogens and endometrial cancer. Postgrad Med 59:66, 1976
37. Hoover R, Gray LA Sr, Cole P, et al: Menopausal estrogens and breast cancer. N Engl J Med 295:401, 1976
38. Hulka BS, Chambless LE, Deubner DC, et al: Breast cancer and estrogen replacement therapy. Am J Obstet Gynecol 143:638, 1982
39. Sartwell PE, Arthes FG, Tonascia JA: Exogenous hormones, reproductive history, and breast cancer. J Natl Cancer Inst 59:1589, 1977
40. Jick H, Walker AM, Watkins RN, et al: Replacement estrogens and breast cancer. Am J Epidemiol 112:586, 1980
41. Hoover R, Glass A, Finkle WD, et al: Conjugated estrogens

and breast cancer risk in women. J Natl Cancer Inst 67:815, 1981

42. Brinton LA, Hoover RN, Szklo M, et al: Menopausal estrogen and risk of breast cancer. Cancer 47:2517, 1981
43. Sobin LH, Sherif M: Relation between male breast cancer and prostate cancer. Br J Cancer 42:787, 1980
44. Crawford JD: Treatment of tall girls with estrogen. Pediatrics 62:1189, 1978
45. Jick H, Slone D, Shapiro S, et al: Reserpine and breast cancer. Lancet ii:669, 1974
46. Mack TM, Henderson BE, Gerkins VR, et al: Reserpine and breast cancer in a retirement community. N Engl J Med 292:1366, 1975
47. Wagner S, Mantel N: Breast cancer at a psychiatric hospital before and after the introduction of neuroleptic agents. Cancer Res 38:2703, 1978
48. Persson BH, Risholm L: Oophorectomy and cortisone treatment as a method of eliminating oestrogen production in patients with breast cancer. Acta Endocrinol 47:15, 1964
49. England PC, Skinner LG, Cottrell KM, et al: Serum oestradiol-17β in women with benign and malignant breast disease. Br J Cancer 30:571, 1974
50. McFadyen IJ, Forrest APM, Prescott RJ, et al: Circulating hormone concentrations in women with breast cancer. Lancet i:1100, 1976
51. McAllister RA, Sim AW, Hobkirk R, et al: Urinary estrogen after endocrine ablation. Lancet i:1102, 1960
52. Siiteri PK, Hammond GL, Nisker JA: Increased availability of serum estrogens in breast cancer: a new hypothesis. In Pike et al, (eds): Banbury Report No. 8: Hormones and Cancer, p 87. Cold Spring Harbor Laboratory, 1981
53. Bruning PF, Bronfrer JMG, Hart AAM: Non-protein bound oestradiol, sex hormone binding globulin, breast cancer and breast cancer risk. Br J Cancer 51:479, 1985
54. Grattarola R: Anovulation and increased androgenic activity as breast cancer risk in women with fibrocystic disease of the breast. Cancer Res 38:3051, 1978
55. Secreto G, Toniolo P, Berrino F, et al: Increased androgen activity and breast cancer risk in premenopausal women. Cancer Res 44:5902, 1984
56. Wang DY, Bulbrook RD, Herian M, et al: Studies on the sulfate esters of dehydroepiandrosterone and androsterone in the blood of women with breast cancer. Eur J Cancer 10:477, 1974
57. Bulbrook RD, Hayward JL, Spicer CC: Relation between urinary androgen and corticoid excretion and subsequent breast cancer. Lancet ii:395, 1971
58. Kodama M, Kodama T, Miura S, et al: Hormonal status of breast cancer. III. Further analysis of ovarian adrenal dysfunction. J Natl Cancer Inst 59:49, 1977
59. Zumoff B: Abnormal plasma hormone levels in women with breast cancer. In Pike et al, (eds): Banbury Report No. 8: Hormones and Cancer, p 143. Cold Spring Harbor Laboratory, 1981
60. Henderson BE, Ross RK, Judd HL, et al: Do regular ovulatory cycles increase breast cancer risk? Cancer 56:1206, 1985
61. Hill P, Wynder EL, Kumar H, et al: Prolactin levels in populations at risk for breast cancer. Cancer Res 36:4102, 1976
62. Rose DB, Pruitt BT: Plasma prolactin levels in patients with breast cancer. Cancer 48:2687, 1981
63. Boyns AR, Cole EN, Griffiths K, et al: Plasma prolactin in breast cancer. Eur J Cancer 9:99, 1973
64. Kwa HG, Engelsman E, DeJong-Bakker M, et al: Plasma prolactin in human breast cancer. Lancet i:433, 1974
65. Levin PA, Malarkey WB: Daughters of women with breast cancer have elevated mean 24-hour prolactin (Prl) levels and a partial resistance of Prl to dopamine suppression. J Clin Endocrinol Metabol 53:179, 1981
66. Fishman J, Bradlow HL, Gallagher TF: Oxidative metabolism of estradiol. J Biol Chem 235:3104, 1960
67. Brown JB, Marian GF: The metabolic reduction of 16α-hydroxyoestrone to oestriol in man. J Endocrinol 15:307, 1957
68. Fishman J: Role of 2-hydroxyestrone in estrogen metabolism. J Clin Endocrinol Metabol 23:207, 1963
69. Lemon HM, Wotiz HH, Parsons L, et al: Reduced estriol excretion in patients with breast cancer prior to endocrine therapy. JAMA 196:1128, 1966
70. Lemon HM: Endocrine influences on human mammary cancer formation. Cancer 23:781,1969
71. Cole P, MacMahon B: Oestrogen fractions during early reproductive life in the aetiology of breast cancer. Lancet i:604, 1969
72. Martucci C, Fishman J: Direction of estradiol metabolism as a control of its hormonal action—uterotropic activity of estradiol metabolism. Endocrinology 101:1709, 1977
73. Anderson JN, Peck EJ, Clark JH: Estrogen-induced uterine responses and growth: Relationship to receptor estrogen binding by uterine nuclei. Endocrinology 96:160, 1975
74. Marmosten J, Crowley LG, Myers SM, et al: Urinary excretion of estrone, estradiol and estriol by patients with breast cancer and benign breast disease. Am J Obstet Gynecol 92:460, 1965
75. Zumoff B, Fishman J, Bradlow HL, et al: Hormone profiles in hormone-dependent cancers. Cancer Res 35:3365, 1975
76. Bulbrook RD, Moore JW, Clark GMG, et al: Plasma oestradiol and progesterone levels in women with varying degrees of risk of breast cancer. Eur J Cancer 14:1369, 1978
77. Pike MC, Cassagrande JT, Brown JB, et al: Composition of urinary and plasma hormone levels in daughters of breast cancer patients and controls. J Natl Cancer Inst 59:1351, 1977
78. Morgan RW, Vakil DV, Brown JB, et al: Estrogen profiles in young women: Effect of maternal history of breast cancer. J Natl Cancer Inst 60:965, 1978
79. Fishman J, Fukushima D, O'Connor J, Rosenfeld RS, et al: Plasma hormonal profiles of young women at risk for familial breast cancer. Cancer Res 38:4006, 1978
80. Fishman J, Fukushima DK, O'Connor J, et al: Low urinary estrogen glucuronides in women at risk for familial breast cancer. Science, 204:1089, 1979
81. Fishman J, Bradlow HL, Fukushima DK, et al: Abnormal estrogen conjugation in women at risk for familial breast cancer at the periovulatory stage of the menstrual cycle. Cancer Res 43:1884, 1983
82. Cole P, Brown JB, MacMahon B: Oestrogen profiles of parous and nulliparous women. Lancet ii:596, 1976
83. Bulbrook RD, Thomas BS, Utsunomiya J, et al: The urinary excretion of 11-deoxy-17-oxosteroids and 17-hydroxycorticosteroids by normal Japanese and British women. J Endocrinol 38:401, 1967
84. MacMahon B, Cole P, Brown JB, et al: Urine oestrogen profiles of Asian and North American women. Int J Cancer 14:161, 1974
85. Buell P: Changing incidence of breast cancer in Japanese-American women. J Natl Cancer Inst 51:147, 1973
86. Miller AB: Role of nutrition in the etiology of breast cancer. Cancer Res 39:2704, 1977
87. Dickerson JW: Nutrition and breast cancer. J Hum Nutr 33:17, 1979
88. Edman CD, MacDonald PC: Effects of obesity on conversion of plasma androstenedione to estrone in ovulatory and anovulatory young women. Am J Obstet Gynecol 130:456, 1978

89. Schneider G, Kirschner MA, Berkowitz R, et al: Increased estrogen production in obese men. J Clin Endocrinol Metabol 48:633, 1979
90. Fishman J, Boyar RM, Hellman L: Influence of body weight on estradiol metabolism in young women. J Clin Endocrinol Metabol 41:989, 1975
91. Schneider J, Bradlow HL, Strain G, et al: Effect of obesity on estradiol metabolism: decreased formation of nonuterotropic metabolites. J Clin Endocrinol Metabol 56:973, 1983
92. de Waard F, Baanders-van Halewijn EA: A prospective study in general practice on breast cancer risk in postmenopausal women. Int J Cancer 14:153, 1974
93. Paffenbarger RS, Kampert JB, Chang H-G: Characteristics that predict risk of breast cancer before and after menopause. Am J Epidemiol 112:258, 1980
94. Donegan WL, Hartz AJ, Rimm AA: The association of body weight with recurrent cancer of the breast. Cancer 41:1590, 1978
95. Anderson KE, Kappas A, Conney AH, et al: The influence of dietary protein and carbohydrate on the principal oxidative biotransformation of estradiol in normal subjects. J Clin Endocrinol Metabol 59:103, 1984
96. Jensen J, Christiansen C, Rødbro P: Cigarette smoking, serum estrogens, and bone loss during hormone-replacement therapy early after menopause. N Engl J Med 313:973, 1985
97. Lesko SM, Rosenberg L, Kaufman DW, et al: Cigarette smoking and risk of endometrial cancer. N Engl J Med 313:593, 1985
98. Vessey M, Baron J, Doll R, McPherson K, et al: Oral contraceptives and breast cancer: Final report of an epidemiological study. Br J Cancer 47:455, 1983
99. Schechter MT, Miller AB, Howe GR: Cigarette smoking and breast cancer: A case-control study of screening program participants. Am J Epidemiol 121:479, 1985
100. Fishman J, Bradlow HL, Schneider J, et al: Radiometric analysis of biological oxidations in man: Sex differences in estradiol metabolism. Proc Natl Acad Sci 77:4957, 1980
101. Fishman J, Schneider J, Hershcopf RJ, et al: Increased estrogen-16α-hydroxylase activity in women with breast cancer and endometrial cancer. J Steroid Biochem 20:1077, 1984
102. Bradlow HL, Hershcopf RJ, Martucci CP, et al: Estradiol 16α-hydroxylation in the mouse correlate with mammary tumor incidence and presence of murine mammary tumor virus. A possible model for the hormonal etiology of breast cancer in humans. Proc Natl Acad Sci 82:6295, 1985
103. Bucala R, Fishman J, Cerami A: Formation of covalent adducts between cortisol and 16α-hydroxyestrone and protein: Possible role in the pathogenesis of cortisol toxicity and systemic lupus erythematosus. Proc Natl Acad Sci 79:3320, 1982
104. Yu S, Fishman J: Interaction of histones with estrogens: Covalent adduct formation with 16α-hydroxyestrone. Biochemistry 24:8017, 1985

Familial Aspects of Breast Cancer: An Overview

Wick R. Williams Michael P. Osborne

A family history of breast cancer is a well-known risk factor for the disease. The risk to a woman with a first-degree relative with breast cancer is generally reported to be two to three times higher than the risk to a woman with a negative family history.[1] This figure represents an average and was obtained by pooling many family histories. It may not accurately reflect the risk that applies to a given individual. In families in which a hereditary form of breast cancer is segregating, the lifetime risk to a first-degree female relative will approach 50%, a much higher figure than the average risk. In other families, the occurrence of breast cancer will reflect a sporadic form of the disease, and the lifetime risk of breast cancer to female relatives will be no greater than that of women in the general population, 9%.[2] In other families, the risk to women will fall between these two bounds, reflecting the fact that relatives share many of the same polygenic and environmental factors that contribute to an individual's multifactorial liability to disease. The variability of risk is thus a reflection of heterogeneity in both genetic mechanisms as well as environmental determinants that interact and contribute differentially to the pathogenesis of breast cancer.

REVIEW OF FAMILY STUDIES

The familial occurrence of breast cancer was known by physicians as early as the year 100 A.D. and pedigrees with striking familial patterns of the disease have been reported for more than a century. The most noted of these is a family described by a French physician, Paul Broca, that was based on his wife's genealogy. Of 24 females who spanned five generations dating back to 1788, 10 deaths were ascribed to breast cancer and another 4 to hepatic carcinoma by 1856.[3] This observation and others like it led to the initiation of studies to determine the role of a family history as a risk factor for cancer. Studies published during the 19th century contrasted the proportion of cancer patients that had a positive family history of cancer to the proportion of noncancerous controls with a positive family history, without adjustment for the size of families and the ages of their members, and consequently left the question of the importance of a family history unanswered.

During the early part of the 20th century, using improved epidemiologic methods, family studies were initiated that focused on site-specific forms of cancer; most of these studies were devoted to breast cancer. Although based on somewhat different experimental designs, the results of studies conducted in Denmark,[4] France,[5] Great Britain,[6–8] Hungary,[9] Iceland,[10,11] Italy,[12] the Netherlands,[13] Norway,[14] Russia,[15] Sweden,[16] and the United States[17–24] demonstrated a consistent and rather uniform two- to threefold increased risk of breast cancer to mothers and sisters of breast cancer patients. Risks of this magnitude, however, can be explained by more than one etiologic hypothesis.

Support for an environmental explanation comes from the fact that the two- to threefold higher risks associated with a positive family history of breast cancer are not very different from those associated with environmentally and physiologically mediated effects such as parity, socioeconomic class, age at first delivery, age at menarche, or age at menopause.[1] Second, studies of migrant populations point to an environmental basis, since the rates of breast cancer in migrants approach the rates of the locale or country to which the women migrate.[25] One possibility not generally considered, however, is that genetic factors could determine the response of the host to specific geographic carcinogens absent in the original country but present in the new locale. For any genetically determined tumor, it is the predisposition that is inherited, not the tumor itself, and some further steps mediated through the environment are then required for the development of cancer.[26] The evidence to support a hereditary component and hence a heterogeneous basis for breast cancer awaited more in-depth pedigree studies.

Contemporary Family Studies

One such study was initiated in 1969 by Dr. David E. Anderson of the M.D. Anderson Hospital and Tumor Institute (MDAH).[27,28] The research plan differed from previous family studies of breast cancer in the following way. Recognizing that breast cancer is a common disease and that most women with breast cancer have a sporadic form of the disease, Anderson used a more stringent selection criterion to ascertain families that would be more likely to reflect a hereditary component if one existed. Pedigrees in his study were ascertained through patients who had a histologically confirmed diagnosis of breast cancer (primary probands) and, in addition, whose medical records indicated the presence of breast cancer in a mother, sister, aunt, grandmother, or cousin (secondary probands). Of the 6550 breast cancer patients admitted to MDAH between 1944 and 1969, 500 (7.6%) satisfied this selection criterion and were recruited into his study. Additional women have been added since 1969, so that presently, his research base comprises more than 600 women with breast cancer and their relatives. As noted by Anderson,[28] not all familial patients could be identified on the basis of information provided by medical records; however, errors in classification should serve to diminish differences between familial and nonfamilial patients.

Anderson has used his resource to demonstrate heterogeneity in familial risk according to age at onset (premenopausal versus postmenopausal), laterality (unilateral versus bilateral), and type of family history (whether the secondary proband was a mother, sister, or second-degree relative of the initial proband).[27–34] The predominant findings are as follows: Compared with an unselected series of breast cancer patients, the frequency of bilateral disease among the familial probands was three to four times higher (2.8% versus 9.6%), and this difference was more pronounced among probands diagnosed at a premenopausal age (younger than 50; 15.5%).[28,32] First-degree relatives of the familial probands had higher rates of breast cancer than first-degree relatives of a control series, and these rates varied according to age at onset and laterality. Relatives of probands with premenopausal onset of disease, for instance, had a three times higher risk of breast disease, whereas relatives of probands with bilateral disease had a five times higher risk.[29] Finally, using survival analysis,[35] when the primary and secondary proband were first-degree relatives (mother-daughter, sister-sister) with premenopausal onset and one had bilateral disease, the lifetime risk as calculated for first-degree relatives was 50%.[32–34] This figure is consistent with what one would expect for an autosomal dominant trait with complete penetrance. In contrast, lifetime risks associated with unilateral and postmenopausal onset were not far removed from the 9% to 10% that applies to women in the general population.

Another recent family study was conducted by Dr. Hans-Olov Adami and his colleagues at the University Hospital, Uppsala, Sweden. This study involved women who had a histologically confirmed breast cancer and who resided in a well-defined geographic region of northern Sweden.[16,36] The large sample size (1423 cases of breast cancer in a 14-month period), the thoroughness of data collection and analysis, and its contemporary reference population make it worthy of review. The Swedish study differs from Anderson's study in two important ways. Patients in the Swedish study were ascertained from a population-based registry, whereas patients in Anderson's study were derived from a large hospital-based registry. Second, all patients with breast cancer were included regardless of whether the disease was known to have developed in a relative. As a consequence, the Swedish sample would be expected to be more representative of the general population of women with breast cancer.

In the Swedish study, the overall risk associated with a positive family history of breast cancer was slightly lower than that reported in most other studies; the relative risk of breast cancer being 1.7 times higher in mothers and sisters of patients with the disease than among mothers and sisters of controls. When patients were classified according to age at diagnosis and laterality, the relative risks associated with premenopausal onset and bilateral disease increased to 2.4 and 2.2, respectively. Although not significantly different from the 1.7 overall, the increase was suggestive of the findings obtained by Anderson.

At least two reasons can be postulated to account for the inability of the Swedish study to confirm the striking familial risks associated with premenopausal/bilateral disease that were observed by Anderson. Anderson's resource of familial pedigrees was much larger (n = 600) than that reported on by Adami and colleagues (n = 149 with at least one additional affected first-degree relative), and in particular, Anderson had a large enough sample of pedigrees in the rarer premenopausal/bilateral categories to test for heterogeneity. The different numbers of familial cases is a direct reflection of the different sampling schemes used in the two studies. Ascertainment of families that have a positive history of breast cancer, as in the case of the Anderson study, served to enrich the sample with hereditary cases. Ascertainment through a single proband, as in the case of the Swedish study, resulted in a sample composed primarily of sporadic cases and fewer hereditary cases, and an association with clinical features that characterize the hereditary subset was more difficult to demonstrate. Second, by 1985, Anderson has been able to follow his resource for approximately 15 years and to document additional cases of breast cancer among relatives. The Swedish study, on the other hand, has had a much shorter follow-up period, and consequently, fewer cases of breast cancer would be expected to have occurred among relatives.

The finding that premenopausal onset is more frequently observed in women with a family history of breast cancer has been verified by other studies on unselected patients,[37–39] and premenopausal onset and bilaterality are characteristics that have been documented in women from other selected pedigrees presenting familial aggregation of breast cancer.[40,41]

Other Clinical Features

In addition to age at onset and laterality, other clinical features that have been investigated for a possible association with a family history of breast cancer include histology and survival. Despite the enormous literature on the subject,[42–44] attempts to determine whether there is an association between histology and a family history of breast cancer have not yielded any conclusive findings. In their review, Mulcahy and Platt[42] report that the weight of evidence suggests that individuals with a medullary form of breast cancer are more likely to have a positive family history of the disease and also that, within pedigrees, there appears to be an association in histologic type. More recently, Rosen and colleagues[45,46] have suggested that a family history of breast cancer is an important risk factor for women with juvenile papillomatosis.

It has also been reported that women with a hereditary form of breast cancer survive longer than women with a nonhereditary form of the disease.[47] Since women with a family history of breast cancer will be more aware of the disease, its early signs and symptoms, and their preconceived risk, they may seek medical attention at an earlier time so that their disease will be diagnosed earlier. To the extent that this lead time is associated with stage at diagnosis and survival, it may explain the association that was observed. Additional evidence is required, with proper adjustment for lead time and stage at diagnosis, to accept this hypothesis.

The Frequency of Hereditary Disease

In an attempt to determine the frequency of hereditary breast cancer, Dr. Henry T. Lynch[48] conducted a family study involving a consecutive series of 225 patients with breast cancer who were seen at the Oncology Clinic of Creighton University (the extent to which this sample of women is representative of the general population is not known). From inspection of family histories, Dr. Lynch determined that 82% of patients had a sporadic form of the disease (i.e., the disease did not occur in a close relative). Of the remaining 18%, 13% were thought to represent polygenic forms of the disease, meaning that although the disease was present in relatives, its distribution and the extent of aggregation were not sufficient to be considered hereditary. The remaining fraction, 5%, were thought to represent examples of hereditary forms of breast cancer. Among the sample of probands diagnosed before 50 years of age, the hereditary fraction was 11.4%, which agrees with Anderson's findings.

Recent developments in genetic epidemiology have provided statistical methodology to formally investigate genetic and environmental models of disease transmission in pedigrees and to determine the most likely explanation for familial aggregation.[49] This method of analysis is referred to as segregation analysis. The application of segregation analysis to breast cancer has confirmed the suspected autosomal dominant mode of inheritance in selected high-risk pedigrees.[50–53] Future application of segregation analysis to population-based cohorts of families that have been ascertained and extended in a known manner will provide a means of resolving the nature of the familial component in the general population and to verify the etiologic composition proposed by Lynch. It will also allow identification of a model that can serve as the basis for genetic counseling.[54]

HEREDITARY FORMS OF BREAST CANCER

On the basis of clinical and epidemiologic features observed in selected pedigrees, a number of different hereditary syndromes that involve breast cancer have been proposed. In one syndrome (site-specific breast cancer), breast cancer represents the predominant phenotypic expression of the gene, whereas in another syndrome (Li-Fraumeni or SBLA [S: sarcoma; B: brain and breast cancer; L: leukemia and lung cancer; A: adrenal cortical cancer]) the gene may be expressed by one of a number of different malignant phenotypes that include breast cancer. In other syndromes, (Cowden disease, Muir syndrome), the gene is predominantly expressed by some unusual clinical feature and the occurrence of breast cancer is more of a secondary feature. The syndromes that have been recognized appear to be inherited as autosomal dominant traits. The extent to which the observed clinical heterogeneity in these syndromes is a reflection of underlying genetic heterogeneity is not known, nor has any molecular defect been defined. A model of carcinogenesis that explains the relationship between hereditary and nonhereditary forms of malignancy was proposed by Knudson.[55] Below we review this model and the hereditary syndromes that have been proposed.

A Model for Hereditary Cancer

The somatic mutation model for the origin of cancer was elaborated on by Knudson and colleagues[55–59] to explain both hereditary and nonhereditary forms of malignant disease. The model is based on the proposition that the majority of cancers are derived from a single cell[60,61] and postulates that at least two mutational events are required

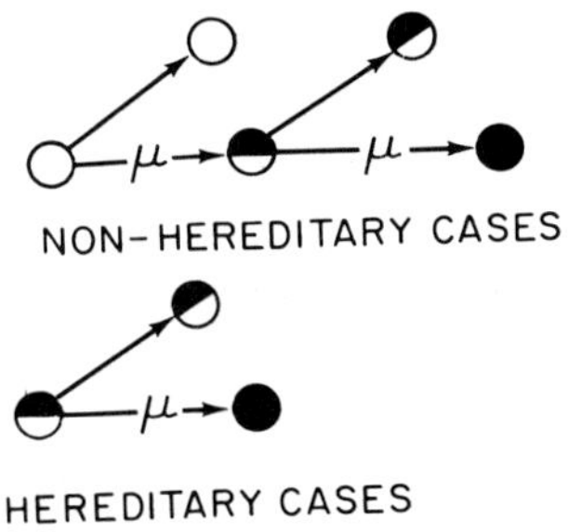

FIGURE 4-2. Two-stage model for carcinogenesis. In nonhereditary cases, normal cells (○) undergo mutation (μ) to produce cells in an intermediate state (◓). A second mutational event is required to transform this cell into a cancer cell (●). In hereditary cases, cells are in an intermediate state as a consequence of inheriting a mutation that is "fixed" in an ancestral germ line. Consequently only a second mutational event is required for such cells to become cancerous.

for the development of cancer (Fig. 4-2). In nonhereditary cases, the first event is a somatic mutation. When cells derived from this clone undergo an additional mutation at the complementary gene of the same locus, the first step toward malignancy may be initiated. Individuals with a hereditary form of the disease, on the other hand, receive the first mutational event from a parental germ cell. All cells in their somatic tissue are therefore in an intermediate or "prone" state and require a second mutational event for cancer to develop. The second mutational event may be in the form of a point mutation, chromosome deletion, somatic recombination, or other event.

Originally, support for this model came from statistical evidence in the form of comparison of age at onset and the numbers of independent tumors observed among individuals with hereditary and nonhereditary forms of two childhood cancers, retinoblastoma and Wilms tumor.[55,56] The model was subsequently extended to incorporate parameters that characterize growth, differentiation and transition rates of normal and intermediate cells.[62,63] As applied to breast cancer, the model was shown to provide a good fit to age-specific incidence data and, in addition, a consistent biologic explanation for other epidemiologic features, including hereditary and endocrine risk factors. As a consequence of developments in molecular biology, there has been recent molecular evidence to support Knudson's model[64–68] for Wilms tumor and retinoblastoma. Knudson[69] has called these loci anti-oncogenes, since the normal allele is in effect anti-oncogenic and it is inactivation or loss of the gene that is associated with the development of cancer.

Site-Specific Forms of Breast Cancer

The most frequent hereditary condition that involves breast cancer is a site-specific form of the disease.[70] Predisposition to breast cancer is inherited as an autosomal dominant trait with high penetrance. It is well documented by case reports of pedigrees that have been published in the literature.[40,70–79] In the pedigree resource of Anderson, the hereditary site-specific form of disease is presumably well represented in the subset of families in which the two probands are first-degree relatives with premenopausal/bilateral disease, as evidenced by the high risk of breast cancer to sisters and daughters.[30,32] In general, these two clinical features, early-premenopausal onset and bilateral disease, are cardinal features of breast cancer in families in which hereditary forms of the disease appear to be segregating. However, in some pedigrees that are thought to present hereditary forms of breast cancer, the disease occurs more frequently at a postmenopausal age (e.g., the pedigree of Woolf and Gardner[75]). Whether differences in age at onset reflect genetic heterogeneity for two different forms of the disease or whether the variation in age at onset is a result of environmentally mediated factors is not known. A pedigree in which a hereditary site-specific form of breast cancer is segregating is shown in Figure 4-3.

Li-Fraumeni or SBLA Syndrome

One of the most unusual of all cancer syndromes has been referred to as the Li-Fraumeni or SBLA syndrome.[80] Individuals with this syndrome are predisposed to a variety of different malignancies including soft tissue sarcomas, breast cancer, brain tumors, leukemias, lung cancer, and adrenal cortical tumors. This syndrome was first identified in 1969, when Li and Fraumeni[81,82] described four families that were ascertained through a pair of relatives who had developed soft tissue sarcomas during childhood. The investigation of cancer among their relatives revealed a dramatic pattern of familial clustering that was consistent with an autosomal dominant mode of transmission. Since the original report, additional families have been identified whose clinical features are consistent with this syndrome.[83,84]

A recent family study involving 161 3-year survivors of childhood soft tissue sarcomas and their first- and second-degree relatives was undertaken to determine the incidence of this syndrome and to formally investigate its mode of inheritance.[85] The suspected autosomal dominant mode of transmission was confirmed, and it was estimated that approximately 8% to 9% of children with soft tissue sarcomas come from families in which susceptibility to cancer may be inherited in the form of an autosomal dominant trait. The early age at onset and the high frequency of second primaries that were observed in these families are consistent features of hereditary forms of cancer. An example of a family with this rare syndrome is presented in Figure 4-4. In the example, the mother of the patient developed bilateral breast cancer at 26 and 27 years of age. Another family in this resource contains a woman who developed bilateral breast cancer at age 23, an extremely rare occurrence. A threefold excess risk of breast cancer among mothers of children with soft tissue sarco-

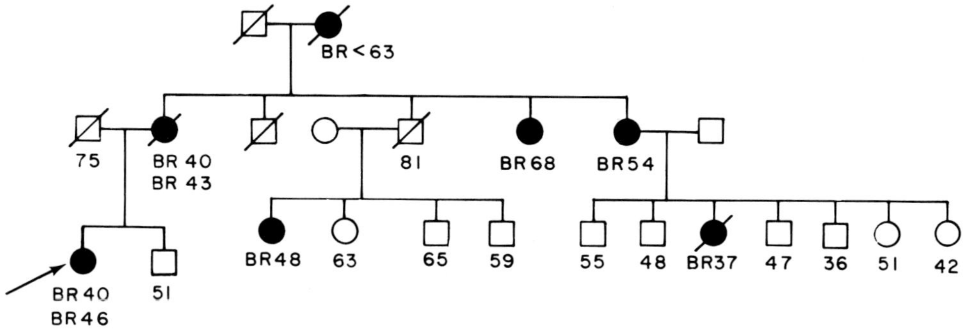

FIGURE 4-3. Pedigree with hereditary breast cancer. Numbers refer to age at diagnosis for individuals with breast cancer (BR) and age at death or last observation for individuals without cancer. See Figure 4-4 for key to other pedigree symbols. (Pedigree is courtesy of David E. Anderson, Ph.D.)

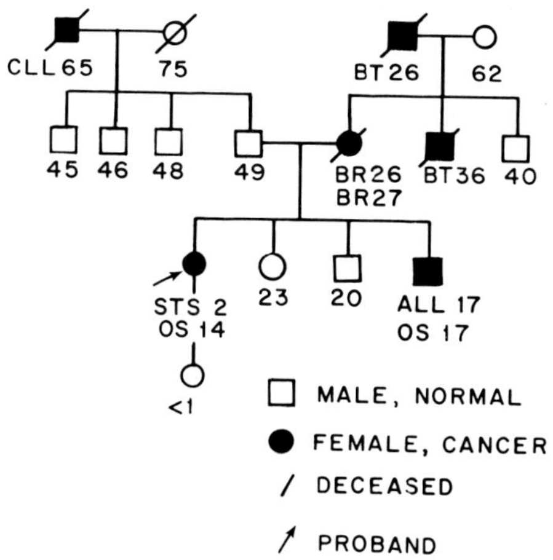

FIGURE 4-4. Pedigree with Li-Fraumeni or SBLA syndrome, in which breast cancer is a predominant phenotype. Numbers refer to age at diagnosis for individuals with cancer and age at death or last observation for individuals without cancer. Cancer abbreviation key: *ALL,* acute lymphocytic leukemia; *BR,* breast cancer; *BT,* brain tumor; *CLL,* chronic lymphocytic leukemia; *OS,* osteosarcoma. (Courtesy of Louise C. Strong, M.D.)

mas was also recently reported,[86] providing additional evidence that breast cancer is a predominant feature of this syndrome.

Cowden Syndrome

Cowden syndrome is a rare disorder that is characterized by hamartomatous lesions of the oral cavity and skin. Oral fibromas and papillomas are frequently observed in patients. Vitiligo, hemangiomas, and other diseases of the skin and subcutaneous tissue have been documented in other individuals.[87]

A recent review of cases revealed a high frequency of breast cancer among female patients with Cowden syndrome.[88] Ten of 21 females, or 47%, had developed breast cancer. This is an underestimate of lifetime risk, since the other 11 may develop breast cancer at a later time. Other breast conditions have been observed among the 11, including fibroadenomas, fibrocystic disease, virginal hypertrophy, and malformations of the nipple and areola.

Individuals suffering from Cowden syndrome are also prone to thyroid problems such as goiter and carcinoma of the thyroid, and some patients have presented with gastrointestinal polyps.

Muir Syndrome

Muir syndrome is characterized by multiple skin tumors (i.e., sebaceous adenomas, keratoacanthomas, and basal and squamous cell carcinomas) in conjunction with polyps and adenocarcinomas primarily of the large bowel, small intestine, and stomach.[89,90] The syndrome is inherited as an autosomal dominant trait with high penetrance. It is a rare disorder, although no firm estimate of the gene frequency exists. Females with Muir syndrome have an excess liability to breast cancer, although the lifetime risk has not been established. The observed cases of breast cancer have, in general, occurred at a postmenopausal age.

Familial Aggregation of Breast Cancer With Other Neoplasms

On the basis of aggregation of breast cancer with other malignant disorders observed for some pedigrees, another group of syndromes has been postulated. Ascertainment-sampling bias has made it difficult to determine whether such families represent unique syndromes or the chance occurrence of different tumors among close relatives. It is also possible that a gene that increases the susceptibility to breast cancer is pleiotropic for susceptibility to other forms of cancer as well. The predominant tumor associations that have been reported involve breast cancer with ovarian cancer and breast cancer with gastrointestinal cancer.

Lynch described three pedigrees and later an additional nine that showed familial clustering of breast cancer and ovarian cancer.[91,92] The lifetime risk of breast cancer or ovarian cancer or both to a first-degree relative of an affected individual was 46%, close to the 50% expected for an autosomal dominant trait with complete penetrance. The mean age at which breast/ovarian cancer was diagnosed was 50.6 years. Additional families showing this tumor aggregation have been reported.[93] A family presenting familial aggregation of breast/ovarian cancer is presented in Figure 4-5.

In 1973, Lynch and colleagues[94] reported an association between breast cancer and gastrointestinal cancer. Among 34 breast-cancer-prone families (at least two affected females), gastrointestinal cancer was observed in 22 families and appeared in subsequent generations in nine of the kindreds. An association between breast cancer and malignant melanoma has also been reported.[80]

THE FAMILIAL COMPONENT IN MALES WITH BREAST CANCER

Thus far, the role of heredity as it relates to breast cancer among females has been reviewed; however, the disease also occurs in males, in whom the incidence is approximately 1% of that observed in females. As a consequence of the low frequency in males, the etiology and role of heredity in male breast cancer have been less thoroughly studied. Nevertheless, there is reason to suspect that hereditary factors contribute to the development of breast cancer in men. One line of evidence comes from families in which a hereditary form of breast cancer is segregating. In such families, despite a preponderance of breast cancer in females, it is not uncommon to observe the disease in males.[4,74,95] There have also been reports of families in which more than one male has developed breast cancer.[96–100]

Williams and Anderson initiated a family study to investigate the relationship between familiality and male breast cancer.[101] Preliminary results have revealed that 33% (22/66) of the Caucasian sample had a family history of breast cancer. This frequency is higher than that recorded on medical records of female patients with breast cancer (15%, David E. Anderson, Ph. D., personal communication). The observed frequencies of disease among mothers and sisters of probands, 10.6% and 11.6%, respectively, were twice the frequencies that were expected on the basis of age. Twenty-five percent (4/17) of the twenty-four probands who reported a family history of breast cancer in a first-degree relative had at least two relatives (first- or second-degree) with the disease, which would suggest a hereditary form of the disease. These results are thus consistent with the notion that hereditary factors may play an etiologic role in the development of breast cancer in males. Future investigation of this resource will determine whether the hereditary contribution is the same as or different from that in females.

The risk of breast cancer is also enhanced in males with certain constitutional chromosomal anomalies. In 1955, there was a report of a male with Klinefelter syndrome, an XXY karyotype, who had developed breast cancer.[102] This led to a number of investigations of sex chromatin in series of males with breast cancer.[96,103–106] A summary of these data indicates that the breast cancer risk of males with Klinefelter syndrome is approximately 20 times that of men with a normal XY karyotype.[107] Breast cancer has also been reported in a phenotypic male with an XX karyotype.[108] The breast cancer risk of males with XXY and XX karyotypes may reflect the altered hormonal profiles that are associated with these chromosomal abnormalities. The breast cancer risk of the relatives of males with Klinefelter syndrome is not expected to be elevated in comparison to the general population.

FIGURE 4-5. Pedigree segregating for hereditary breast cancer demonstrating pleiotropy for susceptibility to ovarian cancer (*OV*). *U* denotes an unknown phenotype. Other notation is the same as given in Figures 4-3 and 4-4. (Courtesy of David E. Anderson, Ph.D.)

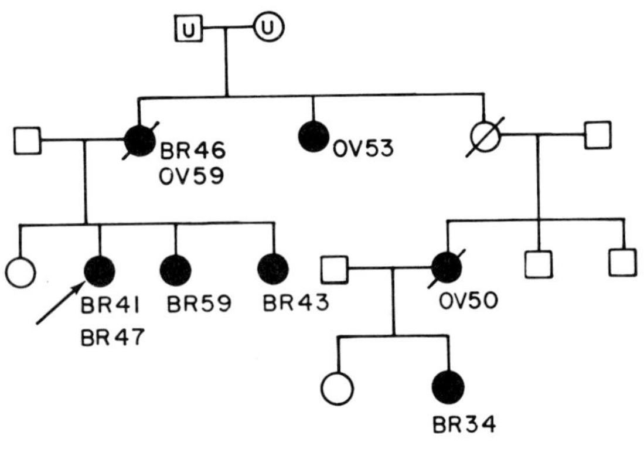

RISK OF BREAST CANCER BASED ON A FAMILY HISTORY

Genetic counseling for breast cancer emphasizes a broad range of medical skills. The first step involves diagnosis of disease, which is followed by taking a medical history of the patient and his or her relatives. The third step involves interpretation of this information and determination of the risk to various categories of relatives. Finally, this information must be conveyed to the patient and his or her relatives in a manner that enables them to have a clear understanding of their risk as well as knowledge of the various options for medical treatment to which they have access.

In procuring a family history, it should be kept in mind that patients' recollection of disease among their relatives is not always reliable; for example, what is reported as breast cancer in a relative may in reality have been a benign breast condition. Thus, in some cases, it may prove useful for a physician to attempt to verify malignant conditions that have been reported. Second, it is not sufficient to obtain information only on the frequency of malignant disease, since the risk of cancer will depend on the number of normal and affected relatives, their distribution within a pedigree, the sites and histologies of the malignancies that have occurred, the ages at which cancer developed, and (for breast cancer) whether the

Table 4-7
Empiric and Analytic Risks for Women with Frequently Observed Family Histories of Breast Cancer

Affected Relatives	*Clinical Features*	*Empiric Risk*	*Analytic Risk**
Mother	Premenopausal (pre)	0.18-0.27†	0.14
	Postmenopausal (post)		0.12
Sister	Pre/unilateral (uni)	0.08‡	0.14
	Pre/bilateral (bil)	0.56‡	
	Post/uni	0.18‡	0.12
	Post/bil		
Grandmother or aunt	Pre	-	0.10
	Post	-	0.09
Mother and sister	Both Pre, 1 bil	0.51§	0.23
	Both pre, 1 uni	0.33§	
	1 Pre, 1 post, 1 bil	0.23§	0.20
	1 Pre, 1 post, both uni	0.10§	
	Both post, 1 bil	0.28§	0.17
	Both post, both uni	0.16§	
Two sisters	Both pre, 1 bil	0.50§	0.23
	Both pre, both uni	0.18§	
	1 pre, 1 post, 1 bil	0.11§	0.20
	1 pre, 1 post, both uni	0.08§	
	Both post, both uni	0.05§	0.17
Mother and grandmother	Both pre		0.18
	1 pre, 1 post	0.27‖	0.16
	Both post		0.14
Mother and aunt	Both pre		0.18
	1 pre, 1 post	0.14‖	0.16
	Both post		0.14

* Based on a multifactorial model with heritability of 0.28.[54]
† Based on the general finding that women with a first-degree relative have a two- to threefold greater risk of the disease.
‡ Based on figures in Ottman[109]
§ Based on figures in Anderson[33]
‖ Based on figures in Anderson [32]

disease presented with unilateral or bilateral involvement. Once a reliable and complete medical history of the patient and his or her relatives is at hand, the physician is ready to make an assessment of risk.

The risk to a woman of developing breast cancer, based on a family history, can be determined by two methods. An empiric risk represents the observed incidence of disease that occurs in relatives with a given family history of disease—for example, the frequency of disease among women whose sisters have breast cancer. It is thus a reflection of ignorance about the mode of transmission of breast cancer among relatives. In Table 4-7, empiric risks for breast cancer for different family histories of affliction are summarized. These risks are based on family studies by Ottman and colleagues[109] and Anderson and colleagues.[27–34] Only studies that published results in terms of lifetime risk of breast cancer have been included. This criterion excludes studies that summarized results in the form of relative risks or odds ratios, because for such studies to be valid it is necessary to demonstrate that both the case and the control sample are representative of the general population.

Ottman's figures[109] were derived from a population-based cohort of Caucasian females. Lifetime risks of breast cancer were computed for mothers and sisters of patients who were classified by age at diagnosis (premenopause versus postmenopause) and laterality (unilateral versus bilateral) in an attempt to resolve genetic heterogeneity by these two risk factors.

Anderson's figures[27–34] are based on a hospital-based

resource and apply to women who report a family history of breast cancer in at least two relatives. Resolution of genetic heterogeneity was provided by partitioning pedigrees according to age at diagnosis, laterality, and type of pedigree involvement (whether the primary and secondary probands were first-degree relatives or second-degree relatives). Risks were derived for sisters and daughters.

The alternative to an empiric risk is an analytic or modular risk.[110] An analytic risk is a prediction of affliction that is based on an underlying model that defines how the disease is transmitted or shared by relatives. An analytic risk is obtained by computing the probability that the phenotype of an individual is affected, given the observed distribution of disease among his or her relatives. It is represented by the standard Bayesian expression:

$$P(PH_I = \text{Affected}/\ PH_R, \theta) = \frac{P(PH_I = \text{Affected},\ PH_R\ /\ \theta)}{P(PH_I = \text{Affected},\ PH_R\ /\theta) + P(PH_I = \text{Normal},\ PH_R\ /\ \theta)}$$

where PH_I refers to the phenotype of the individual at risk, Ph_R to the phenotypes of relatives, and θ to the model of disease transmission. (The algebraic decomposition of this equation in the context of likelihood calculations in pedigrees under genetic models is discussed in detail by Lalouel.[111,112])

Analytic risks form the basis for genetic counseling for most inherited disorders; however, they have not been readily available for breast cancer because a generally accepted model of disease transmission has not been established. With the exclusion of those families in which a hereditary form of breast cancer can be recognized, the most appropriate model from which to base analytic risks is a multifactorial model. Such a model refers to the cumulative influence of numerous genetic and environmental effects, none of which has a sufficient effect on liability to be recognized individually. A strong argument can be made for the aptness of such a model for breast cancer, in view of the large number of risk factors for the disease (i.e., age at menarche, parity, age at first pregnancy, height, weight), which no doubt reflect the interaction of numerous genetic and environmental variables. The parameter of importance for a multifactorial model is the heritability, which reflects the proportion of total phenotypic variation that is attributable to shared genetic and environmental factors. An estimate of the heritability of liability to breast cancer is 0.28, a figure that was derived from genetic analysis of 200 randomly selected families of Danish origin.[54] Risks based on this figure are given in Table 4-7 for the various pedigree situations described, and provide an alternative to the empiric risks for genetic counseling.

Given the large number of family studies that have been performed, the presently available empiric and analytic risks for breast cancer can be faulted for being nonspecific, prone to sampling error, and of questionable applicability. Rather than dismissing the question *in toto,* the recurrence risks have been given to serve as a rough guide for genetic counseling. In the future, application of segregation analysis to family material that is more representative, incorporating attempts to resolve heterogeneity according to clinical features of patients (e.g., laterality, age at onset) should remedy these problems by defining a model that more explicitly characterizes the familial component of breast cancer in the general population. This model in turn can be used to generate a specific analytic recurrence risk for a given individual, taking into consideration the unique pedigree history and the associated clinical demographic features that characterize that person's relatives. In general, the derivation of analytic recurrence risks will require a computer-assisted approach, since for complex models the calculus is too tedious for simple hand calculation and for even simple models the calculations are prone to human error. (Computer-assisted genetic counseling and COUNSEL, a computer program that was developed to provide a practical solution to this problem, have been discussed by Williams and Lalouel.[113,114])

FUTURE AREAS FOR RESEARCH

Three research strategies are currently being used to elucidate the underlying molecular defects that predispose an individual to breast cancer. Two of the strategies take advantage of pedigrees in which a hereditary form of breast cancer is segregating, since they provide a method for identifying a cohort of women at unusually high risk.

One approach is to start with a suspected biomarker and investigate its joint mode of inheritance with breast cancer in families with a hereditary form of the disease. If the trait is a true biomarker, the following predictions should hold: In women with breast cancer, the biomarker should be abnormally distributed, whereas in women who reach an advanced age without developing breast cancer the biomarker should present normal variation. Second, in offspring of women with the hereditary form of breast cancer who have not yet reached an age at which breast cancer normally occurs, the distribution of the biomarker should be bimodal, with one-half of the women presenting abnormal variation and the other half normal variation. Third, women with abnormal levels of the biomarker should proceed to develop breast cancer at higher rates than their relatives with normal levels. The joint mode of inheritance of breast cancer and the biomarker in such families can be investigated using a bivariate model for segregation analysis to determine whether the two traits are transmitted in a dependent fashion and whether this association may reflect the action of a pleiotropic major gene, a multifactorial contribution, or shared environmental determinants.[115] This approach is currently being investigated to a limited extent for the suspected biomarker 16 α-hydroxylation of estrogens.[116]

The other two strategies take advantage of the recent availability of hundreds of DNA polymorphisms defined by restriction enzymes (restriction fragment length polymorphism [RFLP]) that are becoming available and that will soon span the human genome.[117] Using a battery of

RFLPs that cover the genome, the heterozygosity of RFLPs in DNA from normal tissue is compared with that in DNA from the tumor of the same patient. In accordance with the model proposed by Knudson,[55] RFLP markers showing a consistent loss of heterozygosity would suggest that they flank a mutant gene that has become homozygous and for which loss of the normal gene has an important role in the development of cancer. Since the chromosomal location of the RFLPs is known or can be determined without difficulty, this approach can be used to identify a region of the genome that harbors a gene for breast cancer. This in turn can be used for more refined genetic mapping and ultimately for identification of the gene itself, which can be cloned and sequenced, so that the molecular defect can be determined. This approach has been successfully used to determine the chromosomal location of genes that are important for the development of a variety of tumors,[64–68,118–120] and efforts are under way to determine the biochemical defect.

The third strategy combines features of the first two approaches, namely information provided by pedigrees in conjunction with that proffered by DNA markers. Known as a *linkage study,* it is based on the premise that two genes that are located close together on the same chromosome will segregate together in a family whereas two genes that are located on different chromosomes will segregate independently. Examination of the joint segregation pattern of a battery of RFLPs and breast cancer in families with a hereditary form of the disease provides a method for identifying a linked marker that is in proximity to a "breast cancer" locus. Recently there have been reports of linkage of breast cancer to different loci; however, these findings have not been confirmed at this time.[121–123]

Linkage investigation of breast cancer will also serve other purposes.[124] First, it will provide a method for resolving genetic heterogeneity in breast cancer—for example, for determining whether the same or different loci are involved in the various hereditary and nonhereditary forms of the disease. Linkage will also provide a method for refining the clinical definition of hereditary syndromes that involve breast cancer and other cancer/clinical phenotypes. Third, in the short interim between localization of the chromosome and identification of the molecular defect in families in which hereditary forms of cancer are segregating, linked polymorphic markers provide a method of identifying individuals who have inherited a genetic susceptibility to cancer, before onset of the disease, when intervention may be able to reduce or eliminate their risk.[125] Developments in genetic epidemiology and molecular biology promise, in the near future, to clarify the role of heredity in the pathogenesis of breast cancer and to reduce the heritable burden of this disease in human populations.

REFERENCES

1. Kelsey HL, Hildreth NG: Breast and Gynecologic Cancer Epidemiology, pp 5–79. Boca Raton, CRC Press, 1983
2. Young JL, Percy CL, Asire AJ: Surveillance, Epidemiology, and End Results: Incidence and Mortality Data, 1973–1977. NCI Monograph 57, pp 1–1082, Washington, D.C., U.S. Dept. of Health and Human Services, 1981
3. Lynch HT: Introduction to breast cancer genetics. In Lynch HT (ed): Genetics and Breast Cancer, pp. 1–13. New York, Van Nostrand Reinhold, 1981
4. Jacobsen O: Heredity in Breast Cancer: A Genetic and Clinical Study of Two Hundred Probands. London, HK Lewis & Co, 1946
5. Richardson S, Gerber M, Pujol H: Familial risk in a case-control study on breast carcinoma. In Muller HJ, Weber W, Kuttapa T (eds): Familial Cancer, pp. 31–33. New York, S Karger, 1985
6. Lane-Claypon JE: A further report on cancer of the breast, with special reference to its associated antecedent conditions. In Rep Min Health No. 32, London, HM Stationery Office, 1926
7. Penrose LS, MacKenzie HJ, Karn MNA: Genetical study of human mammary cancer. Ann Eug 14:234–266, 1948
8. Smithers DW: Family histories of 459 patients with cancer of the breast. Br J Cancer 2:163–167, 1948
9. Juhasz L: Familial occurrence of breast cancer in North-East Hungary. In Muller HJ, Weber W, Kuttapa T (eds): Familial Cancer, pp 27–30. New York, S Karger, 1985
10. Tulinius H, Day NE, Sigvaldason H, et al: A population-based study on familial aggregation of breast cancer in Iceland. Taking some other risk factors into account. In Gelboin et al (eds): Genetic and Environmental Factors in Experimental and Human Cancer, pp. 303–312. Tokyo, Japan Scientific Society Press, 1980
11. Tulinius H, Day NE, Bjarnason O, et al: Familial breast cancer in Iceland. Int J Cancer 29:365–371, 1982
12. Bucalossi P, Veronesi U, Pandolfi A: Il problema dell'ereditarieta neoplastica nell'uomo. Il cancro della mammela. Tumori 40:365–402, 1954
13. Wassink WF: Cancer et heredite. Genetika 17:103–144, 1935
14. Waaler GHM: Ueber die Erblichkeit des Krebses. Shrifter Utgitt av det Norske Videnskaps-Akademie i Oslo, I. Mat.-Nature. Klasse, 2 (abstract by M Greenwood), Cancer Rev, 7:464, 1932
15. Martynova RP: Studies in the genetics of human neoplasms. Cancer of the breast, based on 201 family histories. Am J Cancer 29:530–540, 1937
16. Adami HL, Hansen J, Jung B, et al: Familiality in breast cancer: A case-control study in a Swedish population. Br J Cancer 42:71–77, 1980
17. Wainwright JM: Comparison of conditions associated with breast cancer in Great Britain and America. Am J Cancer 15:2610–2645, 1931
18. Crabtree JA: Observations on familial incidence of cancer. Am J Public Health 31:49–56, 1941
19. Woolf CM: Investigations on genetic aspects of carcinoma of the stomach and breast. University of California Publ in Public Health 2:1–265, 1955
20. Macklin MT: Comparison of the number of breast cancer deaths observed in relatives of breast cancer patients, and the number expected on the basis of mortality rates. J Natl Cancer Inst 22:927–951, 1959
21. Anderson VE, Goodman HO, Reed SC: Variables Related to Human Breast Cancer. Minneapolis, University of Minnesota Press, 1950
22. Murphey DP, Abbey H: Cancer in Families: A Study of the Relatives of 200 Breast Cancer Probands. Cambridge, Harvard University Press, 1959
23. Bain C, Speizer FE, Rosner B, et al: Family history of breast

cancer as a risk indicator for the disease. Am J Epidemiol 111:301–308, 1980
24. Sattin RW, Rubin GL, Webster LA, et al: Family history and the risk of breast cancer. JAMA 253:1908–1913, 1985
25. Haenszel W, Kurihara M: Studies of Japanese migrants. I. Mortality from cancer and other diseases among Japanese in the United States. J Natl Cancer Inst 40:43–68, 1968
26. Knudson AK, Strong LC, Anderson DE: Heredity and cancer in man. Prog Med Genet 9:113–158, 1973
27. Anderson DE: Genetic considerations in breast cancer. In Breast Cancer: Early and Late, pp. 27–36. Chicago, Year Book Medical Publishers, 1970
28. Anderson DE: Some characteristics of familial breast cancer. Cancer 28:1500–1504, 1971
29. Anderson DE: A genetic study of human breast cancer. J Natl Cancer Inst 48:1029–1034, 1972
30. Anderson DE: Genetic study of breast cancer—identification of a high risk group. Cancer 34:1090–1097, 1974
31. Anderson DE: Genetic predisposition to breast cancer. Recent results. Cancer Res 57:10–20, 1976
32. Anderson DE: Breast cancer in families. Cancer 40:1855–1860, 1977
33. Anderson DE, Williams WR: Implications of a family history of breast or colon cancer. In Chaganti RSK, German JL (eds): Genetics in Clinical Oncology, pp. 241–256. Oxford University Press, 1985
34. Anderson DE, Badzioch MD: Risk of familial breast cancer. Cancer 56:383–387, 1985
35. Gehan EA: Estimating survival functions from the Life Table. J Chronic Dis 21:629–644, 1969
36. Adami HO, Hansen J, Jung B, et al: Characteristics of familial breast cancer in Sweden: Absence of relation of age and unilateral versus bilateral disease. Cancer 48:1688–1695, 1981
37. Brinton LA, Williams RR, Hoover RN, et al: Breast cancer risk factors among screening program participants. J Natl Cancer Inst 62:37–44, 1979
38. Bain C, Speizer FE, Rosner B, et al: Family history of breast cancer as a risk indicator for the disease. Am J Public Health 111:301–308, 1980
39. Lubin JH, Burns PE, Blot WJ, et al: Risk factors for breast cancer in women in Northern Alberta, Canada, as related to age at diagnosis. J Natl Cancer Inst 68:211–217, 1982
40. Lynch HT, Guirgis H, Brodkey F, et al: Early age of onset in familial breast cancer. Arch Surg 111:126–131, 1976
41. Harris RE, Lynch HT, Guirgis HA: Familial breast cancer: Risk to the contralateral breast. J Natl Cancer Inst 60:955–960, 1978
42. Mulcahy GM, Platt R: Pathologic aspects of familial carcinoma of the breast. In Lynch HT (ed): Genetics and Breast Cancer, pp. 65–97. New York, Van Nostrand Reinhold, 1981
43. Adami HO, Jung B, Lindgren A, et al: Histopathological malignancy grading and familiality in an unselected series of 1303 women with breast carcinoma. Ann Clin Res 14:76–82, 1982
44. Rosen PP, Lesser ML, Senie RT, et al: Epidemiology of breast carcinoma. III. Relationship of family history to tumor type. Cancer 50:171–179, 1982
45. Rosen PP, Lyngholm B, Kinne DW, et al: Juvenile papillomatosis of the breast and family history of breast carcinoma. Cancer 49:2591–2595, 1982
46. Rosen PP, Holmes G, Lesser ML, et al: Juvenile papillomatosis and breast carcinoma. Cancer 55:1345–1352, 1985
47. Lynch HT, Albano W, Recerbaren J, et al: Prolonged survival as a component of hereditary breast and nonpolyposis colon cancer. Med Hypotheses 7:1201–1209, 1981
48. Lynch HT, Albano WA, Heieck JJ, et al: Genetics, biomarkers, and control of breast cancer: A review. Cancer Genet Cytogenet 13:43–92, 1984
49. Morton NE, Rao DC, Lalouel JM: Methods in Genetic Epidemiology, pp. 1–261. New York, S Karger, 1983
50. Hill JR, Carmelli D, Gardner EJ, et al: Likelihood analysis of breast cancer predisposition in a Mormon pedigree. In Morton NE, Chung CS (eds): Genetic Epidemiology, pp. 304–310. New York, Academic Press, 1978
51. Bishop DT, Gardner EJ: Analysis of the genetic predisposition to cancer in individual pedigrees. In Cairns J, Lyon JL, Skolnick M (eds): Cancer Incidence in Defined Populations, Banbury Report No. 4, pp. 389–408. New York, Cold Spring Harbor Laboratory, 1980
52. Elston RC, Go RCP, King MC, et al: A statistical model for study of familial breast cancer. In Lynch HT (ed): Genetics and Breast Cancer, pp. 49–64. New York, Van Nostrand Reinhold, 1981
53. Go RCP, King MC, Bailey-Wilson J, et al: Genetic epidemiology of breast and associated cancers in high risk families. I. Segregation analysis. J Natl Cancer Inst 71:455–462, 1983
54. Williams WR, Anderson DE: Genetic epidemiology of breast cancer: Segregation analysis of 200 Danish pedigrees. Genet Epidemiol 1:7–20, 1984
55. Knudson AG: Mutation and cancer: Statistical study of retinoblastoma. Proc Natl Acad Sci USA 68:820–823, 1971
56. Knudson AG, Strong LC: Mutation and cancer: A model for Wilms' tumor of the kidney. J Natl Cancer Inst 48:313–324, 1972
57. Knudson AG, Strong LC: Mutation and cancer: Neuroblastoma and pheochromocytoma. Am J Hum Genet 24:514–532, 1972
58. Knudson AG, Hethcote HW, Brown BW: Mutation and childhood cancer: A probabilistic model for the incidence of retinoblastoma. Proc Natl Acad Sci USA 72:5116–5120, 1975
59. Hethcote HW, Knudson AG Jr: Model for the incidence of embryonal cancers: Application to retinoblastoma. Proc Natl Acad Sci USA 75:2253–2457, 1978
60. Fialkow PJ, Gartler SM, Yoshida A: Clonal origin of chronic myelocytic leukemia in man. Proc Natl Acad Sci USA 58:1468–1471, 1967
61. Fialkow PJ: Clonal origin of human tumors. Cancer Rev 458:283–321, 1976
62. Moolgavkar SH, Knudson AG Jr: Mutation and cancer: A model for human carcinogenesis. J Natl Cancer Inst 66:1037–1052, 1981
63. Moolgavkar SH, Day NE, Stevens RG: Two-stage model for carcinogenesis: Epidemiology of breast cancer in females. J Natl Cancer Inst 65:559–569, 1980
64. Cavenee WK, Dryja TP, Phillips RA, et al: Expression of recessive alleles by chromosomal mechanisms in retinoblastoma. Nature (Br) 305:779–784, 1983
65. Fearon ER, Vogelstein B, Feinberg AP: Somatic deletion and duplication of genes on chromosome 11 in Wilms' tumours. Nature (Br) 309:176–178, 1984
66. Koufos A, Hansen MF, Lampkin BC, et al: Loss of alleles at loci on human chromosome 11 during genesis of Wilms' tumour. Nature (Lond) 309:170–172, 1984
67. Orkin SH, Goldman DS, Sallan SE: Development of homozygosity for chromosome 11p markers in Wilms' tumor. Nature (Am) 309:172–174, 1984
68. Reeve AE, Housiaux PJ, Gardner RJM, et al: Loss of Harvey ras allele in sporadic Wilms' tumour. Nature (Br) 309:74–176, 1984
69. Knudson AG: Hereditary cancer, oncogenes, and anti-oncogenes. Cancer Res 45:1437–1443, 1985

70. Lynch HT, Mulcahy GM, Lybnch P, et al: Genetic factors in breast cancer: A survey. Pathol Annu **11**:77–**101,** 1976
71. Handley WS: Chronic mastitis and breast cancer: A family history of five sisters. Br Med J 2:113–116, 1938
72. Wood DA, Darling HH: A cancer family manifesting multiple occurrences of bilateral carcinoma of the breast. Cancer Res 3:509–514, 1943
73. Smithers DW: Family histories of 459 patients with cancer of the breast. Br J Cancer 2:163–167, 1948
74. Gardner EJ, Stephens FE: Breast cancer in one family group. Am J Hum Genet 2:30–40, 1950
75. Woolf CM, Gardner EJ: The familial distribution of breast cancer in a Utah kindred. Cancer 4:515–520, 1951
76. Papadrianos E, Haagensen CD, Cooley E: Cancer of the breast as a familial disease. Ann Surg 165:10–19, 1967
77. Cady B: Familial bilateral cancer of the breast. Ann Surg 172:264–272, 1970
78. Dmytryk ET: Familial breast carcinoma. JAMA 216:1350, 1971
79. Armstrong AE, Davies JM: Familial breast cancer: Report of a family pedigree. Br J Cancer 37:294–307, 1978
80. Lynch HT: Genetic heterogeneity and breast cancer. In Lynch HT (ed): Genetics and Breast Cancer, pp 134–173. New York, Van Nostrand Reinhold, 1981
81. Li FP, Fraumeni JF Jr: Soft-tissue sarcomas, breast cancer, and other neoplasms: A familial syndrome? Ann Intern Med 71:747–751, 1969
82. Li FP, Fraumeni JF Jr: Rhabdomyosarcoma in children: Epidemiologic study and identification of a familial cancer syndrome. J Natl Cancer Inst 43:1365–1373, 1969
83. Bottomley RH, Condit PT: Cancer families. Cancer Bull 20:22–24, 1968
84. Lynch HT, Mulcahy GM, Harris RE, et al: Genetic and pathologic findings in a kindred with hereditary sarcoma, breast cancer, brain tumors, leukemia, lung, laryngeal, and adrenal cortical carcinoma. Cancer 41:2055–2064, 1978
85. Williams WR, Strong LC: Genetic epidemiology of soft tissue sarcomas in children. In Muller HJ, Weber W, Kuttapa T (eds): Familial Cancer, pp 151–153. New York, S Karger, 1985
86. Birch JM, Hartley AL, Marsden HB, et al: Excess risk of breast cancer in the mothers of children with soft tissue sarcoma. Br J Cancer 49:325–331, 1984
87. Brownstein MH: Cowden's disease. A possible new symptom complex with multiple system involvement. Ann Intern Med 48:136–142, 1978
88. Brownstein MH: Breast cancer in Cowden's syndrome. In Lynch HT (ed): Genetics and Breast Cancer, pp. 187–195. New York, Van Nostrand Reinhold, 1981
89. Muir EG, Yates-Bell AJ, Barlow KA: Multiple primary carcinomata of the colon, duodenum, and larynx associated with keratoacanthomata of the face. Br J Surg 54:191–195, 1966
90. Anderson DE: An inherited form of large bowel cancer, Muir's syndrome. Cancer 45:1103–1107, 1980
91. Lynch HT, Krush AJ: Carcinoma of the breast and ovary in three families. Surg Gynecol Obstet 133:644–648, 1971
92. Lynch HT, Harris RE, Guirgis HA, et al: Familial association of breast/ovarian carcinoma. Cancer 41:1543–1549, 1978
93. Fraumeni JF Jr, Grundy GW, Creagan ET, et al: Six families prone to ovarian cancer. Cancer 36:364–369, 1975
94. Lynch HT, Krush AJ, Guirgis H: Genetic factors in families with combined gastrointestinal and breast cancer. Am J Gastroenterol 59:31–40, 1973
95. Haagensen CD: Carcinoma of the male breast. In Haagensen CD: Diseases of the Breast, pp 779–792. Philadelphia, WB Saunders, 1971
96. Schottenfeld D, Lilienfeld AM, Diamond H: Some observations on the epidemiology of breast cancer among males. Am J Public Health 53:890–897, 1963
97. Marger D, Urdaneta N, Fischer JJ: Breast cancer in brothers: Case reports and a review of 30 cases of male breast cancer. Cancer 36:458–461, 1975
98. Everson RB, Li FP, Fraumeni JF Jr, et al: Familial male breast cancer. Lancet 1:9–12, 1976
99. Teasdale C, Holleb AI: Cancer of the male breast: A report of 146 cases. Cancer 8:1239–1250, 1955
100. Schwarz RM, Newell RB, Hauch JF, et al: A study of familial male breast cancer and a second report. Cancer 46:2697–2701, 1980
101. Williams WR, Badzioch MD, Anderson DE: Epidemiology of male breast cancer. In Ames FC, Blumenschein GR, Montague ED (eds): Current Controversies in Breast Cancer, pp 589–601. Austin, University of Texas Press, 1984
102. Bauer DF, Erickson RL: Male breast cancer. Klinefelter syndrome with prostatic, adrenal and mammary tumors. Northwest Med 54:472–476, 1955
103. Jackson AW, Muldol S, Ockey CH, et al: Carcinoma of the male breast in association with Klinefelter syndrome. Br Med J 23:223–225, 1965
104. Nadel M, Koss LG: Klinefelter's syndrome and male breast cancer. Lancet 2:366, 1967
105. Harnden DG, MacLean N, Langlands AO: Carcinoma of the breast and Klinefelter's syndrome. J Med Genet 8:460–461, 1971
106. Scheike O: Factors provoking male breast cancer. In Stoll BA (ed): Risk Factors in Breast Cancer, New Aspects of Breast Cancer, Vol. 2, pp 173–192. London, William Heinemann, 1976
107. Scheike O, Visfeldt J, Petersen B: Breast carcinoma in association with the Klinefelter syndrome. Acta Pathol Microbiol Scand A81:352–358, 1973
108. Giammarini A, Rocchi M, Zennaro W, et al: XX male with breast cancer. Clin Genet 18:103–108, 1980
109. Ottman R, Pike MC, King MC, et al: Practical guide for estimating risk for familial breast cancer. Lancet 3:553–558, 1983
110. Murphy EA, Chase GA: Principles of Genetic Counseling. Chicago, Year Book Medical Publishers, 1975
111. Lalouel JM: Recurrence risks as an outcome of segregation analysis. In Morton NE, Chung CS (eds): Genetic Epidemiology, pp 255–284. New York, Academic Press, 1978
112. Lalouel JM: Probability calculations in pedigrees under complex modes of inheritance. Hum Hered 30:320–323, 1980
113. Williams WR: Computer-Assisted Genetic Counseling, pp 1–310. Ph.D. dissertation, University of Hawaii, 1981
114. Williams WR, Lalouel JM: Genetic risks. In Morton NE, Rao DC, Lalouel JM (eds): Methods in Genetic Epidemiology, pp 188–206. New York, S Karger, 1983
115. Lalouel JM, Le Mignon L, Simon M, et al: Genetic analysis of idiopathic hemochromatosis using both qualitative (disease status) and quantitative (serum iron) information. Am J Hum Genet 37:700–718, 1985
116. Osborne MP, Crowe JP: The identification of enhanced risk patients and their management in a special surveillance breast clinic. In Ariel IM, Cleary JB (eds): Breast Cancer: Diagnosis, Management and Therapeutics, New York, McGraw-Hill, (in press)
117. Botstein D, White RL, Skolnick M, et al: Construction of a genetic linkage map using restriction fragment length polymorphisms. Am J Hum Genet 32:314–331, 1980
118. Fearon ER, Feinberg AP, Hamilton SH, et al: Loss of genes

on the short arm of chromosome 11 in bladder cancer. Nature 318:377–380, 1985
119. Hansen MF, Koufos A, Gallie BL, et al: Osteosarcoma and retinoblastoma: A shared chromosomal mechanism revealing recessive predisposition. Proc Natl Acad Sci USA 82:6216–6220, 1985
120. Koufos A, Hansen MF, Copeland NG, et al: Loss of heterozygosity in three embryonal tumours suggests a common pathogenetic mechanism. Nature 316:330–334, 1985
121. King MC, Go RCP, Lynch HT, et al: Genetic epidemiology of breast cancer in high-risk families. II. Linkage analysis. J Natl Cancer Inst 71:463–467, 1983
122. Skolnick MH, Thompson EA, Bishop DT, et al: Possible linkage of a breast cancer-susceptibility locus to the ABO locus: Sensitivity of LOD scores to a single new recombinant observation. Genet Epidemiol 1:363–374, 1984
123. Anderson DE, Ferrell RE, Williams WR: A linkage study of breast cancer susceptibility (abstr). Cytogenet Cell Genet 40:568–569, 1985
124. Williams WR, Anderson DE: Genetic epidemiology of breast cancer: Further clarification and a response to King and Elston. Genet Epidemiol 2:170–176, 1985
125. Lathrop GM, Lalouel JM: Easy calculations of lod scores and genetic risks on small computers. Am J Hum Genet 36:460–465, 1984

Prophylactic Mastectomy

Michael P. Osborne

Prophylactic mastectomy is the only known means by which breast cancer can be prevented. Total mastectomy would appear to be the most thorough way of eliminating risk, although as in all areas of medicine, no procedure can give an absolute assurance of freedom from risk. It is clear from anatomic and clinical evidence that complete removal of all breast tissue cannot be accomplished. The use of subcutaneous mastectomy has usually required that significant amounts of breast tissue be left in the subareolar region. This can be regarded as an unacceptable compromise in high-risk individuals. Apart from technical considerations, the indications for these procedures can be debated. The definition of risk as merely a diagnosis of fibrocystic disease or family history is untenable, and a more detailed and refined approach is required.

INDICATIONS

Prophylactic total mastectomy should be reserved for those rare individuals with a defined major risk factor that is unacceptable to the patient.[1] In the absence of a phenotypic marker other than cancer, nonaffected subjects for consideration for this procedure are those with either (1) hereditary breast cancer or (2) carcinoma *in situ*. These categories require detailed discussion between patient and physician in addition to expert genetic or pathologic analysis. It is essential to provide psychological assessment and support before any decision is reached. Evaluation is best conducted in a special surveillance breast clinic[2] where the appropriate multidisciplinary approaches can be coordinated. Women with fibrocystic disease of the breasts, a family history of sporadic breast cancer, or hyperplasia with atypia on biopsy are frequently given unsolicited advice to have prophylactic mastectomy. Such advice is disturbing to the patient and is often given without adequate preparation or discussion. The patient's lack of adequate understanding of the relative risks, coupled with evaluation of the potential physical and psychological morbidity of mastectomy, may render this advice inappropriate. It is therefore essential that, before prophylactic mastectomy is recommended, a complete review of the patient's genetic and pathologic factors is undertaken. In addition, the patient should undergo appropriate psychological counseling. In the event of a severe cancer phobia, the patient may be crippled by anxiety; however caution is required lest the phobia be translated to the postoperative sequelae of bilateral mastectomy.

TECHNIQUES

The choice of procedures recommended lies between subcutaneous and total mastectomy[3] with or without immediate or delayed reconstruction. Subcutaneous mastectomy is frequently advised but poses the problem of retained breast tissue. The results of 12 subcutaneous mastectomies that were performed on six cadavers through a long inframammary incision have been studied with regard to residual breast tissue.[4] The dissection extended from the rectus abdominus muscle to the clavicle and from the midsternum to the midaxillary line. The pectoral fascia was removed, and the anterior skin flap was thinned to full-thickness skin. Following this procedure, multiple samples were taken from the remaining peripheral fibrofatty tissue, from all borders of the resection, from the undersurface of the nipple and areola, and from skin flaps. In all instances, breast tissue was found under the areola. In addition, breast tissue was found in other locations in 83% of the cases. It appears that any procedure less than a total mastectomy will not adequately remove breast tissue, particularly if the nipple-areola complex is left in place. It is unknown whether removing 80% of the breast tissue will yield an equivalent reduction in risk of cancer. In such a subset of patients at high risk for the development of breast cancer, leaving islands of breast tissue with a potential risk for cancer is unsatisfactory. This view is supported by a study in which 285 patients had a breast biopsy that revealed fibrocystic disease. Sixteen of them, with severe epithelial hyperplasia of large and small ducts, had a subcutaneous mastectomy performed. Subsequently, nodules of breast carcinoma developed under the mastectomy flaps in three of the patients.[5] This problem has also been described after prophylactic total mastectomy. Two patients who were treated by simple mastectomy for noncancerous pathologic conditions of the breast and who subsequently developed carcinoma in residual breast tissue have been described.[6] It is therefore suggested that prophylactic mastectomy be of the total type, particular care being taken to raise the skin flaps to minimize leaving residual breast tissue. The pectoral fascia, nipple-areola complex, as well as the axillary tail must also be removed. Techniques of subcutaneous mastectomy have been described to overcome problems relating to retained subareolar tissue. The use of the "cored" nipple areola complex[7] as a free full-thickness skin graft and mastectomy accomplished through wide exposure and reconstituted using an inferiorly based dermal pedicle with a subpectoral silicone implant or tissue expander may lead to a more complete procedure.[8] It is advisable to sample lower axillary lymph nodes at this time, but a complete axillary dissection is unnecessary. Banking the complete nipple-areola complex on the anterior abdominal wall has been described, but the high potential for retained breast tissue at the base of the areola with the possibility for subsequent development of carcinoma makes this procedure inadvisable. Current reconstructive surgical techniques allow satisfactory nipple reconstruction by alternative methods. Claims made by protagonists of various prophylactic procedures have not yet been substantiated. At least 0.5% of those undergoing prophylactic subcutaneous mastectomy developed subsequent breast cancer.[9] It has not been shown that the observed versus expected incidence for the time frame of such studies has been favorably influenced.

Questions relating to the physical and psychological pros and cons in the timing of reconstruction are unanswered at the present time. However, substantial advances in reconstructive techniques have made immediate reconstruction more feasible.[10]

REFERENCES

1. Buehler PK: Patient selection for prophylactic mastectomy: Who is at high risk? Plast Reconstr Surg 72:324–334, 1983
2. Osborne MP, Crowe J: The Identification of High Risk Patients and Their Management in a Special Surveillance Clinic. In Ariel IM, Cleary JB (eds): Breast Cancers: Their Diagnosis and Management. New York, McGraw-Hill (in press)
3. Freeman BS, Wiemer DR: Total glandular mastectomy: Modifications of the subcutaneous mastectomy for use in premalignant disease of the breast. Plast Reconstr Surg 62:167–172, 1978
4. Goldman LD, Godwyn RM: Some anatomical considerations of subcutaneous mastectomy. Plast Reconstr Surg 51:501–505, 1973
5. Humphrey LJ: Subcutaneous mastectomy is not a prophylaxis against carcinoma of the breast: Opinion or knowledge? Am J Surg 145:311–312, 1983
6. Holleb AI, Montgomery R, Farrow J: The hazard of incomplete mastectomy. Surg Gynecol Obstet 121:819–822, 1965
7. Randall P, Dabb R, Loc N: "Apple coring" the nipple in subcutaneous mastectomy. Plast Reconstr Surg 64:800–803, 1978
8. Hyland WT: Subcutaneous mastectomy. Promises and pitfalls. Surg Clin North Am 65:373–381, 1985
9. Pennisi VR: The prevention of breast cancer by subcutaneous mastectomy. Surg Clin North Am 57:1023–1034, 1977
10. Osborne MP, Chaglassian T, Kinne DW: Mastectomy and immediate reconstruction for preinvasive breast cancer. Video Movie, American College of Surgeons Film Library, 1983

Early Detection of Breast Cancer

5

Anthony B. Miller

In the absence of major advances in treatment and because there is a potentially long delay before primary prevention of breast cancer will have a major impact, screening seems to have the most immediate potential for control of breast cancer. In light of the potential importance of screening in the control of breast cancer, much effort has been undertaken in evaluating its impact, including several large controlled trials. Although some of these have not yet reported results, the information now available on the effectiveness of breast cancer screening is considerable, which enables some assessment of its impact on control of breast cancer. In this chapter, the problems and pitfalls in evaluating the effectiveness of early detection are discussed first. Then the results that are now available or anticipated from completed and ongoing studies are presented. Finally, some practical recommendations based on current knowledge are provided.

PROBLEMS IN THE EVALUATION OF SCREENING FOR BREAST CANCER

In screening for breast cancer, one is seeking the cancer as distinct from an identified precursor. However, the currently available screening tests for breast cancer tend to result in detection of the cancer at a fairly late stage in its natural history. Except when a small cancerous area is found in what is largely a benign lesion, a breast cancer has to reach a size of 0.5 cm or more to be detectable. By then it has already been through many cell divisions, may have become intimately related to the vasculature and lymph channels, and, if invasive, may have had opportunities to metastasize.

Because of this, we cannot assume that the mere "early" detection of a breast cancer by the application of a screening test will be beneficial, even though a series of such cases may have a much better distribution by stage of disease than a series diagnosed in the absence of screening.[2] Further, it is not possible to conclude that screening is effective because survival from the time of diagnosis is better than in a clinical series. This is because of four biases that are inseparable from screening for any cancer—lead time, length time, (self) selection, and overdiagnosis bias.

Lead time is the time that the point of diagnosis has been advanced by the application of a screening test. Clearly, survival will inevitably be improved by at least this interval. Therefore, if survival of a group of screen-detected cases is compared with the survival of a group of cases diagnosed clinically the comparison will be biased. Improved survival of the screen-detected cases can be anticipated, but this will be seen even if the time of death or the number of deaths has not been influenced in any way. Lead time will vary from case to case, depending on the rate of growth of that particular case and the time in relation to that case's natural history that the test has been applied. When screening tests are applied in a population, there will therefore be a range or distribution of lead times, ranging from a day or so to several years. Early estimates of lead time for breast cancer screening were a mean of around 1 year.[3] More recent estimates using more modern screening tests suggest longer periods, with distributions of as long as 4 or more years, the mean lead time being shorter for younger than for older women.[4]

Length bias relates to the fact that fast-growing tumors will progress rapidly through the preclinical detectable phase of their natural history and will thus be less likely to be detected by screening tests applied relatively infrequently (e.g., annually or less often) than slow-growing tumors. Hence the tumors detected by screening tests will have a better prognosis than those detected by more conventional methods.

Selection bias relates to the inevitable self-selection for attendance at breast screening programs. The factors that cause people to volunteer for such programs are various. They include a perception of increased risk for the disease (such as a positive family history) and some awareness of approaches that can be taken to improve health care. Informed individuals may be more likely to present themselves promptly for treatment if they develop symptoms. In the absence of screening, therefore, their outcome is likely to be better than that of the general population. Part of this effect is offset by the self-selection of individuals with increased risk. It has been well documented that women who accept invitations for breast screening are at higher risk of developing breast cancer but at lower risk of dying of other causes than those who decline the invitations.[5]

Overdiagnosis bias results from the detection by screening of lesions of questionable malignancy that might never have been diagnosed in its absence. This has been a particular concern for some of the small or *in situ* cancers detected on mammography. Although it is clear that these lesions have a very good prognosis, it is not clear how many cancers that would otherwise result in death go through such a detectable phase. Further, many, in the absence of screening, might never have progressed. Therefore, the extent to which they should be actively sought by screening will probably only be determined by a controlled trial, such as the one now going on in Canada.[6]

Because of these four biases, there is great difficulty in assessing the effectiveness of breast screening unless a control group is an integral part of the design of the study, with mortality (the number of deaths occurring in the population screened) as the end point rather than survival or case fatality.[2]

It should be noted that surrogate measures that are known in the clinical situation to relate to outcome, such as distribution of cases by stage of disease, lymph node involvement, or size of tumor, are all influenced by the same biases. The closest of these measures to mortality is the rate or absolute number of cases of advanced disease occurring in the total population to whom screening is offered.[7] Evaluation of any approach to breast screening therefore has to be performed by a method that avoids these biases. No one has yet devised a method that takes note of the biases and corrects for them, although they are avoided in a controlled trial.[2]

It is important to bear in mind the distinction between evaluation of screening tests for breast cancer and evaluation of screening programs. Screening tests are evaluated by their ability to detect cancer, using measures such as sensitivity (the proportion of persons detected who have the disease), specificity (the proportion of those who do not have the disease, regarded as negative), acceptability, and cost. Their performance in a population is measured by the test's predictive value positive (the proportion of persons with positive tests found to have disease) and negative (the proportion of those with negative tests found not to have disease). It is unlikely that a screening program would be effective unless a good screening test as defined by these measures was used. Yet, although good screening tests are necessary for a successful screening program, effectiveness in reducing mortality from breast cancer cannot be assumed from them—it has to be determined directly.

As described elsewhere in this volume, some screening tests for breast cancer may have potential to detect the disease before the mass is palpable (diaphanography, ultrasonography), but they will not be considered further in this chapter because there is no evidence available for their effectiveness in reducing mortality. Thermography, as used in the Breast Cancer Detection Demonstration Projects, had too low sensitivity and specificity to justify further consideration.[5] The remaining screening tests (breast self-examination, physical examination, and mammography) will be considered here.

EVALUATION OF BREAST SELF-EXAMINATION

As part of their educational approaches to the problem of cancer, the Cancer Societies of North America have provided information to the public on breast cancer, in the hope that women will not delay seeing their physician if they find a breast lump. In addition, they have urged women to practice breast self-examination (BSE) on a regular basis in the hope that if a change does occur, women will detect it promptly. Neither the general public education messages nor BSE has ever been appropriately evaluated. Some investigators have evaluated the stage distribution of cases found on BSE,[8,9] but for the reasons already discussed, it is impossible to equate these measures with eventual reduction in deaths due to breast cancer. Cole and Austin[10] concluded that BSE may contribute more in situations where women do not use other screening modalities, but this conclusion was based on a review of studies that used surrogate measures to assess outcome. On a worldwide basis, BSE may have more potential applicability than other screening tests for breast cancer because it does not involve high technology.[11] It is currently being evaluated in a study of breast screening in the United Kingdom (see below) and in a randomized study based on cluster sampling in the USSR.[12] Nevertheless, it is clear that the reinforcement of training is necessary in order for an appreciable proportion of women to practice BSE well, even when they are initially taught on an individual basis.[13] Hence, costs associated with its use are not negligible, and it cannot yet be advocated as public health policy until more information on its effectiveness is available.[14]

EVALUATION OF PHYSICAL EXAMINATION

No one has yet evaluated the extent to which regular examination by physicians of well women on an annual basis results in reduction of mortality from breast cancer. Hence this procedure, in common with many other examinations routinely performed by physicians,[15] still requires evaluation.

As will be apparent later in this chapter, there are no ongoing studies that will determine unequivocally the effectiveness of physical examination of the breast as a screening test for breast cancer. This is unfortunate, as there is some indirect evidence that physical examination of the breast contributed to reduction in mortality from breast cancer in the Health Insurance Plan (HIP) study (see below). Nevertheless, as emphasized by Bassett,[16] physical examination of the breasts by physicians is often conducted poorly or not at all. It is conceivable that without extensive physician education, the potential benefits of physical examination, maximal under study conditions, may not be realizable in practice.

EVALUATION OF MAMMOGRAPHY

Mammography, or soft tissue x-ray examination of the breast, has come to be regarded as the most important screening test for breast cancer. Since the HIP study, all programs evaluating screening for breast cancer (other than those specifically evaluating BSE mentioned above) have included mammography, either alone or in combination with physical examination of the breasts and sometimes with BSE. Yet, as will become apparent, it is by no means certain that mammography is a necessary part of an effective screening program for breast cancer. In order to assess the evidence, it is appropriate to discuss this on a study-by-study basis.

The Health Insurance Plan Study

The HIP study, conducted with participants in the HIP of Greater New York, was the first randomized controlled trial to evaluate screening for any site of cancer.[17,18] The screening modalities evaluated were the combination of mammography using the Eagan technique[19] and physical examination of the breasts by skilled examiners. BSE was not taught. Sixty-two thousand women were included in the study and were randomized to study or control groups by a pairwise allocation procedure. Of the 31,000 women allocated to the study group, 65% attended one or more of the four annual screening examinations scheduled. The investigators evaluated the outcome in the total study group in comparison with the control group, as they could not have identified within the control group those who would have refused screening if it had been offered to them. Hence a policy of inviting women to attend for screening was evaluated. All women received the routine care available in the HIP. Follow-up was through the HIP and other mechanisms. The wisdom of the controlled trial approach, and as a corollary the difficulty of evaluating screening without an appropriate control group, was emphasized when it became apparent that mortality from causes other than breast cancer was substantially lower in those who accepted the invitation to attend for screening than in the control group.[5] Indeed, the percentage reduction in mortality from breast cancer in those screened compared with the controls was less than the reduction in mortality from all causes other than breast cancer. This apparent paradox was resolved when it was appreciated that the women who accepted the invitation to attend for screening had a higher incidence of breast cancer than those who refused.[5] In assessing the results of this trial, many observers have tended to assume that the benefit obtained was largely due to the use of mammography. This impression was heightened by the early reports of the trial, which showed much better survival in the cases detected on mammography alone than in those detected on physical examination alone or detected by both modalities. However, there was bound to be a differential lead time between those cases identified on mammography, those identified on physical examination, and those identified on both modalities. Such a differential confounds attempts to use survival as a measure of outcome in determining the relative contribution of the modalities used in screening programs. Its presence has been largely confirmed in the long-term follow-up of the study by the increasing juxtaposition, after about a 5-year interval, of the survival of the cases detected by mammography alone compared with those detected on physical examination alone or physical examination plus mammography.[20]

Confining our attention therefore to comparisons of mortality between the study and control groups, two striking features emerged as a result of the analyses. The first was that although there were no differences between study and control groups in deaths from breast cancer in the first 2 years after initiating screening, a differential was seen from 3 years, and it became maximal at 7 years.[20] Walter and Day[4] modeled the lead time distribution and found a best fit with an exponential distribution. This gave an estimate of a mean lead time of 1.7 years (20 months), approximately 44% of cases having a duration less than 1 year and 5% having a duration greater than 5 years. It seems unlikely that cases with a much longer than average lead time, many of whom were probably identified by mammography, could have contributed to an early mortality reduction. The implication is that screening for breast cancer improves the prognosis of cases detected somewhat late in their natural history.

Two other observations support the inference that the reduction in mortality was due to the earlier detection of advanced disease. The first is that the survival in the Stage II (involved node) cases in the study group was better than the survival of those with the same stage in the control group. The second is the progressive erosion of the survival advantage of the cases detected by mammography alone in the study group with increasing duration of follow-up.[20] Thus the physical examination component of the screening probably made an important contribution to the overall reduction in mortality. It has been calculated that this contribution might amount to as much as 70% of the mortality reduction.[21,22]

The other striking aspect of the study was an initial apparent differential in effectiveness of screening at different ages. The initial analyses of the study related to breast cancer deaths in the first 5 years following entry. All of the mortality reduction occurred in women older than 50 years, there being no difference between the study

Table 5-1
Breast Cancer Deaths by Age at Entry 5 and 14 Years From Entry in the HIP Study

Age at Entry	*Number of Deaths* Through Year After Entry:*			
	5 years		*14 years*	
	Study	*Control*	*Study*	*Control*
40–49	19	20	46	61
50–59	15	33	53	68
60+	5	10	19	24
Total	39	63	118	153

*From breast cancer as underlying cause of death among breast cancers diagnosed during the first 5 years after entry. (Shapiro S, Venet W, Strax P, et al: Ten to fourteen-year effects of screening on breast cancer mortality J Natl Cancer Inst 69:349, 1982)

Table 5-2
Cumulative Numbers of Deaths due to Breast Cancer to 14 Years After Entry and Cases of Breast Cancer Diagnosed Within 5 Years of Entry by Age at Diagnosis, Subdivided by Age on Entry

Age at Diagnosis	*Deaths due to Breast Cancer*		*Breast Cancer Cases*	
	Study	*Control*	*Study*	*Control*
Age 40–44 on entry				
40–44	7	11	17	15
45–49	11	15	32	31
Total 40–49	18	26	49	46
Age 45–49 on entry				
45–49	18	12	40	30
50–54	10	23	28	38
Total 45–54	28	35	68	68

(Shapiro S, Venet W, Strax P, et al: Ten to fourteen-year effects of screening on breast cancer mortality. J Natl Cancer Inst 69:349, 1982)

and control groups in breast cancer deaths for women between the ages of 40 and 49 (Table 5-1). However, by 14 years this had changed (Table 5-1). The numbers of deaths due to breast cancer until 14 years from entry and the numbers of cases of breast cancer diagnosed within 5 years of entry in women between the age of 40 and 49 are examined in more detail in Table 5-2. Shapiro and colleagues[20] suggested that some of the benefit in the study group age 45 to 49 on entry could have been due to screening after age 50, and they tended to discount the mortality differential in this group at age 50 to 54 on diagnosis. Instead, they pointed out that there were similar numbers of deaths in study and control groups for all those between the ages of 40 and 49 on diagnosis (36 in each group). However, the larger number of deaths in the study group compared with the control group in women 45 to 49 years of age entry and on diagnosis is at least in part due to the larger numbers of cases diagnosed in the study group, with a corresponding deficit in those 50 to 54 years old on diagnosis. This could be a "lead time" effect of screening, although it is hardly noted in the age group 40 to 44 years on entry. In practice, the mortality differential between study and control group is larger in those 40 to 44 years old on entry than in those age 45 to 49 (31% and 20%, respectively).

The HIP study was not designed to assess a possible differential effect of screening at different ages, and the differences observed could be due to chance. The investigators concluded, "for ages under 50 years, the HIP study does not provide evidence that screening has an effect on mortality."

However, there are explanations other than chance for the apparent difference in effectiveness by age. The age of 50 roughly corresponds to the menopause, and it is known that premenopausal women have denser breasts than postmenopausal women, in whom much of the glandular tissue is replaced by fat. Fat is more radiolucent, and thus early cancers are easier to detect on mammography in postmenopausal women than in premenopausal women. Mammography in the early 1960s was relatively inefficient compared with now, especially in younger women. Only 19% of the cases of breast cancer identified on screening in women age 40 to 49 in the HIP study were found on mammography alone, compared with 44% in women age 50 to 59.[17] However, an alternative explanation for a differential effectiveness at younger compared with older ages is a difference in biologic aggressiveness of breast cancer in premenopausal compared with postmenopausal women. Such differences have been noted in response to therapy in early disease.[23] Further, physical examination of the breasts was equally applied in the two ages, and if it was effective at older ages, why not at younger? The growth rate of cancers premenopausally may be faster than in postmenopausal women, a supposition that may be in part related to the steeper increase of incidence with age premenopausally than postmenopausally (see Chapter 4).

The question of an age differential effect of screening must therefore be regarded as having been raised by the HIP study, but it remains a question to be solved by other investigations. However, any attempt to capitalize on the results of the HIP study should appreciate the possibility of an age differential.

The Breast Cancer Detection Demonstration Projects

In 1973, the American Cancer Society initiated the concept of centers designed to assess the extent to which women would attend for breast cancer screening. This idea was taken up by the National Cancer Institute and eventually extended to include 28 centers in 27 cities throughout the United States. In each city, 10,000 women between the ages of 35 and 74 years were to be recruited. They were to be given information on risk factors for breast cancer and to be screened using physical examination, thermography, and mammography.

In their recruitment drives, the centers were eminently successful. Recruitment was facilitated by the publicity surrounding the development of breast cancer in the wives of the then president and vice president.

Unfortunately, the organizers of this program did not take into account the age differential in the HIP study. However, even at the time the project was initiated, some were advising caution.[24] One of the concerns, namely over radiation-induced breast cancers in an age-group in which benefit had not yet been demonstrated, came to the fore when Bailar[21] predicted that at the mammography dosage then operating, the Breast Cancer Detection Demonstration Project (BCDDP) might be responsible for as many radiation-induced cancers as the number of deaths that might be prevented by the program. Mammography for women younger than 50 years was therefore withdrawn in the BCDDP except for those who had a personal history of breast cancer.[5,22] In the absence of defined populations from which the women who volunteered for the projects were drawn and the lack of a suitable control group, it is not possible to determine effectiveness in terms of mortality reduction.[5]

A review of cancers classified as minimal by a special pathology panel suggested that a number might not have been cancer at all.[5] Although too high a false-positive rate was initially reported because of difficulties in collecting material,[26] the specter was raised of women treated by mastectomy for noncancer abnormalities. Further, some minimal cancers might never have progressed, and they might never have become clinically detectable in the absence of screening.

However, to the extent that earlier diagnosis of abnormalities identified on screening results in less extensive treatment, screening can be regarded as beneficial. The increasing information that suggests the appropriateness of conservative therapy for early breast cancer[23,26] suggests that women with screen-detected early cancer should in general be managed conservatively. At the same time, particular care should be taken by pathologists to ensure that overdiagnosis is avoided.

An analysis of the cancers identified during the five years of the BCDDP[27] confirmed that the ability of mammography to detect lesions in women younger than 50 years was much higher than in the HIP study (Table 5-3). However, many of the projects concentrated on mammography, and it is possible that some of the apparent in-

Table 5-3
Modality of Detection of Breast Cancer in the HIP Study Compared With That in the BCDDPs

Suspicious Modality	HIP Study				BCDDPs			
	Age 40–49		Age 50–59		Age 40–49		Age 50–59	
	Number	%	Number	%	Number	%	Number	%
Mammography alone	6	19	27	42	270	35	540	42
Physical examination alone	19	61	26	40	100	13	86	7
Both	6	19	12	18	381	50	638	50
Unknown	0	0	0	0	11	1	19	2
Total	31	99	65	100	762	99	1283	101

Baker LH: Breast cancer detection demonstration project: Five-year summary report. CA 32:194, 1982) creased sensitivity of mammography compared with physical examination may have been due to less efficient physical examinations.

The apparent improvement in the detection ability of mammography and the favorable stage distribution of the cancers detected led to the publication by the American Cancer Society of guidelines for mammography[28] that updated the Society's previous guidelines and those of the American College of Radiology.[29] These were again updated in 1983.[30] The difficulty with these guidelines is that they are based on assumptions about benefit using end points that are suggestive but that do not prove that mortality reduction can be attributed to mammography, as discussed above. Table 5-4 summarizes the guidelines and the evidence that was available from the only controlled trial then reported at the time they were released.[20] The advocacy of mammography on a routine basis for women requires the availability of facilities and personnel to conduct such examinations.[31] Thus, in the absence of proof that mammography really does contribute substantially to the mortality reduction that was noted in the HIP study, it is difficult to justify routine mammographic screening for breast cancer. This consideration led directly to the design of one of the components of the Canadian randomized trial of breast screening (see below).

The Kaiser Permanente Study

The use of mammography was evaluated as part of a controlled trial of multiphasic screening in the Kaiser Permanente Program in California in women age 45 or older, with follow-up from 1964 to 1975.[32] The results of this trial showed no mortality differential for breast cancer. Fourteen deaths due to breast cancer were reported in each of the two groups compared. Nevertheless, three-quarters of the subjects were younger than 50 years when the study began. Thus, although this study does not have sufficient power to refute the HIP findings, it does reinforce the desirability of not extrapolating from the HIP findings without further study.

Table 5-4
Summary of the American Cancer Society Guidelines on Mammography for Asymptomatic Women and Evidence Relating to These Guidelines Derived From Controlled Trials

Age-group (year)	*Recommendation*	*Evidence From Controlled Trials*
40–49	Mammography performed at intervals of 1–2 years	No early but possible delayed benefit from *combination* of mammography + physical examination
50 or older	Annual mammography	Benefit from *combination* of mammography + physical examination

(Shapiro S, Venet W, Strax P, et al: Ten to fourteen-year effects of screening on breast cancer mortality. J Natl Cancer Inst 69:349, 1982)

Studies in the Netherlands

Two screening projects were initiated in the Netherlands. In Utrecht, all women older than 50 years on the population register were invited to attend a center at which they were offered mammography and physical examination. Mammography used the Xerographic process and was a standard two-view examination; physical examination was performed by the radiology technicians.[33] In another city in the Netherlands, Nijmegen, single-view (lateral) mammography was used alone in a similar population study. In this study, women 35 years of age and older were recruited. In both cities, approximately 70% of those invited attended, but after four screens, attendance fell to a little over 50%.[7]

It was initially planned to assess mortality differentials in comparison to control towns. However, results from both studies have now been published using the case-control approach to analysis. In Utrecht, the breast cancer mortality among those presenting at least once for screening was 70% less than those who refused (relative risk 0.30, 95% confidence interval 0.13 to 0.70).[34] In Nijmegen, a 52% reduction in risk of death was seen (relative risk 0.48, 95% confidence interval 0.23 to 1.00).[35]

The case-control approach is a relatively new way of analyzing the results of screening,[2] and it is not as valid as a randomized controlled trial. Case-control studies essentially mimic the approach that would be taken in a cohort study, and questions have to be raised about the comparability of the cases and controls. The analysis essentially compares the screening history in those who die of breast cancer with comparable persons drawn from the source population who have not. In both cities, it was found that breast cancer mortality was higher among women who refused to attend screening than among women selected as controls. If this approach had been used in analyzing the results of the HIP study, the cases and controls would both have been drawn from the study group (those allocated to screening). We know from that study that the incidence of breast cancer in the refusers was lower than in the acceptors, so that a case-control analysis would not have been valid, although it presumably would have been more likely to have shown a false-negative than a false-positive result.

In the Utrecht study, it was possible to show that the women who declined screening invitations had a breast cancer incidence and stage distribution similar to that seen immediately before screening started and in a control town,[34] so that little bias seemed to be operating in terms of incidence of breast cancer. Nevertheless, it is still possible that some selection bias may have been operating in terms of the factors that influence mortality from breast cancer. If unknown factors led to a higher probability of death from breast cancer if breast cancer occurred in those who refused to enter the screening program than in those who accepted the invitation to be screened, then the result that was seen could have been anticipated.

Although the numbers of deaths were small when considered by age, both studies suggest different effects of screening by age. In Utrecht, a lower effect of screening was noted in women aged 50 to 59 than in older women, the reverse effect to that seen in the HIP study. The Utrecht study provides confirmation of the effectiveness of screening women aged 60 or older. In Nijmegen, in a further analysis using a different control group and including deaths up to 1982, those younger than 50 years at first invitation to screening had no reduction in breast cancer mortality (relative risk 1.23, 95% confidence interval 0.31 to 4.81).[36]

The United Kingdom Study

In the United Kingdom, a geographically based comparative study has been mounted.[37] In two districts, population screening has been initiated; in two others, BSE teaching in clinics or groups is offered; and in four more, data are being gathered for comparative purposes, but no screening or BSE teaching is offered. Women are recruited for screening by letters written to them from their family physicians, after age–sex registers had been created in the practices in the area. In both centers offering screening, mammography is done biennially, a single view in one and two-view examinations in the other. Annual physical examinations are offered, however. In one of the two screening districts, some of the practices have been randomized to a control group. Although response has been of the order of 70% in the screening centers, there was a lower response to invitations for BSE teaching.[7] It may be some years before results are available from the study, and screening is scheduled to continue for 7 years. As indicated above, this is one of the two major studies that may provide evidence on the effectiveness of BSE.

The Swedish Trials

In Sweden, three large trials of mammography alone have been in progress for some years, and a fourth (in Stockholm) has recently been started. In two, single-view mammography is being used with control groups selected by randomization on a cluster sampling basis.[38] When single-view mammography is used alone, the oblique projection is the only view, an approach for which an adequate sensitivity is claimed.[39] Two examinations of the population were planned at 35- to 36-month intervals during a 5-year period that commenced in 1977, but it proved possible to offer three screening rounds to younger women at an interval of about 21 months. At 5 years, the absolute numbers of advanced (Stage II+) breast cancers were less in the screened group than in the control.[7] The third project (in Malmo, in southwestern Sweden) uses two-view mammography and is based on randomization of individuals.[40] In this study, it is known that the controls have access to mammography outside the screening center, and there is some concern over dilution. In the fourth study recently started in Stockholm, randomization is also based on individuals, and single-view mammography is used.

Results have now been reported on mortality from the first two trials using single-view mammography, conducted in the counties of Kopparberg and Ostergotland.[41] All women 40 years or older and resident in the two counties were entered into the study, a total of 162,981 women. Enrollment into the study began in 1977. Participation by women age 75 or older was less than 50%, and this group was excluded from the analysis. Among women 40 to 74 years old at the date of randomization, participation by those invited to screening was approximately 90% at the first screening round and only slightly lower at the second round. In this group, the estimate of relative risk from the two counties combined was 0.69 (95% confidence interval 0.51 to 0.92). However, there was no reduction in mortality in women 40 to 49 years old. In women age 50 to 74 years on entry, breast cancer mortality was 40% less in the screened group than in the control (Table 5-5).

Clearly the Swedish results (and those from Nijmegen) confirm that reduction in mortality from breast cancer can be achieved in women older than 50 years using mammography alone. However, they leave unanswered the question of the amount that mammography adds to the benefit of physical examination, and there has to be concern that the relatively high interval cancer rates noticed are at least partly due to the absence of physical examination.

The Canadian National Breast-Screening Study

The Canadian National Breast-Screening Study (NBSS) commenced in January, 1980,[42] with the following objectives:

1. To determine in volunteers age 40 to 49 on entry to the study whether unselective annual screening by mammography and physical examination, when used as an adjunct to the highest standard of care in the Canadian health care system, reduces the mortality from breast cancer.
2. To determine in volunteers age 50 to 59 on entry to the study the additional contribution of routine annual mammographic screening to screening by physical examination alone.
3. To assess whether an appropriate combination of risk factors for breast cancer can be derived to permit restricting screening to those at highest risk of the disease.
4. To provide the data necessary for an analysis of the cost-effectiveness of breast cancer screening in Canada using current mammography techniques.
5. To provide data on the natural history of breast cancer for incorporation into computer simulation approaches to determine the age at which screening should ideally

Table 5-5
Deaths From Breast Cancer by Age at Entry Over 7 Years From Entry in the Kopparberg and Ostergotland County Project

Age at Entry and Study Group	*Kopparberg County* Deaths	*Kopparberg County* Population	*Ostergotland County* Deaths	*Ostergotland County* Population	*Combined Relative Risk (and 95% Confidence Intervals)*
Age 40–49					
Study	8	9,625	8	10,312	1.26
Control	3	5,053	7	10,625	(0.56, 2.84)
Age 50–74					
Study	43	29,426	28	28,722	0.61
Control	36	13,793	40	27,311	(0.44, 0.84)

(Tabar L, Fagenberg CJG, Gad A, et al: Reduction in mortality from breast cancer after mass screening with mammography. Randomized trial from the breast cancer screening working group of the Swedish National Board of Health and Welfare. Lancet 1:829, 1985)

commence and what its periodicity should be at different ages.

It was planned to recruit 90,000 women into the project, 50,000 age 40 to 49 and 40,000 age 50 to 59 years. This required 15 screening centers across the country, with an individual recruitment target ranging from 1,000 to 15,000 women. It was originally planned to conduct five annual screening examinations but in order to set a termination date to the study, women recruited toward the end of the recruitment phase were offered only four annual screens, as in the HIP study. After cessation of screening, follow-up will be performed by computerized record linkage with the Canadian Cancer Incidence and Mortality files and can therefore be continued indefinitely.[6]

Initially there were some difficulties because it was necessary to adopt general publicity mechanisms in order to recruit participants.[43] There were four issues that tended to keep women away from the NBSS. One was simply ignorance, not knowing that the project existed; a second was a feeling that they were adequately cared for already by their family physicians; a third was a concern over radiation; a fourth was a feeling of fear and "not wishing to know." Many women are frightened of the idea that an examination might reveal breast cancer, even though there is some understanding that earlier diagnosis results in improved probability of cure.

Controversy over mammography and radiation largely relates to the validity of the extrapolations from high-dose level exposure to estimated risk at low-dose levels.[44] When it became clear that the dosages used in film-screen mammography in the NBSS were very much less than had been the norm for the BCDDP, we computed the overall risk-benefit for screening using mammography.[45] Even if the mortality reduction from the use of mammography was as low as 20%, our calculations suggested a clear excess of benefit over risk for women included in the NBSS at all ages.

There is a substantial variation in susceptibility of the breast to the effects of radiation at different ages, with maximum susceptibility when women are first irradiated in their teens or twenties and substantial reduction in risk for women first irradiated after the age of 30 (see Table 4-5 in Chapter 4). With this information, it is possible to reassure women who are considering participating in breast cancer screening. If mammography is only offered to women age 40 or older, the risk of inducing breast cancer is negligible.

It is still too early to expect results from the NBSS. Recruitment was completed at the end of March, 1985, but screening will continue until March, 1988. Thus early mortality results cannot be expected until about 1990. A total of 89,968 women were allocated, 26,653 age 40 to 44, 23,819 age 45 to 49, 22,903 age 50 to 54, and 16,593 age 55 to 59 years. The detection rates by age on initial and repeat screening are of the order anticipated from the BCDDP, although with slightly higher proportions of cancers detected on physical examination alone, possibly a reflection of more efficient physical examination.

One of the features of the NBSS is that all women are taught BSE and that this teaching is reinforced for those who return for rescreening. In addition, the frequency of practice is self-assessed by annual questionnaires and the efficiency of practice is assessed during the screening physical examination. It is therefore planned to attempt to assess the effectiveness of BSE by a case-control approach within the strata formed by randomization in the study.

FUTURE APPLICATION OF BREAST CANCER SCREENING

Existing Technology

Several issues must be borne in mind when decisions are made about whether and how breast cancer screening should be introduced in the general population. The first concerns whether screening for breast cancer is effective in reducing mortality and which screening modalities might contribute to this. The second concerns the groups in the population to be offered screening and the need to demonstrate that screening does result in the mortality reduction anticipated from controlled trials. Associated with this are questions on the age at which screening should start, the periodicity of rescreening, and the age at which screening should end.

There is already substantial information on mortality reduction following breast cancer screening. The Utrecht study[34] provided, for the first time, confirmation of the HIP study finding[20] that the combination of mammography and physical examination of the breasts reduces mortality in women older than 50 years. The Swedish[41] and Nijmegen[35,36] studies have shown that benefit follows the use of mammography alone, although there is a suggestion that the degree of benefit is less than that achieved by the combination of mammography and physical examination. The benefit from mammography over and above that to be obtained from physical examination, a question of particular relevance to North American practice, will be precisely determined in women age 50 to 59 on entry to the Canadian trial.[6] However, the benefit from physical examination alone will not be determined precisely from any study, and comparisons between studies will be needed to produce an estimate of its effect.

Currently, the information available does not support the introduction of population screening for breast cancer in women younger than 50 years. Paradoxically, only the HIP study now shows any evidence of benefit from screening women less than this age, and this only appeared after long follow-up—that is, the benefit is largely restricted to reduction of deaths when these women were in their 50s and is, in any case, not statistically significant. It would seem, therefore, that even if such a benefit were real, it could be substantially overshadowed by the benefit that would be achieved by *starting* screening these same women when they reached their 50s. Unless further follow-up of the Swedish studies provides evidence on this issue, it will be necessary to wait for the results of the United Kingdom and Canadian studies before making recommendations on population screening for younger women.

More information is, however, now available on periodicity of rescreening and the ages to continue with screening. The studies in the Netherlands and in Sweden have demonstrated effectiveness of screening even when conducted every 2 years or less often still. In practice, in the Swedish trials, the periodicity of rescreening in women age 50 or older was closer to 2 than 3 years. Whether greater benefit would be achieved in women older than 50 by annual rescreening will probably be determined by the United Kingdom and Canadian trials. Clearly, however, if 40% reduction in mortality can be achieved by screening with mammography alone every 2 years, screening with mammography and physical examination every year would have to be justified on cost benefit grounds, an issue that is addressed in more detail below.

As far as age of cessation of screening is concerned, information is now available to confirm effectiveness of screening up to the age of 74, after which compliance with screening becomes of increasing concern. More data and possibly computer simulation studies will be required to determine whether rescreening up to this age can be gradually reduced in frequency (as was incorporated in the Utrecht study[33]).

New Technology

Currently, all new devices will have to be evaluated in comparison with mammography and preferably the combination of mammography and physical examination. If devices that appear to be usable for screening are developed, it will probably be unnecessary to mount additional large-scale controlled trials to determine whether mortality reduction would follow from their use. This is because if it can be demonstrated that the new devices have equivalent or preferably superior sensitivity and specificity to mammography and physical examination in a healthy population under screening circumstances, it can be assumed that they will result in at least equivalent mortality reduction. Thus, although substantial numbers of healthy women, as distinct from women who present with possible symptoms of breast cancer, would have to be studied in order to reach a decision with precision, the investigation would not be as expensive as a long-term controlled trial and could be completed relatively rapidly. Nevertheless, difficulty will be encountered if a device that is advocated for screening does not identify a subset of the cases found on mammography, such as those cases in which the only radiologic sign is a cluster of fine calcifications. As it is unlikely that any screening study using mammography can separate the effect of the early detection of such cancers from the other effects of mammography in the reduction in mortality, we will be driven to assess the importance of their early detection by surrogate measures. Nevertheless, with existing studies enabling us to assess benefits in terms of mortality reduction and with their also providing inferences on natural history, there is some hope that survival data in well-conducted screening studies in the future can be assessed in relation to potential mortality reduction using mathematical models.[46]

Barriers in Applying Advances in Screening Detection Technology to Everyday Practice

Screening is not well adapted to application in a purely private medical care environment. Cost-benefit and cost-effectiveness calculations generally presuppose that the screening test is applied in a population in a manner that achieves optimal specificity and sensitivity with sufficient prevalence of the disease to ensure that an appropriate proportion of positive tests will be found to represent disease, i.e., high predictive value positive. This relates to what some have called screening in the public health sense, which is the application of a screening test in an asymptomatic population with a benefit that will not be immediately realizable nor immediately apparent to those screened or those who apply the screen. All screening tests for cancer require at some stage equipment that has to be procured and housed at somewhat substantial capital costs and that involves fairly costly maintenance and the provision of staff who have been adequately trained in the procedures they are applying. Screening programs involving mammography for cancer of the breast need mammography machines that will deliver images of high quality but with low radiation dosage. In my opinion, this requires film-screen technology, since the xerographic process results in nearly 10 times as much midbreast radiation. But in order to maintain high quality at low dosage, periodic monitoring of the machines and skilled maintenance are required. Physical examinations of the breast have to be conducted by skilled practitioners. Most physicians have not had the appropriate training and do not acquire the necessary experience. Nurse examiners, however, can be trained to a high level of competence over a 2- to 3-month period,[16] and the best continue to maintain this skill from year to year. Breast cancer screening also results in high costs in applying the definitive diagnostic procedure, a biopsy, and for nonpalpable lesions requires the provision of skilled practitioners to avoid biopsies that are mutilating.

These requirements for the introduction of mammography in a community, emphasized in a Union Internationale Contre le Cancer (UICC) workshop,[31] have recently been reinforced from experience in the United States.[47] Mammography tends to substantially increase the number of biopsies performed in a community, and thus the cost of health care. In the NBSS, the benign-to-malignant ratio in the first screening year was 3.5 for those allocated to physical examination alone but 5.9 for those allocated to mammography plus physical examination. In the second year, the same differential persisted, but at a lower level for both (1.8 and 4.6, respectively).

In addition to these difficulties, physicians sometimes compound the problem by demanding fees for a service for screening examinations at the same level as for diagnostic examinations.[48,49] This problem has in general been solved for cervical cytology, for which the primary screener is the specially trained cytotechnician whose function it is to recognize abnormalities but not necessarily reach a diagnosis. Similar technicians could be trained to act as the initial screeners for physical and radiologic examination of the breast. It will almost certainly be impossible to justify screening in economic terms unless such individuals are used.

In various cultures, different taboos may interfere with the application of screening tests. Although the effect of these taboos is lessening, they can interfere with the willingness of women to present themselves for breast screening. Currently they seem to be greater at older than younger ages. Thus in two of the Swedish trials, compliance with screening invitations by women older than 75 years was so poor that the findings in this age-group were not reported.[41] It is important to recognize that the social barriers to acceptability of screening tests do not only apply to the person to whom the test is being offered. Spouses at times seem to have a disproportionate influence. However, they may also be an asset. For example, it seems possible that the relative failure of BSE, which can be partly attributed to the necessity for women to dissociate themselves from their own body sensations in carrying out the examinations,[50] might be overcome if their spouse or other partner was trained to carry out the examination and understood the abnormalities that were being sought. With the increasing availability of teaching models, it should be possible to ensure that training sessions incorporate both husband and wife.

In an American Cancer Society survey,[49] 95% of the physicians sampled agreed with the Society's guidelines[30] on physical examination, but only 41% with those on mammography. The most important reasons given for not agreeing completely were that it was too expensive (39%), unnecessary in the absence of symptoms (29%), was not necessary to do annually (28%), caused too much radiation exposure (25%), had a low yield (16%), and, somewhat surprisingly, was unnecessary in the absence of family history (14%). Of the group who regarded mammography as too expensive, nearly one-third also explained their disagreement as a function of concern about radiation, patient fear, and questions about the reliability of the mammogram. Of these factors, radiation was mentioned most often, by one-fifth of the group. Clearly if mammography is to be introduced as a general procedure, much professional education will be required. In addition, the expertise a radiologist requires for mass screening is different from that required for a diagnostic service, and special training should be obligatory.[51] Reference has already been made to the expertise required in the community to diagnose and treat nonpalpable lesions and to diagnose histologically the many abnormalities detected on mammographic screening.

These requirements are not inconsiderable, and so far only Sweden has decided to mount a breast cancer screening program based on mammography for women age 50 or older. However, in the United States, it has been accepted as an objective that, by the year 2000, 80% of women between the ages of 50 and 70 years should be receiving annual physical examinations and annual mammography, substantial increases from the 1983 estimates of 45% and 15%, respectively.[52] Such policies could be expected to have major impacts after only about a 5-year delay, in comparison with the much delayed impact of primary prevention.[1]

ECONOMIC FACTORS

As implied earlier, in reaching decisions about modalities to use for screening, periodicity, and ages to start and stop, detailed consideration of economic issues will become very relevant. I have computed the costs and benefits of screening 100,000 women between the ages of 40 and 59 with physical examination and mammography annually for 5 years.[53] The net costs of screening were related to the expected years of lives saved as a result of screening, assuming a 40% reduction in mortality. The total years of life saved amount to 1855. Relating this to the net costs of screening resulted in a cost per year of life saved of Can$5697 (approximately U.S. $4100). By a sensitivity analysis, I tested the extent to which the assumptions underlying these calculations influenced the conclusions drawn. It was clear that the extent of mortality reduction had the most influence on them.

However, with more information now available on effectiveness—particularly evidence from Utrecht[34] and Sweden[41] that annual screening in women older than 50 may not be needed—it has been possible to revise the earlier calculations examining the effect of different screening policies, costs of different modalities, and so on. All calculations are now based on screening women 50 to 59 years old, as there is insufficient evidence about effectiveness before the age of 50. Three levels of costs for screening procedures have been used—an estimate of $12 for single-view mammography from Sweden,[41] $8 for physical examination of the breasts by trained nurse practitioners derived from the NBSS, and $22 for double-view mammography derived from the NBSS actual costs for 1984–1985. An administrative cost of $11 per examination is added to each (also derived from NBSS 1984–1985 costs). From the Swedish studies, an estimate of 40% reduction in mortality for single-view mammography every 2 years is derived, and from Utrecht a 60% reduction using two-view mammography plus physical examination at approximately 2-year intervals. These figures are then compared with the costs of annual physical examination, making the assumption that 70% of the benefit in Utrecht was obtained from the physical examination component of the screen. The costs and benefits have been applied to a cohort of 100,000 women—55,000 between the ages of 50 and 54 and 45,000 from 55 to 59 years. The basic method was the same I used previously.[54] In addition to determining the costs of screening, it is necessary to estimate the costs of the extra biopsies generated as a result of screening and the potential savings in health care expenditure from reduction in health care costs, as it would not be necessary to pay for treatment of women who would otherwise die of advanced breast cancer.

In determining costs of biopsies, the assumption was made that screening identifies five times more abnormalities than would otherwise come to light if mammography is used either alone or in combination with physical examination, and two times as many if physical examination alone is used. For each biopsy, a cost of $500 was applied to those identified on physical examination, as such lesions are all palpable and no special procedure is required to locate them, but a cost of $1000 was allocated for those identified on mammography. This doubling of cost is an approximation to the additional costs required to locate and remove nonpalpable abnormalities diagnosed on mammography. These costs were then added to the costs of screening to estimate a total cost of the program. Screening examinations were assumed to be applied in years one and three, when mammography was used, and annually, years one to four, when physical examination alone was used. Costs beyond year one were discounted to the present day at a rate of 10% per annum.

The benefit from screening in terms of reduction in mortality was assumed to commence at year three and cumulate through to year seven, as in the HIP study. The degree of mortality reduction permits an estimate of the numbers of deaths that would have otherwise occurred during these years, and it was assumed that on average, each death would have otherwise resulted in an expenditure of $27,500. These amounts were also discounted to the present day. Subtraction from the total costs of the

Table 5-6
Costs and Benefits From Screening 100,000 Women age 50 to 59

	Program		
Item	*Single-View Mammography Alone Biennially*	*Double-View Mammography Plus Physical Examination Biennially*	*Physical Examination Alone Annually*
Mortality reduction years 3–7	40%	60%	42%
Cost of screens	$3,976,700	$7,088,900	$6,086,935
Cost of extra biopsies	$2,261,956	$2,261,956	$ 738,500
Total costs	$6,238,656	$9,350,856	$6,825,435
Savings from averted deaths	$2,918,307	$4,377,461	$3,064,223
Net cost	$3,320,349	$4,973,925	$3,761,212
PYLS*	1,705	2,558	1,790
Cost per PYLS*	$ 1,947	$ 1,944	$ 2,101

*Person years of life saved to age 70

program provides the net cost of the program. This was then related to the potential years of life saved to age 70 to provide a cost per year of life saved. The results are displayed in Table 5-6.

From this analysis, it is apparent that there is very little economic advantage to any one of the three programs. Many would doubt however, that under North American circumstances, it would be possible to achieve the low costs of single-view mammography as in Sweden. It may also, of course, be difficult to achieve in practice the relatively low costs actually expended in Canada in the NBSS. Further, assumptions are built into the calculations about the degree of benefit from screening, and some of these still need to be confirmed. The 40% reduction in mortality observed in the Swedish studies in this age-group is very compatible with the similar order of effectiveness found in the earlier HIP study. The increased order of effectiveness in the Utrecht program for the combination of physical examination and double-view mammography, which in the calculation has counteracted the additional cost of the screen, needs confirmation from the NBSS or the United Kingdom study. Further, the assumption that physical examination alone can achieve 70% of the benefit of the combination of mammography and physical examination also needs confirmation from the NBSS. If it does, however, then skilled physical examination is likely to result in a level of cost-effectiveness similar to programs involving mammography and would not require the expertise and capital expenditures for mammography, costs that have in fact been largely ignored in these calculations. If the additional capital expenditures required for providing mammography were factored in, then physical examination alone, if established as effective, would clearly be a viable rival if the necessary training of physicians or their assistants could be achieved.

Nevertheless, it is clear that effective breast screening will result in a relatively low expenditure per year of life saved. It is here that the computations cease, and we have to determine whether an expenditure of this order per year of life saved is justifiable. This of course is a moral judgment to which the public should contribute.

CONCLUSION

There is clearly still room for controversy about whether breast cancer screening requires further evaluation or whether it can be adopted as population policy. Many radiologists, especially in North America, will not be prepared to abandon double-view mammography, nor will they be able to offer the low-cost mass approach developed in Sweden or even in the NBSS in Canada. It remains to be seen whether the current American Cancer Society guidelines[30] will be revised in the light of new evidence of lack of effectiveness of single-view mammography in screening women younger than 50 years, or whether continued assumptions will be made of a possible greater effectiveness of double-view mammography plus physical examination in this younger age-group. Perhaps the most important lesson to be derived from the experience of the past decade is that we are beyond the stage when large-scale population screening programs for cancer or indeed any disease can be introduced on the basis of assumed benefits. Benefits will have to be established in large-scale studies. The studies that are necessary to fully evaluate breast cancer screening are now in place, and the answers we need should be available by the end of the current decade. However, there has to be one final note of caution. If, as I have inferred, the major benefit in women age 50 or older in the HIP study derived from the physical examination component of the screen, the benefit to be derived from the addition of mammography to annual physical examinations of the breasts may be delayed, because the additional benefit could largely relate to those women with cancers with a relatively good prognosis already. Thus it could be many years before a significant difference is detected in women older than 50 in the NBSS, if at all. In the meantime, physicians will have to weigh the evidence and decide whether to screen using regular and efficient physical examinations of the breast by themselves or by trained nurse practitioners and by the practice of BSE or whether to substitute single-view mammography (if available) or use the more costly double-view mammography on the assumption of additional benefits. Whatever decision they take, it is now clear that all women older than 50 years should be offered regular breast screening in some form or other.

REFERENCES

1. Miller AB: Approaches to the control of breast cancer. In Rich M, Hager JC, Furmanski P (eds): Understanding Breast Cancer: Clinical and Laboratory Concepts, pp 3-25. New York, Marcel Dekker, 1983
2. Prorok PC, Chamberlain J, Day NE, et al: UICC workshop on the evaluation of screening programmes for cancer. Int J Cancer 34:1, 1984
3. Hutchison GB, Shapiro S: Lead time gained by diagnostic screening for breast cancer. J Natl Cancer Inst 41:665, 1968
4. Walter SD, Day NE: Estimation of the duration of a pre-clinical disease state using screening data. Am J Epidemiol 118:865, 1983
5. Beahrs O, Shapiro S, Smart C: Report of the Working Group to review the National Cancer Institute American Cancer Society Breast Cancer Detection Demonstration Projects. J Natl Cancer Inst 62:640, 1979
6. Miller AB, Howe GR, Wall C: The national study of breast cancer screening. Clin Invest Med 4:227, 1981
7. Miller AB, Van Slooten EA: Screening and diagnosis in breast cancer: Workshop report. Eur J Cancer Clin Oncol 19:1711, 1983
8. Foster RS, Lang SP, Costanza MC, et al: Breast self-examination practices and breast cancer stage. N Engl J Med 299:265, 1978
9. Greenwald P, Nasca PC, Lawrence CE, et al: Estimated effect of breast self-examination and routine physician examinations on breast-cancer mortality. N Engl J Med 299:271, 1978
10. Cole P, Austin H: Breast self-examination: An adjuvant to early cancer detection. Am J Public Health 71:572, 1981
11. Miller AB, Chamberlain J, Tsechkovski M: Self-examination in

the early detection of breast cancer. A review of the evidence, with recommendations for further research. J Chronic Dis 38:527, 1985
12. World Health Organization: Role of breast self-examination in reduction of mortality from breast cancer (Protocol of the study). (in press) 1986
13. Baines CJ, Wall C, Risch HA, et al: Changes in breast self-examination behaviour in a cohort of 8214 women in the Canadian National Breast Screening Study. Cancer 57:1209, 1986
14. Miller AB: Editorial: Breast self-examination. (in preparation) 1986
15. Canadian Task Force on the Periodic Health Examination: The periodic health examination. Can Med Assoc J 121:1193, 1979
16. Bassett AA: Physical examination of the breast and breast self-examination. In Miller AB (ed): Screening for Cancer, pp 271-291. New York, Academic Press, 1985
17. Shapiro S, Strax P, Venet W, et al: Changes in 5-year breast cancer mortality in a breast cancer screening program, pp 663-678. Proceedings of the Seventh National Cancer Conference. American Cancer Society, January, 1974
18. Shapiro S: Evidence on screening for breast cancer from a randomized trial. Cancer 39:2772, 1977
19. Eagan RL: Mammography. Springfield, IL, Charles C Thomas, 1964
20. Shapiro S, Venet W, Strax P, et al: Ten to fourteen-year effects of screening on breast cancer mortality. J Natl Cancer Inst 69:349, 1982
21. Bailar JC: Mammography: A contrary view. Ann Intern Med 84:77, 1976
22. Breslow L, Thomas LB, Upton AC (Chairmen): Final reports of the National Cancer Institute ad hoc working groups on mammography in screening for breast cancer and summary report of their joint findings and recommendations. J Natl Cancer Inst 59:467, 1977
23. Canellos GP, Hellman S, Veronesi U: The management of early breast cancer. N Engl J Med 306:1430, 1982
24. Leger JL, Naimark AP, Beique RA, et al: Report of the "Ad Hoc" committee on mammography. J Can Assoc Radiol 25:3, 1974
25. Beahrs OH, Smart CR: Diagnosis of minimal breast cancers in the BCDDP. The 66 questionable cases. Cancer 43:848, 1979
26. Fisher B, Bauer M, Margolese R, et al: Five-year results of a randomized clinical trial comparing total mastectomy and segmental mastectomy with or without radiation in the treatment of breast cancer. N Engl J Med 312:665, 1985
27. Baker LH: Breast cancer detection demonstration project: Five-year summary report. CA 32:194, 1982
28. American Cancer Society: Mammography 1982. CA 32:226, 1982
29. American College of Radiology: Board approves mammography policy, summary of current opinion. Bull Am Coll Radiol 32:1, 1976
30. American Cancer Society: Mammography guidelines 1983: Background statement and update of cancer—related checkup guidelines for breast cancer detection in asymptomatic women age 40 to 49. CA 33:255, 1983
31. Miller AB, Bulbrook RD: Screening, detection and diagnosis of breast cancer. Lancet 1:1109, 1982
32. Dales LG, Freidman GD, Collen MF: Evaluating periodic multi-phasic health check-ups: A controlled trial. J Chronic Dis 32:385, 1979
33. de Waard F, Collette HJA, Rombach JJ, et al: The DOM project for the early detection of breast cancer, Utrecht, the Netherlands. J Chronic Dis 37:1, 1984
34. Collette HJA, Day NE, Rombach JJ, et al: Evaluation of screening for breast cancer in a non-randomized study (the DOM project) by means of a case-control study. Lancet 1:1224, 1984
35. Verbeek ALM, Hendriks JHCL, Holland R, et al: Reduction of breast cancer mortality through mass screening with modern mammography: First results of the Nijmegen project 1975–1981. Lancet 1:1222, 1984
36. Verbeek ALM, Hendriks JHCL, Holland R, et al: Letter: Mammographic screening and breast cancer mortality age specific effects in Nijmegen project, 1975–1982. Lancet 1:865, 1985
37. U.K. Trial of Early Detection of Breast Cancer Group: Trial of early detection of breast cancer: Description of method. Br J Cancer 44:618, 1981
38. Tabar L, Gad A: Screening for breast cancer: The Swedish trial. Radiology 138:219, 1981
39. Lundgren B: Efficiency of single-view mammography: Rate of interval cancer cases. J Natl Cancer Inst 62:799, 1979
40. Andersen I, Andren L, Hildell J, et al: Breast cancer screening with mammography. A population-based, randomized trial with mammography as the only screening mode. Radiology 132:273, 1979
41. Tabar L, Fagerberg CJG, Gad A, et al: Reduction in mortality from breast cancer after mass screening with mammography. Randomized trial from the breast cancer screening working group of the Swedish National Board of Health and Welfare. Lancet 1:829, 1985
42. National Cancer Institute of Canada: National breast-cancer screening study gets underway. Can Med Assoc J 122:243, 1980
43. Baines CJ: Impediments to recruitment in the Canadian National Breast Screening Study: Response and resolution. Controlled Clin Trials 5:129, 1984
44. Bross IDJ: Mammography. Can Med Assoc J 123:94, 1980
45. Howe GR, Sherman GJ, Seminciew RM, et al: Estimated benefits and risks of screening for breast cancer. Can Med Assoc J 124:399, 1981
46. Prorok PC: Methodological issues in randomized controlled trials of screening. In Prorok PC, Miller AB (eds): Screening for Cancer, UICC Technical Report Vol. 78, p 1828. Geneva, International Union Against Cancer, 1984
47. Hall FM: Screening mammography—potential problems on the horizon. N Engl J Med 314:53, 1986
48. Dodd GD: The continuing challenge of mammography. CA 34:57, 1984
49. American Cancer Society: Survey of physicians' attitudes and practices in early cancer detection. CA 35:197, 1985
50. Baines CJ: Some thoughts on why women don't do breast self-examination. Can Med Assoc J 128:255, 1983
51. Editorial: Screening for breast cancer. Lancet 1:851, 1985
52. Greenwald P, Sondik E: Division of Cancer Prevention and Control: Cancer Control Objectives for the Nation 1985–2000. NCI, National Cancer Institute Monograph No. 2, September 1986. Bethesda, MD, National Cancer Institute, 1986
53. Miller AB: Screening for breast cancer. Breast Cancer Research and Treatment 3:143, 1983
54. Miller AB: Risk benefit in mass screening programs for breast cancer. Semin Oncol 5:351, 1978

Biology of Breast Cancer *In Vivo* and *In Vitro*

6

Stephen P. Ethier
Gloria H. Heppner

Experimental carcinogenesis has for more than 50 years been an area of intense interest in cancer research. The broad objective of this research has been to improve our ability to prevent, diagnose, and treat the many forms of human cancer by understanding the nature of the process that culminates in the emergence of a malignant neoplasm. Throughout much of the history of experimental carcinogenesis research, the emphasis was placed on observations of the histopathologic processes associated with cancer development in experimental animals and on obtaining a better understanding of the agents that cause cancer.[1] Consequently, a large research effort has been put forth toward the study of the ability of radiation (both ionizing and ultraviolet), carcinogenic chemicals, and oncogenic viruses to cause a variety of types of neoplasms. This work has resulted in an improved understanding of the mechanisms by which carcinogenic agents act on living cells. Recently, however, with the increasing development of techniques in cell and molecular biology, research is focusing not only on the agents that cause cancer but on the cells themselves. This kind of work is already improving our understanding of how normal cells regulate growth and differentiation. This will allow a new understanding of the specific altered phenotypes that are acquired by cells during the course of neoplastic progression and that are necessary for the development of neoplastic disease.

EXPERIMENTAL MAMMARY CARCINOGENESIS

One of the most important areas in experimental carcinogenesis research has been the study of mammary tumorigenesis in rodents. This has been an important model system for several reasons. First, the three basic types of carcinogens (i.e., viruses, chemicals, and radiation) all can influence breast cancer development in rodents, depending on the species and strain of the animal studied. Second, many of the factors that are known to influence human cancer development, such as hormones and dietary factors, play important roles in mammary tumorigenesis in rodents.

The first account of the chemical induction of mammary tumors in mice was published in 1941.[2] In this study, mice were exposed to the polycyclic hydrocarbon methylcholanthrene (MCA) by weekly painting of a 0.5% solution on the skin of the animals for 23 weeks. This treatment was highly toxic and resulted in the death of many animals; however, 100% of the animals that survived the treatment developed mammary tumors. The first report of the induction of mammary tumors in mice by oral administration of a chemical carcinogen (MCA) was published by Andervant and Dunn.[3] In these studies, animals given weekly 1-mg gastric instillations of MCA developed mammary adenocarcinomas and sarcomas. This treatment regimen also resulted in severe toxicity.

A significant improvement in the area of chemical induction of mammary tumors was made when Huggins and colleagues [4] published the first account of the induction of mammary carcinomas in rats by the synthetic polycyclic hydrocarbon 7,12-dimethylbenz(*a*)anthracene (DMBA). The most important aspect of DMBA as an experimental carcinogen is that high incidences of mammary tumors can be achieved in a short time after a single administration of this compound rather than the repeated instillations that had been required for MCA. Thus, DMBA is not severely toxic at doses that yield high incidences of mammary tumors. Furthermore, unlike other agents that have carcinogenic activity in several tissues, DMBA is more specific for mammary gland tumors. In addition, mammary tumors induced in rats by DMBA are histologically adenocarcinomas and exhibit hormone response patterns that are similar to those of human breast cancer. Since the original work of Huggins and colleagues, [4] DMBA has also been shown to be a potent and relatively specific mammary gland carcinogen in several mouse strains including the BALB/c,[5] BD2F,[6] and C3H/StWi strains.[7] Interestingly, unlike DMBA-induced rat mammary carcinomas, which tend to be hormone dependent (i.e., regress on ovariectomy), DMBA-induced mouse mammary tumors are almost uniformly hormone independent. In mice, DMBA treatment results in the development of different histologic types of tumors, depending on the dose of the agent that is administered. High doses result in development of adenoacanthomas, whereas low doses (doses at which induction is dose responsive) result in development of adenocarcinomas almost exclusively.[8]

One disadvantage of DMBA-induced mammary carcinomas, particularly as they occur in rats, is that the tumors themselves are not highly aggressive. Thus, although these tumors are malignant adenocarcinomas by histologic criteria, extensive invasion into surrounding musculature or metastases to lungs are only rarely observed.[9] These observations have recently led workers to begin using a different carcinogen, namely methylnitrosourea (MNU), to induce mammary tumors with biologic characteristics that more closely resemble those of human breast cancer. Gullino and colleagues[10] reported that administration of a three-dose regimen of MNU results in development of mammary adenocarcinomas in BUF/N rats, with high frequency and with little toxicity. Further, the MNU-induced tumors are hormone dependent. Unlike DMBA-induced tumors, MNU-induced tumors tend to metastasize to spleen, liver, and lung. More recently, McCormick and colleagues[11] characterized the dose-response relationship for MNU-induced tumors in Sprague-Dawley rats following a single intravenous administration. Metastatic foci were observed in the lungs of these animals in these experiments; however, metastases to other sites were not seen.

In addition to the extensive studies on the chemical induction of mammary tumors in rodents, the influence of ionizing radiation on mammary carcinogenesis has also received a great deal of attention. This is of importance because epidemiologic evidence indicates ionizing radiation to be an agent involved in the etiology of human breast cancer.[12-15] These data came from studies of the survivors of the atomic bomb blasts at Hiroshima and Nagasaki and also from studies of women who were given therapeutic x-irradiation for postpartum mastitis. Data from studies of the exposed groups indicate not only excess incidences of breast cancer, but also dose-dependent increases in breast cancer incidence.

Although the human data on the influence of radiation on breast cancer development clearly indicate it to be an etiologic agent, animal studies have shed relatively little light on the phenomenon. It has been shown by a number of investigators that exposure of rats to ionizing radiation result in a dose-dependent increase in tumor incidence. At high dose levels, greater than 90% of the treated animals develop mammary tumors during their first year of life. Histologic evaluation of the radiation-induced tumors reveals that the vast majority are benign fibroadenomas. Adenocarcinomas are also observed, but at fairly low frequencies.[16] The rat strain that is routinely used for radiation carcinogenesis studies, the Sprague-Dawley rat, develops spontaneous fibroadenomas at very high incidences. However, these tumors almost always occur late in the life of the animals. With this in mind, Shellabarger and co-workers[17] performed a large-scale study of mammary tumor development of irradiated and nonirradiated Sprague-Dawley rats over their entire life span and employed rigorous statistical methods to analyze the dose- and time-dependent incidence of mammary tumors in these animals. The results of these studies indicated that radiation exposure of Sprague-Dawley rats results primarily in acceleration of the development of the benign fibroadenomas that occur spontaneously in these rats and does not result in significant induction of new tumors.

Ullrich and associates[18] have studied the development of mammary tumors in BALB/c mice following radiation exposure. BALB/c mice have a very low spontaneous incidence of mammary carcinomas (7% to 10% lifetime) and develop fibroadenomas only rarely. Exposure of these mice to varying doses of radiation results in a dose-dependent increase in the incidence of adenocarcinomas; however, the highest observed incidence of tumors is only 20%, or approximately double the spontaneous incidence. Thus the data obtained with BALB/c mice are in agreement with those obtained with Sprague-Dawley rats in that they both indicate that, although radiation can elevate the incidence of adenocarcinomas, its potency as a mammary carcinogen is low, especially when compared with a chemical carcinogen such as DMBA.

Histopathogenesis of Experimental Mammary Tumor Development

One facet of experimental mammary carcinogenesis that has received a good deal of attention concerns the histopathogenesis of mammary neoplasms, with particular emphasis on putative preneoplastic lesions. Some of the earliest work in experimental mammary carcinogenesis made use of strains of mice that carried the so-called "milk-agent," later shown to be the murine mammary tumor virus (MMTV).[19–21] MMTV-bearing mice were studied because of their high incidence of spontaneous mammary adenocarcinomas. Subgross examination of mammary tissues of animals that bore the milk agent revealed the presence of discrete focal areas of alveolar differentiation against a background of ductal mammary tissue. These lesions were referred to as hyperplastic alveolar nodules (HANs). At the histologic level, the HANs are composed of acini lined by a single layer of cuboidal epithelium and thus are not different from lobules found in midpregnant mice. The incidence of HANs increases with age, and HANs are more prevalent in mammary tissues of parous animals than in those of age-matched virgin mice. These observations provide suggestive evidence for the preneoplastic nature of HANs.

It is now known that there are many different forms of MMTV.[22] Some forms, such as MTV-S, are transmitted from mother to offspring via the milk, whereas others, such as the MTV-L, are transmitted via the germ cells as proviral DNA integrated into the host cell genome. The tumorigenic potential of the different MMTV forms varies widely. The MTV-S carried by the C3H strain results in a virtual 100% incidence of mammary tumors, the MTV-L carried by C3H/Sm mice results in a 40% to 50% incidence of tumors, and the MTV-O carried by the BALB/c mouse strain is defective and probably plays little or no role in mammary tumor development.

In 1959, DeOme and co-workers[23] provided the first conclusive evidence that HANs are indeed preneoplastic lesions. These workers developed a technique in which the mammary rudiments of weanling mice could be surgically removed while leaving within the animal most of the mammary fat pad, which had not yet been filled with mammary epithelium. This gland-free mammary fat pad provided an optimal site for transplantation of mammary tissue from a syngeneic donor animal. Using this method, individual HANs were isolated from mammary tissues of mice bearing MMTV-S and transplanted into gland-free mammary fat pads of syngeneic mice. Transplantation of HANs resulted in the development of mammary outgrowths that completely filled the mammary fat pad within 10 weeks of transplantation. Interestingly, HAN-derived outgrowths exhibited a lobuloalveolar morphology when transplanted into virgin hosts, in contrast to the pure ductal morphology of similarly derived outgrowths resulting from transplantation of a piece of normal mammary duct. In addition to the altered morphology, the incidence of mammary carcinomas was significantly higher in HAN-derived outgrowths than in control outgrowths derived from normal ductal tissue. These findings were interpreted to indicate that MMTV "infection" results in mammary cells that have a higher than normal probability of acquiring neoplastic potential—that is, HANs are preneoplastic lesions.

Since the development of the mammary fat pad transplantation technique and the demonstration of the preneoplastic nature of HANs, much work has been done to characterize some of the biologic properties of nodule-transformed cells. For example, the development of HANs is dependent on the presence of ovarian hormones; however, some HANs acquire hormone independence early and will grow when transplanted into mammary fat pads of ovariectomized hosts.[24] Additionally, some HAN outgrowths acquire the ability to stimulate angiogenesis, a characteristic usually associated with the acquisition of neoplastic potential.[25] One of the most interesting studies concerning the biology of preneoplastic HANs was performed by Daniel and colleagues.[26] These workers demonstrated that the proliferative life span of normal mammary tissue was finite in that serial transplantation of mammary ducts into gland-free mammary fat pads resulted in outgrowth development for approximately six transplant generations, after which the proliferative potential of the cells was lost. In contrast, serial transplantation of HAN-derived tissue resulted in continuous proliferation without loss of growth potential. In fact, some HAN-derived outgrowth lines have been serially transplanted *in vivo* for many years.

The studies of HANs demonstrate that overt mammary neoplasia can be preceded by a nonneoplastic lesion, the cells of which have a higher than normal probability of progressing to malignancy. These preneoplastic cells have also acquired some characteristics associated with neoplastic development, including the ability to stimulate angiogenesis and an enhanced proliferative life span.

The discovery of the role of HANs in the pathogenesis of MMTV-induced mammary carcinoma led to other studies aimed at determining the importance of these lesions in spontaneous and chemical carcinogen–induced mammary neoplasia. In mice that do not carry oncogenic forms of the MMTV, HANs can be induced by chemical carcinogens but only when these are given in combination with intense hormonal stimulation.[27–29] In most such studies, pituitary isografts are transplanted under the kidney or spleen capsule of mice (ectopic pituitary glands secrete prolactin constitutively) followed by treatment with DMBA or MCA. The intense prolactin stimulation results in lobuloalveolar differentiation of the mammary glands. Several weeks after carcinogen administration, the pituitary isografts are removed and most of the gland regresses to a ductal architecture; however, some carcinogen-altered lobules fail to regress, resulting in the presence of HANs in these tissues. HANs derived in this fashion are preneoplastic and are biologically similar to MMTV-induced lesions.

HANs also arise in mammary tissues of rats, both spontaneously and in response to carcinogen treatment. However, in this species there is little evidence that these lesions are preneoplastic. Their incidence, both in non-treated and carcinogen-treated rats, does not correlate with the incidence of neoplasia.[30] Furthermore, transplantation of HANs into gland-free mammary fat pads of syngeneic rats usually does not result in tumor development within the outgrowths,[31,32] although there are at least two reports that indicate that transplantation of these lesions to gland-free mammary fat pads does result in tumor development.[33,34]

Although HANs are the only mammary lesions observed in MMTV-infected mice, in MMTV-negative mouse strains and in rats, mammary lesions of ductal origin predominate and are the more likely precursors of spontaneous and carcinogen-induced mammary tumors. Medina[35] described a variety of ductal lesions that resulted from carcinogen treatment of MMTV-negative BALB/c mice. The lesions observed ranged from mild ductal hyperplasias to severe ductal and lobular dysplasias. Similar ductal lesions, including intraductal papillomas and lesions that resemble carcinoma *in situ,* have been observed in mammary outgrowths derived by transplantation of mammary cells from carcinogen-treated donor animals into gland-free mammary fat pads of syngeneic hosts.[36] The evidence that ductal hyperplasias or dysplasias are important precursors of mammary carcinoma is largely correlative. The incidence of these lesions increases with carcinogen dose and correlates with the final incidence of carcinomas. There is also one report of mammary ductal dysplasias transplanted into gland-free mammary fat pads of syngeneic hosts.[37] Transplantation of abnormal mammary ducts results in mammary outgrowths with a variety of abnormalities. Furthermore, these outgrowths progress to overt neoplasia with high frequency. The data from this study must be interpreted with caution, however, in that unlike HANs, ductal dysplasias are difficult to locate *in vivo* and transplantation studies are more difficult. In Medina's study, mammary tissues were examined 8 months after high-dose carcinogen administration, and dysplastic ducts were localized by the presence of extravascularization within the mammary fat pad. Given these two factors, it is possible that cells that had already progressed to the neoplastic state were transplanted and were thus responsible for tumor development within the outgrowths. Nevertheless, taken together the data suggest strongly that carcinogen-induced mammary tumors in the mouse are preceded by hyperplastic/dysplastic lesions of the mammary ducts.

The pathogenesis of mammary carcinoma development in the rat is similar to that of MMTV-free mice. Chemically induced rat mammary adenocarcinomas are preceded by the development of ductal hyperplasias, the incidence of which correlates with the final incidence of tumors.[38–40] However, there is also evidence that indicates that mammary carcinoma in the rat can arise without passing through a preneoplastic stage.[41]

Russo and co-workers have studied the development of mammary carcinoma in the Sprague-Dawley rat following treatment with DMBA.[42,43] Their data indicate that an important site of origin of rat mammary tumors are the terminal end buds that are found on actively growing mammary ducts. Thus, young virgin rats are highly susceptible to tumor induction by DMBA, and the mammary glands of these animals have numerous terminal end buds. The mammary tissues of old virgin rats have far fewer terminal end buds, since these structures differentiate to alveolar buds. Old virgin rats are also less susceptible to chemical induction of mammary tumors than are young virgins. Parous rats are the least susceptible to chemically induced mammary tumors, and mammary tissues of these animals consist of alveolar buds and fully differentiated lobules. Terminal end buds are absent in parous females. Kinetic analysis of the various mammary gland structures indicates that cells within terminal end buds have a higher labeling index and a shorter cell cycle time than cells in alveolar buds or lobules. Further, cells within alveolar buds of parous rats have a longer cycle time than cells in alveolar buds of virgin rats. The findings from these studies indicate that susceptibility to mammary carcinogenesis in the rat is influenced by the degree of differentiation of the mammary gland. These data also suggest a mechanism for the protective effect of an early first pregnancy on the risk of breast cancer development, a phenomenon that is well known in humans.

It is evident from the preceding discussion that a large research effort has been put forth to understand the histopathogenesis of mammary tumor development in both mice and rats. These studies have revealed that both ductal and alveolar lesions are associated with tumor development. Additionally, the work with the HANs demonstrates that a stable preneoplastic cell population can exist within mammary tissues. There is another aspect of this work, however, that has received relatively little attention but that provides interesting information regarding the biology of cancer development. That aspect concerns the factors that influence the induction and *expression* of preneoplastic and neoplastic phenotypes. This has been examined for both HANs and ductal hyperplasias/dysplasias. It is clear that the emergence of HANs in the mammary tissues of MMTV-carrying mice and of carcinogen-induced ductal dysplasias in the mammary tissues of MMTV-free mice is influenced by the age of the animal. Thus, young animals have few, if any, of either type of lesion. However, after a certain age, both ductal and alveolar lesions begin to emerge, and it is relatively soon after that when overt neoplasia also appears. Thus, the latent periods for the expression of preneoplastic and neoplastic lesions are of the same order. This is important since it has been demonstrated that transplantation of single-cell suspensions of mammary cells derived from very young MMTV-carrying mice into gland-free mammary fat pads results in the development of mammary outgrowths that express HANs with high frequency.[44] Similarly, transplantation of mammary cells of MMTV-free mice into gland-free fat pads 24 hours following low-dose carcinogen administration results in outgrowths expressing ductal hyperplasias/dysplasias with high frequency.[45,46] Thus, the transplantation procedure allows expression of otherwise inapparent transformed cells that are present but unexpressed in young animals. These findings suggest an intriguing possibility: that age-related factors (possibly involving normal cells) can influence the expression of transformed cells and that many more cells are transformed by chemicals and viruses than are normally expressed in the lifetime of the animals. This in turn suggests that the factors that influence the emergence of carcinogen-altered cell populations are of great importance in cancer development and may even represent the rate-determining step in carcinogenesis.

PRENEOPLASTIC LESIONS AND HUMAN BREAST CANCER DEVELOPMENT

The association of both alveolar and ductal hyperplasias in the pathogenesis of mammary carcinoma development in mice and rats led several groups to examine human breast tissue for similar lesions. Wellings and co-workers[47,48] and Squartini and colleagues[49] have published extensively on the subgross pathology of the human breast, with emphasis on proliferative lesions that may be associated with breast cancer development. There appears to be general agreement that human breast cancer arises in the terminal ductal lobular unit (TDLU) of the breast. The lesion most often associated with overt carcinoma is intraductal carcinoma *in situ,* which can be present in 90% of cases. The cells within the noninfiltrating lesions are histologically similar to those present in the infiltrating tissue. These observations have led to the notion that intraductal or intralobular carcinoma *in situ* is the direct precursor of malignant breast disease. In addition to carcinoma *in situ,* a variety of other proliferative, nonneoplastic lesions are found to be associated with breast cancer development. Wellings has classified these proliferative lesions based on their site of origin and degree of epithelial hyperplasia. The majority of these lesions arise in the terminal ducts of the TDLU and have been classified as type A atypical lobules (ALA). Grade 1 ALA are lobules that are greatly enlarged relative to their normal counterparts and are made up of large, distended ducts that are lined by normal-appearing columnar epithelial cells. ALA grade 2 are similar morphologically to grade 1 lesions; however, in ALA-2 the ducts are lined by hyperplastic epithelium that narrows the duct lumen. In ALA grade 3, the ducts within the TDLU are completely occluded with hyperplastic epithelium, which can result in papillary formation. In grade 4 ALA, the hyperplasia is so great as to distend the size of the ducts. Finally, ALA grade 5 is synonomous with carcinoma *in situ* in which the ducts of the TDLU, in addition to being severely hyperplastic, also have epithelial atypia diagnostic of carcinoma *in situ.*

Proliferative lesions of the breast can also arise within the lobules themselves, although this is much more rare, giving rise to what Wellings[48] classifies as type B atypical lobules (ALB). The most severe of these lesions is the lobular carcinoma *in situ.*

It is quite clear that there are a number of proliferative lesions of the breast that are associated with breast cancer development. The preneoplastic significance of these lesions is not clear, however. Circumstantial evidence suggests that these lesions are true precursors of breast cancer. They are more common in cancer-associated breasts than in random autopsy breasts. Their incidence increases with age, and they persist after menopause. They can be arranged in a morphological sequence according to the degree of epithelial hyperplasia associated with the lesions, which ranges from mild hyperplasia to carcinoma *in situ.* Still, the mere presence of these lesions in cancer-associated breasts does not prove that they arise prior to and then give rise to overt neoplasia. However, there is strong evidence that such a phenomenon can occur in the pathogenesis of human cancer, most notably in the development of cervical and colon cancer. Both of these types of neoplastic disease are preceded by dysplastic lesions, which are most likely the site of origin of the overt cancer.

In an attempt to obtain more direct evidence regarding the preneoplastic significance of hyperplastic lesions in human breast tissue, a number of epidemiologic studies have been performed to determine if women who have fibrocystic disease[50] or intraductal papilloma[51] have an elevated risk of breast cancer development. Data obtained from these studies suggest an elevated risk of developing breast cancer for women with fibrocystic disease, particularly in those cases that have associated epithelial hyperplasia. In the latter case, risks in excess of twofold higher than the general population have been reported.

Although it seems very likely that proliferative lesions that arise in the breast can be precursors to overt neoplastic disease, it must be borne in mind that the presence of these lesions does not necessitate their progression to cancer. Furthermore, there is evidence that breast cancer can arise *de novo* without passing through a premalignant phase. Thus, there is probably not a single pathway in the pathogenesis of mammary carcinoma.

CELLULAR HETEROGENEITY OF BREAST NEOPLASMS

One of the most intriguing aspects of breast cancer biology is the extensive phenotypic heterogeneity seen among cancer cells within a single neoplasm. In recent years, this heterogeneity has been the subject of intense experimental and clinical analysis. Work has been directed toward understanding the origin of tumor heterogeneity, as well as its consequences to cancer behavior and response to treatment.

Heterogeneity of Experimental and Human Breast Cancers

Probably the earliest experimental demonstration of breast cancer heterogeneity was that of Henderson and Rous[52] who showed that individual tumors arising in mammary tumor virus-carrying mice contain both benign elements and phenotypically different carcinomatous components. Since then, numerous investigators have been able to isolate distinct clonal tumor cell subpopulations from a variety of mouse and rat mammary cancers, including those induced deliberately by viruses, hormones, and chemicals.[53] Heterogeneity has been seen in newly arisen cancers, as well as in long-term transplants.

Similar in principle to what has been demonstrated in rodent neoplasms is the extensive cellular heterogeneity of human breast cancer.[54] It is important, however, to recognize that the techniques that have been applied to animal tumors are much more difficult, if not impossible, to use with human cancers, so that although human tumors can be shown to be phenotypically heterogeneous, the evidence that this heterogeneity is clonally distributed is slight.[55] Nevertheless, observations on heterogeneity of human breast cancers are consonant with what is known from animal studies, and it is likely that they have a similar basis.

Virtually all characteristics studied have been shown to be distributed differentially within single breast cancers. Thus, both histologic[56] and ultrastructural[57] features of cellular and tissue differentiation have been reported to be nonuniform within breast cancers, as have biochemical markers of differentiation, including casein,[58] keratin, and type IV collagen.[59] Heterogeneity has been described in expression of a variety of differentiation and tumor-associated antigens.[60–62] Hormone dependency[63] has been shown to vary among tumor cell subpopulations of rodent tumors, and hormone receptors may be distributed differentially among cells from both animal and human cancers.[64,65]

Recent advances in cytogenetics and flow cytometry have allowed a detailed look at chromosomal variability within numerous types of cancer.[66] For technical reasons, breast cancer karyology has been particularly difficult to assess, but ploidy differences within single breast cancers have been reported[66,67] and may have prognostic significance.[68]

In addition to histologic, biochemical, and karyotypic characteristics, heterogeneity has been demonstrated in the behavior of tumor subpopulations. Thus, there are several reports of the isolation, from a single rodent tumor, of subpopulations that differ in ability to metastasize.[69–72] Tumor subpopulations can also differ in growth rate, immunogenicity, and, as has been mentioned, hormone dependence. Of particular clinical significance are the numerous studies showing differences among isolated tumor subpopulations in response to chemotherapy[73,74] and to irradiation.[75,76]

Subpopulation Interactions Within Mammary Cancers

Of necessity, most of the reports on cellular heterogeneity of cancers have depended on the ability of investigators to isolate distinct subpopulations from single tumors. The fact, however, that diverse cells can be obtained from tumors that themselves do not display the extreme behaviors of some of their components suggests that the coexistence of clonal subpopulations is not the whole of the tumor heterogeneity story. Although it may be that the techniques used in the isolation procedures or the circumstances of cloning cells may contribute *per se* to tumor cell variability,[77] heterogeneity can be demonstrated in tumor tissue that has not been subjected to such manipulations.[78] A likely explanation is that the characteristics exhibited by subpopulations growing in isolation are modified by the presence of other subpopulations, and indeed there is experimental evidence that tumor subpopulations can interact to affect each other's behavior.[79] In the case of rodent mammary neoplasms, interactions affecting growth,[79,80] immunogenicity,[79] ability to metastasize,[81] hormone responsiveness,[82] and sensitivity to chemotherapy[83] have all ben reported. Similar results have also been found with tumors of nonmammary origin.[77,84] The mechanisms of such tumor subpopulation interactions are diverse but include host-mediated events such as the immune response[81] and metabolism of drugs,[83] as well as the release by one subpopulation of growth factors that affect other subpopulations[78,82] and mechanisms that require physical contact between the interacting cells.[85]

Subpopulation interactions add another level of complexity, beyond the existence of multiple tumor subpopulations, to the tumor heterogeneity phenomenon. The behavior of a neoplasm is not just the "sum" of the characteristics of its component parts, but rather a reflection of an interlocking network of cellular subpopulations. Changes in the distribution of these subpopulations, either as a consequence of therapy or by the addition of new variants (see below), can result in a new equilibrium, or "balance," among the various components. In this sense, a cancer can be thought of as an ecosystem, a cellular society, rather than simply an expanding population of uncontrolled cells.

Origin of Tumor Heterogeneity

One of the current tenets of cancer research is that cancers are clonal in origin; that is, they arise from a single, "transformed" cell.[86] It is sometimes thought that this concept is in conflict with the observations of tumor heterogeneity. However, even if it had been established definitively that breast cancers do, in fact, arise from single cells (and this has not been done[54]) it is well to remember that single-cell origin does not preclude the emergence of variant populations as a cancer develops and grows.

Nowell has hypothesized that the initiation of neoplasia is marked by a predilection for genetic error; that is, that cancer cells are "genetically unstable" in comparison with their normal cell counterparts.[87] There is some, albeit limited, evidence for this hypothesis in breast cancer.[88,89] Genetic instability is hypothesized to be the underlying cause of tumor heterogeneity and, furthermore, to be responsible for the phenomenon of "tumor progression," the evolution, over time, of new phenotypic characteristics by a given cancer. Thus, a cancer may be initially hormone dependent but later become autonomous in regard to the need for hormone stimulation; it may respond initially to chemotherapy and then become resistant; it may grow locally at first and later spread to other parts of the body. These behavioral changes become explicable if one views a cancer as a mixed population of variants, each of which may differ in hormone responsiveness, drug sensitivity, ability to metastasize, and so on. As new variants arise, the behavior of the neoplasm itself can change because of a redistribution of its component parts.

Understanding the underlying mechanisms of genetic instability is clearly important to the eventual control of cancer growth and progression. At this time, however, there is no uniform theory that explains all the many pertinent observations, and, indeed, it is likely that no one mechanism will be found to be responsible. Rather, all sorts of genomic alterations, including point mutations, base-pair shifts, gene amplification, chromosomal rearrangements, ploidy changes, and so on play a part.[87] Furthermore, so-called "epigenetic" changes, those that do not alter the structure of the genome *per se* but rather affect its expression, can be associated with the production of new tumor cell variants.[91] In addition, although it is hypothesized that tumor cells are uniquely unstable, it should be remembered that the production of new cell variants by the processes of differentiation is a key element in normal tissue biology. New tumor cell subpopulations may likewise arise by quite normal mechanisms.[92,93]

The instability of cancer cells is a problem of considerable biologic and clinical significance. However, it should not be overstated. Tumor cells can differ in degree of instability; in some cases new variants arise rapidly, but in others it is a rare event.[78] Furthermore, interactions between tumor subpopulations (see above) can have a moderating influence on the appearance of new variants.[77] Factors in the tumor environment, such as state of nutrition, chemotherapy, and normal host components, may also affect the development of new subpopulations.[87,94] Perhaps the most significant consequence of tumor heterogeneity is the necessity to view cancers, breast cancer included, as dynamic, interacting tissues, the behavior of which is the result of a matrix of factors and influences rather than a series of linear responses or a hierarchy of cause-effect relationships.

IMPORTANCE OF HORMONES AND GROWTH FACTORS ON PROLIFERATION OF NORMAL AND NEOPLASTIC MAMMARY EPITHELIUM

Since the mammary gland is an endocrine target organ, it is not surprising that the growth potential of both normal and neoplastic mammary epithelium can be influenced by hormones. That both the induction and maintenance of mammary neoplasia is, to some extent, under endocrine control has been known for more than 25 years. It has been demonstrated in several experimental systems that the mammary tumorigenic response can be dramatically enhanced by coupling chemical carcinogen administration with exogenous hormone stimulation either by pregnancy,[95] psuedopregnancy,[95,96] ectopic transplantation of pituitary glands,[97,98] or grafting of prolactin-secreting pituitary tumors.[99] Indeed, in some mouse strains, extensive hormone stimulation alone is sufficient to stimulate a tumorigenic response.[100–102]

Just as hormone stimulation can enhance mammary tumorigenesis, endocrine ablation either prior to or immediately after chemical carcinogen administration can completely obliterate the tumorigenic response. This loss of tumorigenic response can be brought about either by ovariectomy or hypophysectomy of carcinogen-treated animals.[103] Both prolactin and ovarian steroids are required for tumor development, since administration of these hormones to carcinogen-treated rats that were ovariectomized and hypophysectomized resulted in development of mammary tumors.[104]

Maintenance and growth of palpable mammary adenocarcinomas is also influenced by hormones. In the rat, the majority of chemically induced mammary tumors regress following hypophysectomy or ovariectomy, and these tumors can be stimulated to regrow by administration of prolactin or estrogen. In contrast, a certain fraction of rat mammary carcinomas and nearly all chemically induced mouse mammary tumors acquire hormone independence early in their development, such that ovariectomy or hypophysectomy has no effect on the continued growth of these tumors.[4,5]

During the past 25 years an enormous amount of literature has accumulated regarding the influence of specific hormones on the induction, expression, and maintenance of carcinogen-induced mammary carcinomas in both mice and rats. A detailed accounting[105,106] of the results of these studies is beyond the scope of this work; however, the weight of the experimental data strongly indicates that prolactin and estrogens play important roles in experimental mammary tumorigenesis. These findings come from studies involving specific loss and subsequent replacement of one or both of these hormones either by hormone ablation or by drugs that inhibit their synthesis or function. What is not at all clear, however, despite an extensive research effort, is the mechanisms by which these hormones act in tumor development. Additionally, other hormones such as adrenal steroids, insulin, and thyroid hormones have been reported to be important in mammary tumorigenesis under certain circumstances.

In vivo studies clearly indicate the importance of hormones in mammary tumorigenesis and have even identified those hormones that appear to be of greatest importance. However, this approach has been of little use for the elucidation of the cellular mechanisms by which hormones act to influence tumor development. In an attempt to understand the role that hormones play in breast cancer development, *in vitro* methods have been applied that allow the study of malignant breast epithelial cells under laboratory conditions. The first human breast cancer-derived cell line to be used in this manner was MCF-7.[107] This line originated from a pleural effusion from a patient with metastatic breast disease. MCF-7 has been used extensively since its development and has several advantages; first, it represents a malignant epithelial cell line of human origin; second, it has been definitively shown to be breast in origin; and third, it produces tumors when inoculated into nude mice, and the tumorigenic potential of these cells is markedly potentiated by estrogen. Thus, inoculation of MCF-7 cells into ovariectomized female or castrated male nude mice does not result in tumor development. Tumors do develop in such animals, however, when they are provided with exogenous estradiol.[108] The estrogen dependence for *in vivo* growth of these cells in nude mice is of particular interest, because many primary human mammary tumors regress on ovariectomy and thus exhibit an estrogen dependence for growth.

The estrogen dependence for *in vivo* growth of MCF-7 cells has resulted in extensive investigation of the interaction of estradiol and MCF-7 cells *in vitro*. The results of these experiments have been equivocal, at best, and there remain serious questions about the role estradiol plays in proliferation of MCF-7 cells. For example, Lippman and colleagues[109] have demonstrated a slight positive effect of estradiol on proliferation of MCF-7 cells in serum-containing media; however, equivalent cell proliferation was seen when estradiol was replaced by insulin. Other workers have reported estradiol to have no effect on MCF-7 proliferation in serum-containing media.[110] Sato and coworkers have defined a serum-free culture medium that supports the growth of MCF-7 cells in a manner equivalent to that obtained in serum-containing media.[111] In this system, Ham's F-12 medium supplemented with insulin, transferrin, prostaglandin $F_{2\alpha}$, epidermal growth factor, serum-spreading factor, and cold-insoluble globulin supports the long-term growth of MCF-7 cells. Under these conditions, estradiol does not significantly alter cell proliferation.

Recently, evidence has been published that indicates that phenol red, the pH indicator commonly used in tissue culture media, has weak estrogenic activity.[112] Subsequently, it was shown that when MCF-7 cells are grown in a phenol red-free medium, a growth response to estradiol is detectable. Furthermore, the proliferative response to estradiol is inhibitable by the anti-estrogen, tamoxifen. Thus, estradiol may indeed have direct growth-promoting activity on human breast epithelial cells.

The requirement of estradiol for MCF-7 tumor growth *in vivo* and the apparent lack of importance of this hormone for MCF-7 cell proliferation *in vitro* have prompted a number of alternate hypotheses regarding the role of estrogen in breast cancer development. One such hypothesis has recently been proposed by Soto and colleagues.[113] This hypothesis proposes that estradiol is not directly mitogenic to MCF-7 cells but rather serves to antagonize an inhibitor of cell proliferation that is present in serum. In support of this hypothesis, these workers have obtained data that indicate that when MCF-7 cells are grown in medium supplemented with human serum, proliferation does not take place unless estradiol is present in the medium. Furthermore, the concentration of estradiol required to stimulate maximum growth of these cells increases proportionately with increases in serum concentration. In contrast, when the MCF-7 cells are grown in a growth factor-supplemented, serum-free medium, cell proliferation is not affected by estradiol.

It is important to note that although estradiol does not appear to play a direct role in stimulating proliferation of MCF-7 cells *in vitro,* the cells do exhibit a physiological response to this hormone. First, MCF-7 cells do have detectable estradiol receptors.[114] Second, addition of the antiestrogen tamoxifen to growth medium has a dramatic effect on cell viability and proliferative potential.[110,115] The action of tamoxifen, which binds to the estradiol receptor, can be inhibited by adding estradiol to the growth medium. Finally, addition of estradiol to growth medium at the same doses that fail to stimulate proliferation of MCF-7 cells does stimulate progesterone receptor activity.[110] These findings suggest that the inability to observe a mitogenic effect of estradiol on MCF-7 cells *in vitro* is not due to an inability of the cells to recognize or otherwise respond to the presence of this hormone.

Another hypothesis that has emerged regarding the influence of estrogens on neoplastic mammary epithelial cells is the estromedin hypothesis of Sirbasku.[116] This hypothesis proposed that since most mitogens that can stimulate DNA synthesis and cell division directly are polypeptides, estradiol—a steroid—might act indirectly by stimulating synthesis of a polypeptide growth factor that is itself the proximal mitogen. Thus, the existence of an estrogen-inducible growth factor or estromedin is postulated. To test this hypothesis, a cell line was developed (MTW9/PL) from a carcinogen-induced mammary adenocarcinoma that arose in a Wistar/Furth rat. This cell line gives rise to mammary adenocarcinomas when transplanted into syngeneic recipients. The tumors are estrogen dependent and develop in intact females and ovariectomized females or castrated males given exogenous estrogen. Despite the estrogen dependence of these cells for *in vivo* growth, when cultured *in vitro,* MTW9/PL cells do not respond mitogenically to estradiol and in this respect resemble MCF-7 cells. Sirbasku[116] has reported the isolation from uterus and kidney of rats and sheep an estrogen-inducible polypeptide that can stimulate cell division of MTW9/PL cells *in vitro.* The same growth factor has also been shown to be mitogenic for MCF-7 cells *in vitro.* Thus, it appears that estradiol can stimulate the synthesis of a growth factor that is active on neoplastic mammary epithelial cells. The precise role that estromedin plays in mammary tumorigenesis or, for that matter, normal mammary growth and differentiation, however, remains to be elucidated.

Danielpour and Sirbasku[82] have recently extended their estromedin hypothesis to account for the difference between estrogen-dependent and estrogen-independent mammary tumors. In these experiments, an estrogen-independent subline of MTW9/PL was developed that reproducibly gives rise to mammary tumors in male rats in the absence of exogenous estrogen stimulation. These tumors were serially transplanted into nonestrogen-treated male rats for several generations and then cloned *in vitro.* They found that 20% to 30% of the clonal cell lines derived from tumors that had been maintained in male rats for up to five transplant generations gave rise to tumors that were estrogen dependent. These findings were interpreted to indicate that estrogen-dependent neoplastic mammary epithelial cells synthesize an estromedin in response to estrogen stimulation, whereas estrogen-independent cells acquire the ability to synthesize this growth factor in the absence of estrogen stimulation. Thus, not all cells within an estrogen-independent tumor need themselves be estrogen independent as long as a sufficient number of cells are present that can synthesize the growth factor. This model explains the presence of estrogen-dependent neoplastic mammary epithelial cells within mammary tumors maintained for several generations in the absence of estrogen (see discussion above on Subpopulation Interactions Within Mammary Cancers).

Experiments using *in vitro* methods to study the interaction of mammary epithelial cells with basement membranes have also provided important information regarding growth control of normal and neoplastic cells. Wicha and colleagues[117] demonstrated that administration of *cis*-hydroxyproline to midpregnant rats inhibits the synthesis of type IV collagen by these cells. This inhibition results in rapid involution of the mammary gland. Thus, mammary epithelial cells play an active role in basement membrane synthesis, and these cells require specific interactions with their extracellular matrix for normal growth and differentiation. Similar, specific epithelial-mesenchymal interactions have been shown to be of importance in other systems as well.[118] David and Bernfield[119,120] have shown that one difference between a tumorigenic and nontumorigenic mouse mammary epithelial cell line is that although the former produces basement membrane glycosaminoglycans, it secretes and degrades them rapidly, whereas the latter cells deposit the glycosaminoglycans into the basement membrane. Thus, the tumorigenic cells retain the ability to proliferate in the absence of a well-formed basement membrane. This is of particular significance since the cells of human infiltrating ductal carcinoma of the breast do not bind antibodies to type IV collagen and thus proliferate in the absence of a well-formed basal lamina. The interaction between epithelial cells and the extracellular matrix may therefore represent an important controlling influence on normal cell proliferation, the escape from which occurs during neoplastic progression.

The preceding discussion demonstrates how *in vitro* systems can be used to study basic mechanisms of growth control at the cellular and molecular level. Yet many of these *in vitro* systems have important limitations that must be kept in mind when interpreting the data. Most *in vitro* experiments make use of immortalized cell lines, which by definition are selected for their propensity for long-term growth in tissue culture. Thus, it is possible that the factors that allow these cells to proliferate *in vitro* are different from those that are operative in growing tumors *in vivo*. In the case of cell lines derived from human breast cancers, the situation is further complicated by the fact that the cells from which these lines were established were obtained from pleural effusions and therefore represent a highly aggressive subpopulation of the primary tumor. Moreover, the patients from which the cells were obtained had often been through courses of radiotherapy or chemotherapy, adding further selection pressures to the population.

A relatively new approach to the study of normal and neoplastic epithelial cells involves the primary culture of cells obtained directly from normal and neoplastic mammary tissues. During the past 5 years, great progress has been made in defining culture conditions that support the long-term growth of normal, diploid epithelial cells. The use of enriched growth media, substrates such as type I and type IV collagen, and addition of specific hormones and growth factors have contributed to recent successes with these *in vitro* systems.[121–124] Both normal human and rat mammary epithelium have been successfully grown in long-term culture, and there are remarkable similarities in the factors that stimulate their proliferation.[125–128] For example, both human and rat mammary epithelium grow well in the presence of insulin, hydrocortisone, epidermal growth factor, and an agent that raises intracellular cyclic adenosine monophosphate levels such as cholera toxin or prostaglandin E_1. Prolactin and progesterone also enhance proliferation of these cells. Interestingly, estradiol has not been found to stimulate proliferation of human or rat mammary epithelium in these culture systems, lending further support to the notion that estradiol stimulates growth of epithelial cells via an indirect mechanism. Although these culture systems have been in use for only a short time, they offer great promise for improving our understanding of the factors that control proliferation of normal epithelial cells. This, in turn, should allow better questions to be asked regarding fundamental differences between normal and neoplastic cells.

Experimental mammary carcinogenesis research has come a long way since the first chemically induced tumors were studied in the 1930s and 1940s. Today we have a thorough descriptive knowledge of the process of breast cancer development as it occurs in rats and mice. What is truly encouraging, however, is that experimental methods continue to be developed that allow studies aimed at determining the cellular and molecular mechanisms involved in the various stages in carcinogenesis. By using these methods, it will be possible to identify and study specific altered cellular phenotypes acquired by cells during neoplastic progression and to determine how these new phenotypes bestow neoplastic potential on cell populations.

REFERENCES

1. Foulds L: The histologic analysis of mammary tumors. I. The histology or responsiveness and progression. The origins of tumors. J Natl Cancer Inst 17:713–753, 1956
2. Englebreth-Holm J: Acceleration of development of mammary carcinomas in mice by methylcholanthrene. Cancer Res 1:109–112, 1941
3. Andervant HB, Dunn TB: Responses of strain DBAf/2 mice, without the mammary tumor agent, to oral administration of methylcholanthrene. J Natl Cancer Inst 14:329–339, 1953
4. Huggins C, Grand LC, Brilantes FP: Mammary cancer induced by a single feeding of polynuclear hydrocarbons and its suppression. Nature 189:204–207, 1961
5. Medina D: Mammary tumorigenesis in chemical carcinogen treated mice. I. Incidence in BALB/c and C57BL mice. J Natl Cancer Inst 53:213–221, 1974
6. Medina D, Butely JS, Socher SH, et al: Mammary tumorigenesis in 7,12-dimethylbenzanthracene-treated C57XDBA/2fF1 mice. Cancer Res 40:368–373, 1980
7. Smith G, Pauley RJ, Socher SH, et al: Chemical carcinogenesis in C3H/StWi mice, a worthwhile experimental model for breast cancer. Cancer Res 36:4504–4509, 1978
8. Ethier SP, Ullrich RL: Induction of mammary tumors in BALB/c mice by single low doses of 7,12-dimethylbenz(a)anthracene. J Natl Cancer Inst 69:1199–1203, 1982
9. Shellabarger CJ: Mammary neoplastic response of Lewis and Sprague-Dawley female rats to 7,12-dimethylbenz(a)anthracene or x-ray. Cancer Res 32:883–885, 1972
10. Gullino PM, Pettigrew HM, Grantham FH: N-Nitrosomethylurea as mammary gland carcinogen in rats. J Natl Cancer Inst 54:401–414, 1975
11. McCormick DL, Adanowski CB, Fiks A, et al: Lifetime dose-response relationships for mammary tumor induction by a single administration of *N*-methyl-*N*-nitrosourea. Cancer Res 41:1690–1694, 1981
12. Tokunaga M, Naman JE, Asano M: Malignant breast tumors among atomic bomb survivors, Hiroshima and Nagasaki, 1950–1974. J Natl Cancer Inst 62:1347–1359, 1979
13. Mettler FA, Hemplemen LH, Dutton HM et al: Breast neoplasms in women treated with x-rays for acute post-partum mastitis. J Natl Cancer Inst 43:803–811, 1969

14. MacKenzie I: Breast cancer following multiple fluoroscopies. Br J Cancer 19:1–8, 1965
15. Land CE, Boice JD, Shore RE, et al: Breast cancer risk from low dose exposures to ionizing radiation: Results of parallel analysis of three exposed populations of women. J Natl Cancer Inst 65:353–376, 1980
16. Shellabarger CJ, Cronkite EP, Bond VP, et al: The occurrence of mammary tumors in the rat after sublethal whole body irradiation. Radiat Res 6:501–512, 1957
17. Shellabarger CJ, Chmelevsky D, Kellerer AM: Induction of mammary neoplasms in the Sprague-Dawley rat by 430 keV neutrons and x-rays. J Natl Cancer Inst 64:821–833, 1980
18. Ullrich RL, Storer JB: Influence of γ-radiation on the development of neoplastic disease in mice. III. Dose-rate effects. Radiat Res 80:325–342, 1979
19. Haaland M: Spontaneous tumors in mice. Fourth Scientific Report, Imperial Cancer Research Fund, p 1–111, 1911
20. Fekety EA: A comparative morphological study of the mammary gland in a high and low tumor strain of mice. Am J Pathol 14:557–578, 1938
21. Huseby RA, Bittner JJ: A comparative morphological study of the mammary glands with reference to known factors influencing the development of mammary carcinoma in mice. Cancer Res 6:240–255, 1946
22. Zotter S, Kemmer C, Muller M: Mammary tumor virus: Investigations in mouse and man. Exp Pathol (Suppl 6), New York Elsevier-Dutton, 1981
23. DeOme KB, Faulkin LJ, Bern HA, et al: Development of mammary tumors from hyperplastic alveolar nodules transplanted into gland free mammary fat pads of female C3H mice. Cancer Res 19:515–520, 1959
24. Medina D, Iramain CA, Clark JH: Hormone dependence and estradiol receptors in the D series of mammary nodule outgrowth lines and tumors. Cancer Res 35:2355–2360, 1975
25. Gullino PM: Natural history of breast cancer—progression from hyperplasia to neoplasia as predicted by angiogenesis. Cancer 39:2697–2703, 1977
26. Daniel CW, DeOme KB, Blair PB, et al: The *in vivo* lifespan of normal and preneoplastic mouse mammary glands: A serial transplantation study. Proc Natl Acad Sci USA 61:52–60, 1968
27. Faulkin LJ: Hyperplastic lesions of mouse mammary glands after treatment with 3-methylcholanthrene. J Natl Cancer Inst 36:289–297, 1966
28. Medina D, DeOme KB: Influence of mammary tumor virus on the tumor-producing capabilities of nodule outgrowth free of mammary tumor virus. J Natl Cancer Inst 40:1303–1308, 1968
29. Medina D, DeOme KB: Effects of various oncogenic agents on tumor-producing capabilities of series D BALB/c mammary nodule outgrowth lines. J Natl Cancer Inst 45:353–363, 1970
30. Faulkin LJ, Shellabarger CJ, DeOme KB: Hyperplastic lesions of Sprague-Dawley rat mammary glands after x-irradiation. J Natl Cancer Inst 39:449–458, 1967
31. Beuving LJ, Bern HA, DeOme KB: Occurrence and transplantation of carcinogen-induced hyperplastic nodules in Fisher rats. J Natl Cancer Inst 39:431–448, 1967
32. Sinha D, Dao TL: Hyperplastic alveolar nodules of the rat mammary gland: Tumor-producing capabilities *in vivo* and *in vitro*. Cancer Lett 2:153–160, 1977
33. Beuving LJ: Mammary tumor formation within outgrowths of transplanted hyperplastic alveolar nodules from carcinogen-treated rats. J Natl Cancer Inst 40:1287–1291, 1968
34. Rivera EM, Hill SD, Taylor M: Organ culture passage enhances the oncogenicity of carcinogen induced hyperplastic mammary nodules. In Vitro 17:159–166, 1981
35. Medina D: Mammary tumorigenesis in chemical carcinogen-treated mice. I. Incidence in BALB/c and C57BL mice. J Natl Cancer Inst 53:213–221, 1974
36. Ethier SP, Ullrich RL: Detection of ductal dysplasias in mammary outgrowths derived from carcinogen-treated virgin female BALB/c mice. Cancer Res 42:1753–1760, 1982
37. Medina D: Serial transplantation of chemical carcinogen-induced mouse mammary ductal dysplasias. J Natl Cancer Inst 62:397–405, 1979
38. Middleton PJ: The histogenesis of mammary tumors induced in the rat by chemical carcinogens. Br J Cancer 19:830–839, 1965
39. Fisher ER, Shoemaker RH, Sabnis A: Relationship of hyperplasia to cancer in 3-methylcholanthrene induced mammary tumorigenesis. Lab Invest 33:33–42, 1975
40. Purnell DM: The relationship of terminal duct hyperplasia to mammary carcinoma in 7,12-dimethylbenz(a)anthracene treated Lew/mai rats. Am J Pathol 98:311–324, 1980
41. Haslam SZ, Bern HA: Histopathogenesis of 7,12-dimethylbenzanthracene induced rat mammary tumors. Proc Natl Acad Sci USA 74:4020–4024, 1977
42. Russo IH, Russo J: Developmental state of the rat mammary gland as determinant of its susceptibility to 7,12-dimethylbenz(a)anthracene. J Natl Cancer Inst, 1978
43. Russo J, Russo IH: Influence of differentiation and cell kinetics on the susceptibility of the rat mammary gland to carcinogenesis. Cancer Res 40:2677–2687, 1980
44. DeOme KB, Miyamoto MJ, Osborn RC, et al: Detection of inapparent nodule-transformed cells in the mammary gland tissues of virgin female BALB/cfC3H mice. Cancer Res 38:2103–2111, 1978
45. Ethier SP, Adams LM, Ullrich RL: Morphological and histological characteristics of mammary dysplasias occurring in cell dissociation-derived mammary outgrowths. Cancer Res 44:4517–4522, 1984
46. Ethier SP, Ullrich RL: Factors influencing expression of mammary ductal dysplasia in cell dissociation-derived murine mammary outgrowths. Cancer Res 44:4523–4527,
47. Wellings SR, Jensen HM, Marcun RG: An atlas of subgross pathology of the human breast with special reference to possible procancerous lesions. J Natl Cancer Inst 55:231–273, 1975
48. Wellings SR: Development of human breast cancer. Adv Cancer Res 31:287–314, 1980
49. Squartini F, Sounelli R: Structure, functional changes, and proliferative pathology of the human mammary lobule in cancerous breasts. J Natl Cancer Inst 67:33–46, 1981
50. Hutchinson WB, Thomas DB, et al: Risk of breast cancer in women with benign breast disease. J Natl Cancer Inst 65:13–20, 1980
51. Onuchi N, Abe R, Kasai M: Possible cancerous change of intraductal papillomas of the breast. Cancer 54:605–611, 1984
52. Henderson JS, Rous P: The plating of tumor components on the subcutaneous expanses of young mice. J Exp Med 115:1211–1254, 1962
53. Heppner GH, Miller BE: Tumor heterogeneity: biological implications and therapeutic consequences. Cancer Metastasis Rev 2:5–23, 1983
54. Parbhoo SP: Heterogeneity in human mammary cancer. In Stoll BA (ed): Systemic Control of Breast Cancer, pp 55–77. London, William Heinemann, 1981
55. Gioanni J, Courdi A, Lalanne CM, et al: Establishment, char-

acterization, chemosensitivity, and radiosensitivity of two different cell lines derived from a human breast cancer biopsy. Cancer Res 45:1246–1258, 1985
56. Sharkey FE: Morphometric analysis of differentiation in human breast carcinoma. Arch Pathol Lab Med 107:411–414, 1983
57. Tseng MT: Ultrastructure of the hormone-dependent *N*-nitrosomethylurea-induced mammary carcinoma of the rat. Cancer Res 40:3112–3115, 1980
58. Johnson ML, Levy J, Rosen JM: Isolation and characterization of casein-producing and nonproducing cell populations from 7,12-dimethylbenz(a)anthracene-induced rat mammary carcinomas. Cancer Res 43:2199–2209, 1983
59. Bano M, Lewko WM, Kidwell WR: Characterization of rat mammary tumor cell populations. Cancer Res 44:3055–3062, 1984
60. Horan Hand P, Nuti M, Colcher D, et al: Definition of antigenic heterogeneity and modulation among human mammary carcinoma cell populations using monoclonal antibodies to tumor-associated antigens. Cancer Res 43:728–735, 1983
61. Natali PG, Giacomini P, Bigotti A, et al: Heterogeneity in the expression of HLA and tumor-associated antigens by surgically removed and cultured breast carcinoma cells. Cancer Res 43:660–668, 1983
62. Ceriani RL, Peterson JA, Blank EW: Variability in surface antigen expression of human breast epithelial cells cultured from normal breast, normal tissue peripheral to breast carcinomas, and breast carcinoma. Cancer Res 44:3033–3039, 1984
63. Macinnes JI, Chan ECM, Percy DH: Mammary tumors from GR mice contain more than one population of mouse mammary tumor virus-infected cells. Virology 113:119–129, 1981
64. Sluyser M, Evers SG, DeGoeij CCJ: Sex hormone receptors in mammary tumors of GR mice. Nature 263:386–389, 1976
65. Oxenhandler RW, McCune R. Subtelney A, et al: Flow cytometric determination of estrogen receptors in intact cells. Cancer Res 44:2516–2523, 1984
66. Wolman SR: Karyotypic progression in human tumors. Cancer Metastasis Rev 2:257–293, 1983
67. Ewers SB, Langstrom E. Baldetorp B, et al: Flow-cytometric DNA analysis in primary breast carcinomas and clinicopathological correlations. Cytometry 5:408–419, 1984
68. Meyer JS, McDivitt RW, Stone KR, et al: Practical breast carcinoma cell kinetics: Review and update. Breast Cancer Res Treatment 4:79–88, 1984
69. Miller FR, Miller BE, Heppner GH: Characterization of metastatic heterogeneity among subpopulations of a single mouse mammary tumor: Heterogeneity in phenotypic stability. Invasion and Metastasis 3:22–31, 1983
70. Lollini PL, de Giovanni C, Eusebi V, et al: High-metastatic clones selected *in vitro* from a recent spontaneous BALB/c mammary adenocarcinoma cell line. Clin Exp Metastasis 2:251–259, 1984
71. Barnett SC, Eccles SA: Studies of mammary carcinoma metastasis in a mouse model system. Clin Exp Metastasis 2:15–36, 1984
72. Neri A, Welch DR, Kawaguchi T, et al: The development and biologic properties of malignant cell sublines and clones of a spontaneously metastasizing rat mammary adenocarcinoma. J Natl Cancer Inst 68:507–517, 1982
73. Heppner GH, Dexter DL, DeNucci T, et al: heterogeneity in drug sensitivity among tumor cell subpopulations of a single mouse mammary tumor. Cancer Res 38:3758–3763, 1978
74. Tsuruo I, Fidler IJ: Differences in drug sensitivity among tumor cells from parental tumors, selected variants, and spontaneous metastasis. Cancer Res 41:3058–3064, 1981
75. Leith JT, Brenner HJ, DeWyngaert JK, et al: Selective modification of the x-ray survival response of two mouse mammary adenocarcinoma sublines by N,N-dimethylformamide. Int J Radiat Oncol Biol Phys 7:943–947, 1981
76. Welch DR, Milas L, Tomasovic SP, et al: Heterogeneous response and clonal drift of sensitivities of metastatic 13762NF mammary adenocarcinoma clones to gamma-radiation *in vitro*. Cancer Res 43:6–10, 1983
77. Poste G, Doll J, Fidler IJ: Interactions among clonal subpopulations affect stability of the metastatic phenotype in polyclonal populations of B16 melanoma cells. Proc Natl Acad Sci USA 78:6226–6230, 1981
78. Heppner GH: Tumor heterogeneity. Cancer Res 44:2259–2265, 1984
79. Heppner GH, Miller GE, Miller FR: Tumor subpopulation interactions in neoplasms. Biochim Biophys Acta 695:215–226, 1983
80. Brodt P, Parhar R, Sankar P, et al: Studies on clonal heterogeneity in two spontaneously metastasizing mammary carcinomas of recent origin. Int J Cancer 35:265–273, 1985
81. Miller FR: Tumor subpopulation interactions in metastasis. Invasion and Metastasis 3:234–242, 1983
82. Danielpour D, Sirbasku DA: New perspectives in hormone-dependent (responsive) and autonomous mammary tumor growth: Role of autostimulatory growth factors. In Vitro 20:975–980, 1984
83. Miller BE, Miller FR, Heppner GH: Interactions between tumor subpopulations affecting their sensitivity to the antineoplastic agents cyclophosphamide and methotrexate. Cancer Res 41:4378–4381, 1981
84. Tofilon PJ, Buckley N, Deen DF: Effect of cell-cell interactions on drug sensitivity and growth of drug-sensitive and resistant tumor cells in spheroids. Science 226:862–864, 1984
85. Miller BE, McInerney DJ, Jackson D, et al: Metabolic cooperation between mouse mammary tumor subpopulations in three-dimensional collagen gel cultures. Cancer Res 46:89–93, 1986
86. Fialkow PJ: Clonal origin of human tumors. Annu Rev Med 30:135–143, 1979
87. Nowell PC: The clonal evolution of tumor cell populations. Science 194:23–28, 1976
88. Peterson JA, Ceriani RL, Blank EW, et al: Comparison of rates of phenotypic variability in surface antigen expression in normal and cancerous human breast epithelial cells. Cancer Res 43: 4291–4296, 1983
89. Yamashina K, Heppner GH: Correlation of frequency of induced mutation and metastatic potential in tumor cell lines from a single mouse mammary tumor. Cancer Res 45:4015–4019, 1985
90. Kerbel RS, Frost P, Liteplo R, et al: Possible epigenetic mechanisms of tumor progression: Induction of high-frequency heritable but phenotypically unstable changes in the tumorigenic and metastatic properties of tumor cell populations by 5-azacytidine treatment. J Cell Physiol [Suppl] 3:87–97, 1984
91. Pierce GB, Cox WF Jr: Neoplasms as caricatures of tissue renewal. *In* Saunders GF (ed): Cell Differentiation and Neoplasia, pp 57–66. New York, Raven Press, 1978
92. Rudland PS, Gusterson BA, Hughes CM, et al: Two forms of tumors in nude mice generated by a neoplastic rat mammary stem cell line. Cancer Res 42:5196–5208, 1982
93. Hager J, Fligiel S, Stanley W, et al: Characterization of a

variant producing tumor cell line from a heterogeneous strain BALB/cfC3H mouse mammary tumor. Cancer Res 41:1293–1300, 1981
94. Fulton AM, Loveless SE, Heppner GH: Mutagenic activity of tumor-associated macrophages. Cancer Res 44:4308–4311, 1984
95. Biancifiori C, Cashera F: The relation between pseudopregnancy and the chemical induction by four carcinogens of mammary and ovarian tumors in BALB/c mice. Br J Cancer 16:722–730, 1962
96. Marchant J: Chemical induction of breast tumors in mice of the C57/Bl strain. The influence of pseudopregnancy, pregnancy and lactation on induction by methylcholanthxene. Br J Cancer 15:568–573, 1961
97. Haran Gliera N: The role of mammotropin in mammary tumor induction in mice. Cancer Res 21:790–795, 1961
98. Medina D: Mammary tumorigenesis in chemical carcinogen-treated mice. II. Dependence on hormone stimulation for tumorigenesis. J Natl Cancer Inst 53: 223–226, 1974
99. Kim U, Furth J: Relation of mammary tumors to mammotropes. Proc Soc Exp Biol Med 103:640–642, 1960
100. Muhlbock O, Boot LM: Induction of mammary cancer in mice without the mammary tumor agent by isografts of hypophyses. Cancer Res 19:402–412, 1959
101. Liebelt AG, Liebelt RA: Effect of a single pituitary isograft on mammary tumorigenesis in mice. Cancer Res 21:86–90, 1961
102. McGrath CM, Jones RF: Hormonal induction of mammary tumor virus and its implications for carcinogenesis. Cancer Res 38:4112–4125, 1978
103. Bern HA, Nandi S: Recent studies on the hormonal influence in mouse mammary tumorigenesis. Prog Exp Tumor Res 2:50–144, 1961
104. Chen CL, Meites J: Effects of estrogen and progesterone on serum and pituitary prolactin levels in ovariectomized rats. Endocrinology 80:503–505, 1970
105. Welsch CW, Nagawasa H: Prolactin and murine mammary tumorigenesis: A review. Cancer Res 37:951–963, 1977
106. Welsch CW: Host factors affecting the growth of carcinogen-induced rat mammary carcinomas: A review and tribute to Charles Brenton Huggins. Cancer Res 45:3415–3443, 1985
107. Soule HD, Vasquez J, Long A, et al: A human cell line from a pleural effusion derived from a breast carcinoma. J Natl Cancer Inst 51:1409–1413, 1973
108. Soule HD, McGrath CM: Estrogen-responsive proliferation of clonal human breast carcinoma cells in athymic mice. Cancer Lett 10:177–189, 1980
109. Lippman ME, Strobl J, Allegra JC: Effects of hormones on human breast cancer cells in tissue culture. *In* McGrath CM, Brennan MJ, Rich MA (eds): Cell Biology of Breast Cancer, p 205–276. New York, Academic Press, 1980
110. Katzenellenbogen BS, Norman MJ, Eckert RL, et al: Bioactivities, estrogen receptor interactions, and plasminogen activator-inducing activities of tamoxifen and hydroxytamoxifen isomers in MCF-7 human breast cancer cells. Cancer Res 44:112–119, 1984
111. Barnes D, Sato G: Factors that stimulate proliferation of breast cancer cells *in vitro* in serum-free medium. *In* McGrath CM, Brennan MJ, Rich MA (eds): Cell Biology of Breast Cancer, p 277–288. New York, Academic Press, 1980
112. Berthois Y, Katzenellenbogen JA, Katzenellenbogen BS: Phenol red in tissue culture media is a weak estrogen: Implications concerning the study of estrogen responsive cells in culture. Proc Natl Acad Sci 83:2496–2500, 1986
113. Soto AM, Sonnenschein C: The role of estrogens on the proliferation of human breast tumor cells (MCF-7). J Steroid Biochem 23:87–94, 1985
114. Brooks SC, Locke ER, Soule HD: Estrogen receptor in a human cell line. J Biol Chem 248:6251–6253, 1973
115. Lippman ME, Bolan G, Huff K: The effects of estrogens and antiestrogens on hormone-responsive human breast cancer in long-term tissue culture. Cancer Res 36:4595–4601, 1976
116. Sirbasku DA: Estrogen induction of growth factors specific for hormone responsive mammary, pituitary and kidney tumor cells. Proc Natl Acad Sci USA 75:3786–3790, 1978
117. Wicha MS, Liotta LA, Vanderhaar BK, et al: Effects of inhibition of basement membrane collagen deposition on rat mammary gland development. Dev Biol 80:253–266, 1980
118. Terzaghi M, Klein-Szanto AJP: Differentiation of normal and cultured preneoplastic tracheal epithelial cells in rats: Importance of epithelial-mesenchymal interactions. J Natl Cancer Inst 65:1039–1048, 1980
119. David G, Bernfield M: Type I collagen reduces the degradation of basal lamina proteoglycan by mammary epithelial cells. J Cell Biol 91:281–286, 1981
120. David G, Bernfield M: Defective basal lamina formation by transformed mammary epithelial cells: A reduced effect of collagen on basal lamina degradation. J Cell Physiol 110:56–62, 1982
121. Rheinwald JG, Green H: Serial cultivation of strains of human epidermal keratinocytes: The formation of keratinizing colonies from single cells. Cell 6:331–344, 1975
122. Gray TE, Thomasson DG, Mass MJ, et al: Quantitation of cell proliferation, colony formation and carcinogen induced cytotoxicity of rat tracheal epithelial cells grown in culture on 3T3 feeder layers. In Vitro 19:559–570, 1983
123. Babcock MS, Marino MR, Cunning WT, et al: Clonal growth and serial propagation of rat esophageal epithelial cells. In Vitro 19:403–415, 1983
124. Hennings H, Michael D, Cheng C, et al: Calcium regulation of growth and differentiation of mouse epidermal cells in culture. Cell 19:245–254, 1980
125. Stampfer M, Hallowes RC, Hackett AJ: Growth of normal human mammary cells in culture. In Vitro 16:415–425, 1980
126. Hammond SL, Ham RG, Stampfer MR: Serum-free growth of human mammary epithelial cells: Rapid clonal growth in defined medium and extended serial passage with pituitary extract. Proc Natl Acad Sci USA 81:5435–5439, 1984
127. Ethier SP: Primary culture and serial passage of normal and carcinogen-treated rat mammary epithelial cells *in vitro*. J Natl Cancer Inst 74:1307–1318, 1985
128. Ethier SP: Development of serum-free culture conditions for the extended growth of normal rat mammary epithelial cells *in vitro*. In Vitro (in press)

7 The Pathology of Breast Carcinoma

Paul Peter Rosen

Mammary carcinoma consists of a diverse group of malignant epithelial neoplasms that exhibit considerable structural heterogeneity. The goal of this chapter is to provide an overview of the pathologic aspects of the disease. Emphasis has been placed on gross and microscopic morphological features that characterize different types of carcinoma because many of the pathologic distinctions have clinical or prognostic significance and may, therefore, influence the treatment of a given patient. The classification of mammary carcinoma used for reference is one proposed by Foote and Stewart,[1] which has been adopted with little change by the Armed Forces Institute of Pathology[2] and the World Health Organization (WHO).[3]

In this chapter, data on prognosis drawn from the literature are considered largely in the context of surgical therapy by mastectomy since this has been, until recently, the most widely used form of treatment. However, these observations should not necessarily be regarded as current therapeutic recommendations. The reader is referred to other chapters in the book for comprehensive discussions of treatment options.

MAMMARY CARCINOMA

In Situ Breast Carcinoma

The epithelial origin of mammary carcinomas was proposed in the mid-19th century. Cornil, who provided some of the earliest illustrations of this process (Fig. 7-1) chose the breast to demonstrate progression from intraepithelial to invasive carcinoma.[4] It is noteworthy that Waldeyer, who coincidentally advocated the same concept in Germany, also referred to the breast as a model (Fig. 7-2),[5] and that both authors used examples of lobular carcinoma to make their point.

As defined in 1932 by Broders, "carcinoma *in situ* is a condition in which malignant epithelial cells and their progeny are found in or near positions occupied by their ancestors before the ancestors underwent malignant transformation."[6] From the descriptions provided in his paper, it is clear that Broders referred specifically to carcinoma in the epithelium of origin—that is, intraepithelial carcinoma. In the context of mammary carcinoma, the term *in situ* became attached to carcinoma originating in lobules, with the introduction in 1941 of the term lobular carcinoma *in situ*.[7] However, it applies equally to intraepithelial carcinoma of the ducts, usually described as intraductal carcinoma.

A variety of alternative, less satisfactory terms have been proposed. The adjective noninvasive suggests that tumor cells have not extended through the basement membrane in so far as can be determined by light microscopy. However, electron microscopy has shown that tumor cells can penetrate the basement membrane even when this cannot be appreciated in routine histologic sections.[8,9] This inconspicuous invasion may account for some of the infrequent instances of metastases developing in a patient diagnosed as having noninvasive carcinoma.[10] The term preinvasive implies evolution of the process to invasive carcinoma. Although this occurs in some cases, it has not been documented to be a consistent property of all intraepithelial or *in situ* breast carcinomas within the limits of clinical study.

Another approach has been to replace the word carcinoma with neoplasia when referring to an *in situ* lesion. This change has been advocated, especially with respect to the lobules, in order to encourage clinical management that does not involve radical surgery.[11] One result has been a tendency to broaden the diagnosis of lobular neoplasia to include lesions that are hyperplastic and that would not ordinarily be regarded as *in situ* lobular carcinoma.

None of the proposed terms is entirely satisfactory. In the present discussion, noninvasive carcinoma will be described as *in situ* lobular, intraductal, or intraepithelial carcinoma, depending on context.

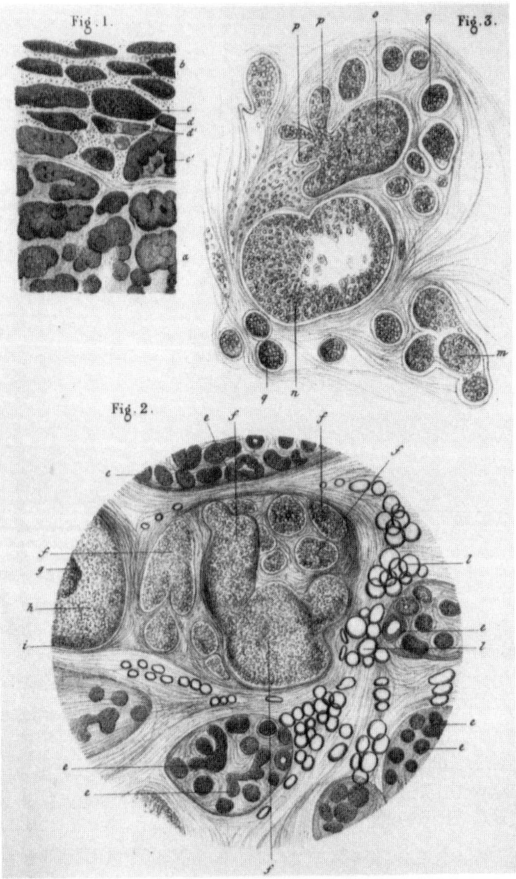

FIGURE 7-1. *In situ* carcinoma. One of a series of illustrations published by Cornil[4] in 1865 to depict stages in the development of mammary carcinoma. Terminal ducts and acini appear to be filled with neoplastic cells.

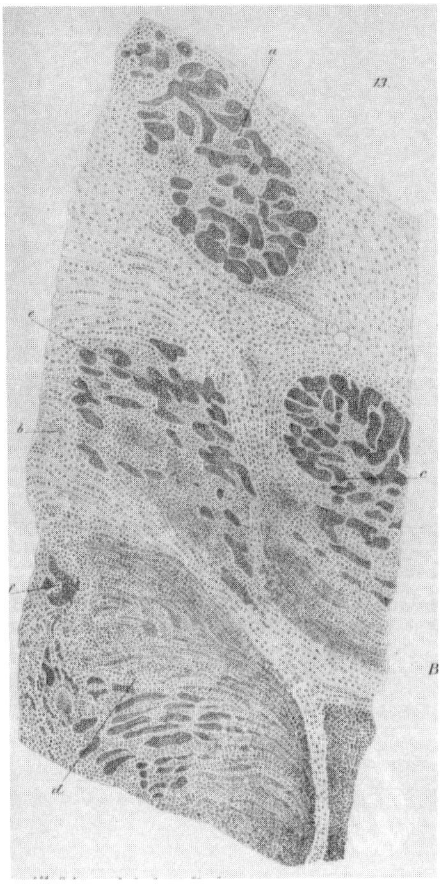

FIGURE 7-2. *In situ* carcinoma. An illustration published by Waldeyer[5] in 1867 showing the progression from *in situ* carcinoma arising in the upper lobule *(a)* to invasive carcinoma in the lower lobules *(d)*.

Until the widespread availability of mammography, intraepithelial carcinoma of the breast was largely a fortuitous, unexpected finding in breast tissue removed because of the presence of a lump. Many lesions are still detected in this fashion, but in a growing number of cases, the presence of a nonpalpable, mammographic abnormality leads to a diagnosis of intraepithelial carcinoma. Among the cases reviewed in a nationwide breast cancer screening program, 143 of 212 intraductal carcinomas (67%) were found in biopsies performed on the basis of mammographic indications alone; 2% were detected in biopsies initiated solely because of clinical abnormalities.[12]

It has been customary to distinguish the two types of intraepithelial carcinoma occurring in the breast on the basis of the anatomic distribution of the lesions in the duct-lobular system, as well as their growth patterns and their cytologic features. Generally accepted histologic criteria serve to distinguish *in situ* lobular from intraductal carcinoma. However, under some circumstances, the distinction is obscured. The two processes may coexist in the breast within a single duct-lobular unit,[13] duct carcinoma may extend into the epithelium of lobules,[14] or lobular carcinoma *in situ* may be observed within ductal epithelium.[15] There is also evidence indicating that the site of origin of many carcinomas may be in the terminal duct epithelium, regardless of histologic type,[16] but this concept has not led to any widely accepted modification of the scheme for classifying breast carcinoma.

Intraductal Carcinoma

The concept of intraductal carcinoma appears to have developed in the early part of the 20th century, largely as a result of studies carried out by surgeons. Of particular interest is the work of J.C. Warren in Boston, Sir G. Lenthal Cheatle of Kings College Hospital in London, and Joseph Colt Bloodgood of the Johns Hopkins Hospital in Baltimore. Warren investigated the pathology of "abnormal involution"(proliferative or fibrocystic disease) and described transitions from duct hyperplasia to intraepithelial carcinoma and progression to invasive carcinoma.[17]

Cheatle conducted a systematic study of the microscopic pathology of whole organ sections of mastectomy specimens. In contrast, Bloodgood examined pathologic findings in individual patients, often dealing in detail with biopsy specimens. As a consequence, Bloodgood was sometimes able to correlate pathologic findings with follow-up in patients who did not undergo mastectomy. He appreciated the problem of predicting the clinical course of patients with atypical intraepithelial proliferative lesions which he described as "border-line breast tumors."[18] The orderly, papillary form of intraductal carcinoma, now referred to as micropapillary carcinoma, was illustrated by Cheatle in 1920[19] and by Bloodgood in 1921.[20] Another intraductal growth pattern, cribriform, was also depicted by Cheatle in 1920.[19]

The early history of comedocarcinoma, as described in 1934 by Bloodgood,[21] is of particular interest:

> In 1893, forty-one years ago, I assisted Dr. Halstead in exploring a clinically benign tumor of the breast. . . . The moment we cut into and pressed on it, there extruded from its surface many grayish white, granular cylinders, which I called at that time comedos. From the gross appearance, the tumor was diagnosed as malignant, and the radical operation was performed. The nodes were not involved. . . . The patient lived nineteen years after the operation, dying at age eighty-six.

Bloodgood reviewed his experience with the "pure comedo tumor"—that is, intraductal comedocarcinoma—and observed that "none of the cases . . . was associated with metastasis to the axillary nodes; not a single patient died of cancer."[21] He recommended treatment by local excision "when the palpable tumor is small and can be completely excised by cutting through normal breast tissue and closing the wound without injury to the symmetry of the breast." Two of his patients were reported to be well 1 and 10 years, respectively, following local excision and radiotherapy for small intraductal lesions.

The frequency of intraductal carcinoma in reported series of carcinomas varies considerably, depending upon clinical circumstances and the manner in which diagnoses are classified. In a review of nearly 1000 women treated consecutively for primary, operable, breast carcinoma at Memorial Hospital in the late 1970s, 5% had intraductal carcinoma.[22] A nationwide review of breast carcinomas based on 1975 data from nine population-based registries, reported that intraductal carcinoma was the primary diagnosis in 2.9% of cases.[23] When mammography screening is employed, the proportion of intraductal carcinomas tends to increase. On initial screening, 8% to 22% of carcinomas detected on mammography were classified as intraductal.[24–27] In populations examined by repeated mammography screening, the proportion of intraductal carcinomas is not appreciably increased in subsequent examinations, but there does appear to be a greater number of small invasive tumors detected.[25,26]

Approximately 5% of male breast carcinomas are intraductal. Men who have intraductal carcinoma are likely to present with nipple discharge that is usually bloody,[28] whereas most women do not have symptoms attributable to the intraductal lesion.

Because intraductal carcinoma is often a lesion of microscopic dimensions, little information is available about its estrogen receptor properties. Biochemical analyses that employ homogenized tissue are likely to be contaminated with a substantial proportion of nonneoplastic tissue, and this may contribute to reports that most specimens analyzed biochemically were receptor-negative.[29–31] In one study, the median level of estrogen receptor in intraductal carcinoma was 5 fmol/mg of cytosol protein, significantly less than a median of 11 fmol for infiltrating ductal carcinomas.[29] Recently available monoclonal antibodies for estrogen receptor protein have made it possible to demonstrate the localization of receptors directly in histologic sections of intraductal carcinoma.[32]

CLINICAL PRESENTATION. Palpable tumors were reportedly present in 50% to 65% of women who had intraductal carcinoma.[33–35] However, in many cases, intraductal carcinoma is a microscopic disease that does not produce a tumor. A study comparing breast carcinomas diagnosed between 1973 and 1974 in Japan and the United States reported a higher frequency of intraductal carcinoma in Japanese patients, and noted that the carcinomas tend to form bulky, palpable tumors in Japanese women.[36]

Intraductal carcinoma may be suspected if a patient with Paget's disease or with a bloody nipple discharge has no palpable breast tumor.[37] The tendency for calcification to develop within intraductal carcinoma may lead to detection of the lesion by mammography. However, the patterns of calcification are not entirely specific; overall, only about 25% of biopsies performed for suspicious calcifications reveal carcinoma, primarily the intraductal type.[38,39] Duct hyperplasia and sclerosing adenosis account for the majority of significant calcifications that do not prove to be carcinoma.

Intraductal carcinoma has the same age distribution as does breast carcinoma generally. The mean age at diagnosis of the patients in five recent studies was between 50 and 59 years, which is quite similar to the mean age of women with invasive ductal carcinoma.[33–35,40,41] Contralateral carcinoma is found in about 10% of patients who undergo concurrent biopsy of both breasts.[42] Contralateral prophylactic mastectomy, performed in a series of 23 women treated for intraductal carcinoma, revealed that 30% of these women had unsuspected carcinoma in the opposite breast.[43]

The diagnosis of intraductal carcinoma requires histologic sections of excised breast tissue. The diagnosis may be made with frozen sections, but if any difficulty is encountered, the decision should be based on permanent sections.[44] Approximately 3% of the biopsies reported to be benign on the basis of frozen sections ultimately reveal carcinoma when paraffin sections are examined.[44] Because sampling of a biopsy is quite limited during surgery, approximately 20% of patients in whom a frozen section diagnosis of intraductal carcinoma is made prove to have invasion when multiple paraffin sections of the same biopsy specimen are examined.[45] A needle biopsy is unsatisfactory for assessing the presence of invasion. Carci-

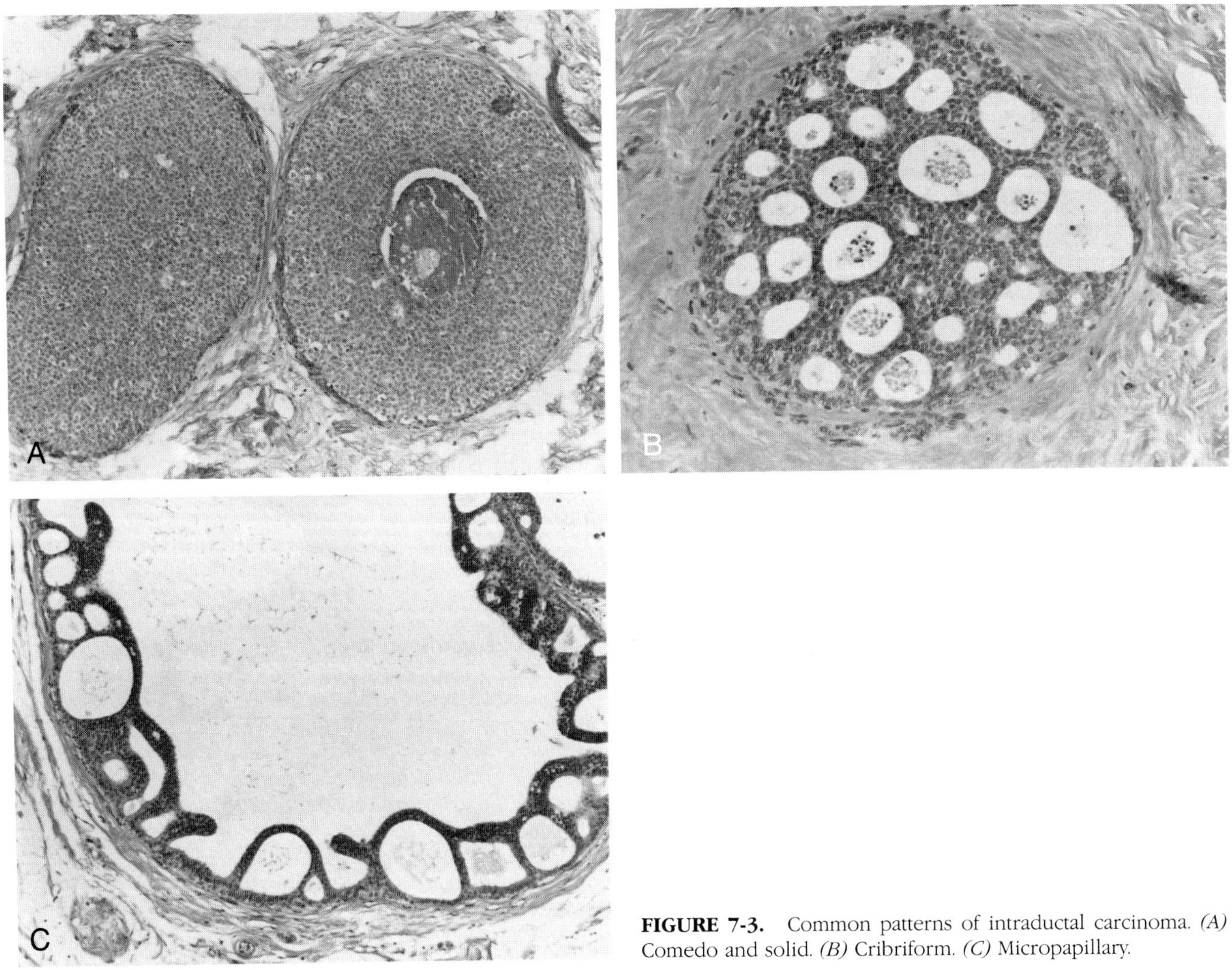

FIGURE 7-3. Common patterns of intraductal carcinoma. *(A)* Comedo and solid. *(B)* Cribriform. *(C)* Micropapillary.

nomatous cells found in spontaneous nipple discharge are not specifically diagnostic of intraductal carcinoma since this material does not provide information about the presence or absence of invasion.

GROSS PATHOLOGY. Intraductal carcinoma is rarely evident on gross examination. Comedocarcinoma involving multiple ducts occasionally produces a firm mass. These lesions tend to be well-defined, tan tumors with white to pale yellow flecks representing necrotic intraductal carcinoma (comedos). These comedos extrude from the cut surface when the lesion is compressed. Abundant calcification in the lesion imparts a gritty sensation upon cutting into the tumor. Although these findings are suggestive of comedocarcinoma, an identical gross appearance is found in some cases of stasis and mastitis.

MICROSCOPIC PATHOLOGY. In standard histologic sections, intraductal carcinoma appears to be confined within the lumens of the ducts involved in the process. It is not practical to employ electron microscopy in routine practice to determine whether there is invasion by individual cells because only very limited samples can be examined by this procedure.[8,46] Intact basement membranes have been demonstrated in intraductal carcinomas with immunohistochemical procedures that utilize antibodies to basement membrane components.[47] Reactivity for basement membrane antigens may be lost in microinvasive foci. Diminished carcinoembryonic antigen (CEA) immunoreactivity in the intraductal component of invasive ductal carcinomas has been described.[48] The distribution of this marker is often so heterogeneous in a given case that it cannot be relied upon as evidence for invasion.

A variety of histologic patterns are encountered in intraductal carcinomas (Fig. 7-3). Except for the smallest foci possibly limited to only a few ducts, more than one pattern is likely to be present in a given case. For example, adjacent ducts in one patient may contain cribriform, papillary, and comedo forms of carcinoma. Differences in the cytologic appearances of intraductal carcinoma cells are

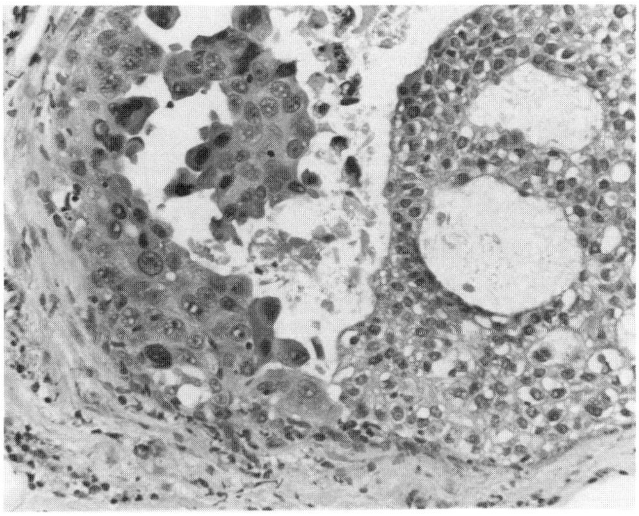

FIGURE 7-4. Cytologic heterogeneity in intraductal carcinoma. The lesion was found in a random biopsy of the left breast of a 62-year-old woman who presented with Stage II carcinoma of the right breast. The tumor in the left part of this duct has a papillary growth pattern and apocrine cytology, including a darkly stained, faintly granular cytoplasm and large, pleomorphic nuclei. The cribriform intraductal carcinoma on the right has small, uniform nuclei in cells with clear or pale cytoplasm.

also encountered. The entire spectrum of nuclear differentiation—from low to high grade—occurs in intraductal, as well as in invasive, carcinoma (Fig. 7-4). An appreciation of this pathologic diversity is of considerable importance for accurate diagnosis, but thus far, these factors have not been shown to correlate with the clinical aspects of disease. The spectrum of histologic patterns of intraductal carcinoma in men does not differ appreciably from the appearance of the disease in women, except for a higher proportion of papillary intraductal carcinoma.

Deposits of precipitated, calcified material may be found in most types of intraductal carcinoma. These calcifications are acellular inert objects, but they are the major reason that these microscopic lesions can be detected by mammography. The calcifications assume many different configurations, varying from minute, round, dense flecks to coarse, granular precipitates in necrotic intraductal carcinoma. Because there is considerable overlap in the histologic appearance of calcifications seen in intraductal carcinoma and in benign lesions, there is little diagnostic benefit derived from the microscopic study of calcifications. However, emerging evidence indicates that differences in the crystalline structure of calcifications may correlate with certain histologic findings.[49]

PROGNOSIS. Confusion about the terminology associated with some histologic types of intraductal carcinoma may have a significant effect on clinical studies of the disease. As noted above, Bloodgood used the name comedocarcinoma to describe noninvasive, as well as invasive, tumors.[21] The former were referred to as pure comedocarcinomas. Failure to separate the two groups clearly is reflected in Haagensen's[50] conclusion that all intraductal carcinomas "are infiltrating and fully malignant even though we do not happen to see actual infiltration." This approach led him "to classify as intraductal only those carcinomas in which at least 50% of the carcinoma grew intraductally." When defined in this fashion, it is not surprising that 24% of his patients with Columbia Stage A "intraductal" carcinoma had axillary metastases when treated with radical mastectomy, and that the 10-year survival rate in this group was 74%.[50]

When data from numerous institutions are combined without a consistent pathologic review, it is impossible to ensure that uniform diagnostic criteria have been employed by all contributing pathologists. The fact that the National Breast Cancer Survey reported a 5-year, disease-free survival rate of 74% for patients with intraductal carcinoma[51] suggests that a number of the cases may have been diagnosed according to criteria similar to those of Haagensen, which classify some invasive tumors as intraductal carcinomas.

To avoid these problems, names such as intraductal, noninfiltrating carcinoma, and preinvasive intraductal carcinoma have been advocated.[41,52] Whether or not these terms are used, if the term is to be clinically meaningful, it is necessary to limit the diagnosis of intraductal carcinoma to cases with no invasion demonstrable on light microscopic study of paraffin sections. When treated with mastectomy, approximately 1% of affected patients prove to have axillary lymph node metastases, even though evidence of invasion cannot be found in the breast.[10,33] After a biopsy diagnosis of intraductal carcinoma, 6% of mastectomies reveal a separate focus of invasive carcinoma elsewhere in the breast, and 64% have additional foci of intraepithelial carcinoma, primarily the intraductal type.[35]

Until recently, the vast majority of patients with noninvasive intraductal carcinoma were treated with mastectomy. Tumor recurrence and death due to breast carcinoma have been reported in about 1% of these patients.[33–35,41,52] In some instances, recurrence was attributable to a contralateral carcinoma.[35,41] A recent review of patients treated with excisional biopsy alone revealed the frequency of recurrence in the breast to vary from 24% to 70% with varying lengths of follow-up.[53] The results of treatment with excision and radiation therapy show promise after short-term follow-up.[54] Patients who receive no treatment after excision of intraductal carcinoma have a higher short-term recurrence rate in the breast than do those who undergo radiation therapy after excisional biopsy.[55]

Lobular Carcinoma In Situ

In 1941, Muir published a lengthy review of the early stages of mammary carcinoma.[56] Lesions were classified on the basis of whether they appeared to originate in ducts or lobules (acini). He noted that location in the duct-lobular system was not, by itself, a sufficient basis on which to establish that a carcinoma arose from lobular epithelium. He stated that, "The question is complicated by the fact that when malignant cells are present within them (*acini*) they may not have developed *in situ*. Intra-acinous carcinoma is often merely the result of the spread of cancer cells from terminal ducts in which the malignant process has started." This brief quotation may well be the first instance in which the words *in situ* were used in relation to lobular carcinoma. Also, it presented the concept that carcinoma could spread within the epithelium from one anatomic unit to another. Muir illustrated examples of duct carcinoma extending to lobules, as well as a lesion that today would qualify as lobular carcinoma *in situ*.

Foote and Stewart introduced the term lobular carcinoma *in situ* (LCIS) in 1941, referring to it as "a disease of small lobular ducts and lobules."[7] The major clinical and pathologic features of the disease were outlined in their report, which established LCIS as a distinct form of mammary carcinoma.

When it occurs alone, lobular carcinoma *in situ* constitutes 1% to 6% of all diagnosed carcinomas and 30% to 50% of noninvasive carcinomas.[22,53,57]

CLINICAL PRESENTATION. Because of the microscopic size of lobules and the fact that they tend to be dispersed in the breast stroma and separated from each other, LCIS does not, by itself, produce a mass lesion that can be detected by palpation or mammography. However, LCIS may be present in breast tissue altered by proliferative disease or in clinically normal tissue that surrounds a benign tumor, such as a fibroadenoma. These associated benign processes may produce clinical or mammographic abnormalities that lead to a biopsy by which LCIS is detected.

Calcifications are rarely produced by LCIS, but they may be present in coexisting lesions, such as sclerosing adenosis.[58] Mammography has not been effective in detecting LCIS[59] and cannot be relied upon to determine whether the disease is multifocal in a given patient. In a report on the Breast Cancer Diagnosis Demonstration Projects,[12] only 4 of 50 patients with LCIS had calcifications seen on pathologic examination; biopsies in these patients were initiated by the mammographic findings.

Lobular carcinoma *in situ* occurs in the same age distribution as does breast carcinoma, but it occurs very infrequently as an isolated lesion in women younger than 35 years or older than 75 years of age. The average age at diagnosis of LCIS ranges from 44 to 54 years in different studies.[60] In one consecutive series of over 1000 patients treated for breast carcinoma, the mean age of women with LCIS (53 years) was not significantly lower than the mean age of patients who had infiltrating duct carcinoma (57 years).[40] Approximately 25% of the women whose only disease is LCIS are postmenopausal at the time of diagnosis. This condition has not been associated with exogenous estrogen usage.[60]

Multicentricity and bilaterality are interrelated characteristics of breast carcinomas in which the reported frequency is influenced by sampling techniques. Foote and Stewart noted that "this lesion occurs in multiple lobules . . . it is always a disease of multiple foci."[7] Multicentric foci of carcinoma reportedly have been found in 60% to 85% of patients undergoing mastectomy for LCIS.[45,61–66] When biopsy results have indicated only LCIS, 93% of the noninvasive carcinoma in the mastectomy specimen was also found to be LCIS, whereas 7% was found to be intraductal carcinoma. Occult, invasive carcinoma was found in 4% to 6% of patients undergoing mastectomy for a biopsy diagnosis of LCIS.[45,65,66] Invasive carcinoma was found in 4 of 38 mastectomy and mammoplasty specimens (11%) obtained within 2 years of a biopsy diagnosis of LCIS, and a fifth specimen contained intraductal carcinoma.[67]

Since LCIS is not detectable clinically, the reported frequency of bilateral involvement is influenced by how often biopsies are obtained from the opposite breast. The first instances of bilaterality were reported by Barnes in 1959.[68] Newman found bilateral disease in 6 of 26 patients (23%) with LCIS; the frequency of bilateral disease among 18 women who actually had a contralateral biopsy was 33%.[69] Lewison and Finney found bilateral carcinoma in 7 of 15 women (47%) who had tissue from both breasts examined.[62] Urban has systematically performed contralateral breast biopsies for all types of breast carcinoma. Concurrent, contralateral carcinoma was found in 10 of 26 patients (38%) who underwent biopsy. Nine of these patients (35%) had bilateral LCIS, and one woman had contralateral invasive carcinoma. Previous contralateral mastectomies had been performed in 4 of the same 26 women (15%).

Ringberg and co-workers studied 16 contralateral subcutaneous mastectomy specimens from patients treated for LCIS.[43] LCIS was found in 11 (69%) of the opposite breasts, intraductal carcinoma was diagnosed in 3 (19%), and invasive carcinoma was found in 1 (6%). LCIS was present in the contralateral breast of 3 of 4 women whose initial diagnosis in the ipsilateral breast was LCIS and intraductal carcinoma.

The status of the contralateral breast was determined histologically in 43 of 59 women (73%) treated for LCIS in one breast.[53] Nine (21%) had previously undergone mastectomy of the other breast. Concurrent, contralateral biopsy in the remaining 34 revealed carcinoma in 16 (47%), with the majority having bilateral LCIS.

GROSS PATHOLOGY. Lobular carcinoma *in situ* does not, by itself, produce any grossly recognizable, pathologic changes in breast tissue. However, the specimen may be altered considerably by a variety of benign proliferative lesions. It is not uncommon for the gross description to record nodular lesions, such as fibroadenomas; areas of firm or hard tissue with various shades of grey and tan; or the presence of cysts. In so far as can be determined, none of the benign proliferative changes bears a specific relationship to LCIS, but as indicated elsewhere, LCIS may occur within the epithelium in a variety of benign lesions.

MICROSCOPIC PATHOLOGY. Foote and Stewart referred to LCIS as "a disease of small lobular ducts and

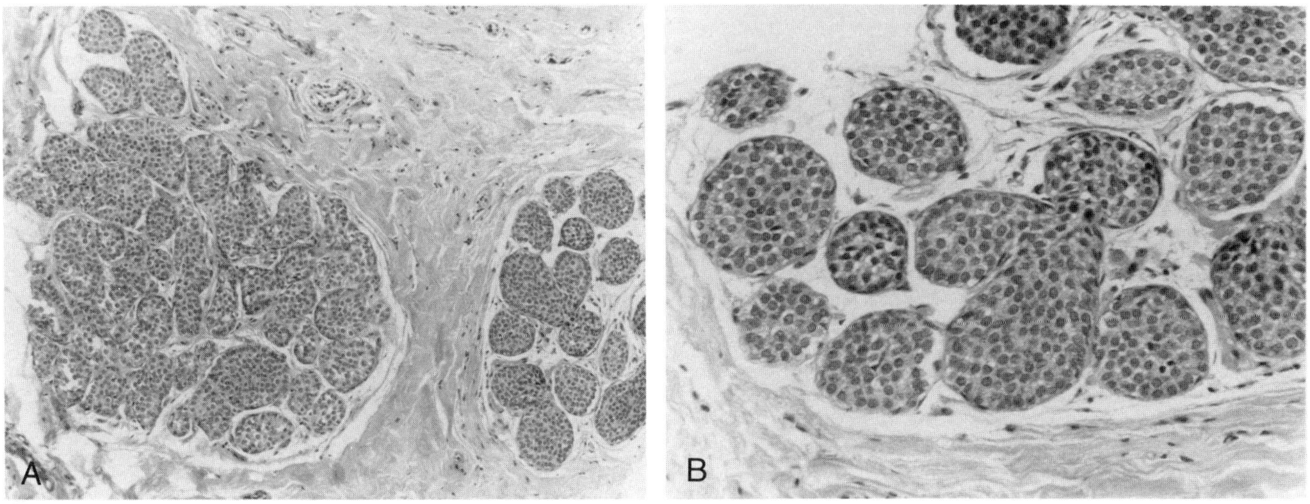

FIGURE 7-5. Lobular carcinoma *in situ*. Patient was a 46-year-old woman who presented with nodularity in the left lower outer quadrant of the breast. *(A)* Low-power view shows involvement of two adjacent lobules. *(B)* Tumor cells that fill and expand individual acinar units have small, uniform nuclei and poorly defined cell borders. Acinar margins are outlined by basement membranes.

lobules."[7] They noted that, in the postmenopausal atrophic breast, the disease arises from the terminal ducts, whereas in the premenopausal patient, the lesion is found in the terminal duct-lobular complex. The distribution of LCIS among lobules and terminal ducts and the alterations in the morphology of these structures have an influence on the histopathology of LCIS in any given case.

The most characteristic microscopic picture is the lobular form (Fig. 7-5), in which a population of neoplastic cells replaces the normal epithelium, filling intralobular ductules and acini. In many, but not all cases, the increased number of cells causes expansion of these structures, resulting in enlargement of the entire lobule. As noted by Foote and Stewart, "large lobules, small lobules . . . and hyalinized lobules may all assume this pattern. Occasionally, only part of a lobule is involved and a sharp line of division between normal epithelium and carcinoma *in situ* is seen . . . distension of the lobule does not assume marked proportions prior to infiltration."[7]

The question of how much lobular involvement warrants a diagnosis of LCIS has not been answered. Partial involvement of one or more lobules is not an uncommon finding in a patient whose biopsy also contains many fully involved lobules. Occasionally, the only evidence of the disease is one lobule in which some, but not all, of the acini contain a neoplastic process (Fig. 7-6). The significance of such minimal evidence remains undetermined. It has been suggested arbitrarily that there be a requirement that at least 75% of a lobule be involved in order to establish a diagnosis of LCIS, and that specimens with lesser lesions be included in the category of atypical lobular hyperplasia.[53] This seems to be a reasonable guideline because the extent of the process may be underrepresented in a particular biopsy owing to sampling error. In a retrospective study, the risk of subsequent carcinoma

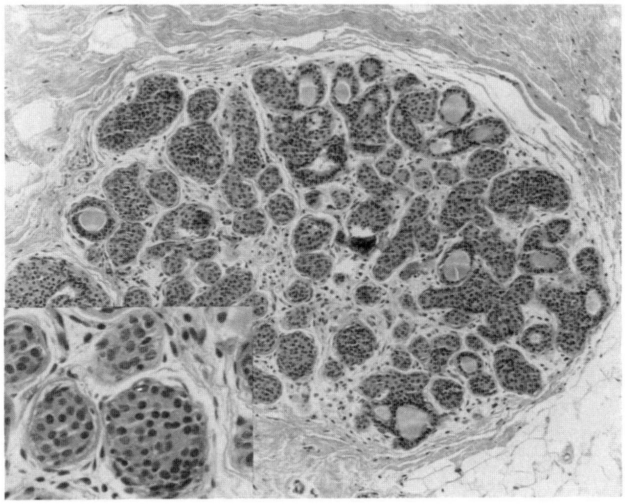

FIGURE 7-6. Lobular carcinoma *in situ* (partial lobular involvement) in a 42-year-old woman. Most acinar units are filled with neoplastic cells, but scattered glands with secretion persist. *Inset* shows cells typical of type A lobular carcinoma *in situ*.

was not significantly related to the number of fully affected lobules found on biopsy in patients who did not undergo mastectomy.[70]

A frequent characteristic of neoplastic cells in LCIS is a lack of cohesion. The cytoplasm may be sparse or indistinct. Although the nuclei of the tumor cells are often small, round, and lacking in nucleoli, considerable cytologic pleomorphism may be encountered. Haagensen and associates referred to the small, round cell pattern as type A (see Figs. 7-6 and 7-7) and the more pleomorphic cells as type B (Fig. 7-7).[11] Type A cells tend to have a diploid

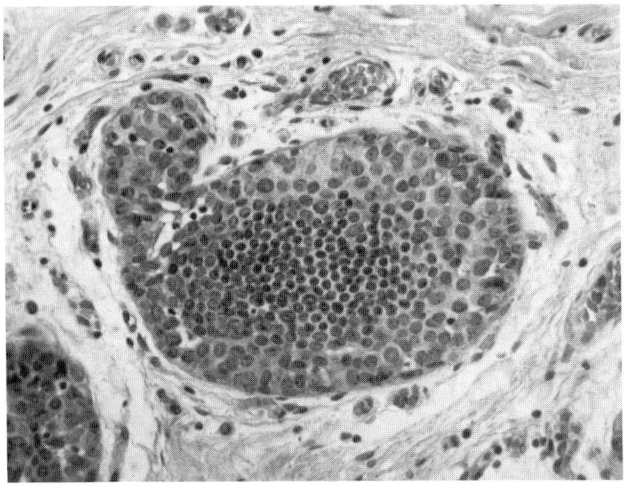

FIGURE 7-7. Lobular carcinoma *in situ* showing type A cytology toward the center of the lobular gland and type B cells at the periphery.

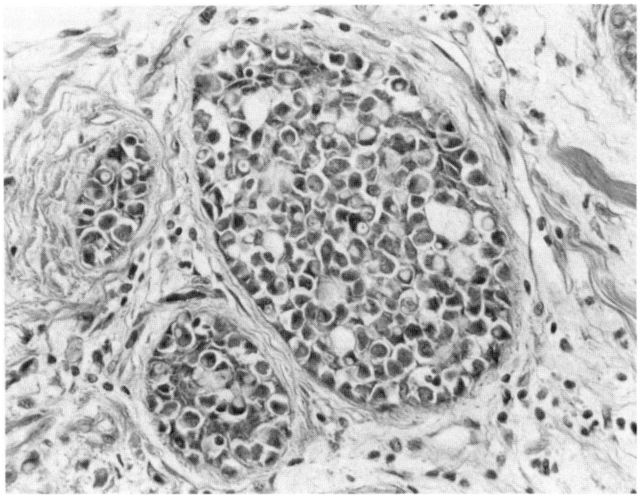

FIGURE 7-8. Lobular carcinoma *in situ,* composed of signet ring cells and with ductal involvement. Patient was a 47-year-old woman who presented with a breast mass that proved to be a Stage II invasive lobular carcinoma. Cytoplasmic vacuoles, which are evident in many cells, stained positively with alcian blue and mucicarmine.

nuclear deoxyribonucleic acid (DNA) content, whereas type B cells are largely hyperdiploid.[71] Follow-up studies suggest that patients with LCIS that comprises both cell types may be at greater risk for the development of invasive carcinoma if not treated by mastectomy than are patients who have LCIS that is composed entirely of either type A or type B cells.[11,70]

Intracytoplasmic vacuoles that contain mucinous secretion are commonly seen in the cells of LCIS.[72,73] Although this feature is generally inconspicuous, an extreme manifestation of this phenomenon is the formation of signet ring cells that have a cytoplasmic vacuole distended by mucin (Fig. 7-8).[74] Casein is also concentrated in this secretion.[75] Because intracytoplasmic mucin vacuoles are found less often in ductal carcinoma and in hyperplastic lesions of lobular or duct epithelium than in other types of carcinoma, their presence is one criterion for the diagnosis of LCIS.[72–74]

Lobular carcinoma *in situ* typically involves intralobular and extralobular, or terminal, ductules, as well as acinar units within the lobule (Fig. 7-9). Tumor cells spreading along the ductal system may replace the normal ductal epithelium, or they may sometimes occur singly within the epithelium in a pattern that resembles Paget's disease of the nipple, so-called pagetoid spread. Extralobular intraepithelial extension of LCIS into ducts occurs in about 75% of patients,[15,76] and does not appear to affect the risk of developing invasive carcinoma.[11,76] In postmenopausal patients with atrophic lobular breast tissue, ductal involvement may be the only manifestation of LCIS.[77] The disease sometimes extends into the epithelium of large lactiferous ducts, and is rarely present in lobules within the nipple.[78] However, Paget's disease of the surface of the nipple is not a feature of LCIS.

Electron microscopic studies have confirmed the light microscopic impression that LCIS originates from epithelial, rather than from myoepithelial, cells.[9,79,80] This observation was recently corroborated by an immunohistochemical investigation. This study demonstrated disordered patterns of myoepithelial cells of LCIS leading to the absence of myoepithelial cells when LCIS was associated with invasive carcinoma.[81] Protrusion of LCIS cells through the basement membrane, described by Ozzello,[9] seems to be an uncommon phenomenon. Discontinuity of basement membranes in patients with LCIS was demonstrated, using histochemical methods, by Andersen, who

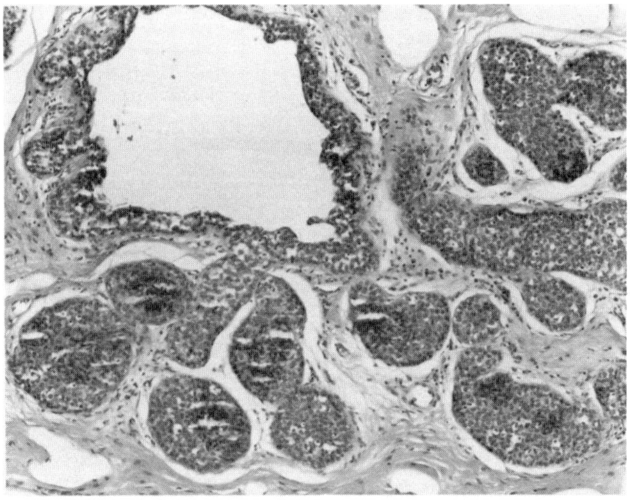

FIGURE 7-9. Ductal involvement in lobular carcinoma *in situ.* Patient was a 57-year-old woman. Tumor cells encircle the open lumen of a terminal duct in the upper left corner and fill the lumens of lobular ductules branching from this duct.

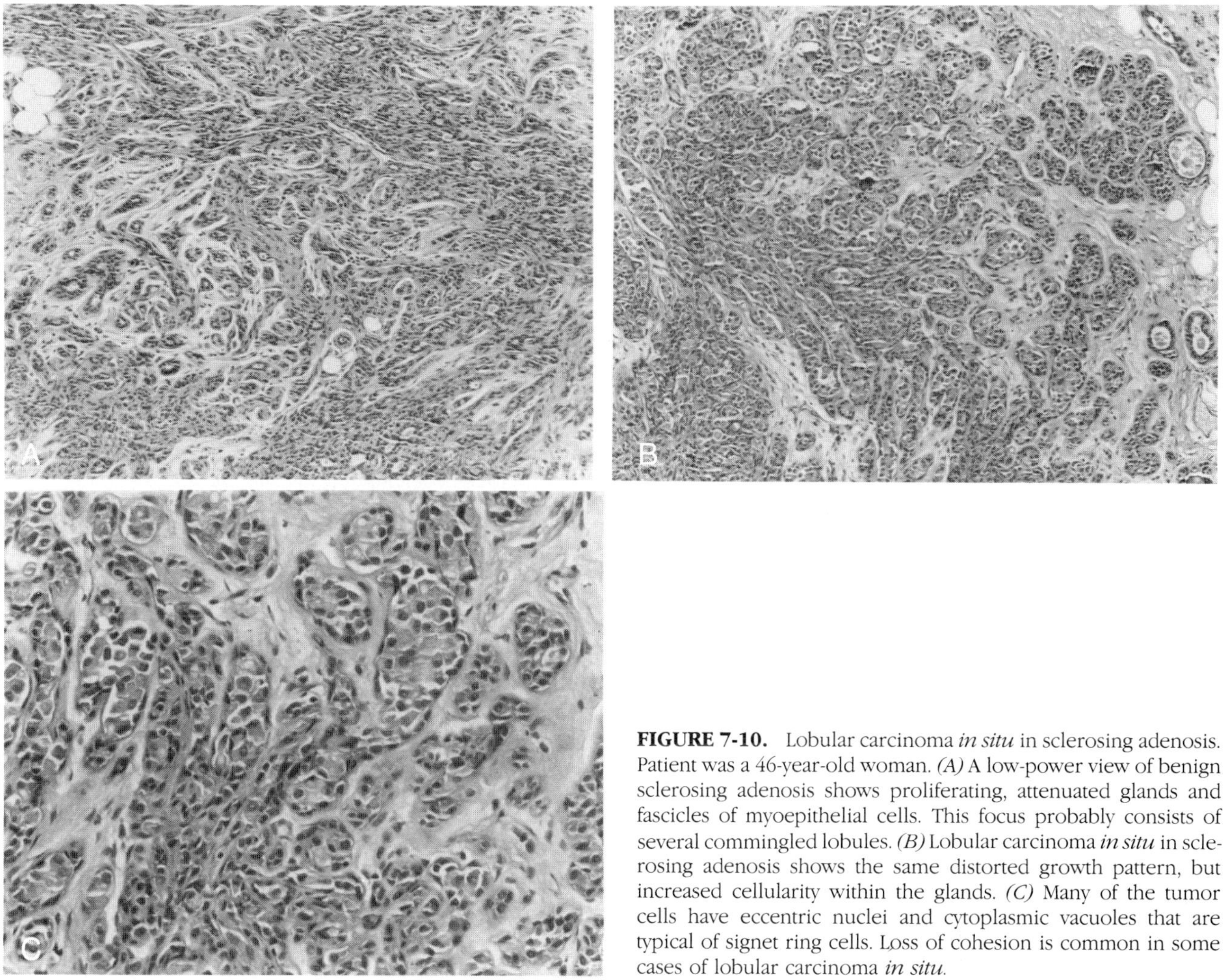

FIGURE 7-10. Lobular carcinoma *in situ* in sclerosing adenosis. Patient was a 46-year-old woman. *(A)* A low-power view of benign sclerosing adenosis shows proliferating, attenuated glands and fascicles of myoepithelial cells. This focus probably consists of several commingled lobules. *(B)* Lobular carcinoma *in situ* in sclerosing adenosis shows the same distorted growth pattern, but increased cellularity within the glands. *(C)* Many of the tumor cells have eccentric nuclei and cytoplasmic vacuoles that are typical of signet ring cells. Loss of cohesion is common in some cases of lobular carcinoma *in situ*.

also noted gaps in the basement membranes of a small number of normal lobules.[82]

Lobular carcinoma *in situ* usually occurs within the architecture of ductules and lobules. However, the disease may develop in lobular tissue that has already been altered by a benign proliferative process. Examples of this include LCIS in fibroadenomas, in sclerosing adenosis (Fig. 7-10), and in sclerosing papillomatosis or radial scar. Because the lobular configuration is radically altered in the sclerosing lesions, it may be difficult to exclude the presence of invasive carcinoma in such foci.[83]

PROGNOSIS. Since LCIS is an intraepithelial carcinoma without access to the bloodstream or lymphatics, a cure rate of nearly 100% is achieved by mastectomy. However, cure in this context must be regarded largely as preventive. The major clinical concerns resolved by immediate mastectomy are the 5% risk that an undetected focus of invasive carcinoma may already have developed in the breast;[45,65] the 1% risk that invasion might have occurred at the submicroscopic level, leading to regional axillary lymph node metastases;[10,84,85] and the possibility that other foci of intraepithelial carcinoma are present in the breast (multicentricity), or that such foci might appear later, leading to the development of an invasive carcinoma.

The reported frequency of subsequent carcinoma in the ipsilateral breast not treated with mastectomy ranges from 10% to 25% in large series involving more than 25 patients with average follow-up periods exceeding 10 years.[11,70,76] The frequency with which carcinoma developed in the unbiopsied contralateral breasts of women with untreated ipsilateral LCIS ranged from 10% to 17%. There is some evidence that biopsy of the opposite breast may help in identifying patients at risk for developing contralateral carcinoma.[86] When compared to normal, age-matched, control populations, the risk that a patient with untreated LCIS would develop invasive carcinoma of one or both breasts ranged from 7.2 to 13.8,[11,70,76] with the highest risk occurring in a subset of women with LCIS who reported a positive family history for breast carcinoma.[11]

Invasive Carcinoma

Invasive Ductal Carcinoma

Invasive ductal carcinoma represents the single largest group of malignant mammary tumors, constituting 70% to 80% of mammary carcinomas.[22] The definition of this category, offered by the WHO, is one of exclusion: "Invasive ductal carcinoma is the most frequently encountered malignant tumour of the breast, not falling into any of the other categories of invasive mammary carcinoma."[87] Included under this heading are lesions characterized variously as ductal carcinoma with productive fibrosis, scirrhous carcinoma, and carcinoma simplex. A generic term sometimes employed is invasive ductal carcinoma, not otherwise specified (NOS). This is a useful designation, since it takes into account the distinction between these tumors and the many other specific forms of ductal carcinoma, such as tubular, medullary, metaplastic, colloid, and adenoid cystic carcinoma.

Invasive ductal carcinoma includes many tumors that express, in part, one or more characteristics of the specific types of breast carcinoma, but that do not constitute pure examples of these individual tumor types. Examples of this phenomenon are invasive ductal carcinomas that have limited microscopic foci of tubular, medullary, papillary, or mucinous differentiation. As noted elsewhere in this chapter, the relatively favorable prognosis associated with specific histologic types has been found to apply only to those tumors composed entirely or mostly of the designated pattern. When these features are less extensively represented, the tumors are relegated to the group designated as invasive ductal carcinoma, NOS. Tumors combining invasive ductal and lobular carcinoma, as well as invasive ductal carcinomas with associated Paget's disease, are also included in this category.

In one detailed review of 1000 carcinomas, approximately one-third of the lesions characterized as invasive ductal carcinoma expressed one or more combined features.[88] Overall, there were 24 subcategories of mixed growth patterns and three subcategories of invasive ductal carcinoma associated with Paget's disease. Slightly more than 50% of the combined tumors were invasive ductal carcinomas with a tubular carcinomatous component. Combinations with invasive lobular carcinoma were detected in 6% of the tumors (Fig. 7-11). Thus far, prognostic differences have not been identified for most of the combined histologic patterns, and as a consequence, they have been grouped together as invasive ductal carcinoma. This section of the chapter considers invasive ductal carcinoma, NOS in the context of this broad definition, and reference will be made to specific, combined, histologic patterns only when relevant.

Breast carcinoma is an extremely heterogeneous disease, both clinically and pathologically. As noted by Sistrunk and MacCarty more than 50 years ago, "It is impossible to foretell the duration of life of all patients with carcinoma of the breast, because the degree of malignancy varies widely, and persons react differently to the disease."[89] Innumerable studies have attempted to assess the prognosis of patients with breast cancer on the basis of clinical and pathologic parameters. Since nearly 75% of the patients have invasive ductal carcinoma, the characteristics of these tumors have a considerable influence on laboratory, clinical, and pathologic studies.

Interval to recurrence and length of survival are the basic measurements of prognosis. In general, these are closely related, so that factors associated with a high frequency of recurrence correlate with reduced survival. However, treatment that delays, but does not reduce, the overall frequency of recurrence may increase the duration of survival without reducing mortality secondary to the disease in the long term. There is also evidence indicating that the prognostic significance of a given pathologic variable does not apply uniformly throughout the course of follow-up. Some variables are effective in predicting short-term outcome, whereas others appear to exert an effect later. The time dependency of prognostic variables has not been thoroughly analyzed.[90,91]

It is also important to consider the impact of primary treatment on the evaluation of prognostic factors. Radical mastectomy has, until fairly recently, been the most widely employed form of primary treatment. A large body of data has been accumulated about the results of this form of treatment with respect to the importance of stage at diagnosis, type of tumor, and other clinical and morphologic parameters. The past 2 decades have witnessed major changes in treatment, with a shift from radical to modified radical or simple mastectomy, and a growing trend toward partial mastectomy, quadrantectomy, or limited resection combined with primary radiation therapy with or without axillary dissection. The scene is further complicated by the introduction of adjuvant chemotherapy, employed largely for women with Stage II disease, but deemed appropriate for selected Stage I patients.

At present, reports documenting the follow-up of patients treated with various modalities suggest that pathologic prognostic variables that are determined to be significant in populations treated with radical mastectomy are also applicable to patients treated with modified radical mastectomy and breast-conserving surgery combined with radiotherapy. The extent to which the assessment of the prognostic significance of pathologic parameters is influenced by adjuvant chemotherapy is less certain.

CLINICAL PRESENTATION. With rare exceptions, there are no clinical features specifically associated with invasive ductal carcinoma. The lesions occur throughout the same age range as breast carcinoma, but are most common in patients in their mid to late 50s. An exception is palpable breast carcinoma associated with Paget's disease of the nipple. The underlying invasive carcinoma in these cases is almost always of the invasive ductal type. However, in exceptional situations, Paget's disease may derive from

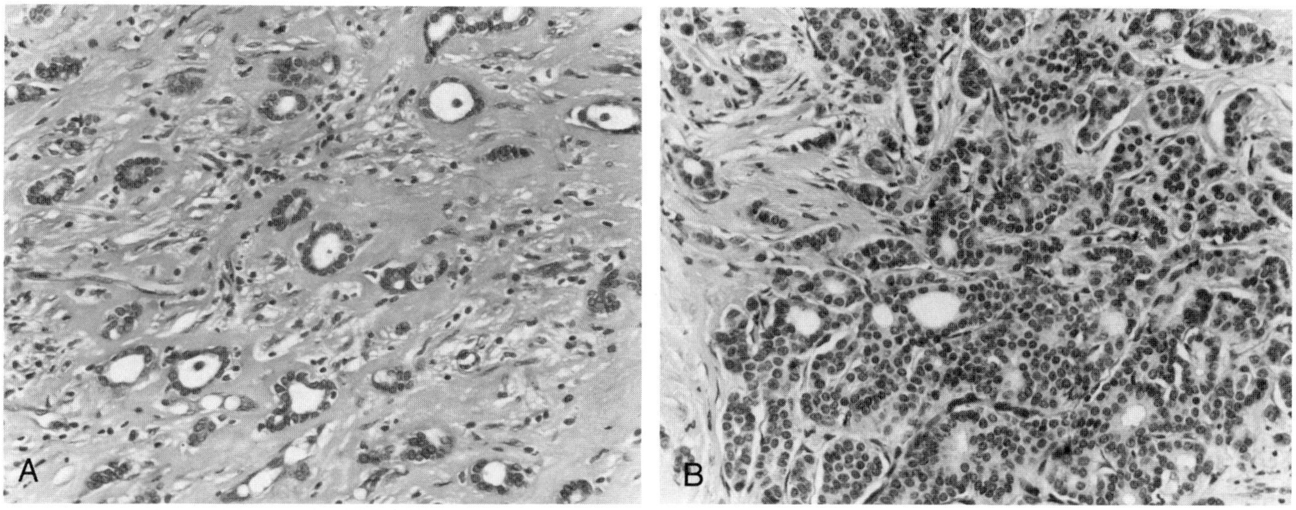

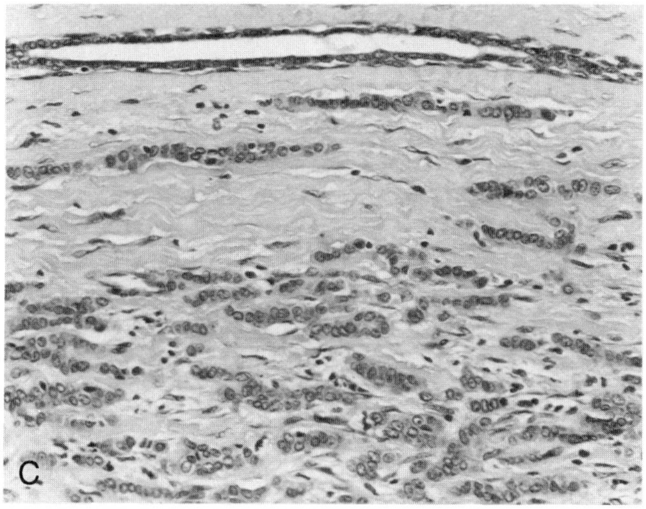

FIGURE 7-11. Infiltrating ductal carcinoma with a heterogeneous histologic appearance. Patient was a 66-year-old woman treated with limited resection, axillary dissection, and radiotherapy. Different microscopic areas exhibited the following patterns: *(A)* tubular; *(B)* moderately differentiated infiltrating duct; and *(C)* infiltrating lobular.

intraductal carcinoma limited to the lactiferous ducts, in which case the palpable lesion is formed by another, separate carcinoma that may be of a specific histologic type, such as a tubular carcinoma.

GROSS PATHOLOGY. Invasive ductal carcinoma invariably forms a solid tumor. The consistency and the appearance of the cut surface vary considerably, depending on the composition of the lesion. Cystic change in this group of lesions is extremely uncommon, but may be a manifestation of necrosis and is usually accompanied by hemorrhage in the degenerated area. Noncystic areas of necrosis tend to be soft and chalky white. Generally, tumors with a relatively abundant scirrhous or fibrotic stroma are extremely firm to hard with a grey to white surface. When there is considerable elastosis of the stroma, a yellow tinge may be observed. Chalky white streaks in the tumor tissue are usually indicative of necrosis, calcification, or elastosis. Tumors with less abundant stroma, which are composed largely of neoplastic cells, tend to be less firm and tan. The cut surfaces of such cellular neoplasms are likely to bulge slightly when bisected.

The measured gross size of a mammary carcinoma is one of the most significant prognostic variables. Numerous studies have shown that survival generally decreases with increasing tumor size, and that there is a coincidental rise in the rate of axillary nodal metastases.[23,90,92–94] Because most carcinomas have irregular shapes, measurement is generally reported in terms of the greatest diameter. It is important that the tumor be submitted intact to the pathologist so that the configuration of the lesion may be assessed by palpation. This makes it possible to bisect the specimen in a plane that exposes the longest diameter. The measurement should be made before any samples are taken for frozen section, estrogen receptor analysis, or any other procedure. When a frozen section is prepared, the grossly measured diameter may be reported with the histologic diagnosis, and it should be entered as part of the frozen section record.

The gross diameter of a carcinoma is only an approx-

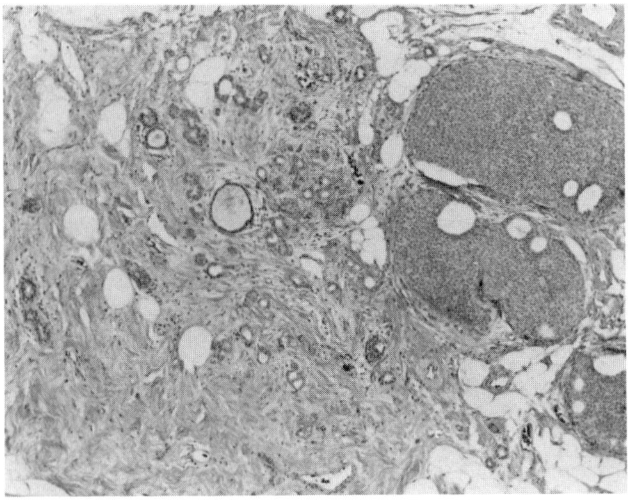

FIGURE 7-12. Microinvasive duct carcinoma in a 64-year-old woman. This 1-cm tumor consisted of numerous clustered ducts with intraductal carcinoma seen on the right. A 1-mm focus of invasive carcinoma, composed of small glands invading the stroma, was also present.

imation of the actual amount of invasive tumor present. Some benign tissue with hyperplastic or reactive changes may contribute to the palpable lesion. In some tumors, a considerable part of the mass is composed of invasive carcinoma, whereas in other lesions of comparable gross size, most of the bulk may be intraductal tumor with only microscopic invasion (Fig. 7-12).

The majority of invasive ductal carcinomas may be assigned, on the basis of gross tumor configuration, to one of two groups: stellate (speculated, infiltrative, radial, serrated) or circumscribed (rounded, pushing, encapsulated, smooth). Approximately one-third of the tumors have grossly circumscribed margins. A minority of tumors have indistinct borders and cannot be described in these terms. In general, the gross appearance of the tumor duplicates the configuration visualized by mammography. However, tumors that appear to have circumscribed margins on gross or mammographic examination may exhibit an invasive growth pattern when studied microscopically. Fisher and associates found invasive margins on microscopic examination in slightly more than 50% of the carcinomas that were described as grossly circumscribed.[88]

Most investigators have observed a more favorable prognosis associated with circumscribed carcinomas, determined by mammography[95] or gross inspection of the tumor,[96] than with stellate carcinomas. Infiltrative tumors tend to be larger,[96,97] and are more likely to have axillary lymph node metastases than those with circumscribed margins.[95,96] Tumors with a stellate configuration in which there is focal necrosis are associated with an especially poor prognosis.[97]

MICROSCOPIC PATHOLOGY AND PROGNOSIS. *Grading* of carcinomas is an estimate of differentiation. Unless otherwise indicated, grade is usually reported for the invasive portion of the tumor. *Nuclear grading* involves a cytologic evaluation in which the structural features of tumor nuclei are compared to the nuclei of normal mammary epithelial cells. Since nuclear grading does not involve an assessment of the growth pattern of the tumor, this procedure is applicable to all types of mammary carcinoma. The most widely employed system for nuclear grading, introduced by Black and co-workers,[98,99] is usually reported in terms of three categories: well-differentiated (grade 3), intermediate (grade 2) and poorly differentiated (grade 1; Fig. 7-13).

Histologic grading takes into consideration the growth pattern of invasive ductal carcinomas, as well as the cytologic features of differentiation.[100,101] The parameters measured are the extent of tubule formation, nuclear hyperchromasia, and mitotic rate. Histologic grade is usually expressed in three categories similar to those employed for nuclear grading (Fig. 7-14). However, by convention, the numerical designations used for histologic grades have been recorded in a sequence that is the reverse of that used in nuclear grading: well-differentiated (grade I), intermediate (grade II), and poorly differentiated (grade III). It has been suggested that the numerical designations employed for nuclear grading be changed to conform with those used in histologic grading.[88]

The histologic and nuclear grades of a given tumor coincide in most, but not all, invasive ductal carcinomas. It has repeatedly been demonstrated that patients with high-grade or poorly differentiated invasive ductal carcinoma have a significantly higher frequency of axillary lymph node metastases, that they develop more recurrences, and that more of them die of metastatic disease than do women with low-grade tumors.[90,98–106] Nuclear and histologic grade have been shown to be significant predictors of prognosis among patients stratified by stage of disease, especially among those without axillary lymph node metastases (Stage I).[18,104,106,107] The absence of tubule formation is a particularly unfavorable histologic feature which, when combined with poorly differentiated nuclear cytology, was associated with a risk of recurrence that was 20 times greater than that in women who had neither variable.[104] In a carefully defined series of patients with T1N1M0 disease, neither histologic nor nuclear grade was significantly correlated with outcome.[108] Others have failed to find nuclear grade to be a significant predictor of prognosis in patients with early breast cancer.[109] However, a case control analysis of patients who survived 25 years after radical mastectomy for invasive carcinoma revealed a significantly higher proportion of histologically grade I tumors (43%) among long-term survivors than among control subjects matched on the basis of tumor size, number of lymph nodes with metastases, and age at diagnosis.[107]

Histologic grade correlates significantly with both the frequency of recurrence and death due to disease, as well as with disease-free interval and overall length of survival,[91] regardless of clinical stage. High-grade carcinomas result in early treatment failures, whereas later recurrences

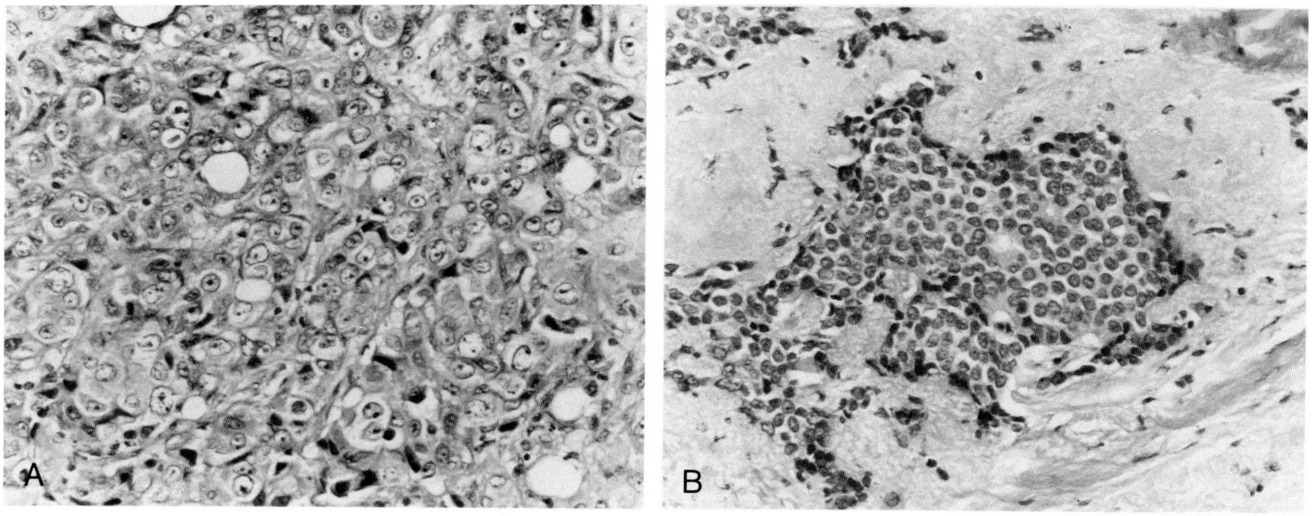

FIGURE 7-13. Nuclear grading. *(A)* Low-grade cytology is characterized by small, round, uniform nuclei lacking nucleoli. *(B)* High-grade nuclei are large, vesicular, and pleomorphic, and have prominent nucleoli.

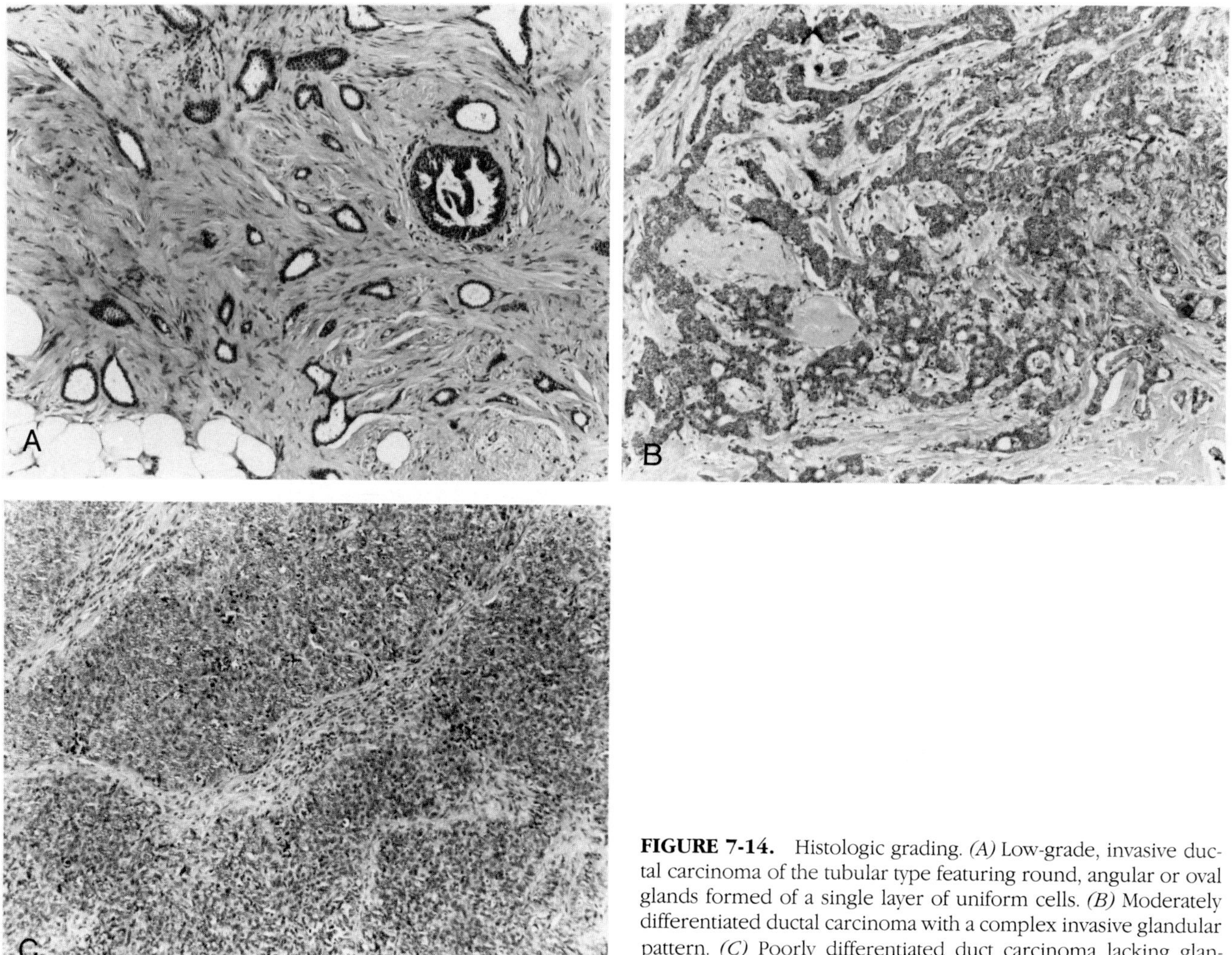

FIGURE 7-14. Histologic grading. *(A)* Low-grade, invasive ductal carcinoma of the tubular type featuring round, angular or oval glands formed of a single layer of uniform cells. *(B)* Moderately differentiated ductal carcinoma with a complex invasive glandular pattern. *(C)* Poorly differentiated duct carcinoma lacking glandular or papillary structures in the invasive tumor.

are observed among low-grade tumors. Consequently, the relative proportions of tumor grade in study populations could significantly influence the results of treatment, especially on a short-term basis.

In an effort to obtain additional prognostic information from breast tumor tissue, studies have been carried out to measure parameters other than those obtained from routine histopathologic procedures. Two methodologies that have been explored most successfully, representing, in effect, attempts to improve tumor grading, are the precise measurement of nuclear DNA content and the precise measurement of the configuration of nuclei, termed *nuclear morphometry.*

In 1979, Atkin and Kay described the relationship of modal DNA values to prognosis in 1465 diverse malignant tumors.[110] The study was based on microspectrophotometric DNA measurements made on Feulgen-stained imprints of fresh tumors. Most tumors exhibited a bimodal distribution of modal DNA values. Generally, patients whose tumors were in the near diploid range had a better survival rate than did those with an aneuploid DNA distribution. These results confirmed an earlier report by Atkin which had described comparable results specifically for breast cancers.[111]

More recently, Auer and colleagues employed fine needle aspiration biopsy of breast cancers to prepare for Feulgen-stained smears, reporting that the resultant DNA histograms correlated with survival time.[112,113] In another study that also used smear material derived from needle aspiration, Auer and co-workers compared the DNA histograms of concurrent primary breast cancers and metastases in 18 patients.[114] With one exception, little difference in DNA patterns was found between the two specimens from a given patient. When related to estrogen receptor content, tumors with a near diploid DNA content tended to be receptor-positive, whereas those with aneuploid DNA were likely to be receptor-negative.[115]

DNA ploidy distributions in breast carcinomas, measured by flow cytometry, have generally confirmed results obtained with the Feulgen-stained smear procedure. The majority of carcinomas in most series had a bimodal distribution of DNA values, with more than 50% of the cells in the hyperdiploid range.[116–120] Tumors with a near diploid DNA distribution tended to be estrogen and progesterone receptor-positive, whereas receptor negativity was associated with aneuploidy.[117,118,121,122] One study reported a significant relationship between ploidy level and age. Older patients were more likely to have hyperdiploid tumors.[118] Pathologic studies have shown a close correlation between cytologic grading of tumor nuclei and DNA ploidy analyzed by flow cytometry.[123] Low-grade tumors exhibited near diploid DNA, whereas aneuploidy was most pronounced in tumors with high-grade nuclei.

Within the past decade, there has been increasing interest in the prognostic value of estimates of the growth rate of breast cancer cells based on statistical models and clinical data. The proliferative proportion of cells in DNA synthesis, as reflected in the thymidine-labeling index, has been shown to correlate significantly with prognosis.[124–128] Flow cytometry provides a simple and precise method of determining the proliferative fraction (S-phase fraction), which is reported to be equivalent to the thymidine-labeling index.[129]

It has been observed that proliferative activity reflected in the S-phase fraction is correlated with ploidy to the extent that diploid carcinomas tend to have a lower S-phase fraction than do aneuploid lesions.[118,130,131] Others have reported finding no correlation between ploidy and S-phase fraction.[16] Tumors with a high S-phase fraction tend to be estrogen receptor-negative.[121,130,132,133] Ploidy and S-phase fraction have been found to correlate with the histologic differentiation of ductal carcinomas and cytologic differentiation.[121,130,133] Although some investigators have reported that ploidy or S-phase fraction, or both, do not correlate with nodal status at the time of initial treatment,[134] others have found a higher S-phase fraction in node-positive patients than in node-negative patients.[122] A reduction in the S-phase fraction was found in nodal metastases from 25% of estrogen receptor-positive tumors.[135] This phenomenon was not apparent when estrogen receptor-negative tumors were compared with their concurrent nodal metastases.[135]

Data relating proliferative activity to prognosis in breast cancer have been based largely on measurements of thymidine-labeling index. Generally, these studies have reported that prognosis decreases with increased labeling, and that thymidine-labeling index is also inversely related to nodal status.[124–126,131] The interrelationships between thymidine-labeling index, DNA ploidy, and S-phase fraction have been extensively reviewed by Meyer, who concluded that "high S-phase fraction and aneuploidy may prove to have prognostic significance like thymidine-labeling index."[127] Human mammary carcinomas implanted in nude mice have exhibited cell cycle changes, monitored by flow cytometry of aspirates from the transplanted tumor, in response to endocrine therapy.[136] To date, a detailed clinical study of the relationship between DNA ploidy and S-phase fraction determined by flow cytometry and long-term prognosis in breast cancer has not been reported.

In 1983, Hedley and co-workers described a method of preparing paraffin-embedded tissues for flow cytometry DNA analysis.[137] DNA histograms of cells from fixed material correlated well with suspensions of unfixed cells from the same tumor. Recently, this method was applied to the short-term prognostic assessment of 165 patients with Stage II disease who participated in a trial of adjuvant chemotherapy.[138] Patients with aneuploid tumors were found to have more extensive axillary nodal metastases than those with diploid tumors, and they were more likely to relapse after 2 years. Patients with diploid lesions tended to remain relapse-free. The difference in curves was statistically different for premenopausal patients, but not for postmenopausal women.

Nuclear morphometry provides a method for obtaining quantitative measurements of the size and shape of tumor cell nuclei. Among the parameters commonly recorded in these studies are nuclear diameter, nuclear area, and nuclear perimeter. Careful counts of mitotic activity have also been obtained in some of these studies. Measurements may be obtained using properly prepared histologic sections[139] and aspiration cytology smears.[140–143] Prognostic correlations have been made with the nuclear morphometry of the primary tumor,[139–143] as well as with morphometric features of tumor cell nuclei in axillary nodal metastases.[144] The morphometric feature that has most often been shown to have a statistically significant association with prognosis has been nuclear area.[139,141–144] Nuclear diameter, a parameter included in the calculation of area, has been shown to be significantly related to prognosis,[140,141] as has the frequency of mitoses.[139,142] Inverse relationships were observed between mean nuclear area, mean nuclear diameter, mitotic index, and prognosis.

Concurrent assessment of nuclear and histologic grading proved prognostically significant in some of these studies.[139,144] It remains to be determined how the more precise observations of morphometry may be used to improve the assessment of prognosis beyond that made possible by nuclear and histologic grading.

The prognostic significance of *lymphoplasmacytic infiltration* in the stroma within and around invasive ductal carcinomas has been a subject of considerable interest and some controversy. A moderate to marked reaction of the intensity observed in medullary carcinoma also occurs in approximately 20% of nonmedullary invasive ductal carcinomas.[88,106] This type of tumor is more common among blacks and the mean age of these patients is relatively young.[145] Invasive ductal carcinoma with a marked lymphoplasmacytic reaction is almost always estrogen and progesterone receptor-negative.[146] A subset of these tumors with some, but not all, of the other features of medullary carcinoma, referred to as atypical medullary carcinoma, had a slightly more favorable prognosis than did infiltrating ductal carcinomas as a group, but the difference was not statistically significant.[147] Marked lymphoplasmacytic reaction generally consists largely of mature lymphocytes with a variable admixture of plasma cells. Rarely, plasma cells predominate. The majority of tumors with such a prominent reaction tend to be poorly differentiated and have a circumscribed, rather than an infiltrative, contour.

Although the favorable prognosis of medullary carcinoma has been ascribed to the lymphoplasmacytic reaction that characterizes these tumors, it is unclear whether the same conclusion may be drawn about nonmedullary invasive ductal carcinomas. Some investigators have found carcinomas with this "host response" to have a relatively favorable prognosis,[90,99,105,148,149] but others have found no significant difference or have reported a less favorable outcome associated with the presence of a prominent lymphoplasmacytic infiltrate.[90,106,107,150]

The intensity of mast cell infiltration in the substance or at the periphery of an invasive breast carcinoma is not significantly related to prognosis.[151]

The presence of lymphatic tumor emboli in the breast is an unfavorable prognostic finding. For this purpose, the lymphatics are defined as vascular channels that are lined by endothelium without supporting smooth muscle or elastica (Fig. 7-15). Most do not contain red blood cells, but undoubtedly, some blood capillaries are included in this definition. Artifactual spaces are commonly formed around nests of tumor cells within an invasive carcinoma as a result of tissue shrinkage during processing. Because it is very difficult to distinguish these artifacts from true lymphatic spaces,[152] assessment for lymphatic invasion is more reliably accomplished in the breast parenchyma adjacent to the invasive tumor margin.[153] Efforts to identify intratumoral lymphatic spaces by using immunoperoxidase reagents associated with endothelial cells (Factor VIII and blood group antigens) have met with only limited success.[154,155] The prognostic significance of intratumoral lymphatic emboli has not been determined.

Extratumoral lymphatic tumor emboli in the breast are associated with approximately 25% of invasive ductal carcinomas. This determination is made on the basis of routine sampling of biopsy and mastectomy specimens. The majority of these patients also have axillary lymph node metastases; it has not yet been determined whether the presence of lymphatic invasion alters their prognosis.

Lymphatic tumor emboli are found in the breast surrounding invasive ductal carcinomas in 10% to 15% of patients who have pathologically negative lymph nodes. Several studies have shown that lymphatic invasion is prognostically unfavorable in node-negative patients treated with mastectomy.[106,150,153,156–159] This deleterious effect is most pronounced in women with T1N0M0 disease. In a 10-year follow-up study of 378 patients treated for T1N0M0 carcinoma, 33% of 30 women with lymphatic invasion died of disease. Death due to breast carcinoma was observed in 10% of the 348 women who did not have lymphatic invasion.[106] Another study comparing similar subsets of patients with TIN0M0 disease found recurrences in 32% of those with lymphatic invasion, compared to 10% of the control subjects.[150] It has not been possible to demonstrate that lymphatic invasion has a statistically significant impact on prognosis in Stage I patients with tumors larger than 2 cm (T2N0M0), although those with lymphatic invasion do experience a higher recurrence rate.[153]

The unfavorable effect of lymphatic invasion in patients with T1N0M0 carcinoma is probably not attributable to occult metastases in the axillary lymph nodes. Serial sections of lymph nodes detected metastases in 9 of 28 patients originally classified as having T1N0M0 disease with lymphatic invasion in the breast. The recurrence rate was no higher among those with occult metastases than among those with truly negative lymph nodes.[160]

Blood vessel invasion is defined as penetration by tumor into the lumen of an artery or vein (Fig. 7-16). These structures may be identified by the presence of a smooth muscle wall supported by elastic fibers. It is usually necessary to employ special histochemical procedures (e.g., orcein or Verhoeff-van Gieson stains), which selectively stain elastic tissue, in order to detect this component of the vascular wall. Elastic fibers are often deposited around ducts with intraductal carcinoma within an invasive tumor; the resulting appearance in an elastic tissue stain prognosis,[170,171,174] or that abundant elastosis had a negative effect on outcome.[175,176]

Recently, attention has been directed to the pattern and distribution of intraductal carcinoma as a prognostic variable in patients with invasive ductal carcinoma. Tumors vary in the relative proportions of their intraductal and invasive components, ranging from those with only microscopic invasion (see Fig. 7-6) to lesions composed entirely of invasive carcinoma. Silverberg and Chitale observed a trend toward decreased nodal metastases and a more favorable prognosis when the intraductal component in the tumor was more abundant.[177] However, it should be noted that the relative quantitative assessment of these components is highly subjective. In one recent report, little or no intraductal carcinoma was detected in sections from 72% of 974 tumors, whereas 11% were described as being composed of at least 66% intraductal carcinoma.[88] These authors noted that patients with lesions having a prominent intratumoral intraductal component also tended to have intraductal carcinoma in surrounding, extratumoral breast tissue, and to have multicentric carcinoma in the breast. Although the distribution of intraductal carcinoma in and around the primary tumor appears to correlate with the risk for recurrence in the breast after lumpectomy and radiation therapy,[178] this feature has no bearing on the risk for systemic recurrence in women treated with mastectomy.[179] There is no clear association between prognosis and the structural pattern of intraductal carcinoma (comedo, cribriform, papillary, and so on) in invasive ductal carcinoma.

Several other histologic variables have been assessed as potential prognostic indicators. Among these are the amount and type of mucin produced by the tumor cells, the mucopolysaccharide content of the tumor stroma, the glycogen content of the tumor cells, the presence of calcifications in the tumor, and the influence of associated benign proliferative changes in the breast. For the most part, none of these variables has been found to correlate strongly with prognosis and to be as useful in making therapeutic decisions as the other observations discussed in detail in this section.

Immunohistochemical markers have attracted some interest as potential indicators of prognosis. Carcinoembryonic antigen is the most extensively studied marker. The frequency of CEA positivity varies considerably in different laboratories, with 90% of tumors showing some reactivity in one study.[180] No consistent relationship has been found to exist between prognosis and the immunohistochemical demonstration of CEA activity in breast cancer. A reduced frequency of axillary lymph node metastases and better prognosis were related to CEA-negative tumors by some authors.[181,182] In other studies, the presence or absence of CEA in tissue has proved to have little or no prognostic value.[180,183,184] Equally conflicting observations have been reported for human chorionic gonadotropin (HCG);[180,183,185] pregnancy-specific, beta-1 glycoprotein;[180,183,185] and placental lactogen.[180,185] The presence or absence of immunohistochemically detected blood group isoantigens has also not been found to be a significant prognostic marker.[186]

Tubular Carcinoma

Tubular (well-differentiated) carcinoma has been recognized as a morphologically distinctive form of mammary carcinoma for more than 100 years.[187] The term *tubular carcinoma*[188,189] describes the distinguishing microscopic feature of the lesion, which is composed of neoplastic elements resembling normal breast ductules. Alternative terms, such as orderly or well-differentiated[190,191] carcinoma, are less specific and have not gained wide acceptance.

The precise pathologic definition of tubular carcinoma has been the subject of some controversy, which has, in turn, influenced the reported frequency of the lesion. Elements of tubular carcinoma may be found in a substantial number of invasive ductal carcinomas, but in relatively few does all or almost all of the tumor have a tubular growth pattern. As used in this section, tubular carcinoma refers to so-called pure tubular carcinoma. Most authors require that at least 75% of the tumor be tubular to qualify for this diagnosis.[192–197]

In its pure form, tubular carcinoma is quite uncommon, constituting not more than 2% of all breast carcinomas in most series.[22,192–194,198] Since tubular carcinomas are generally small, they are found with greater frequency in studies of early breast cancer. In one review of 382 women treated between 1964 and 1969 for T1N1M0 breast carcinoma,[106] tubular carcinoma was present in 5%. This type of lesion occurred in 9% of patients with tumors of 1.0 cm or less in diameter, and in 2% of those with tumors measuring 1.1 to 2.0 cm. Only 1.5% of 142 patients with T1N0M0 disease had tubular carcinoma.[108]

With the widespread use of mammography, emphasis on early breast cancer detection has contributed to an increased interest in tubular carcinoma. These tumors constituted 8% of invasive carcinomas measuring 1.0 cm or less in diameter found in a review of the Breast Cancer Detection Demonstration Projects.[12] Seven percent of 138 carcinomas found in one U.S. screening program were of the tubular variety.[199] All of these tumors were detected on mammography, but only 30% were detected by clinical examination. In Malmo, Sweden, 21.5% of 116 breast carcinomas found on mammography screening were reportedly of the pure tubular variety.[200]

It has recently been suggested that tubular carcinomas are a stage in the evolution of a substantial number of breast cancers.[201,202] Proponents of this theory believe that tubular carcinomas arise from benign proliferative lesions called radial scars, and that, as they enlarge, tubular carcinomas are converted into ordinary invasive ductal carcinomas. This premise remains a subject of considerable controversy.[203,204]

CLINICAL PRESENTATION. With rare exceptions,[196,197,205] most patients with tubular carcinoma have

have also been obtained in some of these studies. Measurements may be obtained using properly prepared histologic sections[139] and aspiration cytology smears.[140–143] Prognostic correlations have been made with the nuclear morphometry of the primary tumor,[139–143] as well as with morphometric features of tumor cell nuclei in axillary nodal metastases.[144] The morphometric feature that has most often been shown to have a statistically significant association with prognosis has been nuclear area.[139,141–144] Nuclear diameter, a parameter included in the calculation of area, has been shown to be significantly related to prognosis,[140,141] as has the frequency of mitoses.[139,142] Inverse relationships were observed between mean nuclear area, mean nuclear diameter, mitotic index, and prognosis.

Concurrent assessment of nuclear and histologic grading proved prognostically significant in some of these studies.[139,144] It remains to be determined how the more precise observations of morphometry may be used to improve the assessment of prognosis beyond that made possible by nuclear and histologic grading.

The prognostic significance of *lymphoplasmacytic infiltration* in the stroma within and around invasive ductal carcinomas has been a subject of considerable interest and some controversy. A moderate to marked reaction of the intensity observed in medullary carcinoma also occurs in approximately 20% of nonmedullary invasive ductal carcinomas.[88,106] This type of tumor is more common among blacks and the mean age of these patients is relatively young.[145] Invasive ductal carcinoma with a marked lymphoplasmacytic reaction is almost always estrogen and progesterone receptor-negative.[146] A subset of these tumors with some, but not all, of the other features of medullary carcinoma, referred to as atypical medullary carcinoma, had a slightly more favorable prognosis than did infiltrating ductal carcinomas as a group, but the difference was not statistically significant.[147] Marked lymphoplasmacytic reaction generally consists largely of mature lymphocytes with a variable admixture of plasma cells. Rarely, plasma cells predominate. The majority of tumors with such a prominent reaction tend to be poorly differentiated and have a circumscribed, rather than an infiltrative, contour.

Although the favorable prognosis of medullary carcinoma has been ascribed to the lymphoplasmacytic reaction that characterizes these tumors, it is unclear whether the same conclusion may be drawn about nonmedullary invasive ductal carcinomas. Some investigators have found carcinomas with this "host response" to have a relatively favorable prognosis,[90,99,105,148,149] but others have found no significant difference or have reported a less favorable outcome associated with the presence of a prominent lymphoplasmacytic infiltrate.[90,106,107,150]

The intensity of mast cell infiltration in the substance or at the periphery of an invasive breast carcinoma is not significantly related to prognosis.[151]

The presence of lymphatic tumor emboli in the breast is an unfavorable prognostic finding. For this purpose, the lymphatics are defined as vascular channels that are lined by endothelium without supporting smooth muscle or elastica (Fig. 7-15). Most do not contain red blood cells, but undoubtedly, some blood capillaries are included in this definition. Artifactual spaces are commonly formed around nests of tumor cells within an invasive carcinoma as a result of tissue shrinkage during processing. Because it is very difficult to distinguish these artifacts from true lymphatic spaces,[152] assessment for lymphatic invasion is more reliably accomplished in the breast parenchyma adjacent to the invasive tumor margin.[153] Efforts to identify intratumoral lymphatic spaces by using immunoperoxidase reagents associated with endothelial cells (Factor VIII and blood group antigens) have met with only limited success.[154,155] The prognostic significance of intratumoral lymphatic emboli has not been determined.

Extratumoral lymphatic tumor emboli in the breast are associated with approximately 25% of invasive ductal carcinomas. This determination is made on the basis of routine sampling of biopsy and mastectomy specimens. The majority of these patients also have axillary lymph node metastases; it has not yet been determined whether the presence of lymphatic invasion alters their prognosis.

Lymphatic tumor emboli are found in the breast surrounding invasive ductal carcinomas in 10% to 15% of patients who have pathologically negative lymph nodes. Several studies have shown that lymphatic invasion is prognostically unfavorable in node-negative patients treated with mastectomy.[106,150,153,156–159] This deleterious effect is most pronounced in women with T1N0M0 disease. In a 10-year follow-up study of 378 patients treated for T1N0M0 carcinoma, 33% of 30 women with lymphatic invasion died of disease. Death due to breast carcinoma was observed in 10% of the 348 women who did not have lymphatic invasion.[106] Another study comparing similar subsets of patients with TIN0M0 disease found recurrences in 32% of those with lymphatic invasion, compared to 10% of the control subjects.[150] It has not been possible to demonstrate that lymphatic invasion has a statistically significant impact on prognosis in Stage I patients with tumors larger than 2 cm (T2N0M0), although those with lymphatic invasion do experience a higher recurrence rate.[153]

The unfavorable effect of lymphatic invasion in patients with T1N0M0 carcinoma is probably not attributable to occult metastases in the axillary lymph nodes. Serial sections of lymph nodes detected metastases in 9 of 28 patients originally classified as having T1N0M0 disease with lymphatic invasion in the breast. The recurrence rate was no higher among those with occult metastases than among those with truly negative lymph nodes.[160]

Blood vessel invasion is defined as penetration by tumor into the lumen of an artery or vein (Fig. 7-16). These structures may be identified by the presence of a smooth muscle wall supported by elastic fibers. It is usually necessary to employ special histochemical procedures (e.g., orcein or Verhoeff-van Gieson stains), which selectively stain elastic tissue, in order to detect this component of the vascular wall. Elastic fibers are often deposited around ducts with intraductal carcinoma within an invasive tumor; the resulting appearance in an elastic tissue stain

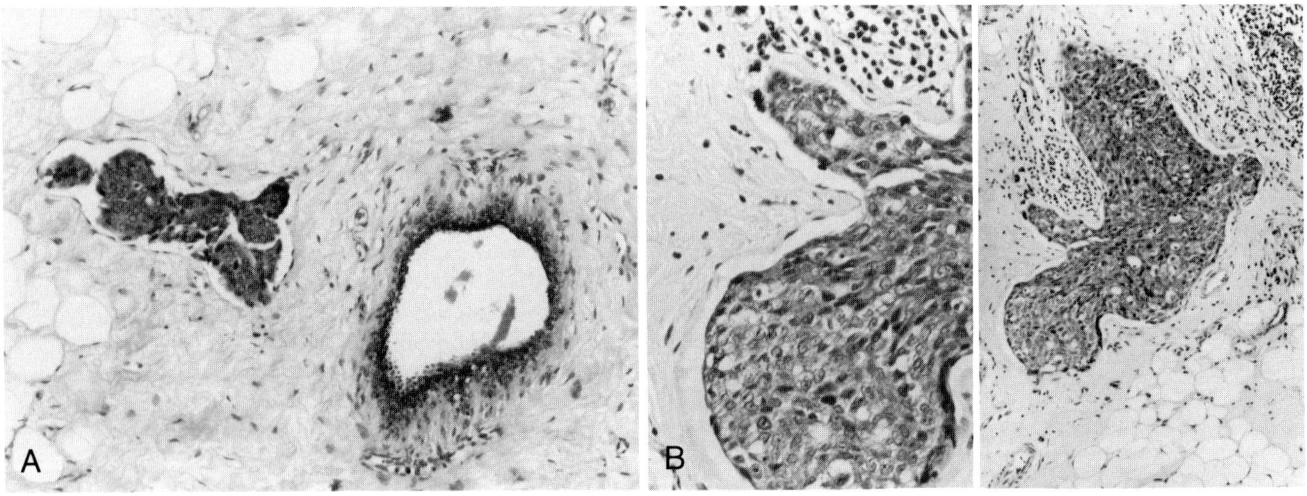

FIGURE 7-15. Lymphatic invasion. *(A)* A cluster of tumor cells in a lymphatic space adjacent to a small duct and at a considerable distance from an invasive carcinoma. Note the nuclei of the endothelial cells lining the vascular channel, which has no discernible, supporting layer of muscle or stroma. *(B)* Composite view of the shrinkage artifact that simulates lymphatic invasion. The mass of invasive tumor cells has separated from the supporting stroma, but retains the same shape. The nuclei of the endothelial cells are absent at high magnification.

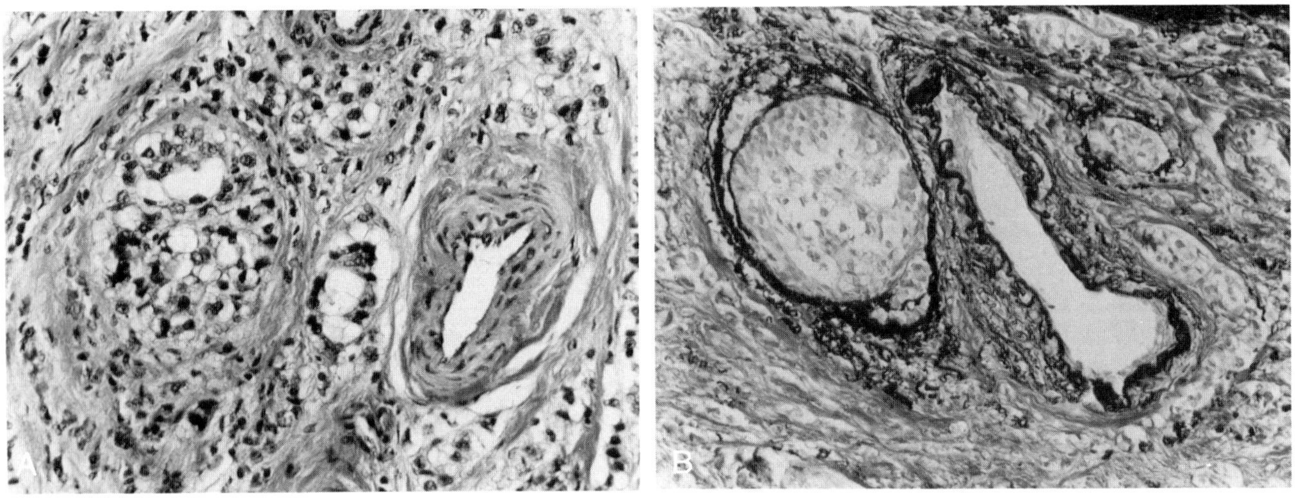

FIGURE 7-16. Blood vessel invasion. *(A)* Routine section stained with hematoxylin and eosin in which vascular invasion can be suspected. A small, unaffected artery is seen on the right. On the left, a vein is filled with tumor cells. *(B)* Comparable section stained for elastic tissue showing vascular structures. Note the presence of invasive carcinoma in the surrounding stroma.

may be indistinguishable from vascular invasion. Since larger vascular components in the breast usually consist of a paired artery and vein, vascular invasion should only be diagnosed with confidence when tumor is demonstrated within one or both of a pair of vessels demonstrated by elastic tissue stain.

The reported frequency of blood vessel invasion varies from 4.7% to 47.2%.[88,106,108,150,161–167] These widely divergent observations reflect major differences in the studies with respect to the number of patients evaluated, clinical and pathologic characteristics of the study population, and the methods by which blood vessel invasion was identified. These variations in study design and methodology are also probably responsible for the widely divergent conclusions reached by these authors with respect to the prognostic significance of blood vessel invasion.

Some have reported that blood vessel invasion denoted a relatively poor prognosis in node-positive patients[163] or only in those with two or more positive lymph nodes.[164] Others concluded that this finding was prognostically significant only in the absence of axillary lymph node metastases.[166]

Recently, 10-year follow-up data were reported for 524 women treated consecutively for invasive carcinomas of 2 cm or less in diameter (T1 with modified or standard radical mastectomy.[106,108] It was possible to evaluate 502 tumors for blood vessel invasion using one section per case stained to demonstrate elastic tissue. Blood vessel invasion was identified in 47 of 362 (13%) T1N0M0 tumors. Recurrence of breast carcinoma occurred more frequently when blood vessel invasion was present (12 of 47 patients, or 26%) than when it was absent (50 of 315 patients, or 16%. Death due to disease also occurred more often among women with blood vessel invasion (9 of 47 patients, or 19%) than among those without blood vessel invasion (38 of 315 patients, or 12%). However, these differences in recurrence and death rates were not statistically significant. Visceral metastases occurred in 67% of patients with blood vessel invasion and in 36% of those without such invasion. Bone recurrences occurred more frequently in the absence of demonstrable blood vessel invasion. Other researchers have also observed a similar, higher, recurrence rate associated with blood vessel invasion in T1N0M0 disease.[150]

Blood vessel invasion was found in 23 of 117 (20%) stage II T1 tumors (T1N0M0).[108] Deaths attributable to metastatic breast carcinoma occurred with significantly greater frequency among women with blood vessel invasion ($P<0.03$), regardless of whether they had a single positive lymph node or two or more affected nodes.

Carcinomas arising in various organs exhibit a capacity and, in some instances, a proclivity for invasion around and into nerves, termed *perineural invasion* (Fig. 7-17). This phenomenon is not frequently observed among invasive mammary carcinomas, perhaps in part because nerves of any notable size are not numerous in mammary tissues and often are not evident. Perineural invasion may be found in approximately 10% of invasive carcinomas. It tends to occur in high-grade tumors, is frequently associated with the presence of lymphatic tumor emboli, and has not been proven to have independent prognostic significance.

A variety of patterns in the connective tissue stroma that is formed in and around invasive ductal carcinomas has been described. Tumors vary considerably with respect to the quantitative and qualitative characteristics of their stroma. The extremes are represented by medullary carcinoma and the very cellular variants of invasive ductal carcinoma, which contain virtually no fibrous stroma, and scirrhous carcinoma, which is characterized by marked collagenization. It is not clear whether the character of stroma in an invasive ductal carcinoma is an independent prognostic variable since there are clear associations between this and other prognostically significant structural features of breast carcinomas. For example, tumors that

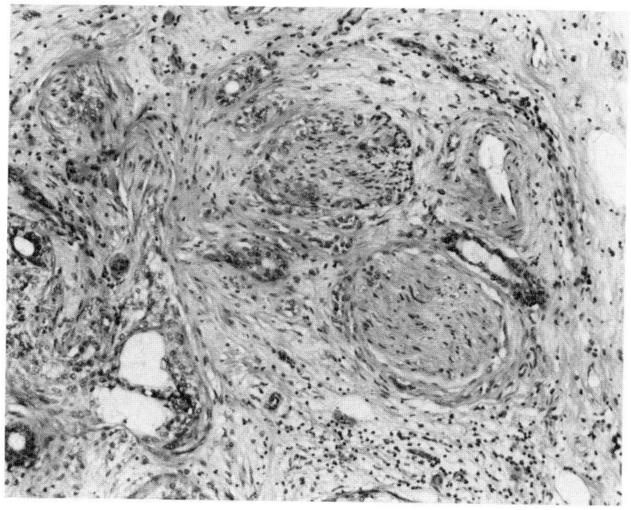

FIGURE 7-17. Perineural invasion. Neoplastic glands surrounding and invading nerves are evident in the center and left parts of this photograph. A tumor gland lies just outside a nerve on the right.

have minimal stromal reaction tend to have the following characteristics: circumscription, poorly differentiated nuclear and histologic grade, and marked lymphoplasmacytic reaction. They also tend to be estrogen receptor-negative. On the other hand, densely fibrotic or scirrhous carcinomas are more likely to be stellate, moderately differentiated, and to have little lymphoplasmacytic reaction. A greater proportion of these lesions are estrogen receptor-positive.

Attempts to assess the character or composition of stroma in invasive ductal carcinomas have focused on the amount of elastic tissue present. Stromal elastic fibers may be detected using the same stains employed to demonstrate the elastic components in blood vessels (orcein or Verhoeff-van Gieson stains). Although rarely found in normal mammary tissue, increased amounts of elastic tissue may be deposited around ducts in benign proliferative breast disease.[168,169] A similar phenomenon occurs quite commonly around intraductal carcinoma, particularly in the invasive portion of the tumor and, to a lesser extent, in the intervening stroma. In the absence of a widely accepted method for describing elastosis, various grading schemes have been adopted in an effort to convey quantitative estimates of the extent of this process. The rate of occurrence of the most extreme or marked degrees of elastosis described in recent reports varied from 17% to 23%;[88,170,171] 12% to 55% of the tumors included in the same studies were characterized by little or no elastosis.

Abundant elastosis is significantly associated with estrogen receptor positivity.[170–172] The significance of elastosis as an independent prognostic variable remains controversial. Although marked elastosis has been described by some investigators as a favorable prognostic feature,[173] others have found that elastosis did not correlate with prognosis,[170,171,174] or that abundant elastosis had a negative effect on outcome.[175,176]

Recently, attention has been directed to the pattern and distribution of intraductal carcinoma as a prognostic variable in patients with invasive ductal carcinoma. Tumors vary in the relative proportions of their intraductal and invasive components, ranging from those with only microscopic invasion (see Fig. 7-6) to lesions composed entirely of invasive carcinoma. Silverberg and Chitale observed a trend toward decreased nodal metastases and a more favorable prognosis when the intraductal component in the tumor was more abundant.[177] However, it should be noted that the relative quantitative assessment of these components is highly subjective. In one recent report, little or no intraductal carcinoma was detected in sections from 72% of 974 tumors, whereas 11% were described as being composed of at least 66% intraductal carcinoma.[88] These authors noted that patients with lesions having a prominent intratumoral intraductal component also tended to have intraductal carcinoma in surrounding, extratumoral breast tissue, and to have multicentric carcinoma in the breast. Although the distribution of intraductal carcinoma in and around the primary tumor appears to correlate with the risk for recurrence in the breast after lumpectomy and radiation therapy,[178] this feature has no bearing on the risk for systemic recurrence in women treated with mastectomy.[179] There is no clear association between prognosis and the structural pattern of intraductal carcinoma (comedo, cribriform, papillary, and so on) in invasive ductal carcinoma.

Several other histologic variables have been assessed as potential prognostic indicators. Among these are the amount and type of mucin produced by the tumor cells, the mucopolysaccharide content of the tumor stroma, the glycogen content of the tumor cells, the presence of calcifications in the tumor, and the influence of associated benign proliferative changes in the breast. For the most part, none of these variables has been found to correlate strongly with prognosis and to be as useful in making therapeutic decisions as the other observations discussed in detail in this section.

Immunohistochemical markers have attracted some interest as potential indicators of prognosis. Carcinoembryonic antigen is the most extensively studied marker. The frequency of CEA positivity varies considerably in different laboratories, with 90% of tumors showing some reactivity in one study.[180] No consistent relationship has been found to exist between prognosis and the immunohistochemical demonstration of CEA activity in breast cancer. A reduced frequency of axillary lymph node metastases and better prognosis were related to CEA-negative tumors by some authors.[181,182] In other studies, the presence or absence of CEA in tissue has proved to have little or no prognostic value.[180,183,184] Equally conflicting observations have been reported for human chorionic gonadotropin (HCG);[180,183,185] pregnancy-specific, beta-1 glycoprotein;[180,183,185] and placental lactogen.[180,185] The presence or absence of immunohistochemically detected blood group isoantigens has also not been found to be a significant prognostic marker.[186]

Tubular Carcinoma

Tubular (well-differentiated) carcinoma has been recognized as a morphologically distinctive form of mammary carcinoma for more than 100 years.[187] The term *tubular carcinoma*[188,189] describes the distinguishing microscopic feature of the lesion, which is composed of neoplastic elements resembling normal breast ductules. Alternative terms, such as orderly or well-differentiated[190,191] carcinoma, are less specific and have not gained wide acceptance.

The precise pathologic definition of tubular carcinoma has been the subject of some controversy, which has, in turn, influenced the reported frequency of the lesion. Elements of tubular carcinoma may be found in a substantial number of invasive ductal carcinomas, but in relatively few does all or almost all of the tumor have a tubular growth pattern. As used in this section, tubular carcinoma refers to so-called pure tubular carcinoma. Most authors require that at least 75% of the tumor be tubular to qualify for this diagnosis.[192–197]

In its pure form, tubular carcinoma is quite uncommon, constituting not more than 2% of all breast carcinomas in most series.[22,192–194,198] Since tubular carcinomas are generally small, they are found with greater frequency in studies of early breast cancer. In one review of 382 women treated between 1964 and 1969 for T1N1M0 breast carcinoma,[106] tubular carcinoma was present in 5%. This type of lesion occurred in 9% of patients with tumors of 1.0 cm or less in diameter, and in 2% of those with tumors measuring 1.1 to 2.0 cm. Only 1.5% of 142 patients with T1N0M0 disease had tubular carcinoma.[108]

With the widespread use of mammography, emphasis on early breast cancer detection has contributed to an increased interest in tubular carcinoma. These tumors constituted 8% of invasive carcinomas measuring 1.0 cm or less in diameter found in a review of the Breast Cancer Detection Demonstration Projects.[12] Seven percent of 138 carcinomas found in one U.S. screening program were of the tubular variety.[199] All of these tumors were detected on mammography, but only 30% were detected by clinical examination. In Malmo, Sweden, 21.5% of 116 breast carcinomas found on mammography screening were reportedly of the pure tubular variety.[200]

It has recently been suggested that tubular carcinomas are a stage in the evolution of a substantial number of breast cancers.[201,202] Proponents of this theory believe that tubular carcinomas arise from benign proliferative lesions called radial scars, and that, as they enlarge, tubular carcinomas are converted into ordinary invasive ductal carcinomas. This premise remains a subject of considerable controversy.[203,204]

CLINICAL PRESENTATION. With rare exceptions,[196,197,205] most patients with tubular carcinoma have been women. Tubular carcinoma constitutes only about 1% of breast carcinomas in men.[28,206] The clinical data presented here deal with women reported to have pure tubular carcinoma.

In patients with tubular carcinoma, the age distribution at diagnosis ranges from 24 to 83 years,[194–197] with a median age in the mid to late 40s (44 to 49 years). The majority of patients present with a palpable lesion which, in most cases, proves to be the carcinoma. The reported duration of symptoms is 1 week to 20 years, with a median duration of 2 months.[195–197] Skin retraction or fixation occurs in about 15% of cases; nipple discharge is rarely reported.[194] Several studies have compared patients treated for pure tubular carcinoma with women who had invasive carcinomas that contained tubular elements (so-called mixed tubular carcinomas).[192–195] Other than a trend toward a younger age at diagnosis in patients with pure tubular carcinoma, no consistent clinical differences have been noted. In one study, 40% of patients with tubular carcinoma reported a positive family history for breast carcinoma among first-degree relatives.[207]

GROSS PATHOLOGY. The reported size of tubular carcinomas ranges from 0.2 cm to 4 cm[190–198] except for one study in which the largest tumor measured 12 cm.[203] In two studies, 80%[196] and 87%[197] of tubular carcinomas were 1 cm or less in diameter; in the latter series, the median size of 90 pure lesions was 0.8 cm. By contrast, these authors described a size range of 0.4 cm to 2.1 cm for 55 mixed tubular carcinomas (with a median size of 1.1 cm) and noted that 52% were 1 cm or less in diameter.[197]

On gross examination, tubular carcinoma produces a firm to hard tumor. The cut surface is grey to white. Rarely, a tan or pale yellow tinge may be found in lesions that have extensive elastosis. Tumor margins are ill-defined or stellate. The cut surface tends to retract and become depressed in relation to the surrounding breast parenchyma. Although the diagnosis of tubular carcinoma might be suggested on gross inspection, the features are not specific enough to exclude some benign lesions or less well-differentiated invasive carcinomas of comparable size.

MICROSCOPIC PATHOLOGY. Tubular carcinoma is a variant of invasive ductal carcinoma. As illustrated in Fig. 7-18, the tumor is characterized microscopically by a proliferation of small glands or tubules that closely resemble nonneoplastic mammary ductules. These invasive tubular structures are haphazardly distributed, and tend to form a stellate tumor with ill-defined boundaries. The stroma within the tumor is formed of dense collagenous tissue with variable, sometimes abundant, amounts of elastic tissue.[208–210, 210A] Calcifications are found in about 50% of cases, sometimes in the lumens of neoplastic tubules or in the stroma. More commonly, calcifications are detected in the intraductal component, which has reportedly been present in 60% to 84% of the tumors.[190,193,196,197,210] Most often, tubular carcinoma arises from papillary and cribri-

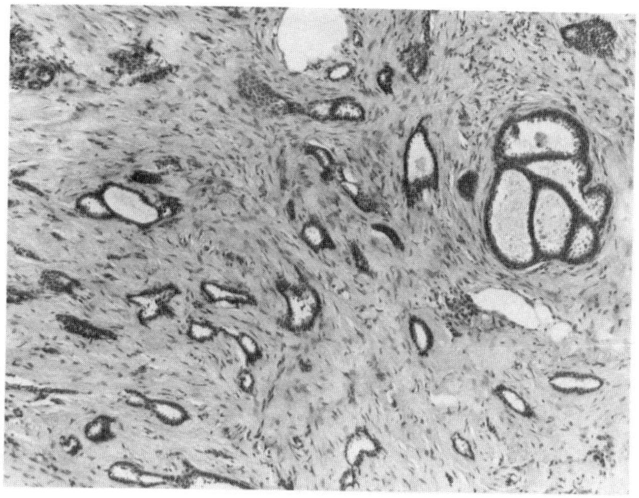

FIGURE 7-18. Pure tubular carcinoma. Patient was a 57-year-old woman who had an asymptomatic lesion detected on mammography. Low-power view shows characteristic angular and oval invasive glands embedded in moderately cellular stroma. Micropapillary intraductal carcinoma fills a duct near the right margin.

form intraductal carcinoma. Lobular carcinoma *in situ* has been found in association with tubular carcinoma in 0.7% to 40% of cases,[193,195–197,211] usually not as part of the primary tumor.

Tubular carcinoma is not often accompanied by an appreciable lymphocytic reaction. Perineural invasion may be observed, but is uncommon, and this form of carcinoma virtually never has lymphatic tumor emboli detectable on histologic sections of the breast.[106]

Microscopically, tubular carcinoma must be distinguished from benign conditions, such as sclerosing adenosis and microglandular adenosis. The proliferative pattern of sclerosing adenosis is lobulocentric; consequently, at low magnification, one can identify multiple, individual, altered lobules even when the process is sufficiently developed to form a coalescent mass or adenosis tumor clinically.[212] In contrast to the haphazardly dispersed, open, often angular glands of tubular carcinoma, the proliferation in sclerosing adenosis tends to be a compact, whorled mixture of elongated and compressed glands interlaced with spindly myoepithelial cells. Histochemical studies have shown preservation of the basement membranes around the glands in sclerosing adenosis; this preservation is, however, absent in tubular carcinoma.[213,214] These differences have been confirmed by electron microscopy.[215,216] The distinction between tubular carcinoma and microglandular adenosis, a very uncommon tumor, is more difficult to establish, and requires a careful assessment of fine cytologic details.[217]

Clinically, tubular carcinoma usually forms a single tumor. However, in an as yet undetermined number of cases, tubular carcinoma may grow as a more diffuse process, with multiple, seemingly separate, foci in one or

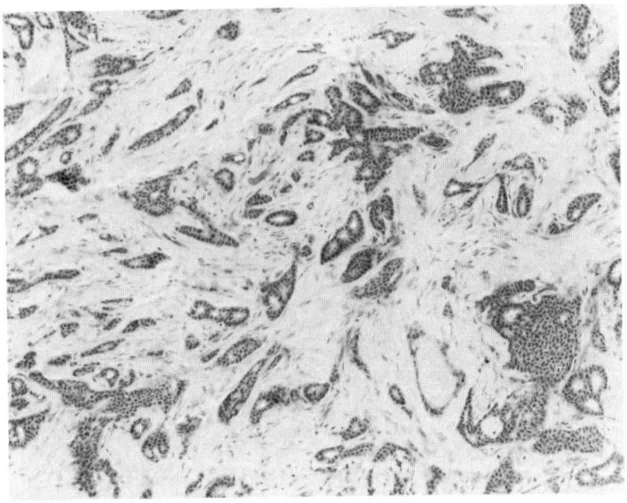

FIGURE 7-19. Mixed tubular carcinoma in a 70-year-old woman. Low-power view showing numerous invasive tubular glands and alveolar masses of invasive tumor with solid and laciform growth patterns.

more quadrants of the breast. Ten percent to 56% of patients with tubular carcinoma have been reported to have independent foci of carcinoma elsewhere in the breast,[193,195,197,207,210] including various types of *in situ* and invasive carcinoma. In one series of 120 patients treated with mastectomy, 20 (16.7%) had residual tubular carcinoma at the biopsy site; 6 (5%) had a second, remote invasive carcinoma; 4 (3.3%) had multicentric intraductal carcinoma; and 3 (2.5%) had multicentric, *in situ* lobular carcinoma.[197] Contralateral carcinoma has been reported in several series, with the percentage of cases varying from 0 to 38.[193,207] The incidence of contralateral cancer in three studies ranged from 9% to 12%.[195–197] Most contralateral carcinomas were of the infiltrating duct type. Rare instances of bilateral tubular carcinoma have been noted.[194,195,210]

The tubular elements, found in varying proportions in mixed tubular carcinomas, are indistinguishable from those in pure tubular carcinomas (Fig. 7-19). Trabecular, alveolar, and papillary growth, as well as nontubular gland formation, are included among the components of infiltrating ductal carcinoma found in mixed tubular lesions.

PROGNOSIS. The favorable prognosis attributed to tubular carcinoma appears to be restricted to tumors composed of at least 75% tubular elements.[192–198] The reported incidence of axillary metastases ranges from 0[194] to 25%,[191] with an average of 9%.[106,108,192,194–197,210] Involved lymph nodes rarely number more than three, are usually located at Level 1, and the metastatic foci tend to have a tubular growth pattern. Axillary lymph node metastases have been reported in 21%[192] and 29%[195] of patients with mixed tubular carcinoma. In one study,[195] 21% of patients with Stage II mixed tubular carcinoma had more than three lymph nodes involved.

The majority of patients with pure or mixed tubular carcinoma described in the literature have been treated with mastectomy, usually of the modified or radical type. Simple mastectomy or excisional treatment were employed in less than 10% of patients. Seven follow-up studies describe a total of 341 women with pure tubular carcinoma.[191,193–197,210] Recurrences attributable to tubular carcinoma were reported in 12 patients (3.5%). Six of these were women who developed recurrences in the breast following simple excision. The interval to recurrence in the breast ranged from 2 to 22 years. Only one of these women had axillary nodal metastases at the time of recurrence and none were reported to have systemic spread after mastectomy for the recurrence.

Recurrence of disease following mastectomy was described in six patients, three of whom had had positive axillary lymph nodes at mastectomy. One developed a local recurrence, whereas the other two had systemic metastases that proved to be fatal. Of two patients with negative axillary nodes, one developed systemic spread and another had "persistent carcinoma." The sixth patient, whose nodal status was unreported, developed a local recurrence. There were several patients with bilateral carcinoma whose death from metastatic disease appeared to be attributable to the contralateral lesion.[195,197] Among patients with mixed tubular carcinomas, 32% developed recurrence[193–195] and 6% to 28% died of disease.[193–195]

Medullary Carcinoma

The term medullary has been used to describe mammary carcinomas for nearly a century. For much of this time, the name was employed to describe the clinical or gross pathologic appearance of large, solid, or papillary carcinomas that often produced axillary metastases. None of the various histopathologic patterns included under this heading was regarded as a specific entity. A subset of these tumors with marked lymphoid infiltration and a relatively favorable prognosis was, for many years, classified as bulky adenocarcinoma at Memorial Hospital and as cystic neomammary carcinoma by Geschickter.[218] The name medullary carcinoma has been applied to this specific type of carcinoma since the 1940s.[1,219] Medullary carcinoma has also been referred to as solid, circumscribed carcinoma.[220,221] These uncommon tumors constitute less than 5% of the mammary carcinomas in most series,[222,223] but frequencies of 8%[224] and 9%[22] have been reported.

CLINICAL PRESENTATION. Patients with medullary carcinoma tend to be younger than those with other types of carcinoma. In their initial description of medullary carcinoma, Moore and Foote reported that 59% of affected patients were younger than 50 years old.[219] Others have found 40%,[224] 60%,[40] and 66%[221] of patients with medullary carcinoma to be younger than 50 years of age. The mean age at diagnosis in several series was 46 to 54 years.[40,147,221,223] Medullary carcinoma constitutes 11% of the carcinomas diagnosed in women 35 years of age or younger;[145] it is relatively uncommon in elderly patients.[225]

Early clinical descriptions of patients with medullary carcinoma emphasized large tumor size, circumscription, and a tendency for cystic degeneration.[218,219] Fixation to the skin or chest wall and ulceration have been reported to occur with large tumors.[221] Smaller lesions with well-defined contours and a firm, but not hard, consistency may readily be mistaken clinically for fibroadenomas, especially in young women.

Medullary carcinoma occurs in various parts of the breast with a frequency similar to that of breast carcinoma in general. Because of its histologic and clinical characteristics, medullary carcinoma in the axillary tail of the breast may be mistaken for metastatic carcinoma in a lymph node.[226] Bilateral breast carcinoma has been reported in 3% to 18% of patients who have medullary carcinoma in one breast.[221,223,225,227] However, medullary carcinoma affecting both breasts, whether simultaneous or asynchronous, is quite uncommon.[225,227]

Fewer than 10% of primary medullary carcinomas of the breast contain sufficient levels of estrogen or progesterone receptor to be regarded as positive.[228] Consequently, metastases from these tumors show little response to endocrine therapy.[229] The growth rate of medullary carcinoma, measured by thymidine incorporation, is among the fastest recorded among breast carcinomas,[230] an observation that is consistent with the rapid growth and short duration reported by many patients.

GROSS PATHOLOGY. Medullary carcinomas have a well-defined contour that separates the tumor from the surrounding breast parenchyma. Close inspection of the cut surface of a bisected medullary carcinoma usually reveals that the tumor has a nodular architecture. The tumor is firm, but softer than the average breast carcinoma, and bulges above the surrounding tissue. Other notable features are a pale brown or grey color, and the presence of hemorrhage or necrosis, or both, in some tumors. The extent of necrosis tends to increase in proportion to tumor size, but may be quite prominent even in small lesions. The necrotic tissue may have a granular, almost caseous, appearance in medullary carcinomas. Lesions larger than 5 cm in diameter tend to undergo cystic degeneration. Residual fragments of tumor attached to the cyst wall may resemble a cystic papillary carcinoma.

MICROSCOPIC PATHOLOGY. Medullary carcinoma is defined by a complex constellation of histopathologic features.[219,225] The tumor must exhibit all of these elements in order to be diagnosed as medullary carcinoma. Carcinomas that have most, but not all, of the necessary microscopic components have been referred to as atypical medullary carcinomas. It is imperative that the histologic criteria for the diagnosis of medullary carcinoma be rigorously applied since the prognosis of women with atypical medullary carcinoma is significantly less favorable than that of patients with medullary carcinoma.[225]

In addition to gross and microscopic circumscription, the histopathologic features that define medullary carcinoma are intense lymphoplasmacytic reaction around and within the tumor, poorly differentiated nuclear grade (usually accompanied by a high mitotic rate among tumor cells), and a tendency for tumor cells to grow in broad sheets (syncytial pattern) rather than in the trabecular, alveolar, or gland-forming configuration of ordinary invasive ductal carcinoma (Fig. 7-20). Intraductal carcinoma is commonly present (in 46% of cases) at the periphery of the tumor, often with involvement of the epithelium in adjacent lobules. An intense lymphoplasmacytic reaction occurs around these affected ducts and lobules. This reactive process may also involve lobules and ducts that are somewhat more distant from the tumor and that do not contain recognizable tumor cells. It has been suggested that the expansile growth is at least partly attributable to coalescence of enlarging nodules of carcinoma in these peripheral ducts and lobules, a conclusion supported by the grossly nodular character of medullary carcinoma.[224,225]

Squamous metaplasia occurs in a substantial number of medullary carcinomas (16%), and one may also find osteocartilaginous and anaplastic giant cell formation. Medullary carcinoma is only rarely accompanied by intramammary lymphatic tumor emboli. Multicentricity, defined as carcinoma in the breast outside the primary quadrant, is relatively uncommon in medullary carcinoma, having been found in only 10% of 58 cases in one series.[227]

Electron microscopy has revealed some distinctive ultrastructural features of medullary carcinoma.[231,232] The tumor cells are rich in organelles and have a well-developed Golgi complex. Light and dark cells, which differ in cytoplasmic density, have been described. Mucin secretory vacuoles are virtually absent from the tumor cells. Endothelial cells in the tumor stroma are prominent, and migration of lymphocytes has been observed through the endothelium of these channels.

Immunohistochemical study has shown that IgA plasma cells predominate in medullary carcinomas. The tumor cells contain IgA and secretory component. By contrast, typical infiltrating ductal carcinomas contain little or none of these substances, and their associated plasma cells contain IgG.

PROGNOSIS. Moore and Foote reported that 82.7% of 52 patients with medullary carcinoma were alive and disease-free 5 years after radical mastectomy.[219] Only 11.5% of their patients died of breast carcinoma within 5 years after surgery. They found axillary node metastases in 42% of cases, and observed a five-year survival of 50% in node-positive patients. Nine patients with a single lymph node metastasis survived, without disease, for 5 years. Richardson's series of 99 patients had a disease-free survival rate of 78% at 5 years.[224] Death due to disease was reported in 10%. Survival among 47 patients with 10 years

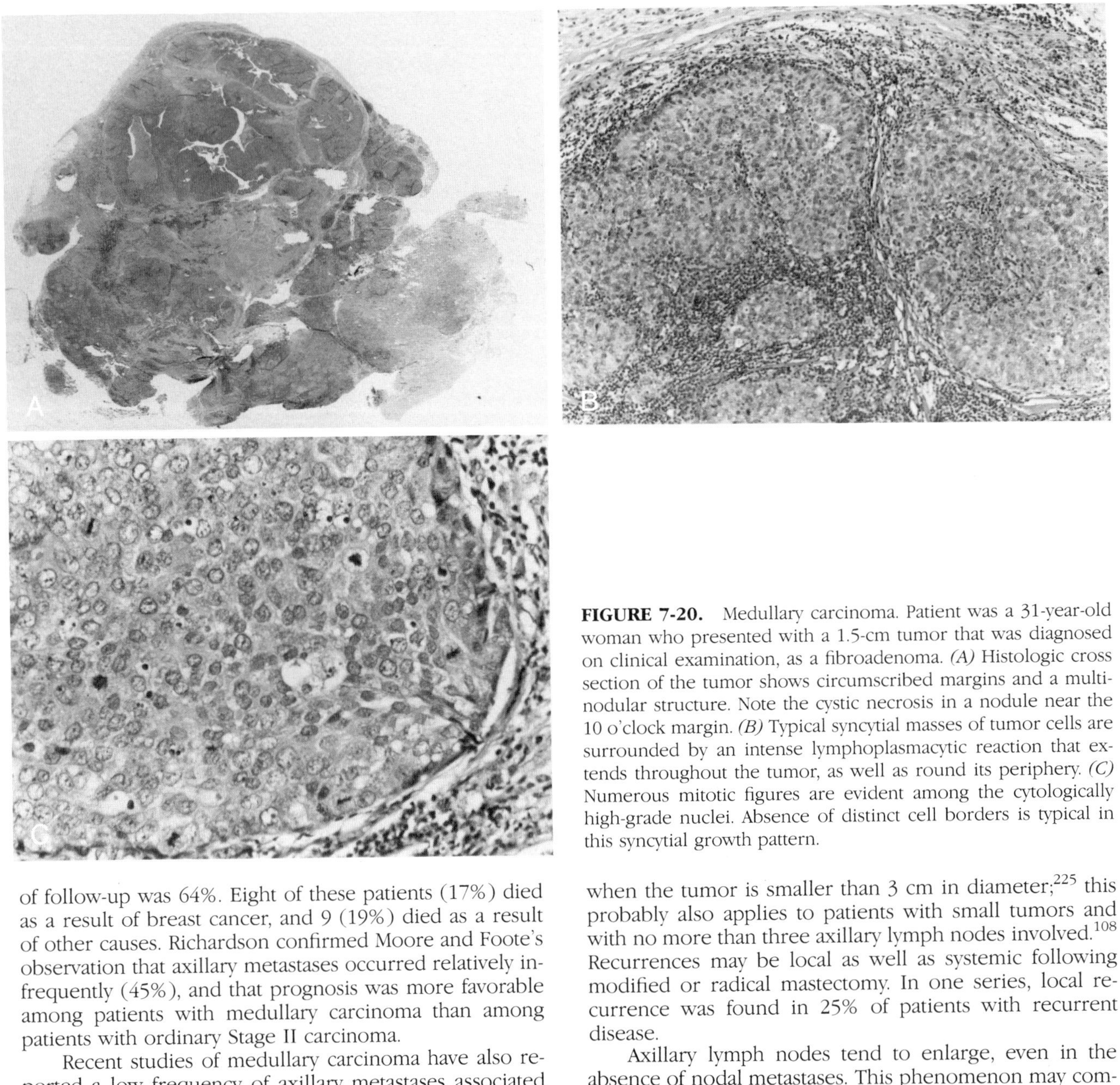

FIGURE 7-20. Medullary carcinoma. Patient was a 31-year-old woman who presented with a 1.5-cm tumor that was diagnosed on clinical examination, as a fibroadenoma. *(A)* Histologic cross section of the tumor shows circumscribed margins and a multinodular structure. Note the cystic necrosis in a nodule near the 10 o'clock margin. *(B)* Typical syncytial masses of tumor cells are surrounded by an intense lymphoplasmacytic reaction that extends throughout the tumor, as well as round its periphery. *(C)* Numerous mitotic figures are evident among the cytologically high-grade nuclei. Absence of distinct cell borders is typical in this syncytial growth pattern.

of follow-up was 64%. Eight of these patients (17%) died as a result of breast cancer, and 9 (19%) died as a result of other causes. Richardson confirmed Moore and Foote's observation that axillary metastases occurred relatively infrequently (45%), and that prognosis was more favorable among patients with medullary carcinoma than among patients with ordinary Stage II carcinoma.

Recent studies of medullary carcinoma have also reported a low frequency of axillary metastases associated with this disease,[221,223,225] and with few exceptions,[221,233] researchers have confirmed the observations regarding a more favorable prognosis than that associated with other types of carcinoma (Fig. 7-21*A*).[223,225] From these data, it now seems clear that the size of the primary tumor and axillary nodal status are significant determinants of survival (Fig. 7-21*B*) for patients with medullary carcinoma.[223,225] Tumors larger than 3 cm in diameter, when accompanied by more than three involved lymph nodes, are associated with recurrence rates that are not appreciably different from those in patients with ordinary types of breast carcinoma. The outcome for women with node-negative medullary carcinoma appears to be especially favorable[106] when the tumor is smaller than 3 cm in diameter;[225] this probably also applies to patients with small tumors and with no more than three axillary lymph nodes involved.[108] Recurrences may be local as well as systemic following modified or radical mastectomy. In one series, local recurrence was found in 25% of patients with recurrent disease.

Axillary lymph nodes tend to enlarge, even in the absence of nodal metastases. This phenomenon may complicate clinical staging.[221] Microscopic examination reveals lymphoplasmacytic infiltration and follicular hyperplasia with variable sinus histiocytosis. Because these hyperplastic lymph nodes are grossly conspicuous, the average number of lymph nodes obtained on pathologic dissection of the axillary contents exceeds that obtained in other types of carcinoma.[234]

Mucinous Carcinoma

In their pure or nearly pure form, mucinous (colloid or gelatinous) tumors constitute 1% to 2% of breast carcinomas.[12] Approximately another 2% of carcinomas have

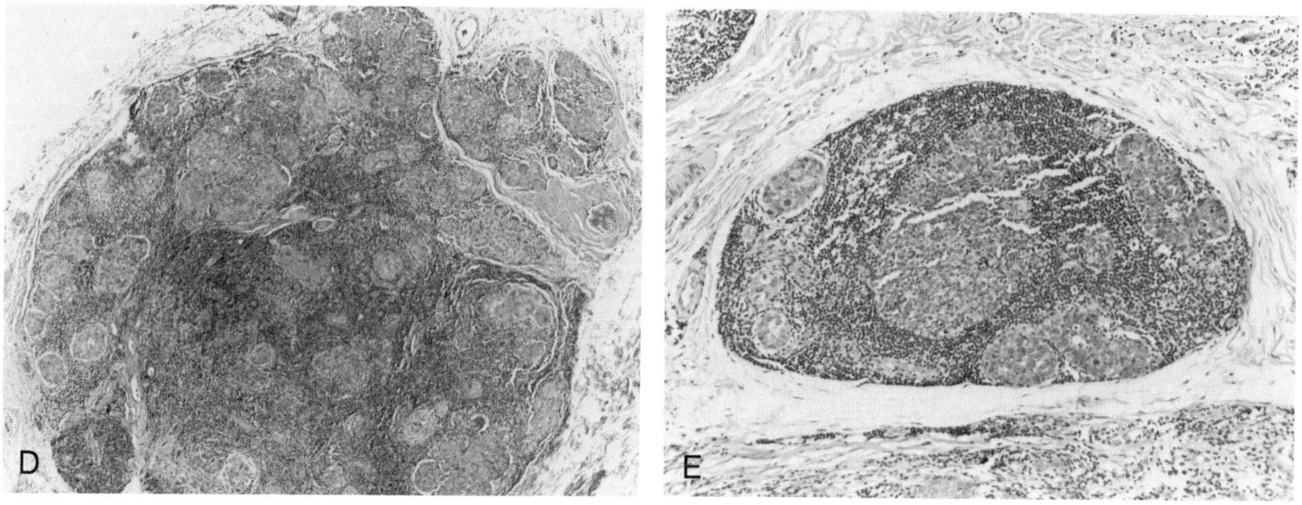

(D) A nodule, visible at the periphery of the tumor in a different section, appears to consist of several coalescent lobules and ducts surrounded by an intense lymphoplasmactic infiltrate. Most, if not all, of the round nests of tumor cells are composed of *in situ* tumor. *(E)* A single lobule in which acinar units are expanded by tumor cells is pictured. Lymphoplasmacytic reaction is confined to the intralobular stroma, resulting in a sharply defined contour.

areas of mucinous differentiation. The unusual microscopic appearance of this tumor, as well as its slow growth rate and favorable prognosis, has been recognized for more than a century.[235–237] Geschickter stressed the importance of distinguishing pure lesions from those containing mucinous and ordinary carcinoma elements.[238] A tendency for metastases to become manifest late in the course of the disease has been reported in many studies.[238–242]

CLINICAL PRESENTATION. Mucinous carcinoma occurs throughout the same age range as does breast carcinoma. Some authors have noted an older mean age for pure mucinous carcinoma,[7–9] but this has not been reported in other studies.[240,243] Mucinous carcinoma constitutes about 7% of the carcinomas occurring in women older than 75 years of age and 1% of those occurring in women younger than 35 years old at diagnosis.[225]

The initial symptom is usually a mass. Accompanying signs, such as nipple discharge, fixation, and skin ulceration, do not occur with exceptional frequency. The palpatory "swish" sign, described by Halstead, is rarely mentioned. A duration of symptoms exceeding one year has been observed in some elderly patients who present with large, pure, mucinous carcinomas.[244] In recent years, small, clinically occult, mucinous carcinomas have been detected on mammography. The calcifications that occur in some mucinous carcinomas may be detected on a mammogram. Mucinous carcinoma is not significantly associated with bilaterality. Approximately 60% of pure mucinous carcinomas are estrogen receptor-positive.[29,30]

GROSS PATHOLOGY. Published studies of mucinous carcinoma have described tumors ranging in size from less than 1 cm in diameter to 20 cm or more. A widely held perception that pure mucinous carcinomas tend to be larger than other types of carcinomas[240,244,246] is based on observations made several decades ago. More recent experience suggests that currently diagnosed mucinous carcinomas are not especially large.

On gross inspection, pure mucinous carcinoma varies in consistency from soft and gelatinous to firm or hard, depending upon the relative proportions of tumor and fibrous stroma present in the tumor. The mucinous character is readily appreciated on the cut surface, which appears moist and glistening. Margins of the tumor tend to be circumscribed, an impression often accentuated by a reddish zone of congested tissue at the periphery. Large mucinous tumors may develop areas of cystic degeneration.

MICROSCOPIC PATHOLOGY. The distinguishing histopathologic feature of mucinous carcinoma is the accumulation of abundant, extracellular, mucinous secretion around clusters of tumor cells. In pure mucinous carcinoma, this pattern is seen in all histologic sections. However, the relative proportions of secretion and tumor cells may vary considerably from one patient to another, and even within a given tumor. One extreme variant is the tumor that is so disproportionately composed of mucin that numerous sections may be necessary to detect any carcinoma cells (Fig. 7-22).

Tumor cells are usually dispersed in the mucinous secretion in slender strands or in papillary clusters. Large sheets of cells and zones of trabecular growth are also encountered. Gland formation is uncommon, and little intracellular mucin is generally evident in routine histologic sections. Signet ring cells containing abundant cytoplasmic mucin, which are characteristic of infiltrating lobular carcinoma,[247] are rarely present in mucinous carcinoma. Mucin may be demonstrated within the cells by electron microscopy.[247,248] The amount of secretion

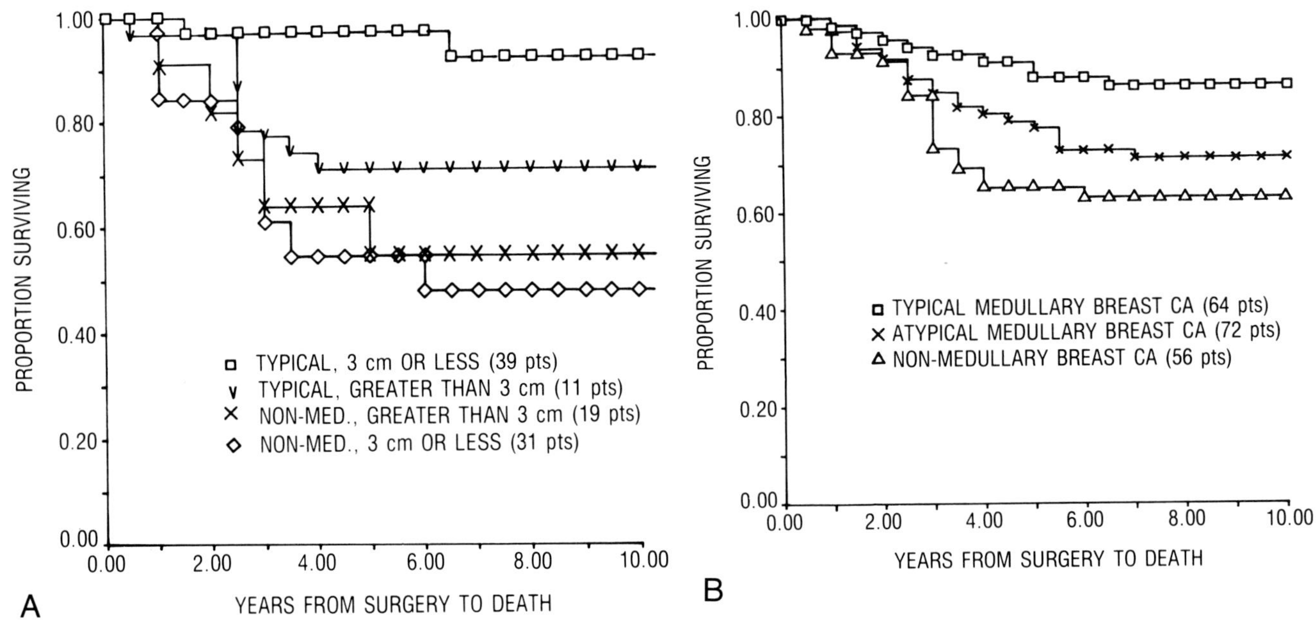

FIGURE 7-21. Prognosis in medullary carcinoma. *(A)* The overall prognosis for patients with medullary carcinoma is significantly more favorable than for patients with ordinary invasive ductal carcinoma and those having invasive ductal carcinoma with medullary features. The survival curves for nonmedullary and atypical medullary carcinoma patients are not significantly different. *(B)* Survival curves of patients with typical medullary carcinoma and those with invasive ductal carcinoma, stratified by tumor size, are depicted. The group with the most favorable prognosis consists of those with typical medullary carcinoma of 3 cm or less in diameter. (Non-med., nonmedullary).

found in most cells of mucinous carcinoma is substantially less than that in signet ring cell carcinomas. However, a small number of cells that appear to accumulate abundant mucin are disrupted, discharging the secretion.[249] Acidic and neutral mucopolysaccharides have been detected in mucinous carcinomas. Generally, the type of mucin is homogeneous within a given tumor.[250,251]

Argyrophilic granules with the ultrastructural features of endocrine granules have been detected in the cytoplasm of 25% to 50% of mucinous carcinoma cells.[253–255] Mucinous carcinomas composed of cells arranged in sheets and trabeculae tend to contain argyrophilic granules, and seem to occur more often in elderly women than do mucinous carcinomas with the papillary or festooned cell pattern. The content of the endocrine secretory granules has not been determined in most cases, but one tumor reportedly contained serotonin.[256] (The prognostic significance of argyrophilic granules in mucinous carcinoma is discussed in the section on mammary carcinomas with endocrine features, below.)

The classification of pure mucinous carcinoma as a variant of ductal carcinoma is supported by finding an intraductal component in a substantial proportion of cases. The intraductal histologic pattern tends to be complementary to the growth pattern in the invasive tumor. Hence, mucinous carcinoma with a festooned or papillary structure usually derives from papillary, micropapillary, or cribriform intraductal carcinoma. Comedocarcinoma is more commonly associated with invasive mucinous carcinomas in which tumor cells form sheets and broad trabeculae in the mucinous secretion.

The diagnosis of mucinous carcinoma may be suggested by material obtained on aspiration biopsy since the smears typically contain clusters of tumor cells and mucin.[6] However, some benign lesions, such as edematous fibroadenomas, some papillomas, and mucin-containing cysts, also must be considered.

PROGNOSIS. Mucinous carcinoma is regarded as a prognostically favorable variant of ductal carcinoma. With certain reservations, this conclusion appears warranted on the basis of the reported data.[238–240,243–246] However, the disease is sufficiently uncommon to prevent any one group of investigators from assembling enough cases to compare patients with mucinous carcinoma to those with nonmucinous carcinoma according to standard staging systems such as TNM. The term TNM has already been used in this chapter, for example, T1N0M0. Because of differences in reporting among published series, combined data cannot readily be assembled.

Most studies have compared the prognosis of patients treated for pure mucinous carcinoma with that of women who had mixed ductal-mucinous carcinoma or ordinary invasive ductal carcinoma. In these comparisons, pure mucinous carcinoma is associated with a lower frequency of metastases in axillary lymph nodes and fewer deaths

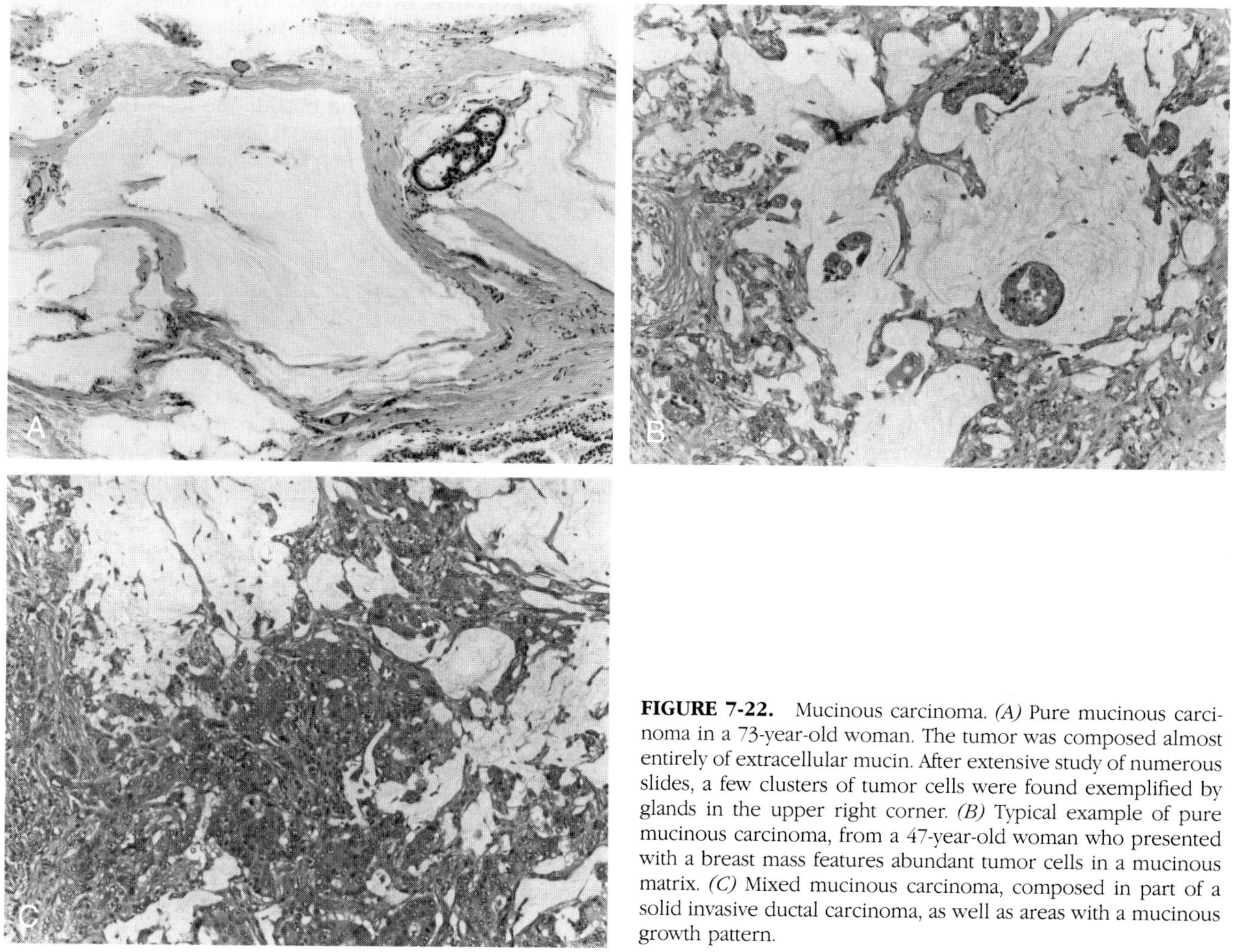

FIGURE 7-22. Mucinous carcinoma. *(A)* Pure mucinous carcinoma in a 73-year-old woman. The tumor was composed almost entirely of extracellular mucin. After extensive study of numerous slides, a few clusters of tumor cells were found exemplified by glands in the upper right corner. *(B)* Typical example of pure mucinous carcinoma, from a 47-year-old woman who presented with a breast mass features abundant tumor cells in a mucinous matrix. *(C)* Mixed mucinous carcinoma, composed in part of a solid invasive ductal carcinoma, as well as areas with a mucinous growth pattern.

attributable to breast carcinoma 5 and 10 years after treatment by mastectomy than are the ductal carcinomas.[240–246]

Systemic recurrences more than 10 years after mastectomy have been described by many investigators.[238–240] Geschickter observed recurrences 6 to 18 years after diagnosis among 14 of 59 patients with pure colloid carcinoma, and he concluded that "a period of 5 to 10 years of freedom from symptoms following treatment does not necessarily indicate permanent cure."[238] In a recent study of 41 patients with pure mucinous carcinoma who underwent follow-up for a mean of 16 years, 11 women (27%) developed recurrences and died of breast carcinoma.[241] Five of these deaths occurred 12 years or more after diagnosis. Most patients described in the literature were treated with radical or modified mastectomy. A few patients treated with simple or partial mastectomy have also done well with limited follow-up. Radiation treatment of a large, unresected, mucinous carcinoma that was diagnosed on incisional biopsy has also been reported.[257]

An unusual, fatal complication of mucinous carcinoma of the breast[258,259] and other organs is mucin embolism. This condition causes cerebral infarction.

Papillary Carcinoma

The problems in terminology associated with the diagnosis of papillary carcinoma have been reviewed by Fisher and associates[260] and Carter.[261] Lesions classified as papillary carcinoma have included intraductal carcinoma with a papillary configuration involving multiple ducts, solitary papillary carcinomas that often have a cystic component, and invasive carcinomas with a papillary growth pattern. The WHO's histological classification of breast tumors defined papillary carcinoma as "a rare carcinoma whose invasive pattern is predominantly in the form of papillary structures. The same architecture is usually displayed in the metastases. Frequently foci of intraductal papillary growth are recognizable."[3]

Separately, the WHO classification states that "papillary

Metaplasia also may occur in the glandular epithelium of benign mammary tumors, such as fibroadenomas and papillomas, and in nonneoplastic breast epithelium (e.g., ducts or cysts). The epithelium of many other glandular organs is also capable of metaplasia.

Two types of metaplastic mammary carcinoma are generally described: squamous and pseudosarcomatous. The former has been referred to as homologous because it retains an epithelial character, whereas the latter is termed heterologous because of its similarity to neoplasms of mesenchymal origin. The fact that squamous metaplasia may undergo further alteration to an undifferentiated spindle cell pseudosarcomatous pattern weakens the usefulness of this traditional distinction.[274]

The relative frequency with which metaplastic carcinoma occurs is difficult to ascertain because these neoplasms are not consistently described in routine pathology reports. Small foci of squamous metaplasia may not be noted in an otherwise typical mammary carcinoma. Some pathologists restrict their diagnoses to neoplasms that exhibit only pseudosarcomatous features, whereas others prefer alternative diagnostic terms, such as carcinosarcoma or mixed tumor of the breast. To some extent, squamous metaplasia occurs in approximately 2% of all mammary carcinomas, but it is a prominent feature in only a small fraction of these tumors. An exception to this is medullary carcinoma, 16% of which exhibit some squamous metaplasia.[147] Pseudosarcomatous metaplasia, which typically features bone, cartilage, or undifferentiated spindle cell elements, generates a greater level of interest and is, therefore usually noted in the diagnosis. Metaplastic carcinomas constitute fewer than 1% of breast carcinomas.

The mechanism by which metaplasia occurs is not well understood. Early concepts, which suggest that pseudosarcomatous metaplasia constitutes an alteration of the stroma induced by the adenocarcinoma, have largely been abandoned, and it is now widely accepted that the process evolves from altered epithelial cells. The strongest support for the current interpretation comes from electron microscopic studies.[274–278]

Uncertainty about the histogenesis of these carcinomas is reflected in confusing diagnostic terminology.[279] Carcinosarcoma is appropriate for malignant neoplasms that can be shown to contain distinct carcinomatous and sarcomatous components derived separately from epithelial and mesenchymal tissues (for example, carcinoma arising in a malignant cystosarcoma phyllodes with sarcomatous stroma). The term mixed tumor is not satisfactory because it creates confusion with neoplasms that more commonly develop in the salivary glands than in the breast.

CLINICAL PRESENTATION. The initial symptom of metaplastic carcinoma is almost always a mass. Secondary manifestations such as fixation of the tumor to the skin or underlying tissues occur, and skin ulceration has been reported with large lesions. The duration of symptoms rarely exceeds a few months. The age distribution and mean age at diagnosis correspond closely to those of breast carcinoma in general. Metaplastic carcinoma is not associated with bilaterality. Bone formation within the tumor may result in calcifications detectable on mammography, but not enough data are available to indicate a radiologic appearance that is specific for this type of carcinoma.

GROSS PATHOLOGY. Tumors ranging in size from less than 1 cm to more than 10 cm in diameter have been reported.[280–283] The size distribution approximates that of mammary carcinoma generally, with a mean size of 2 cm to 3 cm in the reported series. Gross appearance varies with the constituent parts, but most examples are described as hard, nodular, and well circumscribed. Cystic degeneration is common when there is extensive squamous metaplasia.

MICROSCOPIC PATHOLOGY. Squamous metaplasia has been observed in many of the standard histologic variants of breast carcinoma (Fig. 7-24). In these cases, the microscopic description is determined by the basic configuration of the tumor (e.g., medullary carcinoma with squamous metaplasia, or infiltrating ductal carcinoma with squamous metaplasia). Metaplastic epithelium may form a mature, keratinizing tissue with keratohyaline granules. Various gradations of less well-differentiated epithelium usually occur in the same specimen, with transitions to a spindle cell pseudosarcomatous appearance commonly present.[274] Recent reports have drawn attention to a spindle cell variant of squamous metaplastic carcinoma which is composed largely of less well-differentiated spindle cell elements and may, therefore, be mistaken for a sarcoma.

FIGURE 7-24. Squamous metaplasia in invasive ductal carcinoma, manifested in this case by three solid nodules of keratin pearl formation. Also evident are three glandular spaces, containing mucinous secretion, which are indicative of the underlying adenocarcinoma. The patient is a 63-year-old woman who presented with a 2-cm tumor.

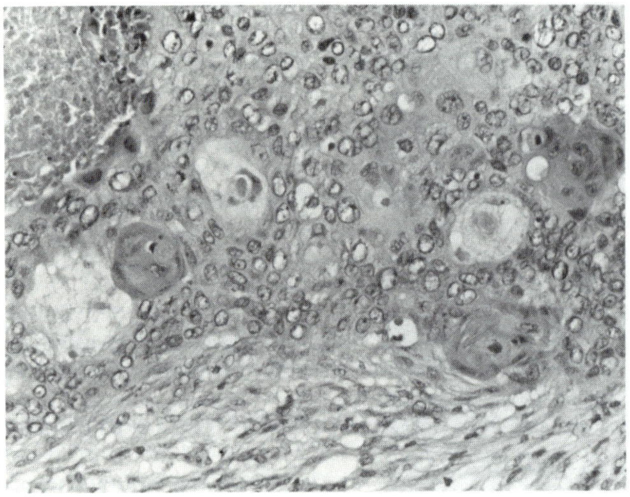

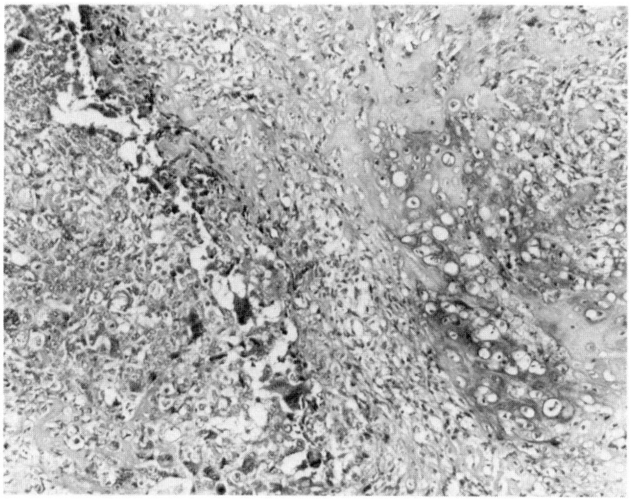

FIGURE 7-25. Sarcomatous metaplasia in invasive ductal carcinoma. Cartilage is evident on the right, and osteoid with osteoclasts is present on the left. A zone of undifferentiated spindle cell growth separates the two areas. At mastectomy, this 37-year-old patient had a 6-cm tumor and metastases in four axillary lymph nodes.

The presence of squamous areas detectable through sampling, as well as epithelial features detected on electron microscopy and immunohistochemistry, may be used to distinguish these lesions from sarcomas.[274,278]

Overt pseudosarcomatous differentiation is manifested by areas of cartilage or bone formation, or both, which may appear to be benign or malignant on histologic examination (Fig. 7-25). Undifferentiated pseudosarcomatous areas with spindle or round cell features, or both, may coexist with osteocartilaginous metaplasia, or they may be the only metaplastic element. Rarely, angiosarcomatous and myosarcomatous metaplasia may also be detectable. Infiltrating ductal carcinomas that develop pseudosarcomatous metaplasia tend to be poorly differentiated, but metaplasia does occur in well-differentiated tumors. Metastases resulting from a metaplastic carcinoma may also have metaplastic foci, generally with the same pattern as the primary tumor, but more often, they are entirely composed of adenocarcinoma.

PROGNOSIS. A proper assessment of prognosis would require a sufficient number of cases to allow consideration of tumor size; histologic type; grade; nodal status; the type, amount, and differentiation of the metaplastic component; and the form of treatment. No published series has been large enough to evaluate these factors independently, and many reports do not provide the necessary data. In general terms, it appears that metaplasia does not confer a favorable prognosis, and it appears likely that pseudosarcomatous metaplasia has an unfavorable impact on outcome, especially in patients with poorly differentiated carcinomas. Squamous metaplasia seems to have little effect prognostically, except for lesions with an extensive spindle cell component. These tend to be especially aggressive.

Data on prognosis are based almost entirely on patients treated with mastectomy. In a recent study of 26 women with pseudosarcomatous metaplasia, overall survival was 44%, with an estimated 5-year survival for TNM Stages I, II, and III of 56%, 26%, and 18%, respectively.[281] Axillary nodal metastases were detected in 25% of the patients. Responsiveness of metaplastic carcinoma to radiation and chemotherapy has not been determined.

Apocrine Carcinoma

The apocrine glands are normal cutaneous appendages that are concentrated in the skin of the axilla, groin, anogenital region, and other sites. Histologically, the cells that form these glands have abundant, pink, finely granular cytoplasm. At the luminal surface, the apical cytoplasm forms tufts or blebs characteristic of merocrine secretion. Nuclei, typically round with a small punctate nucleolus, are located near the base of the cell. Electron microscopy has demonstrated the presence of cytoplasmic secretory granules and abundant mitochondria in apocrine cells.[284]

A variety of benign proliferative breast lesions may contain cells that are cytologically identical to those of the apocrine glands. The phenomenon by which duct or lobular epithelial cells undergo this structural alteration is referred to as apocrine metaplasia. Apocrine metaplasia occurs most often in the lining of cysts and in papillary duct hyperplasia, but it may be encountered in fibroadenomas, sclerosing adenosis, and in other benign lesions. Histochemical and ultrastructural studies have consistently shown that the cells of apocrine metaplasia in the breast have many characteristics in common with the cells of normal cutaneous apocrine glands.[284–287] Because of the pink, variably granular or vacuolated cytoplasm of cells in apocrine metaplasia, they have also been referred to as oncocytes or pale cells.

Apocrine metaplastic epithelium exhibits a spectrum of cytologic appearances ranging from a cell population that is histologically identical to that of normal apocrine glands to extreme atypia. The degree of abnormality is judged on the basis of cytologic criteria, as well as the epithelial growth pattern. Analysis of the DNA content of nuclei in apocrine metaplasia by Izuo and co-workers has shown that tetraploid cells become significantly more numerous with increasing atypia.[288] The authors described one patient with aneuploid apocrine metaplasia who subsequently proved to have mammary carcinoma.

The precancerous significance of apocrine metaplasia has not been determined. Foote and Stewart compared the distribution of benign proliferative changes in the breasts of women with and without carcinoma and, after finding no difference in the distribution of apocrine metaplasia, concluded that it was not a precancerous change.[289] However, others have reported an association between papillary apocrine metaplasia in a benign breast biopsy and an increased risk for subsequent carcinoma.[290]

The cells in a small number of breast carcinomas have

a resemblance to apocrine cells. These lesions have been referred to as apocrine carcinomas. In most of these cases, the noncancerous breast contains areas of apocrine metaplasia that may exhibit varying degrees of atypia, but it is often difficult to demonstrate transitions to carcinoma. Electron microscopy has demonstrated that the cells of apocrine carcinomas have many ultrastructural features in common with the cells found in apocrine metaplasia and in the apocrine glands.[291–292]

Apocrine carcinoma generally has a ductal growth pattern, but rarely, cells with this appearance may be found in lobular carcinoma *in situ*.[293] Apocrine duct carcinoma exhibits a distinct tendency to involve lobular epithelium by direct intraepithelial extension. Apocrine carcinoma has been described arising in the male breast.[294] Until fairly recently, apocrine carcinoma was often classified under the heading of sweat gland carcinoma of the breast.[295,296] Although the latter term may occasionally be applied to breast carcinomas,[297] it is unsatisfactory because sweat gland carcinoma of the skin is a morphologically heterogenous disease in which only a small minority of tumors resemble mammary apocrine carcinoma.

Because many pathologists fail to recognize it as a specific histologic variant, the frequency of apocrine carcinoma is uncertain, and little is known about the clinical features of this tumor. Data from many papers describing "sweat gland" carcinoma are difficult to interpret because of uncertainty as to how many of the lesions were apocrine carcinomas. Frable and Kay compared 18 patients with apocrine carcinoma with 34 control subjects matched for clinicopathologic prognostic parameters and observed no significant difference in outcome between the two groups.[298] Apocrine features were present in 2.2% of carcinomas studied by Fisher and associates,[88] and this finding was not found to correlate significantly with prognosis. Data about pure apocrine carcinomas were not presented in their report.

All six patients with apocrine carcinoma studied by one group of investigators had low levels of estrogen and progesterone receptor protein.[292] *In vitro* studies have demonstrated enhanced metabolism of testosterone precursors by apocrine carcinomas when compared with other types of carcinoma.[299] This observation has not been correlated with levels of androgen receptors or clinical response to hormonal treatment, but is of considerable interest because the growth of cutaneous apocrine glands is stimulated by androgens,[300] and some androgen metabolites have been found to be concentrated in axillary secretions.[301]

Adenoid Cystic Carcinoma

These lesions constitute less than 0.1% of mammary carcinomas. Disproportionate interest in this type of carcinoma stems from its favorable prognosis and distinctive histopathologic appearance, which is identical to that of comparable tumors that originate in the salivary glands. Adenoid cystic carcinoma arising in both sites is prone to microscopic invasion of the perineural spaces.

Cylindroma, a term used synonymously with adenoid cystic carcinoma, was apparently introduced by Billroth to describe his concept that the tumor is composed of entwined cylinders of hyaline stroma and cylinders of tumor cells. Ewing[302] referred to adenoid cystic carcinoma of the salivary glands, and a similar term was first used with reference to mammary tumors by Geschickter in 1945 when he described four breast lesions as "adenocystic basal cell cancer."[303] Foote and Stewart mentioned three examples of adenoid cystic carcinoma of the breast in 1946.[1] Reports of single cases were published in the succeeding two decades until 1966, when Galloway and colleagues summarized data on 9 new cases from the Mayo Clinic and 12 others that had been reported previously.[304]

CLINICAL PRESENTATION. The age distribution of adenoid cystic carcinoma parallels that which is generally observed in breast cancer. Cases may be diagnosed in patients between the ages of 38 and 80 years, with the mean age at diagnosis in studies with five or more cases ranging from 50 to 63 years.[305] The majority of patients are women, but this type of carcinoma has also been described in the male breast.[306,307] There appears to be no predilection for either breast to be affected, and the disease is not associated with bilaterality. However, patients with adenoid cystic carcinoma have been reported to have other types of carcinoma in the opposite breast,[308,309] or rarely, elsewhere in the same breast.[310]

The typical presenting symptom is a tumor which may be painful or tender. Large or superficial lesions may exhibit changes in the overlying skin, such as ulceration, peau d'orange, or dimpling. Although any part of the breast may be affected, adenoid cystic carcinoma occurs with disproportionately high frequency in the central or subareolar region, but is not associated with nipple discharge. Most patients report the tumor to have been present for days or weeks before seeking medical attention, but intervals of from 18 months to 15 years have been described in a number of patients.[304,305] A small number of tumors analyzed have been negative for estrogen and progesterone receptors.[311]

GROSS PATHOLOGY. Reported examples of adenoid cystic carcinoma range in diameter from 2 mm to 12 cm, with the majority measuring between 1 cm and 3 cm.[304,305,308,312] The grey to pale yellow cut surface reveals a neoplasm with well-defined margins that may appear to be circumscribed. Focal cystic areas may occur in tumors less than 5 cm in diameter; larger lesions tend to undergo cystic degeneration.[304,313]

MICROSCOPIC PATHOLOGY. Figure 7-26 illustrates the characteristic microscopic appearance of adenoid cystic carcinoma, which features a mixture of glandular (adenoid component) and stromal or basement membrane material (cystic, pseudoglandular, or cylindromatous component). Within a given tumor, one may find substantial heterogeneity in the organization of these elements. Some microscopic fields will consist entirely of the adenoid elements,

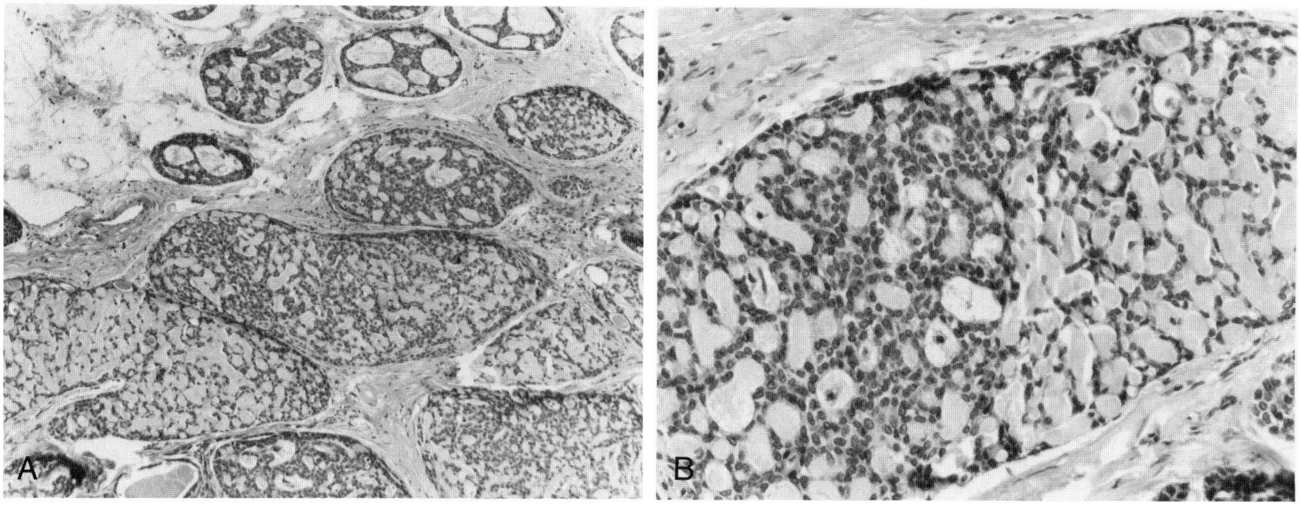

FIGURE 7-26. Adenoid cystic carcinoma. *(A)* The tumor consists of circumscribed masses of tumor cells. Because much of the lesion may have this growth pattern, an intraductal component may be difficult to identify. In the upper central part of the picture, the adenoid structure of the lesion resembles cribriform intraductal carcinoma, whereas in the lower half, a cylindromatous component is more prominent. *(B)* A high-power view shows a cylindromatous area on the left where tumor cells surround cords of basement membrane material. An adenoid pattern is evident on the right where tumor cells encircle round to oval glandular spaces containing mucin.

thereby bearing a close resemblance to cribriform carcinoma.[314] Other portions of the lesion may be highly endowed with the stromal material and lacking in glandular elements. Such areas may be misinterpreted as scirrhous carcinoma. Because of this diversity, adenoid cystic carcinoma may not be recognizable in a small needle biopsy sample unless the typical constellation of features is represented. Adenoid cystic carcinoma may be diagnosed on the basis of a needle aspiration smear when globules of cylindromatous material and adenoid gland clusters are present.[315,316]

Clusters of tumor cells at the invasive edges of adenoid cystic carcinoma tend to shrink and separate from the surrounding stroma. This appearance simulates the pattern of tumor invasion of lymphatics. True lymphatic invasion is extremely uncommon in adenoid cystic carcinoma.

It has been claimed that electron microscopy and mucin histochemistry may be of diagnostic assistance in distinguishing between true glandular lumens and the cylindromatous element.[306,308,310,311,314] However, electron microscopy may be misleading if the cylindromatous component is absent in the small sample studied from an otherwise typical adenoid cystic carcinoma. With an adequate number of histologic sections of an excised lesion, it is rarely necessary to employ histochemical studies to diagnose adenoid cystic carcinoma. The electron microscopic features of adenoid cystic carcinoma of the salivary glands and breast are identical.[317]

PROGNOSIS. With few exceptions, published data on the prognosis of patients with adenoid cystic carcinoma relate to those treated with modified or standard radical mastectomy. Axillary metastases have been described in one case.[318] Recurrence has been reported in the breast as late as 7 years following treatment with local excision alone,[308,312] and tumor recurrence in the chest wall has occurred after simple mastectomy.[319] Distant metastases have been described in seven patients,[320] four of whom died, apparently from adenoid cystic carcinoma with pulmonary involvement.[311,316] Intervals of up to 9 years have been reported before lung lesions have appeared.[316–320]

Squamous Carcinoma

A mammary carcinoma must be composed entirely of squamous carcinoma to be diagnosed as this extremely uncommon neoplasm. Since keratinizing epithelium is not a normal constituent of breast glandular tissue, the presence of squamous carcinoma in this organ must be regarded as a form of metaplasia. However, pure squamous carcinoma of the breast is usually considered to be a pathologic entity that is distinct from the group of metaplastic carcinomas in which adenocarcinoma is found to give rise to squamous or sarcomatous metaplasia.

The histogenesis of squamous carcinoma of the breast remains unexplained. It is likely that two pathways exist for these tumors to arise. Some lesions represent an extreme variant of metaplastic carcinoma. In these tumors, a residual component of the original adenocarcinoma from which the squamous carcinoma arose may be overlooked because of limited sampling, or the adenocarcinoma may have been destroyed by growth of the squamous component.

Metaplasia to histologically benign squamous epithelium probably also occurs as a precursor lesion. Squamous metaplasia has been observed in the glandular epithelium of the breast, and has been associated with benign conditions, such as fibroadenomas,[321] benign cystosarcoma phyllodes, papillomas,[322] and gynecomastia.[323] Benign squamous metaplasia is occasionally found in the epithelium of hyperplastic mammary ducts, in the lining of cysts in ordinary proliferative breast lesions ("fibrocystic disease"), and in extensive duct hyperplasia or papillomatosis.[324] Benign squamous metaplasia may be induced in organ cultures of human breast tissue,[325] a phenomenon enhanced by high concentrations of insulin.[326] Chemical carcinogens cause this alteration in murine mammary[327] and prostate glands[328] *in vitro*. It has recently been suggested that cyclic adenine nucleotide may be the primary mediator of benign squamous metaplasia in human breast epithelium. Tissues from patients who were in the early part of the menstrual cycle at the time of biopsy were less susceptible to the induction of squamous metaplasia than were those obtained in the latter third of the cycle. This observation suggests that progesterone or estrogen, or both, may promote the process.[329]

CLINICAL PRESENTATION. The clinical features of squamous carcinoma of the breast are not distinctive. The age distribution, which is 31 to 83 years, encompasses much the same range as breast carcinoma in general.[330,331] The average age in one review of 20 cases was 57 years, and 50% of the patients were 60 years or older.[330]

Two-thirds of the cases of primary squamous carcinoma occur in the left breast.[331] Large tumors may be fixed to the skin or deep structures, and skin ulceration may occur. No consistent mammographic features have been described.[332,333] Calcification in the squamous tissue may be seen on x-ray examination. These tumors are estrogen receptor-negative.[330,334]

GROSS PATHOLOGY. Squamous carcinomas vary in diameter from 1 cm to more than 10 cm, but tend to be relatively larger than other forms of breast carcinoma. Approximately 50% of the reported cases involve a lesion 5 cm or more in diameter. Cystic degeneration is very common, especially in tumors larger than 2 cm in diameter. Hemorrhage and accumulated necrotic squamous debris fill the cavity. When keratinizing epithelium predominates, the tumor tissue will be relatively soft and granular. Extensive spindle cell metaplasia results in a firm to hard lesion.

MICROSCOPIC PATHOLOGY. The diagnosis of primary squamous carcinoma of the breast may be made only after excluding metastasis from an extramammary primary lesion.[330] Tumors responsible for metastatic squamous carcinoma in the breast have been reported to originate in the lung, uterine cervix, esophagus, and urinary bladder, as well as in other sites. Generally, the existence of an extramammary primary tumor is evident on clinical examination. Unfortunately, this information may not be provided to the pathologist if the physician and surgeon do not consider a metastatic lesion when evaluating a patient with a breast tumor.

The microscopic appearance of squamous carcinoma of the breast is indistinguishable by light microscopy from that of similar carcinomas that arise in numerous other sites. Many of the lesions are histologically well differentiated and produce substantial keratin. Ultrastructural studies have confirmed the squamous character of the tissue,[335] but intracellular canaliculi observed in some cells suggest that glandular features may persist in these tumors.[334] Immunohistochemical markers for intracellular keratin are strongly reactive with squamous mammary carcinoma.

Transformation from a squamous epithelial pattern to spindle cell pseudosarcomatous growth occurs, to some extent, in most squamous carcinomas of the breast. This phenomenon, which is also found in other sites,[336] may produce a tumor that is largely composed of the spindle cell component,[337] currently referred to as spindle cell carcinoma.[274,338] Extreme examples of this process are tumors that are virtually indistinguishable from a fibrosarcoma. Extensive sampling of the tumor, immunohistochemical studies, and electron microscopy may be necessary to determine that the tumor is a carcinoma. A needle or incisional biopsy of such a lesion is likely to be interpreted as sarcoma.

PROGNOSIS. Data describing the treatment and follow-up course of these patients are variable or incomplete in reported cases. Most patients have been treated with mastectomy, usually with an axillary dissection. Postoperative radiotherapy and chemotherapy were administered in some cases. Of 15 women without axillary lymph node metastases, 8 were alive and free of disease with follow-up periods ranging from 1 to 12 years, and 2 died of other causes 7 and 8 years after treatment. Five women who had negative axillary lymph nodes died of metastatic carcinoma 4 to 30 months after diagnosis. One patient with axillary lymph node metastases died 17 months after treatment, whereas two others were alive and well after 16 months and 6 years of follow-up. Local recurrence has been reported. Metastases usually involve the bones and the lungs.

Mammary Carcinoma With Osteoclast-like Giant Cells

Carcinomas containing benign, osteoclast-like, multinucleated, giant cells have been described in the pancreas, thyroid, lung, and breast. Fewer than 50 examples of such breast carcinomas have been reported.[339,340] Although individual cases had been described previously, it was not until 1979 that the first series was reported.[341] The giant cells are found within the stroma of the tumor, and the condition is often associated with hemorrhage, lymphocytic reaction, and increased vascularity.[341] Electron microscopic and immunohistochemical studies have shown that the giant cells have histiocytic properties, and are derived from stroma associated with the tumor.[342–345]

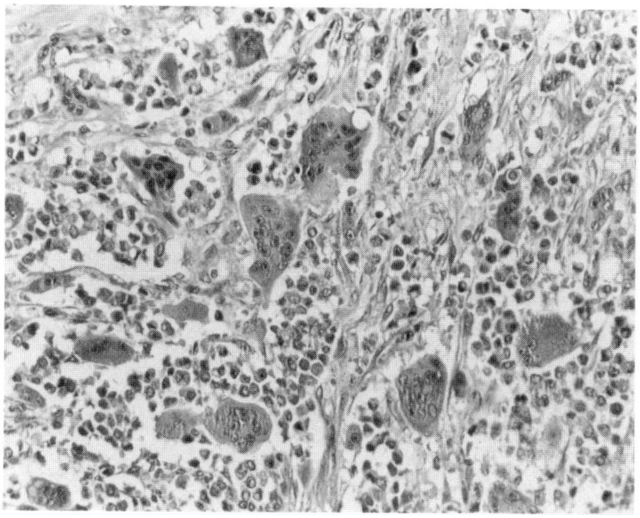

FIGURE 7-27. Infiltrating lobular carcinoma with osteoclast-like giant cells featuring multinucleated cells are distributed among infiltrating small carcinoma cells. The patient was a 43-year-old woman with a 3.5-cm tumor that had been present for 5 months. At mastectomy, a grossly circumscribed, reddish, firm lesion was found. There were no lymph node metastases. The patient died of metastatic disease 7 years after mastectomy.

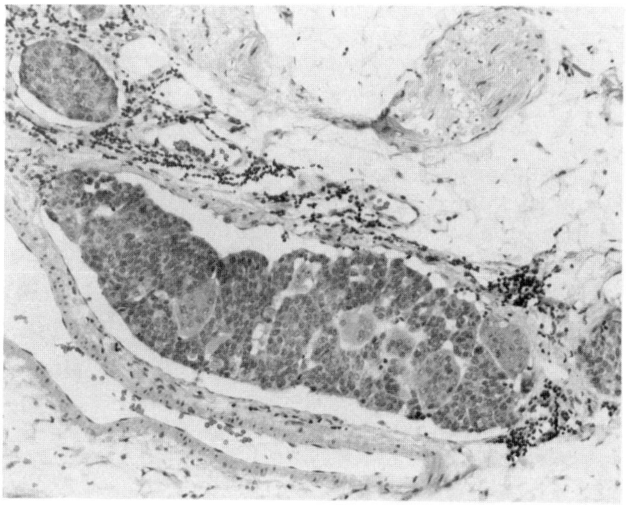

FIGURE 7-28. Intralymphatic tumor embolus with osteoclast-like giant cells. This remarkable phenomenon indicates that histologically benign cells of stromal origin may be transported with metastasizing tumor cells.

Patients with this type of carcinoma range in age from 32 to 84 years. The average age of 20 patients included in three recent reviews was 53 years.[341,343,344] The majority of the tumors occur in the upper outer quadrant of the breast, but the lesion has been found in all quadrants. On mammography, the well-circumscribed contour observed in many cases may suggest a benign lesion, such as a cyst or fibroadenoma.[344]

The excised tumor usually has a striking, characteristic gross appearance when bisected. The dark brown or red-brown tumor tissue tends to bulge slightly above the surrounding breast parenchyma, from which it is generally separated by a rounded, well-defined margin. On gross inspection, the lesion may suggest heavily pigmented metastatic melanoma, but it tends to be brown rather than black. The reported diameter in 22 cases ranged from 0.5 cm to 10 cm, and averaged 3.2 cm. Nine tumors were 2.0 cm or less in diameter.

Microscopically, the majority of these lesions are invasive ductal carcinomas (Fig. 7-27). Uncommon examples of infiltrating lobular,[341] papillary[341] and mucinous[343] carcinomas with osteoclast-like giant cells have been reported. The giant cells are characteristically closely approximated to the periphery of carcinomatous glands, and may be found in the glandular lumens as well. Extravascular erythrocytes, hemosiderin, and lymphocytes are typically present in the surrounding, highly vascular stroma. Erythrophagocytosis by the giant cells is uncommon. Inconspicuous metaplastic foci with spindle cells and squamous or osseous features have been described in a minority of cases.[341]

Osteoclast-like, multinucleated giant cells have been observed within intralymphatic tumor emboli (Fig. 7-28), in regional lymph node metastases, and in distant metastases, but not all metastatic foci contain these giant cells. Absence of Factor VIII activity from giant cells suggests they are not of endothelial origin.[343] It has been postulated that one or more substances produced by the neoplastic cells in these tumors induces the formation of the giant cells, and that that same process is linked to the accompanying vascularity and hemorrhage.

Axillary lymph node metastases have been reported in approximately one-third of cases. Follow-up is relatively short in many cases because this type of carcinoma has not, until recently, been widely recognized. Local recurrence[344] and systemic metastases to the eye, liver, and other organs have been described.[341] Nearly two-thirds of affected patients have been reported to be alive and well, with follow-up rarely exceeding 5 years. Although most of these tumors have demonstrated low levels of estrogen receptor, many have remarkably high levels of progesterone receptors.[344]

Secretory Carcinoma

Although breast carcinoma is extraordinarily uncommon in children, many of the various histologic types found in adults have also been described in children.[346] As one of the least common forms of mammary carcinoma, secretory or juvenile carcinoma is noteworthy for its tendency to occur relatively more frequently, but not exclusively, in children. For this reason, the term secretory carcinoma is preferable to juvenile carcinoma in describing this tumor since its microscopic appearance is identical in children and adults. This is a morphologically distinctive tumor with low-grade clinical features.

The first full description of secretory carcinoma was published in 1966 by McDivitt and Stewart in a report based on seven patients who ranged in age from 3 to 15 years, averaging 9 years.[347] In 1972, Oberman and Stephens[348] referred to secretory carcinoma that was diagnosed in two women aged 25 and 56 years, and Oberman later described four additional instances of this carcinoma in women 22 to 73 years old.[349] A review of the experience at the Armed Forces Institute of Pathology yielded a report on 19 patients in 1980.[350] Their median age was 25 years (ranging from 9 to 69 years), and six were 30 years of age or older. One patient was a 9-year-old boy. Three additional adult cases have been described,[351] and there have been reports of single cases in children.[352–355]

Secretory carcinoma does not occur with especial frequency in any particular part of the breast. A few lesions have been subareolar, and these may present with nipple discharge. In most cases, the primary symptom is a painless mass that may be present for years before biopsy.[349] No clinical evidence of an associated hormonal abnormality has been reported. The development of these tumors has not been related to pregnancy or lactation in children, most of whom have been nulliparous.

The excised tumor appears to be circumscribed or discrete in most cases, but infiltrative margins have been described. Color varies from white to grey or yellow to tan. Most tumors have been less than 3 cm in diameter, but lesions with diameters of up to 12 cm have been reported.

Microscopically, the tumor typically exhibits papillary and solid areas of growth. It is composed of cells with abundant, pale to clear or amphophilic cytoplasm and small, round, cytologically low-grade nuclei (Fig. 7-29). Abundant secretion, which is positive on periodic-acid Schiff (PAS) and mucin stains, is found within tumor cells and glandular spaces formed by the tumor cells. Rarely, portions of the lesion may have granular, eosinophilic cytoplasm and a nuclear cytology suggesting apocrine carcinoma. In most cases, the periphery exhibits a pushing or circumscribed margin microscopically, but invasive foci are not unusual. Intraductal carcinoma, generally with a secretory appearance, may be found within or at the periphery of some tumors.

Coexistence of secretory carcinoma with juvenile papillomatosis has been reported in two cases.[356] In one patient, secretory carcinoma appeared to arise from juvenile papillomatosis in the same breast. The other patient had juvenile papillomatosis in one breast and secretory carcinoma in the other breast.

The prognosis for these patients is exceptionally favorable. Although most children and adults have been treated with mastectomy, a few have been free of disease 7 to 15 years after excisional biopsy.[347,348] Axillary metastases have been described,[350–352,354] but probably occur in no more than 20% of the cases, rarely involving more than three lymph nodes. Most of the patients with positive lymph nodes have been older than 20 years of age. Recurrence in the breast has been described by several authors.[347,348,350,352] In one case, axillary metastases were first evident in a 19-year-old patient at the time of a local recurrence, 7 years after local excision of the primary tumor. Another patient developed a recurrence in the breast 21 years after initial excision, which was performed at 4 years of age.[348] Patients with axillary metastases have been reported to be well for as long as 6 years after primary therapy. One patient who had eight positive lymph nodes developed distant metastases and died less than a year after diagnosis.[350]

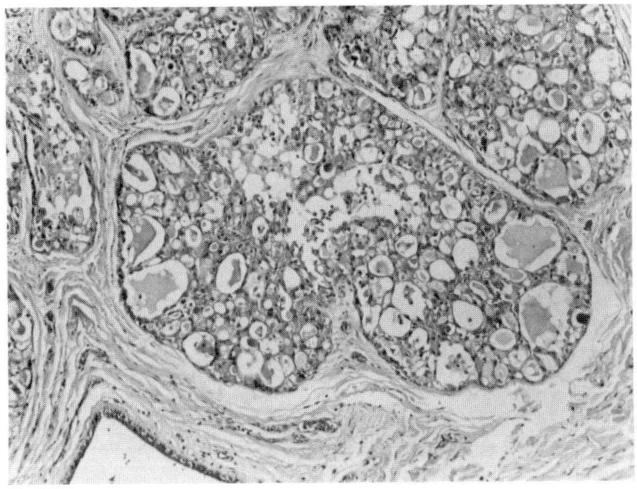

FIGURE 7-29. Secretory carcinoma was found on biopsy of the breast of an elderly woman. The tumor exhibits a typical lobulated, growth pattern composed of expanded ducts filled with small glands that contain secretion.

Wide local excision is the preferred initial treatment in children found to have secretory carcinoma. Since axillary lymph node metastases occur so infrequently in this age group, axillary dissection would be indicated only if the clinical examination suggested nodal involvement. Long-term follow-up is imperative because of the indolent nature of the disease and the risk of later recurrence. In adult patients, local excision may also be appropriate, and should be combined with dissection of the lower axillary lymph nodes. For large tumors or those with unsatisfactory margins, mastectomy or primary radiotherapy should also be considered.

Lipid-Rich Carcinoma

Only a few examples of lipid-rich carcinoma, an extremely rare variant of infiltrating ductal carcinoma, have been described.[357–359] This tumor is composed of cells that contain abundant lipid which, when processed for histologic sections, may be extracted, leaving clear, vacuolated cytoplasm. The tumor cells, which have been described as having small, round, uniform nuclei, resemble those found in clear cell renal carcinoma. The presence of lipid may be demonstrated in frozen sections of fresh tissue, on electron microscopy, or in tissue prepared by special processes that preserve cytoplasmic lipids. The disease was first described by Aboumrad and co-workers in a case report.[357] Subsequently, these authors found one other example among 100 breast carcinomas, and estimated the frequency of lipid-rich carcinoma to be 1%.

Ramos and Taylor described 13 cases which they felt had the characteristic pattern of lipid-rich carcinoma on routine histologic sections.[358] However, they were able to demonstrate lipid in only four cases in which unfixed specimens were available. The other nine were identified retrospectively among 900 cases on the basis of histologic pattern alone. Eleven of the 12 patients treated with radical mastectomy had axillary lymph node metastases. Follow-up studies revealed that six patients died of metastatic disease and two were alive with recurrence. The remainder were alive and disease-free, with the majority undergoing follow-up for less than 2 years.

Additional studies of a larger series are required before it can be determined whether this condition is a morphologically and clinically distinctive type of carcinoma. Cells that appear to have clear vacuolated cytoplasm have been described in histologic reports on sections of benign breast lesions, in various types of breast carcinoma,[360] and in occult mammary carcinoma presenting with axillary lymph node metastases.[226] Thus far, these clear cell forms of breast carcinoma have not been studied for lipid.

Cystic Hypersecretory Carcinoma

Cystic hypersecretory carcinoma is a recently described, multicystic variant of ductal carcinoma of the breast.[361] Affected patients, who have ranged in age from 39 to 78 years (with a mean age of 54 years), have presented with masses of at least 2 cm in diameter, with the diameter of the largest tumor being 10 cm. When examined grossly, the tumors have been composed of numerous cysts containing viscid secretion that has been described variously as thyroid-like, colloid-like, and gelatinous.

Microscopic examination reveals dilated ducts and cysts containing homogeneous, eosinophilic material resembling thyroid colloid (Fig. 7-30). Histochemical study of the secreted material yields positive reactions for mucin, CEA, and α-lactalbumin. The secretion is uniformly negative for thyroglobulin. Many cysts are lined by flat, inconspicuous epithelial cells, but transitions to a micropapillary, intraductal carcinoma growth pattern are found in the tumor. Generally, the best evidence of intraductal carcinoma may be found in nondilated ducts in the stroma between the cysts, rather than in the cysts themselves. When biopsy, rather than excision, of such a tumor is performed, the sample obtained may consist largely of cysts, with few diagnostic foci of intraductal carcinoma. In cases in which these biopsy specimens have been diagnosed as cystic disease, failure to excise the remainder of the tumor has been followed by continued growth of the lesion.

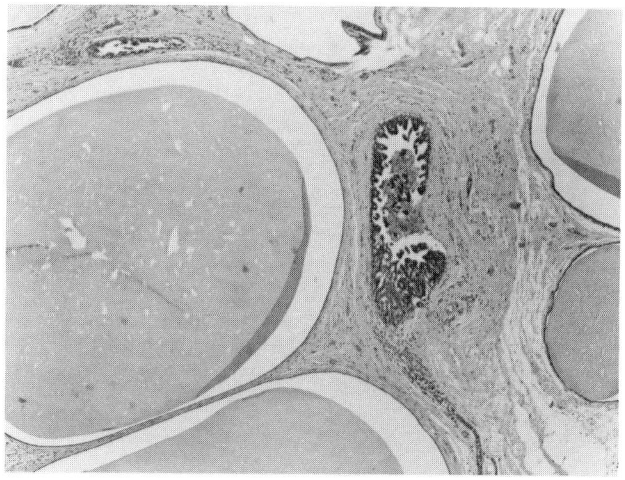

FIGURE 7-30. Cystic hypersecretory carcinoma, characterized by cystically dilated ducts filled with homogeneous eosinophilic secretion and intervening ducts with micropapillary intraductal carcinoma.

Because this very uncommon form of breast carcinoma has only recently been described, little is known about its clinical course. Coexistent invasive carcinoma, appearing to originate in cystic hypersecretory ductal carcinoma, has been observed in 2 of 10 cases. One woman, who presented with the clinical features of inflammatory carcinoma, died of systemic metastases. The other patient had metastasis to a single axillary lymph node detected on mastectomy, and was well 6 months later. Eight patients who had only intraductal carcinoma remained well during a maximum follow-up period of 2 years after mastectomy.

Infiltrating Lobular Carcinoma

The concept that invasive carcinoma could arise from the mammary lobules appears in some of the earliest discussions of the epithelial origin of mammary carcinoma. More than a century ago, Cornil[4] and Waldeyer[5] illustrated invasive carcinomas with the linear growth pattern that is now associated with the diagnosis of invasive lobular carcinoma. They traced the origin of the process to carcinoma within lobules, an observation that was subsequently confirmed by Salomon,[362] (Fig. 7-31) as well as Cheatle and Cutler[363] (Fig. 7-32).

In 1941, Foote and Stewart published a description of lobular carcinoma *in situ,* noting that "when the tumor infiltrates, it is apt to do so in a peculiar fashion which permits one, after some experience, to recognize the high probability of such origin . . ."[7] The "peculiar" characteristics of infiltrating lobular carcinoma include an accompanying desmoplastic stromal reaction, a linear arrangement of tumor cells, and a tendency to grow circumferentially around ducts and lobules. The latter two patterns, now commonly referred to as Indian-file and targetoid growth, respectively, are important histologic features defining this type of invasive mammary carcinoma.

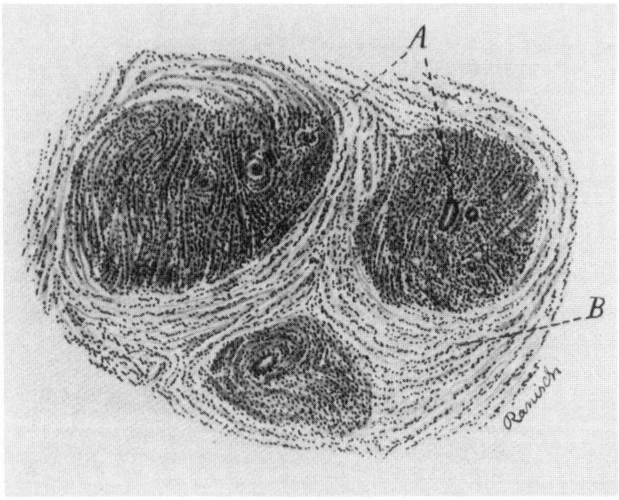

FIGURE 7-31. Classic infiltrating lobular carcinoma exhibits a linear, perilobular, and periductal growth pattern (as illustrated by Salomon in 1913[362].

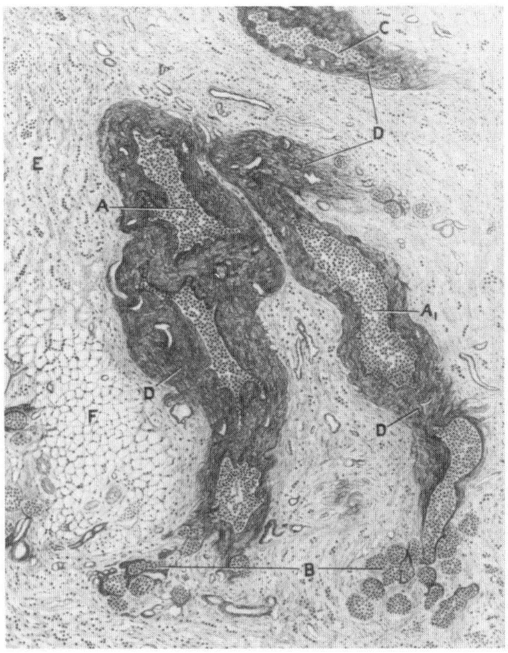

FIGURE 7-32. *In situ* lobular carcinoma in the terminal duct and lobule has given rise to invasive lobular carcinoma in the surrounding breast (*E* and *F*), as illustrated by Cheatle and Cutler.[363]

Foote and Stewart pointed out that invasive lobular carcinoma was not always accompanied by an *in situ* lobular component, but concluded that the histologic pattern was sufficiently distinct to warrant designation as a specific type of mammary carcinoma. In a subsequent description, they noted that the tumor growth featured "thread-like strands of tumor cells rather loosely dispersed throughout a fibrous matrix," with "no tendency for the cells to simulate atypical lobules." They further commented that "sheet-like growth is distinctly uncharacteristic." The presence of "central mucoid globules" (or signet ring cells) and the small size of the tumor cells, which may lead to an incorrect diagnosis of lymphoma, were additional features described by Foote and Stewart.[1,7]

Few studies of infiltrating lobular carcinoma have appeared in the succeeding 25 years, and those few consist largely of case reports documenting progression from *in situ* lobular carcinoma.[68,85,364–366] In 1966, Newman reported that invasive lobular carcinoma constituted 5% of 1436 carcinomas treated during a 17-year period at a single hospital.[367]

A review of over 21,000 breast carcinomas diagnosed in the United States from 1969 to 1971 found that only 3% were classified as infiltrating lobular carcinomas.[368] At Memorial Sloan-Kettering Cancer Center, 4.2% of carcinomas diagnosed from 1956 to 1970 were classified as pure infiltrating lobular carcinomas.[20] With the less restrictive microscopic criteria that have been advocated in recent years, the lesion has been reported to constitute 10% to 14% of all invasive carcinomas.[247,369,370]

CLINICAL PRESENTATION. Infiltrating lobular carcinoma occurs with the same age distribution as breast carcinoma (26 to 86 years) generally. The median age at diagnosis in various series ranges from 45 to 56 years for the pure forms.[367,369,371–373] In a study of carcinoma at the extremes of age, infiltrating lobular carcinoma constituted only 2% of the lesions diagnosed in women 35 years of age or younger, and 11% of the carcinomas found in women 75 years or older.[374] A review of 1024 patients treated at Memorial Sloan-Kettering Cancer Center between 1976 and 1978 yielded a report of 70 infiltrating lobular carcinomas (6.8% of patients). The mean age of these patients was 57 years, which is identical to that of 676 women treated for infiltrating ductal carcinoma.[40] One study, which compared patients with pure and variant forms of the disease, found a younger median age at diagnosis in patients with variant tumors (47 years) than in those with pure forms (53 years).[372] However, others have reported that patients with a solid variant were, on average, older (median of 63 years of age) than were women with classic infiltrating, lobular carcinoma (median of 56 years of age).[369]

Virtually all patients with infiltrating lobular carcinoma present with a tumor, which is located most frequently in the upper outer quadrant of the breast. The lesions tend to have ill-defined margins, and occasionally, the only evidence of a tumor is a subtle thickening or induration. Skin retraction, fixation, and other signs of advanced local disease accompany large lesions. Nipple discharge and Paget's disease are not symptoms of pure infiltrating lobular carcinoma, but may occur when there is a concurrent ductal carcinoma. Rarely, Paget's disease results from direct extension of an underlying infiltrating lobular carcinoma to the nipple.

Calcifications are not ordinarily formed by infiltrating lobular carcinoma; therefore, this feature cannot be relied upon for diagnosis by mammography. Lack of definite margins and a tendency to grow in multiple foci throughout the breast are other features that may obscure the lesion on radiographic studies.

Patients with infiltrating lobular carcinoma are especially prone to bilateral carcinoma. Prior and concurrent carcinoma of the opposite breast has been reported in 6% to 28% of cases.[227,367,373,375] Subsequent contralateral carcinoma occurs in 9% to 14% of patients initially diagnosed as having infiltrating lobular carcinoma.[369,375] The majority of synchronous and metachronous contralateral tumors have a lobular component or are pure lobular carcinomas, with 50% or more being invasive carcinomas.[227,373,375]

Approximately 50% of infiltrating lobular carcinomas are classified as estrogen receptor-positive, a proportion that is not significantly different from that found in infiltrating ductal carcinomas.[29] The median estrogen receptor-positive concentration in 55 tumors was 10 fmol/mg of cytosol protein. The alveolar variant is reported to have especially high concentrations of estrogen receptor protein.[374]

GROSS PATHOLOGY. Infiltrating lobular carcinomas range in size from microscopic lesions to tumors that diffusely infiltrate the entire breast. On average, the size of these lesions does not differ appreciably from that of infiltrating ductal carcinomas.

The excised carcinoma is usually firmer than the surrounding breast parenchyma, but the margins tend to be indistinct in many cases, and the tumor tissue may not be visibly abnormal. Infiltrating lobular carcinoma is not prone to cyst formation, necrosis, hemorrhage, or calcification. Occasional lesions are distinctly tan, a feature associated with the more cellular variants of the disease.

Uncommon and exceptional gross forms of infiltrating lobular carcinoma exist, one of which has been described graphically by Foote and Stewart.[1] They noted that the "specimen may present no distinctly visible lesion and yet contain a palpable area of peculiar induration, the precise limits of which are vague. . . . After the diagnosis of cancer is made, it is well to be prepared for querulousness from the operating surgeon who understandably would like to be operating for something more finite than indistinct induration."[1]

The other gross manifestation of infiltrating lobular carcinoma may be minute, distinct, firm nodules that feel like grains of sand buried in the breast tissue. When such areas are the only evidence of carcinoma, the disease may be difficult to distinguish, both grossly and microscopically, from sclerosing adenosis. Vague induration or minute, sand-like nodules may be the only gross evidence of carcinoma on biopsy of the contralateral breast when the opposite breast is considered to be normal on clinical examination.

MICROSCOPIC PATHOLOGY. Newman, who published the first series of patients with infiltrating lobular carcinoma, found that 142 tumors had features of infiltrating lobular carcinoma.[367] However, on further review, he determined that only 73 fulfilled his criteria for pure disease (Fig. 7-33).[367] In making this distinction, he sought to exclude cases in which there was a prominent, duct-forming component, or in which the growth pattern was not predominantly linear, as originally described by Foote and Stewart.[1]

The difficulty which Newman faced in assigning tumors to the category of invasive lobular carcinoma persists today. The histologic definition of this type of mammary carcinoma has become one of the least precise of the major categories of breast carcinoma listed in present classification schemes. This is because one rarely finds a tumor composed only of the histologic pattern described by Foote and Stewart.[1] Many tumors exhibiting areas of classic infiltrating lobular carcinoma also have components with other features (Fig. 7-34). In the last decade, these variants of infiltrating lobular carcinoma, described as tubular, solid, and alveolar forms of the lesion, have considerably extended this diagnosis to include a larger group of lesions.[369,370,372,373,376]

A tubulolobular form of this carcinoma contains glands of the type usually found in tubular carcinoma, and cells with the growth pattern of invasive lobular carcinoma.[370,377] Fechner described a variant group of tumors composed in part of trabeculae or broad sheets of tumor cells with cytologic features identical to those of cells in other areas growing in the classic pattern.[372] Other than the structural distinction, no outstanding clinical or pathologic differences were found between cases of pure carcinoma and cases of solid variant carcinoma. Other researchers have commented on an alveolar arrangement of tumor cells in groups that appear, on histologic sections, as rounded masses.[369,370,374] Finally, it has been noted that many tumors have combinations or mixtures of the classic and variant patterns. Dixon and co-workers classified 103 cases of infiltrating lobular carcinoma in the following manner: classic, 30%; mixed, 29%; solid, 22%; and alveolar, 19%.[369]

The cytology of cells found within infiltrating lobular carcinomas has received less attention than has the growth pattern of the tumor. In classic lesions, the invasive tumor cells are usually described as having small, round nuclei without prominent nucleoli, and a limited amount of cytoplasm. Intracytoplasmic lumina, containing mucinous secretion that reacts with mucicarmine and alcian blue stains, are found in a variable proportion of the cells.[72,74] When a cell contains a prominent, large, cytoplasmic, mucin vacuole that pushes the nucleus peripherally, the cell has a signet ring cell configuration. The name signet ring cell carcinoma has been applied to a group of tumors composed of such cells. The majority are variants of infiltrating lobular carcinoma,[72,74,247,378] but this cytologic appearance is also found in ductal carcinomas.[215,379,380]

Neurosecretory granules with dense cores have been detected on electron microscopy in invasive lobular carcinoma.[381] It is possible that a recently described, small cell, neuroendocrine (oat cell) carcinoma of the breast is a variant of infiltrating lobular carcinoma.[382,383]

PROGNOSIS. When it metastasizes, infiltrating lobular carcinoma is predisposed to several unusual patterns of

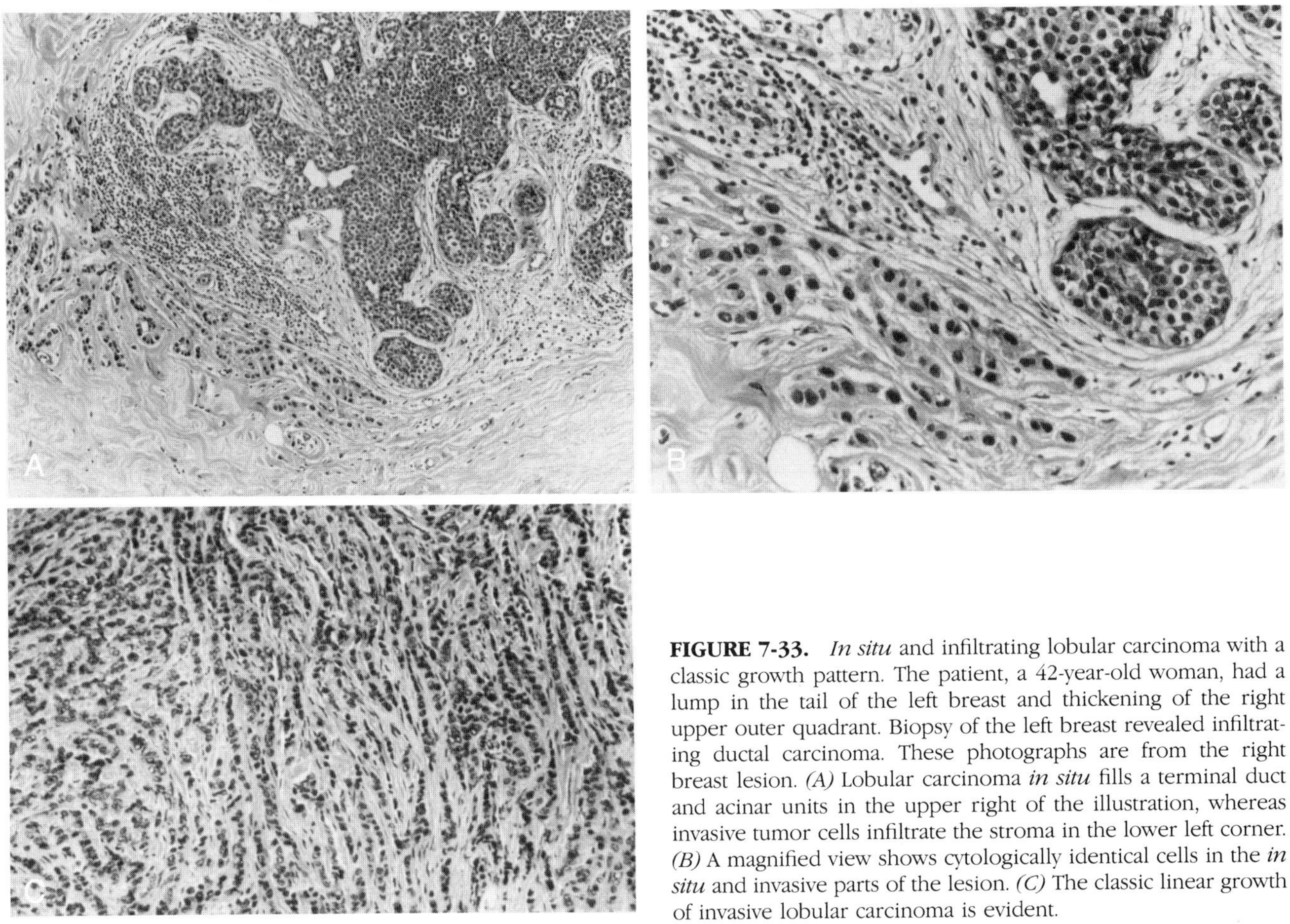

FIGURE 7-33. *In situ* and infiltrating lobular carcinoma with a classic growth pattern. The patient, a 42-year-old woman, had a lump in the tail of the left breast and thickening of the right upper outer quadrant. Biopsy of the left breast revealed infiltrating ductal carcinoma. These photographs are from the right breast lesion. *(A)* Lobular carcinoma *in situ* fills a terminal duct and acinar units in the upper right of the illustration, whereas invasive tumor cells infiltrate the stroma in the lower left corner. *(B)* A magnified view shows cytologically identical cells in the *in situ* and invasive parts of the lesion. *(C)* The classic linear growth of invasive lobular carcinoma is evident.

FIGURE 7-34. Variants of infiltrating lobular carcinoma. *(A)* This invasive carcinoma, which is composed of small uniform cells with cytologic features of lobular carcinoma, is growing in a trabecular pattern on the right, and in a more characteristically linear fashion on the left. *(B)* An area from the same tumor features rounded masses of cells which are characteristic of the alveolar growth pattern.

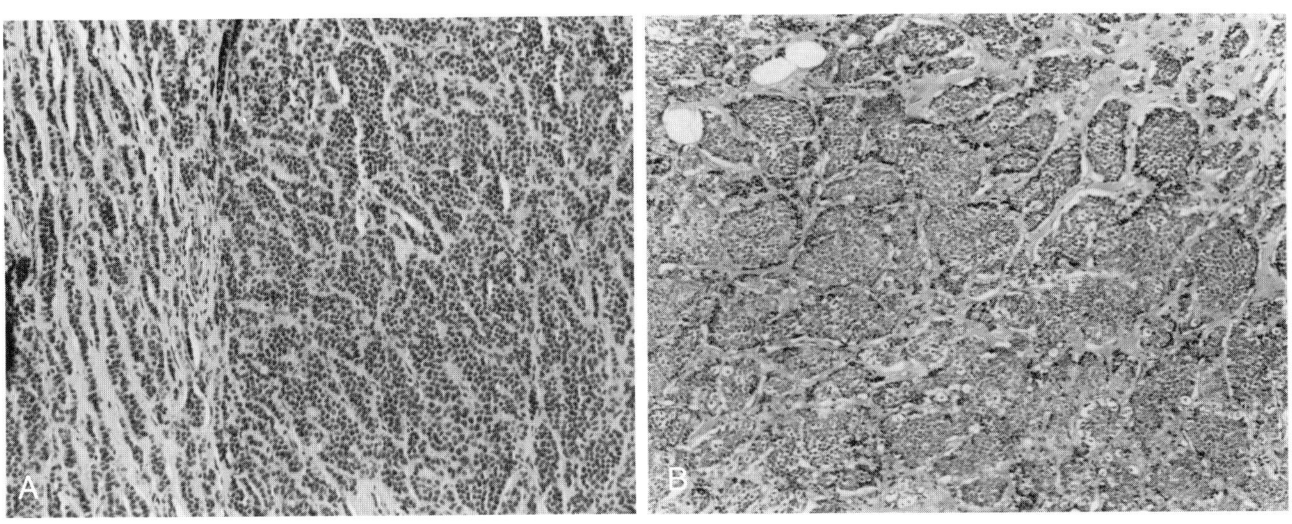

spread. Central nervous system metastases tend to be in the form of meningeal infiltration (carcinomatous meningitis), in contrast to those in ductal carcinoma, which more often result in parenchymal deposits.[384] Intra-abdominal metastases often involve the retroperitoneum and serosal surfaces diffusely.[378,385–387] Intestinal and ureteral obstructions have been reported to occur as a consequence. The operative findings may reveal only thickening of serosal, mesenteric, or retroperitoneal tissue, with no apparent mass.

Tumor invasion of the abdominal organs sometimes occurs coincidentally with diffuse serosal spread or as separate parenchymal metastases. Because the signet ring cells of mammary and other types of carcinoma are morphologically indistinguishable, metastatic lobular carcinoma involving the gastrointestinal tract may cause considerable diagnostic difficulty.[386,388,389] Metastases in the stomach mimic primary gastric carcinoma and, when transmural, the clinical and pathologic findings are those of linitus plastica.[390,391] Under these circumstances, gastric and mammary carcinoma have an identical histologic appearance on gastric biopsy. A positive immunohistochemical reaction for hormone receptor may be a helpful diagnostic procedure, especially if material from the original breast tumor is available for comparison.

Infiltrating lobular carcinoma also has a predilection for spread to the ovaries and uterus. Because the carcinomatous cells tend to blend with the normal cells of the endometrial stroma, they may be overlooked in an endometrial biopsy performed for vaginal bleeding. Neglecting to inform the pathologist of a previously treated breast carcinoma increases the likelihood that metastatic carcinoma will not be recognized in an endometrial or endocervical biopsy.

Metastatic lobular carcinoma has been mistaken for histiocytes. Such lesions in the eyelid may resemble a chalazion.[392,393] Similar diagnostic problems have been encountered in other sites, such as the bone marrow. Histochemical studies for mucin secretion or the immunohistochemical demonstration of epithelial-associated antigens (epithelial membrane antigen or cytokeratins) can usually resolve the issue.[394]

Reported data on prognosis present an incomplete picture. In a series of women who underwent mastectomy for T1N0M0 carcinomas, death as a result of disease within 10 years of treatment occurred in 6% of those with infiltrating lobular carcinoma and in 14% of those with invasive ductal carcinoma.[106] Newman reported that 14% of all node-negative patients with infiltrating lobular carcinoma died of disease, with an average follow-up of approximately 8 years.[367] Death due to disease occurred in nearly 50% of women who had lymph node metastases. Ashikari and colleagues reported the overall 5- and 10-year survival rates in node-negative patients not stratified by tumor size to be 86% and 74%, respectively.[371] They found no significant differences in survival when patients having invasive lobular carcinoma were stratified by nodal status and compared with similar groups treated for infiltrating ductal carcinoma.

Data on the prognostic significance of variant histologic patterns are inconclusive. Fechner reported a lower incidence of axillary nodal metastases in women who had one of the variant forms of infiltrating lobular carcinoma, but he provided no follow-up data.[372] Dixon and associates reported that patients with classic infiltrating lobular carcinoma had a better prognosis than those with variant forms of the disease.[369] In their series, the majority of patients were treated with simple mastectomy, radiation, and in some cases, axillary lymph node biopsy or dissection. On the basis of Manchester clinical staging, there was a great deal of variation in the extent of disease among the histologic types of invasive lobular carcinoma. The small groups of patients who were compared, the limited staging data, and the absence of a uniform approach to treatment weaken the reliability of these data.

Mammary Carcinomas With Endocrine Features

The capacity of some mammary carcinomas to produce or concentrate hormones not ordinarily considered to be normal products of the mammary gland may be regarded as endocrine or biochemical metaplasia. Included in this category are tumors that are found to contain certain substances, such as HCG, calcitonin, adrenal corticotropic hormone (ACTH), and epinephrine. These products, which may be detected by biochemical analysis and morphologically by immunohistochemical study of the tissues, are rarely produced in sufficient amounts to cause clinically apparent effects. In a minority of cases, the microscopic growth pattern may resemble that of extramammary neoplasms that are typically associated with the hormone in question, thus constituting biochemical and structural metaplasia. A particularly striking and extremely uncommon form of such combined metaplasia is mammary carcinoma with choriocarcinomatous differentiation that occurs in the breast[395] and in the gastrointestinal tract.[396] This type of mammary carcinoma contains areas of syncytiotrophoblastic and cytotrophoblastic elements that are strongly reactive for the β unit of HCG. Serum levels of HCG were not reported in a patient with choriocarcinomatous mammary carcinoma, but they were elevated in patients with gastrointestinal adenocarcinoma with choriocarcinomatous metaplasia.[396] Isolated cells that are reactive immunohistologically for α and β HCG may be found in 15% to 21% of ordinary infiltrating ductal carcinomas that do not exhibit choriocarcinomatous metaplasia.[180] These occasional HCG-positive cells do not have prognostic significance.[180]

A more common form of biochemical and structural metaplasia is represented by a heterogeneous group of mammary carcinomas found to contain argyrophilic cytoplasmic granules. The presence of these granules, with their characteristic dense core structure, detectable on electron microscopy, is a feature usually associated with neoplasms of the endocrine organs, particularly those termed carcinoid tumors. Granules with dense cores are the ultrastructural form in which many endocrine secretory products are packaged, but the specific nature of the hormone may be determined only by biochemical or immunohistochemical study of the tissue.

Granules with dense cores may be detected in cells by a variety of routine histochemical techniques. The most widely employed procedures rely on reactions in which ammoniacal silver is reduced to particles of metallic silver that can be visualized with the light microscope.[397] Argentaffin granules, such as those typically formed in midgut carcinoid tumors, contain endogenous reducing substances. In the argyrophilic reaction (e.g., the Grimelius stain), an exogenous reducing agent is added because some granules do not contain endogenous reducing substances. Because most cells with either argentaffin or argyrophilic granules are visualized with the argyrophilic reaction, this is the preferable procedure. Breast neoplasms that contain dense-core, argyrophilic, neurosecretory granules have largely been argentaffin-negative.

There have been few reports on the frequency of argyrophilic mammary carcinoma. Among studies in which more than 50 consecutive tumors have been examined, the frequencies reported were 3 of 67 cases (4.5%), 3 of 90 cases (3.3%), 19 of 92 cases (21%), and 27 of 253 cases (10.7%), respectively.[253,398–400] Carcinomas that contain argyrophilic granules include a variety of histologic types, including infiltrating ductal, infiltrating lobular,[399] mucinous,[253,254,399] intraductal, and papillary carcinomas. One recent study suggested that the presence of argyrophilic granules imparted a less favorable prognosis to mucinous carcinoma,[401] whereas another report stated that the presence of argyrophilic granules did not affect the prognosis of patients with mucinous carcinoma.[255] Presently, the data are not conclusive and the prognostic significance of these granules remains undetermined. An association with estrogen receptor positivity has been observed in a limited number of cases.[402–404] Argyrophilic granules have also been described in breast carcinoma in men.[405–406]

Histochemical studies to determine the nature of the secretory products contained in argyrophilic granules have been carried out in relatively few cases. Positive reactions have been reported for ACTH,[407,408] HCG,[408–410] prolactin,[407] neurotensin,[407] and norepinephrine.[406] In the latter case, a male patient was found to have elevated levels of urinary catecholamine. However, a substantial number of tumors with argyrophilic granules have not reacted positively for these or other polypeptide hormones and biogenic amines.[253,403,411] Recently, evidence has been presented suggesting that some argyrophilic, dense-core, secretory granules may contain lactalbumin.[403,412]

As noted, argyrophilic granules have been detected in various types of breast carcinomas. Some of these tumors, particularly some of those categorized as mucinous and infiltrating ductal carcinomas, have endocrine growth patterns similar to those of carcinoid tumors that arise in other organs.[413] These patterns initially provided the impetus for seeking argyrophilic granules, and with their detection, the diagnostic term carcinoid tumor of the breast was introduced.[413] However, this appellation has not been widely accepted for several reasons.[253,254,398–400,414,415] First, many mammary carcinomas that contain argyrophilic cells do not have a carcinoid growth pattern. Second, given the relatively high frequency of carcinomas with argyrophilic cells, one would not expect difficulty in detecting progenitor argyrophilic cells in normal mammary epithelium. However, such cells have only rarely been described.[254,416] Despite the efforts of many investigators to find them, therefore, their existence remains in doubt. Third, it has not been possible thus far to detect hormonal substances in many so-called carcinoid tumors, and there is evidence that at least some argyrophilic granules are associated with nonhormonal secretory products. Consequently, the term carcinoid tumor of the breast cannot be regarded as a specific histologic diagnosis.

Because some mammary carcinomas with carcinoid-like differentiation are morphologically similar to extramammary carcinoid tumors, a metastatic lesion in the breast may be mistaken for a primary tumor.[417–419] The presence of an intraductal component may be regarded as definitive evidence of breast origin. When intraductal carcinoma cannot be found, careful assessment of the patient's clinical history and clinical findings is necessary to rule out an extramammary primary tumor.

In summary, it may be concluded that there is a group of mammary carcinomas capable of producing a variety of hormonal substances. In some instances, the microscopic morphology of the tumor resembles that of extramammary neoplasms typically associated with these hormones. These neoplasms all should be regarded as variants of mammary carcinoma. Presently, these morphologically distinctive tumors may be referred to as mammary carcinomas with endocrine features so that their clinical and pathologic characteristics may be defined in the future. To the extent that they can be determined, the endocrine features should be described (for example, "infiltrating ductal carcinoma with endocrine features, argyrophil- and HCG-positive"). Until more data are available, it should be presumed that prognosis may be determined by the grade and stage of the lesion.

Unusual Diagnostic Problems

Inflammatory Carcinoma

The earliest clinical description of inflammatory carcinoma has been attributed to Charles Bell who, in 1807, noted that "when a purple color is on the skin over the tumor it is a very unpropitious beginning."[420] A variety of names, such as mastitis carcinomatosa and carcinoma mastitoides, were subsequently proposed to describe the clinical characteristics of the disease. Leitch observed subdermal lymphatic spread in acute mammary carcinoma and attributed peau d'orange to prominent pores in the skin made edematous by lymph stasis.[421] Lee and Tannenbaum proposed the term inflammatory carcinoma in 1924.[422]

The clinical features of this condition have been discussed in detail elsewhere. Typically, the patient presents with warm, cutaneous erythema of the breast. Dermal thickening or a ridge is palpable, especially at the margin of the red zone. Edema is usually present, and is accompanied by peau d'orange, especially over the dependent part of the breast.[423–425] Induration or a palpable mass is noted in the breast of most patients, but early in the disease, no tumor may be evident.[426] At this stage, primary inflammatory carcinoma may be misdiagnosed as a nonneoplastic inflammatory condition. The rapidly progressive breast carcinoma found in Tunisia has the clinical features of inflammatory carcinoma in most cases.[427]

The clinical findings in primary inflammatory carcinoma represent a superficial manifestation of an underlying invasive carcinoma. The primary carcinoma tends to be indistinct clinically and, on gross inspection of a mastectomy specimen, an exact size is frequently not recorded because the gross margins are not easily defined. The lesion may be described as diffusely involving the breast or simply as a large tumor.[428,429]

The WHO's report on the histological typing of breast tumors states that "inflammatory carcinoma does not constitute a histological type but rather a clinical entity."[430] Microscopically, a poorly differentiated, infiltrating ductal carcinoma is usually evident. Rarely, the primary lesion is an invasive lobular or mucinous carcinoma. In virtually every case, there is some invasion of the intramammary vascular spaces within and at the perimeter of the tumor. Usually, this invasion is an extensive process occurring throughout the breast, but in a few patients, parenchymal vascular invasion is inconspicuous. Because the vascular channels typically lack erythrocytes, they are usually regarded as lymphatic vessels. However, tumor emboli may be found in vascular spaces containing red blood cells. Lymphoplasmacytic reaction to the tumor occurs with varying intensity, but is generally inconspicuous. Paget's disease of the nipple may be present[429] in association with intraductal carcinoma of the main lactiferous ducts.

Because of the striking clinical cutaneous findings, a great deal of attention has been directed to the pathology of the skin. This is especially important because a biopsy of the skin is usually one of the first diagnostic procedures to be performed. In the typical case, microscopic examination of the skin reveals dilated, dermal, lymphatic channels; intralymphatic tumor emboli; and a lymphocytic reaction in the dermis that tends to localize around the dilated vascular spaces (Fig. 7-35).

There is considerable variation in the clinical and pathologic features of inflammatory carcinoma. The intensity of erythema and edema do not correlate well with the amount of vascular dilatation or lymphoplasmacytic reaction, or with the number of intravascular tumor emboli seen on microscopic sections of the skin. Biopsies of skin within and outside the zone of erythema may have identical histopathologic features, including intralymphatic tumor emboli. It has not been possible to detect intralymphatic tumor emboli in the skin of all patients who present with the typical clinical appearance of inflammatory carcinoma.[424–426,429,431] In one study, 8 of 16 patients had negative results on skin biopsy.[425] A small group of long-term survivors among women treated for clinically diagnosed inflammatory carcinoma did not have dermal lymphatic tumor emboli demonstrated on skin biopsy.[431] Consequently, no specific histologic picture is consistently associated with the diagnosis of inflammatory carcinoma clinically, or with the clinical findings in a particular case.

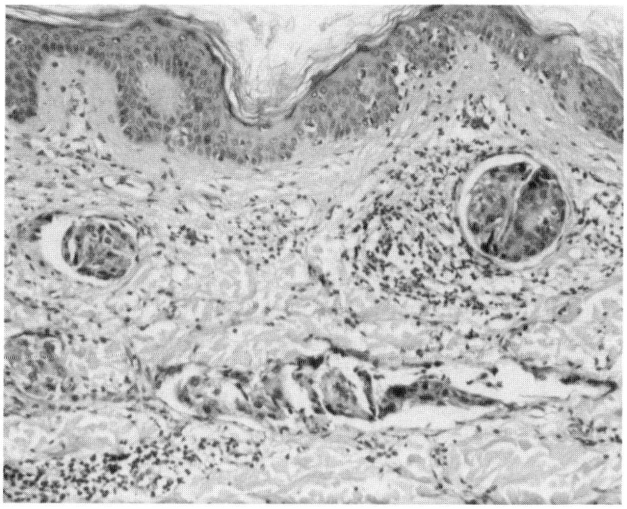

FIGURE 7-35. Inflammatory carcinoma. A skin biopsy was performed in a patient who presented with a breast mass and inflammatory carcinoma clinically. Three dilated lymphatic channels contain tumor emboli. Note the lymphocytic infiltrate in the dermis which is frequently found in the skin of patients with inflammatory carcinoma.

A group of patients with cutaneous lymphatic tumor emboli in the absence of the clinical findings of inflammatory carcinoma (especially erythema) also exists.[429] In general, their presenting signs are otherwise similar to those associated with inflammatory carcinoma in terms of tumor size, nodal involvement, and pathologic features of the underlying carcinoma. The prognosis in this condition, termed occult inflammatory carcinoma,[432] appears to be a bit more favorable than that observed in women with the typical clinical features of inflammatory carcinoma.[429–433]

Invasion of the dermis and dermal lymphatics was encountered in 4% (38 of 946) of primary operable patients treated with mastectomy for invasive carcinoma who did not have inflammatory features demonstrated on clinical examination. Dermal lymphatic involvement alone was encountered in 1%. These tumors tended to be centrally located, were generally larger than 4 cm in diameter, and were frequently multicentric.

When lymphatic tumor emboli are present in a skin biopsy from a patient with inflammatory carcinoma, the tumor cells constitute a small percentage of the volume of the specimen. The majority of these biopsies have been reported to be estrogen receptor-negative,[30] as have biopsies of the more cellular primary tumors.[434]

Recurrent mammary carcinoma involving the skin may also have inflammatory features clinically.[423,425] This type of recurrence generally occurs on the chest wall near the area of primary therapy, or in the opposite breast.

Distant skin metastases may also have an inflammatory presentation,[435] but this appearance is not specific for mammary carcinoma.[436–438] The majority of these skin lesions exhibit the same pattern of inflammation and dermal lymphatic tumor emboli observed in the skin of patients with primary inflammatory carcinoma, but nodular or plaque-like solid infiltrates of tumor are also often evident in the skin. A review of the primary lesions in a series of patients with recurrent inflammatory carcinoma revealed that all were ductal in origin.[423] A relatively high proportion of the original tumors had the cytologic features of apocrine carcinoma. There were single examples of medullary and mucinous carcinoma. Intralymphatic tumor emboli were frequently present in the breast, nipple, or skin at the time of mastectomy, but in most cases, the clinical presentation of the primary tumors did not have the typical appearance of inflammatory carcinoma.

Metastases to the Breast From Extramammary Malignant Tumors

Nearly one-third of metastatic tumors in the breast represent the presenting manifestation of an otherwise occult, extramammary, malignant tumor (usually, a carcinoma). The single most common primary site of an occult tumor presenting in this fashion is the lungs.[439–441] Clinically inapparent carcinoma of the ovaries, stomach, and uterus, and intestinal carcinoid tumors may present as metastases in the breast. Malignant melanoma and carcinomas of the lung, prostate, cervix, ovaries, and urinary bladder are among the most common, previously diagnosed lesions to give rise to metastases in the breast that are detectable clinically or at autopsy. The distinction between a metastasis from pulmonary oat cell carcinoma and a primary lymphoma of the breast may be a particularly difficult diagnostic problem. Adenocarcinoma of the colon and rectum is rarely the source of metastatic carcinoma in the breast, despite its relatively frequent occurrence in the population at large. In children, metastases to the breast from medulloblastoma[442] and rhabdomyosarcoma[443] have been reported.

For the pathologist, one of the most important aspects of metastatic tumor in the breast is that he or she should consider it as a possible diagnosis when faced with a morphologically unusual breast lesion (Fig. 7-36). This requires sensitivity to morphologic patterns that are atypical for breast carcinomas. The pathologist cannot depend upon receiving a complete history of previously treated neoplasms, and even when this is provided, the primary tumor may be a new, occult tumor. The preoperative clinical work-up for a patient with a "breast tumor" who appears to be in good health is often perfunctory, and cannot be relied upon to exclude an extramammary primary tumor.

In addition to an unusual histologic pattern and pertinent clinical information, there are a few other clues that may help to identify a metastatic tumor in the breast. *In situ* carcinoma of the ducts and lobules should be carefully sought since such a finding provides definitive evidence of a mammary origin. Because an *in situ* component is not detectable in a substantial number of primary breast carcinomas, absence of this finding is not conclusive. Metastases may produce solitary or multiple tumor nodules in the breast. The latter should lead one to suspect metastatic tumor since primary breast carcinoma only rarely presents with two or more palpable tumors. Tumor emboli within intramammary lymphatic spaces have been observed to be associated with metastases to the breast, as well as with primary breast carcinomas. Metastatic tumor is suggested by the following combination of microscopic findings: a tumor composed of a rather homogeneous population of neoplastic cells without desmoplastic stromal reaction, no detectable *in situ* carcinoma of the lobules or ducts, and a sharp transition at the periphery between tumor and entirely normal breast tissue with no benign proliferative breast disease. In some particularly difficult cases, electron microscopy, lymphocyte markers, immunohistochemical studies, and estrogen receptor analysis may be helpful in assessing a tumor suspected to be metastatic in the breast. The problems of distinguishing between mammary carcinoma with carcinoid features and metastatic carcinoid in the breast are discussed elsewhere in this chapter.

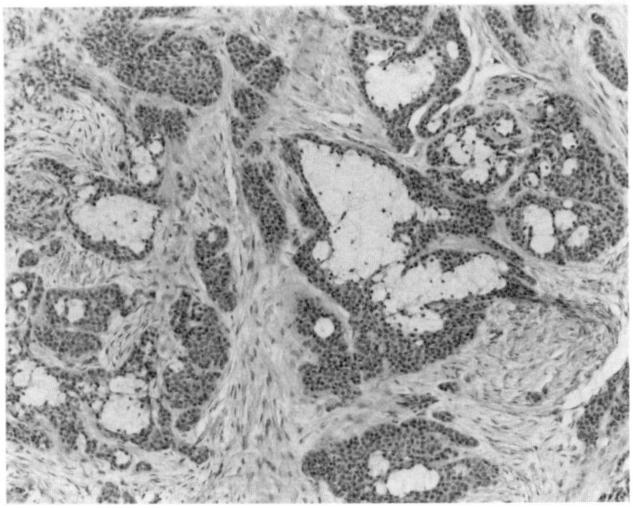

FIGURE 7-36. Metastatic mucoepidermoid carcinoma of the parotid gland in the breast, showing characteristic, vacuolated, mucin-containing cells. The primary salivary gland tumor was resected several years before the breast metastasis became apparent.

Distinguishing between a primary tumor of the breast and a metastasis to the breast is important in determining both a therapeutic regimen and a prognosis. When an occult, extramammary neoplasm presents with a breast metastasis, work-up of the patient will be influenced by the morphologic features of the tumor that may suggest particular primary sites. Only in exceptional circumstances would mastectomy be appropriate for metastatic tumor in the breast, and emphasis should necessarily be placed on systemic treatment appropriate to the primary lesion.

Carcinomas Arising in Fibroadenomas and Cystosarcomas

Fibroadenoma and cystosarcoma phyllodes are fibroepithelial neoplasms composed of proliferating epithelial and stromal tissues of the breast. The distinction between these lesions depends upon qualitative and quantitative features of the stromal component. Generally, in a cystosarcoma, there is more stroma relative to the epithelial component, and the stroma is more cellular than in a fibroadenoma. In a malignant cystosarcoma, the stroma has the histologic features of a soft tissue sarcoma, usually fibrosarcoma.

The epithelium in fibroepithelial neoplasms may exhibit many of the proliferative changes observed throughout the breast. Lactational hyperplasia occurs during pregnancy, sometimes with infarction of the fibroadenoma. Cysts, adenosis, sclerosing adenosis, apocrine metaplasia, and epithelial hyperplasia are not uncommon in patients with fibroadenomas. Proliferative changes consisting of epithelial hyperplasia, squamous metaplasia, and cysts may be found in cystosarcomas.

Florid epithelial hyperplasia, initially linked to oral contraceptive use,[444] has been shown on further study not to be related specifically to these agents.[445] The term *juvenile fibroadenoma* has recently been adopted to describe fibroadenomas that exhibit florid, atypical hyperplasia with features resembling *in situ* carcinoma.[446] Lesions of this type occur in patients of age groups that are significantly younger than those associated with ordinary fibroadenomas. With follow-up of 1 to 19 years, none of 49 patients studied developed carcinoma of the breast following excision of such a lesion.

Carcinoma arising in a fibroadenoma was illustrated by Cheatle and Cutler in 1931,[447] and similar lesions were mentioned in 1940 by Harrington and Miller.[448] The first reported series, which described 26 patients with follow-up, appeared in 1967,[449] and with the cases described subsequently, the total number of affected patients is now approximately 100.[450–454] The occurrence of carcinoma in less than 0.5% of fibroadenomas[453,454] is low enough to indicate that this is a chance event. Carcinoma occurs in 1% to 2% of patients with cystosarcoma phyllodes.[454,455]

CLINICAL PRESENTATION. The ages of patients found to have carcinoma arising in a fibroadenoma range from 15 to 70 years, with a mean age of 42 to 44 years in two recent reviews.[453,454] The range in the ages of women with *in situ* lesions (42 to 45 years) is somewhat lower than that for patients with invasive lesions (47 to 51 years). In view of this age distribution, an elevated index of suspicion may be warranted when a woman 40 years of age or older is found to have a lesion with the clinical features of a fibroadenoma.

There are no clinical or radiographic clues to the diagnosis of *in situ* carcinoma within a fibroadenoma. Invasive carcinoma arising in a fibroadenoma may be suspected on mammography when part of the margin of the tumor is poorly circumscribed or ill-defined. There are no clinical signs indicative of carcinoma arising in a cystosarcoma.

GROSS PATHOLOGY. These tumors have the usual gross appearance of fibroadenomas; when *in situ* carcinoma is present, it will not be suspected on gross inspection of the tumor. Small, invasive carcinomas that are confined to fibroadenomas are generally not appreciated on gross examination, but invasion into the adjacent breast distorts the tumor sufficiently to suggest carcinoma. The presence of carcinoma in a cystosarcoma is generally not evident on gross inspection.

MICROSCOPIC PATHOLOGY. About 50% of affected patients have lobular carcinoma *in situ* that is confined to the fibroadenoma in about half of the patients who undergo mastectomy. Intraductal carcinoma occurs in nearly 20% of patients, including a small number of patients who also have lobular carcinoma *in situ* in the fibroadenoma. Infiltrating ductal carcinoma arising in a fibroadenoma (Fig. 7-37) accounts for 20% of the cases, and about 10% have invasive lobular carcinoma.

It is difficult to assess the extent of coexistent carcinoma in the breast from published reports because a substantial number of patients were treated only by excisional biopsy. However, data presented in recent reviews suggest that carcinoma is confined to the fibroadenoma in one-third to one-half of those cases in which there is *in situ* lobular, intraductal, or invasive lobular carcinoma.[453,454] The surrounding breast was involved in at least 50% of cases when invasive ductal carcinoma arose within a fibroadenoma. Generally, the same type of carcinoma has been detected within the fibroadenoma and breast. Lobular carcinoma *in situ* may involve multiple

FIGURE 7-37. Invasive duct carcinoma in fibroadenoma. Remnants of benign fibroadenomatous epithelium are seen in the center of this lesion surrounded by nests of invasive tumor. Carcinoma was confined entirely to the fibroadenoma.

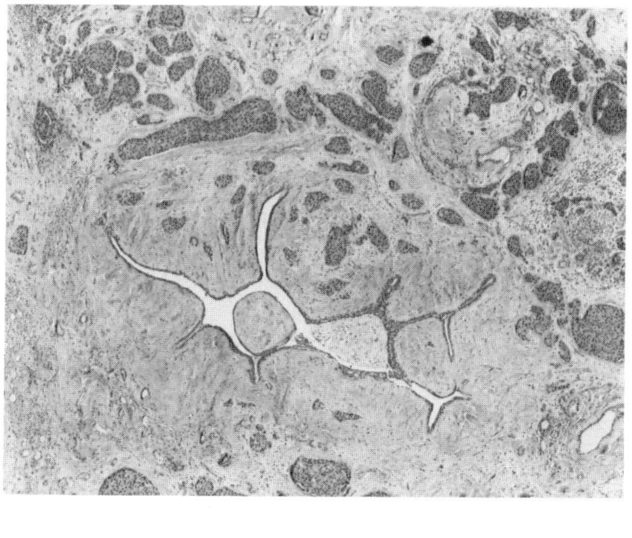

fibroadenomas in the same breast, or may be present in bilateral tumors.[451,452] In 10% to 15% of patients, contralateral carcinomas have occurred concurrently or have previously been treated.[449–452,454] In the majority of cases, the opposite breast contained invasive ductal carcinoma.

Carcinomas arising in cystosarcoma phyllodes have the same histologic features as do carcinomas that develop in fibroadenomas. The majority represent *in situ* lobular carcinomas, but infiltrating ductal carcinomas have also been described.[454,455] Carcinomas may also develop concurrently in the surrounding breast tissue, even when there is no carcinoma in the cystosarcoma, and carcinoma has also been reported subsequent to excision of cystosarcomas.[455]

PROGNOSIS. Whether treated with mastectomy or simple excision of the affected fibroadenoma, very few deaths have been reported in patients with carcinoma arising in a fibroadenoma. Those that have been reported have been attributable to invasive ductal carcinoma.[453,454] Rarely, recurrence in the breast following excisional biopsy has occurred. It may be concluded that carcinomas arising within fibroadenomas and cystosarcomas are not intrinsically different from lesions of the same histologic appearance that develop in the breast and that are unrelated to fibroadenomas.

Breast Carcinoma and Florid Papillomatosis of the Nipple

Florid papillomatosis is an uncommon, benign, proliferative lesion of the nipple.[456,457] Other terms applied to this condition include adenoma of the nipple and papillomatosis of the subareolar ducts.[458,459] The lesion usually presents as a firm, tumorous thickening of the nipple, which is often accompanied by erosion of the nipple surface, suggesting Paget's disease clinically. In many respects, the histopathologic features of this lesion duplicate those observed in proliferative duct lesions that occur elsewhere in the breast,[458] including the entire spectrum of benign and atypical ductal hyperplasia, which may be accompanied by cysts, adenosis, and other hyperplastic changes. When the sample obtained in a small biopsy exhibits considerable atypia, a mistaken diagnosis of carcinoma may be made.

The relationship of florid papillomatosis of the nipple to breast carcinoma was recently reviewed. Of 173 patients with florid papillomatosis who had been reported previously, 24 (14%) also had breast carcinoma. This finding also occurred in 9 of 51 patients (18%) included in a new series.[460] Nineteen of a total of 33 patients had a concurrent carcinoma in the same breast that arose separately from the nipple lesion. Two other patients developed subsequent carcinoma in the ipsilateral breast 7 and 10 years after excision of florid papillomatosis of the nipple. All of the carcinomas were of the ductal variety. In a series of patients whose carcinoma was treated with mastectomy, florid papillomatosis of the nipple was detected in 1.2% (12 of 967) of the nipples examined.[88]

Carcinoma has been found to arise directly in florid papillomatosis in eight patients. Two of these patients were men whose lesions contained intraductal carcinoma and microscopic changes of Paget's disease in the overlying epidermis. Another man had invasive ductal carcinoma. The five women included in the study all had invasive ductal carcinoma arising in florid papillomatosis.

Carcinoma of the contralateral breast has been described in seven patients. Three of these patients were women with bilateral breast carcinoma who also had florid papillomatosis as a separate, coincidental lesion in one breast. The other four patients had florid papillomatosis involving the nipple of one breast and carcinoma that was limited to the contralateral breast.

It is clear from these data that florid papillomatosis rarely gives rise directly to mammary carcinoma, and that very few patients subsequently develop carcinoma in the breast from which the lesion is excised. However, it is necessary to remove the entire tumor for diagnosis in order to exclude carcinoma within the lesion, especially since this determination cannot readily be made on the basis of a small, superficial biopsy. Demonstration of Paget's disease of the epidermis or invasive carcinoma is a critical factor in establishing a diagnosis of carcinoma arising in florid papillomatosis of the nipple. Patients who are found to have florid papillomatosis of the nipple should undergo clinical and mammographic examination to rule out a separate, coincidental carcinoma in either breast.

CYTOLOGIC DIAGNOSIS OF BREAST CANCER

For decades, very small samples of lesions obtained by needle puncture have been used for the diagnosis of lesions in many anatomic locations. Breast tumors are especially suited to this method of diagnosis because they are accessible with minimal preparation. The specimens obtained may be an aspirate of cells or fluid suitable for cytologic examination or a needle biopsy of tissue for histologic study.

Aspiration biopsy has been practiced for more than 50 years.[461] In 1933, Stewart described his experience with aspiration smears from approximately 2500 specimens, including nearly 500 breast lesions.[462] Among the lesions that he found difficult to distinguish from carcinoma were atypical epithelial hyperplasia, gynecomastia, and lactating breast. Stewart concluded that, "It must not be inferred that diagnosis is always simple and that no errors have been made. Until the pathologist has familiarized himself with the various pitfalls, errors are certain to occur."[462]

Martin and Ellis described 280 breast cancers among 1405 malignant tumors diagnosed prior to 1934 at Memorial Hospital.[463] They emphasized several advantages of the procedure, which are equally applicable today: the relative simplicity of the procedure, which can be performed in an office setting; the ease of sample preparation and prompt diagnosis which, if positive, make it possible to discuss therapeutic options; and the advantage of avoiding surgical biopsy of patients who have clinically advanced disease.

Technical problems that were encountered early in

the use of aspiration biopsy were described by McLean.[464] The quality of needles was a particular concern:

> The steel of the needle should also be of the nonrusting variety, as well as stainless. Rust formation destroys the sharp cutting edge of the point and bevel, and pits and clogs the bore .... such a needle is difficult to clean. Certainly, syringing air or water through a rust-lined needle, after use in biopsy, cannot be trusted to remove all cancer tissue.

Fortunately, the availability of disposable needles and other technical advances have eliminated many of the problems faced by Drs. Martin and McLean and their colleagues. However, skill in performing aspirations and expertise in their interpretation depend upon continued experience with substantial numbers of cases. As noted by Christopherson, "The method is most successful in institutions dealing with a large number of cancer patients. Experience is the *sine qua non* of success."[465]

Aspiration biopsy was initially introduced as an alternative to incisional surgical biopsy because of concern that trauma associated with the latter procedure could result in vascular dissemination of tumor cells.[465] The presence of circulating tumor cells has repeatedly been documented in patients with a variety of cancers, including mammary carcinoma.[466–470] This phenomenon has been observed when there has been no manipulation of the tumor, but there is evidence that more cells may be dispersed after palpation or biopsy.[469] The prognostic significance of circulating tumor cells remains uncertain. Some investigators have reported no demonstrable effect on survival,[467,469] whereas others have ascribed a less favorable prognosis to the finding of tumor cells in the blood.[471,472] The extent to which needle aspiration biopsy may contribute, to a greater or lesser extent than surgical biopsy, to the hematogenous dispersal of tumor cells has not specifically been determined. However, two studies failed to find any difference between the survival rates of patients with breast cancer whose diagnosis was based on needle aspiration and the rates of those who underwent surgical biopsy.[473,474]

Cystic Lesions

One of the most important practical uses of aspiration biopsy is to distinguish between a fluid-filled cyst and a solid tumor of the breast.[475,476] In most instances, aspiration of the cyst contents is a therapeutic, as well as a diagnostic, procedure. During this procedure, the cyst collapses, and in most cases, much of the epithelium that lines a benign cyst, stripped from the supporting stroma, is removed in the aspirate. Since reaccumulation of fluid rarely occurs in such cases, it may be presumed that the epithelium contributed to fluid formation, and that in the absence of the epithelium, the cystic space is effaced by the adherent, exposed, apposing surfaces of stroma.

It is generally agreed that cytologic examination of cyst fluid is appropriate in some circumstances. A bloody or serosanguinous aspirate should be examined microscopically. Bright red blood may be indicative of a traumatic aspiration, with hemorrhage into the cyst resulting in a persistent mass. Regardless of the character of the fluid obtained, the presence of a residual mass immediately after aspiration requires examination of the specimen. Reaccumulation of fluid within a cyst, particularly within a short period of time, is an indication for cytologic study of the second aspirate. In some cases, regardless of the cytologic findings, excisional biopsy will be necessary, especially for aspirates that yield bloody fluid or are associated with a mass.

The necessity for the routine cytologic examination of cystic fluid aspirated from the breast is the subject of some controversy. In three recent studies, the incidence of carcinoma in cystic lesions from which material was submitted for cytology was 2% of 1714 specimens (Table 7-1). The majority of the carcinomas were associated with bloody fluid or a mass, or both, all of which require cytologic study. As a consequence, it would appear that, in the absence of such clinical indications, microscopic examination is not mandatory. However, consideration should also be given to other factors, such as a family history for the disease or a previous biopsy that demonstrated significant atypia or carcinoma of the contralateral breast, that may indicate the patient is at increased risk for the development of breast carcinoma.

The results of microscopic examination of breast cyst fluid vary considerably. Many specimens are nearly acellular, especially if no effort has been made to concentrate the material by centrifugation or filtration. When cells are present, benign epithelial cells occurring singly or in small groups, histiocytes (foam cells), lymphocytes, and epithelial cells exhibiting apocrine metaplasia are found in varying proportions. Clustered cells generally indicate papillary proliferation of the epithelial lining of the cyst, an especially common finding when there is apocrine metaplasia, a benign process. Standard cytologic criteria are applied to the diagnosis of cells obtained in a cyst aspirate.

Solid Tumors

Needle aspiration biopsy of solid breast tumors has become an established diagnostic procedure. Numerous studies have been conducted to evaluate the accuracy and clinical utility of diagnoses of breast carcinoma established

Table 7-1
Aspiration Diagnosis of Carcinoma in Cystic Lesions

Study	*Cystic Lesions (No.)*	*Carcinomatous Lesions (No./%)*
Kline et al.[477]	354	8/2
Strawbridge et al[485]	834	10/1
Bell et al.[478]	526	14/3
Total	1714	32/2

Table 7-2
*Correlation of Aspiration Cytology Diagnosis with Incidence of Breast Carcinoma**

	Aspiration Diagnosis				
	Carcinoma	*Atypia*			
		Marked	*Moderate*	*Mild*	*None*
No. of patients (Total of 986)	76	16	41	46	807
No. of patients with carcinoma (Total of 109)	76	14	10	4	5
% of patients with carcinoma	100	88	24	9	0.6

* Adapted from Rimsten A, Stenkvist B, Johanson H, et al: The diagnostic accuracy of palpation and fine-needle biopsy and evaluation of their combined use in the diagnosis of breast lesions. Report of a prospective study in 1244 women with symptoms. Ann Surg 182:1, 1975.

by aspiration cytology. The primary role of this procedure is to provide a prompt diagnosis of a palpable breast tumor. The frequency with which carcinoma has been diagnosed in various series depends on the selection of patients, as well as on the skill of the personnel who perform and interpret the aspiration. The percentage of true-positive diagnoses (the proportion of histologically proven carcinomas detected cytologically) ranges from 69% to 96% in some of the larger series reported.[477–485] The corresponding false-negative reports (the proportion of carcinomas that are not detected cytologically) are the result of scanty, improperly prepared, or poorly preserved samples of the lesion; aspirates of lesions that present inherent diagnostic problems (e.g., differentiation between papillary carcinoma and papilloma); and aspirates that have missed the lesion entirely.[486] Attempts to aspirate palpable tumors that are indistinct, smaller than 2 cm in diameter, or located deep in large breasts, or nonpalpable lesions that are detected on mammography are more likely to result in false-negative diagnoses. A surgical biopsy should be performed whenever the clinical features of the lesion indicate any possibility of carcinoma despite a nondiagnostic aspiration cytology report to the contrary. Atypical cells found in an aspirate may be a clue to the presence of carcinoma (Table 7-2).[483] Although carcinomatous cells are much more likely to be present in the aspirate from a tumor regarded clinically to be a carcinoma, Bell and co-workers recently reported the detection of carcinoma in 36% of aspirated, clinically suspicious lesions; in 20% of those lesions identified as clinically significant; and in 3% of specimens from lesions diagnosed clinically as benign (Table 7-3).[478]

The incidence of false-positive diagnoses has been remarkably low in larger series,[477,479,480,484,487] ranging from 0% to 3%. In most institutions, the frequency of error is the same for both frozen sections in general and frozen sections of breast tumors.[44,488–490] Inexperience is a significant contributing factor when a false-positive diagnosis is made, and it is essential that a high threshold for the diagnosis of cancer based on stringent diagnostic criteria, be maintained to minimize such errors. It is also important to require that diagnostic material be abundant and be present on at least two separate slides. However, cellularity is not by itself sufficient for diagnosis since substantial amounts of benign epithelium may be obtained from papillomas, fibroadenomas, and other benign lesions. The epithelium from a benign lesion usually forms cohesive sheets or clusters, whereas cells from carcinomas tend to separate and to appear to be dispersed. Aspirates from patients with lactating breasts, gynecomastia, and various proliferative ductal lesions (atypical papillomatosis) constitute significant diagnostic hazards. The aspirate obtained from a granular cell tumor, which clinically simulates carcinoma, may easily be misdiagnosed as carcinoma if the cytologist does not notice the granules dispersed on the slide from disrupted cells. Finally, technically imperfect preparations, particularly those with drying artifacts, should be interpreted with extreme caution.

It may be possible to identify some specific histologic types of carcinoma in an aspiration biopsy. The aspirate from infiltrating lobular carcinoma may be relatively scanty and is generally composed of small, isolated cells with sparse cytoplasm. Occasionally, the cells are arranged in the characteristic linear fashion seen in tissue sections. Abundant extracellular mucin distinguishes the aspirate obtained from mucinous carcinoma, whereas a specimen from medullary carcinoma typically has poorly differentiated tumor cells scattered among numerous lymphocytes and plasma cells. However, there are benign lesions that can mimic each of the patterns associated with different tumor types, and it is, therefore, essential to establish the presence of carcinomatous cells before attempting to classify the lesion.

In the past decade, there has been growing interest in the use of needle biopsy as an alternative to needle aspiration for the diagnosis of solid tumors. This diagnostic method has become especially attractive with the availability of the disposable Tru-cut® needle (Travenol Laboratories) which has obviated the need for the cumbersome drill biopsy. The specimen obtained by this method consists of one or more slender, cylindrical fragments or cores of tissue that may be used to make frozen as well as paraffin sections.

The reported range of true-positive diagnoses of carcinoma obtained by needle biopsy (67% to 89%) is slightly lower than that reported with drill biopsy (75% to 99%)

Table 7-3
Correlation of Clinical Diagnosis with Findings on Biopsy and Aspiration Cytology

		Carcinoma Found On Biopsy		*Carcinoma Found on Aspiration*		
Clinical Diagnosis	***Number of Patients Undergoing Biopsy***	*Number*	*(Percent)*	*Number*	*(Percent of All Patients)*	*(Percent of Patients With Carcinoma)*
Benign	174	21	(12)	6	(3)	(29)
Significant	142	41	(29)	28	(20)	(67)
Suspicious	73	36	(49)	26	(36)	(70)
Carcinoma	104	102	(98)	82	(79)	(81)

Adapted from Bell DA, Hajdu SI, Urban JA, et al: Role of aspiration cytology in the diagnosis and management of mammary lesions in office practice. Cancer 51:1182, 1983.

or aspiration cytology.[491–498] Studies that have demonstrated a higher frequency of true-positive diagnoses associated with needle biopsy than with aspiration cytology have had remarkably poor results with the latter procedure (positive rates of 52% and 42%, respectively) and have included very few patients (119 and 60 patients, respectively).[491,499] In a third study of 50 women with malignant breast tumors, the frequency of positive diagnosis by aspiration cytology (76%) was slightly higher than that obtained with needle biopsy (69%).[492]

False-negative diagnoses obtained with needle biopsy reflect problems in sampling and tissue preservation that are comparable to those encountered in the use of aspiration biopsy. In addition to a possible failure to enter the lesion, diagnostic material may not be obtained from carcinomas in which there is considerable necrosis or desmoplastic fibrosis. Neoplastic cells in some tumors are particularly susceptible to distortion by the biopsy procedure (termed crush artifact), and may be unable to be interpreted.

Although false-positive diagnoses have not been described in published reports of needle biopsy diagnosis, the potential for this to occur is at least as great as it is for aspiration cytology. The lesions of particular concern are sclerosing adenosis and sclerosing ductal proliferations, such as the so-called radical scar. Mingling of proliferating epithelium and stroma in these tumors often simulates the appearance of invasive carcinoma. Although this process, referred to as pseudoinvasion, can generally be appreciated in a tissue section of the entire lesion, the small sample represented by a needle core biopsy could easily lead to a misdiagnosis of carcinoma. The risk of a false-positive diagnosis is especially great when dealing with frozen section material in which the quality of cytologic detail is, of necessity, less than that obtained in paraffin sections.

PATHOLOGIC EXAMINATION OF BREAST SPECIMENS

The purpose of this section is to highlight clinically important factors, not discussed elsewhere in this chapter, relating to the gross pathologic examination of breast specimens. Although some technical aspects of the laboratory processing of tissues are addressed, this discussion is not intended to be a comprehensive presentation of differing points of view, nor should this material be regarded as sufficiently detailed to serve as a laboratory workbook. Additional information may be found in recent comprehensive reviews.[500,501]

The Biopsy

Needle or Incisional Biopsy Specimens

Small needle or incisional biopsy specimens will generally be processed for histologic examination in their entirety. The operator who performs the biopsy should exercise care not to crush the specimens. *A cautery type of scalpel must not be used in obtaining such a biopsy (see below).* These samples are suitable for frozen section, but it should be remembered that only limited information about the characteristics of a lesion may be obtained from such small specimens. The samples are generally too small to permit standard biochemical assays of hormone receptors, but they may be suitable for immunohistochemical receptor analysis (see Chapter 8). Unless frozen section analysis or some other study that requires fresh tissue is intended, small biopsy specimens should immediately be placed in fixative for transport to the laboratory.

Excisional Biopsy Specimens

Many factors influence the manner in which excisional biopsies are handled in a given situation. Paramount among these are the logistical considerations relating to when and where the biopsy is performed and under what particular clinical circumstances. Hence, the material presented in this section should be regarded as a series of guidelines which may need to be modified in some situations.

GROSS EXAMINATION OF EXCISIONAL BIOPSY SPECIMENS. The pathologist is responsible for describing the dimensions and character of the tissue removed from the patient. This can be accomplished most accurately if the excised specimen is delivered intact, promptly, and unfixed to the pathology laboratory.

The size of an excisional biopsy specimen should be recorded in centimeters in three dimensions, as should the general shape (e.g., ovoid or spherical) of the specimen. Because the overall dimensions of an excisional biopsy specimen cannot be determined after the tissue has been sliced open and dissected, the specimen should be intact when delivered to the laboratory. It is also useful to record specimen weight in grams.

Whenever feasible, the intact specimen should be delivered to the pathology laboratory immediately. It is preferable that the tissue be unfixed in order not to preclude the possibility of performing a frozen section or of obtaining material for receptor analysis, electron microscopy, or other studies. If a delay is anticipated, the tissue may be chilled, but freezing the entire specimen will compromise histologic examination. Even if a frozen section is not requested, the tissue should be dissected promptly by a pathologist to determine whether any grossly identifiable tumor is present. If such a lesion is found, its size should be recorded in centimeters in three dimensions. Because of the critical prognostic significance of tumor size, this measurement should be made before tissue is removed for frozen section or other studies, such as hormone receptor analysis. It may be difficult to measure the tumor accurately if the specimen is received after being previously sliced by the operator. The gross character of the tumor including its shape, consistency, and the appearance of its cut surface, should be described. Whether or not a distinct lesion is found, the appearance of the breast parenchyma, including its consistency, the relative proportions of fat and fibrous tissue, and the presence or absence of cysts or other lesions, should be noted.

In some laboratories in which frozen sections are not routinely performed, it is customary to freeze and store a portion of any lesion suspected to be carcinomatous until paraffin sections have been prepared. If the lesion proves to be a carcinoma, the frozen sample is then submitted for biochemical analysis. If the diagnosis proves to be difficult, the reserved, frozen sample may be submitted for histologic study. Unfortunately, the thawed tissue is often somewhat distorted, and these specimens may not help to resolve a diagnostic problem.

The number of samples taken from an excisional biopsy for histologic examination varies greatly according to the clinical circumstances, the gross appearance of the tissue, and the results of frozen section studies, if performed. No fixed rule designating the appropriate number of specimens per a specific amount (e.g., 5 grams) of tissue can reasonably be applied. The tissue used for frozen section is routinely saved, processed into a paraffin section, and identified by a term such as the frozen section control. If a sample is removed for hormone receptor analysis, a corresponding specimen should be examined histologically as a receptor control. Distinct tumors that appear on gross examination to be carcinomas of 2 cm or less in diameter can generally be submitted in their entirety for histology. Some sections should be taken to demonstrate the margin of the tumor and surrounding breast; these are examined microscopically for evidence of lymphatic emboli and *in situ* carcinoma outside the lesion. When no distinct tumor is present, some laboratories advocate processing the entire specimen. This may be appropriate in some situations owing to clinical or pathologic findings, or both. However, the cost of applying this approach indiscriminately may become prohibitive, and judgment must be exercised in these cases, as well as in the selection of other clinical or laboratory diagnostic procedures.

The description of the gross appearance of a biopsy, mastectomy, or other specimen becomes part of the pathology report. Included in this section of the report should be a list of the tissue samples taken for microscopic examination, indicating the number of tissue blocks and providing an explanation of the abbreviations used to designate individual samples. This information serves as an index and is particularly important in assisting pathologists who are called upon to review slides from other institutions when patients are referred for treatment. The majority of pathology reports presently prepared in the United States do not provide any of this information, or do so in a cursory, often confusing, manner.

ASSESSMENT OF THE MARGINS OF EXCISION. It may be useful to assess accurately the margins of an excision by microscopic examination. Because the contours and orientation of tissue slices may be altered in the course of preparing histologic sections, it is necessary to mark the surfaces so that they may be identified microscopically. This is most easily accomplished with finely particulate reagents, such as India ink or tattoo dyes, which remain adherent to the tissue throughout processing and which are visible through the microscope (Fig. 7-38). These pigments adhere better to fresh tissue that has been blotted free of surface blood and moisture than to fixed tissue. If properly applied, the surface pigment should not contaminate the interior of the specimen; otherwise, misleading conclusions about the margins could result. With experience, it is possible to ink the surface of an excisional biopsy in less than 5 minutes. Hence, this procedure is not a significant impediment to performing a frozen section, nor does it appreciably delay obtaining tissue for receptor analysis.

An excisional biopsy specimen that has been sliced by the operator cannot reliably be reassembled in order to ink the margins. This is another reason why it is necessary for excisional biopsy specimens to be submitted intact to the pathologist.

Once inked, the specimen should be split in a plane that will bisect a palpable tumor, if present. It is possible to remove portions immediately for frozen section or receptor analysis, or both. The practice of obtaining frozen sections of the margins should be discouraged unless the tumor appears to be close to a margin and intraoperative confirmation of this will have an immediate impact on treatment.

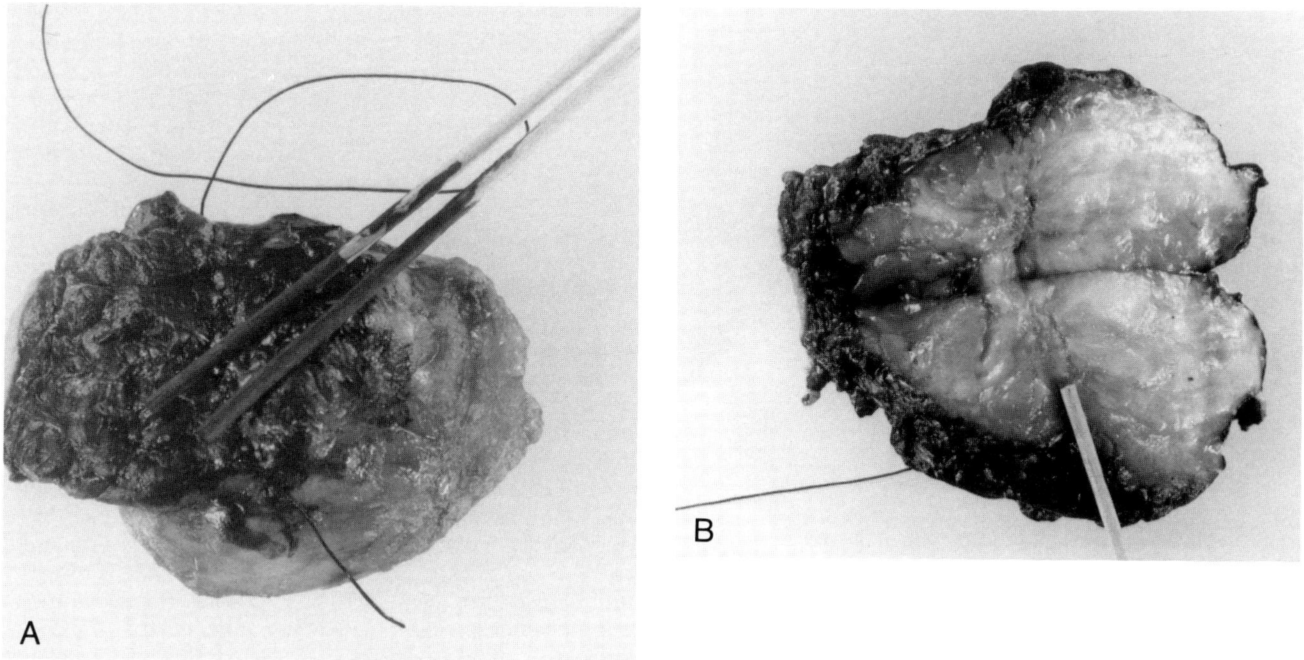

FIGURE 7-38. Procedure for inking the margins of an excisional biopsy specimen. *(A)* Intact excisional biopsy specimen with short and long sutures indicating the superior and lateral margins, respectively. India ink has been applied with wooden applicators. *(B)* Specimen that has been bisected after completion of the inking process. The applicator points to a carcinoma that does not extend to the margins.

It is not possible to orient an excisional biopsy specimen without guidance from the surgeon. This can easily be accomplished if the operator places a short suture at the superior margin and a long stitch laterally. At least two sections should be taken perpendicular to each of the six inked surfaces (superior, inferior, medial, lateral, superficial, and deep); additional samples of margins may be obtained on the basis of the gross findings.

There is no standardized system for reporting the microscopic appearance of excisional margins. Tumor that is transected at an inked surface represents a clearly positive margin (Fig. 7-39). This criterion applies equally to *in situ* and to invasive carcinoma, but the type of tumor must be specified. Borderline situations occur in which tumor very closely approaches the margin, but is not truly transected. One useful convention in these situations is to regard foci within one high-power microscopic field as being close to the margin. The nature and amount of the tumor, as well as the character of the tissue intervening to the margin, should be specified. To date, it has not been determined whether transection of tumor at the margin or close to the margin, as defined here, is clinically significant.

SPECIMEN RADIOGRAPHY. The radiologic examination of excised breast tissue, termed specimen radiography, has been performed for nearly 75 years.[502] As early as 1913, Salomon, a surgeon at the University of Berlin, reported on the use of x-ray films to study mastectomy specimens.[362] Salomon used serial sections of specimens to correlate the histologic and radiologic features of breast carcinoma. He described calcifications in breast carcinomas that were detected on radiography. However, the clinical significance of these calcifications was not appreciated until several decades later, when clinical mammography had been improved substantially.[503] In 1951, Leborgne commented on a case in which "roentgenographic study of the operative specimen also permitted the localization of the tiny calcifications for histopathologic study, and thus aided in finding a small cancer. . . ."[504]

With the increasingly widespread use of mammography, considerable interest in specimen radiography of lesions that contain calcifications has developed. This interest reflects the fact that many mammographic features attributable to soft tissue alterations in the breast may be distorted in the excised specimen, rendering them unsuitable for specimen radiography. Changes in the interrelationships of structures in the compressed breast at the time of mammography and the changed orientation in an excised specimen make it difficult to compare these features accurately in clinical and specimen radiographs. The clinical mammographic findings that do not lend themselves to specimen radiography include alterations in parenchymal pattern, skin changes, vascular abnormalities, and ill-defined mass lesions.[505,506]

The presence of calcifications in the lesion or close

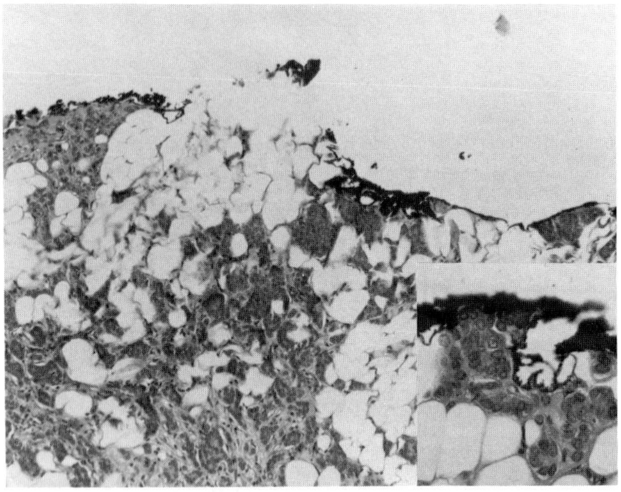

FIGURE 7-39. A positive inked margin in invasive carcinoma. Clusters of poorly differentiated tumor cells infiltrating through fat extend to the ink-covered surface (*inset*) of this excisional biopsy specimen taken from the breast of a 66-year-old woman.

to it provides an intrinsic marker that may be visualized in clinical and specimen radiographs. Specimen radiography is extremely useful in the management of nonpalpable lesions with calcifications detected on mammography because it provides a method for proving that the lesion has been removed, and it is an efficient technique for pinpointing the appropriate area for histologic examination.[507,508] Carcinoma is found in approximately 25% of nonpalpable lesions examined by biopsy because the mammogram reveals a pattern of calcification that suggests carcinoma.[505,506]

In order to evaluate a breast specimen radiograph effectively, the clinical mammogram should be available for simultaneous interpretation. A variety of procedures for specimen radiography have been described in the literature; this presentation will not, therefore, address their advantages or disadvantages, which often depend on the availability of personnel and other resources within a given institution. The processing or interpretation of specimen radiographs may be the responsibility of a pathologist or a radiologist. Film, Polaroid, or xerographic imaging may be used. However, certain principles apply in most situations.

An x-ray film of the intact excisional biopsy should be made, and the film should be compared with the mammogram before the specimen is moved or dissected. If the tissue were to be dissected prior to obtaining a specimen radiograph, a fortuitous cut might disrupt the pattern of calcifications and interfere with the comparison of the clinical and specimen films. Changes in the position of the specimen also make it difficult to pinpoint the location of calcifications.

When a lesion is not apparent on gross examination, it is unwise to select a random sample for frozen section prior to specimen radiography. This would not only result in problems in dissecting the tissue, as detailed earlier, but would also necessitate radiography of the frozen section sample if the specimen x-ray film failed to show the calcifications. Theoretically, it is possible that calcification could be lost in tissue trimmed away in the process of preparing the frozen section.

The first goal of specimen radiography is to confirm that a nonpalpable lesion with calcifications has been excised. This should be determined intraoperatively because if the lesion is not present in the specimen, the surgeon may then elect to perform an additional biopsy. A variety of procedures are available for marking areas in the breast preoperatively in order to assist the surgeon in excising the lesion and to minimize the size of the specimen required. These methods, described in Chapter 3, may also assist the pathologist in locating the lesion for pathologic study. Before the position of the specimen is changed, the site of the calcifications should be identified grossly. This portion of the tissue should be excised from the specimen and labeled. The remainder of the tissue should also be dissected in the event that calcifications prove to be located in a benign process near an unanticipated carcinoma that has fortuitously been included in the excisional biopsy.

The decision as to whether to obtain a frozen section of the area of calcification depends on the customary practice in a given institution and the specific clinical circumstances of a given case. Many of the lesions are quite small, and they often present diagnostic problems. Unless there is a compelling clinical need, it is preferable not to do frozen sections in most of these cases. If a decision is made to attempt a frozen section and the diagnosis is not readily apparent on examination of the initial slides from the tissue block, further sectioning should not be done. Rather, the remaining tissue should be fixed for paraffin sections. In making these decisions, the surgeon must defer to the pathologist's judgment regarding the feasibility of obtaining a diagnosis by frozen section. With few exceptions, pathology laboratories are equipped to process tissue rapidly for paraffin sections so that a report may be obtained within 24 hours.

INTRAOPERATIVE THERMAL DAMAGE TO BIOPSY SPECIMENS. Electrocautery instruments, used for the excision of tissue from the urinary bladder, prostate gland, the breast, and other sites, decrease blood loss from dissected tissues by coagulating the tissue surfaces as they are separated by the cutting edge. When used to perform an excisional breast biopsy, these instruments reduce the risk of hematoma formation in the biopsy cavity and allow the operation to be completed in a shorter period of time.

The thermal effect of electrocautery may produce significant changes in the tissues. Reduced estrogen receptor activity attributable to this procedure has been described,[509–511] which decrease has been sufficient to produce a false-negative report.[512] Histochemical study of prostate and breast specimens after electrocautery has also

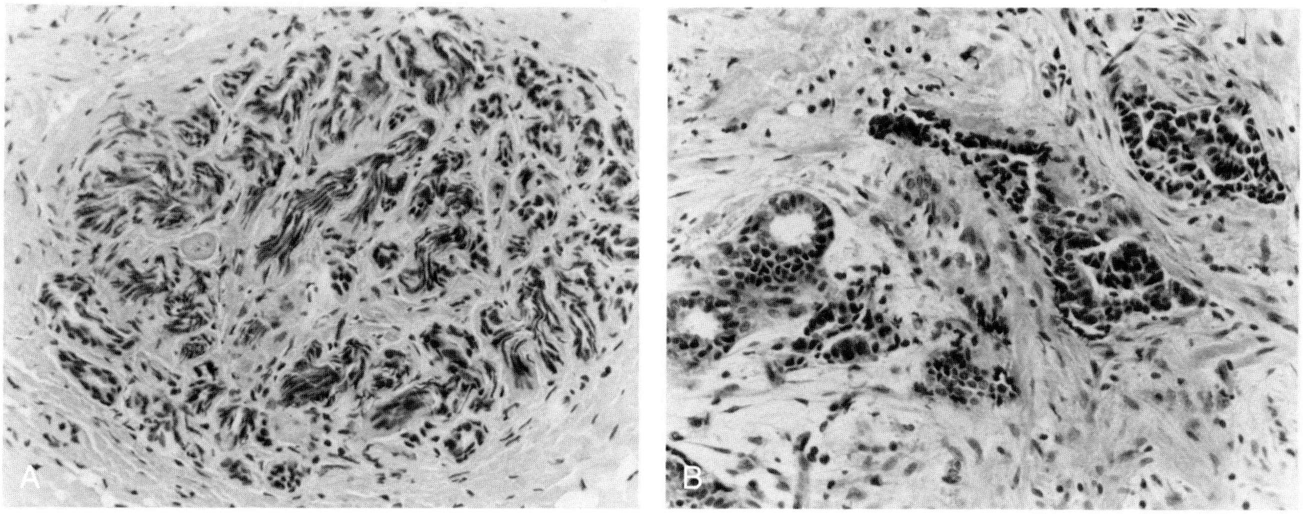

FIGURE 7-40. Thermal damage from electrocautery in an excision biopsy in a 40-year-old woman. *(A)* Views of a lobule showing considerable distortion, particularly smudging of nuclei. *(B)* The lesion was a sclerosing tumor composed of small glands in proliferating stroma. This picture demonstrates sheeding of cells, which is another effect of thermal damage. Disruption of the glandular elements made it impossible to distinguish between sclerosing adenosis and tubular carcinoma.

revealed a decrease in cytoplasmic fluorescent steroid binding and a concomitant increase in fluorescent nuclear activity.[509–510]

The histologic effects of thermal damage from electrocautery on biopsy tissue are well known to pathologists. These changes may create substantial diagnostic problems in biopsies of the prostate and urinary bladder. Because breast biopsies usually consist of a single piece of tissue, thermal damage is usually limited to the surface of the specimen, and generally penetrates no more than 1 mm. The manner in which the instrument is used, the character of the tissue, and the size of the specimen removed influence the intensity and depth of the effect.

The histologic changes in the breast caused by thermal injury are similar to those seen at other sites (Fig. 7-40). The most significant effect is a severe alteration in cytologic detail. Microscopic architecture may be so distorted that a distinction between normal, hyperplastic, and neoplastic tissues may become impossible. Because the damage is maximal at the edges or marginal surfaces of the tissues, electrocautery artifacts severely limit the assessment of the margins of excision when mammary carcinoma is to be treated with limited resection and primary radiotherapy.

If an excision is carried out without taking much, if any, breast parenchyma surrounding a carcinoma, thermal damage to the tumor itself may occur. This is a serious problem in the excision of recurrent or metastatic lesions. In addition to altering receptor activity, the histologic artifacts interfere with the assessment of microscopic prognostic features of the primary tumor, such as nuclear and histologic grade. As a result of damage to cells within ducts, it may be impossible to determine whether intraductal carcinoma is present in tissue outside the tumor mass.

Mastectomy Specimens

The purpose of the gross description of a mastectomy specimen is to document the extent of the operation and the amount and nature of the tissue removed. A standard radical mastectomy can usually be oriented anatomically on the basis of landmarks in the specimen, especially the position of the muscle segments. This may not be accomplished so easily with various types of modified radical mastectomy which have, for the most part, replaced the radical mastectomy. It is important that the surgeon indicate whether there is anything unusual about the specimen, and that important landmarks, such as the levels of axillary lymph nodes and segments of muscle, if present, be identified. Tumor tissue may be taken for receptor analysis at the time of mastectomy if the specimen is submitted immediately to the laboratory and the pathologist has been alerted.

The external description of the specimen should include the following: overall size of the specimen; dimensions and appearance of the skin, with measurement of scars or incisions; the appearance of the nipple and areola; the presence of muscle and axillary tissue; and the location of any distinct, palpable lesion.

Dissection of the specimen is most easily accomplished by placing it, skin side down, in an anatomical orientation in order to identify the quadrants. The findings can thus be visualized as if one were looking through the patient from back to front. The deep surface of the specimen should be inspected and palpated for evidence of tumor involvement and inked as deemed appropriate. In a standard radical mastectomy, the cut edge of the sternal attachment of the pectoralis major muscle marks the medial side. In such a specimen, the fascia between the major and minor pectoralis muscles should be dissected to identify Rotter's node.

The breast is dissected by a series of parallel incisions through the posterior surface up to the skin. A tumor, if present, should be described in the same fashion as a biopsy specimen. The size and character of a biopsy site should be noted, including any areas of induration. It is preferable that these areas not be identified as tumor since the tissue reaction in a healing biopsy cavity may be grossly indistinguishable from carcinoma. The appearance of the remaining breast parenchyma is also recorded, including relative proportions of fat and fibrous parenchyma; the size, location, and character of any discrete lesions; and the presence or absence of cysts. Samples for histologic examination are taken from the tumor or biopsy site, or both, and from the nipple, skin quadrants, and deep margin under the tumor.

One vertical section of the nipple will suffice to detect Paget's disease even when this condition is not suspected on the basis of clinical findings. More elaborate sectioning schemes may be employed in special circumstances, but their routine use is not cost-efficient in view of the low incidence of occult Paget's disease, which is not a clinically significant finding in a patient treated with mastectomy. Generally, two sections per quadrant are taken randomly, but more extensive sectioning may be indicated by the gross findings or when mastectomy is performed for *in situ* lobular or intraductal carcinoma.

Axillary Lymph Nodes

With the exception of standard radical mastectomy specimens, it is virtually impossible to determine the position or level of axillary lymph nodes from axillary contents received with a mastectomy specimen. If this information is desired for clinical reasons, the lymph node groups should be tagged or submitted as separately identified specimens.

Careful, manual dissection of the unfixed axillary fat is the most cost-effective method for isolating the lymph nodes for microscopic study. In using this process, firm bits of fat and other tissue may be mistaken for lymph nodes. Although the gross description should include a count of the tissue samples thought to be lymph nodes, which are submitted for histology, the final number of nodes is determined from those counted in the tissue sections. The overall character and dimensions of the lymph nodes should be described. It is generally advisable to avoid stating that metastases are grossly present or absent since uncertainty arises when the results of microscopic study differ from the gross impression. Lymph nodes that are distorted by inflammation or hyperplasia or, in some cases, enlarged by fatty infiltration are a common cause of false-positive interpretations on gross pathologic and clinical examination.

A number of other elaborate procedures are available to identify lymph nodes in the fat. These methods include obtaining x-ray films of the fat;[513,514] fixing the fat in Bouin's solution, which stains fat intensely yellow but leaves the lymph nodes white; and clearing the fat by a process that renders it relatively transparent so that solid structures, such as lymph nodes, stand out when the tissue is placed over a light source.[515]

These procedures will generally increase the number of lymph nodes obtained by locating very small lymph nodes that might otherwise be missed on palpation. In a study of 42 axillary dissections, the mean number of lymph nodes found was increased, by clearing, from 20 to 26 in patients with Stage I disease and from 22 to 30 in patients with Stage II disease.[516] Additional positive lymph nodes were found in the latter group, but not in those patients originally assigned to Stage I on the basis of manually dissected nodes. Hartveit and colleagues cleared axillary tissue from 63 node-negative patients and found one node containing a micrometastasis that had not been found on routine processing.[517] Although it is possible that a patient may occasionally be incorrectly staged because a positive node was missed in manual dissection, the likelihood of this is so small that the considerable time and expense required for clearing is not justified.

REFERENCES

1. Foote FW Jr, Stewart FW: A histologic classification of carcinoma of the breast. Surgery 19:74, 1946
2. McDivitt RW, Stewart FW, Berg JW: Tumors of the Breast. Atlas of Tumor Pathology, Series 2, Fascicle No 2. Washington, DC, Armed Forces Institute of Pathology, 1968
3. World Health Organization: Histological typing of breast tumors. Tumori 68:181, 1982
4. Cornil A-V: Contributions a l'histoire du developpement histologique des tumeurs epitheliales (squirrhe, encephaloide, etc). J Anat Physiol 2:266, 1865
5. Waldeyer W: Die Entwickelung der Carcinome. Arch Pathol Anat Phys Klin Med 41:470, 1867
6. Broders AC: Carcinoma *in situ* contrasted with benign penetrating epithelium. JAMA 99:1670, 1932
7. Foote FW Jr, Stewart FW: Lobular carcinoma *in situ:* A rare form of mammary cancer. Am J Pathol 17:491, 1941
8. Ozzello L: The behavior of basement membranes of intraductal carcinoma of the breast. Am J Pathol 35:887, 1959
9. Ozzello L: Ultrastructure of intra-epithelial carcinomas of the breast. Cancer 28:1508, 1971
10. Rosen PP: Axillary lymph node metastases in patients with occult noninvasive breast carcinoma. Cancer 46:1298, 1980
11. Haagensen CD, Lane N, Lattes R et al: Lobular neoplasia (so-called lobular carcinoma *in situ*) of the breast. Cancer 42:737, 1978
12. Beahrs O, Shapiro S, Smart C: Report of the working group to review the National Cancer Institute—American Cancer Society Breast Cancer Detection Demonstration Projects. J Natl Cancer Inst 62:640, 1979

13. Rosen PP: Coexistent lobular carcinoma *in situ* and intraductal carcinoma in a single lobular-duct unit. Am J Surg Pathol 4:241, 1980
14. Fechner RE: Ductal carcinoma involving the lobule of the breast. A source of confusion with lobular carcinoma *in situ*. Cancer 28:274, 1971
15. Fechner RE: Epithelial alterations in extralobular ducts of breasts with lobular carcinoma. Arch Pathol 93:164, 1972
16. Wellings SR, Jensen HM: On the origin and progression of ductal carcinoma in the human breast. J Natl Cancer Inst 50:1111, 1973
17. Warren JC: Abnormal involution of the mammary gland with its treatment by operation. Am J Med Sci 134:521, 1907
18. Bloodgood JC: Border-line breast tumors. Ann Surg 93:235, 1931
19. Cheatle GL: Cysts and primary cancer in cysts of the breast. Br J Surg 8:149, 1920–21
20. Bloodgood JC: The pathology of chronic cystic mastitis of the female breast. Arch Surg 3:445, 1921
21. Bloodgood JC: Comedo carcinoma (or comedo-carcinoma) of the female breast. Am J Cancer 22:842, 1934
22. Rosen PP: The pathological classification of human mammary carcinoma: Past, present and future. Ann Clin Lab Sci 9:144, 1979
23. Smart CR, Myers MH, Gloeckler LA: Implications from SEER data on breast cancer management. Cancer 41:787, 1978
24. Hendricks JHCL: Population screening for breast cancer by means of mammography in Nijmegen, 1975–1982. MD thesis, Nijmegen University, 1982
25. Tabar L, Akerlund E, Gad A: Five year experience with single-view mammography randomized controlled screening in Sweden. Recent Results Cancer Res 90:105, 1984
26. Andersson I: Breast cancer screening in Malmo. Recent Results Cancer Res 90:114, 1984
27. Andersson I, Andren L, Hildell J, et al: Breast cancer screening with mammography. A population-based randomized trial with mammography as the only screening mode. Radiology 132:273, 1979
28. Heller KS, Rosen PP, Schottenfeld D, et al: Male breast cancer. A clinicopathologic study of 97 cases. Ann Surg 188:60, 1978
29. Lesser ML, Rosen PP, Senie RT, et al: Estrogen and progesterone receptors in breast carcinoma: Correlations with epidemiology and pathology. Cancer 48:299, 1981
30. Rosen PP, Menendez-Botet CJ, Senie RT, et al Estrogen receptor protein (ERP) and the histopathology of human mammary carcinoma. In WL McGuire (ed): Hormones, Receptors and Breast Cancer, pp 71–83. New York, Raven Press, 1978
31. Silfversward C, Gustafsson J-A, Gustafsson SA, et al: Estrogen receptor concentrations in 269 cases of histologically classified human breast cancer. Cancer 45:2001, 1980
32. King WJ, DeSombre ER, Jensen EV, et al: Comparison of immunocytochemical and steroid-binding assays for estrogen receptor in human breast tumors. Cancer Res 45:293, 1985
33. Westbrook KC, Gallager HS: Intraductal carcinoma of the breast. A comparative study. Am J Surg 130:667, 1975
34. von Rueden DG, Wilson RE: Intraductal carcinoma of the breast. Surg Gynecol Obstet 158:105, 1984
35. Ashikari R, Hajdu SI, Robbins GF: Intraductal carcinoma of the breast (1960–1969). Cancer 28:1182, 1971
36. Rosen PP, Ashikari R, Thaler H, et al: A comparative study of some pathologic features of mammary carcinoma in Tokyo, Japan and New York, USA. Cancer 39:429, 1977
37. Gibbons CP: Intraductal breast cancer. Lancet 11:462, 1984
38. Rosen PP, Snyder RE, Robbins G: Specimen radiography for non-palpable breast lesions found by mammography: Procedures and results. Cancer 34:2028, 1974
39. Strax P, Venet L, Shapiro S: Value of mammography in reduction of mortality from breast cancer in mass screening. Am J Roentgenol 117:686, 1973
40. Rosen PP, Lesser ML, Senie RT, et al: Epidemiology of breast carcinoma IV: Age and histologic tumor type. J Surg Oncol 19:44, 1982
41. Brown PW, Silverman J, Owens E, et al: Intraductal "noninfiltrating" carcinoma of the breast. Arch Surg 111:1063, 1976
42. Urban JA: Biopsy of the "normal" breast in treating breast cancer. Surg Clin North Am 49:291, 1969
43. Ringberg A, Palmer B, Linell F: The contralateral breast at reconstructive surgery after breast cancer operation—A histological study. Breast Cancer Res Treat 2:151, 1982
44. Rosen PP: Frozen section diagnosis of breast lesions. Recent experience with 556 consecutive biopsies. Ann Surg 187:17, 1978
45. Rosen PP, Senie R, Schottenfeld D, et al: Noninvasive breast carcinoma. Frequency of unsuspected invasion and implications for treatment. Ann Surg 189:377, 1979
46. Tulusan AH, Grunsteidel W, Ramming I, et al: A contribution to the natural history of breast cancer III. Changes in the basement membranes in breast cancers with stromal microinvasion. Arch Gynecol 231:209, 1982
47. Barsky SH, Siegal GP, Jannotta F, et al: Loss of basement membrane components by invasive tumors but not by their benign counterparts. Lab Invest 49:140, 1983
48. Wells S, Hasleton PS: A dilutional immunoperoxidase study of proliferative ductal lesions and carcinomata of the breast. Histopathology 5:517, 1981
49. Frappart L, Boudeulle M, Boumendil J, et al: Structure and composition of microcalcifications in benign and malignant lesions of the breast: Study by light microscopy, transmission and scanning electron microscopy, microprobe analysis and x-ray diffraction. Hum Pathol 15:880, 1984
50. Haagensen CD: Diseases of the Breast, 2nd ed, pp 586–590. Philadelphia, WB Saunders, 1971
51. Rosner D, Bedwani RN, Vana J, et al: Noninvasive breast carcinoma. Results of a national survey by the American College of Surgeons. Ann Surg 192:139, 1980
52. Gillis DA, Dockerty MB, Clagett OT: Preinvasive intraductal carcinoma of the breast. Surg Gynecol Obstet 110:555, 1960
53. Rosen PP: Lobular carcinoma *in situ* and intraductal carcinoma of the breast. In McDivitt RW, Oberman HA, Ozzello L, et al (eds): The Breast, pp 59–105. Baltimore, Williams & Wilkins, 1984
54. Recht A, Danoff BS, Salin LJ, et al: Intraductal carcinoma of the breast: Results of treatment with excisional biopsy and irradiation. J Clin Oncol 3:1339, 1985
55. Fisher E, Sass R, Fisher B, et al: Pathologic findings from the National Surgical Adjuvant Breast Project (Protocol 6). I. Intraductal carcinoma (DCIS). Cancer 57:197, 1986
56. Muir R: The evolution of carcinoma of the mamma. J Pathol Bacteriol 52:153, 1941
57. Farrow JH: Clinical considerations and treatment of *in situ* lobular breast cancer. Am J Roentgenol 102:652, 1968
58. Hutter RVP, Snyder RE, Lucas J, et al: Clinical and pathologic correlation with mammographic findings in lobular carcinoma *in situ*. Cancer 23:826, 1969
59. Morris DM, Walker AP, Coker DC: Lack of efficacy of xeromammography in preoperatively detecting lobular carcinoma *in situ* of the breast. Breast Cancer Res Treat 1:363, 1982
60. Rosen PP, Senie RT, Farr GH, et al: Epidemiology of breast

carcinoma: Age, menstrual status, and exogenous hormone usage in patients with lobular carcinoma *in situ*. Surgery 85:215, 1979
61. Farrow JH: Current concepts in the detection and treatment of the earliest of the early breast cancers. Cancer 25:468, 1970
62. Lewison EF, Finney GG: Lobular carcinoma *in situ* of the breast. Surg Gynecol Obstet 126:1280, 1968
63. Warner NE: Lobular carcinoma of the breast. Cancer 23:840, 1969
64. Anderson JA: Multicentric and bilateral appearance of lobular carcinoma *in situ* of the breast. Acta Pathol Microbiol Scand [A] 82:730, 1974
65. Carter D, Smith AL: Carcinoma *in situ* of the breast. Cancer 40:1189, 1977
66. Shah JP, Rosen PP, Robbins GF: Pitfalls of local excision in the treatment of carcinoma of the breast. Surg Gynecol Obstet 136:721, 1973
67. Tulusan AH, Egger H, Schneider ML, et al: A contribution to the natural history of breast cancer. IV. Lobular carcinoma *in situ* and its relation to breast cancer. Arch Gynecol 231:219, 1982
68. Barnes JP: Bilateral lobular carcinoma *in situ*. Report of two cases. Texas State J Med 55:581, 1959
69. Newman W: *In situ* lobular carcinoma of the breast. Ann Surg 151:520, 1963
70. Rosen PP, Lieberman PH, Braun DW Jr, et al: Lobular carcinoma *in situ* of the breast. Detailed analysis of 99 patients with average follow-up of 24 years. Am J Surg Pathol 2:225, 1978
71. Zippel HH, Hematsch HJ, Kunze WP: Morphometric and cytophotometric investigations of lobular neoplasia of the breast with ductal involvement. J Cancer Res Clin Oncol 93:265, 1979
72. Gad A, Azzopardi JG: Lobular carcinoma of the breast: A special variant of mucin secreting carcinoma. J Clin Pathol 28:711, 1975
73. Andersen JA, Vendelhoe ML: Cytoplasmic mucous globules in lobular carcinoma *in situ*. Diagnosis and prognosis. Am J Surg Pathol 5:251, 1981
74. Breslow A, Brancaccio ME: Intracellular mucin production by lobular breast carcinoma cells. Arch Pathol Lab Med 100:620, 1976
75. Eusebi V, Pich A, Macchiorlatti E, et al: Morphofunctional differentiation in lobular carcinoma of the breast. Histopathology 1:301, 1977
76. Andersen, JA: Lobular carcinoma *in situ* of the breast with ductal involvement. Frequency and possible influence on prognosis. Acta Pathol Microbiol Scand [A] 82:655, 1974
77. Haagensen CD, Lane N, Lattes R: Neoplastic proliferation of the epithelium of the mammary lobules: Adenosis, lobular neoplasia and small cell carcinoma. Surg Clin North Am 52:497, 1972
78. Rosen PP, Tench W: Lobules in the nipple. Frequency and significance for breast cancer treatment. Pathol Annu 20(Pt 2):217, 1985
79. Tobon H, Price HM: Lobular carcinoma *in situ*. Some ultrastructural observations. Cancer 30:1082, 1972
80. Nesland JM, Johannessen JV: Malignant breast lesions. J Submicrosc Cytol 14:553, 1982
81. Bussolati G: Actin-rich (myoepithelial) cells in lobular carcinoma *in situ* of the breast. Virchows Arch [Cell Pathol] 32:165, 1980
82. Andersen JA: The basement membrane and lobular carcinoma *in situ* of the breast. A light microscopical study. Acta Pathol Microbiol Scand [A] 83:245, 1975
83. Fechner RE: Lobular carcinoma *in situ* in sclerosing adenosis. A potential source of confusion with invasive carcinoma. Am J Surg Pathol 5:233, 1981
84. Andersen JA: Lobular carcinoma *in situ:* A long term follow-up in 52 cases. Acta Pathol Microbiol Scand [A] 82:519, 1974
85. Benfield JR, Jacobson M, Warner NE: *In situ* lobular carcinoma of the breast. Arch Surg 91:130, 1965
86. Rosen PP, Braun DW Jr, Lyngholm B, et al: Lobular carcinoma *in situ* of the breast: Preliminary results of treatment by ipsilateral mastectomy and contralateral breast biopsy. Cancer 47:813, 1981
87. World Health Organization: Histological Typing of Breast Tumours, 2nd ed. International Histological Classification of Tumours No 2, p 19. Geneva, World Health Organization, 1981
88. Fisher ER, Gregorio RM, Fisher B, et al: The pathology of invasive breast cancer. A syllabus derived from findings of the National Surgical Adjuvant Breast Project (No 4). Cancer 36:1, 1975
89. Sistrunk WE, MacCarty WC: Life expectancy following radical amputation for carcinoma of the breast: A clinical and pathologic study of 218 cases. Ann Surg 75:61, 1922
90. Stenkvist B, Bengtsson E, Dahlqvist B, et al: Predicting breast cancer recurrence. Cancer 50:2884, 1982
91. Freedman LS, Edwards DN, McConnell EM, et al: Histological grade and other prognostic factors in relation to survival of patients with breast cancer. Br J Cancer 40:44, 1979
92. Adair F, Berg J, Joubert L, et al: Long-term follow-up of breast cancer patients. The 30 year report. Cancer 33:1145, 1974
93. Fisher B, Slack NH, Bross IDJ, et al: Cancer of the breast: Size of neoplasm and prognosis. Cancer 24:1071, 1969
94. Say CC, Donegan WL: Invasive carcinoma of the breast: Prognostic significance of tumor size and involved axillary lymph nodes. Cancer 34:468, 1974
95. Gold RH, Main G, Zippin C, et al: Infiltration of mammary carcinoma as an indicator of axillary metastases. A preliminary report. Cancer 29:35, 1972
96. Lane N, Goksel H, Salerno RA, et al: Clinicopathologic analysis of the surgical curability of breast cancers. A minimum ten year study. Ann Surg 153:483, 1961
97. Carter D, Pipkin RD, Shepard RH, et al: Relationship of necrosis and tumor border to lymph node metastases and 10 year survival in carcinoma of the breast. Am J Surg Pathol 2:39, 1978
98. Black MM, Speer FD: Nuclear structure in cancer tissues. Surg Gynecol Obstet 105:97, 1957
99. Cutler SJ, Black MM, Mork T, et al: Further observations on prognostic factors in cancer of the female breast. Cancer 24:653, 1969
100. Bloom HJG: Prognosis in carcinoma of the breast. Br J Cancer 4:259, 1950
101. Bloom HJG, Richardson WW: Histological grading and prognosis in breast cancer. A study of 1049 cases, of which 359 have been followed 15 years. Br J Cancer 11:359, 1957
102. Thoresen S: Histological grading and clinical stage at presentation in breast carcinoma. Br J Cancer 46:457, 1982
103. Andersen JA, Fischermann K, Hou-Jensen K, et al: Selection of high risk groups among prognostically favorable patients with breast cancer. An analysis of the value of prospective grading of tumor anaplasia in 1048 patients. Ann Surg 194:1, 1981
104. Parl FF, Dupont WD: A retrospective cohort study of histologic risk fctors in breast cancer patients. Cancer 50:2410, 1982
105. Black MM, Barclay THC, Hankey BF: Prognosis in breast

cancer utilizing histologic characteristics of the primary tumor. Cancer 36:2048, 1975
106. Rosen PP, Saigo PE, Braun DW Jr, et al: Predictors of recurrence in Stage I (T1N0M0) breast carcinoma. Ann Surg 193:15, 1981
107. Dawson PJ, Ferguson DJ, Karrison T: The pathologic findings of breast cancer in patients surviving 25 years after radical mastectomy. Cancer 50:2131, 1982
108. Rosen PP, Saigo PE, Braun DW Jr, et al: Prognosis in Stage II (T1N1M0) breast cancer. Ann Surg 194:576, 1981
109. Kister SJ, Sommers SC, Haagensen CD, et al: Nuclear grade and sinus histiocytosis in cancer of the breast. Cancer 23:570, 1969
110. Atkin NB, Kay R: Prognostic significance of modal DNA value and other factors in malignant tumors, based on 1465 cases. Br J Cancer 40:210, 1979
111. Atkin NB: Modal deoxyribonucleic acid value and survival in carcinomas of the breast. Br Med J 1:271, 1972
112. Auer GU, Caspersson TO, Wallgren AS: DNA content and survival in mammary carcinomas. Anal Quant Cytol 2:162, 1980
113. Auer GU, Eriksson E, Azavedo E, et al: Prognostic significance of nuclear DNA content in mammary adenocarcinomas in humans. Cancer Res 44:394, 1984
114. Auer GU, Fallenius AG, Erhardt KY, et al: Progression of mammary adenocarcinomas as reflected by nuclear DNA content. Cytometry 5:420, 1984
115. Auer GU, Caspersson TO, Gustafsson SA, et al: Relationship between nuclear DNA distribution and estrogen receptors in human mammary carcinomas. Anal Quant Cytol 2:280, 1980
116. Bedrossian CWM, Raber M, Barlogie B: Flow cytometry and cytomorphology in primary resectable breast carcinomas. Anal Quant Cytol 3:112, 1981
117. Bichel P, Paulsen HS, Andersen J: Estrogen receptor content and ploidy of human mammary carcinomas. Cancer 50:1771, 1982
118. Taylor IW, Musgrove EA, Friedlander ML, et al: The influence of age on the DNA ploidy levels of breast tumors. Eur J Cancer 19:623, 1983
119. Sven-Borje E, Langstrom E, Baldetorp B, et al: Flow-cytometric DNA analysis in primary breast carcinomas and clinicopathologic correlations. Cytometry 5:408, 1984
120. Chassevent A, Daver A, Bertrand G, et al: Comparative flow DNA analysis of different cell suspensions in the breast carcinomas. Cytometry 5:263, 1984
121. Raber MN, Barlogie B, Latreille J, et al: Ploidy, proliferative activity and estrogen receptor content in human breast cancer. Cytometry 3:36, 1982
122. Cornelisse CJ, de Koning HR, Moolenaar AJ, et al: Image and flow cytometric analysis of DNA content in breast cancer. Relation to estrogen receptor content and lymph node involvement. Anal Quant Cytol 6:9, 1984
123. Patek E, Johannisson E, Krauer F, et al: Microfluorometric grading of mammary tumors. Anal Quant Cytol 2:264, 1980
124. Gentili C, Sanfilippo O, Silvestrini R: Cell proliferation and its relationship to clinical features and relapses in breast cancers. Cancer 48:974, 1981
125. Meyer JS, Friedman E, McCrate M, et al: Prediction of early course of breast carcinomas by thymidine labeling. Cancer 51:1879, 1983
126. Tubiana M, Pejovic JM, Renaud A, et al: Kinetic parameters and the course of the disease in breast cancer. Cancer 47:937, 1981
127. Meyer JS, McDivitt RW, Stone KR, et al: Practical breast carcinoma cell kinetics: Review and update. Breast Cancer Res Treat 4:79, 1984
128. Tubiana M, Pejovic MH, Chavaudra N, et al: The long-term prognostic significance of the thymidine labeling index in breast cancer. Int J Cancer 33:441, 1984
129. Fossa SD, Thorud E, Vaage S, et al: DNA cytometry of primary breast cancer. A comparison of microspectrophotometry and flow cytometry and different preparation methods for flow cytometric measurements. Acta Pathol Microbiol Immunol Scand [A] 91:235, 1983
130. Moran RE, Black M, Alpert L, et al: Correlation of cell-cycle kinetics, hormone receptors, histopathology and nodal status in human breast cancer. Cancer 54:1586, 1984
131. Meyer JS, Hixon B: Advanced stage and early relapse of breast carcinomas associated with high thymidine labeling indices. Cancer Res 39:4042, 1979
132. Olszewski W, Darzynkiewicz Z, Rosen PP, et al: Flow cytometry of breast carcinoma: I. Relation of DNA ploidy level to histology and estrogen receptor. Cancer 48:980, 1981
133. Olszewski W, Darzynkiewicz Z, Rosen PP, et al: Flow cytometry of breast carcinoma: II. Relation of tumor cell cycle distribution to histology and estrogen receptor. Cancer 48:985, 1981
134. McDivitt RW, Stone KR, Craig B, et al: A proposed classification of breast cancer based on kinetic information derived from a comparison of risk factors in 168 primary operable breast cancers. Cancer 57:269, 1986
135. Olszewski W, Darzynkiewicz Z, Rosen PP, et al: Flow cytometry of breast carcinoma: III. Possible altered kinetics in axillary lymph node metastases. Anal Quant Cytol 4:275, 1982
136. Brunner N, Spang-Thomsen M, Vindelv A, et al: Detection of endocrine responsiveness by flow cytometric DNA analysis in experimental human breast cancer. Recent Results Cancer Res 90:200, 1984
137. Hedley DW, Friedlander ML, Taylor IW, et al: Method for analysis of cellular DNA content of paraffin-embedded pathological material using flow cytometry. J Histochem Cytochem 31:1333, 1983
138. Hedley DW, Rugg CA, Ng ABP, et al: Influence of cellular DNA content on disease-free survival of Stage II breast cancer patients. Cancer Res 44:5395, 1984
139. Baak JPA, VanDop H, Kurver PHJ, et al: The value of morphometry to classic prognosticators in breast cancer. Cancer 56:374, 1985
140. Zajdela A, DeLaRiva LS, Ghossein NA: The relation of prognosis to the nuclear diameter of breast cancer cells obtained by cytologic aspiration. Acta Cytol 23:75, 1979
141. Kuenen-Boumeester V, Hop WCJ, Blonk DI, et al: Prognostic scoring using cytomorphometry and lymph node status of patients with breast carcinoma. Eur J Cancer Clin Oncol 20:337, 1984
142. Stenkvist B, Bengtsson E, Eriksson O, et al: Correlation between cytometric features and mitotic frequency in human breast carcinoma. Cytometry 1:287, 1981
143. Stenkvist B, Bengtsson E, Eriksson O, et al: A morphometric expression of differentiation in fine-needle biopsies of breast cancer. Cytometry 1:292, 1981
144. Maehle B, Thoresen S, Skjaerve R, et al: Mean nuclear area and histological grade of axillary node tumor in breast cancer. Relation to prognosis. Br J Cancer 46:95, 1982
145. Rosen PP, Lesser ML, Kinne DW, et al: Breast carcinoma in women 35 years of age or younger. Ann Surg 199:133, 1984
146. Contesso JC, Delarue J, Mouriesse H, et al: Correlation between hormone receptors and histological characters in human breast tumours. Pathol Biol 31:747, 1983

147. Ridolfi R, Rosen P, Port A, et al: Medullary carcinoma of the breast. A clinicopathologic study with 10 year follow-up. Cancer 40:1365, 1977
148. Alderson MR, Hamlin I, Staunton MD: The relative significance of prognostic factors in breast carcinoma. Br J Cancer 25:646, 1971
149. Berg JW: Morphological evidence for immune response to cancer—An historical review. Cancer 28:1453, 1971
150. Roses DF, Bell DA, Flotte TJ, et al: Pathologic predictors of recurrence in Stage I (T1N0M0) breast cancer. Am J Clin Pathol 78:817, 1982
151. Fisher ER, Sass R, Watkins G, et al: Tissue mast cells in breast cancer. Breast Cancer Res Treat 5:285, 1985
152. Gilchrist KW, Gould VE, Hirschl S, et al: Interobserver variation in the identification of breast carcinoma in intramammary lymphatics. Hum Pathol 13:170, 1982
153. Rosen PP: Tumor emboli in intramammary lymphatics in breast carcinoma: Pathologic criteria for diagnosis and clinical significance. Pathol Annu 18(Pt: 2):215, 1983
154. Bettelheim R, Mitchell D, Gusterson BA: Immunocytochemistry in the identification of vascular invasion in breast cancer. J Clin Pathol 37:364, 1984
155. Saigo PE, Rosen PP: The application of immunohistochemical stains to identify endothelial lined channels in mammary carcinoma. Cancer (in press)
156. Nime F, Rosen PP, Thaler H, et al: Prognostic significance of tumor emboli in intramammary lymphatics in patients with mammary carcinoma. Am J Surg Pathol 1:25, 1977
157. Fracchia AA, Rosen PP, Ashikari R: Primary carcinoma of the breast without axillary lymph node metastases. Surg Gynecol Obstet 151:375, 1980
158. Merlin C, Gloor F, Hardmeier T, et al: Hat die intramammarare lymphangiosis carcinomatosa bein nodal—negativen Mammakarzion eine prognostische Bedeutung? Schweiz Med Wochenschr 110:605, 1980
159. Bettelheim R, Penman HG, Thornton-Jones H, et al: Prognostic significance of peritumoral vascular invasion in breast cancer. Br J Cancer 50:771, 1984
160. Rosen PP, Saigo PE, Braun DW Jr, et al: Occult axillary lymph node metastases from breast cancers with intramammary lymphatic tumor emboli. Am J Surg Pathol 6:639, 1982
161. Sampat MB, Sirsat MV, Gangadharan P: Prognostic significance of blood vessel invasion in carcinoma of the breast in women. J Surg Oncol 9:623, 1977
162. Teel P, Sommers SC: Vascular invasion as a prognostic factor in breast carcinoma. Surg Gynecol Obstet 118:1006, 1964
163. Kister SJ, Sommers SC, Haagensen CD, et al: Reevaluation of blood vessel invasion and lymphocytic infiltrates in breast carcinoma. Cancer 19:1213, 1966
164. Weigand RA, Isenberg WM, Russo J, et al: Blood vessel invasion and axillary lymph node involvement as prognostic indicators for human breast cancer. Cancer 50:962, 1982
165. Friedell GH, Betts A, Sommers SC: Prognostic value of blood vessel invasion and lymphocytic infiltrates in breast carcinoma. Cancer 18:164, 1965
166. Bell JR, Friedell GH, Goldenberg IS: Prognostic significance of pathologic findings in human breast carcinoma. Surg Gynecol Obstet 129:258, 1969
167. Sato E, Kumagai N, Abe R: Significant prognostic factors in breast cancer of Japanese women: Special reference to nuclear grade and sinus histiocytosis. Tohoku J Exp Med 120:135, 1976
168. Davies JD: Hyperelastosis, obliteration and fibrous plaques in major ducts of the human breast. J Pathol 110:13, 1973
169. Reyes MG, Bazile DB, Tosch T, et al: Periductal elastic tissue of breast cancer. Arch Pathol Lab Med 106:610, 1982
170. Humeniuk V, Forrest APM, Hawkins RA, et al: Elastosis and primary breast cancer. Cancer 52:1448, 1983
171. Rasmussen BB, Pedersen BV, Thorpe SM, et al: Elastosis in relation to prognosis in primary breast carcinoma. Cancer Res 45:1428, 1985
172. Masters JRW, Sangster K, Hawkins RA, et al: Elastosis and estrogen receptors in human breast cancer. Br J Cancer 33:342, 1976
173. Shivas AA, Douglas JG: The prognostic significance of elastosis in breast carcinoma. J R Coll Surg Edinb 17:315, 1972
174. Robertson AJ, Brown RA, Cree IA, et al: Prognostic value of measurement of elastosis in breast carcinoma. J Clin Pathol 34:738, 1981
175. Glaubitz LC, Bowen JH, Cox ED, et al: Elastosis in human breast cancer. Correlation with sex steroid receptors and comparison with clinical outcome. Arch Pathol Lab Med 108:27, 1984
176. Anastassiades OT, Bouropoulou V, Kontogeorgos G, et al: Duct elastosis in infiltrating carcinoma of the breast. Pathol Res Pract 165:411, 1979
177. Silverberg SG, Chitale AR: Assessment of significance of proportions of intraductal and infiltrating tumor growth in ductal carcinoma of the breast. Cancer 32:830, 1978
178. Schnitt SJ, Connolly JL, Harris JR, et al: Pathologic predictors of early local recurrences in Stage I and II breast cancer treated by primary radiation therapy. Cancer 53:1049, 1984
179. Rosen PP, Kinne DW, Lesser ML, et al: Are prognostic factors for local control of breast cancer treated by primary radiotherapy significant for patients treated by mastectomy? Cancer 57:1415. 1986
180. Lee AK, Rosen PP, DeLellis RA, et al: Tumor marker expression in breast carcinomas and relationship to prognosis. An immunohistochemical study. Am J Clin Pathol 84:687, 1985
181. Shousha S, Lysiottis T, Godfrey VM, et al: Carcinoembryonic antigen in breast cancer tissue: A useful prognostic indicator. Br Med J 1:777, 1979
182. Kuhajda FP, Offutt LE, Mendelsohn G: The distribution of carcinoembryonic antigen in breast carcinoma. Cancer 52:1257, 1983
183. Walker RA: Immunohistochemistry of biological markers of breast carcinoma. In DeLellis RA (ed): Advances in Immunohistochemistry, pp. 223–241. New York, Masson Publishing, 1984
184. Gilchrist KW, Kalish L, Gould VE, et al: Immunostaining for carcinoembryonic antigen does not discriminate for early recurrence in breast cancer. The ECOG experience. Cancer 56:351, 1985
185. Horne CHW, Reid IN, Milne GD: Prognostic significance of inappropriate production of pregnancy proteins by breast cancers. Lancet 2:279, 1976
186. Lee AK, DeLellis RA, Rosen PP: ABH blood group isoantigens in breast carcinomas—An immunohistochemical evaluation using monoclonal antibodies. Am J Clin Pathol 83:308, 1985
187. Cornil V, Ranvier L: Manuel d'Histologie Pathologique, pp 1167–1170. Paris, Germer Bailliere, 1869
188. Foote FW Jr: Surgical pathology of cancer of the breast. In Parsons WH (ed): Cancer of the Breast, pp 37–38. Springfield, Charles C Thomas, 1959
189. McDivitt RW, Stewart FW, Berg JW: Tumors of the Breast. Atlas of Tumor Pathology, Series 2, Fascicle No 2, pp 89–90. Washington, DC, Armed Forces Institute of Pathology, 1968

190. Taylor HB, Norris HJ: Well differentiated carcinoma of the breast. Cancer 25:687, 1970
191. Kouchoukos NT, Ackerman LV, Butcher HR: Prediction of axillary nodal metastases from the morphology of primary mammary carcinomas. Cancer 20:948, 1967
192. Carstens PHB: Tubular carcinoma of the breast. A study of frequency. Am J Clin Pathol 70:204, 1978
193. Cooper HS, Patchefsky AS, Krall RA: Tubular carcinoma of the breast. Cancer 42:2334, 1978
194. Peters GN, Wolff M, Haagensen CD: Tubular carcinoma of the breast. Clinical pathologic correlations based on 100 cases. Ann Surg 193:138, 1981
195. Deos PH, Norris HJ: Well-differentiated (tubular) carcinoma of the breast. Am J Clin Pathol 78:1, 1982
196. Oberman HA, Fidler WJ Jr: Tubular carcinoma of the breast. Am J Surg Pathol 13:387, 1979
197. McDivitt RW, Boyce W, Gersell D: Tubular carcinoma of the breast. Clinical and pathological observations concerning 135 cases. Am J Surg Pathol 6:401, 1982
198. Carstens PHB, Greenberg RA, Francis D, et al: Tubular carcinoma of the breast. A long term folow-up. Histopathology 9:271, 1985
199. Feig SA, Shaber GS, Patchefsky A, et al: Analysis of clinically occult and mammographically occult breast tumors. Am J Roentgenol 128:403, 1977
200. Andersson I: Radiographic screening for breast carcinoma. II. Prognostic considerations on the basis of short-term follow-up. Acta Radiol [Diagn] 22:227, 1982
201. Linell F, Ljungberg O: Breast carcinoma, progression of tubular carcinoma and a new classification. Acta Pathol Microbiol Scand [A] 88:59, 1980
202. Linell F, Ljungberg O, Anderson I: Breast carcinoma: Aspects of early stages, progression and related problems. Acta Pathol Microbiol Scand [A] (suppl) 272:1, 1980
203. Andersen JA, Carter D, Linell F: A symposium on sclerosing duct lesions of the breast. Pathol Annu 21 (2):145, 1986
204. Wellings SR, Alpers CE: Subgross pathologic features and incidence of radial scars in the breast. Hum Pathol 15:475, 1984
205. Taxy JB: Tubular carcinoma of the male breast: Report of a case. Cancer 36:462, 1975
206. Norris HJ, Taylor HB: Carcinoma of the male breast. Cancer 23:1428, 1969
207. Lagios MD, Rose MR, Margolin FR: Tubular carcinoma of the breast: Association with multicentricity, bilaterality and family history of mammary carcinoma. Am J Clin Pathol 73:25, 1980
208. Tremblay G: Elastosis in tubular carcinoma of the breast. Arch Pathol 98:302, 1974
209. Eggor H, Dressler W: A contribution to the natural history of breast cancer 1. Duct obliteration with periductal elastosis in the centre of breast cancers. Arch Gynecol 231:191, 1982
210. Carstens PHB, Huvos AG, Foote FW Jr, et al: Tubular carcinoma of the breast: A clinicopathologic study of 35 cases. Am J Clin Pathol 58:231, 1972
210A. Tremblay G: Elastosis in tubular carcinoma of the breast. Arch Pathol 98:302, 1974
211. Eusebi V, Betts CM, Bussolati G: Tubular carcinoma: A variant of secretory breast carcinoma. Histopathology 3:407, 1979
212. Haagensen CD: Diseases of the Breast, 2nd ed, pp 177–185. Philadelphia, WB Saunders, 1971
213. Ekblom P, Miettinen M, Forsman L, et al: Basement membrane and apocrine epithelial antigens in differential diagnosis between tubular carcinoma and sclerosing adenosis of the breast. J Clin Pathol 37:357, 1984
214. Flotte TJ, Bell DA, Greco MA: Tubular carcinoma and sclerosing adenosis. The use of basal lamina as a differential feature. Am J Surg Pathol 4:75, 1980
215. Erlandson RA, Carstens PHB: Ultrastructure of tubular carcinoma of the breast. Cancer 29:987, 1972
216. Harris M, Ahmed A: The ultrastructure of tubular carcinoma of the breast. J Pathol 123:79, 1977
217. Rosen PP: Microglandular adenosis. a benign lesion simulating invasive mammary carcinoma. Am J Surg Pathol 7:137, 1983
218. Geschickter CF: Disease of the Breast: Diagnosis, Pathology, Treatment, 2nd ed, pp 565–575. Philadelphia, JB Lippincott, 1945
219. Moore OS Jr, Foote FW Jr: The relatively favorable prognosis of medullary carcinoma of the breast. Cancer 2:635, 1949
220. Haagensen CD: Diseases of the Breast, 2nd ed, pp 570–575. Philadelphia, WB Saunders, 1971
221. Schwartz GF: Solid circumscribed carcinoma of the breast. Ann Surg 169:165, 1969
222. Bloom HJG, Richardson WW, Fields JR: Host resistance and survival in carcinoma of breast: A study of 104 cases of medullary carcinoma in a series of 1411 cases of breast cancer followed for 20 years. Br Med J 3:181, 1970
223. Maier WP, Rosemond GP, Goldman LI, et al: A ten year study of medullary carcinoma of the breast. Surg Gynecol Obstet 144:695, 1977
224. Richardson WW: Medullary carcinoma of the breast. A distinctive tumor type with a relatively good prognosis following radical mastectomy. Br J Cancer 10:415, 1956
225. Rosen PP, Lesser ML, Kinne DW: Breast carcinoma at the extremes of age: A comparison of patients younger than 35 years and older than 75 years. J Surg Oncol 28:90, 1985
226. Haupt HM, Rosen PP, Kinne DW: Breast carcinoma presenting with axillary lymph node metastasis: An analysis of specific histopathologic features. Am J Surg Pathol 9:165, 1985
227. Lesser ML, Rosen PP, Kinne DW: Multicentricity and bilaterality in invasive breast carcinoma. Surgery 1:234, 1982
228. Rosen PP, Menendez-Botet CJ, Nisselbaum JS, et al: Pathological review of breast lesions analyzed for estrogen receptor protein. Cancer Res 35:3187, 1975
229. Patel JK, Nemoto T, Dao TL: Is medullary carcinoma of the breast hormone-dependent? J Surg Oncol 24:290, 1983
230. Meyer JS, Bauer WC, Rao BR: Subpopulations of breast carcinoma defined by S-phase fraction, morphology and estrogen receptor content. Lab Invest 39:225, 1978
231. Fisher ER: Ultrastructure of human breast and its disorders. Am J Clin Pathol 66:291, 1976
232. Ahmed A: The ultrastructure of medullary carcinoma of the breast. Virchows Arch [Pathol Anat] 388:175, 1980
233. Black CL, Morris DM, Goldman LI: The significance of lymph node involvement in patients with medullary carcinoma of the breast. Surg Gynecol Obstet 157:497, 1983
234. Rosen PP, Lesser ML, Kinne DW, et al: Discontinuous or "skip" metastases in breast carcinoma. Ann Surg 197:276, 1983
235. Robinson RR: Gelatinous cancer of the breast. Trans Pathol Soc London 4:275, 1852
236. Lange F: Der Gallertkrebs der Brustdruse. Beitr Klin Chir 16:1, 1896
237. Larrey M: Tumeur gelatiniforme ou colloide de la mamelle. Bull Soc Chir Paris 3:545, 1853
238. Geschickter CF: Gelatinous mammary cancer. Ann Surg 108:321, 1938
239. Cheatle GL, Cutler M: Gelatinous carcinoma of the breast. Arch Surg 20:568, 1930

240. Lee BJ, Hauser H, Pack GT: Gelatinous carcinoma of the breast. Surg Gynecol Obstet 59:841, 1934
241. Rosen PP, Wang T-Y: Colloid carcinoma of the breast. Analysis of 64 patients with long-term follow up. Am J Clin Pathol 73:30, 1980
242. Veronesi U, Gennari L: Il carcinoma gelatinoso della mammella. Tumori 46:119, 1960
243. Melamed MR, Robbins GF, Foote FW Jr: Prognostic significance of gelatinous mammary carcinoma. Cancer 14:699, 1961
244. Silverberg SG, Kay S, Chitale AR, et al: Colloid carcinoma of the breast. Am J Clin Pathol 55:355, 1971
245. Wulsin JH, Schreiber JT: Improved prognosis in certain patterns of carcinoma of the breast. Arch Surg 85:791, 1962
246. Snyder M, Tobon H: Primary mucinous carcinoma of the breast. Breast 3:17, 1977
247. Steinbrecher JS, Silverberg SG: Signet ring cell carcinoma of the breast. The mucinous variant of infiltrating lobular carcinoma. Cancer 37:828, 1976
248. Jao W, Lao IO, Chowdhury LN, et al: Ultrastructural aspects of mucinous (colloid) breast carcinoma. Diagn Gynecol Obstet 2:83, 1980
249. Harris M, Vasudev KS, Anfield C, et al: Mucin producing carcinomas of the breast: Ultrastructural observations. Histopathology 2:177, 1978
250. Walker RA: Mucoid carcinomas of the breast: A study using mucin histochemistry and peanut lectin. Histopathology 6:571, 1982
251. Tellem M, Nedwick A, Amenta PS, et al: Mucin-producing carcinoma of the breast: Tissue culture, histochemical and electron microscopic study. Cancer 19:573, 1966
252. Capella C, Eusebi V, Mann B, et al: Endocrine differentiation in mucoid carcinoma of the breast. Histopathology 4:613, 1980
253. Fetissof F, Dubois MP, Arbeille-Brassart B, et al: Argyrophilic cells in mammary carcinoma. Hum Pathol 14:127, 1983
254. Fisher ER, Palekar AS: Solid and mucinous varieties of so-called mammary carcinoid tumors. Am J Clin Pathol 72:909, 1979
255. Rasmussen BB, Rose C, Thorpe SM, et al: Argyrophilic cells in 202 human mucinous breast carcinomas. Relation to histopathologic and clinical features. Am J Clin Pathol 84:737, 1985
256. Feyrter F, Hartmann G: Uber die carcinoide Wuchsform des Carcinoma mammae, insbesondere das Carcinoma solidum (gelatinosum) mammae. Frandf Z Pathol 73:24, 1963
257. Wasserman TH, Sickles EA, Phillips TL: Primary radiation treatment of colloid carcinoma: A case report. Cancer 48:1972, 1981
258. Towfighi J, Simmonds MA, Davidson EA: Mucin and fat emboli in mucinous carcinomas causing hemorrhagic cerebral infarcts. Arch Pathol Lab Med 107:646, 1983
259. Deck JHN, Lee MA: Mucin embolism to cerebral arteries: A fatal complication of carcinoma of breast. Can J Neurol Sci 5:327, 1978
260. Fisher ER, Palekar AS, Redmond C, et al: Pathologic findings from the National Surgical Adjuvant Breast Project (Protocol No. 4). VI. Invasive papillary cancer. Am J Clin Pathol 73:313, 1980
261. Carter D, Orr SL, Merino MJ: Intracystic papillary carcinoma of the breast after mastectomy, radiotherapy or excisional biopsy alone. Cancer 52:14, 1983
262. Haagensen CD: Diseases of the Breast, 2nd ed, pp 528–544. Philadelphia, WB Saunders, 1971
263. Czernobilsky B: Intracystic carcinoma of the female breast. Surg Gynecol Obstet 124:93, 1967
264. Devitt JE, Barr JR: The clinical recognition of cystic carcinoma of the breast. Surg Gynecol Obstet 159:130, 1984
265. Hunter CE Jr, Sawyers JL: Intracystic papillary carcinoma of the breast. South Med J 73:1484, 1980
266. Schaefer G, Rosen PP, Lesser ML, et al: Breast carcinoma in elderly women: Pathology prognosis and survival. Pathol Annu 19(Pt: 1):195: 1984
267. Rosen PP: A.P. Stout, M.D. and papilloma of the breast. Comments on the occasion of his 100th birthday. Am J Surg Pathol 10 (suppl 1): 100, 1986
268. Papotti M, Gugliotta P, Eusebi V, et al: Immunohistochemical analysis of benign and malignant papillary lesions of the breast. Am J Surg Pathol 7:451, 1983
269. Papotti M, Gugliotta P, Ghiringhello B, et al: Association of breast carcinoma and multiple intraductal papillomas: An histological and immunohistochemical investigation. Histopathology 8:963, 1984
270. Ohuchi N, Abe R, Kasai M: Possible cancerous change in intraductal papillomas of the breast. A 3-D reconstruction study of 25 cases. Cancer 54:605, 1984
271. Ohuchi N, Abe R, Takahashi T, et al: Three-dimensional atypical structure in intraductal carcinoma differentiating from papilloma and papillomatosis of the breast. Breast Cancer Res Treat 5:57, 1985
272. Tsuchiya S, Takayama S, Higashi Y: Electron microscopy of intraductal papilloma of the breast. Ultrastructural comparison of papillary carcinoma with normal large duct. Acta Pathol Jpn 33:97, 1983
273. Ahmed A: Ultrastructural aspects of human breast lesions. Pathol Annu 15(Pt. 2):411, 1980
274. Gersell DJ, Katzenstein A-L: Spindle cell carcinoma of the breast. A clinicopathologic and ultrastructural study. Hum Pathol 12:550, 1981
275. Llombart-Bosch A, Peydro A: Malignant mixed osteogenic tumours of the breast. An ultrastructural study of two cases. Virchows Arch [Pathol Anat] 366:1, 1975
276. An T, Grathwohl M, Frable WJ: Breast carcinoma with osseous metaplasia: An electron microscopic study. Am J Clin Pathol 80:127, 1983
277. Kahn LB, Vys CJ, Dale J, et al: Carcinoma of the breast with metaplasia to chondrosarcoma: A light and electron microscopic study. Histopathology 2:93, 1978
278. Battifora H: Spindle cell carcinoma. Ultrastructural evidence of squamous origin and collagen production by the tumor cells. Cancer 37:2275, 1976
279. Rottino A, Wilson K: Osseous, cartilaginous and mixed tumors of the human breast: A review of the literature. Arch Surg 50:184, 1945
280. Huvos AG, Lucas JC Jr, Foote FW Jr: Metaplastic breast carcinoma. NY State J Med 73:1078, 1973
281. Kaufman MW, Morti JR, Gallager HS, et al: Carcinoma of the breast with pseudosarcomatous metaplasia. Cancer 53:1908, 1984
282. Smith BH, Taylor HB: The occurrence of bone and cartilage in mammary tumors. Am J Clin Pathol 51:610, 1969
283. Haagensen CD: Diseases of the Breast, 2nd ed, pp 600–605. Philadelphia, WB Saunders, 1971
284. Charles A: An electron microscopic study of the human axillary apocrine gland. J Anat 93:226, 1959
285. Archer F, Omar M: Pink cell (oncocytic) metaplasia in a fibroadenoma of the human breast: Electron microscope observations. J Pathol 99:119, 1969

286. Pier WJ Jr, Garancis JC, Kuzma JF: The ultrastructure of apocrine cells in intracystic papilloma and fibrocystic disease of the breast. Arch Pathol 89:446, 1970
287. Ahmed A: Apocrine metaplasia in cystic hyperplastic mastopathy. Histochemical and ultrastructural observations. J Pathol 115:211, 1975
288. Izuo M, Okagaki T, Richart RM, et al: DNA content in "apocrine metaplasia" of fibrocystic disease of the breast. Cancer 27:643, 1971
289. Foote FW Jr, Stewart FW: Comparative studies of cancerous versus noncancerous breasts. Ann Surg 121:6; 197, 1945
290. Page DL, Vander Zwaag R, Rogers LW, et al: Relation between component parts of fibrocystic disease complex and breast cancer. J Natl Cancer Inst 61:1055, 1978
291. Roddy HJ, Silverberg SG: Ultrastructural analysis of apocrine carcinoma of the human breast. Ultrastruct Pathol 1:385, 1980
292. Mossler J, Barton TK, Brinkhous AD, et al: Apocrine differentiation in human mammary carcinoma. Cancer 46:2463, 1980
293. Eusebi V, Betts C, Haagensen DE, et al: Apocrine differentiation in lobular carcinoma of the breast: A morphologic, immunologic and ultrastructural study. Hum Pathol 15:134, 1984
294. Bryant J: Male breast cancer: A case of apocrine carcinoma with psammoma bodies. Hum Pathol 12:751, 1981
295. Lee BJ, Pack GT, Scharnagel I: Sweat gland cancer of the breast. Surg Gynecol Obstet 54:975, 1933
296. Wald M, Kakulas BA: Apocrine gland carcinoma (sweat gland carcinoma) of the breast. Aust NZ J Surg 33:200, 1964
297. Hamperl H: The so-called sweat gland carcinoma of the human breast: A review. Z Krebsforsch 88:105, 1977
298. Frable WJ, Kay S: Carcinoma of the breast: Histologic and clinical features of apocrine tumors. Cancer 21:756, 1968
299. Miller WR, Telford J, Dixon JM, et al: Androgen metabolism and apocrine differentiation in human breast cancer. Breast Cancer Res Treat 5:67, 1985
300. Wales NAM, Ebling FJ: The control of apocrine glands of the rabbit by steroid hormones. J Endocrinol 51:763, 1971
301. Labows JN, Preti G, Hoelzle E, et al: Steroid analysis of human apocrine secretion. Steroids 34:249, 1979
302. Ewing J: Neoplastic Diseases, 3rd ed, p 780. Philadelphia, WB Saunders, 1919
303. Geschickter CF: Diseases of the Breast: Diagnosis, Pathology Treatment, 2nd ed, p. 824. Philadelphia, JB Lippincott, 1945
304. Galloway JR, Woolner LB, Clagett OT: Adenoid cystic carcinoma of the breast. Surg Gynecol Obstet 122:1289, 1966
305. Anthony PP, James PD: Adenoid cystic carcinoma of the breast: Prevalence, diagnostic criteria and histogenesis. J Clin Pathol 28:647, 1975
306. Qizilbash AH, Patterson MC, Oliveira KF: Adenoid cystic carcinoma of the breast. Arch Pathol Lab Med 101:302, 1977
307. Hjorth S, Magnusson PH, Blomquist P: Adenoid cystic carcinoma of the breast. Acta Chir Scand 143:155, 1977
308. Peters GN, Wolff M: Adenoid cystic carcinoma of the breast: Report of 11 new cases. Cancer 52:680, 1982
309. Friedman BA, Oberman HA: Adenoid cystic carcinoma of the breast. Am J Clin Pathol 54:1, 1970
310. Koss LG, Brannan CD, Ashikari R: Histologic and ultrastructural features of adenoid cystic carcinoma of the breast. Cancer 26:1271, 1970
311. Zaloudek C, Oertel YC, Orenstein JM: Adenoid cystic carcinoma of the breast. Am J Clin Pathol 81:297, 1984
312. Cavanzo FJ, Taylor HB: Adenoid cystic carcinoma of the breast. An analysis of 21 cases. Cancer 24:740, 1969
313. Lerner AG, Molnar JJ, Adam YG: Adenoid cystic carcinoma of the breast. Am J Surg 127:585, 1974
314. Harris M: Pseudoadenoid cystic carcinoma of the breast. Arch Pathol Lab Med 101:307, 1977
315. Oertel YC, Golblum LI: Fine needle aspiration of the breast. Diagnostic criteria. Pathol Annu 18(Pt. 1):375, 1983
316. Nayer HR: Cylindroma of the breast with pulmonary metastases. Dis Chest 31:324, 1957
317. Orenstein JM, Dardick I, van Nostrand AWP: Ultrastructural similarities of adenoid cystic carcinoma and pleomorphic adenoma. Histopathology 9:623, 1985
318. Verani RR, Vander Bel-Kahn J: Mammary adenoid cystic carcinoma with unusual features. Am J Clin Pathol 59:653, 1976
319. Wilson WB, Spell JP: Adenoid cystic carcinoma of breast: A case with recurrence and regional metastases. Ann Surg 166:861, 1967
320. Lim SK, Kovi J, Warner OG: Adenoid cystic carcinoma of breast with metastasis: A case report and review of the literature. J Natl Med Assoc 71:329, 1979
321. Salm R: Epidermoid metaplasia in mammary fibro-adenoma with formation of keratin cysts. J Pathol Bacteriol 74:221, 1957
322. Flint, A, Oberman HA: Infarction and squamous metaplasia of intraductal papilloma: A benign breast lesion that may simulate carcinoma. Hum Pathol 15:764, 1984
323. Hassan MO, Olaizola MY: Ultrastructural observations on gynecomastia. Arch Pathol Lab Med 103:624, 1979
324. Soderstrom K-O, Toikkanen S: Extensive squamous metaplasia simulating squamous cell carcinoma in benign breast papillomatosis. Hum Pathol 14:1081, 1983
325. Van Bogaert LJ: Squamous metaplasia in human mammary epithelium in long-term organ culture. Experientia 33:1450, 1977
326. Elias JJ, Armstrong RC: Hyperplastic and metaplastic response of human mammary fibroadenoma and dysplasias in organ culture. J Natl Cancer Inst 51:1341, 1973
327. Tonelli QT, Custer RP, Sorof S: Transformation of cultured mouse mammary glands by aromatic amines and amides and their derivatives. Cancer Res 39:1784, 1979
328. Lasnitziki I: Precancerous changes induced by 20-methylcholanthrene in mouse prostates grown *in vitro*. Br J Cancer 5:345, 1951
329. Schaefer FV, Custer RP, Sorof S: Squamous metaplasia in human breast culture: Induction by cyclic adenine nucleotide and prostaglandins and influence of menstrual cycle. Cancer Res 43:279, 1983
330. Rostock RA, Bauer TW, Eggleston JC: Primary squamous carcinoma of the breast: A review. Breast 10:27, 1984
331. Shousha S, James AH, Fernandez MD, et al: Squamous cell carcinoma of the breast. Arch Pathol Lab Med 108:893, 1984
332. Hasleton PS, Misch KA, Vasudev KS, et al: Squamous carcinoma of the breast. J Clin Pathol 31:116, 1978
333. Bogomoletz WV: Pure squamous cell carcinoma of the breast. Arch Pathol Lab Med 106:57, 1982
334. Woodard BH, Brinkhaus AD, McCarty KS, et al: Adenosquamous differentiation in mammary carcinoma. Arch Pathol Lab Med 104:130, 1980
335. Toikkonen S: Primary squamous cell carcinoma of the breast. Cancer 48:1629, 1981
336. Lane N: Pseudosarcoma (polypoid sarcoma-like masses) associated with squamous cell carcinoma of the mouth, fauces and larynx. Report of 10 cases. Cancer 10:19, 1957

337. Willis RA: Squamous cell mammary carcinoma of predominantly fibrosarcoma-like structure. J Pathol Bacteriol 76:511, 1958
338. Bauer TW, Rostock RA, Eggleston JC, et al: Spindle cell carcinoma of the breast: Four cases and review of the literature. Hum Pathol 15:147, 1984
339. Leroux R: Reaction giganto cellulaire du stroma dans un epithelioma mammaire. Bull. Cancer 20:692, 1971
340. Duboucher H, Montpellier J, Laffarque F: Epithelioma mammaire avec reaction de type myeloplaxique. Ann Anat Pathol (Paris) 70:787, 1933
341. Agnantis NT, Rosen PP: Mammary carcinoma with osteoclast-like giant cells. Am J Clin Pathol 72:383, 1979
342. Sugano I, Nagao K, Kondo Y, et al: Cytologic and ultrastructural studies of a rare breast carcinoma with osteoclast-like giant cells. Cancer 52:74, 1983
343. Nielsen BB, Kiaer HW: Carcinoma of the breast with stromal multinucleated giant cells. Histopathlolology 9:183, 1985
344. Holland R, VanHaelst VJGM: Mammary carcinoma with osteoclast-like giant cells. Additional observations on six cases. Cancer 53:1963, 1984
345. Factor FM, Biempica L, Ratner I, et al: Carcinoma of the breast with multinucleated reactive stromal giant cells. A light and electron microscopic study of two cases. Virchows Arch [Pathol Anat] 374:1, 1977
346. Ashikari H, Jun MY, Farrow JH, et al: Breast carcinoma in children and adolescents. Clin Bull 7:55, 1977
347. McDivitt RW, Stewart FW: Breast carcinoma in children. JAMA 195:388, 1966
348. Oberman HA, Stephens PJ: Carcinoma of the breast in childhood. Cancer 30:420, 1972
349. Oberman HA: Secretory carcinoma of the breast in adults. Am J Surg Pathol 4:465, 1980
350. Tavassoli FA, Norris HJ: Secretory carcinoma of the breast. Cancer 45:2404, 1980
351. Akhtar M, Robinson C, Ali MA, et al: Secretory carcinoma of the breast in adults. Light and electron microscopic study of three cases with review of the literature. Cancer 51:2245, 1983
352. Botta G, Fessia L, Ghiringhello B: Juvenile milk protein secreting carcinoma. Virchows Arch [Pathol Anat] 395:145, 1982
353. Sullivan JJ, Magee JJ, Donald KJ: Secretory (juvenile) carcinoma of the breast. Pathology 9:341, 1977
354. Byrne MP, Fahey MM, Gooselaw JG: Breast cancer with axillary metastasis in an 8½-year-old girl. Cancer 31:726, 1972
355. Masse SR, Rioux A, Beauchesne C: Juvenile carcinoma of the breast. Hum Pathol 12:1044, 1981
356. Rosen PP, Holmes G, Lesser ML, et al: Juvenile papillomatosis and breast carcinoma. Cancer 55:1345, 1985
357. Aboumrad MH, Horn RC Jr, Fine G: Lipid secreting mammary carcinoma. Report of a case associated with Paget's disease of the nipple. Cancer 16:521, 1963
358. Ramos CV, Taylor HB: Lipid-rich carcinoma of the breast. A clinicopathologic analysis of 13 examples. Cancer 33:812, 1974
359. Lin-Co RY, Gisser SD: Unusual variant of lipid-rich mammary carcinoma. Arch Pathol Lab Med 102:193, 1978
360. Barwick KW, Kashgarian M, Rosen PP: Clear cell change within duct and lobular epithelium of the human breast. Pathol Annu 17(Pt. 1):319, 1982
361. Rosen PP, Scott M: Cystic hypersecretory duct carcinoma of the breast. Am J Surg Pathol 8:31, 1984
362. Salomon A: Beitrag zur Pathologie und Klinik der mammacarcinome. Arch Klin Chir 101:573, 1918
363. Cheatle GL, Cutler M: Tumors of the Breast. Philadelphia, JB Lippincott, 1931
364. Godwin JT: Chronology of lobular carcinoma of the breast: Report of a case. Cancer 5:259, 1952
365. Miller HW Jr, Kay S: Infiltrating lobular carcinoma of the female mammary gland. Surg Gynecol Obstet 102:661, 1956
366. Haagensen CD: Lobular carcinoma of the breast: A precancerous lesion? Clin Obstet Gynecol 5:1093, 1962
367. Newman W: Lobular carcinoma of the female breast. Report of 73 cases. Ann Surg 164:305, 1966
368. Henson D, Tarone R: A study of lobular carcinoma of the breast based on the Third National Cancer Survey in the United States of America. Tumori 65:133, 1979
369. Dixon JM, Anderson TJ, Page DL, et al: Infiltrating lobular carcinoma of the breast. Histopathology 6:149, 1982
370. Martinez V, Azzopardi JG: Invasive lobular carcinoma of the breast: Incidence and variants. Histopathology 3:467, 1979
371. Ashikari R, Huvos AG, Urban JA, et al: Infiltrating lobular carcinoma of the breast. Cancer 31:110, 1973
372. Fechner RE: Histologic variants of infiltrating lobular carcinoma of the breast. Hum Pathol 6:373, 1975
373. Fechner RE: Infiltrating lobular carcinoma without lobular carcinoma *in situ*. Cancer 29:1539, 1972
374. Shousha S, Backhous CM, Alaghband-Zadeh J, et al: Alveolar variant of invasive lobular carcinoma of the breast. Am J Clin Pathol 85:1, 1986
375. Dixon JM, Anderson TJ, Page DL, et al: Infiltrating lobular carcinoma of the breast: An evolution of the incidence and consequence of bilateral disease. Br J Surg 70:513, 1983
376. Van Bogaert L-J, Maldaque P: Infiltrating lobular carcinoma of the female breast. Deviations from the usual histopathologic appearance. Cancer 45:979, 1980
377. Fisher ER, Gregorio RM, Redmond C, et al: Tubulolobular invasive breast carcinoma: A variant of lobular invasive cancer. Hum Pathol 8:679, 1977
378. Merino MJ, LiVolsi VA: Signet ring carcinoma of the female breast: A clinicopathologic analysis of 24 cases. Cancer 48:1830, 1981
379. Hull MT, Seo IS, Battersby JS, et al: Signet-ring cell carcinoma of the breast: A clinicopathologic study of 24 cases. Am J Clin Pathol 73:31, 1980
380. Battifora H: Intracytoplasmic lumina in breast carcinoma. Arch Pathol 99:614, 1975
381. Gould VE, Chejfec G: Lobular carcinoma of the breast with secretory features. Ultrastruct Pathol 1:151, 1980
382. Jundt G, Schulz A, Heitz PU, et al: Small cell neuroendocrine (oat cell) carcinoma of the male breast. Virchows Arch [Pathol Anat] 404:213, 1984
383. Wade PM, Mills SE, Read M, et al: Small cell neuroendocrine (oat cell) carcinoma of the breast. Cancer 52:121, 1983
384. Smith DB, Howell A, Harris M, et al: Carcinomatous meningitis associated with infiltrating lobular carcinoma of the breast. Eur J Surg Oncol 11:33, 1985
385. Harris M, Howell A, Chrissohou M, et al: A comparison of the metastatic pattern of infiltrating lobular carcinoma and infiltrating duct carcinoma of the breast. Br J Cancer 50:23, 1984
386. Klein M, Sherlock P: Gastric and colonic metastases from breast cancer. Am J Dig Dis 17:881, 1972
387. Feun L, Drelichman A, Singhakowinta A, et al: Ureteral obstruction secondary to metastatic breast carcinoma. Cancer 44:1164, 1979
388. Hartman S, Schliftman R, Bennett B: Correlation conferences in radiology and pathology: Gastric rigidity and breast masses. NY State J Med 77:1120, 1977

389. Hartmann WH, Sherlock P: Gastroduodenal metastases from carcinoma of the breast. An adrenal steroid induced phenomenon. Cancer 14:426, 1961
390. Cormier WJ, Gaffey TA, Welch JM, et al: Linitis plastica caused by metastatic lobular carcinoma of the breast. Mayo Clin Proc 55:747, 1980
391. Yoshida Y: Metastases and primary neoplasms of the stomach in patients with breast cancer. Surgery 125:738, 1973
392. Weinstein GW, Goldman JN: Metastatic adenocarcinoma of the breast masquerading as chalazion. Am J Ophthalmol 69:259, 1970
393. Hood CL, Font RL, Zimmerman LE: Metastatic mammary carcinoma in the eyelid with histiocytoid appearance. Cancer 31:793, 1973
394. Dearnaley DP, Sloane JP, Ormerod MG, et al: Increased detection of mammary carcinoma cells in marrow smears using antisera to epithelial membrane antigen. Br J Cancer 44:85, 1981
395. Saigo PE, Rosen PP: Mammary carcinoma with "choriocarcinomatous" features. Am J Surg Pathol 5:773, 1981
396. Saigo PE, Brigati JJ, Sternberg SS, et al: Primary gastric choriocarcinoma. An immunohistological study. Am J Surg Pathol 5:333, 1981
397. Smith DM Jr, Haggitt RC: A comparative study of generic stains for carcinoid secretory granules. Am J Surg Pathol 7:61, 1983
398. Azzopardi JG, Muretto P, Goddeeris P, et al: Carcinoid tumors of the breast: The morphological spectrum of argyrophil carcinomas. Histopathology 6:549, 1982
399. Partanen S, Syrjanen K: Argyrophilic cells in carcinoma of the female breast. Virchows Arch [Pathol Anat] 391:45, 1981
400. Toyoshima S: Mammary carcinoma with argyrophil cells. Cancer 52:2129, 1983
401. Cubilla AL, Woodruff JM, Erlandson RA: Comparative clinicopathologic study of endocrine-like and ordinary mucinous carcinomas of the breast. Lab Invest 50:14A, 1984
402. Chabon AB, Costales F: Estrogen receptor activity in primary argyrophil carcinoma of the breast. Diagn Gynecol Obstet 2:93, 1980
403. Clayton F, Sibley RK, Ordonez NG, et al: Argyrophilic breast carcinomas. Evidence of lactational differentiation. Am J Surg Pathol 6:323, 1982
404. Chen KTK: Breast carcinomas with carcinoid features. Breast 7:2, 1981
405. Kaneko H, Sumida T, Sekiya M, et al: A breast carcinoid tumor with special reference to ultrastructural study. Acta Pathol Jpn 32:327, 1982
406. Kaneko H, Hojo H, Ishikawa S, et al: Norepinephrine-producing tumors of bilateral breasts. A case report. Cancer 41:2002, 1978
407. Cross AS, Azzopardi JG, Krausz T, et al: A morphological and immunocytochemical study of a distinctive variant of ductal carciinoma *in situ* of the breast. Histopathology 9:21, 1985
408. Juntti-Berggen L, Pitkanen P, Wilander E: Argyrophil endocrine cells with ACTH and HCG immunoreactivity in a carcinoma of the breast. Virchows Arch [Cell Pathol] 43:37, 1983
409. Raju U, Fine G: The controversial mammary carcinoid tumor. Lab Invest 48:69A, 1983
410. Sariola H, Lehtonen E, Saxen E: Breast tumors with a solid and uniform carcinoid pattern. Ultrastructural and immunohistochemical study of two cases. Pathol Res Pract 178:405, 1985
411. Min K-W: Argyrophilia in breast carcinomas: Histochemical, ultrastructural and immunocytochemical study. Lab Invest 48:58A, 1983
412. Memoli VA, Nesland J, Warren WH, et al: Immunohistochemical and ultrastructural observations concerning the issue of neuroendocrine differentiation in breast carcinomas. Lab Invest 50:39A, 1984
413. Cubilla AL, Woodruff JM: Primary carcinoid tumor of the breast: A report of eight patients. Am J Surg Pathol 1:283, 1977
414. Santini D, Bazzocchi F, Pileri S, et al: Mammary carcinoma with argyrophilic cells: An immunochemical and ultrastructural study. Tumori 71:331, 1985
415. Taxy JB, Tischler AS, Insalaco SJ, et al: "Carcinoid" tumor of the breast. A variant of conventional breast cancer? Hum Pathol 12:170, 1981
416. Bussolati G, Gugliotta P, Sapino A, et al: Chromogranin-reactive endocrine cells in argyrophilic carcinomas ("carcinoids") and normal tissue of the breast. Am J Pathol 120:186, 1985
417. Kashlan RB, Powell RW, Nolting SF: Carcinoid and other tumors metastatic to the breast. J Surg Oncol 20:25, 1982
418. Hawley PR: A case of secondary carcinoid tumours in both breasts following excision of primary carcinoid tumour of the duodenum. Br J Surg 53:818, 1966
419. Harrist TJ, Kalisher L: Breast metastasis: An unusual manifestation of a malignant carcinoid tumor. Cancer 40:3102, 1977
420. Bell C: A System of Operative Surgery. 1:180, 1807
421. Leitch A: Peau d'orange in acute mammary carcinoma: Its cause and diagnostic value. Lancet 2:861, 1909
422. Lee BJ, Tannenbaum E: Inflammatory carcinoma of the breast: A report of twenty-eight cases from the breast clinic of the Memorial Hospital. Surg Gynecol Obstet 39:580, 1924
423. Robbins GF, Shah J, Rosen P: Inflammatory carcinoma of the breast. Surg Clin North Am 54:801, 1974
424. Barker JL, Nelson AJ III, Montague ED: Inflammatory carcinoma of the breast. Radiology 121:173, 1976
425. Droulias CA, Sewell CW, McSweeney MB, et al: Inflammatory carcinoma of the breast: A correlation of clinical radiologic and pathologic findings. Ann Surg 184:217, 1976
426. Nussbaum H, Kagan AR, Gilbert H, et al: Management of inflammatory breast carcinoma. Breast 3:25, 1977
427. Mourali N, Muenz LR, Tabbane F, et al: Epidemiologic features of rapidly progressing breast cancer in Tunisia. Cancer 46:2741, 1980
428. Meyer AC, Dockerty MB, Harrington SW: Inflammatory carcinoma of the breast. Surg Gynecol Obstet 87:417, 1948
429. Lucas FV, Perez-Mesa C: Inflammatory carcinoma of the breast. Cancer 41:1595, 1978
430. World Health Organization: International Histological Classification of Tumours, No. 2. Histological Typing of Breast Tumours, 2nd ed, p 21. Geneva, World Health Organization, 1981
431. Ellis DL, Teitelbaum SL: Inflammatory carcinoma of the breast. A pathologic definition. Cancer 33:1045, 1974
432. Saltzstein SL: Clinically occult inflammatory carcinoma of the breast. Cancer 34:382, 1974
433. Levine PH, Steinhorn SC, Ries LG: Inflammatory breast cancer: The experience of the Surveillance, Epidemiology, and End Results (SEER) Program. J Natl Cancer Inst 74:291, 1985
434. Harvey HA, Lipton A, Lawrence BV, et al: Estrogen receptor status and inflammatory carcinoma. J Surg Oncol 21:42, 1982
435. Tschen EH, Apisarnthanarax P: Inflammatory metastatic carcinoma of the breast. Arch Dermatol 177:120, 1981
436. Mehregan A: Metastatic carcinoma to the skin. Dermatologica 123:311, 1961

437. Hazelrigg DC, Rudolph AH: Inflammatory metastatic carcinoma. Arch Dermatol 113:69, 1977
438. Brownstein MH, Helwig EB: Spread of tumors to the skin. Arch Dermatol 107:80, 1973
439. Nielsen M, Andersen JA, Henriksen FW, et al: Metastases to the breast from extramammary carrcinomas. Acta Pathol Microbiol Scand [A] 89:251, 1981
440. Hajdu SI, Urban JA: Cancers metastatic to the breast. Cancer 29:1691, 1972
441. McCrea ES, Johnston C, Haney PJ: Metastases to the breast. Am J Roentgenol 141:685, 1983
442. Brutschin P, Culver GJ: Extracranial metastases from medulloblastoma. Radiology 107:359, 1973
443. Howarth GB, Caces JN, Pratt CB: Breast metastases in children with rhabdomyosarcoma. Cancer 46:2520, 1980
444. Goldenberg VE, Wiegenstein L, Mason NK: Florid breast fibroadenomas in patients taking hormonal oral contraceptives. Am J Clin Pathol 49:52, 1968
445. Fechner RE: Fibroadenomas in patients receiving oral contraceptives: A clinical and pathologic study. Am J Clin Pathol 53:857, 1970
446. Mies C, Rosen PP: Juvenile fibroadenoma: A study of 49 patients. Lab Invest 54:42A, 1986
447. Cheatle GL, Cutler M: Tumours of the Breast. Their Pathology, Symptoms, Diagnosis and Treatment, pp 483–484. London, Edward Arnold & Co, 1931
448. Harrington SW, Miller JM: Malignant changes in fibro-adenoma of the mammary gland. Surg Gynecol Obstet 70:615, 1940
449. McDivitt RW, Stewart FW, Farrow JH: Breast carcinoma arising in solitary fibroadenomas. Surg Gynecol Obstet 125:572, 1967
450. Goldman RL, Friedman NB: Carcinoma of the breast arising in fibroadenomas, with emphasis on lobular carcinoma. Cancer 23:544, 1969
451. Buzanowski-Konakry K, Harrison EGJ, Payne WS: Lobular carcinoma arising in fibroadenoma of the breast. Cancer 35:450, 1975
452. Fondo EY, Rosen PP, Fracchia AA, et al: The problem of carcinoma developing in a fibroadenoma. Recent experience at Memorial Hospital. Cancer 43:563, 1979
453. Pick PW, Iossifides IA: Occurrence of breast carcinoma within a fibroadenoma. A review. Arch Pathol Lab Med 108:590, 1984
454. Ozzello L, Gump FE: The management of patients with carcinomas in fibroadenomatous tumors of the breast. Surg Gynecol Obstet 160:99, 1985
455. Rosen PP, Urban JA: Coexistent mammary carcinoma and cystosarcoma phyllodes. Breast 1:9, 1975
456. Jones DB: Florid papillomatosis of the nipple ducts. Cancer 8:315, 1955
457. Nichols FC, Dockerty MD, Judd ES: Florid papillomatosis of the nipple. Surg Gynecol Obstet 107:474, 1958
458. Perzin KH, Lattes R: Papillary adenoma of the nipple (florid papillomatosis adenoma, adenomatosis). A clinicopathologic study. Cancer 29:996, 1972
459. Goldman RL, Cooperman H: Adenoma of the nipple. A benign lesion simulating carcinoma clinically and pathologically. Am J Surg 119:322, 1970
460. Rosen PP, Caicco J: Florid papillomatosis of the nipple: A study of 51 patients including nine having mammary carcinoma. Am J Surg Pathol 10:87, 1986
461. Martin HE, Ellis EB: Biopsy by needle puncture and aspiration. Ann Surg 92:169, 1930
462. Stewart FW: The diagnosis of tumors by aspiration. Am J Pathol 9:801, 1933
463. Martin HE, Ellis EB: Aspiration biopsy. Surg Gynecol Obstet 59:578, 1934
464. McLean J: An instrument for needle (aspiration) biopsy of tumors and a technic for its use. Surg Clin North Am 19:519, 1939
465. Christopherson WM: Cytologic detection and diagnosis of cancer. Its contributions and limitations. Cancer 51:1201, 1983
466. Engell HC: Cancer cells in the circulating blood. A clinical study on the occurrence of cancer cells. Acta Chir Scand [Suppl] 201:1, 1955
467. Engell HC: Cancer cells in the blood. A five- to nine-year follow-up study. Ann Surg 104:457, 1959
468. Romsdahl MM, Valaitis J, McGrath RG, et al: Circulating tumor cells in patients with carcinoma. JAMA 193:1087, 1965
469. Roger V, Brennhovd I, Hoeg K: Tumor cells in blood: The prognostic significance of tumor cells in blood during palpation and biopsy. Acta Cytol 16:557, 1972
470. Shibata HR, Ritchie AC, Hopkirk JF, et al: Tumor cells in the circulating blood of patients with carcinoma of the breast and the gastrointestinal tract. Can Med Assoc J 89:863, 1963
471. Watne AL, Sandberg AA, Moore GE: The prognostic value of tumor cells in the blood. Arch Surg 83:190, 1961
472. Roberts S, Jonasson O, Long L, et al: Relationship of cancer cells in the circulating blood to operation. Clin Oncol 15:232, 1962
473. Robbins GF, Brothers JH III, Eberhart WF, et al: Is aspiration biopsy of breast cancer dangerous to the patient? Cancer 7:774, 1954
474. Berg JW, Robbins GF: A late look at the safety of aspiration biopsy. Cancer 15:826, 1962
475. Rosemond GP: Differentiation between the cystic and solid breast mass by needle aspiration. Surg Clin North Am 43:1433, 1963
476. Abramson DJ: A clinical evaluation of aspiration of cysts of the breast. Surg Gynecol Obstet 139:531, 1974
477. Kline TS, Joshi LP, Neal HS: Fine needle aspiration of the breast. Diagnosis and pitfalls: A review of 3545 cases. Cancer 44:1458, 1979
478. Bell DA, Hajdu SI, Urban JA, et al: Role of aspiration cytology in the diagnosis and management of mammary lesions in office practice. Cancer 51:1182, 1983
479. Webb AJ: A cytological study of mammary disease. Ann R Coll Surg Engl 56:181, 1975
480. Franzen S, Zajicek J: Aspiration biopsy in diagnosis of palpable lesions of the breast. Acta Radiol 7:241, 1968
481. Rosen P, Hajdu SI, Robbins G, et al: Diagnosis of carcinoma of the breast by aspiration biopsy. Surg Gynecol Obstet 134:837, 1972
482. Gardecki TIM, Hogbin BM, Melcher DH, et al: Aspiration cytology in the preoperative management of breast cancer. Lancet 2:790, 1980
483. Rimsten A, Stenkvist B, Johanson H, et al: The diagnostic accuracy of palpation and fine-needle biopsy and evaluation of their combined use in the diagnosis of breast lesions. Report of a prospective study in 1244 women with symptoms. Ann Surg 182:1, 1975
484. Zajdela A, Ghossein NA, Pilleron JP, et al: The value of aspiration cytology in the diagnosis of breast cancer: Experience at the Fondation Curie. Cancer 35:499, 1975
485. Strawbridge HTG, Bassett AA, Foldes I: Role of cytology in management of lesions of the breast. Surg Gynecol Obstet 152:1, 1981
486. Kreuzer G, Zajicek J: Cytologic diagnosis of mammary tumors from aspiration biopsy smears. III. Studies on 200

carcinomas with false negative or doubtful cytologic reports. Acta Cytol 16:249, 1972
487. Koivuniemi AP: Fine needle aspiration biopsy of the breast. Ann Clin Res 8:272, 1976
488. Nakazawa H, Rosen P, Lane N, et al: Frozen section experience in 3000 cases. Accuracy, limitations and value in residency training. Am J Clin Pathol 49:41, 1968
489. Ackerman LV, Ramirez GA: The indications for and limitations of frozen section diagnosis. A review of 1269 consecutive frozen section diagnoses. Br J Surg 46:336, 1959
490. Winship T, Rosvoll RV: Frozen sections. An evaluation of 1810 cases. Surgery 45:462, 1959
491. Elston CW, Cotton RE, Davies CJ, et al: A comparison of the use of the "Tru-Cut" needle and fine needle aspiration cytology in the pre-operative diagnosis of carcinoma of the breast. Histopathology 2:239, 1978
492. Shabot MM, Goldberg IM, Schick P, et al: Aspiration cytology is superior to "Tru-Cut" needle biopsy in establishing the diagnosis of clinically suspicious breast masses. Ann Surg 196:122, 1982
493. Roberts JG, Preece PE, Bolton PM, et al: The "tru-cut" biopsy in breast cancer. Clin Oncol 1:297, 1975
494. Millis RR: Needle biopsy of the breast. In McDivitt RW, Oberman HA, Ozzello L, et al (eds): The Breast, pp 186–303. Baltimore, Williams and Wilkins, 1984
495. McCormick J St C, Shivas AA: Drill biopsy of the breast—-A critical analysis. Br J Surg 60:953, 1973
496. Sieinski W, Dabska M: Usefulness of drill biopsy in the diagnosis of breast tumors. Cancer 38:2567, 1976
497. Meyerowitz BR: Drill biopsy confirmation of breast cancer. Arch Surg 111:826, 1976
498. Minkowitz S, Moskowitz R, Khafif RA, et al: TRU-CUT needle biopsy of the breast. An analysis of its specificity and sensitivity. Cancer 57:320, 1986
499. Owen AWMC, Anderson TJ, Forrest APM: Closed biopsy for breast cancer. JR Coll Surg Edinb 25:237, 1980
500. National Cancer Institute: Standardized management of breast specimens. Recommended by Pathology Working Group, Breast Cancer Task Force. Am J Clin Pathol 60:789, 1973
501. Schmidt WA: The breast. In Principles and Techniques of Surgical Pathology, pp 362–388. Stoneham, MA, Butterworth, 1983
502. Rosen PP: Specimen radiography and the diagnosis of clinically occult mammary carcinoma. Pathol Annu 15(Pt. 1):225, 1980
503. Gershon-Cohen J, Colcher AE: An evaluation of the roentgen diagnosis of early carcinoma of the breast. JAMA 108:867, 1937
504. Leborgne R: Diagnosis of tumors of the breast by simple roentgenography: Calcifications in carcinoma. Am J Roentgenol 65:1, 1951
505. Rosen PP, Snyder RE, Urban JA, et al: Correlation of suspicious mammograms and x-rays of breast biopsies during surgery. Results in 60 cases. Cancer 31:656, 1973
506. Snyder RE, Rosen PP: Radiography of breast specimens. Cancer 28:1608, 1971
507. Bauermeister DE, Hall MH: Specimen radiography—A mandatory adjunct to mammography. Am J Clin Pathol 59:782, 1973
508. Gallager HS: Breast specimen radiography: Obligatory, adjunct, investigative. Am J Clin Pathol 64:749, 1975
509. Bloom ND, Johnson F, Pertshuck L, et al: Electrocautery: Effects on steroid receptors in human breast cancer. J Surg Oncol 25:21, 1984
510. Pertshuck LP, Tobin EH, Tanapat P, et al: Histochemical analyses of steroid hormone receptors in breast and prostate carcinoma. J Histochem Cytochem 28:799, 1980
511. Rosenthal LJ: Discrepant estrogen receptor protein levels according to surgical technique. Am J Surg 138:680, 1979
512. Rosen PP: Electrocautery-induced artifacts in breast biopsy specimens: An iatrogenic source of diagnostic difficulty. Ann Surg (in press).
513. Anderson J, Jensen J: Lymph node identification: Specimen radiography of tissue predominated by fat. Am J Clin Pathol 68:511, 1977
514. Groote AD, Oosterhuis JW, Molenaar WM, et al: Radiographic imaging of lymph nodes in lymph node dissection specimens. Lab Invest 52:326, 1985
515. Durkin K, Haagensen CD: An improved technique for the study of lymph nodes in surgical specimens. Ann Surg 191:419, 1980
516. Morrow M, Evans J, Rosen PP, et al: Does clearing of axillary lymph nodes contribute to accurate staging of breast carcinoma? Cancer 53:1329, 1984
517. Hartveit F, Samonsen G, Tanqen M, et al: Routine histological investigation of the axillary lymph nodes in breast cancer. Clin Oncol 8:121, 1982

8 Receptors

C. Kent Osborne

There have been several advances in the management of patients with breast cancer in the past decade. One of these advances stems from laboratory observations that have led to a greater understanding of the mechanisms by which hormones regulate cellular growth. It is now clear that hormones influence cells by first binding to high-affinity receptor proteins that are specific for a given hormone and are located either on the cell surface or in the cell interior. This receptor-hormone interaction then initiates a series of biochemical steps that eventually lead to an alteration in cellular metabolism or growth. Whether a hormone exerts biologic activity for an individual cell or tissue is determined largely by the presence or absence of specific receptors for that hormone. Thus, the breast and the uterus, which possess estrogen receptor proteins, are target tissues for estrogen whereas muscle tissue, which lacks these receptors, is not.

It has been known for many years that growth of certain breast cancers can be modulated by changes in the hormonal environment. The recognition that these hormonal effects are mediated through specific hormone receptors led to at least two important ideas. The first was speculation that the presence of receptors in a breast cancer specimen might be used as a biologic marker for hormone responsiveness and the degree of differentiation of the tumor. The second idea was to develop pharmacologic agents to bind to and functionally block cell receptors, thereby preventing stimulatory effects from normal hormones in the cell's environment. The birth of the compounds known as antiestrogens followed. Further understanding of the biochemical events required for hormone action may yield equally important hypotheses.

HORMONAL REGULATION OF BREAST TISSUE

Normal Breast

The adult female breast is composed of epithelial lactiferous ducts terminating in secretory alveoli embedded in a fibrous tissue framework and fat. Breast growth and development are regulated by the complex interaction of many hormones (Fig. 8-1). Effects of each of these hormones are triggered by binding to specific receptors. Polypeptide hormone receptors are located on the cell membrane. Steroid hormone receptors are found in the interior of the cell. Whether they are normally in the cytoplasm or in the nucleus is debatable (see below). Thyroid hormone receptors reside in the nucleus of the cell.

Several of these hormones have been shown to play active or permissive roles in breast development or in lactation.[1] Estrogen and progesterone together are important in breast development. Estrogen primarily stimulates ductal growth, whereas progesterone is responsible for lobuloalveolar development. Insulin and growth hormone are permissive factors for mammary epithelial stem cell division. Prior exposure to cortisol and insulin allows prolactin to complete the final differentiation of alveolar cells into milk secretory cells. Thyroid hormone stimulates the metabolic activity of the breast cell. The role of other hormones such as androgens, insulin-like growth factor, or epidermal growth factor is less clear. In view of the importance of a variety of hormones for normal breast growth, it is not surprising that malignant cells arising from this tissue might express receptors for these

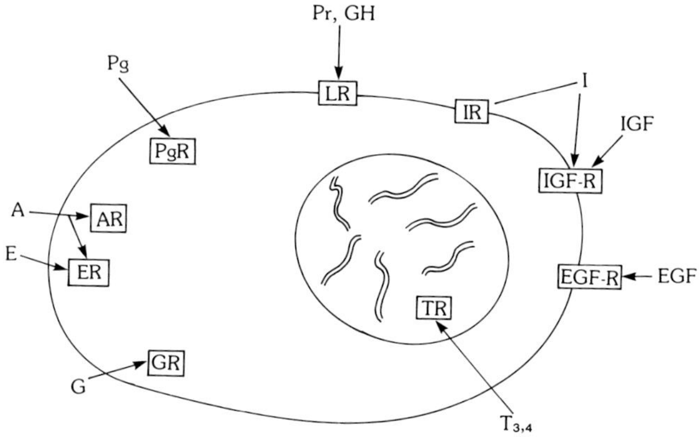

FIGURE 8-1. Breast cell. Potential hormonal interactions with breast epithelial cells. *E,* estrogen; *ER,* estrogen receptor; *A,* androgens; *AR,* androgen receptor; *G,* glucocorticoids; *GR,* glucocorticoid receptor; *Pg,* progesterone; *PgR,* progesterone receptor; *Pr,* prolactin; *GH,* growth hormone; *LR,* lactogenic receptor; *I,* insulin; *IR,* insulin receptor; *IGF,* insulin-like growth factor; *IGF-R,* insulin-like growth factor receptor; *EGF,* epidermal growth factor; *EGF-R,* epidermal growth factor receptor; $T_{3,4}$, thyroid hormones; *TR,* thyroid hormone receptor.

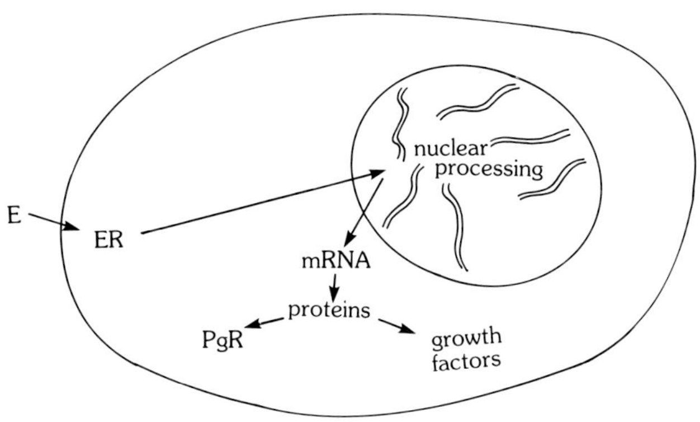

FIGURE 8-2. Breast cancer cell. Biochemical mechanism of estrogen action in human breast cancer cells. *E,* estrogen; *ER,* estrogen receptor; *PgR,* progesterone receptor.

hormones and might retain some degree of hormonal dependence.

Breast Cancer

Numerous research studies using *in vivo* and *in vitro* model systems have demonstrated the presence of receptors for a variety of hormones in human breast cancer cells and have begun to unravel the complex mechanisms by which these hormones regulate breast cancer growth. The greatest volume of work has been with the female sex steroid hormone estrogen.

Estrogen

The proposed biochemical mechanism by which estrogens regulate breast cancer growth is shown schematically in Figure 8-2. The lipid-soluble estrogen molecules (estrone, estradiol, or estriol) diffuse through the cell membrane to the interior of the cell. The traditional two-step hypothesis speculates that estrogen receptors (ER) are located primarily in the cytoplasm of the cell and that, after binding to estrogen, they undergo a transformation step prior to translocation of the entire complex to the nucleus.[2] There is growing evidence, however, that unbound ER actually resides *de novo* in the nucleus and that "cytoplasmic ER" may be an artifact of tissue processing.[3] In any event, the hormone receptor complex binds to nuclear chromatin and then, by poorly defined mechanisms, alters transcription of messenger ribonucleic acid (mRNA). Specific mRNA leaves the nucleus and codes for the translation of specific proteins. Certain estrogen-induced proteins, such as progesterone receptor (PgR), may be important for control of critical metabolic processes in the cell. Other estrogen-induced proteins may be involved in regulating events leading to cell proliferation. These latter proteins have not been definitively identified or characterized. Interestingly, two growth factors, insulin-like growth factor (IGF-I) and transforming growth factor (TGF) have been reported to be secreted products found in the media of cultured human breast cancer cells.[4] Synthesis of these factors may be controlled by estrogen in hormone-dependent tumors. Whether these or other estrogen-regulated proteins are the primary mediators of estrogen-stimulated growth requires additional study.

ER dynamics in response to estrogen or antiestrogens have been studied in detail using cultured human breast cancer cells.[5,6] Within minutes after the addition of estradiol, all ER tightly bound in the nucleus. Shortly thereafter, the cellular ER level declines, with the eventual loss of 50% to 70% of detectable ER by 5 hours after estrogen treatment. This event has been termed receptor processing.

ER dynamics in response to antiestrogen treatment are more complex. Antiestrogens can bind ER and fix receptor in the nucleus. Then, depending on the antiestrogen used, ER processing may be totally or only partially blocked. This observation led to speculation that ER processing was an integral step in the biologic activity of estrogens.[5] However, later work showed that there is a poor correlation between the level of ER processing and subsequent biologic activity of estrogens and antiestrogens.[6] Thus, the nuclear events controlling the activity of these compounds remain poorly defined.

Estrogen or antiestrogen treatment of human breast cancer cells results in a variety of biologic consequences.[7] RNA, DNA, and protein synthesis, the activity of key regulatory enzymes, and cell proliferative activity can be modulated by the direct addition of estrogens or antiestrogens to cultured cells. With physiological or pharmacologic concentrations, these effects are limited to ER-positive cells, supporting the hypothesis that these events are mediated through the ER.

Antiestrogens influence a variety of functions. The rates of RNA and DNA synthesis are reduced,[8] enzymes such as thymidine kinase,[9] carbamoylphosphate synthetase, aspartate transcarbamoylase, orotidine pyrophosphorylase, orotidine decarboxylase, and DNA polymerase are inhibited,[10,11] and cell proliferation is slowed.[12] Cell kinetic studies demonstrate that cells are blocked in G_1 phase in response to antiestrogens.[12] All of these effects can be prevented or reversed by the addition of a 100-fold lower concentration of estradiol, paralleling estradiol's greater affinity for ER compared with the affinity of tamoxifen.[8,11,13] These data illustrate the importance of ER in mediating the effects of these hormones.

Despite these data, controversy remains concerning the mechanisms by which estrogens stimulate breast cancer growth. Direct effects of estrogen on growth of cultured cells have been inconsistent in published reports,[8,11,14,15] leading some investigators to speculate that estrogen's effects are indirect and are mediated through the secretion of another growth factor or estromedin,[16] or by blocking certain inhibitory factors present in serum.[15] Nevertheless, the bulk of evidence suggests that estrogen can stimulate cell proliferation by direct interaction with ER-positive breast cancer cells.

Progesterone, Androgen, and Glucocorticoids

Androgen receptors, glucocorticoid receptors, and PgRs have been found in a substantial proportion of breast cancer specimens, although their function is not known. Presumably they mediate specific hormonal effects on normal breast growth and development. Conceivably, the effects of endocrine therapy with pharmacologic doses of these agents are also mediated through their respective specific receptors. As discussed later, the presence of these receptors along with ERs in a breast tumor specimen may be more indicative of an endocrine-responsive tumor than the presence of ERs alone. In fact, measurement of PgR together with ER has become standard clinical practice, and these tests are available in laboratories throughout the world.

Polypeptide Hormones and Growth Factors

Normal breast epithelial cells as well as breast cancer cells may be target tissues for a variety of polypeptide hormones and growth factors. Membrane receptors for prolactin,[17] insulin,[18] IGF-I,[19] and epidermal growth factor (EGF)[20,21] have been identified in cultured human breast cancer cells or in actual human breast cancer biopsy specimens. The role of these hormones in regulating breast cancer growth is not clear, but the presence of specific receptors and reports of proliferative effects on cultured cells[17–23] suggest that these factors may be important. In particular, insulin, IGF-I, and EGF in physiologic concentrations have been reported to stimulate a variety of metabolic processes including cell proliferation. Prolactin may modulate the level of ER in breast cancer cells. A recent report of the secretion by human breast cancer cells into the culture medium of IGF-I and a protein with TGF activity raises the interesting possibility of autocrine or paracrine growth regulation.[4] Knowledge of the presence or absence of receptors for polypeptide hormones has not yet proved useful clinically. However, if additional research identifies a critical role in growth regulation for one or more of these hormones, then new treatment strategies using receptor-blocking agents or agents that inhibit later biochemical events may emerge.

Thyroid Hormone

Normal breast development and growth are influenced by thyroid hormone. It is of interest that specific nuclear thyroid hormone receptors have been identified in several cultured human breast cancer cell lines.[24] Furthermore, proliferation of human breast cancer cells is stimulated by triiodothyronine. The importance of these observations to breast cancer growth *in vivo* remains to be defined.

ESTROGEN AND PROGESTERONE RECEPTOR ASSAYS

General Considerations

At the present time, among the hormone receptors discussed above, only ER and PgR are used clinically. Numerous methods have been developed to detect the presence and amount of ER and PgR in human breast cancer.[25] The steroid hormone receptor assays can be listed as follows:

Conventional assays
- Sucrose density gradient centrifugation
- Dextran-coated charcoal (DCC)
- Tissue slice uptake
- Gel filtration
- Agar gel electrophoresis
- Protamine sulfate
- Hydroxylapatite
- Isoelectric focusing

New methods
- Histochemical and immunohistochemical
- Dual label assays
- Receptor monoclonal antibodies
- Flow cytometry

Today most laboratories use either the dextran-coated charcoal assay, often with Scatchard analysis, or the sucrose density gradient centrifugation method. Most other methods are also satisfactory if performed and interpreted expertly. Almost all of these methods are based on the binding of a radiolabeled steroid to receptor in tissue slices or, more commonly, to receptor present in soluble proteins extracted in the supernatant of a tissue homogenate. The methods differ primarily in the technique used to separate receptor-bound from unbound hormone. Most of the methods are complicated by contamination of tissue extracts with plasma proteins such as albumin or sex-hormone-binding globulin, which may also bind to the labeled steroid. Appropriate techniques to distinguish true receptor from these plasma binders are critical.

Several other general points deserve emphasis. First, results of all of these assays correlate with patient response to endocrine therapy as shown by the data from several institutions reviewed at the international workshop on ER held in 1974.[26] Second, absolute values for receptor may be expressed differently from laboratory to laboratory, and the cutoff values for positive and negative are not uniform among laboratories but are based on the assay sensitivity of a particular laboratory or on results of correlations with clinical information. This may confuse some physicians, since an absolute value for receptor in one laboratory may not be equivalent to that obtained in another. Finally, the assays themselves require considerable experience from a technical and interpretive point of view. Valid results depend on proper handling of the specimen by the surgeon and pathologist, proper transport to and storage in the laboratory, and precise methodology. The 5% to 10% response rate to endocrine therapy in ER-negative tumors may partially reflect false-negative assays as a result of undetected procedural errors. Finally, specimens should be sent to laboratories providing evidence for assay quality control.

Specimen Handling and Preparation

The volume of malignant tissue obtained by the surgeon is very important. Small specimens, needle biopsies, or malignant effusions generally do not provide sufficient protein for a valid assay by standard methods, and false-negative values may result. Between 200 mg and 1 g of tissue, depending on the amount of contaminating fat or connective tissue, provides sufficient material for assay of ER and PgR by either sucrose gradient or dextran-coated charcoal (DCC) methods. Smaller tissue samples (as little as 50 mg) can be analyzed by special methods usually not available except in research laboratories.

Improper tissue processing after the biopsy specimen is taken will lead to invalid results, primarily because of the heat lability of receptor proteins. Tumor tissue for receptor assay must not be placed in fixative but, instead, should be chilled immediately on ice and either processed within hours or quickly frozen in liquid nitrogen. Frozen specimens should be stored at −70°C or below and shipped, if necessary, in dry ice. This has permitted the development of centralized laboratories nationwide and has brought receptor assay technology to all patients with breast cancer.

Prior to assay, frozen tissue is first pulverized to break up fibrous tissue and to permit thorough mixing. Pulverization is followed by homogenization in buffer. Care must be taken to keep the sample cold at all times to prevent loss of receptor. A cytosol extract is then obtained by collecting the supernatant after ultracentrifugation. The cytosol is used for the receptor assay, as well as for total protein determination, which is used to normalize receptor values. Alternatively, DNA content of the specimen can be measured in the pellet following centrifugation to normalize results.

Conventional Receptor Assays

Only the commonly used methods or methods of special interest will be discussed here. The reader is referred to the review by Chamness and McGuire[25] for details of other methods. The conventional assays used in most clinical laboratories measure only free (unbound) cytosol receptor; bound nuclear receptor is missed with these techniques.

Sucrose Density Gradient Centrifugation

This assay was among the first used for quantitative assay of ER. The cytosol is first incubated with [^{3}H] estradiol and is then layered on a continuous sucrose gradient. A parallel gradient is layered with cytosol incubated with excess unlabeled competitor (usually diethylstilbestrol) along with [^{3}H] estradiol to determine nonspecific binding. The gradients are ultracentrifuged, and then radioactivity in collected fractions is counted to determine peaks of bound [^{3}H] estradiol (Fig. 8-3). Unbound hormone remains at the top of the gradient. The sedimentation velocity of the peaks is determined by comparison with a standard (usually bovine serum albumin, 4.6S). True ER sediments at 8S under these conditions, whereas other nonreceptor binding proteins sediment at 4S. Some specimens also contain competible 4S binding, suggesting that ER may appear in two molecular forms,[27] but the clinical importance of this 8S/4S fractionation remains controversial.[28] The sucrose gradient method accurately measures and quantifies ER, but it is cumbersome and time-consuming and requires expensive equipment.

The sucrose gradient method can also be used, after appropriate modifications, to measure PgR. This receptor is less stable than ER. Many laboratories add sodium molybdate to the assay to stabilize the receptor. Usually the synthetic progestin ORG 2058 or R5020 is used to detect PgR, since progesterone itself has a lower affinity for receptor and also has a relatively high affinity for glucocorticoid receptor and corticosteroid binding globulin. R5020 does cross-react with glucocorticoid and androgen receptors, but hydrocortisone and dihydrotestosterone can be used to prevent binding to these receptors. True PgR sediments at 7S to 8S on sucrose gradients. Frequently a 4S competible peak is also present, although this may not represent true PgR.[29]

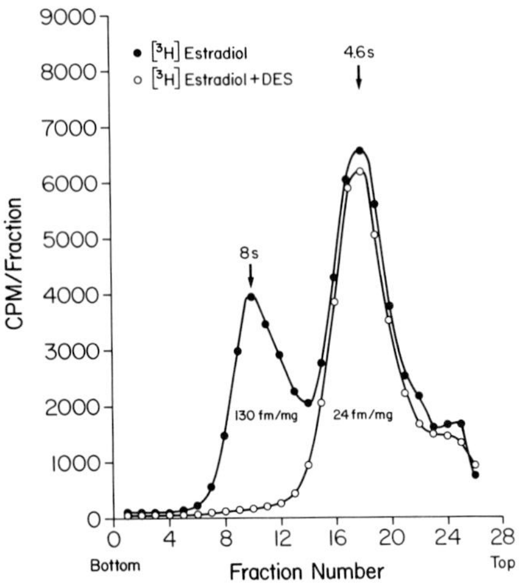

FIGURE 8-3. Typical sucrose gradient analysis of specific ([^{3}H] estradiol) and nonspecific ([^{3}H] estradiol + DES) binding to estrogen receptor in a human breast cancer cytosol. Nearly all of the competible binding is in the 8S fraction.

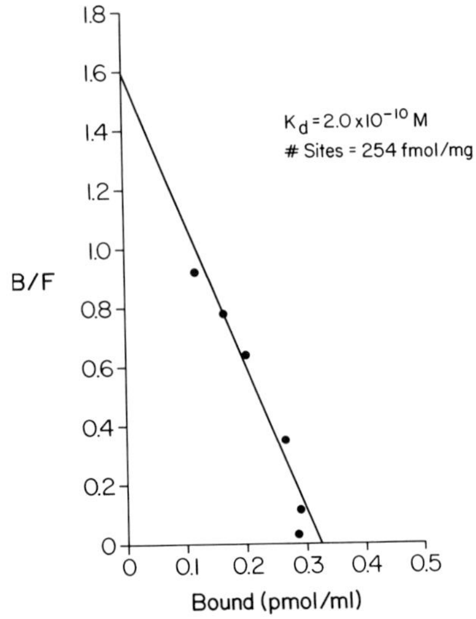

FIGURE 8-4. Typical Scatchard analysis of [^{3}H] estradiol binding to estrogen receptor in a human breast cancer cytosol determined by the multipoint DCC assay. The calculated binding affinity (K_d) and the quantitative receptor content are shown.

Dextran-Coated Charcoal Assay

The DCC method takes advantage of the property of charcoal to adsorb unbound steroid hormones. Cytosol is first incubated with [^{3}H] steroid. Dextran-coated charcoal is added, and the incubation mixture is shaken for 30 minutes in the cold. The dextran reduces adsorption of proteins to the charcoal without interfering with adsorption of free steroids, although some protein loss still occurs at low cytosol protein concentrations. Bovine serum albumin or 0.1% gelatin may also be added to reduce adsorption of cytosol proteins. DCC should be made fresh at regular intervals and each batch checked in a controlled assay to ensure consistency of results. After incubation with DCC, receptor-bound hormone is separated from free hormone bound to charcoal by centrifugation, and an aliquot of the supernatant is counted to determine receptor-bound [^{3}H] steroid. A parallel tube using excess unlabeled hormone is used to determine nonspecific binding. The duration of the cytosol incubation with DCC is important. If it is too short, [^{3}H] steroid will not be adsorbed from albumin and other low-affinity nonreceptor binders, and the level of measured receptor will be artificially increased; if it is too long, then some receptor-bound steroid may dissociate from receptor and be adsorbed onto the charcoal, reducing the measured receptor concentration.

Most laboratories using the DCC assay employ a range of [^{3}H] steroid concentrations in order to produce Scatchard plots for data interpretation (Fig. 8-4). This technique permits quantification of receptor number as well as an estimate of the binding affinity. A few laboratories have used a single-point assay with a single "saturating" concentration of ligand.[30,31] This variation does not allow an estimate of affinity. If this assay is done carefully, results correlate well with results from the standard multipoint DCC assay and with the sucrose gradient method. However, because the potential for error using this method is great it is not recommended for general use. Finding an appropriate binding affinity by Scatchard analysis or an 8S peak by sucrose gradient assay provides additional assurance that true receptor is present. The multipoint DCC assay, because of its simplicity, is now widely used for measurement of both ER and PgR.

Other Assays

Numerous other methods have been developed to measure steroid hormone receptors.[25] None of these offers major advantages over sucrose gradient or DCC assays, although a few are used for special situations. Sephadex LH20 gel filtration has been used to measure receptors in tissues with very low receptor concentrations.[32] Agar gel electrophoresis distinguishes receptor from other nonreceptor proteins on the basis of size and electrophoretic mobility.[33] Despite the high resolution attained, this more cumbersome method has not been used widely. The protamine sulfate assay may be used for special situations in which interference from nonreceptor proteins and degradation by proteolytic enzymes are potential problems. Protamine sulfate precipitates receptor protein, thereby stabilizing and protecting it. This assay has been useful in measuring nuclear receptor by exchange techniques requiring elevated temperature.[34] Receptor assays using small hydroxylapatite columns to adsorb [^{3}H] steroid-charged receptor may possibly be more reliable than the standard DCC assay at low cytosol protein concentrations.[35] This method has also been used to measure nuclear ER in human breast cancer.[36]

Nuclear Receptor Assays

Measurement of nuclear receptors might be important in situations in which high concentrations of endogenous hormones exist. For instance, patients undergoing postmenopausal estrogen therapy may have a false-negative cytosol ER assay since all receptors will be bound in the nucleus. Furthermore, quantifying nuclear receptors might provide additional evidence for the integrity of the hormone-response pathways. Methods to measure nuclear receptors have been developed,[25,36] but these assays are not widely available for clinical purposes, despite the potential advantages.

Newer Methods

Double-Label Assays for Simultaneous Measurement of ER and PgR

Both the ER and PgR assays provide useful clinical information, and both assays are now routine practice. However, sufficient tissue may not always be available to perform both assays. Furthermore, two separate assays are required, increasing working time and cost. The availability of radioiodinated estradiol with binding properties similar to unlabeled or [^{3}H]-labeled hormone has facilitated the development of a double-label assay for the simultaneous determination of both ER and PgR. The standard multipoint DCC assay has been modified to incorporate [^{125}I] estradiol and [^{3}H] R5020 in a single assay.[37] Unlabeled DES and R5020 are used as competitors to determine nonspecific binding. Preliminary experience supports the validity of this assay, which may help to reduce the amount of tissue required for a multipoint assay as well as time and expense.

Histochemical and Immunohistochemical Assays

Although biochemical assays are reliable and reproducible and correlate reasonably well with important clinical parameters, they have several drawbacks. First, although lack of ER usually indicates a hormone-unresponsive tumor, the presence of receptors as determined biochemically does not guarantee a response to hormone therapy. In fact, 40% of ER-positive tumors fail to respond, indicating the need for improvements in the assay or the development of alternative predictive assays. Second, biochemical assays can only be performed on relatively large tumor samples, precluding the use of malignant effusions or needle biopsy specimens for routine assay. Third, these assays as usually performed do not recognize bound nuclear receptors, which may lead to inaccurate estimates of receptor content in premenopausal women with high estrogen or progesterone levels or in women on estrogen therapy. Finally, these assays do not permit assessment of receptor status in individual tumor cells and do not address the problem of tumor heterogeneity. In an attempt to address these problems, several histochemical or immunohistochemical assays have been developed over the past 10 years. However, significant questions regarding the validity of many of these assays have been raised.

Several investigators have claimed detection of ER in human breast cancer specimens immunohistochemically using antiestradiol antibody.[38–42] After incubation with antibody, the putative antibody-hormone-ER complex is then detected either by incubation with a second fluoresceinated antibody or by incubation with unlabeled second antibody followed by reaction with a peroxidase-antiperoxidase complex. These methods reveal predominantly cytoplasmic staining. Correlations of these immunohistochemical assays with the conventional biochemical assay have shown 60% to 90% agreement. These methods also show tumor cell heterogeneity, with the majority of tumors being composed of variable proportions of positively stained and negative cells.

Results of cytochemical ER assays using estrogen conjugated directly or through bovine serum albumin to fluorescein have also been published.[43–48] Like the immunohistochemical techniques, these methods demonstrate some specificity for estrogen target tissues, cytoplasmic as well as some nuclear staining in certain tumors, partial qualitative agreement with conventional receptor determinations, and tumor heterogeneity. One study even reported a reasonably good correlation between the presence of ER determined histochemically and response to endocrine therapy.[45] Initially these techniques appeared to be new and promising methods for detecting and studying steroid hormone receptors.

More recent studies, however, suggest that these immunohistochemical and histochemical assays may not be measuring true ER.[49–57] The antiestradiol antibodies used in the immunohistochemical assays probably do not recognize receptor-bound estradiol. Preincubation with extremely high concentrations of estradiol is required for positive staining. Suprapharmacologic concentrations of the estrogen conjugates used for the histochemical assays are also required, indicating very low affinity for ER. In addition, binding with these conjugates is not saturable, and there is either no competition or, at best, incomplete competition of the binding of the conjugates even by large excess concentrations of diethylstilbestrol or other active estrogens. Thus, critical criteria for receptor binding have not been met. These observations suggest that these techniques may be detecting lower affinity type 2 or even type 3 estrogen binders, which are of questionable biologic significance.

If these histochemical assays are not measuring true ER, it is still possible that they might somehow be detecting the estrogen-sensitive cell population. However, a recent study comparing a standard biochemical ER assay with three different histochemical assays casts some doubt.[58] In 72 patients treated with endocrine therapy, only the standard biochemical assay correlated significantly with clinical response. Thus, the histochemical techniques discussed above do not measure true ER and do not predict response to endocrine therapy.

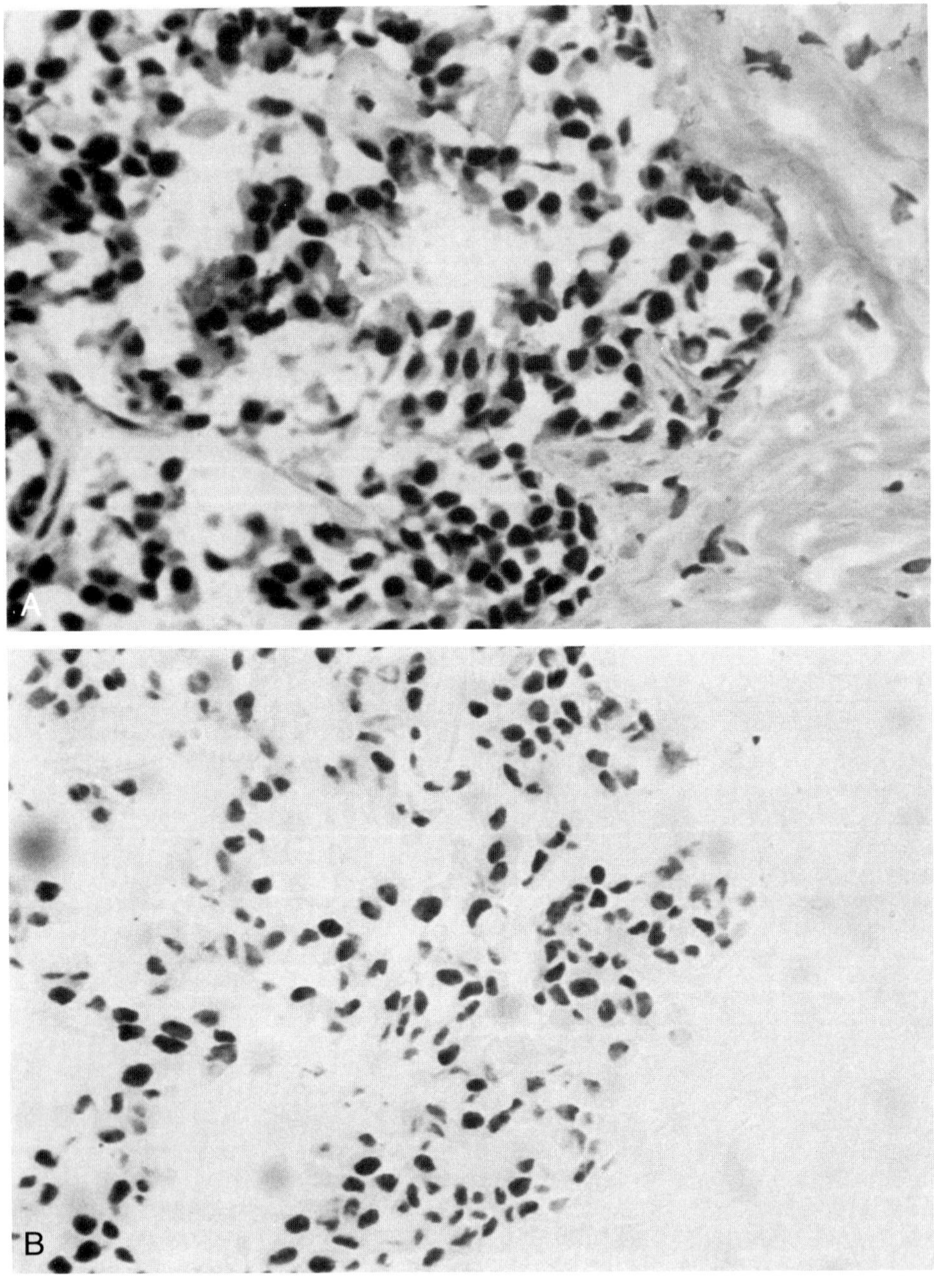

FIGURE 8-5. Immunohistochemistry using anti-ER antibody. *(A)* Photomicrograph of a primary breast cancer specimen incubated with anti-ER antibody followed by the peroxidase antiperoxidase procedure with DAB used as the chromogen. Hematoxylin counterstain was used (× 312). *(B)* Same specimen and processing as in *A* except no counterstain was used. Note that the majority of nuclei are stained, and the staining intensity is relatively homogeneous.

Immunohistochemistry With Monoclonal Antireceptor Antibodies

Using standard hybridoma technology, a panel of monoclonal antibodies has been produced that recognizes different determinants of human ER.[59,60] Immunohistochemical assays have been developed using these antireceptor antibodies, hopefully avoiding many of the pitfalls described above for assays using antiestradiol antibodies or those using fluoresceinated estrogen conjugates. Immunochemical staining using these new antireceptor antibodies is dependent on the antibody concentration, and it is competitively inhibited by purified ER, supporting the validity of the assay. Interestingly, nuclear but not cytoplasmic staining has consistently been observed, suggesting that all forms of ER may reside in the nucleus *in vivo*. This technique has also identified mixed populations of receptor-positive and receptor-negative cells within the same tumor specimen, as well as heterogeneity of staining intensity (Fig. 8-5). Preliminary data showing a relatively

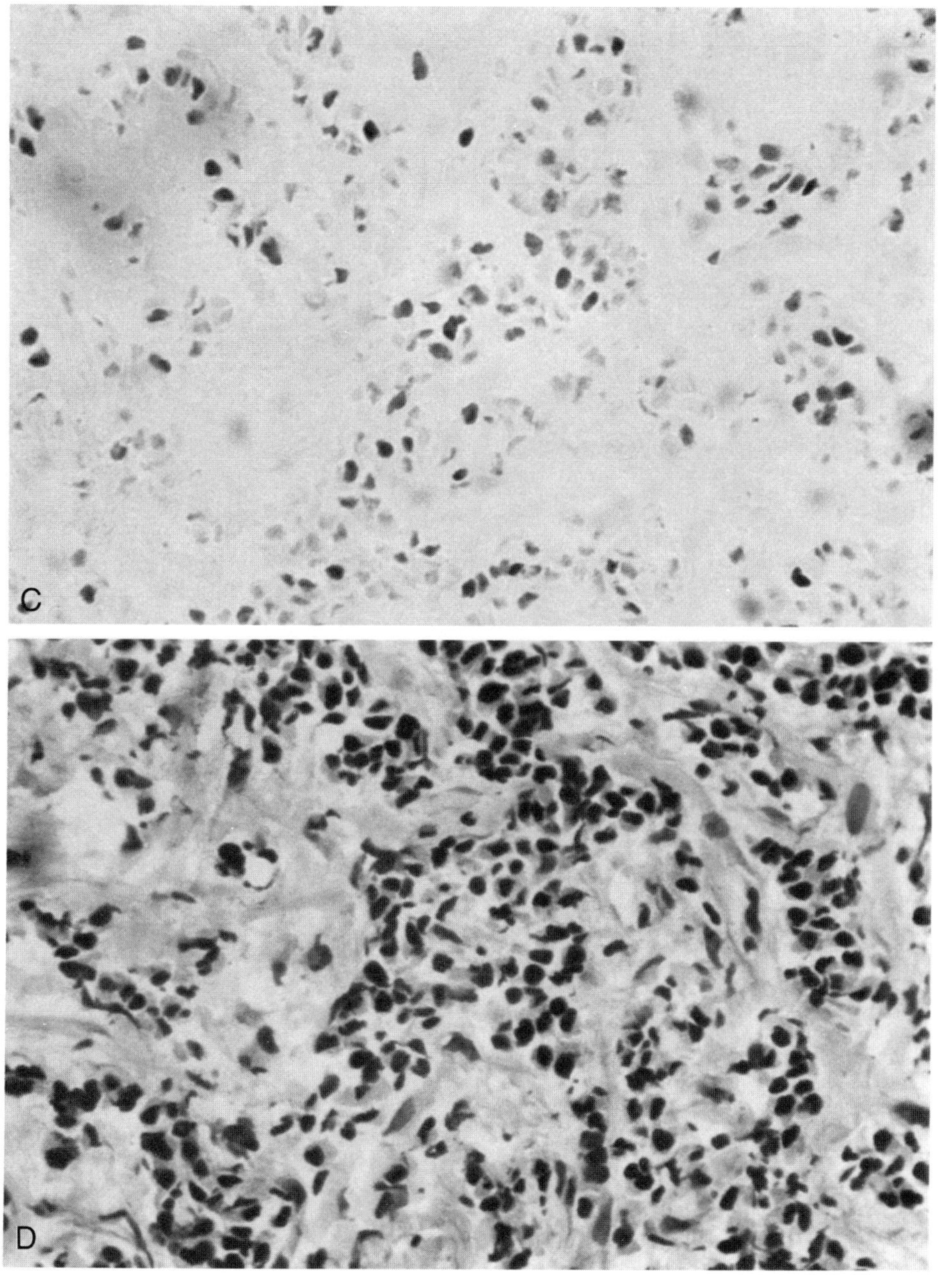

(C and D) Another breast cancer specimen processed as described on page 216, with and without counterstain. Note the heterogeneity of positive staining and staining intensity.

good correlation between this immunohistochemical method and standard biochemical ER assays, as well as with clinical response to treatment, are encouraging.[56] This assay will probably not replace biochemical assays for routine clinical use, but it will provide helpful complementary information. Furthermore, estimates of ER may be made on small biopsy specimens.

Monoclonal anti-ER antibody also has permitted the development of more quantitative immunoassays. Both the enzyme-linked immunochemical assay (ER-EIA) and the immunoradiometric assay (IRMA) are assays based on a sandwich technique using two antibodies.[61] In the ER-EIA assay, the second antibody is labeled with the enzyme horseradish peroxidase, which serves as a colorimetric marker. In the IRMA assay, the second antibody is labeled with ^{125}I to quantify bound receptor. Although field trials of these assays are in progress, preliminary studies suggest that there is excellent correlation with the conventional DCC assay.[61] Simplicity, consistency, accuracy, and low cost are potential advantages of these assays.

Receptor Analysis by Flow Cytometry

The newest technique for measuring ER involves flow cytometry of cells labeled with fluorescent estradiol.[62–64] The sensitivity of flow cytometry is superior to that of fluorescence microscopy; a few thousand molecules of fluorescein can be detected by this technique. Thus, fluorescent estrogens, like those used in the histochemical assays in huge concentrations, can be employed in more physiological concentrations capable of detecting type 1 ER binding. These assays are in the early stages of development, and certain problems need to be addressed. Furthermore, there are as yet no reports of the use of this assay in a large number of human breast cancer specimens. However, the potential value of the flow cytometry assay for studying ER is enormous.

Reliability and Quality Control of Steroid Hormone Receptor Assays

Reliability of receptor assays has been assessed in several ways. Using two randomly selected tissue blocks from the same primary tumor, a coefficient of variation of 17% for ER level was obtained.[65] These differences could be explained by procedural assay errors or by differences in tumor cellularity between two different areas of the same tumor. No specimens were positive for ER in one block but negative in another; differences were quantitative, not qualitative. Major discordant rates (clearly positive in one assay but negative in another) were only 3%, even when simultaneous assays from different sites in the same patient were performed.[66] Standard deviations of 5% to 16% were found for multiple determinations of a single cytosol dilution performed on the same or different days.[67] The reproducibility of ER and PgR assays was also monitored in a multi-institutional international study.[68] Tissue reference powders with low, intermediate, and high receptor content were shipped to laboratories throughout the world and assayed repeatedly. In general, receptor content decreased slightly during storage and transit, but all laboratories were able to correctly assign specimens to the three categories of receptor content for ER. Furthermore, intralaboratory variation in receptor content was good, with standard errors consistently less than 10% of the means. PgR concentrations were more variable, with standard errors ranging as high as 20%. Several laboratories had difficulty distinguishing between the powders with intermediate and high PgR content. In any event, from these studies it is clear that experienced laboratories have no difficulty in distinguishing between a receptor-positive and receptor-negative specimen. Agreement regarding the actual receptor concentration is also good for ER. Agreement for PgR is less satisfactory, perhaps because of the inherent lability of this receptor protein as well as other methodologic variables.

It is clear that daily quality control checks within laboratories are essential to detect contamination of buffers and reagents and to monitor the integrity of the radiolabeled ligand. Periodic quality control by an impartial organization is also helpful in maintaining accuracy, as well as in helping to make quantitative assay results more uniform across laboratories. Most of the large cooperative research groups involved in clinical breast cancer trials in this country and elsewhere have established quality control programs with outside monitoring. In the Southwest Oncology Group, frozen powders, not lyophilized cytosol, are sent twice a year to participating laboratories. Powders are used so that tissue preparation and homogenization are monitored in addition to the actual assay itself. Receptor-positive and negative powders are sent with each quality control check. Powders with different receptor levels (low, intermediate, or high) are sent periodically to assess the accuracy at different receptor concentrations. Results are returned to a central laboratory and are compared with the target values obtained in the reference laboratory, as well as with those obtained in the other participating laboratories. The reference laboratory also assays powders that are shipped elsewhere on ice and then returned, to account for receptor degradation that might occur during transit. Laboratories with consistent problems are notified and methodology is reviewed.

This system has been helpful in reducing differences in quantitative receptor values among laboratories and in identifying problem laboratories. Such a system, however, is not without problems. Questions such as which laboratory or which methodology should serve as the "gold standard" are encountered. Furthermore, changes or improvements in methodology are sometimes difficult to implement when many research and commercial laboratories are involved. Quality control monitoring is also costly and time-consuming, and just because a laboratory performs well on an occasional quality control assay does not necessarily mean that the laboratory performs well on a daily basis. Nevertheless, quality control programs are bound to improve laboratory performance, thereby improving the quality of the clinical trials themselves.

Recommended Assay Procedures

Many of the assays described above provide valid quantitative receptor information if tissue handling and assay technique are performed meticulously. It is difficult to recommend one specific methodology over another. For routine clinical purposes, simplicity, reliability, and cost of the assay should also be considered. For these reasons, the DCC multipoint assay with Scatchard analysis has been chosen most often for measurement of both ER and PgR. The additional information provided by calculation of binding affinity is helpful in assuring that true ER, and not a low-affinity binder, has been detected. A single-point assay is not recommended for routine purposes because of the potential problems discussed above. The sucrose gradient method is also used by a few laboratories, and it provides equivalent quantitative information as well as additional assurance (sedimentation velocity) that true receptor has been measured. Sodium molybdate should probably be used in all PgR assays to stabilize receptor. Dual-label ([^{125}I]estradiol, [^{3}H]R5020) DCC assays are becoming increasingly popular because both receptors can be determined on a single cytosol, thus reducing the tissue requirement and also reducing labor time and expense. Comparison of this or any new method with standard or proven assays is always important. The laboratory performing the assay should develop strict quality control procedures internally and should participate in an outside quality control program. The immunohistochemical assay using monoclonal anti-ER antibody may also be used for small tissue specimens or effusions or to assess heterogeneity. Commercial assay kits are now available.

Immunohistochemical assays using monoclonal antireceptor antibody appear promising for measurement of ER. Currently these assays provide only semiquantitative information, although they have the advantage of requiring only small tissue samples or body fluids. Furthermore, an assessment of tumor cell heterogeneity regarding receptor content can be made. These assays should provide a useful adjunct to conventional methods in the near future. Other histochemical methods using antiestradiol antibody or fluoresceinated estrogens are not recommended since they do not correlate well with conventional assays or, more importantly, with the clinical parameters of interest.

Problems in Interpretation of Receptor Assays

Proper interpretation of ER and PgR assays is critical for optimal decision making in the clinic. Major problems in the interpretation of assay results may come from at least two sources: (1) tumor cellularity and heterogeneity and (2) the blood level of estrogen and progesterone.

Tumor Cellularity

ER and PgR are found only in the epithelial component of breast cancer tissue. Supporting stromal tissues or adjacent fatty tissues are devoid of these proteins. The epithelial cellularity of a tumor varies widely. Some breast cancers are densely cellular, whereas others have a sparse epithelial component with the major portion of the tumor being composed of a fibrous stroma. Other tumors have large necrotic areas or infiltration with mononuclear cells. Conventional biochemical assays measure receptors on a tumor cytosol extract that includes all of these elements and not just the epithelial component. Thus, differences in epithelial cellularity could affect the measured receptor concentration. Tumors with a sparse but receptor-positive epithelial component might be measured as low positive or even receptor negative by biochemical assay. This question has been addressed by several investigators, with contradictory results. It has been reported that the quantitative ER level varies according to the density of the epithelial component and that discordant ER results from simultaneous biopsies can be minimized by correcting for the fraction of nontumor tissue in the sample.[65,69–72] Others have been unable to document a relationship between ER content and tumor cellularity.[73,74] The development of valid histochemical assays will permit more accurate assessments of tumor cellularity and ER content and may provide an explanation for these discrepant results. Meanwhile, detailed histopathologic review for a quantitative assessment of tumor cell density to provide a "correction factor" for ER results is not routine in most laboratories. However, histologic sections of tissue sent for ER analysis should be reviewed to ensure that the specimen does contain tumor tissue.

Size of the Biopsy Specimen

False-negative receptor assays can occur when insufficient material is provided to the receptor laboratory. Initial biopsy specimens may be divided, and tissue sent to different laboratories for histology, cell kinetic analysis, and receptor assays. If the biopsy is not done carefully, one or more laboratories may receive a specimen that is not representative of the main tumor mass itself or that may not even contain tumor cells. Hull and colleagues[66] studied a large number of patients who had an ER determination on the primary breast tumor and a subsequent ER assay performed later on a metastatic lesion. Only 13% of all tumors that were initially ER negative were clearly ER positive at the second assay. However, if the initial primary tumor size was less than 2 cm, the discordance rate was 50%. This suggests that an inadequate amount of tissue may have been submitted from the small primary lesion for the initial ER analysis. Thus, ER results from small biopsy specimens can be falsely negative and should be interpreted with caution.

Endogenous Hormone Levels

ER and PgR content may be influenced by the blood concentration of estrogen and progesterone. Since the conventional biochemical assays only measure unbound receptor present in cytosol preparations, measurements performed in the face of high blood hormone levels may be falsely negative; under these conditions all receptors may be occupied by hormone and retained in the nucleus, where they are unavailable for routine assay. The PgR level may be artificially low or even absent when biopsy specimens are taken from premenopausal women during the luteal phase of the menstrual cycle, when endogenous progesterone levels are high.[75] ER level is probably not influenced greatly by the endogenous estrogen concentration, since it is doubtful that physiologic estrogen concentrations ever reach levels sufficient to saturate all of the available receptor sites and cause a negative ER assay.[76] Furthermore, an inverse correlation between measured ER content and the concentration of estrogen in serum, or even in tumor tissue itself, has not been observed.[75,77]

PgR synthesis is induced by estrogen in target tissues, including breast cancer. One might speculate that some postmenopausal women with very low estrogen levels may have inadequate estrogen to increase PgR to detectable levels. A report that administration of estrogen to postmenopausal women converted several PgR-negative tumors to PgR positive supports this idea.[78]

Exogenous Hormones

The administration of exogenous hormones to patients undergoing receptor analysis can have profound effects on ER and PgR concentration. Although endogenous physiologic concentrations of estrogen do not saturate all receptors, estrogens used to treat menopausal symptoms or those used to treat breast cancer may mask all ER, resulting in a falsely negative assay. Antiestrogens such as tamoxifen have a similar effect on the ER assay. PgR levels might not be affected or may actually be increased under stimulation with estrogen or tamoxifen, but administration of progestational agents might mask PgR. A common clinical problem is posed by the patient undergoing biopsy of a new breast lump when she has been taking postmenopausal estrogens or the patient with advanced breast cancer undergoing a second biopsy for receptor analysis after having failed estrogen or antiestrogen therapy. Even if these drugs are discontinued prior to obtaining the tissue specimen, the potential for a false-negative ER assay exists because of the prolonged half-life of some of these agents. In one study, of those patients with ER-positive tumors who had a repeat biopsy for ER within 2 months of stopping tamoxifen, 78% converted to ER-negative status (Fig. 8-6).[66] This apparent conversion was not seen when the repeat biopsy was performed more than 2 months after stopping tamoxifen or with ablative forms of endocrine therapy, suggesting that many of the repeat assays were falsely negative because of receptor occupancy by the drug. Thus, a negative ER assay from a patient recently undergoing estrogen or antiestrogen therapy is not interpretable. More emphasis should be placed on the result of the PgR assay in these circumstances.

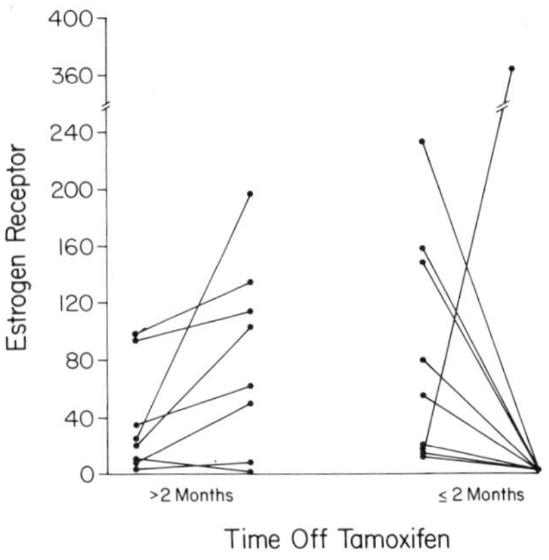

FIGURE 8-6. Changes in ER content with sequential assays in patients with intervening tamoxifen therapy. Patients were classified into two groups depending on the duration of time off tamoxifen at the time of the repeat biopsy. (Hull, DF, Clark GM, Osborne CK, et al: Multiple estrogen receptor assays in human breast cancer. Cancer Res 43:413–416, 1983)

CLINICAL USE OF RECEPTORS

History and Rationale

For nearly 90 years it has been recognized that human breast cancer may respond favorably to endocrine manipulations such as oophorectomy, adrenalectomy, or the pharmacologic administration of certain hormones.[79] About one-third of breast cancers demonstrate this endocrine dependence. Prior to the development of steroid hormone receptor assays, physicians relied on a variety of clinical criteria in selecting the proper breast cancer patients for endocrine therapy. Parameters such as age, menopausal status, disease-free interval after mastectomy, and sites of metastatic disease were thought to correlate with the likelihood of clinical response to therapy. Unfortunately, even with these criteria, only 30% to 40% of patients chosen for endocrine treatment responded.

Over the past 15 years, the discovery of active cytotoxic drugs has caused a therapeutic dilemma: which patients should receive chemotherapy and which patients should receive endocrine therapy as initial treatment for metastatic disease. Combination chemotherapy has an objective remission rate between 50% and 70%, compared with the 30% response rate for hormone therapy. Consequently, many physicians began to routinely prescribe cytotoxic chemotherapy as the initial approach to patients with advanced disease because of the higher response rate. Thus, patients who might have responded to endocrine therapy received, instead, cytotoxic drugs with their potentially severe untoward side effects. A more accurate method of selecting patients for chemotherapy or hormone manipulation was urgently needed.

Around the year 1960, the synthesis of high-specific-activity radioactive estrogens, [^{3}H] hexestrol or [^{3}H] estradiol, provided the necessary tools for further studies of tumor hormone dependence.[80,81] Glascock and Hoekstra reported the selective accumulation of [^{3}H] hexestrol in the normal estrogen target organs of animals injected with the hormone.[80] Several years later this observation was extended to show the accumulation of labeled estrogens by breast cancer tissue from both humans and animals.[82–92] Of special interest were the reports that patients or experimental animals whose tumors contained excess [^{3}H] hexestrol after *in vivo* injection responded to later endocrine treatment, whereas those whose tumors did not concentrate the hormone failed to respond. The mechanisms by which these tumors concentrated radioactive estrogen then became the focus of study.

Later studies eventually revealed that a protein present in normal estrogen target tissues and certain breast tumors was responsible for the intracellular accumulation of estrogen.[2,93] This protein became known as estrogen receptor or estrophilin because of its high affinity and specificity for estrogens. This discovery led to speculation that the presence of ER might signal hormone dependence of a tumor. Since ER is required for estrogenic biologic activity, absence of receptor would preclude a direct effect of the hormone on the cell, leading to hormone independence.

Table 8-1
Association Between ER Status, Menopausal Status, and Patient Age

Group	*No. of Patients*	*ER+ (%)**	*Median ER†*
Premenopausal	625	64	8
Postmenopausal	2152	79	46
Age < 50	765	62	8
Age ≥ 50	2212	80	44

* ER+: at least 3 fmol/mg protein
† Median ER concentration in fmol/mg protein
(Clark GM, Osborne CK, McGuire WL: Correlations between estrogen receptor, progesterone receptor, and patient characteristics in human breast cancer. J Clin Oncol 2:1102–1109, 1984)

As discussed below, numerous studies have now confirmed the utility of ER assays in predicting tumor hormone dependence, and they have revealed other uses for the ER assay as well.

Correlation of Estrogen Receptors With Clinical Parameters

Age and Menopausal Status

Several investigators have reported that postmenopausal patients have tumors that are more frequently ER positive and have a higher ER concentration than those in premenopausal women. Whether the higher ER level is related more to menopausal status (endogenous estrogen concentration) or to the age of the patient independent of menopausal status is controversial. Some reports conclude that age has no or little effect on ER level within menopausal groups.[94,95] Others conclude that there is a stronger correlation between ER status and age than with menopausal status.[96–98] A large study with nearly 3000 ER assays performed on primary breast tumors confirmed that tumors from older women or postmenopausal women were more likely to be ER positive and contain a higher ER concentration (Table 8-1).[99] However, further analysis revealed that ER level was associated primarily with age but not with menopausal status independent of age. No difference in ER concentration between premenopausal and postmenopausal women of the same age was found, suggesting that the lower ER levels found in younger women are not due to higher circulating estrogen levels binding to and masking ER. The differences must be related to other unknown biologic factors that distinguish breast cancers found in younger women from those in the elderly population.

Biopsy Site

Tumor ER content may depend partially on the type of tissue sent for assay. A slightly greater proportion of primary tumor samples are ER positive than are specimens from metastatic sites.[26] This may reflect a selective increase in ER-negative cells over time from a heterogeneous primary tumor, a greater risk for the development of metastatic disease in patients with ER-negative tumors (see below), or even contamination of the biopsy specimen from metastatic sites with normal receptor-negative cells, resulting in a falsely low ER value. Positive assays may be obtained less frequently from visceral sites such as lung or liver than from other metastatic sites including skin, soft tissue, or lymph nodes.[95] This may be explained by the fact that ER-negative primary tumors have a significantly higher propensity for recurring in a visceral site than do ER-positive tumors.[100]

Histopathology

Early studies reported no correlation between ER content and the histologic type of breast cancer, but they did suggest that the presence of ER was associated with histologic features of tumor differentiation.[26] A later study suggested that lobular carcinoma is more frequently ER positive.[101] This study failed to show a relationship between tumor ER and histologic grade or other features of tumor differentiation. However, more recent larger studies demonstrated a significant correlation between ER content and a variety of histologic features including histologic grade, nuclear grade, elastosis, necrosis, and lymphoid infiltration.[102–106] Tumors demonstrating histologic evidence of poor tumor differentiation such as high histologic or nuclear grade, extensive necrosis, little or no elastosis, and a prominent lymphoid infiltrate are frequently ER negative. In fact, nearly all ER-negative tumors display at least one of these unfavorable histologic characteristics, and the majority demonstrate at least three. ER-positive tumors are more likely to demonstrate low grade, little or no necrosis, marked elastosis, and absent lymphoid infiltrate, all features of well-differentiated tumors. These histologic characteristics have also been associated with improved prognosis of patients with primary breast cancer. No consistent associations between ER and other histologic features such as tumor size, stroma, nipple involvement, vascular or lymphatic invasion, intraductal component, axillary node involvement, or lymph node sinus histiocytosis have been found. These studies suggest that ER content is a biochemical marker for the degree of differentiation of human breast cancer. It is a more convenient and reproducible marker than the histologic variables, which require careful and expert pathologic review not available in all centers. Further study will be required to determine whether these histologic parameters of differentiation and ER status are independent variables with a high degree of association or that one is dependent on the other for its expression.

Cell Cycle Kinetics

Several investigators have applied cell kinetic parameters to the study of ER in breast cancer. If ER content is a biochemical marker for the degree of tumor differentiation, it is reasonable to speculate that it might correlate with an index of proliferative activity. Meyer and colleagues[107] used the technique of measuring the tritiated thymidine labeling index (TLI) to study the proliferative activity of human breast cancer. The TLI estimates the proportion of tumor cells that are engaged in replication of DNA (S-phase fraction) during a brief incubation with [^{3}H] thymidine. As such the TLI is a measure of the rate of replication or proliferative potential of the tumor cells. An excellent correlation between TLI and ER content in primary breast tumors was observed. Tumors with a low TLI were more frequently ER positive, whereas those with a high TLI infrequently contained ER. These studies were later extended to show that low TLIs were associated with older age, minimal nuclear anaplasia histologically, ER positivity, and prolonged patient survival.[108] The TLI was the only variable to have independent prognostic significance.

In Italy, Silvestrini's group later confirmed and extended the observations of Meyer.[109] They studied the relationship between ER, TLI, and menopausal status in patients with primary breast cancer and identified three groups with different cell kinetic activity. A very low TLI included ER-positive cancers from postmenopausal women. An intermittent TLI was observed in ER-positive tumors from premenopausal patients or ER-negative tumors from postmenopausal patients. A high TLI was associated with ER-negative tumors from premenopausal women.

Cell kinetic analyses using flow cytometry have also been applied to the study of ER in human breast cancer.[110] ER-positive tumors were found to have a lower mean percent of cells in S-phase of the cell cycle than ER-negative tumors. Furthermore, receptor-positive tumors were more likely to express a diploid, rather than aneuploid, DNA content.

It is clear from these data that ER content not only is associated with histologic features of differentiation but that it is also associated with evidence of low proliferative potential. These results provide a rationale for the use of ER level as a prognostic factor for recurrence and survival of patients with operable breast cancer.

Estrogen Receptors as a Predictor of Response to Therapy

Qualitative Estrogen Receptor Assay

When binding to ER was recognized as the first step in the mechanism of estrogen action in human breast cancer cells and after methods were devised to conveniently measure ER content, numerous investigators throughout the world began measuring ER and correlating its presence with tumor response to endocrine treatment. The hypothesis that ER might be a marker for endocrine responsiveness was soon confirmed by cumulative data from an international meeting held in 1974.[26] Numerous laboratories using various methodologies to measure ER content came to the same conclusion, that the presence of ER was associated with clinical response to all types of endocrine therapies (Table 8-2). Of 423 patients with outside review to assess response, 55% to 60% responded to surgical ablative or additive hormonal therapies. More importantly, only 8% of patients with ER-negative tumors responded to endocrine therapy. It is important to emphasize that ER content did not predict for response to any specific type of hormonal therapy; it predicted as well for response to adrenalectomy or androgens as it did for ovariectomy. More recent studies have confirmed these observations and extended them to include clinical response to new endocrine therapies such as antiestrogens, the aromatase inhibitors, or progestin therapy.[111–113]

Table 8-2
Cumulative Data on the Response to Endocrine Therapy by Tumor ER Status

Treatment	*ER-Positive*	*ER-Negative*
Ablative	59/107 (55%)	8/94 (8%)
Adrenalectomy	32/66	4/33
Oophorectomy	25/33	4/53
Hypophysectomy	2/8	0/8
Additive	51/85 (60%)	7/82 (8%)
Androgen	12/26	2/24
Estrogen	37/57	5/58
Glucocorticoid	2/2	—
Antiestrogens	8/20	5/27

(McGuire WL, Vollmer EP, Carbone PP (eds): Estrogen Receptors in Human Breast Cancer. New York, Raven Press, 1975)

Thus, patients with ER-negative tumors infrequently benefit from endocrine therapy and can be spared the morbidity of major ablative surgery or the long delays waiting for a response to additive hormone treatment. With a few exceptions, such patients are generally considered candidates for cytotoxic chemotherapy. (See Chapter 13.) On the other hand, one-half to two-thirds of patients with ER-positive tumors respond to endocrine therapy. In another large multi-institution study, ER content was found by multivariate analysis techniques to be the most significant predictor for tumor response to endocrine treatment.[114] However, other clinical variables including site of visceral metastasis and disease-free interval were also found to be important. Receptor status as well as these clinical variables should be used to optimize the proper selection of patients for endocrine treatment. Since as many as 40% of patients with ER-positive tumors fail to benefit from endocrine treatment, other techniques have been studied to improve the predictive accuracy of the test. ER status does not correlate with response duration.

Nuclear Estrogen Receptor Assay

One attempt to improve the predictive ability of the ER assay is to measure both cytosol and nuclear ER content. Finding nuclear receptors might indicate that the binding *and* translocation steps are functional; absence of nuclear ER, in contrast, might indicate defective steps in estrogen action leading to hormone independence. To examine this possibility, two studies measured receptor in both cytosol extracts and in nuclear pellets.[115,116] Tumors with ER in both fractions had a high regression rate (71%) compared with those with no receptor (9%) or those with cytoplasmic receptor only (24%). Despite these encouraging data, nuclear ER assays have received little attention and, in the absence of confirming studies, they have not become routine in clinical laboratories.

Quantitative Estrogen Receptor Assay

Another method of increasing the predictive accuracy of the ER assay in receptor-positive tumors is to examine the quantitative receptor concentration. If breast cancers contain variable proportions of ER-positive and ER-negative cells, tumors with more ER-positive cells and, thus, a higher ER concentration might be more responsive to endocrine therapy. Early studies failed to show a correlation between ER level and response to therapy.[26] Later studies, however, convincingly demonstrate that the higher the ER level the greater the chance for response.[117–120] In our own experience of 198 trials of various endocrine therapies for advanced breast cancer, only 9% of patients with low to absent tumor ER responded, compared with 42% of those with intermediate ER levels (3 to 100 fmol/mg proteins), or 64% of those with high levels (> 100 fmol/mg protein) (Table 8-3). Thus, quantifying ER in a breast cancer specimen may further improve the selection of patients for endocrine therapy.

Predictive Accuracy of an Estrogen Receptor Assay on the Primary Tumor

Many of the studies reviewed above were based on the result of an ER assay performed on a metastatic biopsy specimen obtained just prior to a trial of endocrine therapy. However, many patients with advanced breast cancer do not present with disease easily accessible to biopsy for receptor determination. Two obvious questions are raised. Does ER status change over time or with interval treatment, and does an ER result from the primary tumor predict as well as a metastatic biopsy for endocrine responsiveness at the time of recurrence. If breast cancers are composed initially of receptor-positive (hormone-sensitive) and receptor negative (hormone-insensitive) cells, then shifts in the majority cell population are possible as a result of natural selection processes such as differences in proliferation kinetics between clones or as a result of the selective pressure of therapy. These questions have been addressed by analyzing patients who have had sequential tumor biopsies for ER.[66,70,121–124] In the absence of intervening therapy, discordance rates for ER are about 15% to 20% between sequential biopsies, and no significant difference in receptor concentration is observed. These discordance rates are no larger than those for multiple simultaneous biopsies. Intervening chemotherapy does not have a major effect on discordance rates, which are similar to those for untreated patients. Intervening endocrine therapy may result in a higher proportion of ER-positive tumors converting to ER-negative, as well as a reduction in the ER concentration. Although this may in part reflect a loss of ER-positive cells with treatment, it could also be explained by false-negative ER assays resulting from receptor occupancy in patients treated with additive hormone therapy. Discordance rates similar to untreated patients are observed if patients recently receiving tamoxifen therapy are excluded from analysis.[66] As discussed earlier, residual tamoxifen may bind to and mask receptor sites. Thus, there is no convincing evidence that ER content changes significantly over time, even with intervening therapy.

Table 8-3
ER Concentration and Response to Endocrine Therapy

ER (fmol/mg protein)	*Response (%)*
0–2	5/53 (9%)
3–100	43/103 (42%)
> 100	27/42 (64%)

Data from clinical trials support this conclusion.[118,125] In patients receiving endocrine therapy for advanced breast cancer, an ER assay from the primary tumor at the time of mastectomy was as predictive for response as was an assay from a metastatic specimen at the time of recurrence. This does not necessarily mean that a single ER assay from the primary tumor is sufficient; patients should have repeat biopsies for receptor if accessible disease is present. If not, the primary tumor ER assay can be used to guide treatment.

Estrogen Receptors and Response to Chemotherapy

The association between tumor ER status and response to chemotherapy is controversial. Since ER-negative tumors tend to have high proliferative indices, one might speculate that they would respond better to chemotherapy. Reported studies reveal a wide spectrum of results (Table 8-4). Some studies claim a higher response rate to chemotherapy for ER-negative tumors, whereas others claim higher response rates with ER-positive tumors. The explanation for these contradictory results is not clear, but it may be due to problems inherent in retrospective analyses, to differences between chemotherapy regimens, or to differences among studies regarding the chronological sequence of the ER biopsy and the administration of chemotherapy. A prospective clinical trial is needed to answer this question.

Progesterone Receptors

General Characteristics

Synthesis of PgR is increased by estrogen in target tissues including breast cancer. Being an end product of

Table 8-4
ER and Response to Chemotherapy

Study	ER-Negative	ER-Positive
Lippman[127]	34/45 (76%)	3/25 (12%)
Jonat[128]	20/28 (71%)	6/14 (43%)
King	8/12 (67%)	11/19 (58%)
Bonadonna	7/16 (44%)	14/28 (50%)
Samal	35/69 (51%)	24/37 (65%)
Webster[129]	17/45 (38%)	12/20 (60%)
Nomura	3/22 (13%)	6/14 (42%)
Kiang[130]	14/40 (35%)	16/20 (80%)
Block[124]	0/11 (0%)	3/4 (75%)

(Osborne CK, McGuire WL: The use of steroid hormone receptors in the management of patients with breast cancer. In Hoogstraten B, McDivitt RW (eds): Breast Cancer, pp 155–169. Boca Raton, CRC Press, 1981)

Table 8-5
Distribution of ER and PgR in Human Breast Cancer

Receptor Status	Number of Patients (%)
ER−, PgR−	171/638 (27%)
ER−, PgR+	15/638 (2%)
ER+, PgR−	189/638 (30%)
ER+, PgR+	263/638 (41%)

Cumulative data from several institutions.
(Clark GM, McGuire WL: Progesterone receptors and human breast cancer. Breast Cancer Res Treat 3:157–163, 1983)

Table 8-6
Association Between PgR Status, Menopausal Status, and Patient Age

Group	Number of Patients	PgR+ (%)*	Median PgR†
Premenopausal	503	58	8
Postmenopausal	1698	53	6
Age < 50	626	53	6
Age ≥ 50	1749	54	6

* PgR+: at least 5 fmol/mg protein
† Median PgR concentration in fmol/mg protein
(Clark GM, Osborne CK, McGuire WL: Correlations between estrogen receptor, progesterone receptor, and patient characteristics in human breast cancer. J Clin Oncol 2:1102–1109, 1984)

estrogen action, PgR was proposed to be a better indicator of tumor endocrine responsiveness than ER.[131] Detection of PgR in a human breast cancer specimen would suggest that not only was ER present, but that the biochemical events distal to the binding step were functional.

Techniques for measuring PgR levels were optimized and clinical correlative studies were begun in the mid-1970s. The distribution of ER and PgR in a large number of human breast cancer specimens is shown in Table 8-5. Twenty-seven percent of tumors lack receptors. Not surprisingly, ER-negative, PgR-positive tumors are rare, as one might have predicted if PgR synthesis is an estrogen-dependent process. This group probably reflects falsely negative ER assays. More than 40% of tumors contain both receptors, whereas 30% lack PgR despite having detectable ER.

Unlike ER content, PgR level appears to have no significant relationship with either age or menopausal status when these variables are analyzed separately (Table 8-6).[99] But premenopausal patients have higher PgR concentrations than postmenopausal women when patients of the same age are compared. This may reflect greater estrogen-mediated synthesis of PgR in younger women. Large tumors tend to be less frequently PgR positive and to have a lower median PgR concentration.[132] Furthermore, well-differentiated tumors are more likely to be PgR-positive than poorly differentiated tumors.[102,133]

Sequential assays

Changes in PgR content over time with or without intervening therapy may be more important clinically than changes in ER content, since, as discussed below, PgR may be a better marker for tumor hormone responsiveness. In contrast to ER, significant discordance rates for PgR are evident in patients undergoing sequential repeat biopsies for receptor analysis.[134] Tumors that are PgR negative on initial biopsy usually remain so on a repeat biopsy; only 9% convert to PgR positive. Tumors that are initially PgR positive, on the other hand, frequently convert to PgR negative by the time of the second biopsy. The discordance rate for this group is 44%. This high discordance rate is largely due to intervening endocrine therapy. Tumors from more than half of patients receiving endocrine therapy convert from PgR positive to negative. This loss of PgR with endocrine therapy may be explained by the gradual elimination of the hormone-sensitive population and the emergence of resistant cells lacking PgR. It is interesting that the survival duration of patients whose tumors convert to PgR negative is significantly shorter than those whose tumors remain PgR positive. This emphasizes the potential importance of repeated receptor analyses in patients with accessible tumor for biopsy.

Progesterone Receptors in Predicting Response to Endocrine Therapy

Numerous studies have examined the value of PgR as a predictor of response to endocrine therapy (Table 8-7). Most of these studies are small retrospective analyses. Nevertheless, the pooled data suggest that PgR may be an important marker for hormone dependence. As predicted from the hypothesis discussed above, tumors lacking both receptors are usually endocrine independent and regress infrequently (9%) with hormone treatment. ER-negative, PgR-positive tumors are rare, but responses to endocrine therapy are common (42%). The highest response rate

Table 8-7
Cumulative Data on the Response to Endocrine Therapy by Tumor ER and PgR Status

Study	*ER+, PgR+*	*ER+, PgR−*	*ER−, PgR+*	*ER−, PgR−*
Matsumoto[135]	12/20	9/25	0/1	2/20
Degenshein[136]	26/33	3/14	1/1	0/14
Young[137]	20/29	3/14	1/2	2/9
Brooks[138]	4/6	2/7	—	—
Stewart[139]	31/62	11/41	3/11	2/33
Manni[140]	15/24	3/5	—	0/2
McCarty[141]	33/40	2/20	1/3	3/35
Nomura[142]	7/10	8/12	—	—
Osborne[118]	16/20	14/45	—	3/20
Skinner[143]	9/12	2/6	2/3	3/30
Bloom[78]	23/30	3/14	1/1	0/10
Holdaway[144]	7/10	11/15	1/1	2/16
Johnson[145]	14/23	1/5	1/3	1/8
Total	217/319 (68%)	72/223 (32%)	11/26 (42%)	18/197 (9%)

(68%) is observed in tumors containing both receptors. This lends credence to the hypothesis that PgR may be a good marker for hormone dependence. According to the hypothesis, ER-positive, PgR-negative tumors should be autonomous and should not respond to hormone treatment, yet the response rate in this group is 32%. Perhaps PgR synthesis is not linked sufficiently to the pathway of tumor growth to be an accurate predictor of response in all cases. Alternatively, the PgR assay in some of these cases could be "falsely" negative as a result of the conditions described in an earlier section. In any event, these cumulative data suggest that the PgR assay may improve our ability to select patients likely to respond to endocrine therapy.

Quantitative Estrogen Receptor Versus Progesterone Receptor Assays

The quantitative ER assay and the PgR assay are useful markers of hormone dependence. An important question is whether or not the time and expense required for both assays is necessary. Possibly, these assays are selecting the same set of patients, since tumors with high ER content are more likely to have PgR (Table 8-8). In fact, more than three-fourths of tumors containing greater than 100 fmol/mg protein of ER, those with the highest response rate to endocrine therapy, also contain PgR. Thus, a positive PgR assay might simply be a marker for those tumors with high ER content. This question has not been rigorously addressed. In a small series, clinical response to endocrine therapy was assessed in 65 ER-positive patients for whom both quantitative ER and PgR data were available.[118] In this limited study, PgR appeared to be a better discriminant for objective response than quantitative ER alone (Table 8-9). However, there has not been a large prospective study with patients treated with a uniform approach designed to address the relative significance of tumor ER and PgR content. The Southwest Oncology Group is currently carrying out such a study, which should provide conclusive information on the prognostic value of PgR for endocrine responsiveness in advanced breast cancer.

Androgen and Glucocorticoid Receptors

Androgen receptors (AR) have been found in 35% to 50% and glucocorticoid receptors (GR) in up to 77% of human breast cancers assayed.[146–149] AR and GR are associated with the presence of ER and PgR. Perhaps these receptors are also biochemical markers of tumor differentiation. AR and GR have not been studied as well as other steroid hormone receptors in breast cancer. However, there is some evidence that their presence may correlate with response to endocrine therapy and with patient survival. Whether knowledge of AR or GR status improves the predictive index beyond that provided by ER and PgR has not been answered definitively. At the present time, these receptor assays remain a research tool, and they have not been incorporated into routine clinical practice.

Estrogen Receptors and Progesterone Receptors as Prognostic Factors in Primary Breast Cancer

The rationale for the use of receptor assays as prognostic factors is summarized in Table 8-10. As described previously, ER-positive tumors tend to show morphological evidence for tumor differentiation, they are associated with a low proliferative potential as measured by cell kinetic analyses, they have a low propensity for visceral recurrence especially in liver and brain, and they are frequently hormone dependent. ER-negative tumors are frequently poorly differentiated histologically, they have a higher proliferative potential, they frequently recur in visceral sites,

Table 8-8
*PgR Status According to ER Content**

ER (fmol/mg)	PgR-positive (%)
0-2	9%
3-10	40%
11-100	70%
> 100	77%

* Data from 2943 primary tumor assays

Table 8-9
Response to Endocrine Therapy by Quantitative ER and PgR

Receptor Status	Objective Response
ER (fmol/mg)	
3–100	13/38 (34%)
>100	17/27 (63%)
PgR	
Negative	14/45 (31%)
Positive	16/20 (80%)

(Osborne CK, Yockmowitz MG, Knight WA, et al: The value of estrogen and progesterone receptors in the treatment of breast cancer. Cancer 46:2884–2888, 1980)

Table 8-10
Rationale for ER As a Prognostic Factor in Primary Breast Cancer

Variable	ER +	ER −
Degree of differentiation	High	Low
Proliferative potential	Low	High
Visceral recurrence	Low	High
Hormone dependence	High	Low

and response to endocrine treatment is unusual. Cumulative data from numerous clinical trials demonstrate that receptor-positive tumors have a more indolent natural history, which is reflected in a longer disease-free interval and survival in women with primary breast cancer.

Estrogen Receptors As a Prognostic Factor

The first evidence that ER might be a useful prognostic marker came from a study of women with advanced breast cancer who had a receptor assay performed either on their primary tumor or on a metastatic lesion at the time of recurrence.[150] Two important observations suggested that the clinical aggressiveness of ER-positive and ER-negative tumors might be different. First, patients with ER-positive tumors were more likely to have bone or soft tissue involvement as their dominant site of metastasis; in contrast, more life-threatening visceral involvement predominated with ER-negative tumors. Second, the median survival from original diagnosis was shorter with ER-negative tumors (21 months) than with ER-positive tumors (46 months). Although this was a select group of patients (all had recurrent breast cancer), the data suggested that inherent biologic differences that could directly influence prognosis may exist between endocrine-dependent and -independent tumors.

In 1977, another report suggested that patients with operable breast cancer could be segregated into two prognostic subgroups by ER status.[151] During an analysis of patients who had receptor assays on their primary tumor, it became evident that patients with ER-negative tumors had recurrences and were dying at a faster rate than those with ER-positive tumors. After a short median follow-up time, patients with receptor-negative tumors had recurrences at twice the rate of those with tumors containing ER. Furthermore, this difference was independent of other potential prognostic factors such as age or menopausal status, size of the primary tumor, location of the primary axillary lymph node status, or treatment delivered after surgery.

This study was updated later with the inclusion of additional patients (288 total), with longer follow-up and with the exclusion of patients who had received any systemic adjuvant therapy, so that the natural history of primary breast cancer could be observed.[152] Again the recurrence and survival rates for the ER-negative group were inferior to those for the ER-positive group (Figs. 8-7 and 8-8). Similar patterns were observed when patients were subgrouped by axillary node status, indicating that the prognostic influence of ER status is independent of this important variable. Of special interest was the observation that patients without axillary node involvement had a surprisingly poor prognosis if their tumors lacked ER.

Numerous other studies have evaluated the prognostic significance of ER status. The majority of reports confirm the observations described above, although in some the prognostic significance is confined to certain subgroups of patients.[153–164] Many of these studies suffer because they were retrospective, because they included relatively small patient numbers, and because of relatively short follow-up. Nevertheless, the more aggressive natural history of ER-negative tumors is a constant feature. An especially poor prognostic group is composed of patients with more than three involved axillary lymph nodes and with a negative ER assay; these patients have a very high relapse rate, with as many as two-thirds suffering recurrence only 2 years after mastectomy.[152]

Other studies with longer follow-up suggest that the improved prognosis in patients with ER-positive tumors may not be sustained.[165,166] Both of these reports found prolonged disease-free and overall survival in patients with ER-positive tumors at early follow-up times. However, the difference in disease-free survival disappeared with longer follow-up, although the survival advantage persisted. This suggests that ER status is not a factor associated with metastatic potential but that it is related to those factors contributing to the growth rate and, thus, the time lag until

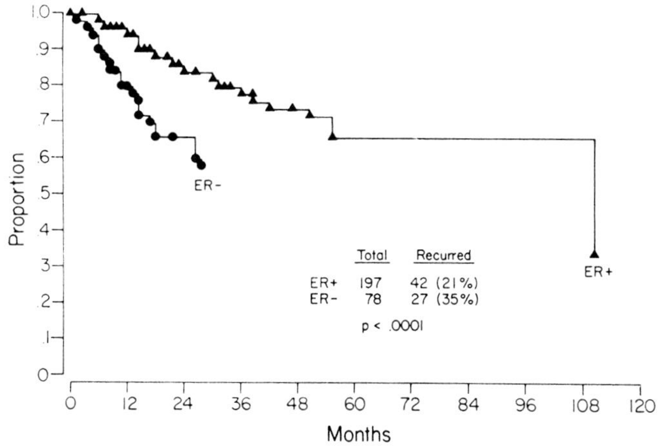

FIGURE 8-7. Recurrence rate among patients with Stage I or II breast cancer according to ER status. (Osborne CK, Knight WA III, Yochmowitz MG, et al: Estrogen receptor and prognosis in breast cancer. In McGuire WL (ed); Breast Cancer. Vol 4, Advances in Research and Treatment, pp 33–49. New York, Plenum, 1981)

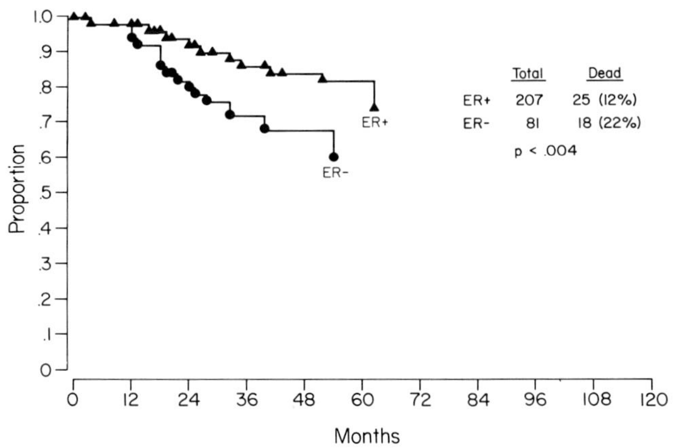

FIGURE 8-8. Overall survival rates for patients with Stage I or II breast cancer according to ER status. (Osborne CK, Knight WA III, Yochmowitz MG, et al: Estrogen receptor and prognosis in breast cancer. In McGuire WL (ed); Breast Cancer. Vol 4, Advances in Research and Treatment, pp 33–49. New York, Plenum, 1981)

these metastases make their clinical appearance. This is further supported by the consistent observation that receptor status does not correlate with the presence or absence of axillary lymph node involvement. Another report argued that the prolonged survival of patients with ER-positive tumors is related to their increased chance of responding to endocrine therapy after relapse, rather than to some other intrinsic biologic property of the tumor.[167]

A few studies fail to show even a temporary improvement in relapse rate or survival in patients with ER-positive tumors.[168–170] In one small study, patients with ER-positive tumors even had a slightly worse prognosis.[170] The explanation for these disparate results is not clear, but it may be related to problems inherent in retrospective evaluations. The bulk of evidence, however, does suggest that biologic differences between ER-positive and ER-negative tumors do exist and that these differences are manifest clinically by differences in natural history and patient outcome.

Progesterone Receptors As a Prognostic Factor

Since PgR may be a better marker for tumor endocrine dependence than ER, one might also presume that PgR might be a valuable predictor of time to recurrence and survival for patients with primary breast cancer, especially those undergoing adjuvant endocrine therapy. Several studies have recently addressed this question.

Pichon and colleagues[171] reported that the presence of PgR was associated with favorable prognosis in patients with operable breast cancer (none of whom received adjuvant endocrine therapy), including those with positive or negative axillary nodes. An inverse relationship between the concentration of PgR and frequency of metastases was also found. Knowledge of ER status did not add prognostic information when PgR status was known. Similar results were reported by Saez and colleagues.[172] After 5 years of follow-up of 148 patients with Stage I and II breast cancer, many of whom received adjuvant chemotherapy or chemo-endocrine therapy, the disease-free survival was shorter in patients with PgR-negative tumors. Again, PgR appeared to be a more significant criterion than ER for long-term prognosis. Mason and colleagues[173] examined the value of ER and PgR in nearly 400 node-negative or -positive breast cancer patients, most of whom did not receive adjuvant hormone therapy or chemotherapy. Both ER and PgR status predicted overall survival, but only PgR was predictive for prolonged disease-free survival. Both receptors were believed to be important complementary prognostic factors. Clark and colleagues[174] analyzed ER and PgR data from patients in a prospective randomized adjuvant therapy study. Stage II patients were randomized to combination chemotherapy alone, chemotherapy plus tamoxifen, or chemotherapy plus tamoxifen plus immunotherapy with BCG. Regardless of the type of adjuvant therapy received, the presence of ER or PgR was positively correlated with disease-free survival. However, when ER and PgR were analyzed together in a multivariate analysis, the presence of PgR was more significant than ER in predicting time to recurrence, regardless of what other potential prognostic variables were included in the model. In a more recent similar analysis of 1529 patients with Stage II breast cancer in San Antonio, the multivariate analysis has shown that nodal status, tumor size, PgR content, the administration of adjuvant endocrine therapy or chemotherapy, but not ER status or age are all significant predictors of prolonged time to first recurrence (personal communication, WL McGuire).

Not all studies agree that PgR is an important prognostic factor. Stewart and colleagues[175] studied 447 Stage I or II patients and found that neither ER nor PgR content significantly correlated with disease-free survival, although there was a trend in favor of receptor-positive tumors. Survival was prolonged in patients with receptor-positive tumors, but the effect was most closely related to ER content; PgR added relatively little information. Allegra and colleagues[154] also did not find an association between disease-free survival and PgR status. However, nearly one-third of their patients had receptor analysis performed on a metastatic lesion rather than the primary tumor, which clouds interpretation of their data. Although there is not total consistency in studies of PgR, the cumulative evidence strongly suggests that PgR content is an important prognostic factor and that it should be measured routinely in studies of patients with primary breast cancer.

REFERENCES

1. Ceriani RL: Hormones and other factors controlling growth in the mammary gland: A review. J Invest Dermatol 63:93–108, 1974
2. Jensen EU, DeSombre ER: Mechanism of action of the female sex hormones. Ann Rev Biochem 41:203–230, 1972
3. King WJ, DeSombre ER, Jensen EV, et al: Comparison of immunocytochemical and steroid-binding assays for estrogen receptor in human breast tumors. Cancer Res 45:293–304, 1985
4. Lippman ME: Growth regulation of human breast cancer. Clin Res 33(3):375–382, 1985
5. Horwitz KB, McGuire WL: Nuclear mechanisms of estrogen action. J Biol Chem 253:8185–8191, 1978
6. Eckert RL, Katzenellenbogen BS: Effects of estrogens and antiestrogens on estrogen receptor dynamics and the induction of progesterone receptor in MCF-7 human breast cancer cells. Cancer Res 42:139–144, 1982
7. Lippman ME, Osborne CK, Knazek R, et al: In vitro model systems for the study of hormone-dependent human breast cancer. N Engl J Med 296:154–159, 1977
8. Lippman ME, Bolan G, Huff K: The effects of estrogens and antiestrogens on hormone-responsive human breast cancer in long-term tissue culture. Cancer Res 36:4595–4601, 1976
9. Osborne CK, Lippman ME: Human breast cancer in tissue culture: The effects of hormones. *In* McGuire WL (ed): Breast Cancer, Advances in Research and Treatment, Vol 2, pp 103–154. New York, Plenum, 1978
10. Aitken SC, Lippman ME: Hormonal regulation of *de novo* pyrimidine synthesis and utilization in human breast cancer cells in tissue culture. Cancer Res 43:4681–4690, 1983
11. Edwards DP, Murthy SR, McGuire WL: Estrogen and antiestrogen effects on DNA polymerase in breast cancer. Cancer Res 40:1722–1726, 1980
12. Osborne CK, Boldt DH, Clark GM, et al: Effects of tamoxifen on human breast cancer cell cycle kinetics: Accumulation of cells in early G_1 phase. Cancer Res 43:3583–3585, 1983
13. Osborne CK, Boldt DH, Estrada P: Human breast cancer cell cycle synchronization by estrogens and antiestrogens in culture. Cancer Res 44:1433–1439, 1984
14. Shafie SM: Estrogen and the growth of breast cancer: New evidence suggests indirect action. Science 209:701–702, 1980
15. Soto AM, Sonnenschein C: The role of estrogen on the proliferation of human breast tumor cells (MCF-7). J Steroid Biochem 23:87–94, 1985
16. Sirbasku DA: Estrogen-induction of growth factors specific for hormone-responsive mammary, pituitary and kidney tumor cells. Proc Natl Acad Sci USA 74:3786–3790, 1978
17. Shiu RP: Processing of prolactin by human breast cancer cells in long term tissue culture. J Biol Chem 255:4278–4281, 1980
18. Osborne CK, Monaco ME, Lippman ME, et al: Correlation among insulin binding, degradation, and biological activity in human breast cancer cells in long-term tissue culture. Cancer Res 38:94–102, 1978
19. Furlanetto RW, DiCarlo JN: Somatomedin-C receptors and growth effects in human breast cells maintained in long-term tissue culture. Cancer Res 44:2122–2128, 1984
20. Osborne CK, Hamilton B, Nover M: Receptor binding and processing of epidermal growth factor by human breast cancer cells. J Clin Endocrinol Metab 55:86–93, 1982
21. Fitzpatrick SL, Brightwell J, Wittliff JL, et al: Epidermal growth factor binding by breast tumor biopsies and relationship to estrogen receptor and progestin receptor levels. Cancer Res 44:3448–3453, 1984
22. Osborne CK, Bolan G, Monaco ME, et al: Hormone responsive human breast cancer in long-term tissue culture: Effect of insulin. Proc Natl Acad Sci USA 73:4536–4540, 1976
23. Osborne CK, Hamilton B, Titus G, et al: Epidermal growth factor stimulation of human breast cancer cells in culture. Cancer Res 40:2361–2366, 1980
24. Burke RE, McGuire WL: Nuclear thyroid hormone receptors in a human breast cancer cell line. Cancer Res 38:3769–3773, 1978
25. Chamness GC, McGuire WL: Methods for analyzing steroid receptors in human breast cancer. *In* McGuire WL (ed), Breast Cancer, Advances in Research and Treatment, Vol 3, pp 149–197. New York, Plenum, 1979
26. McGuire WL, Vollmer EP, Carbone PP (eds): Estrogen Receptors in Human Breast Cancer. New York, Raven Press, 1975
27. Wittliff JL: Steroid receptor interactions in human breast carcinoma. Cancer 46:2953–2960, 1980
28. Wang G, Vogel CL, Hilsenbeck SG, et al: Value of 8S/4S fractionation of estrogen receptors (ER) for prediction of response to hormonal manipulation in metastatic breast cancer. Breast Cancer Res Treat 4:283–288, 1984
29. Powell B, Garola RE, Chamness GC, et al: Measurement of progesterone receptor in human breast cancer biopsies. Cancer Res 39:1678–1682, 1979
30. Leung BS, Fletcher WS, Lindell TD, et al: Predictability of response to endocrine ablation in advanced breast carcinoma. Arch Surg 106:515–519, 1973
31. McGuire WL, De La Garza M, Chamness GC: Evaluation of estrogen receptor assays in human breast cancer tissue. Cancer Res 37:367–387, 1967
32. Ginsburg M. Greenstein BD, Maclusky NJ, et al: An improved method for the study of high-affinity steroid binding: Oestradiol binding in brain and pituitary. Steroids 23:773–792, 1974
33. Jungblut PW, Hughes S, Hughes A, et al: Evaluation of various methods for the assay to cytoplasmic oestrogen receptors in extracts of calf uteri and human breast cancer. Acta Endocrinol 70:185–195, 1972
34. Chamness GC, Huff K, McGuire WL: Protamine-precipitated estrogen receptor: A solid phase ligand exchange assay. Steroids 25:627–635, 1975
35. Garola RE, McGuire WL: A hydroxylapatite micro-method for measuring estrogen receptor in human breast cancer. Cancer Res 38:2216–2220, 1978
36. Garola RE, McGuire WL: An improved assay for nuclear estrogen receptor in experimental and human breast cancer. Cancer Res 37:3333–3337, 1977
37. Grill HJ, Manz B, Pollow K: Double-labeling assay system for

estrogen and progesterone receptors. Lancet i:679–681, 1982
38. Nenci I, Beccati MD, Piffanelli A, et al: Detection and dynamic localization of estradiol-receptor complexes in intact target cells by immunofluorescence technique. J Steroid Biochem 7:505–510, 1976
39. Pertschuk LP, Tobin EH, Brigati DJ, et al: Immunofluorescent detection of estrogen receptors in breast cancer. Cancer 41:907–911, 1978
40. Taylor CR, Cooper CL, Kurman RJ, et al: Detection of estrogen receptor in breast and endometrial carcinoma by the immunoperoxidase technique. Cancer 47:2634–2640, 1981
41. Ghosh L, Ghosh DC, Das Gupta TK: Immunocytological localization of estrogen in human mammary carcinoma cells by horseradish–anti-horseradish peroxidase complex. J Surg Oncol 10:221–224, 1978
42. Mercer WD, Lippman ME, Wahl TM, et al: The use of immunocytochemical techniques for the detection of steroid hormones in breast cancer cells. Cancer 46:2859–2868, 1980
43. Lee SH: Cytochemical study of estrogen receptor in human mammary cancer. Am J Clin Pathol 70:197–203, 1978
44. Dandliker WB, Brawn RJ, Hsu ML, et al: Investigation of hormone-receptor interactions by means of fluorescence labeling. Cancer Res 38:4212–4224, 1978
45. Pertschuk LP, Tobin EH, Gaetjens E, et al: Histochemical assay of estrogen and progesterone receptors in breast cancer: Correlation with biochemical assays and patients' response to endocrine therapies. Cancer 46:2896–2901, 1980
46. Rao BR, Fry CG, Hunt S, et al: A fluorescent probe for rapid detection of estrogen receptors. Cancer 46:2902–2906, 1980
47. Walker RA, Cove DH, Howell A: Histological detection of oestrogen receptor in human breast carcinomas. Lancet i:171–173, 1980
48. Hanna W, Ryder DE, Mobbs BG: Cellular localization of estrogen binding sites in human breast cancer. Am J Clin Pathol 77:391–395, 1982
49. Chamness GC, Mercer WD, McGuire WL: Are histochemical methods for estrogen receptor valid? J Histochem Cytochem 28:792–798, 1980
50. Panko WB, Mattioli CA, Wheeler TM: Lack of correlation of a histochemical method for estrogen receptor analysis with the biochemical assay results. Cancer 49:2148–2152, 1982
51. Penney GC, Hawkins RA: Histochemical detection of oestrogen receptors: A progress report. Br J Cancer 45:237–246, 1982
52. Daxenbichler G, Weiss P, Ortner A, et al: Microscopic visualization of steroid receptor sites: A mirage? Recent Results Cancer Res 92:75–85, 1984
53. McCarty KS, Woodard BH, Nichols DE, et al: Comparison of biochemical and histochemical techniques for estrogen receptor analyses in mammary carcinoma. Cancer 46:2842–2845, 1980
54. Morrow B, Leav I, Delellis RA, et al: Use of polyestradiol phosphate and anti-17β estradiol antibodies for the localization of estrogen receptors in target tissues: A critique. Cancer 46:2872–2879, 1980
55. Nenci I: Estrogen receptor cytochemistry in human breast cancer: Status and prospects. Cancer 48:2674–2686, 1981
56. Pertschuk LP, Eisenberg KB, Carter AC, et al: Heterogeneity of estrogen binding sites in breast cancer: Morphologic demonstration and relationship to endocrine response. Breast Cancer Res Treat 5:137–147, 1985
57. Berns EMJJ, Mulder E, Rommerts FFG, et al: Fluorescent ligands, used in histocytochemistry, do not discriminate between oestrogen receptor positive and negative humor tumour cell lines. Breast Cancer Res Treat 4:195–204, 1984
58. McCarty KS, Hiatt KB, Budwit DA, et al: Clinical response to hormone therapy correlated with estrogen receptor analyses. Arch Pathol Lab Med 108:24–26, 1984
59. Green GL, Sobel NB, King WJ, et al: Immunochemical studies of estrogen receptors. J Steroid Biochem 20:51–56, 1984
60. King WJ, Green GL: Monoclonal antibodies localize oestrogen receptor in the nuclei of target cells. Nature 307:745–747, 1984
61. Mirecki DM, Jordan VC: Steroid hormone receptors and human breast cancer. Lab Med 16:287–294, 1985
62. Van NT, Raber M: Estrogen receptor analysis by flow cytometry. Science 224:876–879, 1984
63. Oxenhandler RW, McCune R, Subtelney A, et al: Flow cytometric determination of estrogen receptor in intact cells. Cancer Res 44:2516–2523, 1984
64. Kute TE, Linville C, Barrows G: Cytofluorometric analysis for estrogen receptors using fluorescent estrogen probes. Cytometry 4:132–140, 1983
65. Hawkins RA, Hill A, Freedman B, et al: Reproducibility of measurements of oestrogen-receptor concentration in breast cancer. Br J Cancer 36:355–361, 1977
66. Hull DF, Clark GM, Osborne CK, et al: Multiple estrogen receptor assays in human breast cancer. Cancer Res 43:413–416, 1983
67. Hahnel R, Vivian AB: Biochemical and clinical experience with the estimation of estrogen receptors in human breast carcinoma. In McGuire WL, Carbone PP, Vollmer EP (eds): Estrogen Receptors in Human Breast Cancer, pp 205–235. New York, Raven Press, 1975
68. Jordan VC, Zava DT, Uppenburger U, et al: Reliability of steroid hormone receptor assays: an international study. Eur Cancer Clin Oncol 19:357–363, 1983
69. Silfversward C, Skoog L, Humla S, et al: Intratumoral variation of cytoplasmic and nuclear estrogen receptor concentrations in human mammary carcinoma. Eur J Cancer 16:59–65, 1980
70. Kiang DT, Kennedy BJ: Factors affecting estrogen receptors in breast cancer. Cancer 40:1571–1576, 1977
71. Hoehn JL, Plotka ED, Dickson KB: Comparison of estrogen receptor levels in primary and regional metastatic carcinoma of the breast. Ann Surg 190(1):69–71, 1979
72. Mumford CJ, Elston CW, Campbell FC, et al: Tumour epithelial cellularity and quantitative oestrogen receptor values in primary breast cancer. Br J Cancer 47:549–552, 1983
73. Davis BW, Zava DT, Locher GW, et al: Receptor heterogeneity of human breast cancer as measured by multiple intratumoral assays of estrogen and progesterone receptor. Eur J Cancer Clin Oncol 20:375–382, 1984
74. Rosen PP, Menendez-Botet CJ, Nisselbaum JS, et al: Pathological review of breast lesions analyzed for estrogen receptor protein. Cancer Res 35:3187–3194, 1975
75. Saez S, Martin PM, Chouvet CD: Estradiol and progesterone receptor levels in human breast adenocarcinoma in relation to plasma estrogen and progesterone levels. Cancer Res 38:3468–3473, 1978
76. Sakai F, Saez S: Existence of receptors bound to endogenous estradiol in breast cancer of premenopausal and postmenopausal women. Steroids 27:99–110, 1976
77. Fishman J, Nisselbaum JS, Menendez-Botet CF, et al: Estrone and estradiol content in human breast tumors: Relationship to estradiol receptors. J Steroid Biochem 8:893–896, 1977
78. Bloom ND, Tobin EH, Schreibman B, et al: The role of progesterone receptors in the management of advanced breast cancer. Cancer 45:2992–2997, 1980
79. Beatson GT: On the treatment of inoperable cases of carcinoma of the mamma: Suggestions for a new method of treatment with illustrative cases. Lancet 3:104–107, 1896
80. Glascock RF, Hoekstra WG: Selective accumulation of tritium-

labeled hexoestrol by the reproductive organs of immature female goats and sheep. J Biochem 72:673–682, 1959
81. Jensen EV, Jacobson HI: Basic guides to the mechanism of estrogen action. Recent Prog Horm Res 18:387–414, 1962
82. Folca PJ, Glascock RF, Irvine WT: Studies with tritium-labeled hexoestrol in advanced breast cancer. Lancet 2:796–802, 1961
83. Ellis FG, Berne TV, Deshpande N, et al: The uptake of tritiated steroids by human breast carcinoma. Surg Gynecol Obstet 28:975–984, 1969
84. Pearlman WH, DeHertogh R, Laumas KR, et al: Metabolism and tissue uptake of estrogen in women with advanced carcinoma of the breast. J Clin Endocrinol 29:707–720, 1969
85. King RJB, Cowan DM, Inman DR: The uptake of (6,7-^{3}H)oestradiol by dimethylbenzanthracene-induced rat mammary tumours. J Endocrinol 32:83–90, 1965
86. King RJB, Gordon J, Cowan DM, et al: The intranuclear localization of (6,7-^{3}H)oestradiol-17β in dimethylbenzanthracene-induced rat mammary adenocarcinoma and other tissues. J Endocrinol 34:139–146, 1966
87. Mobbs BG: The uptake of tritiated oestradiol by dimethylbenzanthracene-induced mammary tumours of the rat. J Endocrinol 36:409–414, 1966
88. Sander S, Attramadal A: The *in vivo* uptake of oestradiol-17β by hormone responsive and unresponsive breast tumors of the rat. Acta Pathol Microbiol Scand 74:169–178, 1968
89. Terenius L: Parallelism between oestrogen binding capacity and hormone responsiveness of mammary tumours in GR/A mice. Eur J Cancer 8:55–58, 1972
90. Mobbs BG: Uptake of [^{3}H]oestradiol by dimethylbenzanthracene-induced rat mammary tumours regressing spontaneously or after ovariectomy. J Endocrinol 44:463–464, 1969
91. Jensen EV, DeSombre ER, Jungblut PW: Estrogen receptors in hormone-responsive tissues and tumors. In Wissler RW, Dao TL, Woods S Jr (eds): Endogenous Factors Influencing Host-Tumor Balance, pp 15–30. Chicago, University of Chicago Press, 1967
92. Terenius L: Selective retention of estrogen isomers in estrogen dependent breast tumors of rats demonstrated by *in vitro* methods. Cancer Res 28(1):328–337, 1968
93. Gorski J, Toft DO, Shyamala G, et al: Hormone receptors: Studies on the interaction of estrogen with uterus. Recent Prog Horm Res 24:45–80, 1968
94. Martin PM, Rolland PH, Jacquemier J, et al: Multiple steroid receptors in human breast cancer. II. Estrogen and progestin receptors in 672 primary tumors. Cancer Chemother Pharmacol 2:107–113, 1979
95. Allegra JC, Lippman ME, Thompson EB, et al: Distribution, frequency, and quantitative analysis of estrogen, progesterone, androgen, and glucocorticoid receptors in human breast cancer. Cancer Res 39:1447–1454, 1979
96. Fisher ER, Redmond CK, Liu H, et al: Correlation of estrogen receptor and pathologic characteristics of invasive breast cancer. Cancer 45:349–353, 1980
97. Elwood JM, Godolphin W: Oestrogen receptors in breast tumors: Associations with age, menopausal status and epidemiological and clinical features in 735 patients. Br J Cancer 42:635–644, 1980
98. McCarty KS Jr, Silva JS, Cox EB, et al: Relationship of age and menopausal status to estrogen receptor content in primary carcinoma of the breast. Ann Surg 197:123–127, 1983
99. Clark GM, Osborne CK, McGuire WL: Correlations between estrogen receptor, progesterone receptor, and patient characteristics in human breast cancer. J Clin Oncol 2:1102–1109, 1984
100. Qazi R, Chuang J-L, Drobyski W: Estrogen receptors and the pattern of relapse in breast cancer. Arch Intern Med 144:2365–2367, 1984
101. Rosen PP, Menendez-Botet CJ, Nisselbaum JS, et al: Pathological review of breast lesions analyzed for estrogen receptor protein. Cancer Res 35:3187–3194, 1975
102. Millis RR: Correlation of hormone receptors with pathological features in human breast cancer. Cancer 46:2869–2871, 1980
103. Fisher ER, Osborne CK, McGuire WL, et al: Correlation of primary breast cancer histopathology and estrogen receptor content. Breast Cancer Res Treat 1:37–41, 1981
104. Maynard PV, Davies CJ, Blamey RW, et al: Relationship between oestrogen-receptor content and histological grade in human primary breast tumours. Br J Cancer 38:745–748, 1978
105. Fisher ER, Redmond CK, Liu H, et al: Correlation of estrogen receptor and pathologic characteristics of invasive breast cancer. Cancer 45:349–353, 1980
106. Glaubitz LC, Bowen JH, Cox EB, et al: Elastosis in human breast cancer. Correlation with sex steroid receptors and comparison with clinical outcome. Arch Pathol Lab Med 108:27–30, 1984
107. Meyer JS, Rao BR, Stevens SC, et al: Low incidence of estrogen receptor in breast carcinomas with rapid rates of cellular replication. Cancer 40:2290–2298, 1977
108. Meyer JS, Lee JY: Relationships of S-phase fraction of breast carcinoma in relapse to duration of remission, estrogen receptor content, therapeutic responsiveness, and duration of survival. Cancer Res 40:1890–1896, 1980
109. Silvestrini R, Daidone MG, Fronzo GD: Relationship between proliferative activity and estrogen receptors in breast cancer. Cancer 44:665–670, 1979
110. Kute TE, Muss HB, Anderson D, et al: Relationship of steroid receptor, cell kinetics, and clinical status in patients with breast cancer. Cancer Res 41:3524–3529, 1981
Allegra JC, Lippman ME, Thompson EB, et al: Estrogen receptor status: An important variable in predicting response to endocrine therapy in metastatic breast cancer. Eur J Cancer 16:323–331, 1980
112. Rubens RD, Hayward JL: Estrogen receptors and response to endocrine therapy and cytotoxic chemotherapy in advanced breast cancer. Cancer 46:2922–2924, 1980
113. Young PCM, Ehrlich CE, Einhorn LH: Relationship between steroid receptors and response to endocrine therapy and cytotoxic chemotherapy in metastatic breast cancer. Cancer 46:2961–2963, 1980
114. Byar DP, Sears ME, McGuire WL: Relationship between estrogen receptor values and clinical data in predicting the response to endocrine therapy for patients with advanced breast cancer. Eur J Cancer 15:299–310, 1979
115. Macfarlane JK, Fleiszer D, Fazekas AG: Studies on estrogen receptors and regression in human breast cancer. Cancer 45:2998–3003, 1980
116. Leake Re, Laing L, Calman KC, et al: Oestrogen-receptor status and endocrine therapy of breast cancer: Response rates and status stability. Br J Cancer 43:59–66, 1981
117. Lippman ME, Allegra JC: Quantitative estrogen receptor analyses: The response to endocrine and cytotoxic chemotherapy in human breast cancer and the disease-free interval. Cancer 46:2829–2834, 1980
118. Osborne CK, Yochmowitz MG, Knight WA, et al: The value of estrogen and progesterone receptors in the treatment of breast cancer. Cancer 46:2884–2888, 1980
119. Paridaens R, Sylvester RJ, Ferrazzi E: Clinical significance of

the quantitative assessment of estrogen receptors in advanced breast cancer. Cancer 46:2889–2895, 1980
120. Campbell FC, Blamey RW, Elston CW, et al: Quantitative oestradiol receptor values in primary breast cancer and response of metastases to endocrine therapy. Lancet ii: 1317–1319, 1981
121. Allegra JC, Barlock A, Huff KK, et al: Changes in multiple or sequential estrogen receptor determinations in breast cancer. Cancer 45:792–794, 1980
122. Rosen PP, Menendez-Botet CJ, Urban JA, et al: Estrogen receptor protein (ERP) in multiple tumor specimens from individual patients with breast cancer. Cancer 39:2194–2200, 1977
123. Taylor RE, Powles TJ, Humphreys J, et al: Effects of endocrine therapy on steroid-receptor content of breast cancer. Br J Cancer 45:80–85, 1982
124. Holdaway M, Bowditch JV: Variation in receptor status between primary and metastatic breast cancer. Cancer 52:479–485, 1983
125. Block GE, Ellis RS, DeSombre E, et al: Correlation of estrophilin content of primary mammary cancer to eventual endocrine treatment. Ann Surg 188:372–376, 1978
126. Osborne CK, McGuire WL: The use of steroid hormone receptors in the management of patients with breast cancer. In Hoogstraten B, McDivitt RW (eds): Breast Cancer, pp 155–169. Boca Raton, CRC Press, 1981
127. Lippman ME, Allegra JC, Thompson EB, et al: Lack of estrogen receptor predicts response to chemotherapy in breast cancer. N Engl J Med 298:1223–1228, 1978
128. Jonat W, Maass H: Some comments on the necessity of receptor determination in human breast cancer. Cancer Res 38:4305–4306, 1978
129. Webster DJT, Bronn DG, Minton JP: Estrogen receptors and response of breast cancer to chemotherapy. N Engl J Med 299:604, 1978
130. Kiang DT, Frenning DH, Goldman AI, et al: Estrogen receptors and response to chemotherapy and hormonal therapy in advanced breast cancer. N Engl J Med 299:1330–1334, 1978
131. Horwitz KB, McGuire WL, Pearson O, et al: Predicting response to endocrine therapy in human breast cancer: A hypothesis. Science 189:726–727, 1975
132. Clark GM, McGuire WL: Progesterone receptors and human breast cancer. Breast Cancer Res Treat 3:157–163, 1983
133. McCarty KS Jr, Barton TK, Fetter BF, et al: Correlation of estrogen and progesterone receptors with histologic differentiation in mammary carcinoma. Cancer 46:2851–2858, 1980
134. Gross GE, Clark GM, Chamness GC, et al: Multiple progesterone receptor assays in human breast cancer. Cancer Res 44:836–840, 1984
135. Matsumoto K, Ochi H, Nomura Y, et al: Progesterone and estrogen receptors in Japanese breast cancer. In McGuire WL (ed): Hormones, Receptors, and Breast Cancer, pp 43–57. New York, Raven Press, 1978
136. Degenshein GA, Bloom N, Robin E: The value of progesterone receptor assays in the management of advanced breast cancer. Cancer 46:2789–2793, 1980
137. Young PCM, Ehrlich CE, Einhorn LH: Relationship between steroid receptors and response to endocrine therapy and cytotoxic chemotherapy in metastatic breast cancer. Cancer 46:2961–2963, 1980
138. Brooks C, Saunders DE, Singhakowinta A, et al: Relation of tumor content of estrogen and progesterone receptors with response of patient to endocrine therapy. Cancer 46:2775–2778, 1980
139. Stewart J, King R, Hayward J, et al: Estrogen and progesterone receptors: Correlation of response rates, site and timing of receptor analysis. Breast Cancer Res Treat 2:243–250, 1982
140. Manni A, Arafah B, Pearson OH: Estrogen and progesterone receptors in the prediction of response of breast cancer to endocrine therapy. Cancer 46:2838–2841, 1980
141. McCarty KS Jr, Cox C, Silva JS, et al: Comparison of sex steroid receptor analyses and carcinoembryonic antigen with clinical response to hormone therapy. Cancer 46:2846–2850, 1980
142. Nomura Y, Yamagata J, Takenaka K, et al: Steroid hormone receptors and clinical usefulness in human breast cancer. Cancer 46:2880–2883, 1980
143. Skinner LG, Barnes DM, Ribeiro GG: The clinical value of multiple steroid receptor assays in breast cancer management. Cancer 46:2939–2945, 1980
144. Holdaway IM, Skinner SJM: Predicting treatment response in breast cancer using urinary discriminant ratio and receptor assay. Eur J Cancer Clin Oncol 17:1295–1300, 1981
145. Johnson PA, Bonomi PD, Anderson KM, et al: Megestrol acetate (MA) in advanced breast cancer: Response rate related to estrogen receptor (ER) and progesterone receptor (PR) levels. Proc Am Soc Clin Oncol 1:89, 1982
146. Allegra JC, Lippman ME, Thompson EB, et al: Relationship between progesterone, androgen, and glucocorticoid receptor and response rate to endocrine therapy in metastatic breast cancer. Cancer Res 39:1973–1979, 1979
147. Bryan RM, Mercer RJ, Bennett RC, et al: Androgen receptors in breast cancer. Cancer 54:2436–2440, 1984
148. Ochi H, Hayashi T, Nakao K, et al: Estrogen, progesterone, and androgen receptors in breast cancer in the Japanese: Brief communication. J Natl Cancer Inst 60:291–293, 1978
149. Teulings FAG, Van Gilse HA: Demonstration of glucocorticoid receptors in human mammary carcinoma. Horm Res 8:107–116, 1977
150. Walt AJ, Singhakowinta A, Brooks SC, et al: The surgical implications of estrophile protein estimations in carcinoma of the breast. Surgery 80:506–512, 1976
151. Knight WA III, Livingston RB, Gregory EJ, et al: Estrogen receptor as an independent prognostic factor for early recurrence in breast cancer. Cancer Res 37:4669–4671, 1977
152. Osborne CK, Knight WA III, Yochmowitz MG, et al: Estrogen receptor and prognosis in breast cancer. In McGuire WL (ed): Breast Cancer, Advances in Research and Treatment, Vol 4, pp 33–49. New York, Plenum, 1981
153. Samaan NA, Buzdar AU, Aldinger KA, et al: Estrogen receptor: A prognostic factor in breast cancer. Cancer 47:554–560, 1981
154. Allegra JC, Lippman ME, Simon R, et al: Association between steroid hormone receptor status and disease-free interval in breast cancer. Cancer Treat Rep 63:1271–1277, 1979
155. Westerberg H, Gustafson SA, Nordenskjold B, et al: Estrogen receptor level and other factors in early recurrence of breast cancer. Int J Cancer 26:429–433, 1980
156. Rich MA, Furmanski P, Brooks SC, et al: Prognostic value of estrogen receptor determinations in patients with breast cancer. Cancer Res 38:4296–4298, 1978
157. Bishop HM, Blamey RW, Elston CW, et al: Relationship of oestrogen-receptor status to survival in breast cancer. Lancet ii: 283–284, 1979
158. Cooke T, George D, Shields R, et al: Oestrogen receptors and prognosis in early breast cancer. Lancet 1:995–997, 1979.
159. Kinne DW, Ashikari R, Butler A, et al: Estrogen receptor protein in breast cancer as a predictor of recurrence. Cancer 47:2364–2367, 1981

160. Godolphin W, Elwood JM, Spinelli JJ: Estrogen receptor quantitation and staging as complementary prognostic indicators in breast cancer: A study of 583 patients. Int J Cancer 28:677–683, 1981
161. Nicholson RI, Campbell FC, Blamey RW, et al: Steroid receptors in early breast cancer: Value in prognosis. J Steroid Biochem 15:193–199, 1981
162. Leake RE, Laing L, McArdle C, et al: Soluble and nuclear oestrogen receptor status in human breast cancer in relation to prognosis. Br J Cancer 43:67–71, 1981
163. Stewart JF, King RJB, Winter PJ, et al: Oestrogen receptors, clinical features and prognosis in stage III breast cancer. Eur J Cancer Clin Oncol 18:1315–1320, 1982
164. Crowe JP, Hubay CA, Pearson OH, et al: Estrogen receptor status as a prognostic indicator for stage I breast cancer patients. Breast Cancer Res Treat 2:171–176, 1982
165. Aamdal S, Bormer O, Jorgensen O, et al: Estrogen receptors and long-term prognosis in breast cancer. Cancer 53:2525–2529, 1984
166. Hahnel R, Woodings T, Vivian AB: Prognostic value of estrogen receptors in primary breast cancer. Cancer 44:671–675, 1979
167. Howell A, Barnes DM, Harland RNL, et al: Steroid-hormone receptors and survival after first relapse in breast cancer. Lancet 1:588–591, 1984
168. Howat JMT, Barnes DM, Harris M, et al: The association of cytosol oestrogen and progesterone receptors with histological features of breast cancer and early recurrence of disease. Br J Cancer 47:629–640, 1983
169. Hilf R, Feldstein ML, Gibson SL, et al: The relative importance of estrogen receptor analysis as a prognostic factor for recurrence or response to chemotherapy in women with breast cancer. Cancer 45:1993–2000, 1980
170. Bloom ND, Degenshein GA: Estrogen receptors and disease-free interval: A dissenting opinion. Breast 6:25–27, 1980
171. Pichon MF, Pallud C, Brunet M, et al: Relationship of presence of progesterone receptors to prognosis in early breast cancer. Cancer Res 40:3357–3360, 1980
172. Saez S, Cheix F, Asselain B: Prognostic value of estrogen and progesterone receptors in primary breast cancer. Breast Cancer Res Treat 3:345–354, 1983
173. Mason BH, Holdaway IM, Mullins PR, et al: Progesterone and estrogen receptors as prognostic variables in breast cancer. Cancer Res 43:2985–2990, 1983
174. Clark GM, McGuire WL, Hubay CA, et al: Progesterone receptors as a prognostic factor in stage II breast cancer. N Engl J Med 309:1343–1347, 1983
175. Stewart JF, Rubens RD, Millis RR, et al: Steroid receptors and prognosis in operable (stage I and II) breast cancer. Eur J Cancer Clin Oncol 19:1381–1387, 1983

Natural History and Staging of Breast Cancer

9

Jay R. Harris
I. Craig Henderson

Breast cancer is characterized by a long natural history and by a wide variation in its clinical course. This chapter reviews information related to these features of the disease and factors affecting outcome and summarizes the staging system used to describe its course.

NATURAL HISTORY OF UNTREATED BREAST CANCER

By documenting the natural history of untreated breast cancer, one can establish a baseline by which to judge the effects of treatment. Since breast cancer has been considered a treatable disease for at least the past several hundred years, series of untreated but well-documented patients are not generally available. One such series is from Middlesex Hospital in England, where one of the first cancer wards was established in 1792. Bloom and colleagues reported on a group of 250 patients seen at Middlesex Hospital between 1805 and 1933.[1] When patients were admitted to the hospital, they generally had advanced disease. Seventy-four percent were in Stage IV, 23% in Stage III, and only 2% in Stage II. There were no Stage I cases. Sixty-eight percent had ulceration when first seen in the hospital. No patient was treated with any form of surgery, radiotherapy, or hormone therapy. It is important to note that patients were not admitted to the hospital at the clinical onset of the disease but for terminal care. In all cases, a postmortem examination was performed. Because of the meticulous medical records kept, it was possible to determine the alleged onset of the disease with a fair degree of accuracy. Only 7% of the patients presented within 6 months of the initial symptom of the disease, and only 29% within 1 year. Figure 9-1*A* shows the percentage of patients surviving, plotted from the time of the first onset of symptoms. The median survival time from the alleged onset of symptoms was 2.7 years. Eighteen percent of untreated patients survived 5 years, and 4% survived 10 years. These figures are comparable to those seen from other series and indicate that survival of breast cancer patients can be lengthy even if the disease is untreated.

The usefulness of plotting survival curves semilogarithmically is shown by Figure 9-1*B*. In this figure, the same survival data from the Middlesex Hospital given in Figure 9-1*A* are replotted semilogarithmically. The approximately straight line in this figure indicates that the force of mortality (i.e., the likelihood of dying per year) is constant. In this group of patients, 25% died each year.

Comparing the results in these untreated patients with the results seen in treated patients is fraught with difficulties. The Middlesex Hospital results clearly represent a highly selected group of patients, since only 250 patients were collected over 128 years, or approximately 2 per year. It is not clear how these patients were selected, but selection appears to be related to their need for care of locally advanced breast cancer using dressings and opiates. Of note, these patients were identified for inclusion in the series only if a postmortem examination had been performed, not at the onset of their disease. Given these caveats, it is interesting to compare these results with results seen in modern times. Figure 9-2 shows the survival results collected by the End Results Section of the Biometry Branch of the National Cancer Institute on a large group of patients treated for histologically confirmed breast cancer.[2] The results are corrected for causes of death other than breast cancer. This survival curve suggests that there are two subgroups of patients. One subgroup is manifested by the curve past 10 years and represents patients who have a force of mortality of 2.5% per year. By backward extrapolation of this portion of the curve to time 0, one can estimate that this subgroup represents approximately 60% of the total group. The other subgroup has more aggressive disease, with a force of mortality of 25% per year, similar to that observed for untreated patients seen at Middlesex Hospital. These results indicate that breast cancer is not a homogeneous disease and that its

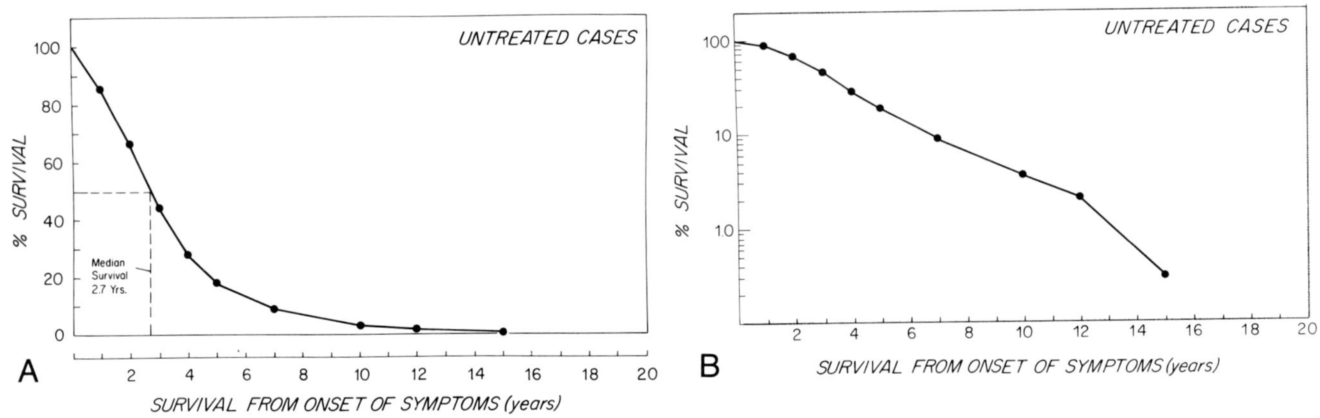

FIGURE 9-1. Survival of untreated breast cancer patients, Middlesex Hospital (250 cases). *(A)* Plotted linearly. *(B)* Plotted semilogarithmically. (Bloom HJG, Richardson WW, Harrier EJ: Natural history of untreated breast cancer [1805–1933]. Br Med J 2:213–221, 1962)

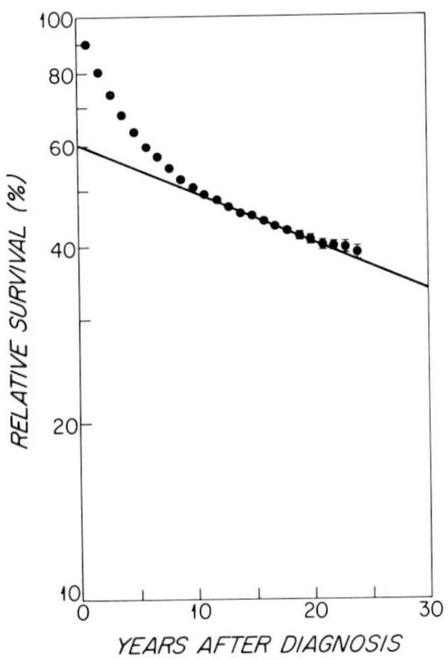

FIGURE 9-2. Relative survival of breast cancer patients (all stages) from the End Results Section, Biometry Branch, National Cancer Institute, 1977. (Fox MS: On the diagnosis and treatment of breast cancer. JAMA 241:489–494, 1979)

natural history is even more protracted than was apparent in the Middlesex series. A subgroup of patients constituting 60% of the entire group has a more indolent course, with a continued risk of death from breast cancer up to 20 years after treatment. It is difficult to assess the impact of treatment from a comparison of Figures 9-1 and 9-2. It suggests, however, that there is a subgroup of patients with aggressive breast cancer who die at an annual rate of 25%, with or without treatment.

The nature of the survival curve after breast cancer treatment has implications for mammographic screening programs. The long natural history of breast cancer suggests the possibility that screening may simply detect the disease earlier in its course without altering its outcome. This effect is referred to as lead-time bias. The heterogeneity of the disease suggests the possibility that periodic screening (performed annually, for example) might detect slow-growing or more favorable tumors rather than fast-growing or less favorable tumors. This effect is known as length-time bias. These effects, described in greater detail in Chapter 5, raise the possibility that although screening may appear to improve survival, it may in fact simply identify patients with favorable tumors earlier in the course of their disease and not alter the long-term survival rate for the entire screened population.

CURABILITY OF BREAST CANCER

The protracted nature of the survival curve shown in Figure 9-2 raises the question of whether a patient with breast cancer is ever truly cured of her disease. There are a number of reasons why it is difficult to answer this question. Breast cancer has a relatively late age of onset and an extremely long natural history, with death due to the disease occurring long after diagnosis. As a result, a large group of patients must be observed a very long time in order to begin to address this question. Furthermore, the definition of "cure" is not straightforward. It is possible to describe cure in a number of different ways. Haybittle has summarized these ways and the evidence for cure of the disease.[3] Of note, these various definitions of cure do not allow an assessment of the impact of treatment. Given the heterogeneity of breast cancer as described above, it is possible that long-term survival after treatment may relate principally to the inherent biology of the patient's disease rather than to the treatment.

The most common concept of cure is referred to as *statistical* cure. A group of treated patients can be considered statistically cured if their subsequent death rate due to all causes is similar to that of a normal population group with the same age and sex distribution. *Clinical* cure for an individual refers to the complete eradication of the disease. Clinical cure for a group occurs when long-term follow-up of the causes of death for the group reveals that the risk of dying of breast cancer is the same as for females of the same age in the general population. An assessment of the likelihood of clinical cure involves determining the cause of death for treated patients. The unreliability of the information recorded on death certificates, however, greatly limits the usefulness of this definition of cure. The third possible definition of cure is the likelihood of a patient's living free of symptoms of breast cancer and dying of other causes. This is referred to as a *personal* cure.

Statistical cure is the usual method for assessing outcome in cancer treatment. Attempts to assess statistical cure in breast cancer patients have all indicated a persistent excess risk of mortality. Brinkley and Haybittle reported on a group of 704 breast cancer patients from the Cambridge, England, area first diagnosed between 1947 and 1950 and observed for at least 31 years.[4] Figure 9-3 shows the survival curves calculated by the life-table method and the expected curves for the normal population of the region with the same age distribution. The survival curves for breast cancer patients never became parallel to those for the normal population. There were eight deaths due to breast cancer more than 25 years after treatment—15 times the number that would be expected. Hibberd and colleagues followed 2019 cases for 30 years and found a small excess of observed over expected deaths even between 25 and 30 years.[5] Rutqvist and Wallgren presented follow-up on 458 patients 40 years of age or younger at diagnosis and found an excess mortality that persisted for at least 40 years.[6] All of these studies indicate a persistent excess risk of mortality after treatment for breast cancer.

Despite the lack of evidence for a statistical cure, a significant percentage of patients will experience a personal cure as defined above. In the Brinkley and Haybittle report, 176 (26%) of the 683 deaths fell in this category.[4] In the experience from Memorial Sloan-Kettering Cancer Center reported by Adair and colleagues, 300 of the 1458 patients (21%) with operable breast cancer had a personal cure of their disease.[7] This means that many patients treated for breast cancer will live out their normal life expectancy free of further evidence of the disease.

GROWTH RATE OF BREAST CANCER

The long natural history of breast cancer has been evaluated in terms of the clinical growth rate of the disease. The growth rate of breast cancer can be assessed by the time required for a tumor to double its diameter, an amount equivalent to an eightfold increase in volume. Determination of clinical growth rate can provide information regarding the heterogeneity of the disease, and it has been used to estimate the time from oncogenesis to clinical presentation.

In 1956, Collins and colleagues described the clinical growth rates of several human tumors, including carcinoma of the breast.[8] Collins assumed an exponential model for tumor growth—that is, tumor cells divide at a constant rate over time. According to this hypothesis, a single cancer cell 10.0 μm in diameter will grow to a nodule 1 mm in diameter in 20 doublings. Another 10 doublings would produce approximately 1 kg of tumor tissue, an amount commonly observed at the time of death due to the disease. Collins plotted the clinical doubling time for a group of 24 patients who had metastatic cancer involving the lungs and in whom measurements of tumor size could be performed on serial chest x-rays. The observed doubling times ranged from 28 to 164 days for patients with tumors of epithelial origin. The median volume-doubling time for this group was 78 days. This study helped to establish the heterogeneity of clinical growth

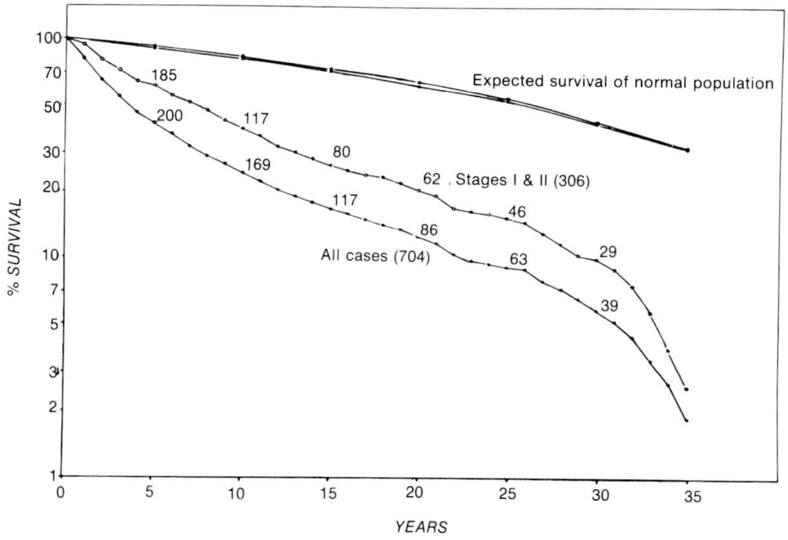

FIGURE 9-3. Survival curve for 704 breast cancer patients treated between 1947 and 1950 and observed for at least 31 years, compared with survival curve of the normal population. (Brinkley D, Haybittle JL: Long term survival of women with breast cancer. Lancet 1:1118, 1984)

rates for human tumors and to provide an estimate of the duration of the preclinical phase of the disease. If one assumes this exponential model, a doubling time of 100 days, and that a primary and metastatic tumor have similar growth rates, then the time required for a single malignant cell to grow to a clinically detectable 1-cm mass would be slightly more than 8 years. The time at which metastasis occurs is not known, but this analysis suggests that there is ample time for spread even before the earliest possible time of detection. The validity of these various assumptions has been questioned and will be discussed below.

These observations on the clinical growth rates of breast cancer have been confirmed by other investigators. Gershon-Cohen and colleagues reported on the growth rate of breast cancer in 18 patients calculated from serial mammographic studies.[9] The distribution of doubling times varied from 23 to 209 days, with a median of 120. Fournier and colleagues studied serial mammograms in 147 cases of breast cancer and found a range of doubling times from 44 to 1869 days, with a median of 212 days.[10] Kusama and associates calculated the volume-doubling time in 199 patients based on serial measurements of either the primary tumor, skin recurrences, or axillary or lung metastases and found a range from 6 to 540 days, with a median of 105 days.[11]

There appears to be an inverse relationship between doubling time and prognosis. Pearlman calculated volume-doubling times in 82 breast cancer patients with mastectomy scar recurrence and assumed that there was a single cell present at the time of mastectomy.[12] Fifty-three percent of patients had rapid growth (doubling times less than or equal to 25 days) and had a 5-year survival rate of 5%. Fourteen percent of patients had slow growth (doubling time equal to or greater than 76 days) and had a 5-year survival rate of 100%. The remainder of the patients were classified as having an intermediate growth rate and had a 5-year survival rate of 62%. Primary tumors with a more rapid growth rate have been associated with a greater likelihood of axillary node involvement. Fournier found that the mean volume-doubling time (as determined by serial mammograms) was 179 days for 14 premenopausal patients with positive axillary nodes compared with 226 days for 31 premenopausal patients with negative nodes ($p<0.05$).[10] The mean diameter of the primary was 15 mm in both groups. Gershon-Cohen similarly found that primary breast tumors associated with axillary metastasis had an average doubling time of 85 days, compared with 128 days when axillary nodes were negative.[9] Based on these observations, it would be reasonable to consider such doubling times as a measure of prognosis. In clinical practice, however, it is rare to have two measurements of a primary on which to calculate a doubling time. Charlson and Feinstein have developed a clinical index of growth rate based on history, which can be used to provide a guide to prognosis.[13] This will be discussed in greater detail below in the section on prognostic factors.

It is important to emphasize certain deficiencies in the concept of the volume-doubling time. As noted above, this concept assumes a constant growth rate or an exponential model. In fact, tumor growth is better described by a gompertzian rather than an exponential model. In a gompertzian model, tumor growth at every instant is exponential, but with a growth constant that is simultaneously exponentially slowing. Therefore, as the tumor mass increases in size, its doubling time becomes progressively longer. In addition, more recent *in vitro* and *in vivo* studies have indicated that the human tumor cell cycle time is on the order of 2 days, not 100 days.[14] Gross tumor doubling times, in fact, represent a complex relationship between cell cycle time, the percent of cells cycling ("growth fraction"), and the likelihood that a newly divided cell will not contribute to the tumor mass ("cell loss factor"). For breast cancer, the growth fraction is approximately 5% and the cell loss factor is on the order of 75%. Thus, the majority of a tumor is made of cells that are not cycling. Furthermore, those cells that are cycling do so at a very rapid rate, but the majority of their progeny do not survive. In this light, it is necessary to interpret volume-doubling times as only a rough index of the aggressiveness of the tumor.

THE PRIMARY CANCER IN THE BREAST

The spread of primary cancer through the breast occurs (1) by direct infiltration into the breast parenchyma, (2) along mammary ducts, and (3) by way of breast lymphatics. Direct infiltration of the cancer tends to occur by ramifying projections, which give a characteristic stellate appearance on gross examination and on mammography. If the condition is untreated, direct involvement of overlying skin or deep pectoral fascia can be seen. Involvement along ducts is observed frequently and may include wide segments of the breast. It is unclear, however, whether this intraductal involvement represents true spread of a primary cancer along previously uninvolved ducts or a field cancerization that results in simultaneous transformation along entire lengths of ducts. Spread also can occur by the extensive network of breast lymphatics. Investigators have emphasized lymphatic spread vertically down to the lymphatic plexus in the deep pectoral fascia underlying the breast. In addition, spread to the central subareolar region has been described. These multiple mechanisms of spread through the breast emphasize the likelihood that cancer will be present in the breast well beyond the palpable primary mass.

The primary site of breast cancer is usually described by its location by quadrant in the breast. In one series of 696 cases, 48% were located in the upper outer quadrant, 15% in the upper inner quadrant, 11% in the lower outer quadrant, 6% in the lower inner quadrant, and 17% in the central region (designated as within 1 cm of the areola).[15] An additional 3% were termed diffuse because of multifocal origin or massive involvement of the entire breast. The reason for the increased frequency of breast cancer in the upper outer quadrant is thought to be simply related to the greater amount of breast tissue in that quadrant. In this series of patients, no differences in survival based on

Table 9-1
Five-Year Recurrence Rates (RR) by Tumor Size, Tumor Location, and Axillary Node Involvement

Tumor Size (cm)	Nodes Negative *				Nodes Positive			
	Medial		Lateral		Medial		Lateral	
	Number of Patients	RR	Number of Patients	RR	Number of Patients	RR	Number of Patients	RR
0.1–1.0	141	12%	408	10%	19	32%	83	21%
1.1–2.0	471	16%	1357	12%	102	41%	411	34%
2.1–3.0	347	19%	1034	13%	114	43%	424	36%
3.1–5.0	227	20%	721	17%	102	47%	406	45%
≥ 5.1	54	34%	191	21%	46	33%	166	57%
All	1240	18%	8711	14%	383	42%	1490	39%

(Nemoto T, Vana J, Bedwani RN, et al: Management and survival of female breast cancer: Results of a national survey by the American College of Surgeons. Cancer 45:2917–2924, 1980)

quadrant location were noted. The relationship between the location of the breast primary and prognosis has also been examined in large series of patients from the 1978 National Survey of the American College of Surgeons (ACS)[16] and the National Surgical Adjuvant Breast Project (NSABP).[17] In the ACS study, the 5-year results in 9401 women were examined in relation to the size of the primary, the location of the primary, and involvement of axillary nodes. The results of this study for patients treated with mastectomy without radiotherapy are shown in Table 9-1. The distribution of tumor sizes for patients with medial and lateral tumors was nearly identical. Patients with medial tumors and negative nodes, however, did somewhat worse than patients with lateral tumors and negative nodes (recurrence rates 18% versus 14%, $p<0.005$). The results for patients with positive nodes were not statistically different based on tumor location. The results obtained in the NSABP study were similar. Patients with medial tumors and negative nodes also did somewhat worse than patients with lateral tumors and negative nodes (recurrence rates 24% versus 19%). The number of patients in this study was smaller, however, and the results did not reach statistical significance. Patients with positive nodes had the same prognosis regardless of location. The results from the ACS and NSABP studies suggest that patients with inner-half tumors and negative nodes have a somewhat worse prognosis than patients with outer-half tumors and negative nodes. This observation will be discussed further below.

The clinical size of the primary lesion is highly correlated with prognosis. The data from Koscielny and colleagues of the Institut Gustave-Roussy illustrates this point.[18] They examined the relationship between the size of the primary tumor and the likelihood of distant metastasis in 2648 breast cancers treated at their institution between 1954 and 1972 (Fig. 9-4). Follow-up ranged from 10 years to more than 25 years. The data are plotted using a log-probit coordinate system and indicate a direct relationship between tumor size and the probability of metastasis. Of note, patients who presented with metastatic disease were included in the analysis. These data illustrate the direct relationship between tumor size and prognosis and are consistent with other studies that have investigated this point.[7,19–21] The relative importance of tumor size and involvement of axillary nodes will be discussed below.

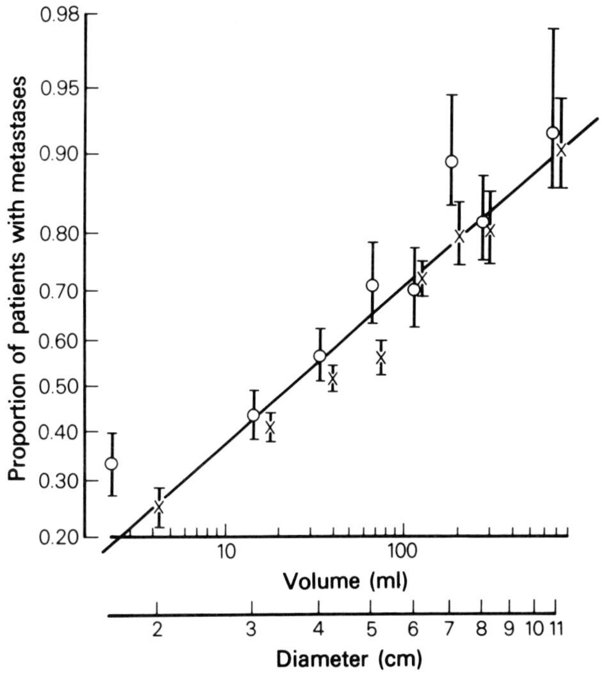

FIGURE 9-4. Relationship between clinical size of the tumor and the likelihood of distant metastasis for patients treated during the period 1954–1958 (o) and 1959–1972 (x). (Koscielny S, Tubiana M, Le MG, et al: Breast cancer: Relationship between the size of the primary tumour and the probability of metastatic dissemination. Br J Cancer 49:709, 1984)

The data above presented by Koscielny and colleagues have important implications regarding the time at which metastases occur in breast cancer. The linearity of the relationship between tumor size and the likelihood of metastasis (when both are plotted logarithmically) indicates a log-normal distribution, with a median diameter of 3.56 cm. This implies that metastasis does not occur in half the cases until the tumor exceeds 3.56 cm in diameter. This observation is at odds with prior studies, which suggested that metastasis occurs very early in the life of the tumor. These prior studies were based on the observed growth rate of metastatic disease and back-extrapolation of this rate to the time when the metastasis contained one cell.[8,9,22] Koscielny and colleagues point out that these prior studies assume an exponential model and that the growth rate of the tumor and its metastasis are equal. It has subsequently been noted that the doubling time for primary tumors is generally greater than that for metastases.[23,24] The interpretation by Koscielny and colleagues provides a more optimistic view regarding the importance of early detection and is in keeping with the positive findings on the value of mammographic screening.[25,26] These results suggest that in many patients metastases occur within the range of clinical detectability of the primary tumor.

REGIONAL NODE INVOLVEMENT

The most common sites of regional involvement of breast cancer are the axillary, internal mammary, and supraclavicular lymph node regions. Knowledge of the likelihood of involvement of these sites and their significance is critical for planning treatment for patients with breast cancer.

Axillary Node Involvement

The axillary lymph node region is the major regional drainage for the breast. Approximately 50% of patients with breast cancer have histologic evidence of involvement of axillary nodes. The likelihood of axillary node involvement is related directly to the size of the primary lesion (Table 9-2). The larger the primary tumor, the greater the risk for axillary node involvement. Even for the smallest tumors (less than 1 cm), the risk of axillary involvement is approximately 25%.

Table 9-2
Frequency of Axillary Node Involvement by Tumor Size

	Frequency of Axillary Node Involvement		
Tumor Size (cm)	*Nemoto et al*[20]	*Haagensen*[27]	*Fisher et al*[21]
<1	24%	29%	20%
1–2	34%	27%	39%
2–3	43%	29%	57%
3–4	50%	41%	54%
4–5	57%	50%	56%
>5	65%	49%	62%

There is evidence that the location of the primary tumor in the breast influences the likelihood of axillary lymph node involvement. Several studies have indicated that axillary nodes are more commonly involved when tumors are located in the lateral portion of the breast than when they are in the medial portion. In the 1978 national survey by the ACS, 43% of patients with lateral-half tumors had positive nodes compared with 35% of patients with medial-half tumors.[20] Haagensen[28] described similar results on the frequency of axillary node metastasis from his personal series of 917 patients treated with radical mastectomy. Positive nodes were found in 47% of patients with upper outer quadrant tumors, 38% with lower outer quadrant tumors, 30% with upper inner quadrant tumors, and 23% with lower inner quadrant tumors. In particular, Haagensen found that tumors located in the extreme medial portion of the breast (defined as within 3 cm of the edge of the sternum) had the lowest frequency of axillary involvement (20%), although this may in part be related to the smaller size of tumors found in that location. Similarly, Fisher and colleagues found that 52% of patients with lateral-half tumors had positive nodes, compared with 39% of patients with medial-half tumors.[17] In the ACS study noted above, the results were examined in relation to tumor size as well as location (Table 9-3). In each tumor size category, patients with medial tumors were less likely to have positive axillary nodes compared with patients with lateral tumors.

The increased likelihood of axillary involvement for lateral compared with medial primary tumors is most likely related to preferential drainage of medial tumors to internal mammary nodes (IMNs) and lateral tumors to axillary nodes. (The frequency of IMN involvement in patients with breast cancer will be discussed in greater detail below). As will be shown, involvement of IMNs is more likely for patients with medial tumors than for patients with lateral tumors. As a result, regional lymph node involvement (either axillary or IMN) is similar for medial and lateral tumors. This observation would also explain the difference in prognosis noted in the ACS study based

Table 9-3
Percentage of Patients with Positive Axillary Nodes by the Location and Size of the Primary Tumor

Tumor Size (cm)	*Medial*		*Lateral*	
	Number of Patients	*% positive*	*Number of Patients*	*% positive*
0.1–1.0	219	18%	578	25%
1.1–2.0	820	28%	2212	35%
2.1–3.0	691	35%	1951	43%
3.1–5.0	522	44%	1651	53%
>5	165	58%	592	63%
Total	2417	35%	6984	43%

(Nemoto T, Vana J, Bedwani RN, et al: Management and survival of female breast cancer: Results of a national survey by the American College of Surgeons. Cancer 45:2917–2924, 1980)

on location (Table 9-1), since IMN involvement as well as axillary node involvement is associated with a worse prognosis. These results suggest that location does not affect the likelihood of regional node involvement or prognosis but does affect which regional nodes will be involved.

To some extent, the incidence of histologic involvement of axillary nodes is dependent on the type of surgery performed and the extent of the pathologic analysis of the axillary specimen. Radical mastectomy allows for the most complete dissection of the axillary contents and yields the greatest number of axillary nodes. Lesser surgical procedures, such as the modified radical mastectomy, typically give a less complete axillary dissection and yield fewer axillary nodes. As a result of this variable extent of axillary dissection, the likelihood of histologic involvement must be viewed in terms of the surgical procedure performed. In one pathologic study of axillary specimens, it was noted that axillary node involvement would have been reduced by 29% if the axillary dissection had been extended only to the lower border of the pectoralis minor muscle.[29] The incidence of histologic involvement also is related to the degree of pathologic analysis. Pickren was among the first to show that a more thorough clearing and sectioning of the axillary specimen results in a greater yield of positive nodes.[30] In his study of 51 specimens routinely analyzed and found to be negative, 11 (22%) showed evidence of involvement on more careful analysis.

Detection of axillary involvement by physical examination has both a high false-positive and false-negative rate (Table 9-4). When axillary lymph nodes are palpable and are suspicious for cancer, histologic evidence of metastatic disease is found in approximately 70% of cases. Conversely, when axillary nodes are not palpable, histologic involvement is detected in approximately 30% of cases. These figures indicate the shortcomings of clinical evaluation in predicting histologic involvement. These results are of particular importance because histologic involvement of axillary nodes has a high correlation with prognosis. Table 9-5 shows 10-year survival figures related to axillary involvement from six separate series of patients treated with radical mastectomy. Patients with histologically negative axillary nodes have markedly better survival rates than do patients with histologic involvement. Furthermore, patients with one to three positive nodes do better than patients with four or more positive nodes. In fact, prognosis is directly related to the number of positive axillary nodes. This is illustrated in the results obtained in the ACS survey (Table 9-6).[20] Prognosis showed a progressive decline with increasing numbers of positive nodes. Patients with one positive node had a 63% 5-year likelihood of survival and a 33% risk of recurrence, compared with a 22% 5-year likelihood of survival and an 82% risk of recurrence for patients with 21 or more positive nodes. These data suggest that any comparison of prognosis based on dividing patients by a certain number of positive nodes is somewhat artificial since there is no clear dividing point. However, such a division is of practical use. The NSABP and others have divided patients into groups having one to three positive nodes or four or more positive nodes. The International Union Against Cancer (UICC) and the American Joint Commission on Cancer Staging and End Results Reporting (AJC) have recently divided patients into groups having one to four positive nodes or five or more positive nodes.

Table 9-4
Accuracy of Physical Examination in Predicting Histologic Involvement of Axillary Nodes

Study	*False-Positive (percent)*	*False-Negative (percent)*
Butcher[31]	25	32
Haagensen[32]	31	28
Schottenfeld et al[19]	26	27
Bucalossi et al[33]	29	29

For purposes of analysis, the axilla is commonly divided into three levels: *level I* or *proximal,* defined as tissue inferior and lateral to the lower border of the pectoralis minor muscle; *level II* or *middle,* tissue directly beneath the pectoralis minor; and *level III* or *distal,* tissue superior and medial to the pectoralis minor. Prognosis has been shown to be related to the level of axillary involvement.[19] Involvement of the distal level nodes carries a worse prognosis than involvement of the proximal level nodes. In a study of 182 mastectomy specimens examined by clearing, involvement of nodes in the distal portion of the axilla was found in 15.[39] All 15 patients suffered relapse, indicating the grave prognosis associated with involvement high in the axilla. In this group of 15 patients, the mean number of involved nodes was 16.2 (range, 4 to 37). In general, involvement of the distal level nodes is associated with a high total number of lymph nodes involved. In another study, axillary node involvement and survival were examined in 385 patients to determine whether the total number of involved nodes or the level of axillary node involvement was a better indicator of prognosis.[24] They found that for any given number of involved nodes, survival was independent of the level of involvement, and they concluded that prognosis was related more directly to the total number of nodes involved.

Prognosis has been shown to be related to both the size of the primary tumor and to axillary node involvement. The question whether these two factors independently predict for prognosis has been addressed in a number of studies (Table 9-7). The results indicate that when axillary nodes are involved, the size of the primary tumor is still of prognostic value. For example, in the data from Valagussa and colleagues,[34] the 5-year relapse rate was 37% for patients with positive nodes and small (2 cm or less) primary tumors and 79% for patients with positive nodes and large (greater than 5 cm) primary tumors. In the data by Fisher and colleagues,[36] this relationship was analyzed further by the number of positive axillary nodes (one to three versus four or more). Within each subgroup of positive axillary nodes, the size of the primary lesion was still an independent prognostic factor. When axillary nodes are

Table 9-5
Ten-Year Survival by Axillary Node Status for Patients Treated With Radical Mastectomy

Study	Nodes Negative	Nodes Positive	1–3 Positive	4 or More Positive
Valagussa et al[34]	80%	38%	50%	24%
Haagensen[35]	76%	48%	63%	27%
Schottenfeld et al[19]	72%	43%	—	—
Fisher et al[36]	65%	25%	38%	13%
Spratt and Donegan[37]	68%	27%	—	—
Payne et al[38]	76%	35%	—	—

Table 9-6
Five-Year Results by the Number of Pathologically Positive Axillary Nodes

Number of Positive Axillary Nodes	Number of Patients	Survival Rate (percent)	Recurrence Rate (percent)
0	12,299	72	19
1	2,012	63	33
2	1,338	62	40
3	842	59	43
4	615	52	44
5	478	47	54
6–10	1,261	41	63
11–15	562	29	72
16–20	301	29	75
≥ 21	225	22	82

(Nemoto T, Vana J, Bedwani RN, et al: Management and survival of female breast cancer: Results of a national survey by the American College of Surgeons, Cancer 45:2917–2924, 1980)

Table 9-7
Five-Year Relapse Rate By Primary Tumor Size and Axillary Node Involvement

	Size of Primary Tumor		
Axillary Node Involvement	< 2 cm	2–5 cm	> 5 cm
Axillary Nodes Negative			
Fisher et al[36]	12%	24%	27%
Nemoto et al[20]	13%	19%	25%
Valagussa[34]	8%	24%	19%
Axillary Nodes Positive			
Fisher	50%	60%	79%
Nemoto	39%	50%	65%
Valagussa	37%	64%	74%

negative, the relationship between prognosis and tumor size is not linear. The prognosis for patients with small (2 cm or less) primary tumors and negative nodes is exceptionally good, with a 5-year relapse rate of approximately 10%. For women with primary tumors larger than 2 cm, the prognosis is not quite as good, with a 5-year relapse rate of approximately 20% to 25%. Of note, however, is that the prognosis for patients with a large (greater than 5 cm) primary tumor and negative nodes is not significantly worse than for patients with primary tumors between 2 cm and 5 cm and negative nodes. These results are corroborated by results of studies having longer follow-up. Adair and colleagues reported that for patients with negative nodes, the 30-year relative survival rate was

61% when the primary tumor was 2 cm or smaller, 46% for primary tumors between 2 cm and 5 cm, and 50% for primary tumors larger than 5 cm.[7] For patients with involvement of proximal level axillary nodes, the 30-year relative survival rate was 40% when the primary was 2 cm or smaller, 31% for primaries between 2 cm and 5 cm, and 14% for primaries larger than 5 cm. The results seen at the Institut Gustave-Roussy are also in general agreement.[18]

In summary, the axilla is a major lymph node region for carcinoma of the breast, and a histologic analysis of the axillary nodes provides a useful guide for prognosis.

Internal Mammary Node Involvement

The second major site of node involvement in carcinoma of the breast is the IMN chain. This chain lies at the anterior end of the intercostal spaces by the side of the internal thoracic artery. Because of the intrathoracic location and the uncommon clinical presentation of IMN involvement, the frequency was not appreciated as early as axillary node involvement. One of the first to document this second route of spread was Sampson Handley, who reported his results of internal mammary node biopsy in 1000 patients in 1975 (Table 9-8).[40] These results indicated that (1) overall, axillary lymph node involvement is more likely than IMN involvement (54% versus 22%); (2) internal mammary node involvement is more common when axillary nodes are involved than when uninvolved (35% versus 8%); and (3) internal mammary node involvement is more common for inner quadrant or central primary tumors than for outer quadrant primary tumors. However, even in patients with inner or central primary lesions, axillary involvement was more common than IMN involvement (42% versus 28%). Furthermore, when axillary nodes were uninvolved, IMN involvement was uncommon even with inner or central primaries.

Another large series of patients treated with internal mammary node biopsy has been reported by Veronesi and colleagues.[41] In this series of 1119 patients, axillary involvement was seen in 50% of patients and IMN involvement was seen in 19%. They found that the likelihood of IMN involvement was related to axillary involvement (axillary nodes positive, 29% versus negative 9%, $p<0.01$), tumor size (less than 2 cm, 16% versus larger than 2 cm 25%, $p<0.01$) and to patient age (40 years of age or younger, 28%; 41 to 50 years, 20%; and older than 50 years, 16%; $p = 0.01$). In contrast to the findings of Handley, however, IMN involvement was not related to the location of the primary tumor in the breast (inner, 19% versus outer 18%). Veronesi and colleagues found that axillary involvement, tumor size, and patient age influence the likelihood of IMN involvement independently. For a patient less than 40 years old with positive axillary nodes and a primary larger than 2 cm, the risk of IMN involvement was 44.3%. For a patient older than 50 years with negative axillary nodes and a primary smaller than 2 cm, the risk of IMN involvement was only 6.8%. In this study, the prognostic implication of IMN involvement was similar to that for axillary node involvement (Fig. 9-5). The 10-year rate of disease-free survival was 73% when both axillary and IMNs were negative, 47% when axillary nodes alone were positive, 52% when IMNs alone were positive, and only 25% when both areas were positive.

Other investigators have examined the relation between tumor location and IMN involvement and, like Handley, have found that IMN involvement is more common for medial or central tumors. Haagensen performed IMN biopsy on 1007 patients and found IMN involvement in 29% of patients with medial tumors, compared with 17% of patients with lateral tumors.[42] Patients with central tumors had a 43% risk of IMN involvement. Patients with tumors in the extreme medial portion of the breast (defined as within 3 cm of the sternal edge) had a risk of IMN involvement similar to that of patients with tumors in other medial portions of the breast (approximately 29% in both situations). Similarly, LaCour and colleagues[43] reported on a group of 703 patients and found IMN involvement in 24% of patients with medial or central tumors and in 16% of patients with lateral tumors. These results were from an international randomized trial testing the value of IMN dissection in which half of the patients were entered from Milan.

Overall, roughly 50% of patients have axillary node involvement and 20% of patients have IMN involvement.

Table 9-8
Internal Mammary Node (IMN) Involvement Related to Primary Tumor Location and Axillary Node Involvement

Axillary Node Status	*Location of Primary Tumor*					
	UIQ	*LIQ*	*Central*	*UOQ*	*LOQ*	*All*
Negative	20/143	2/36	5/76	7/170	2/40	8%
	14%	6%	7%	4%	5%	
Positive	47/105	18/25	65/140	47/212	10/53	35%
	45%	72%	46%	22%	19%	
All	27%	33%	32%	14%	13%	22%

(Handley RS: Carcinoma of the breast. Ann R Coll Surg Engl 57:59–66, 1975)

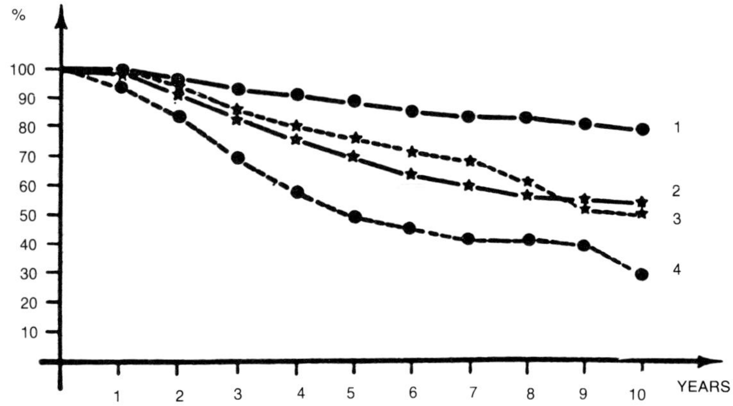

FIGURE 9-5. Ten-year overall survival in patients without node metastases (1), with axillary node metastases only (2), with internal mammary node metastases only (3), and with both groups involved (4) ($p = 10^{-9}$). (Veronesi U, Cascinelli N, Greco M, et al: Prognosis of breast cancer patients after mastectomy and dissection of internal mammary nodes. Ann Surg 202:702–707, 1985)

The most consistent finding regarding IMN involvement is its relation to axillary node involvement. When axillary nodes are negative, IMN involvement is uncommon (approximately 10%). When axillary nodes are positive, IMN involvement is approximately 30%. Furthermore, the greater the extent of axillary node involvement, the greater the likelihood of IMN involvement.[44] However, the prognostic significance of IMN involvement is still apparent even when adjusted for the extent of axillary node involvement.[44] These results indicate that the axilla is the major site of node involvement in breast cancer and that the IMN region is generally a secondary site of involvement.

Supraclavicular Lymph Node Involvement

Supraclavicular lymph node involvement is associated with extensive axillary node involvement. In one series of patients undergoing routine supraclavicular dissection, involvement of the supraclavicular region was found in 23 (18%) of 125 patients who had positive axillary nodes and none of 149 patients who did not have positive axillary nodes.[45] The significance of supraclavicular node involvement was first shown by Halsted, who performed a supraclavicular dissection in 119 patients. Forty-four patients were found to have involvement of these nodes, and only two of the patients were free of cancer at 5 years.[46] Supraclavicular node involvement represents a late stage of axillary node involvement and carries a grave prognosis.

Clinical Implications of Regional Node Involvement

The previous discussion describes the frequency and prognostic significance of regional node involvement in patients with carcinoma of the breast. The critical issue of whether or not treatment of these nodal areas is important is discussed in detail in Chapter 10. In brief, the available data indicate that treatment of regional nodal areas has, at most, only a small impact on the likelihood of long-term survival. As a result, the determination of axillary and internal mammary node involvement is useful chiefly as a means of assessing prognosis. Axillary lymph node involvement can be easily and safely assessed by axillary dissection. An internal mammary node dissection, on the other hand, is a considerably more extensive and morbid procedure and is rarely performed now. Other methods for the detection of IMN involvement, such as lymphoscintigraphy, are being developed, but their value has not been established. As discussed below in this chapter, the presence and extent of axillary node involvement are the most important means of assessing prognosis. This is best achieved by a complete axillary dissection. It remains controversial, however, whether the increased prognostic data gained by a complete axillary dissection outweigh the increased morbidity compared with a subtotal (level I and II) dissection. In practice in the United States at this time, most patients undergo an axillary dissection that is less than complete.

DISTANT METASTASES

Metastasis from carcinoma of the breast can be noted in a variety of organs. The likelihood of organ involvement has been studied in a number of autopsy series (Table 9-9).[47–49] The most common sites of metastatic spread are bone, lung, and liver. The time course to the appearance of distant metastases can be extremely long. It is not uncommon for metastases to first become manifest 10 years or more after initial diagnosis. The time course to distant metastases is influenced by the size of the primary tumor, the number of positive axillary nodes, and the histologic grade of the tumor. Figure 9-6 shows the time course to the appearance of distant metastases related to the size of the primary lesion. For patients with the smallest primary tumors (1 cm to 2.5 cm), the time course to the appearance of distant disease is the greatest. The cumulative proportion of patients with metastases reached half its ultimate value ("median delay" or median interval) 42 months after initial treatment. In contrast, the median interval was only 4 months for patients with tumors 8.5 cm or larger. The median interval between diagnosis and detection of first distant metastasis was 69 months when axillary nodes were negative, 43 months when one to three axillary nodes were positive, and 30 months when four or more axillary nodes

Table 9-9
Sites of Metastases from Breast Cancer in Three Collected Series

Organ	*160 Cases*	*43 Cases*	*100 Cases*
Lung	59%	65%	69%
Liver	58%	56%	65%
Bone	44%	—	71%
Pleura	37%	23%	51%
Adrenals	31%	41%	49%
Kidneys	Not recorded	14%	17%
Spleen	14%	23%	17%
Pancreas	—	11%	17%
Ovaries	9%	16%	20%
Brain	—	9%	22%
Thyroid	—	—	24%
Heart	—	—	11%
Diaphragm	—	—	11%
Pericardium	5%	21%	19%
Intestine	—	—	18%
Peritoneum	12%	9%	13%
Uterus	—	—	15%
Lymph nodes	72%	—	76%
Skin	34%	7%	30%
Reference	Warren[47]	Saphillo[48]	Haagensen[49]

were positive. Similarly, the median interval was 65 months for patients with histologic grade 1 primary tumors, 44 months for grade 2 primaries, and 21 months for grade 3 primaries. These data illustrate that distant metastases can first appear long after diagnosis and that this is particularly so for well-differentiated, early stage breast cancers.

STAGING

Staging refers to the grouping of patients according to the extent of their disease. It is useful in determining the choice of treatment for individual patients, estimating their prognosis and comparing the results of different treatment programs. Breast cancer is staged initially on a clinical basis—that is, based on the physical examination as well as on laboratory and radiologic evaluation. Staging can also be performed on a pathologic basis based on the findings of the resection of the primary tumor and on axillary dissection. Factors other than stage, including tumor histology, patient age, and delay, also influence prognosis, and these will be discussed below.

One of the first widely accepted staging systems was developed at the Christie Hospital and Holt Radium Institute in Manchester, England. It has been called the Manchester system and uses four stages based on the clinical features of the disease, as shown in Table 9-10.

Another clinical staging system of historical importance is the Columbia Clinical Classification (CCC), given in Table 9-11.

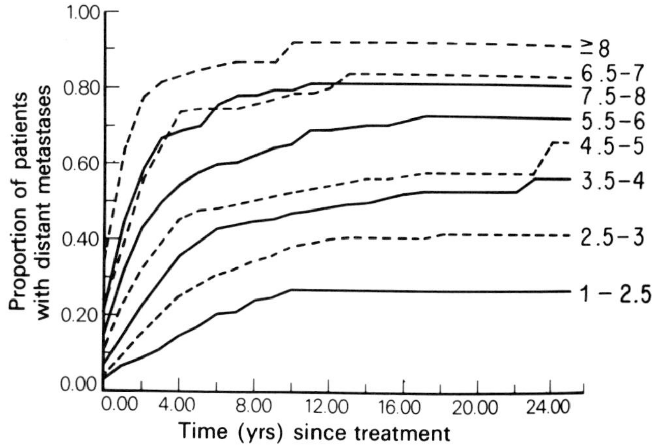

FIGURE 9-6. The cumulated proportions of patients with metastases as a function of the time after treatment in the different groups of patients defined by the clinical size of the tumor in centimeters. (Koscielny S, Tubiana M, Le MG, et al: Breast cancer: Relationship between the size of the primary tumour and the probability of metastatic dissemination. Br J Cancer 49:709–715, 1984)

Currently, the most widely used staging system is the one adopted by both the UICC and the AJC. This is a clinical staging system based on the findings prior to surgery. It is based on the TNM system (T, tumor; N, nodes; M, metastases), and the 1983 (second edition) version is given in Table 9-12.

Basis for the UICC-AJC Clinical Staging System

Beginning in the late 1950s, both the UICC and the AJC attempted to formulate standard systems to be used by physicians for the clinical staging of cancer based on the TNM system. The UICC system was first published in 1960 and the AJC system in 1962. To compare these two systems, the results from 2039 breast cancer patients from 12 hospitals in the United States were evaluated. Cutler and colleagues[50] used these results to substantiate the importance of the clinical assessment of the axillary lymph nodes (Fig. 9-7). Patients with nonpalpable axillary nodes had the best prognosis, and patients with fixed nodes had the worst prognosis. Patients who had mobile axillary nodes had an intermediate prognosis. Of note, the original AJC system allowed any size tumor in Stage I, whereas the UICC restricted Stage I to tumors smaller than 5 cm. Zippin evaluated the validity of these two systems by examining the results from 556 patients (of the total study group of 2039) who had no palpable axillary nodes and no skin involvement (Fig. 9-8).[51] Two hundred and three of these patients had tumors 2 cm or smaller, 287 patients had tumors between 2 cm and 5 cm, and 66 patients had tumors larger than 5 cm. These 66 patients were classified as Stage I in the AJC system and Stage III in the UICC. Figure 9-8 shows that the prognosis for these 66 patients

Table 9-10
Manchester Staging System

Stage I	The growth is confined to the breast. Involvement of the skin directly over and in continuity with the tumor does not affect staging, provided that the area involved is small in relation to the size of the breast.
Stage II	As in Stage I, but there are palpable mobile nodes in the axilla.
Stage III	The growth extends beyond the breast as shown by (A) involvement of a large portion of skin or by ulceration (B) fixation to the underlying muscle or fascia
Stage IV	Any of the following features: (A) fixation or matting of the axillary nodes (B) fixation of the tumor to the chest wall (C) supraclavicular involvement (D) opposite breast involvement (E) satellite skin nodules

(Patterson R: The Treatment of Malignant Disease by Radium and X-Rays. London, Edward Arnold, 1948)

Table 9-11
Columbia Clinical Classification

Stage A	No skin edema, ulceration, or solid fixation of the tumor to the chest wall. Axillary nodes are not involved clinically.
Stage B	No skin edema, ulceration, or solid fixation of the tumor to the chest wall. Clinically involved nodes, but less than 2.5 cm in transverse diameter and not fixed to overlying skin or deeper structures of the axilla.
Stage C	Any one of the five grave signs of advanced breast carcinoma: (1) edema of the skin of limited extent (involving less than one-third of the skin over the breast) (2) skin ulceration (3) solid fixation of the tumor to the chest wall (4) massive involvement of axillary lymph nodes (measuring 2.5 cm or more in transverse diameter) (5) fixation of the axillary nodes to overlying skin or deeper structures of the axilla.
Stage D	All other patients with more advanced breast carcinoma, including: (1) a combination of any two or more of the five grave signs listed under Stage C (2) extensive edema of the skin (involving more than one-third of the skin over the breast) (3) satellite skin nodules (4) the inflammatory type of carcinoma (5) clinically involved supraclavicular lymph nodes (6) internal mammary metastases as evidenced by a parasternal tumor (7) edema of the arm (8) distant metastases

(Haagensen CD: Diseases of the Breast, 3rd ed. Philadelphia, WB Saunders, 1986)

was worse than that for other Stage I patients and was between that of Stage II and Stage III patients. These results substantiated the UICC view that tumor size is an important prognostic variable even when axillary nodes are clinically negative. Figure 9-8 shows that for patients with clinically negative nodes, prognosis is best for patients with tumors 2 cm or smaller, intermediate with tumors between 2 and 5 cm, and worst with tumors larger than 5 cm. In a later study by Cutler and colleagues,[52] the relative importance of axillary node status and tumor size was evaluated in a group of 1252 patients treated with radical mastectomy at Memorial Hospital, New York City, between 1950 and 1952 (Fig. 9-9). Survival of subgroups was characterized in terms of the average annual mortality ($\hat{q}$) over a period of 10 years after diagnosis. Calculation of $\hat{q}$ was done by dividing the observed number of deaths in 10 years by the sum of the number of patients at risk at the beginning of each year. Figure 9-9 shows the average annual mortality ($\hat{q}$) in relation to tumor size and clinical axillary node status. These data provide strong support for the current UICC-AJC staging system. Patients with T1N0 breast cancer have a singularly good prognosis and are therefore classified as Stage I. Patients with fixed axillary nodes (N2) have a generally poor prognosis and are clas-

Table 9-12
UICC-AJC Clinical Staging System

T Primary Tumor

T0	No evidence of primary tumor
Tis	*In situ* cancer
T1	Tumor 2 cm or less in its greatest dimension
T1a	No fixation to underlying pectoral fascia or muscle
T1b	Fixation to underlying pectoral fascia or muscle
T2	Tumor more than 2 cm but not more than 5 cm in its greatest dimension
T3	Tumor more than 5 cm in its greatest dimension
T3a	No fixation to underlying pectoral fascia or muscle
T3b	Fixation to underlying pectoral fascia or muscle
T4	Tumor of any size with direct extension to chest wall or skin
T4a	Fixation to chest wall
T4b	Edema (including peau d'orange), ulceration of the skin of the breast, or satellite skin nodules confined to the same breast
T4c	Both of above

Notes: (1) Chest wall includes ribs, intercostal muscles, and serratus anterior muscle, but not pectoral muscle. (2) Dimpling of the skin, nipple retraction, or any other skin changes except those in T4b may occur in T1, T2, or T3 without affecting classification. (3) Inflammatory carcinoma of the breast is considered a histologic subtype, not a separate stage. It is defined as a clinicopathologic entity characterized by diffuse, brawny induration of the skin with an erysipeloid edge, usually with no underlying palpable mass. This clinical presentation is due to tumor embolization of dermal lymphatics. (4) When multiple, simultaneous ipsilateral breast tumors are present, the largest one should be used for staging. These cases should be recorded as such and analyzed separately: When there are simultaneous bilateral breast tumors, each should be staged independently.

N Regional Lymph Nodes

N0	Homolateral axillary nodes not considered to contain growth
N1	Movable homolateral axillary nodes considered to contain growth
N2	Homolateral axillary nodes containing growth and fixed to one another or to other structures
N3	Homolateral supraclavicular or infraclavicular nodes containing growth or edema of the arm

M Distant Metastasis

M0	No evidence of distant metastasis
M1	Distant metastasis present, including skin involvement beyond the breast area

Clinical Stage Grouping

Stage I	T1	N0	M0
Stage II	T0	N1	M0
	T1	N1	M0
	T2	N0	M0
	T2	N1	M0
Stage IIIA	T3	N0	M0
	T3	N1	M0
	T0–3	N2	M0
IIIB	T4	any N	M0
	any T	N3	M0
Stage IV	any T	any N	M1

American Joint Committee on Cancer: Manual for Staging of Cancer, 3rd ed. Philadelphia, JB Lippincott, 1987)

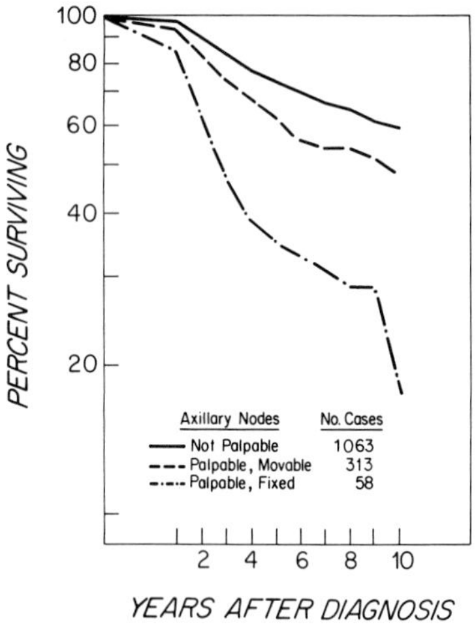

FIGURE 9-7. Survival related to the clinical assessment of the axillary nodes. (Cutler SJ, Zippin C, Asire AJ: The prognostic significance of palpable lymph nodes in cancer of the breast. Cancer 23:243–250, 1969)

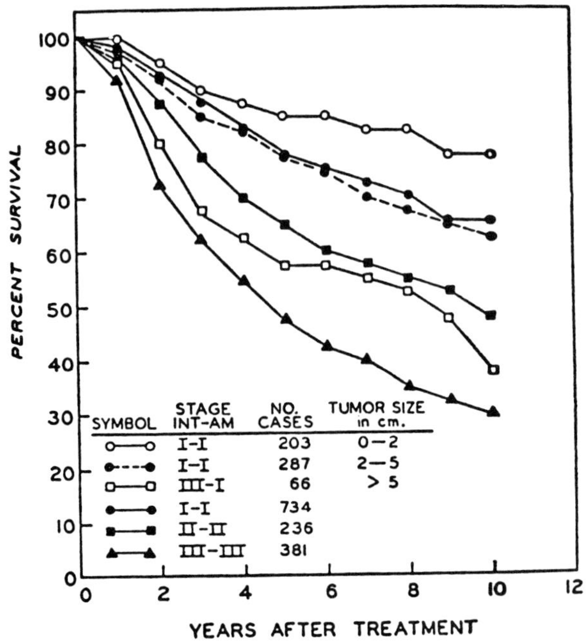

FIGURE 9-8. Survival related to clinical staging according to the original UICC (Int) and AJC (Am) systems. Patients with tumors larger than 5 cm were originally classified as Stage I in the AJC system and Stage III in the UICC system. (Zippin C: Comparison of the International and American Systems for the staging of breast cancer. J Natl Cancer Inst 36:53–62, 1966)

sified as Stage III. Patients with large primaries (T3) have a poor prognosis, as previously shown by Zippin. This is primarily related to the fact that these patients more commonly have microscopic axillary node involvement than do patients with T1 or T2 tumors. In the data analyzed by Cutler, the likelihood for nodal metastases was 32% for T1N0 tumors, 46% for T2N0 tumors, and 57% for T3N0 tumors. The prognosis for patients who have T3 primary tumors and negative axillary nodes pathologically is only slightly worse than that for patients with T2 primaries and negative nodes. Patients with T1N1 and T2N0 breast cancer have a good prognosis and are reasonably classified as early Stage II (IIA).

Cutler and colleagues also evaluated the prognostic significance of skin changes in this study.[52] Three categories of skin status were defined: (1) no involvement, (2) dimpling or retraction, and (3) edema or ulceration. The average annual mortality was evaluated in relation to the skin status and the clinical assessment of the axillary nodes (Fig. 9-10). Figure 9-10 shows that dimpling or retraction does not have a significant impact on prognosis, whereas ulceration or edema does have a significant impact on prognosis. Of note, patients with ulceration or edema and clinically negative nodes had a 55% likelihood of having pathologically evident axillary metastases. The prognosis for this group when nodes were histologically negative was similar to that for other patients with negative nodes. These observations suggest that ulceration and edema are important elements in clinical staging but that they become less important when the pathologic status of the axillary nodes is known.

FIGURE 9-9. Average annual mortality ($\hat{q}$) related to the clinical assessment of axillary nodes and tumor size. (Adapted from Cutler SJ, Axtell LM. Schottenfeld D: Clinical assessment of lymph nodes in carcinoma of the breast. Surg Gynecol Obstet 131:41–52, 1970)

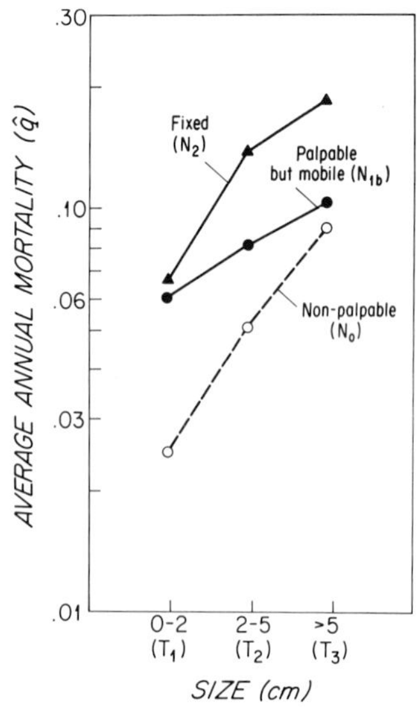

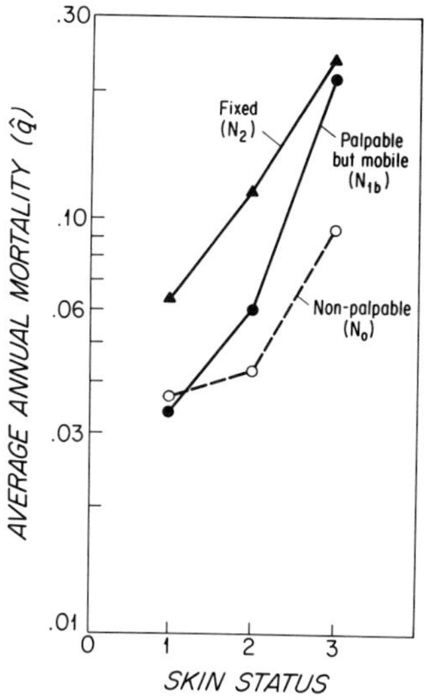

FIGURE 9-10. Average annual mortality (q̂) related to the clinical assessment of axillary nodes and the status of the skin. Skin status; 1, no involvement; 2, dimpling or retraction; and 3, edema or ulceration. (Adapted from Cutler SJ, Axtell LM, Schottenfeld D: Clinical assessment of lymph nodes in carcinoma of the breast. Surg Gynecol Obstet 131:41–52, 1970)

Pathologic Staging

Since clinical evaluation of spread to the axilla has a high false-positive and false-negative rate, pathologic staging based on the histologic evaluation of the axillary specimen is preferable in judging prognosis for the individual patient. This is illustrated in the data given by Haagensen (Table 9-13).[53] For patients who have clinically suspicious nodes but in whom the histologic evaluation is negative, 10-year survival (72%) is comparable to that of the entire group of patients with histologically negative nodes (76%) and not to the group with histologically positive nodes (48%). Similarly, if a patient does not have clinical evidence of axillary involvement but microscopic involvement is detected pathologically, 10-year survival (57%) is comparable to that of the entire group of patients with microscopic involvement (48%).

Pathologic stage is commonly given as Stage I (axillary nodes not involved) or Stage II (axillary nodes involved). This simple staging format has been refined by subdividing Stage II by the number of positive axillary nodes. Because prognosis is clearly related to the extent of axillary involvement, it has become convention to subdivide axillary involvement into one to three nodes positive or more than four nodes positive. It is important to note, however, that prognosis for patients with four or more positive nodes will vary depending on the precise number of positive nodes (see Table 9-6).

A system for pathologic staging has also been given by the UICC-AJC. It requires, at a minimum, gross excision of the tumor and the resection of at least four axillary nodes. A case can be included in a UICC-AJC pathologic stage if there is microscopic, but not gross, involvement of a margin. If there is tumor at a margin of resection by gross examination, the case is classified as Tx. The tumor size is a measurement of the *invasive* component as determined by the pathologist. Another important refinement of the UICC-AJC pathologic staging system is based on the data that show that micrometastatic involvement of axillary lymph nodes is not associated with the poor prognosis seen with macrometastatic involvement. A comparison of the significance of axillary node micro- and macrometastases has been the subject of a number of clinical-pathologic studies. In one study noted above,[30] occult metastases were demonstrated in axillary lymph nodes by an extended histopathologic technique in 22% of 51 cases that would have been regarded as pathologic Stage I (absent nodal metastases) after "routine" pathologic examination. The prognosis for these node-positive patients was similar to that for patients with negative nodes. In another study from the NSABP,[54] the results for patients with axillary metastases measuring only 2 mm or less in greatest diameter (micrometastases) were compared with results for patients with metastases larger than 2 mm (macrometastases) and those without nodal metastases. Life-table analysis revealed that the survival rates for patients with micrometastases and for those without nodal metastases were similar, and that both of these groups exhibited a significantly higher likelihood of survival than did patients with macrometastases. In another study by Huvos and coworkers from Memorial Hospital in New York City,[55] prognosis also was related to the micrometastatic involvement of axillary nodes. For the 62 patients with no involvement of axillary nodes, the 8-year survival rate was 82% (51 of 62). When micrometastatic involvement (defined as less than 2 mm) of level I axillary nodes was found, the 8-year survival rate was 94% (17 of 18). In comparison, the survival rate was 62% (28 of 45) for patients with macrometastatic involvement of level I axillary nodes. These results all suggest that patients with micrometastases have a prognosis that is more similar to that of patients with negative nodes than to that of patients with positive nodes.

Table 9-13
Relationship of Clinical and Pathologic Axillary Assessment to 10-Year Survival Rates

Clinical Assessment of Axillary Nodes	*Pathologic Assessment of Axillary Nodes* N −	N +	All
N0	77%	57%	71%
N1	72%	34%	44%
All	76%	48%	

(Haagensen CD: Treatment of curable carcinoma of the breast. Int J Radiat Oncol Biol Phys 2:975–980, 1977)

Table 9-14

UICC-AJC Postsurgical Treatment Pathologic Classification

T Primary Tumor

Definitions for the primary tumor for postsurgical-pathologic classification are the same as those for clinical classification.

N Node Involvement

Nx	Criteria to assess regional lymph node metastasis cannot be met
N0	No metastatic regional lymph nodes
N1	Metastasis to movable homolateral axillary nodes, not fixed to one another or to other structures
N1a	Micrometastasis only (none larger than 0.2 cm)
N1b	Gross Metastasis (larger than 0.2 cm)
	I Metastasis more than 0.2 cm but less than 2.0 cm in 1 to 3 nodes.
	II Metastasis more than 0.2 cm but less than 2.0 cm in 4 or more nodes.
	III Extension beyond the lymph node capsule (less than 2.0 cm)
	IV Metastasis in lymph node 2.0 cm or more in dimension
N2	Metastasis to homolateral axillary lymph nodes that are fixed to one another or to other structures
N3	Metastasis to homolateral supraclavicular or infraclavicular lymph notes

Note: If inflammatory carcinoma is diagnozed clinically and the skin biopsy is negative in the absence of palpable mass, the proper T category is Tx.

(American Joint Committee on Cancer: Manual for Staging of Cancer, 3rd ed. Philadelphia, JB Lippincott, 1987)

The post-surgical treatment pathologic classification of the UICC-AJC in 1983 is shown in Table 9-14.

Relationship Between Clinical and Pathologic Staging

Both clinical and pathologic staging provide effective discriminants for the prognosis of treated patients. For the individual patient, prognosis is better determined by the pathologic stage than by the clinical stage; for comparison of results between groups of patients, it is reasonable to use either clinical or pathologic staging. In order to use pathologic staging, however, it is essential that patients in each group have similar degrees of axillary dissection and pathologic analysis. For example, if one group of patients had complete axillary node dissections with clearing of the specimen and multiple sections taken of each cleared lymph node and another group of patients had only lower axillary dissections without clearing of the specimen and only one section taken of each lymph node, it would not be reasonable to compare the results between these two groups using pathologic staging. Many patients would be node positive in the first group and node negative in the second group simply because of the differences in the type of surgery and pathologic analysis. In this setting, the use of clinical staging is preferred.

The results of clinical and pathologic studies have indicated that the single most important prognostic indicator is the number of positive axillary lymph nodes. This is illustrated in data from the ACS[20] (see Table 9-6) and from the NSABP, in which the 10-year results in 614 patients treated with radical mastectomy were related to 38 pathologic and 6 clinical features.[56] The likelihood of treatment failure was most closely correlated with the number of positive axillary nodes (Table 9-15). Among the other clinical features examined, only tumor size was also found to influence the likelihood of treatment failure. This was particularly true in patients with positive nodes as previously shown in other studies. Other factors investigated for their possible influence on prognosis in breast cancer include histopathologic features, tumor growth rate, delay in instituting treatment, patient age, and patient race. These will be discussed in the section that follows.

OTHER FACTORS POSSIBLY INFLUENCING PROGNOSIS IN BREAST CANCER

Histologic Features

The influence of histopathology on prognosis is discussed in Chapter 8. The relationship between staging and histopathology and their combined effect on prognosis will be presented here. Among the first to systematically investigate the relationship between tumor grade and staging were Bloom, Richardson, and Field,[57] from the Middlesex and Royal Marsden Hospitals in London. They examined the 20-year results from 1411 patients treated with radical or modified radical mastectomy at the Middlesex Hospital between 1936 and 1949. They used a system of histologic grading that evaluated the degree of tubule formation and nuclear pleomorphism, and the frequency of hyperchromatic and mitotic figures. Considering the histologic picture as a whole, each tumor was classified as being of high, low, or intermediate malignancy. Tumors were clinically staged using the Manchester

Table 9-15

Relationship Between Number of Positive Nodes and Likelihood of Treatment Failure by the 10th Year

Number of Positive Nodes	*Number of Patients*	*% With Treatment Failure*
0	279	20%
1–3	160	47%
4–6	65	59%
7–12	55	69%
≥ 13	55	87%

(Fisher ER, Sass R, Fisher B, et al: Pathologic findings from the National Surgical Adjuvant Project for breast cancers. Cancer 53:712–723, 1984)

system. The 5- and 15-year survival results according to the clinical stage and grade are shown in Table 9-16 and indicate that the histopathologic features of the tumor influence outcome independent of clinical stage. Of note, the importance of tumor grade was more apparent at 5 years than at 15 years, suggesting that tumor grade is principally a reflection of the pace of the disease rather than an indicator of the likelihood of metastasis. These histopathologic features were interpreted by Bloom and Richardson to indicate the inherent virulence of the tumor, aside from its anatomic extent.

Bloom and co-workers also examined the impact of the relationship between tumor grade and pathologic stage on prognosis (Table 9-17). Tumor grade was found to be correlated with node involvement. Seventy-one percent of grade 3 tumors had node involvement compared with only 44% of grade 1 tumors. Table 9-17 indicates that tumor grade independently influences prognosis apart from stage, particularly at 5 years. The results at 15 years, however, indicated poor outcome for all groups with positive nodes, irrespective of tumor grade. It should be stressed that lymph node involvement in this study was not assessed quantitatively—that is, by the number of positive nodes. Involvement was scored only as positive or negative, since complete axillary dissection and pathologic analysis were not routinely performed in this series.

Investigators at the Institut Gustave-Roussy in France have also evaluated the effect of pathologic stage and grade on prognosis.[58] Full axillary dissections and analysis were performed, and the tumor grade was assessed by Bloom's rules. Multivariate analysis indicated that nodal status and histologic grade were the main prognostic features but that tumor size also had some independent effect on prognosis. The influence of nodal status and grade on the 7-year relapse-free survival rate among 528 patients treated with radical mastectomy is shown in Table 9-18. Tumor grade was significantly correlated with node involvement. Only 15% of grade 1 patients had four or more positive nodes, compared with 34% of grade 3 patients. The results are similar to those obtained by Bloom at 5 years, in that both tumor grade and pathologic stage appear to influence outcome. Long-term results are not yet available from this study.

The findings from the NSABP study on prognostic factors[56] also confirm the importance of tumor grade on outcome. In this study, tumor grade was based on assessment of both tubule formation and nuclear grade, similar to Bloom's grading. The NSABP results indicate that tumor grade is significantly correlated with involvement of axillary nodes but is also an important prognostic factor. It should be noted, however, that the quantitative assessment of axillary node involvement was a much stronger predictive factor than tumor grade. The Cramer V scale (a measure of predictive value) was 0.45 for lymph node involvement and only 0.10 for grade.

Haybittle and colleagues from Nottingham also evaluated the importance of tumor grade in a multivariate analysis in which a number of other clinical and histopathologic features were also assessed.[59] They studied 500 patients who were treated with total mastectomy and triple-node biopsy (low axilla, axillary apex, and internal mammary region). Complete axillary dissection was not performed. Histologic grade was assessed by the rules of Bloom and Richardson. Follow-up was only 1 to 6 years. The results of the multivariate analysis were summarized for each prognostic factor in terms of the beta score. The beta score for lymph node stage was 5.29; for tumor size, 2.92; and for histologic grade, 4.56. All of these beta values were statistically significant. These results also indicate that tumor grade is an important prognostic indicator for short-term survival.

Another aspect of histopathology relates to the influence of manifestations of host defenses on survival. Black and associates, from the United States, and Hamlin and co-workers, from England, have emphasized that in addition to the extent of the disease (staging) and its inherent

Table 9-16
Corrected 5- and 15-Year Survival by Clinical Stage and Grade

Grade	*Clinical Stage* I	II	III
5-Year Results			
Grade 1	91%	76%	74%
Grade 2	76%	46%	32%
Grade 3	74%	28%	21%
15-Year Results			
Grade 1	62%	40%	37%
Grade 2	61%	23%	11%
Grade 3	57%	13%	11%

(Bloom HJG, Field JR: Impact of tumor grade and host resistance on survival of women with breast cancer. Cancer 28:1580–1589, 1971)

Table 9-17
Corrected 5- and 15-Year Survival by Axillary Node Involvement and Grade

Grade	*Node Involvement* Negative	Positive
5-Year Results		
Grade 1	86%	68%
Grade 2	68%	33%
Grade 3	64%	19%
15-Year Results		
Grade 1	49%	15%
Grade 2	29%	11%
Grade 3	25%	7%

(Bloom HJG, Field JR: Impact of tumor grade and host resistance on survival of women with breast cancer. Cancer 28:1580–1589, 1971)

Table 9-18
Seven-Year Relapse-Free Survival by Axillary Node Involvement and Grade

	Number of Positive Axillary Nodes							
Grade	*n=0*	*Number of Patients*	*n=1–3*	*Number of Patients*	*n≥4*	*Number of Patients*	*All*	*Number of Patients*
Grade 1	93%	61	84%	27	83%	15	89%	103
Grade 2	75%	105	70%	101	41%	62	65%	268
Grade 3	70%	57	48%	46	40%	54	54%	157
All grades	79%	223	67%	174	45%	131	60%	528

(Sarrazin D, Le M, Mouriesse H, et al: Radiotherapeutic studies on breast cancer at Villejuif. Cancer Bull 34:242–249, 1982)

virulence (grading), the finding of histopathologic evidence of host defense also influences outcome. Black and Spur investigated the importance of the extent to which the sinusoids of the axillary nodes are distended by elongated histiocytes (sinus histiocytosis) as a manifestation of host defense.[60] Sinus histiocytosis is a well-recognized nonspecific immunologic response observed in lymph nodes. Black and Spur noted a direct relationship between the detection of sinus histiocytosis and survival. In a later study, Cutler and colleagues attempted to evaluate the relative effect of sinus histiocytosis, nuclear grade, and stage on outcome.[61] They studied the results of 879 patients from the Norwegian Radium Hospital treated with radical mastectomy between 1951 and 1959. Both nuclear grade and sinus histiocytosis were correlated with node involvement, but they also independently influenced outcome for both node-negative and node-positive patients, although this influence was more obvious for node-positive patients. Since node status was the most significant prognostic feature, the influence of these other features was examined in relation to the extent of node involvement. Figure 9-11 indicates that nuclear grade and sinus histiocytosis each have a small influence on the 5-year survival rates independent of the degree of node involvement. Cutler and colleagues also examined the interrelationship between nuclear grade, sinus histiocytosis, and node involvement. Within groups of node involvement (nodes negative, 0 to one-third of nodes positive, or more than one-third positive), both nuclear grade and sinus histiocytosis influenced 5-year survival. In particular, patients with more than one-third of nodes positive but with sinus histiocytosis and good nuclear grade had survival at 5 years comparable to patients with negative nodes but without sinus histiocytosis and with poor nuclear grade. These data provide the strongest support for sinus histiocytosis as an independent prognostic factor.

Alderson and colleagues also evaluated the relative significance of prognostic factors in a group of 258 patients treated with radical mastectomy at the Royal Marsden Hospital between 1935 and 1945.[62] Follow-up of 15 years or longer was available on all patients. Of note, during this time, patients presented with more advanced disease than in more recent series; the large majority had Manchester Stage III disease and had positive nodes. A multivariate analysis was performed in which the influence of various clinical and histopathologic features was assessed and was summarized as a percentage of the total variance influencing survival. Clinical and pathologic stage were the most significant factors in outcome, but both tumor grade and host-defense response influenced survival. Tumor grading (similar to Bloom's) contributed 3.4% of the total variance ($p<0.01$) and "host-defense response" contributed 2.9% of the total variance ($p<0.01$). Host-defense response was derived from a combined score of five items, including lymphatic and plasmacytic infiltration around and within the tumor; the number, size, and activity of germinal centers in the axillary nodes; the immunoblast content of the axillary nodes; and the plasma cell content in the axillary nodes. None of these individual items significantly contributed to outcome. The presence of sinus histiocytosis was also not significantly related to outcome.

The importance of host-defense manifestation as a prognostic feature has not been consistently noted. In the NSABP study, sinus histiocytosis was correlated with the extent of lymph node involvement but was not an independent prognostic feature.[56] Also, neither the degree nor the type of cell reaction to the tumor influenced outcome. Kister and colleagues, from Columbia, evaluated the importance of sinus histiocytosis among 318 patients with Stage A breast cancer treated with radical mastectomy and followed for at least 10 years.[63] No relationship between sinus histiocytosis and survival was noted. Similarly, in the multivariate analysis by Haybittle and associates, sinus histiocytosis was not found to influence outcome.[59] These results indicate that host defense has not been consistently found to be an important prognostic factor.

In considering the possible importance of these various histopathologic features, it is important to stress that the level of concordance between different observers in assessing these features is often low. In a study from the Eastern Cooperative Oncology Group (ECOG), 11 surgical pathologists evaluated specimens for nuclear grade, lymphoid reaction, and sinus histiocytosis.[64] Their findings were compared, and agreement on these various items was quite low. For example, among three reviewers of nuclear grade, there was complete agreement in only 34%

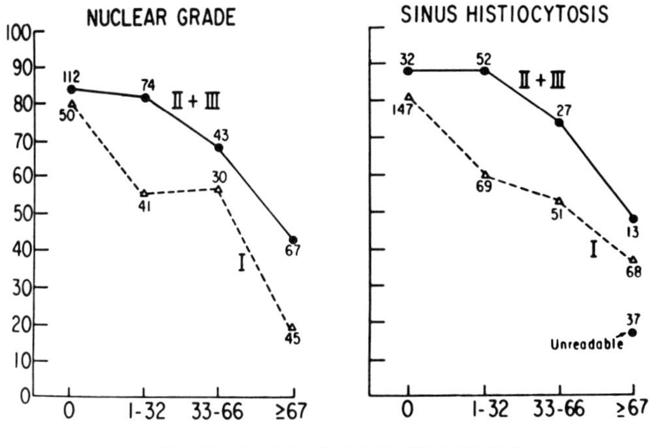

FIGURE 9-11. Five-year relative survival related to the degree of node involvement and nuclear grade and sinus histiocytosis. (Cutler SJ, Black MM, Mork T, et al: Further observations on prognostic factors in cancer of the female breast. Cancer: 24:653–667, 1969)

of cases; among five reviewers, there was complete agreement in only 17% of cases. This difficulty in assigning reproducible scores poses a significant practical problem to the use of those histopathologic features.

In assessing the impact of histopathologic features on outcome, it appears that tumor grade but not host-defense response has been consistently found to affect prognosis. However, this effect of grade is more obvious in relation to clinical stage. Tumor grade is significantly correlated with node involvement, so that the influence of tumor grade in the context of full pathologic staging is diminished. Furthermore, this influence of grade is more prominent in studies with shorter follow-up, suggesting that grade may exert a greater effect on the initial force of mortality than on the ultimate mortality rate. Patients with positive nodes appear to have a poor long-term prognosis regardless of tumor grade.

Delay

The importance of prompt treatment for breast cancer has generally been accepted without question. Since the disease is believed to run a uniformly progressive course, it is natural to assume that prompt treatment offers the best hope for long-term survival. However, the data supporting this view are somewhat tenuous.

There are significant practical problems in assessing the importance of delay as a prognostic factor. One problem is that the extent of delay is not always clearly discernible. Patients who delay seeking treatment may also have denied the existence of their problem in the first place. A more important methodologic problem relates to integrating the combined effects of delay and stage. Within a given stage, patients with the longest delay may have the most indolent disease and those with the shortest delay may have the most aggressive disease. As a result, examining results within a given stage may be misleading. An example of this problem is illustrated in the results reported by Robbins and Bross, from Memorial Hospital.[65] They examined the results of 1281 patients treated with radical mastectomy between 1940 and 1943. In a multivariate analysis of tumor size, axillary node involvement, and delay, delay did not have a statistically significant impact on survival.

Bloom attempted to demonstrate the importance of delay by evaluating results in relation to histologic grade (a measure of the inherent aggressiveness of the tumor) as well as stage.[66] When he first looked at survival in terms of delay, there was no apparent relation; survival was independent of the extent of delay. Bloom then related the likelihood of a patient's presenting with a Stage I cancer to delay and grade (Table 9-19). It is clear from these data that the likelihood of presenting with a Stage I cancer is directly related to both grade and delay. Since the cure rate of Stage I cancers is high, Bloom concluded that delay was a significant factor in prognosis.

The problem of demonstrating the value of prompt treatment is similar to the difficulties in demonstrating the value of mammographic screening, discussed in Chapter 5. There are potential serious biases in comparing the outcome of groups of varying delay. The only scientific method of verifying the importance of delay would be to perform a randomized trial in which some patients were allocated to delayed treatment and others to prompt treatment. Such a trial is obviously unethical. The demonstration in randomized trials that mammographic screening is of value[25,26] and the data presented above by Koscielny and colleagues[18] provide strong evidence that prompt local treatment is of value.

Growth Rate

One attempt to improve the estimation of prognosis has been to incorporate some factor related to tumor growth rate, as demonstrated by the patient's history. Charlson and Feinstein[13] described such a method, which involved identifying the first clinical manifestation of the disease observed by the patient or physician and then noting the progression interval before treatment and the occurrence of prognostically unfavorable transition events during that

Table 9-19
Incidence of Stage I Tumors Related to Delay and Grade

Delay (Months)	*Grade 1*	*Grade 2*	*Grade 3*
≤3	56%	37%	26%
6–12	39%	34%	22%
>24	25%	20%	8%

(Bloom HJG: The influence of delay on the natural history and prognosis of breast cancer. Br J Cancer 19:228, 1965)

interval. By the use of these two features (progression interval and transition events), tumors were classified as slow, intermediate, or rapid. Slow tumors had a progression interval of 4 months or longer without a transition event. Rapid tumors had some transition event, regardless of progression interval. Intermediate tumors had a progression interval of less than 4 months without a transition event. Any number of local or regional events (such as a change in the size or consistency of the breast or the appearance of nodes) were classified as transition events. They examined the results of 685 patients treated at Yale-New Haven Hospital between 1962 and 1969 in relation to TNM stage or axillary involvement, and the growth rate class as defined above. Within each TNM stage, the use of the growth rate class improved prognosis. Similarly, within groups based on lymph node status, growth rate class improved prognosis (Fig. 9-12).

The utility of the growth rate classification was also assessed by Boyd and colleagues, from the Princess Margaret Hospital.[67] They examined the results of 756 patients treated at their institution between 1965 and 1972. Patients were classified by tumor growth rate as described by Charlson and Feinstein, except that patients with a transition event and an interval of 4 months or longer were classified as intermediate rather than rapid. Like Charlson and Feinstein, they found that the ability to estimate survival was improved by use of the growth rate class in addition to either clinical or pathologic staging (Table 9-20). They also related tumor growth to histologic grade and found a positive correlation. For example, 33% of grade 3 tumors were classified as fast, but only 12% of grade 1 tumors were classified as fast. In addition, the use of the tumor growth rate classification improved the prognostic value of the histologic grade. These results confirm the utility of using a tumor growth classification in addition to stage as an aid in the determination of prognosis.

With the use of mass screening by mammography, it is also possible to estimate growth rates by the findings obtained in serial mammograms.[9,10] The relation between the mammographic findings and prognosis is illustrated in the data of Lundgren, from Sweden.[68] In his county in Sweden, 91% of women 40 to 69 years of age participate in a breast cancer screening program. Between 1974 and 1981, there were 280 evaluable cases of breast cancer in which doubling times could be calculated. When a prior screening mammogram did not reveal any evidence of malignancy, it was assumed that the tumor measured 0.1 mm at that time. One hundred thirty-nine cases were diagnosed by repeat screening and had an average doubling time of 5.0 months. Twenty-seven cases were diagnosed by repeat screening, but in retrospect an obvious cancer had been overlooked on the prior mammogram. These cases had an average doubling time of 12.4 months. One hundred fourteen cases were diagnosed during the interval between scheduled mammographic screenings, and they had an average doubling time of 2.2 months. There was a clear relation between doubling time and 5-year survival. Of the seven cases with doubling times less than 1 month, only one (14%) was alive at 5 years, and of the 32 cases with doubling times between one and three months, 21 (66%) were alive at 5 years. Of the 12 cases with doubling times greater than 3 months, all 12 (100%) were alive at 5 years. Similar findings relating growth rate estimates based on serial mammograms to prognosis have been obtained in the United States in the Breast Cancer Detection Demonstration Project.[69,70]

FIGURE 9-12. Survival by histologic status of the axillary nodes and growth rate class. (Charlson ME, Feinstein AR: A new clinical index of growth rate in the staging of breast cancer. Am J Med 69:527–536, 1980)

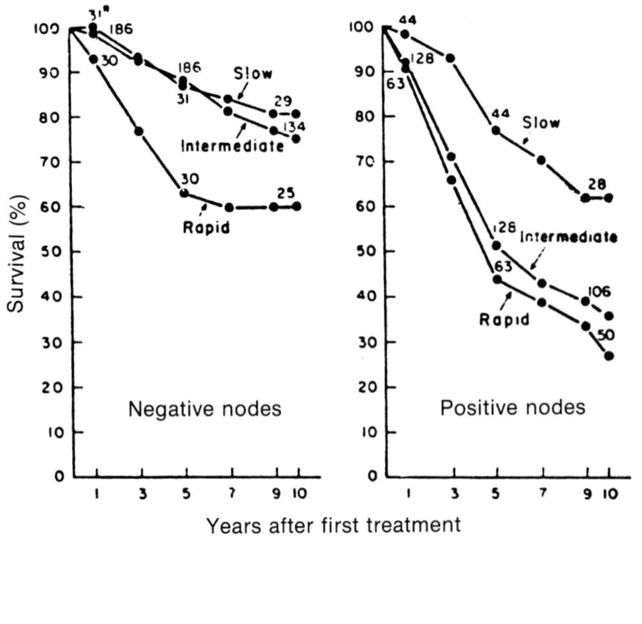

Cell Kinetics As a Prognostic Factor

Recent studies have suggested that cell kinetics and the DNA content of the tumor are important prognostic factors.[71] The parameter of cell kinetics that has been studied most extensively is the labeling index (LI). The LI can be determined by incubating tumor cells with 3H-thymidine and counting the percentage of cells that take up the 3H-thymidine by autoradiography. Since thymidine is primarily taken up by cells in the DNA synthetic or S-phase of the cycle, the LI is a measure of the percentage of cells in S-phase. More recently, the LI has been determined by the use of DNA flow cytometry. By flow cytometry, the entire partition of the cell cycle can be evaluated using DNA-specific fluorescent stains. In addition, flow cytometry can determine the degree of abnormality of DNA content (aneuploidy) in the tumor cells.

The LI has been shown to be an important prognostic factor. This is illustrated by the data of Tubiana and colleagues, from the Institut Gustave-Roussy.[72] They studied tumor samples from 128 breast cancer patients seen at the institution between 1972 and 1973, 96 of whom had diagnostic axillary dissections. The likelihood of relapse and death was analyzed by the LI level among the 125 patients

Table 9-20
Influence of Nodal Status and Growth Rate Class on the Relative Death Rate

Growth Rate Class	*Lymph Node Status*		
	N = 0	*N = 1–3*	*N ≥ 4*
Slow	0.20	0.58	0.99
Intermediate	0.61	0.84	1.97
Fast	0.62	1.23	1.87

(Boyd NF, Meakin JW, Hayward JL, et al: Clinical estimation of the growth rate of breast cancer. Cancer 48:1037–1042, 1981)

Table 9-21
Ten-Year Results Related to Labeling Index

Labeling Index Levels	*Number of Patients*	*Number of Relapses*	*Number of Deaths*
Low (< 0.25)	20	5 (25%)	6 (30%)
Intermediate (0.25–3.83)	84	45 (53%)	44 (52%)
High (≥ 3.84)	21	13 (62%)	12 (37%)

(Tubiana M, Pejovic MH, Chavaudra N, et al: The long term prognostic significance of the thymidine labeling index in breast cancer. Int J Cancer 33:441–445, 1984)

evaluable at 10 years (Table 9-21). The results indicate that the LI is highly predictive of both relapse and death. Similar findings have been described by Meyer and colleagues[73] and by Silvestrini and associates.[74]

The relation between LI and other prognostic factors was also investigated by Meyer and co-workers.[73] They found that LI was significantly correlated with the histologic features of the tumor but not with tumor size or the number of positive axillary nodes. A multivariate analysis was performed on the results of 186 patients with a median follow-up of approximately 2 years. This analysis indicated that axillary node involvement ($x^2 = 18.4$, $p<0.0001$), LI ($x^2 = 10.6$, $p=0.001$) and nuclear grade ($x^2 = 7.8$, $p=0.005$) had an independent influence on the likelihood of relapse-free survival. Tubiana and colleagues similarly found that LI was not correlated with node involvement and that LI was an important prognostic factor independent of clinical and pathologic staging.[72] They found in a multivariate analysis of their results that LI, tumor size, and tumor grade (and not axillary node involvement) were the main independent prognostic factors. Silvestrini and associates[74] also did not find any correlation between LI and tumor size or node involvement. LI was found to be a highly significant prognostic factor for node-negative patients. All these results indicate that LI is correlated with tumor grade and is an important prognostic factor independent of clinical or pathologic staging.

LI has been shown to be inversely related to the level of steroid hormone receptors. Steroid hormone receptors (estrogen receptor protein [ERP] and progesterone receptor protein [PRP]) have both been investigated as prognostic factors. At the present time, the relative prognostic importance of LI and steroid hormone receptors has not been clearly delineated. (This issue is discussed in greater detail in Chapter 8.) It is also important to note that LI is not a readily obtainable study in most institutions. Its determination by autoradiography is tedious, and flow cytometry is not generally available at this time. This limits the utility of LI as a prognostic factor in clinical practice.

More recently, flow cytometry has been used to investigate the relation between aneuploidy and prognosis. Patients with aneuploid tumors have been found to have a worse short-term prognosis than patients with diploid tumor.[75,76] The relation between DNA content, LI, and steroid hormone receptors as independent prognostic factors remains to be elucidated. McDivitt and colleagues found that DNA content, S-phase fraction (SPF) as measured by flow cytometry, and estrogen receptor protein were all correlated.[77] It should also be noted that flow cytometry offers the possibility of even more sophisticated characterization of a tumor by the use of monoclonal antibody probes.

Age

The effect of age on prognosis has been investigated in a number of studies, but the results have not been consistent.[78–86] There are a number of reasons for this failure to determine clearly if age is a prognostic factor. Many of the studies on age fail to adjust the results by stage. This is important, since it is possible that patients in different age-groups may present at different stages. In some studies, young patients appear to present at later stages than older patients. This is perhaps so because they and their physicians are less suspicious of the disease in the younger age-group. It is also somewhat more difficult to detect abnormalities in young women because their breasts are firmer and more cystic than those of older women. There is also the problem of adjusting for intercurrent deaths. If intercurrent deaths are not accounted for fully, the breast cancer mortality in older patients may be overestimated. An additional problem is that the various studies select different age-groups to examine. These methodologic problems in relating age and prognosis probably account for the wide variation in reported results.

The evidence available from a number of recent large studies supports the view that, overall, the disease has a more favorable prognosis in younger women. In the study by Hibberd and colleagues,[5] the long-term prognosis (given as relative survival) of women registered in the National Cancer Registry of New Zealand between 1950 and 1954 was evaluated (Table 9-22). Relative survival was calculated by dividing the observed survival rate for a given age-group by the expected survival rate for a group of persons of similar age from the normal population. These data suggest that breast cancer has a more favorable prognosis in younger patients, particularly with follow-up beyond 10 years. Relative survival was fairly constant beyond 10 years in women 20 to 34 years of age but showed an increasingly progressive decline with advancing age-groups. This study did not adjust for the stage of the disease.

Another long-term study was performed by Langlands and associates,[87] from Edinburgh, on 3878 patients treated between 1954 and 1964. Patients were subdivided into three groups: 1064 who were premenopausal, 450 who were menopausal (less than 5 years past the menopause), and 2166 who were postmenopausal. They examined the annual percentage of patients dying (of all causes) according to their menopausal status (excluding Stage IV) and found that premenopausal patients had the best prognosis overall. Menopausal patients had the worst prognosis during the first 5 years, but after 5 years, postmenopausal patients had the worst prognosis. These results were not corrected for death from other causes or for differences in stage but also suggest that younger patients (i.e., premenopausal patients) have a more favorable prognosis than other patients.

Similar findings have been noted in cancer registry studies of Norway, Sweden, and the United States. The Norwegian study[88] evaluated 14,731 cases of breast cancer that had been reported to the registry between 1953 and 1967. Follow-up times ranged from 5 to 18 years. These results were adjusted for stage, using a staging system similar to the Manchester system. There was a correlation between age and stage, in that older patients presented with more advanced stages. Among the patients younger than 45 years of age, 8% presented as Stage III or IV, compared with 11% of patients between 45 and 54 years, 17% of patients between 55 and 74 years, and 43% of patients 75 or older. The authors found that the distribution of time to death was best fit by a log-normal model that contained a term for a cured population. The results, however, did not indicate that a cured population actually existed, so that "percent cured" can only be taken as an indication of long-term survival corrected for deaths due to other causes. Table 9-23 shows the results of this study subdivided by age and stage. These results indicate that younger patients not only have a better prognosis overall but a better prognosis within each stage. The Swedish study[89] evaluated the records of 12,319 women who had breast cancer and who had been registered in the Swedish National Registry between 1959 and 1963. The relative 20-year survival rates were 51%, 41%, 34%, and 16% for age-groups 40 to 44, 50 to 54, 60 to 69, and 70 to 79 years, respectively. Patients younger than 40 years diverged from the general trend, with a 20-year survival rate of 44%. Similar findings were noted in the American study.[90]

The above results suggest that younger women (generally defined in relation to the menopause) have a better prognosis than older women. There is some evidence to suggest that the small subset of very young patients, younger than 30 years, does worse as a group than other

Table 9-22
Relative Survival of Women with Breast Cancer by Age (New Zealand)

Age	*Number of Patients*	*Relative Survival*		
		10 Years	*20 Years*	*30 Years*
20–34	60	0.37	0.35	0.36
35–44	276	0.41	0.32	0.27
45–54	463	0.41	0.31	0.27
55–64	452	0.34	0.22	0.19
≥65	760	0.34	0.21	0.00

(Hibberd AD, Harwood LJ, Wells JE: Long term prognosis of women with breast cancer in New Zealand: Study of survival to 30 years. Br Med J 286:1777–1779, 1983)

Table 9-23
Prognosis by Stage and Age Expressed as "percent cured"

Stage	*Age (Years)* < 55	*Age (Years)* ≥ 55
I	64 ± 3%	45 ± 6%
II	32 ± 2%	20 ± 2%
III	28 ± 4%	14 ± 3%
IV	0%	2 ± 1%
Total	44 ± 1%	26 ± 2%

(Rutqvist LE, Wallgren A, Nilsson B: Is breast cancer a curable disease? Cancer 56:898–902, 1985)

patients. Noyes and colleagues,[91] from the M.D. Anderson Hospital, performed a retrospective study of 125 patients who were 30 years of age or younger and who had localized invasive breast cancer treated at their institution between 1945 and 1977, and they compared their results with 3380 similar patients 31 years of age or older. The 5-year rate of disease-free survival of the younger women was 43%, compared with 59% for the older women ($p<0.01$). When the results were analyzed by pathologic nodal status, the younger patients did significantly worse than the older patients when nodes were negative (5-year rate of disease-free survival 54% versus 77%, $p < 0.05$). When nodes were positive, the outcome was similar for the two age-groups. Haagensen[92] compared the 10-year rate of survival of 46 patients 30 years of age or younger with Stage A breast cancer to the entire group of 727 patients with Stage A breast cancer. The results were somewhat worse for the younger patients, both in the node-negative (60% versus 78%) and node-positive (48% versus 59%) subgroups. Ribeiro and Swindell analyzed the long-term results of 803 patients less than 40 years old treated at the Christie Hospital.[93] The rate of survival was lower for patients 30 years old or younger, compared with patients between 31 and 39 years of age. This was true for both Stage I and II cancers.

These findings on the relation between prognosis and age need to be examined in light of the kinetic analysis described above. Kinetic analyses have generally revealed that younger patients have a higher LI. This finding was most obvious in the Milan experience, in which the median LI was 4.7 for patients 50 years old or younger, compared with 1.9 for patients older than 50 ($p< 0.001$).[74] This finding is also in keeping with the observation that younger women are less likely to have ERP-positive tumors. Since high LI and ERP-negative tumors have been associated with a poor prognosis, it is surprising that these tumors are more common in younger patients, a group reported to have a more favorable prognosis. There is no clear explanation for these apparently conflicting observations. It may be related to the fact that the prognostic value of LI is only available on short-term follow-up. It is possible that these tumors may be more lethal in the short run but have a better prognosis in the long run. This explanation is suggested by the data from Hibberd (Table 9-22) and from the National Cancer Institute's End Results Program.[94] In this latter study, the relative survival segregated by stage over the first 5 years was worst for the patients younger than 35, but at 20 years their relative survival was the best (Fig. 9-13).

Race

Breast cancer appears to be a more lethal disease in black women than in white women in the United States.[95–97] This is shown in the data obtained in the 1982 National Survey of Breast Cancer by the American College of Surgeons.[98] In this survey, the disease was diagnosed at a later stage in blacks than in whites. Forty-five percent of whites

FIGURE 9-13. Conditional 5-year relative survival for patients with localized *(A)* or regional *(B)* breast cancer analyzed by age (NCI End Results). (Hankey BF, Steinhorn SC: Long term patient survival for some of the more frequently occurring cancers. Cancer 50:1904–1912, 1982)

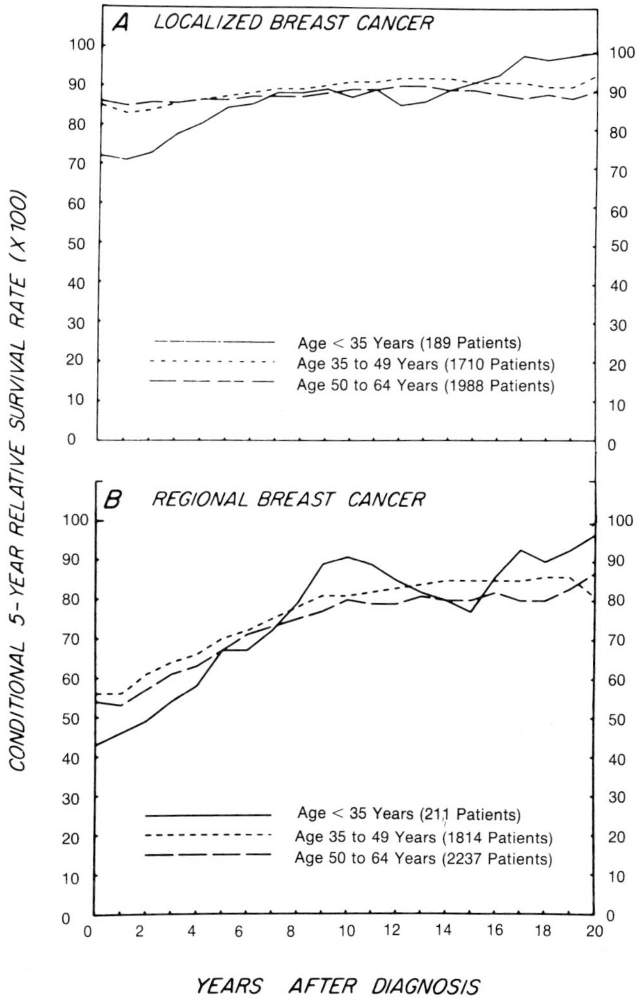

had T1 lesions, compared with 34% of blacks. Similarly, 58% of whites had negative nodes, compared with 48% of blacks. Survival was analyzed within groups by nodal status: negative nodes, one to three positive nodes, and four or more positive nodes. Within each group, the rate of survival was worse for blacks than for whites. In addition, a multivariate analysis of race, clinical stage, age, estrogen receptor status, nodal status, and tumor location showed that race was a significant factor ($p=0.01$).

Obesity

Obesity has been implicated as a prognostic factor in breast cancer survival.[99,100] Donegan evaluated survival rates in relation to obesity in 83 patients treated with mastectomy. Obesity was based on a ratio of weight to height according to an obesity index. Thirty-four patients had indices above 2.45 and were similar to other patients in regard to age. They had a small increased likelihood of positive axillary nodes (44% versus 35%) but a significantly greater likelihood of recurrence (41% versus 8%), with a mean follow-up of approximately 2 years. The effect of obesity was evaluated in two later studies,[101,102] but it was not found to be a statistically significant factor when adjusted for stage.

ASSESSMENT

The data presented in this chapter demonstrate that breast cancer is a disease with a long natural history and a high propensity for systemic involvement. Because of the long natural history and onset typically at middle age, it is difficult to demonstrate, in a strict sense, that breast cancer is a curable disease. It is clear, however, that a significant percentage of patients with treated breast cancer will live out their lives without further evidence of the disease. A number of factors have been shown to influence the prognosis of the disease, the most important being stage. Clinical staging can provide an excellent guide to prognosis for groups of patients, but the use of pathologic staging provides a more exact guide to prognosis for the individual patient. The number of positive axillary lymph nodes appears to be the single most important prognostic factor. In the experience of most investigators, the histologic appearance of the tumor (tumor grade) can also be used to estimate prognosis and is useful even as an adjunct to staging. The use of tumor grading, however, is limited by the lack of agreement between pathologists in its scoring. More recently, flow cytometry has been used to measure the S-phase fraction of the tumor and its DNA content, and in the future, this may be used to provide a more reproducible method to judge tumor grade.

REFERENCES

1. Bloom HJG, Richardson WW, Harrier EJ: Natural history of untreated breast cancer (1805–1933). Br Med J 2:213–221, 1962
2. Fox MS: On the diagnosis and treatment of breast cancer. JAMA 241:489–494, 1979
3. Haybittle JL: Commentaries on research in breast disease. 3:181–194, 1983
4. Brinkley D, Haybittle JL: Long term survival of women with breast cancer. Lancet 1:1118, 1984
5. Hibberd AD, Harwood LJ, Wells JE: Long term prognosis of women with breast cancer in New Zealand: Study of survival to 30 years. Br Med J 286:1777–1779, 1983
6. Rutqvist LE, Wallgren A: Long term survival of 458 young breast cancer patients. Cancer 55:658–665, 1985
7. Adair F, Berg J, Joubert L: Long term follow-up of breast cancer patients: The thirty year report. Cancer 33:1145–1150, 1974
8. Collins V, Loeffler RK, Tivey H: Observations on growth rates of human tumors. Am J Roentgenol 76:988–1000, 1956
9. Gershon-Cohen J, Berger SM, Klickstein HS: Roentgenography of breast cancer moderating concept of "biological predeterminism." Cancer 16:961–964, 1963
10. Fournier DV, Weber E, Hoeffken W, et al: Growth rate of 147 mammary carcinomas. Cancer 45:2198–2207, 1980
11. Kusama S, Spratt JS, Donegan WL, et al: The gross rates of growth of human mammary carcinoma. Cancer 30:594–599, 1972
12. Pearlman AW: Breast cancer—influence of growth rate on prognosis and treatment evaluation. Cancer 38:1826–1833, 1976
13. Charlson ME, Feinstein AR: A new clinical index of growth rate in the staging of breast cancer. Am J Med 69:527–536, 1980
14. Tubiana M, Malaise EP: Growth rate and cell kinetics in human tumors. In Symington T, Carter RL (eds): On Scientific Functions of Oncology, pp 126–136. Chicago, Year Book Medical Publishers, 1976
15. Spratt JS, Donegan WL: Cancer of the Breast, pp 133–134. Philadelphia, WB Saunders, 1971
16. Nemoto T, Natarajan N, Bedwani R, et al: Breast cancer in the medial half: Results of the 1978 national survey of the American College of Surgeons. Cancer 51:1333–1338, 1983
17. Fisher B, Slack NH, Ausman RK, et al: Location of breast carcinoma and prognosis. Surg Gynecol Obstet 129:705–716, 1969
18. Koscielny S, Tubiana M, Le MG, et al: Breast cancer: Relationship between the size of the primary tumour and the probability of metastatic dissemination. Br J Cancer 49:709–715, 1984
19. Schottenfeld D, Nash AG, Robbins GF, et al: Ten-year results of the treatment of primary operable breast carcinoma. Cancer 38:1001–1007, 1976
20. Nemoto T, Vana J, Bedwani RN, et al: Management and survival of female breast cancer: Results of a national survey by the American College of Surgeons. Cancer 45:2917–2924, 1980
21. Fisher B, Slack NH, Bross IDJ, et al: Cancer of the breast: Size of neoplasm and prognosis. Cancer 24:1071–1080, 1969
22. Igot JP, LeGal Y: Age des andeopathies metastiques dans le cancer mammaire. Ann Anat Pathol 13:449–459, 1968
23. Charbit A, Malaise EP, Tubiana M: Relation between the pathological nature and the growth rate of human tumors. Eur J Cancer 7:307–315, 1971
24. Steel GG: Growth Kinetics of Tumours. New York, Oxford University Press, 1977
25. Tabar L, Fagerberg CJ, Gad A, et al: Reduction in mortality from breast cancer after mass screening with mammography. Lancet 1:829–832, 1985

26. Shapiro S, Venet W, Strax P, et al: Ten to fourteen year effect of screening on breast cancer mortality. J Natl Cancer Inst 69:349–355, 1982
27. Haagensen CD: Diseases of the Breast, 3rd ed, p 656. Philadelphia, WB Saunders, 1986
28. Haagensen CD: Diseases of the Breast, 3rd ed, p 655. Philadelphia, WB Saunders, 1986
29. Smith JA, Gamez-Araujo JJ, Gallagher HS, et al: Carcinoma of the breast: Analysis of total lymph node involvement versus level of metastasis. Cancer 39:527–532, 1977
30. Pickren JW. Significance of occult metastases. Cancer 14:1266–1271, 1961
31. Butcher HR. Radical mastectomy for mammary carcinoma. Ann Surg 170:833–884, 1969
32. Haagensen CD: Diseases of the Breast, 3rd ed, p 656. Philadelphia, WB Saunders, 1986
33. Bucalossi P, Veronesi V, Zingo L, et al: Enlarged mastectomy for breast cancer: Review of 1213 cases. Am J Roentgenol Radium Ther Nucl Med 111:119–122, 1971
34. Valagussa P, Bonadonna G, Veronesi V: Patterns of relapse and survival following radical mastectomy. Cancer 41:1170–1178, 1978
35. Haagensen CD: Treatment of curable carcinoma of the breast. Int J Radiat Oncol Biol Phys 2:975–980, 1977
36. Fisher B, Slack NH, Katrych D, et al: Ten-year followup results of patients with carcinoma of the breast in a cooperative clinical trial evaluating surgical adjuvant chemotherapy. Surg Gynecol Obstet 140:528–534, 1975
37. Spratt JS, Donegan WL; Carcinoma of the Breast, p 136. Philadelphia, WB Saunders, 1971
38. Payne WS, Taylor WF, Khonsari S, et al: Surgical treatment of breast cancer: Trends and factors affecting survival. Arch Surg 101:105–113, 1970
39. Haagensen CD: Diseases of the Breast, 2nd ed, p 405. Philadelphia, WB Saunders, 1971
40. Handley RS: Carcinoma of the breast. Ann R Coll Surg Engl 57:59–66, 1975
41. Veronesi U, Cascinelli N, Greco M, et al: Prognosis of breast cancer patients after mastectomy and dissection of internal mammary nodes. Ann Surg 202:702–707, 1985
42. Haagensen CD: Diseases of the Breast, 2nd ed, p 423. Philadelphia, WB Saunders, 1971
43. LaCour J, Le M, Caceres E, et al: Radical mastectomy versus radical mastectomy plus internal mammary dissection. Cancer 51:1941–1943, 1983
44. Veronesi U, Cascinelli N, Buffalino R, et al: Risk of internal mammary lymph node metastasis and its relevance on prognosis in breast cancer patients. Ann Surg 198:681–684, 1983
45. Dahl-Iversen E: Recherches sur les metastases microscopiques des cancers du sein dans les ganglions lymphatiques parasternaux et susclaviculaires. Mem Acad Clin 78:651–663, 1952
46. Halsted WS: The results of radical operations for the cure of cancer of the breast. Ann Surg 46:1–19, 1907
47. Warren S, Witman EM: Studies on tumor metastases: The distribution of metastases in cancer of the breast. Surg Gynecol Obstet 57:81, 1937
48. Saphillo O, Parker ML: Metastases of primary carcinoma of the breast with special reference to spleen, adrenal glands and ovaries. Arch Surg 42:1003, 1941
49. Haagensen CD: Diseases of the Breast, 2nd ed, p 426. Philadelphia, WB Saunders, 1971
50. Cutler SJ, Zippin C, Asire AJ: The prognostic significance of palpable lymph nodes in cancer of the breast. Cancer 23:243–250, 1969
51. Zippin C: Comparison of the International and American Systems for the staging of breast cancer. J Natl Cancer Inst 36:53–62, 1966
52. Cutler SJ, Axtell LM, Schottenfeld D: Clinical assessment of lymph nodes in carcinoma of the breast. Surg Gynecol Obstet 131:41–52, 1970
53. Haagensen CD: Treatment of curable carcinoma of the breast. Int J Radiat Oncol Biol Phys 2:975–980, 1977
54. Fisher ER, Swamidoss S, Lee CH, et al: Detection and significance of occult axillary node metastases in patients with invasive breast cancer. Cancer 42:2025–2031, 1978
55. Huvos AG, Hutter RVP, Berg JW: Significance of axillary macrometastases and micrometastasis in mammary cancer. Ann Surg 173:44–46, 1971
56. Fisher ER, Sass R, Fisher B, et al: Pathologic findings from the National Surgical Adjuvant Project for breast cancers. Cancer 53:712–723, 1984
57. Bloom HJG, Field JR: Impact of tumor grade and host resistance on survival of women with breast cancer. Cancer 28:1580–1589, 1971
58. Sarrazin D, Le M, Mouriesse H, et al: Radiotherapeutic studies on breast cancer at Villejuif. Cancer Bulletin 34:242–249, 1982
59. Haybittle JL, Blamey RW, Elston CW, et al: A prognostic index in primary breast cancer. Br J Cancer 45:361–366, 1982
60. Black MM, Spur FD: Sinus histiocytosis of lymph nodes in cancer. Surg Gynecol Obstet 106:163–175, 1950
61. Cutler SJ, Black MM, Mork T, et al: Further observations on prognostic factors in cancer of the female breast. Cancer 24:653–667, 1969
62. Alderson MR, Hamlin I, Staunton MD: The relative significance of prognostic factors in breast carcinoma. Br J Cancer 25:646–656, 1971
63. Kister SJ, Sommers SC, Haagensen CD, et al: Nuclear grade and sinus histiocytosis in cancer of the breast. Cancer 23:570–575, 1969
64. Gilchrist KW, Kalish L, Gould VE, et al: Interobserver reproducibility of histopathological features in stage II breast cancer. Breast Cancer Res Treat 5:3–10, 1985
65. Robbins GF, Bross I: The significance of delay in relation to prognosis of patients with primary operable breast cancer. Cancer 10:338–344, 1957
66. Bloom HJG: The influence of delay on the natural history and prognosis of breast cancer. Br J Cancer 19:228, 1965
67. Boyd NF, Meakin JW, Hayward JL, et al: Clinical estimation of the growth rate of breast cancer. Cancer 48:1037–1042, 1981
68. Lundgren B: The growth rate of breast cancer as a dynamic indicator of prognosis. Australas Radiol 27:178–180, 1983
69. Spratt JS, Heuser L, Kuhns JG, et al: Association between the actual doubling times of primary breast cancer with histopathological characteristics and Wolfe's parenchymal mammographic patterns. Cancer 47:2265–2268, 1981
70. Heuser LS, Spratt JS, Kuhns JG, et al: The association of pathologic and mammographic characteristics of primary human breast cancers with "slow" and "fast" growth rates and with axillary lymph node metastases. Cancer 53:96–98, 1984
71. McGuire WL, Dressler LG: Emerging impact of flow cytometry in predicting recurrence and survival in breast cancer patients. J Natl Cancer Inst 75:405–410, 1985
72. Tubiana M, Pejovic MH, Chavaudra N, et al: The long term prognostic significance of the thymidine labeling index in breast cancer. Int J Cancer 33:441–445, 1984
73. Meyer JS, Friedman E, McCrate MM, et al: Prediction of early course of breast carcinoma by thymidine labeling. Cancer 51:1879–1886, 1983
74. Silvestrini R, Daidone MG, Gasparini G: Cell kinetics as a

prognostic marker in node negative breast cancer. Cancer 56:1982–1987, 1985
75. Hedley DW, Rugg CA, Ng ABP, et al: Influence of cellular DNA content on disease free survival of Stage II breast cancer patients. Cancer Res 44:5395–5398, 1984
76. Coulson PB, Thornthwaite JT, Woolley TW, et al: Prognostic indicators including DNA histogram type, receptor content, and staging related to human breast cancer patient survival. Cancer Res 44:4187–4196, 1984
77. McDivitt RW, Stone KR, Craig RB, et al: A proposed classification of breast cancer based on kinetic information. Cancer 57:269–276, 1986
78. Birks DM, Crawford GM, Ellison LG, et al: Carcinoma of the breast in women 30 years of age or less. Surg Gynecol Obstet 137:21–25, 1973
79. Brightmore TGJ, Greening WP, Hamlin I: An analysis of clinical and histopathological features in 101 cases of carcinoma of the breast in women under 35 years of age. Br J Cancer 24:644–669, 1970
80. de Cholnoky T: Mammary cancer in youth. Surg Gynecol Obstet 77:55–60, 1943
81. Gogas J, Skalkeas G: Prognosis of mammary carcinoma in young women. Surgery 78:339–342, 1975
82. Horsely JS, Alrich EM, Wright CG: Carcinoma of the breast in women 35 years of age or younger. Ann Surg 169:839–842, 1969
83. MacDonald I, Wilcox NE: Prognosis of mammary carcinoma in young women. Cancer 9:281–287, 1966
84. Skalkeas G, Gogas J, Katsikas D, et al: Carcinoma of the breast in young women. Int Surg 54:286–289, 1970
85. Tepas JH III, Carr RE, Mullen JT: Breast cancer in young women. Am J Surg 129:289–291, 1975
86. Treves N, Holleb AI: A report of 549 cases of breast cancer in women 35 years of age or younger. Surg Gynecol Obstet 107:271–283, 1958
87. Langlands AO, Popock SJ, Kerr GR, et al: Long term survival of patients with breast cancer: A study of the curability of the disease. Br Med J 2:1247–1251, 1979
88. Rutqvist LE, Wallgren A, Nilsson B: Is breast cancer a curable disease? Cancer 53:1793–1800, 1984
89. Adami H, Malker B, Meirik O, et al: Age as a prognostic factor in breast cancer. Cancer 56:898–902, 1985
90. Mueller CB, Ames F, Anderson GD: Breast cancer in 3558 women, age as a significant determinant in the rate of dying and causes of death. Surgery 83:123–132, 1978
91. Noyes RD, Spanos WJ, Montague ED: Breast cancer in women aged 30 and under. Cancer 49:1302–1307, 1982
92. Haagensen CD: Diseases of the Breast, 3rd ed, p 921–924. Philadelphia. WB Saunders, 1986
93. Ribeiro GG, Swindell R: The prognosis of breast carcinoma in women aged less than 40 years. Clin Radiol 32:231–236, 1981
94. Hankey BF, Steinhorn SC: Long term patient survival for some of the more frequently occurring cancers. Cancer 50:1904–1912, 1982
95. Silverberg E, Poindexter CE, Garfinkel L: Cancer in black Americans. CA 30:39–44, 1980
96. Mittra NK, Rush BF, Verner E: A comparative study of breast cancer in black and white populations of two inner-city hospitals. J Surg Oncol 15:11–17, 1980
97. Mohla S, Sampson CC, Khan T, et al: Estrogen and progesterone receptors in black Americans. Cancer 50:552–559, 1982
98. Natarajan N, Nemoto T, Mettlin C, et al: Race-related differences in breast cancer patients. Cancer 56:1704–1709, 1985
99. Donegan WL, Hartz AJ, Rimm AA: The association of body weight with recurrent cancer of the breast. Cancer 41:1590–1594, 1978
100. Donegan WL, Jayich S, Koehler MR, et al: The prognostic implications of obesity for the surgical cure of breast cancer. Breast 4:14–17, 1978
101. Tartter PI, Papatestas AE, Ivannovich J, et al: Cholesterol and obesity as prognostic factors in breast cancer. Cancer 47:2222–2227, 1981
102. Sohrabi A, Sandoz J, Spratt JS, et al: Recurrence of breast cancer: Obesity, tumor size and axillary lymph node metastases. JAMA 244:264–265, 1980

Primary Treatment of Breast Cancer

10

Surgery

David W. Kinne

HISTORICAL BACKGROUND

Breast diseases, both benign and malignant, have been recorded since ancient times. The earliest documented cases appear in the Edwin Smith papyrus, which dates back to approximately 3000 BC and which may have been written by the famous Egyptian physician, Imhotep.[1] Eight references to breast disease are described in the Smith papyrus; some of these diseases are clearly attributable to abscess, trauma, or infected wounds. Almost certainly, Case 45, and perhaps Case 39 (described as a tumor that produced cysts and pus), represented malignant breast tumors. Translations of these cases, as well as their modern interpretations, may be found in *Silvergirl's Surgery: The Breast.*[2]

After describing the subjective and objective findings of the examination, the physician would make a diagnosis that included the prognosis. One of three courses of treatment was then recommended. A decision to treat the patient implied that the disease was curable and represented a contract to do so, whereas an ailment that was not to be treated carried a certain fatal outcome. Alternatively, a lesion of uncertain outcome could be observed or treated for a period of time. Case 45, a bulging tumor of the breast, was declared untreatable, whereas Case 39 was considered of uncertain prognosis and treated with a fire drill (a type of cauterization used for incision and drainage and, in this case, burning of remaining tumors).

Several historical reviews have documented the management of breast cancer throughout the preanesthetic and preantiseptic era.[3–7] Treatment was considered to be palliative, and ranged from no therapy at all to the application of salves, ointments, or caustics, or to cauterization, or even amputation. Amputation, usually done only for smaller tumors, was carried out rapidly with a wide variety of instruments designed for that purpose. Hemostasis was achieved by a combination of pressure, cauterization, or, from the time of the 16th-century surgeon Ambrose Pare onward, by the use of ligatures. These reviews attest to the ubiquitous nature of breast cancer throughout recorded time, and to its incurability. Sir James Paget, known for his description of Paget's disease of the nipple, reported 235 cases of breast carcinoma with a 10% operative mortality rate.[8] Most importantly, neither he nor any of his associates had ever seen a case in which recurrence was delayed beyond 8 years.

The first surgeon to form a unified concept of an operative approach for breast cancer was Jean Louis Petit (1674–1750), Director of the French Surgical Academy. His work, published 24 years after his death, described the importance of wide excision, en bloc resection, axillary dissection, and evaluation of the pectoral fascia. As detailed in *Silvergirl's Surgery: The Breast,*[9] these concepts were extended in the 1800s by a number of surgeons, including Velpeau, Pancoast, Moore, Banks, Lister, Sweeting, von Volkmann, and Gross. Heidenhain's pathologic documentation of involvement of the pectoralis major muscle by cancer and the demonstration by Rotter of interpectoral lymph node metastases established the rationale for a wide excision.

William S. Halsted is credited with devising and perfecting the radical mastectomy, which was to become the universal approach to resectable breast cancer for several decades. His first published report is included at the end of his paper "The Treatment of Wounds," published in 1890–91.[10] He performed his first radical mastectomy in 1882, while he was still at the Roosevelt Hospital in New York City. He described full axillary dissection, resection of the pectoralis major muscle, as well as wide skin excision. In 1894, Halsted published his results with 50 patients who underwent radical mastectomy,[11] reporting only three recurrences. This degree of improvement in local control,

Table 10-1
Local Recurrence Rates

Surgeon	*Time Period*	*No. of Cases*	*Local Recurrence Rate*
Bergmann	1882–1887	114	51%–60%
Billroth	1867–1876	170	82%
Czerny	1877–1886	102	62%
Fischer	1871–1878	147	75%
Gussenbauer	1878–1886	151	64%
Konig	1875–1885	152	58%–62%
Kuster	1871–1885	228	59.6%
Lucke	1881–1890	110	66%
Von Volkmann	1874–1878	131	60%
Halsted	1889–1894	50	6%

(Halsted WS: The results of operations for the cure of cancer of the breast performed at the Johns Hopkins Hospital from June, 1889 to January, 1894. Johns Hopkins Hosp Bull 4:297, 1894–1895.)

which was remarkable when compared to prior unpublished results, is outlined in Table 10-1.

Also in 1894, Meyer reported on the use of his technique of radical mastectomy in six patients. His approach and Halsted's differed principally in the fact that the axillary dissection in the Meyer operation was done before the removal of the breast and pectoralis muscles from the chest wall. This technique resulted in a less adequate exposure (and perhaps, less adequate dissection) than that achieved with the Halsted mastectomy. However, Meyer removed the pectoralis minor muscle, a procedure that Halsted later adopted. A thorough comparison of these techniques is provided by Haagensen,[13] who documents the theoretical superiority of the Halsted radical mastectomy; its subsequent refinement, including thin skin graft closure of chest wall defects; and many aspects of Halsted's personal life, including his tragic addiction to cocaine, and later, to morphine.

It is noteworthy that the favorable local recurrence rate of 6%, reported in Halsted's first series, was achieved despite the advanced stages of disease in those 50 patients. All of them had involved lymph nodes documented on pathologic studies, and 27 had an unfavorable or hopeless prognosis. In Halsted's last paper in which he published survival rates, 42.3% of 232 patients treated by radical mastectomy survived for 3 years.[14]

Halsted recognized that one common site of recurrence was in the ipsilateral supraclavicular nodes. For a time, he combined supraclavicular node dissection with radical mastectomy, but discontinued this because the morbidity rate was high and results were not improved. However, wider en bloc resections were envisioned, encompassing this nodal basin or the internal mammary lymph node chain, or both. Treatment of the internal mammary lymph node chain was proposed by Handley, who placed radium tubes in the intercostal spaces at the time of radical mastectomy.[15] Surgical approaches to this nodal basin included biopsy of the lymph node in the second intercostal space, a technique advocated by Handley.[16] He later advised postoperative radiation therapy based upon the information derived from such biopsies. Extrapleural dissection of a portion of the lymph node chain, performed in procedures that were not en bloc resections, was described by Dahl-Iversen,[17] as well as by Margottini.[18] Although internal mammary lymph node involvement was documented in a significant number of patients with cancer affecting the central or inner quadrants of the breast, a survival advantage for patients so treated was not proven. Urban described an en bloc in continuity resection of the internal mammary lymph node chain with radical mastectomy.[19] This procedure required an intrapleural dissection and closure of the defect with fascia lata. As will be discussed later, Urban's results were encouraging; however, randomized trials failed to demonstrate a survival advantage for extended radical mastectomy compared to that achieved with radical mastectomy, and the procedure is seldom carried out today. Wangensteen described the super-radical mastectomy, perhaps the widest surgical excision for breast carcinoma, which combined radical mastectomy and supraclavicular lymph node dissection with median sternotomy to resect both internal mammary lymph node chains.[20] This procedure was associated with an unacceptable morbidity and mortality rate, but was typical of an era when surgeons, encouraged by improved anesthesia techniques and intraoperative and postoperative care, as well as by the support of blood banks and the availability of antibiotic coverage, designed wide-ranging, en bloc dissections.

For the first 75 years of this century, the Halsted radical mastectomy was the operation of choice for patients with breast carcinoma. Haagensen, one of its strongest proponents, perfected this approach, utilizing a vertical incision with wide skin excision which required a skin graft for closure, dissection of thin skin flaps, and en bloc removal of the breast, pectoralis muscles, and axillary lymph nodes.[21] He developed the Columbia Clinical Staging System as an aid to selecting patients with more favorable prognoses for mastectomy, considering patients with more advanced stages of disease to be inoperable.

During this same period, radical mastectomies, usually through an oblique incision and without skin grafting, were being carried out at Memorial Sloan-Kettering Cancer Center. Fewer lesions were considered unresectable; indeed, between 1940 and 1943, only 11% of 1640 patients had breast cancer that was considered to be inoperable, and 89% underwent radical mastectomy.[22] The 30-year survival rate in this series, as well as in other series in which there was long-term follow-up of patients who had undergone radical mastectomy, showed significant cure rates, especially for patients with axillary lymph nodes that were uninvolved on pathologic examination. However, as has been discussed in Chapter 9, and as will be discussed in more detail later in this chapter, several factors have brought into question the supremacy of radical mastectomy.

1. A better understanding of the natural history of the disease has been gained. It is now understood that patients in whom subsequent metastatic disease develops after radical mastectomy actually had micrometastases at the time of, or before, surgery. The procedure offered no survival advantage for these patients, although local-regional control probably contributed to palliation. However, it is possible that this result could have been achieved with a less radical surgical approach. Patients with axillary lymph nodes that are shown to be pathologically involved are candidates for adjuvant systemic therapy in most centers, undertaken in the hope of controlling distant micrometastases and improving cure rates. An insidious extension of this concept is the premise that perhaps less extensive local-regional treatment is necessary. We at Memorial Sloan-Kettering Cancer Center do not support this premise, but believe there are adequate alternative approaches to radical mastectomy that may be offered to patients.
2. There is a growing awareness on the part of physicians and patients alike that early diagnosis through breast self-examination, periodic examination by physicians, and mammography is possible. An increasing number of cancers are being detected in nonpalpable stages, making possible less extensive surgical approaches. The risk of multicentric disease occurring elsewhere in the breasts of such patients must be understood, however, and appropriate treatment initiated.
3. Initially documented in retrospective studies and more recently supported by ongoing, prospective, randomized trials, alternative approaches to radical mastectomy have been found to offer equivalent disease-free survival rates. This is true for modified radical mastectomy (or total mastectomy), axillary dissection, and preservation of the pectoralis major muscle, and a growing body of evidence suggests that this is also true for breast preservation with radiation therapy.
4. The improved cosmetic result achieved with preservation of the pectoralis major muscle is appreciated by patients, even if breast reconstruction is not done. Should patients subsequently become candidates for breast reconstruction, good surgical results are more easily accomplished when the pectoralis major muscle has been preserved than when it is absent. Patients who have undergone breast preservation procedures thus enjoy a cosmetic advantage over those who have had radical mastectomies, provided there is no significant surgical deformity or poor cosmetic effect from radiation therapy.
5. Patients' awareness of their options and the fact that radical mastectomy has not proved to be clearly superior in randomized trials has led to an increased demand for alternative forms of therapy.

These factors and many others have led to the development of our present policies. Based upon our interpretation of the available data, we believe that most patients with primary operable breast cancer are best treated with either a modified radical mastectomy or a breast preservation approach entailing wide excision of the primary tumor, with clean margins histologically, axillary dissection, and radiation therapy to the remaining breast. Potential candidates for breast preservation procedures should be seen by surgeons and radiation therapists prior to treatment, as some patients are more appropriately treated with mastectomy. In patients treated by either approach who have axillary lymph nodes that are pathologically involved, a course of adjuvant systemic therapy is advised. A small percentage of patients with more advanced local-regional disease are best treated by radical mastectomy. There is little, if any, role for adjuvant radiation therapy in these patients, with the possible exception of those with cancer involving the central or medial breast quadrants and with extensive axillary nodal disease. In these patients, sequential treatment with chemotherapy and irradiation of the internal mammary lymph node chain and base of the neck is recommended.

SURGICAL PROCEDURES

As has been discussed, a few decades ago, virtually every patient with primary operable breast cancer underwent a radical mastectomy. Postoperatively, therapy consisted of irradiation (usually for patients with pathologically involved axillary lymph nodes) or no treatment at all. No systemic therapy was given. This approach to treatment of breast cancer has since evolved to include more than 20 different local-regional therapeutic approaches (with some of these differences in treatment being semantic in nature). Many systemic treatment regimens are now also available, with or without radiation therapy, resulting in more than 100 possible treatment programs for breast cancer patients. This section will describe the most common surgical procedures, in terms of both techniques and indications, which are recommended in various clinical settings, as well as the results achieved in terms of local control and survival rates.

To put these many choices in perspective, it is helpful to note the frequency with which they are used. A large survey conducted in 1982 by the American College of Surgeons includes data from several hundred hospitals in the United States and reports about one-fifth of the incident cases of breast cancer for that year.[23] When the results of this survey are compared to those of similar surveys conducted in 1972 and 1977, significant differences between 1977 and 1981, summarized in Table 10-2, are evident. The incidence of modified radical mastectomy increased from 55.6% to 78.2%, whereas the incidence of radical mastectomy decreased from 27.5% to only 3.4%. Use of partial mastectomy procedures increased from 2.8% to 7.2%. Figure 10-1 shows the 1972 data also, indicating that modified radical mastectomy became the standard operation in the mid 1970s. It must be recognized that a certain "lag time" is reflected in these figures, and it is likely that the percentage of breast-sparing procedures

Table 10-2
Operations Performed for Carcinoma of the Breast in 1977 and 1981

Operation	*1977* *Number*	*(%)*	*1981* *Number*	*(%)*
Partial mastectomy	693	(2.8)	1,283	(7.2)
Total mastectomy only	1,920	(7.8)	916	(5.2)
Total mastectomy with low axillary dissection	1,274	(5.2)	960	(5.4)
Modified radical mastectomy	13,721	(55.6)	13,827	(78.2)
Radical mastectomy	6,793	(27.5)	603	(3.4)
Extended radical mastectomy	271	(1.1)	103	(0.6)
Total	24,672	(100.0)	17,692	(100.0)

(Wilson RE, Donegan WL, Mettlin C, et al: The 1982 survey of carcinoma of the breast in the United States by the American College of Surgeons. Surg Gynecol Obstet 159:309, 1984. By permission of SURGERY, GYNECOLOGY & OBSTETRICS)

being done in many parts of the country today has increased. At Memorial Sloan-Kettering Cancer Center, 817 patients with breast cancer were treated by the Breast Service staff in 1984 (Table 10-3). Seventy-six percent of these patients underwent modified radical mastectomy, whereas only 6% had a radical mastectomy. Breast preservation techniques (partial mastectomy, axillary dissection followed by radiation therapy) were performed in 111 patients (14%). This figure represents an increase from 8% (in 1983) and from 1% (in 1982) in the total number of patients so treated.

Of interest in this regard is a recent report from the United Kingdom.[24] In September of 1983, Gazet and associates conducted a survey by mail of 766 consultant surgeons who were Fellows of the Association of Surgeons of Great Britain and Ireland. Questionnaires were completed by 454 surgeons who had an interest in or who treated breast diseases in a total of 17,000 new patients a year. Eighty-four percent of these surgeons treated most of their patients with breast cancer by mastectomy (usually, total mastectomy with or without axillary dissection, followed in frequency by modified radical mastectomy). Only 16% of the surgeons who practiced breast preservation techniques performed a biopsy of the axillary nodes, and adjuvant systemic therapy was not commonly advised.

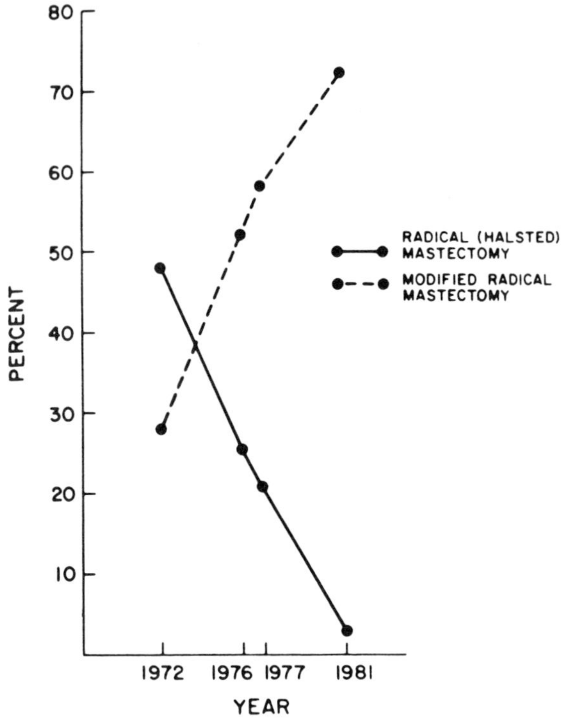

FIGURE 10-1. Trends in the type of operation performed on patients with breast cancer in the United States. (Wilson RE, Donegan WL, Mettlin C, et al: The 1982 survey of carcinoma of the breast in the United States by the American College of Surgeons. Surg Gynecol Obstet 159:309, 1984.)

Modified Radical Mastectomy

Modified radical mastectomy, also termed total mastectomy with axillary lymph node dissection and preservation of the pectoralis major muscle, is not as precisely defined or standardized as is radical mastectomy. Considerable variation is possible in both the procedure used to dissect the pectoralis minor muscle (preservation of the muscle leaving the neurovascular bundle intact; division at the muscle's rib origins or insertion at the coracoid process, with or without preservation of the neurovascular supply; or excision of the muscle with the specimen) and, more importantly, in the extent of axillary lymph node dissection (ranging from a sampling procedure to full dissection of levels I, II, and III).

Most patients with operable breast cancer are candidates for modified radical mastectomy, including those with Stage I, II, and III breast cancer that is not fixed to the pectoralis major muscle or accompanied by bulky axillary lymph node involvement. (In the latter clinical settings, radical mastectomy is indicated.) We consider the Patey procedure to be preferable, with removal of the pectoralis minor muscle and complete axillary dissection.[25]

In the Patey procedure, the entire breast, axilla, and arm are prepared and draped free in a sterile manner for subsequent mobilization of the arm. At a minimum, a 4-cm skin margin is outlined around the tumor (or biopsy site); an elliptical incision encompassing the tumor (or biopsy site) and nipple-areolar complex is preferable (Fig. 10-2). This allows a slightly oblique scar, producing an optimal cosmetic result and facilitating possible subsequent breast reconstruction. Thin skin flaps are dissected to the outer limit of the breast in all directions, with the

Table 10-3
Surgical Procedures Performed by the Memorial Sloan-Kettering Cancer Center Breast Service—1984

Operation	*No. of Patients (%)*
Modified radical mastectomy	619 (76)
Partial mastectomy with axillary dissection and radiotherapy	111 (14)
Radical mastectomy	50 (6)
Total mastectomy	36 (4)
Extended radical mastectomy	1
Total	817 (100)

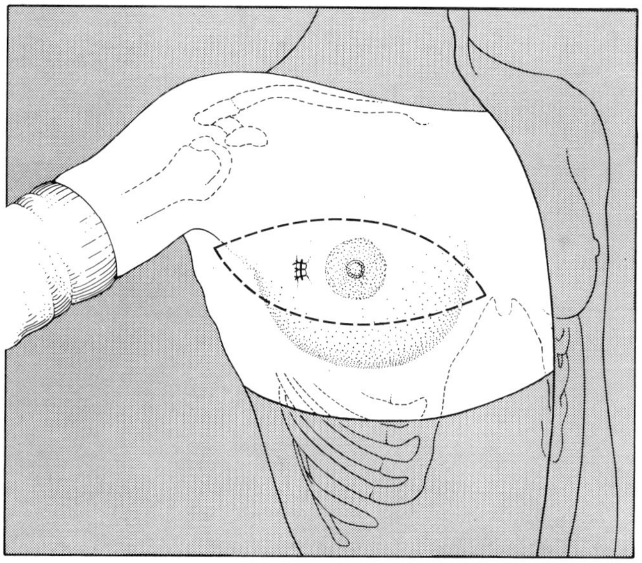

FIGURE 10-2. The outline of the oblique skin incision for modified radical mastectomy is shown to encompass the biopsy site by at least 4 cm on each side. (Kinne DW, DeCosse JJ: Modified radical mastectomy for carcinoma of the breast. Am Surg 48:543, 1982.)

latissimus dorsi muscle identified laterally and traced superiorly to the axillary vein. Then, the breast and pectoralis major muscle fascia are removed together in a medial to lateral direction, affording access to the axilla with the breast at the patient's side (Fig. 10-3). During this step, care must be taken in patients who have had an incisional or excisional biopsy of their breast cancer elsewhere and are having mastectomy as a second-stage procedure. The surgeon may be uncertain as to whether or not the pectoralis major muscle (or its fascia) were entered during the biopsy, with possible implantation of tumor cells. Such an assessment is difficult on clinical examination and even during mastectomy. If tumor implantation is suspected, saucerization of the pectoralis major muscle (or en bloc removal of a portion of the muscle beneath the biopsy site) is indicated to ensure a clean, deep margin.[26] Although some advise radical mastectomy in such cases, if the tumor (or biopsy wound) is relatively small, little is to be gained by sacrificing the entire pectoralis major muscle.

The clavipectoral fascia, investing the axillary contents and the pectoralis minor muscle, is then incised and the pectoralis minor muscle is divided near the coracoid process (Fig. 10-4). The lateral pectoral nerve, which arises from the medial cord of the brachial plexus and which is the smaller of the two nerves supplying the pectoralis major muscle, sweeps around the lateral border of the pectoralis minor muscle in 38% of patients and comes through the belly of the muscle in 62% of patients. It supplies the lower one-third of the pectoralis major muscle, and its preservation has been advocated to avoid atrophy of this portion of the muscle and shoulder stiffness.[27] Although this is possible in procedures in which the pectoralis minor muscle is preserved, during the Patey procedure, the lateral pectoral nerve is usually sacrificed. However, with preservation of the medial pectoral nerve and early adequate shoulder exercises, the above problems can usually be minimized.

The arm is then mobilized, with care being taken to avoid damage to the medial pectoral nerve (either from the dissection or retraction). Axillary node dissection of levels III (from the subclavian muscle laterally), II, and I is then carried en bloc in a medial to lateral fashion. At this point, assessment and biopsy of interpectoral (Rotter's) nodes may be undertaken. In the series of 301 such biopsies reported by Cody and associates, nodes (positive and negative) were found in 73% of cases.[28] The incidence of interpectoral node metastasis was 8% in patients with positive axillary nodes and 0.5% in those without axillary node metastases. Frequently, conversion to radical mastectomy was made owing to the involvement of these nodes and their proximity to pectoralis major muscle fascia. Durkin and Haagensen reported a 19% incidence of positive interpectoral nodes in 42 patients with Columbia Clinical Stage A breast cancer who were treated by radical mastectomy and in whom nodes were identified by clearing.[29] Long-term follow-up showed that only 2 of 14 patients with concomitant axillary node metastases survived 10 years, whereas 3 patients with Rotter's node involvement only were disease-free at 10 years. (None of these patients underwent systemic therapy.) Kay's study yielded similar results; four patients with interpectoral node involvement only were free of disease 5 years later.[30]

It is advisable to return the patient's arm to her side while dissecting level I nodes in order to avoid injuring the neurovascular structures that course to the arm (Figs. 10-5 and 10-6). In these illustrations, the thoracodorsal nerve and vessels are shown being sacrificed, a procedure that is recommended if the patient has suspicious axillary lymph nodes. Many surgeons prefer to spare this neurovascular bundle if a clinically normal axilla is encountered during the dissection. However, proximity of the lymph nodes to this bundle, as determined by clearing of axillary specimens, makes this a questionable routine practice.

(Text continues on p. 266)

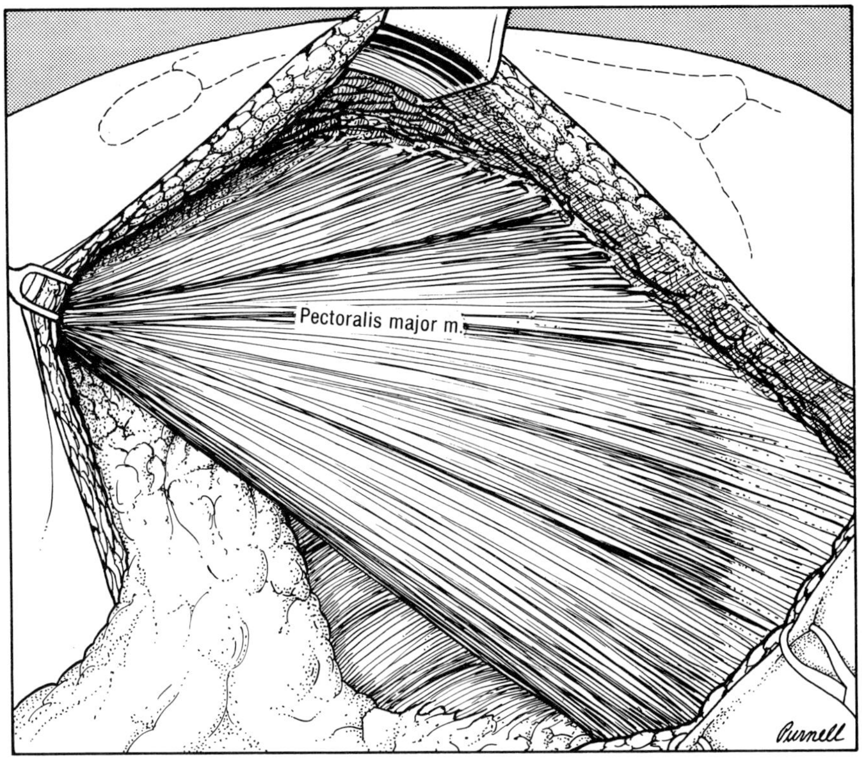

FIGURE 10-3. The breast and pectoralis major muscle fascia are dissected from the muscle and lie laterally. (Kinne DW, DeCosse JJ: Modified radical mastectomy for carcinoma of the breast. Am Surg 48:543, 1982.)

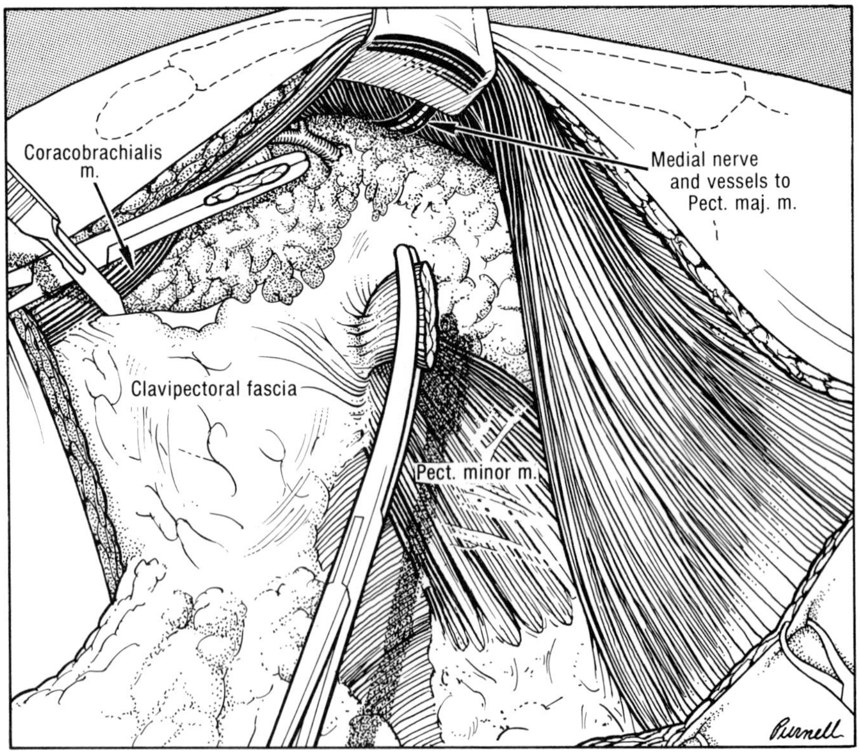

FIGURE 10-4. The clavipectoral fascia is incised and reflected caudad. The pectoralis minor muscle is divided near the coracoid process. (Kinne DW, DeCosse JJ: Modified radical mastectomy for carcinoma of the breast. Am Surg 48:543, 1982.)

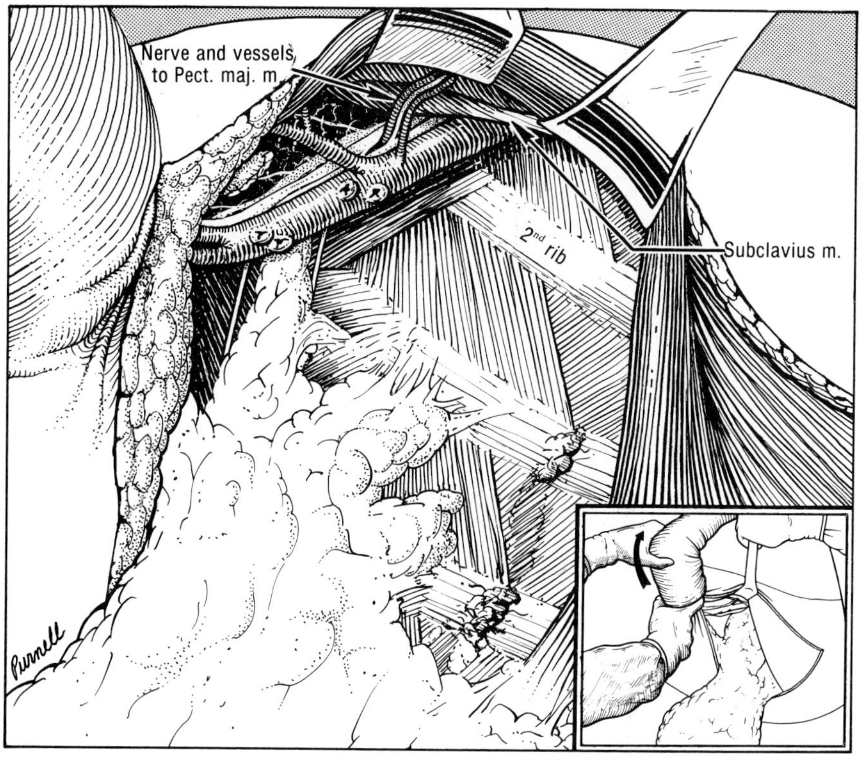

FIGURE 10-5. The pectoralis minor muscle is dissected from the chest wall in a medial-to-lateral direction, and lies laterally with the breast. The inset in the far right corner shows the arm mobilization that facilitates exposure to the apex of the axilla. (Kinne DW, DeCosse JJ: Modified radical mastectomy for carcinoma of the breast. Am Surg 48:543, 1982.)

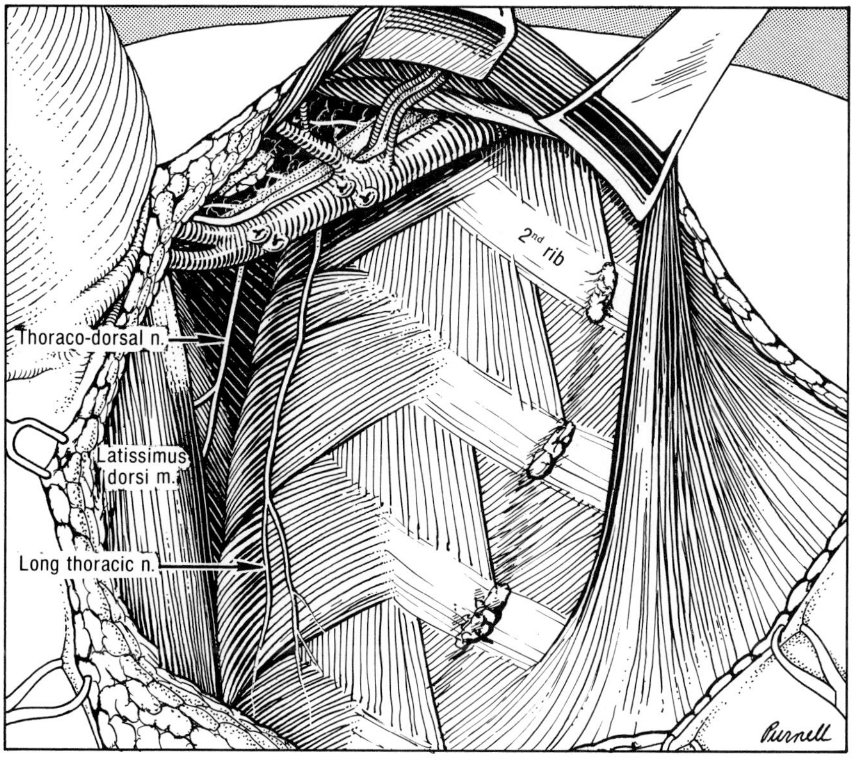

FIGURE 10-6. Axillary dissection is completed. (Kinne DW, DeCosse JJ: Modified radical mastectomy for carcinoma of the breast. Am Surg 48:543, 1982.)

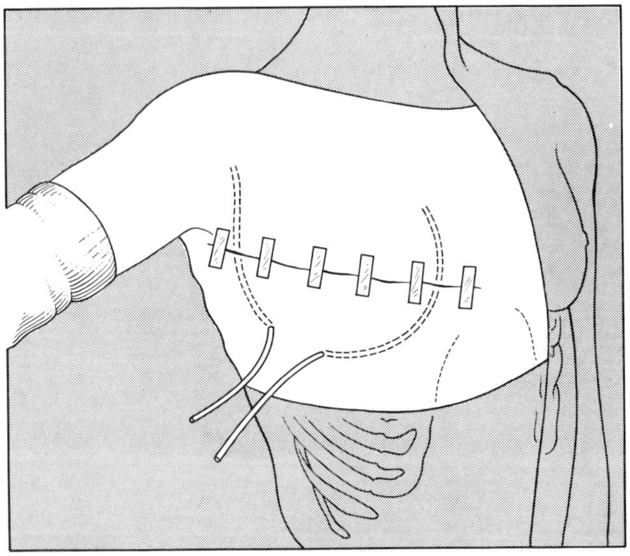

FIGURE 10-7. Subcuticular closure is done over suction drains. (Kinne DW, DeCosse JJ: Modified radical mastectomy for carcinoma of the breast. Am Surg 48:543, 1982.)

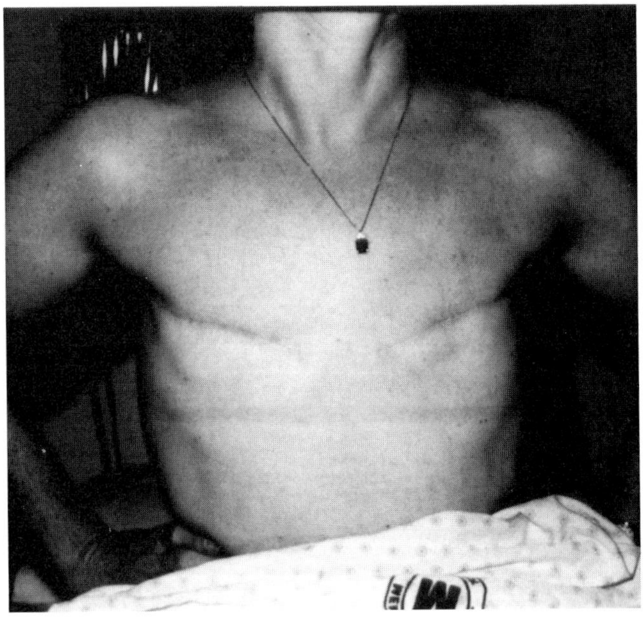

FIGURE 10-8. Patient who has undergone bilateral modified radical mastectomy, showing contraction of the pectoralis major muscle.

(Text continued from p. 263)

Finally, after removal of the specimen, a subcuticular closure over suction drains affords the best cosmetic appearance of the scar (Fig. 10-7). An illustration of a patient who underwent bilateral modified radical mastectomy is shown in Figure 10-8. The modified radical mastectomy yields a cosmetic result that facilitates breast reconstruction, as illustrated in Figure 10-9. Variations of the modified radical mastectomy procedure have been described by Handley and Thackray[31] and Maier and colleagues.[32] The pectoralis major muscle may also be split transversely below its clavicular portion to allow access to the upper axilla.[33] Roses and co-workers divide and resuture the pectoralis major tendon near the humerus.[34]

The second major type of modified radical mastectomy preserves the pectoralis minor muscle. As described by Auchincloss, dissection of the apex of the axilla may be accomplished in most patients with gentle retraction of the pectoralis minor muscle.[35] One disadvantage of this approach is that the interpectoral (Rotter's) node area cannot be assessed or examined by biopsy. Other modified radical mastectomy procedures that involve preservation of the pectoralis minor muscle have been described.[36] One potential limitation of these approaches, in comparison with the Patey procedure, is that preservation of the pectoralis minor muscle and its neurovascular supply at the lateral pectoral nerve may result in a less than complete axillary dissection. Removal of level I nodes with some level II nodes is frequently the extent of the dissection; the upper portion of levels II and III may be left in place. The risk of leaving micrometastases behind, especially if nodes in level I or II prove to have disease on pathologic examination, is high enough to question the adequacy of this approach.

Radical Mastectomy

Radical mastectomy, which involves en bloc removal of the breast and skin overlying the tumor and the pectoralis major and minor muscles, as well as complete axillary dissection, is a more standardized procedure than are the many procedures that may be called modified radical mastectomies. The indications for this procedure have diminished for a variety of reasons: (1) retrospective studies have shown that good local-regional control may be achieved using a modified radical mastectomy procedure; (2) patients have presented with smaller cancers, even with nonpalpable lesions detected by mammography, negating the need to remove the pectoralis major muscle for better local control; (3) an increasing number of patients have opted to undergo breast reconstruction, which is facilitated by modified radical mastectomy; and (4) patients have become increasingly aware of the improved cosmetic results achieved with modified radical mastectomy compared to those achieved with radical mastectomy, without apparent sacrifice in local control or overall survival rate. However, radical mastectomy is the procedure of choice in patients with large, bulky tumors involving the pectoralis major muscle or fascia, those with bulky axillary lymph node involvement, or those with grossly involved interpectoral nodes in whom the posterior fascia of the muscle is also involved.

The dissection technique for radical mastectomy is quite similar to that described for modified radical mastectomy in terms of incision placement and flap dissection.

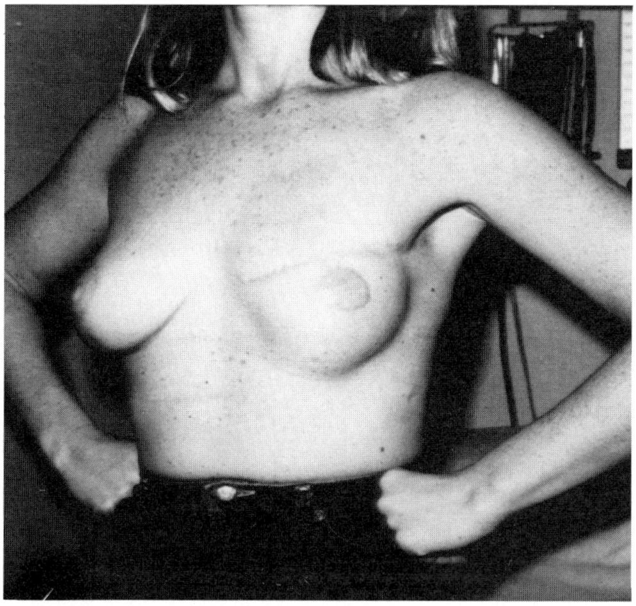

FIGURE 10-9. Patient who has undergone left breast reconstruction, including placement of a nipple-areolar complex. The oblique mastectomy scar is noted superior to the nipple.

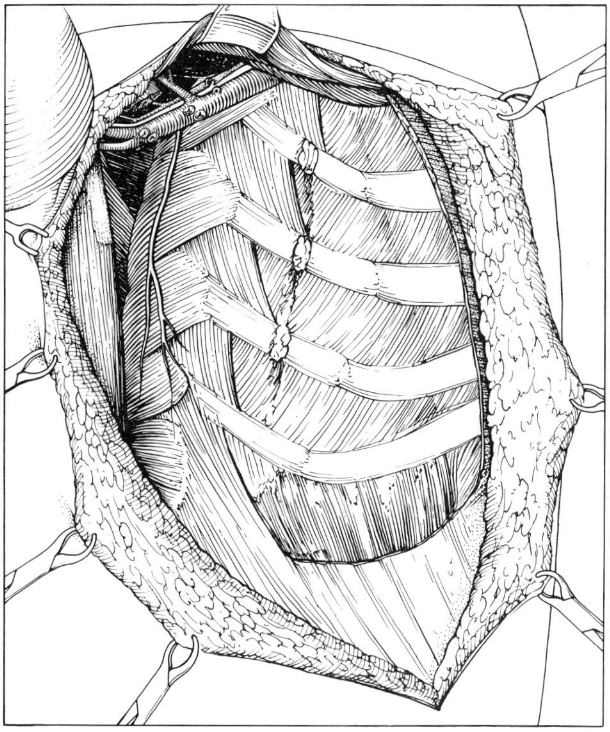

FIGURE 10-10. The operative field after removal of the radical mastectomy specimen. The clavicular head of the pectoralis major muscle has been preserved.

However, the breast and pectoralis major muscle fascia are not removed from the muscle as is shown in Figure 10-3. Instead, at this point, the area between the clavicular and sternal heads of the pectoralis major muscle is entered, preserving the clavicular head. As described by Urban, the muscle is then divided at its humeral attachment.[37] The operation proceeds in a lateral to medial direction in this plane, with elevation of the breast and pectoralis major muscle to reach its sternal attachment (Fig. 10-10). The pectoralis major muscle is divided at its sternal attachment, and the dissection is carried laterally until the pectoralis minor muscle is encountered. By dividing this muscle near the coracoid process and at its rib attachments (in a medial to lateral fashion), the interpectoral node area is removed en bloc. Axillary dissection proceeds in much the same way as described for the modified radical mastectomy, although the exposure is better because the pectoralis major and minor muscles have been removed. The patient shown in Figures 10-11 and 10-12 underwent a right radical mastectomy 20 years prior to the taking of these photographs, and, more recently, a left modified radical mastectomy for contralateral breast carcinoma. The difference in the cosmetic result of these procedures is apparent, especially as revealed by the vertical scar and the axillary hollow resulting from the radical mastectomy.

Haagensen's description of Halsted's radical mastectomy procedure reveals several important differences.[38] The incision is vertically placed, with a large skin excision that requires a split-thickness skin graft for closure (Fig. 10-13). The clavicular head of the pectoralis major muscle is not preserved, and this muscle is divided at the clavicle.

Extended Radical Mastectomy

En bloc excision of the internal mammary lymph node chain and vessels, as described by Urban,[19] involves an intrapleural resection of these structures with a portion of the sternum and adjacent ribs. This oval-shaped defect may be closed with a fascial graft or Marlex mesh (Fig. 10-14), and requires chest tube drainage for a few days. An extrapleural dissection may be done, although only the first three interspaces may be removed predictably. It is generally not an en bloc procedure, it entails the removal of the costal cartilage of ribs 1, 2, and 3, and it does not require stabilization of the chest wall or a chest tube.

Total (Simple) Mastectomy

This procedure involves removal of the entire breast, including the nipple-areolar complex with the pectoralis major muscle fascia, but without axillary lymph node dissection or removal of the pectoralis muscles. Simple mastectomy is an inappropriate term that is misleading to patients and physicians alike. To many patients, the most "radical" change in their appearance after radical mastectomy is the loss of the breast, precisely what occurs with

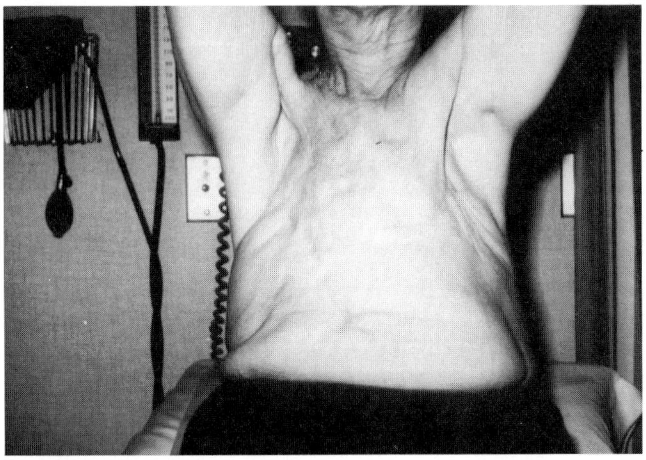

FIGURE 10-11. Patient who underwent a right radical mastectomy years ago, and a left modified radical mastectomy more recently. The right axillary hollow and the more vertical scar on the right, as compared to the left, are evident when the patient's arms are raised.

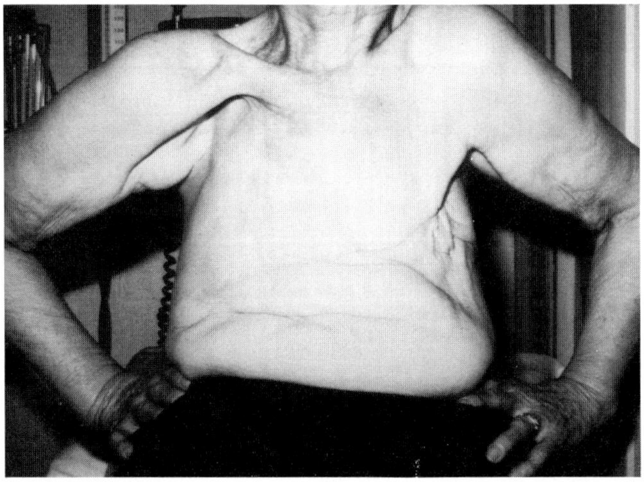

FIGURE 10-12. In the same patient, contraction of the intact pectoralis major muscle can be seen on the left. This photograph demonstrates the difference in the axilla and chest wall defects associated with the two operations.

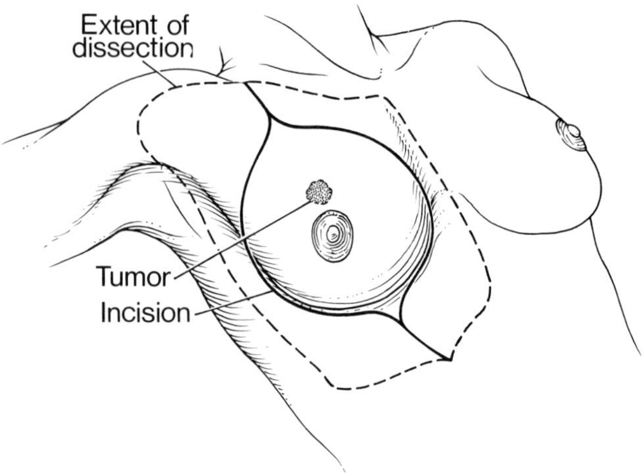

FIGURE 10-13. An outline of the dissection used in the Haagensen technique of the Halsted radical mastectomy shows the vertical scar and skin graft closure.

a "simple" mastectomy. The emotional response to the terms radical and simple in these procedures is best avoided; calling this operation a total mastectomy achieves that objective.

This procedure is indicated in four principal clinical settings: (1) in patients with *in situ* carcinoma (ductal or lobular) with no suspicious axillary lymphadenopathy (in whom metastatic disease to the axillary nodes occurs in less than 1%); (2) in carefully selected patients undergoing prophylactic mastectomy, often of the contralateral breast; (3) in patients who develop breast recurrence after partial mastectomy and axillary dissection (or axillary irradiation), with or without breast irradiation, and who remain free of distant disease (a so-called salvage mastectomy); and (4) as a palliative procedure in patients with bulky breast tumors and distant metastasis in whom local control will be facilitated by removal of the breast.

In each of these clinical settings except the last, it is an operation to be carried out with careful attention to technical details. As in a radical or modified radical mastectomy, thin skin flaps are dissected to appropriate borders, including to the latissimus dorsi muscle laterally and superiorly, to ensure complete breast removal, including the axillary tail of Spence.

Breast Preservation Procedures

It is generally agreed that the principal objective of breast-preserving surgical techniques in patients with breast cancer is a cosmetic one, designed to retain a cosmetically acceptable breast after complete excision of the tumor. Usually, such procedures are accompanied by an axillary dissection of some type, followed by radiation therapy to the remaining breast.

At a consensus conference in New York in June of 1985, which was sponsored jointly by Memorial Sloan-Kettering Cancer Center and the Joint Center for Radiation Therapy, a faculty of surgeons and radiotherapists with some experience in breast preservation techniques, along with pathologists and medical oncologists, met to discuss appropriate techniques. There was an attempt to define procedures and to recommend certain techniques and discourage others.[39] The following terms for the excision of breast cancer were established:

Excision (tumorectomy, lumpectomy)—removal of the tumor grossly without attention to margins

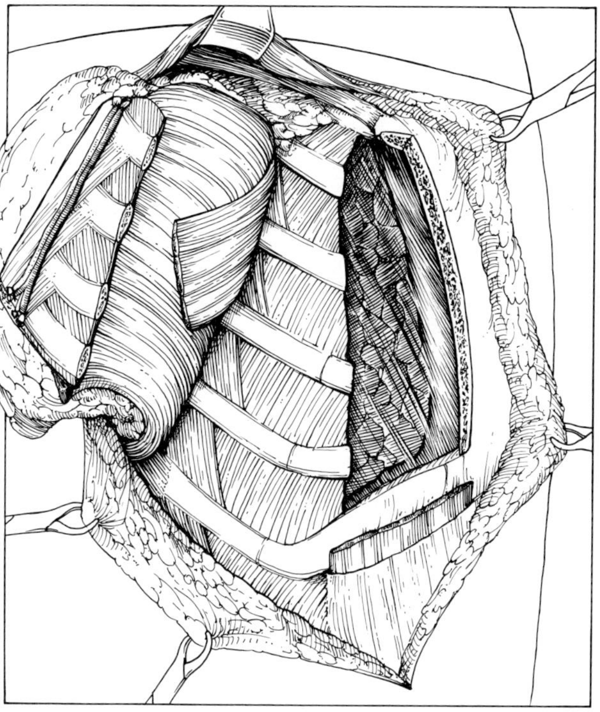

FIGURE 10-14. Extended radical mastectomy, as described by Urban, showing en bloc radical mastectomy specimen with a portion of sternum, ribs, and internal mammary vessels and nodes. Prior to skin closure, the oval chest wall defect is to be closed with fascia or synthetic material over a chest tube.

Wide excision (limited resection, partial mastectomy)—excision of the tumor with grossly normal, clean margins

Quadrantectomy—en bloc excision of the tumor within a quadrant of breast tissue along with the pectoralis major muscle fascia and overlying skin

Most faculty members advocated a wide excision. A simple excision without regard to margins was thought to carry a high risk of local recurrence, and quadrantectomy was considered to be too deforming to permit an acceptable cosmetic result. The terms lumpectomy and segmental mastectomy were considered to be imprecise, and their use was discouraged.

Axillary dissections also have a variety of definitions:

Sampling—removal of an axillary node or nodes from the lower axilla without definition of precise anatomic boundaries

Low axillary dissection—an en bloc excision of level I of the axilla, from the latissimus dorsi muscle laterally to the lateral border of the pectoralis minor muscle medially, and clearing of the axillary vein superiorly.

Level I to II dissection—en bloc excision of the low and mid portions of the axilla, facilitated by elevation of the pectoralis minor muscle and mobilization of the ipsilateral arm to relax the pectoralis major muscle. This dissection proceeds from the latissimus dorsi muscle laterally to the medial border of the pectoralis minor muscle medially, with clearing of the axillary vein.

Full axillary dissection (levels I, II, III)—removal of the entire axillary contents, from the latissimus dorsi muscle laterally to the subclavius muscle (Halsted's ligament) medially, clearing the axillary vein, with preservation of or excision of the pectoralis minor muscle.

In patients with a clinically negative axilla, a level I to II dissection or a full dissection is the optimal approach. Approximately 25% to 40% of the patients so treated will prove to have pathologically involved axillary nodes;[40] these patients would require radiation therapy to the unremoved higher nodes if a less thorough dissection were done. The combination of some surgery and irradiation to the axilla increases the chances of complications, especially edema of the breast or arm, or both. Should irradiation not eliminate disease in the higher nodes, detection and surgical excision may be difficult. The problem of "skip" metastases in axillary nodes is also a consideration. Whereas only 1% of patients with pathologically negative axillary lymph nodes in levels I and II have been shown to have metastases in level III,[41] a less thorough axillary dissection which is negative on pathologic examination will leave micrometastases in the higher axillary nodes in 14% to 24% of patients.[42,43] For these reasons, dissection of at least levels I to II should be done in patients with a clinically negative axilla; for patients with clinically suspicious axillary nodes, a full dissection of the axilla is preferable. Axillary sampling, which helps neither patients nor physicians in planning treatment, is imprecise, both as a term and as a procedure, and should not be used.

Indications

The ideal patients for breast-preserving treatment approaches combining surgery and radiation therapy are those with small, peripheral, infiltrating carcinomas and clinically negative axillae who understand what the treatment entails and who desire breast preservation. Several relative contraindications have delineated certain groups of patients that are not well suited for breast preservation. If the relative size of the tumor to the breast is such that complete surgical excision will cause deformity, patients are better advised to undergo mastectomy and to consider subsequent breast reconstruction. Some patients are severely deformed by the surgical procedure, as depicted in Figure 10-15, which shows a patient who has undergone medial quadrantectomy. Patients with multiple, palpable cancers in different quadrants of the breast, or those with suspicious calcifications detected on mammography in widely separated areas of the breast, should be treated by mastectomy. Other patients for whom breast preservation techniques are not recommended include those who are pregnant or elderly and those who present with the fol-

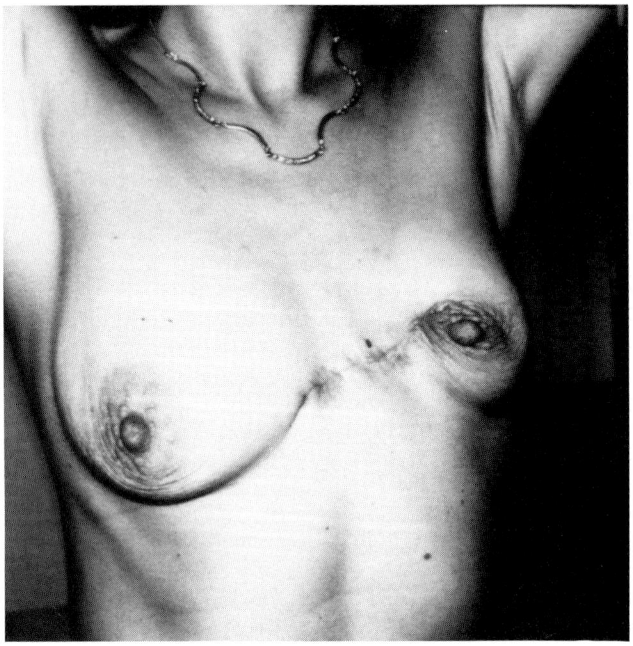

FIGURE 10-15. Patient who underwent medial quadrantectomy for carcinoma, which resulted in severe breast and nipple deformity. Such cosmetic results are to be avoided; either the patient should have a less extensive resection or, if this is not possible owing to the size or location of the tumor, the patient should undergo a mastectomy. This patient was referred for an axillary dissection and breast irradiation, but underwent modified radical mastectomy instead.

lowing clinical backgrounds: central lesions, with or without Paget's disease; margins that are involved histologically with carcinoma, especially multifocal intraductal disease; and very large or pendulous breasts. Treatment recommendations should be made after a joint consultation with the surgeon and radiotherapist prior to initiation of therapy.

Procedure

For wide excision of breast cancers, the best incision is usually a curvilinear one placed over the tumor. Circumareolar incisions, especially for peripheral tumors, should not be done because the surgeon will have difficulty ensuring that the margins are clear, and the tunnel through which the carcinoma is removed will present problems to the radiotherapist in terms of planning a boost dose. In certain cases, radial incisions may provide acceptable cosmetic results in the lower half of the breast (although curvilinear incisions closed in a manner to avoid inferior retraction of the nipple are preferable). Such incisions are also used in quadrantectomy approaches.

Careful histologic assessment of the margins of resection is important to avoid early recurrence of cancer in the irradiated breast. In a retrospective review from the Joint Center for Radiation Therapy, the finding of concomitant intraductal carcinoma with the infiltrating cancer, and its presence in grossly normal adjacent breast tissue, was associated with the development of recurrent cancer in 39% of cases.[44] Therefore, this histologic assessment should be made prior to treatment, and if intraductal carcinoma is present (as it was in 38% of the patients in this series), further surgery should be carried out to obtain clear margins. This surgery could entail either re-excision (if an acceptable cosmetic result can still be achieved) or mastectomy.

It is important to note that this histologic judgment cannot be made on the basis of frozen section analysis. The approach of the Breast Service at Memorial Sloan-Kettering Cancer Center is to carry out a limited resection as the first stage in a breast preservation procedure, with submission of the wide excision specimen for pathologic assessment. The excision of the tumor, which is carried out through a curvilinear incision placed over the tumor, includes the tumor with grossly normal margins of 1 cm to 2 cm (Fig. 10-16). The surgeon then orients the specimen for the pathologist with suture tags (e.g., by delineating the lateral margin as long [L] or the superior margin as short [S]) and submits the entire, uncut specimen to the Pathology Department for inking of the margins. Following this procedure, an incision is made into the tumor for histologic and estrogen/progesterone receptor determinations. If a grossly involved margin is noted by the pathologist, which margin may be identified through the use of sutures, a wider excision of that margin may be carried out prior to closure. Electrocautery should not be used up to this point in the procedure because thermal injury makes histologic interpretation of the margins difficult and possibly inaccurate. Electrocautery also has been shown to decrease estrogen receptor concentration owing to thermal injury. However, once all pathologic material has been submitted, careful hemostasis should be carried out

FIGURE 10-16. This illustration depicts the ideal incisions for limited resection of breast carcinoma (a curvilinear incision placed over the tumor). Through a separate incision, the axillary dissection may be carried out within the skin lines.

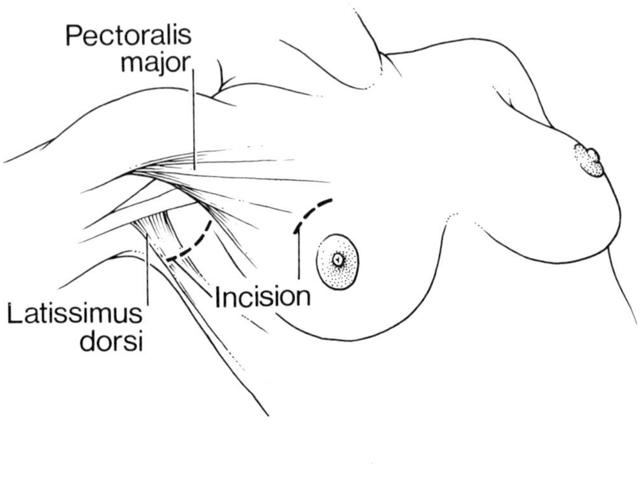

(perhaps with electrocautery) to avoid wound ecchymosis and hematoma, which would make the delivery of a boost dose more difficult. Cosmetic closure is best accomplished when the breast is not reapproximated (except in the case of large defects, such as those caused by quadrantectomy), and when subcutaneous and subcuticular closure is done without drains. This procedure is well-suited for ambulatory (same-day) surgical centers.

The next step is then carefully planned. If the cancer is confined to the specimen, with clear margins, the patient is admitted for axillary dissection and interstitial implantation of the primary site, if indicated. If the surgeon and the radiotherapist believe that the volume and multifocal nature of the cancer in the specimen is great enough to increase the likelihood of local failure, the patient is advised to undergo either re-excision (if cosmetically feasible) or mastectomy. This step-wise approach has a number of advantages over the one-step procedure advocated by the National Surgical Adjuvant Breast Project (NSABP)[45] once the diagnosis has been established by needle biopsy or open biopsy. We have treated patients in whom the NSABP approach has been employed who have so much multifocal disease, even in the re-excision specimen, that mastectomy has been advised (or elected by concerned patients). This has led to a total mastectomy, performed through a transverse or slightly oblique incision, in patients who have a higher transverse scar in the axilla, yielding a result that is suboptimal cosmetically and often, psychologically harmful.

The axillary dissection in breast preservation procedures is best done through a transverse incision in the skin lines (see Fig. 10-16), separate from the excision of the primary lesion (except in certain lesions of the axillary tail, where proximity to the axilla dictates a common incision). In patients with a clinically negative axilla, a level I to II dissection is done with preservation of the medial and lateral pectoral nerves to the pectoralis major muscle. The thoracodorsal nerve and vessels to the latissimus dorsi are spared, and in some cases, it is possible to save the larger or dominant intercostal brachial nerve supplying sensation to the skin of the upper inner arm. Routine division of this nerve may lead to formation of a neuroma and postmastectomy pain syndrome in 4% to 6% of patients.[46] However, the nerve usually bifurcates or trifurcates as it courses through level I, making its preservation difficult and compromising the axillary dissection. It has been our practice to place a metal clip at the high point of the axillary dissection (between levels II and III). If nodes that are pathologically involved are then found at level I or II, or both, radiotherapy to level III (medial to the clip) can be included with breast irradiation.

COMPLICATIONS

Mastectomy (or axillary dissection as part of a breast-sparing procedure) is a relatively superficial operative procedure in which easy and adequate exposure is possible. Intraoperative complications, such as vascular injuries (to the axillary artery or vein) or damage to the long thoracic nerve, are rare occurrences which should easily be identified and repaired. Although intraoperative or postoperative complications leading to mortality (such as myocardial infarction or pulmonary embolism) do occur, they are uncommon. The mortality rate for these procedures is essentially the same as that for anesthesia, which is very low.

Early Complications

INFECTION. Mastectomy procedures are relatively clean, but the use of suction catheters provides a potential portal of entry for infection. Predisposing factors to infection include advanced age, prolonged drainage through a suction catheter, skin flap necrosis or separation, poor nutritional state, and various medical problems, such as diabetes mellitus.[47] The organisms responsible for infection in these patients are usually gram-positive (streptococcus or *Staphylococcus aureus*), causing cellulitis more often than they cause abscess formation. The incidence of wound infection ranges from 5.6% to 14.2%.[48] Treatment with moist warm compresses and antibiotics (usually, penicillin or a cephalosporin) will generally resolve the problem. Rarely are incision and drainage required.

A recent report showed an overall wound infection rate of 8.2% in postmastectomy patients,[49] with a 5.3% and 12.4% wound infection rate associated with one-step and two-step procedures, respectively. The highest wound infection rate (23%) was seen in patients undergoing two-step procedures in which an interval of 4 to 7 days separated the operations. Needle biopsy as an initial step led to a lower infection rate, resulting in the recommendation that this approach be utilized. Administration of prophylactic antibiotics in patients undergoing mastectomy as a second step should be considered.

SKIN NECROSIS. Skin necrosis is a relatively uncommon problem in our experience, but full-thickness losses have been reported in 8% of the patients in one series.[50] Factors that increase the likelihood of this problem in patients who have had thin skin flap dissection include tight pressure dressings, utilization of vertical (as opposed to transverse) incisions, and tight wound closure.[47] It is unusual for re-excision or skin grafting to be required, and routine postoperative wound care facilitates wound healing by secondary intention.

SEROMA. Seroma, one of the most common postoperative problems, is more of an annoyance to patients than a cause of significant morbidity. Frequent wound aspiration during the postoperative period is required. This condition occurs most commonly in obese patients and in those with axillary lymph nodes that are pathologically involved. Prolongation of this complication is associated with a high incidence of wound infection. In a controlled study conducted at the National Cancer Institute, patients who had undergone mastectomy (or axillary dissection) and who had begun shoulder exercises early in the postoperative period had greater total wound drainage, more days of drainage, and a longer hospital stay than did patients who underwent similar operations but who delayed shoulder exercises for one week.[51] The risk of frozen shoulder must be recognized if the latter program is followed, and physicians must ensure that patients continue to exercise and make progress after discharge from the hospital.

Another method for decreasing the risk of seroma formation in postmastectomy patients has been described by Aitken and associates.[52] Prior to wound closure, they advocate tacking the skin flaps to the underlying chest wall with subdermal buried sutures of absorbable material, thereby effectively minimizing dead space. Approximately 25 to 30 sutures are used, and shoulder mobilization is delayed to avoid tearing the sutures.

Seromas are managed by wound aspiration. Our impression is that they occur more commonly after modified radical mastectomy (or axillary dissection) than after radical mastectomy procedures in which the skin is flush against the chest instead of healing against the chest wall around the fold of the pectoralis major muscle border. Pressure dressings are not effective in reducing seromas, and may cause skin necrosis. If the amount of seroma formation remains high (e.g., 150 ml) despite twice-weekly aspirations, placement of a small drain after administration of local anesthesia will facilitate effective drainage into dressings (which may have to be changed frequently).

Late Complications

LYMPHEDEMA. Although it can occur in the early postmastectomy period, lymphedema is usually associated with wound infection. It is rarely seen today, but as described by Halsted, it was a common problem in the preantibiotic era, especially in patients with advanced (sometimes ulcerated and infected) tumors.

The later development of lymphedema is the most distressing long-term complication of mastectomy or axillary dissection. Patients should be instructed that it is a lifetime risk, and that it is almost always attributable to low-grade infection in the extremity. Preventive measures should be stressed; patients should be urged to avoid having blood withdrawn from or injections given into the ipsilateral extremity. Any constricting activity (even blood pressure monitoring) should be done on the contralateral arm. Avoidance of heavy lifting and cuts or burns (by using a rubber glove while gardening, for instance) is encouraged. At the first sign of edema, a course of antibiotics, warm soaks, and elevation of the arm should be instituted in the hope of reversing the process. Once established, the edema often persists and is difficult to manage. Lymphedema is discussed in Chapter 15 in greater detail.

Lymphedema has been reported in 6.7% to 62.5% of patients following radical mastectomy. The incidence is increased with either preoperative or postoperative radiotherapy.[48] The higher rates are associated with wound problems, as discussed by Haagensen,[53] who reports edema in about 5% of his patients.

POSTMASTECTOMY PAIN SYNDROME. Although general tightness of the chest wall and shoulder is frequently reported, a significant and sometimes disabling pain is reported in 4% to 6% of patients owing to division of the inferocostobrachial nerve.[46,54] Frequently, a trigger point on the chest wall may be identified, indicating a neuroma in the stump of this nerve. Management of this condition by injection or excision, or both, has been attempted, but with little success. This complication provides added incentive for preserving the nerve during axillary dissection, despite the difficulty in doing so and the potential for compromising the adequacy of axillary dissection.

RESULTS

Rationale for Treatment

In patients with breast cancer but no evidence of distant disease, the goals of adequate local-regional treatment are to provide optimal local control, to stage the disease so that patients at high risk for recurrence (who are advised to undertake a course of systemic treatment) may be identified, and to provide the best chance of overall survival. Patients who die of breast cancer have distant metastases, indicating the presence of occult disease at the time of local treatment (and presumably, being unaffected by it), or metastases from inadequately treated local or regional disease. In this regard, two principal factors must be addressed.

Multicentricity

The incidence of multicentric breast cancer in sites that are distinct from the biopsy site in mastectomy specimens is reported to range from 9% to 75%.[55] This wide discrepancy is caused by variations in three factors: the precision with which multicentricity is defined, the technique of examination employed, and the extent of tissue sampling. When several sections are taken from each of the three quadrants apart from that containing the cancer, higher rates of multicentricity are reported. This was true in a simulated partial mastectomy series of Rosen and associates, who reported residual cancer in 56% of patients.[56] In patients with clinically occult, nonpalpable breast cancers detected on mammography, Schwartz and co-workers reported a 44% incidence of multicentricity.[57] Of the tumors found to be microinvasive on pathologic examination, 57% were multifocal. In another series from Memorial Sloan-Kettering Cancer Center, 60% of patients in whom mastectomies were performed for *in situ* cancer had multicentric disease.[58] Thus, even in the earliest (nonpalpable) breast cancers treated, multicentricity is frequently seen upon close examination.

Lagios and associates examined mastectomy specimens for cancers with tumor foci outside a 5-cm radius of the reference tumor, the hypothetical border of a breast quadrant.[59] Multifocality was found in 20% of cases. Their findings closely approximated those of Rosen and colleagues, who reported residual tumor in 26% and 38% of patients with reference tumors smaller than and larger than 2 cm in diameter, respectively.[56]

These series analyzed conservative mastectomy specimens. A more recent study by Holland and co-workers excluded the mastectomy specimens of patients who were clearly not candidates for breast-sparing procedures in an attempt to gauge the incidence of multifocal disease left behind if these procedures had been performed.[60] Of 399 mastectomy specimens, 315 (79%), including specimens from 282 patients with invasive cancers smaller than 5 cm and 33 patients with noninvasive cancer, were judged to have been taken from possible candidates for breast preservation and thus were analyzed. Excluded from this series were 84 patients who had multifocal tumors (detected clinically or by mammogram), tumors larger than 5 cm in diameter or extending to the skin or chest wall, diffuse invasive cancers, or clinically and radiographically occult cancers found on "blind" biopsy.

If invasive tumors of 2 cm or less in diameter had been removed with a margin of 4 cm (representing a quadrantectomy) in this study, 5% of these patients would have been found to harbor invasive tumor foci elsewhere in the breast, and another 5% would have had noninvasive cancer detected. However, if these same tumors had been removed with a 2-cm margin, the percentage of patients harboring invasive or noninvasive cancers elsewhere would have increased to 14% and 28%, respectively. These data indicate that a quadrantectomy leaves less multicentric disease in the remaining breast than does wide excision with a 2-cm margin.

Of greater importance is whether or not these histologic findings indicate any biological or clinical activity. As is discussed in Chapter 11, *In Situ Cancers,* long-term follow-up studies of patients with noninvasive breast cancer treated by biopsy alone are available. In a retrospective review at Memorial Sloan-Kettering Cancer Center, Rosen and colleagues reported a series of 99 patients with lobular carcinoma *in situ* detected by biopsy between 1940 and 1950.[61] To identify these patients, a pathologic review of all patients undergoing a biopsy for benign disease during that period was undertaken, and once these patients were identified, follow-up studies were conducted. The median duration of follow-up was 25 years. None of these patients had coexistent infiltrating or intraductal carcinoma on biopsy examination. The average age of these patients at the time of biopsy was in the middle of the fifth decade of life, indicating that the follow-up period approached the life expectancy of this group. As can be seen in Table 10-4, 15 patients were lost to follow-up. Of the remaining 84, 32 developed breast carcinoma, and half of these patients died of breast cancer. More than 50% of the patients who developed breast cancer did so more than 15 years after biopsy, with no intervening cancer, underscoring the need for long-term observation of patients with this disease. The tendency for bilaterality is reflected in the fact that 50% of the patients who developed subsequent breast cancer did so in the contralateral breast. The incidence of subsequent carcinoma in this series was nine times the expected rate, and mortality from breast cancer was 11 times greater than that anticipated in the general population.

Table 10-4

Summary of Follow-up Status of Patients With Lobular Carcinoma in Situ

Follow-up Status	*No. of Patients*
Alive, no carcinoma prior or subsequent to diagnosis of lobular carcinoma in situ	39
Treated for breast carcinoma	32
Died of other causes, no carcinoma prior or subsequent to diagnosis of lobular carcinoma in situ	13
Follow-up status unknown	15
Total	99

(Rosen PP, Lieberman PH, Braun DW, et al: Lobular carcinoma in situ of the breast. Am J Surg Pathol 2:225, 1978.)

Patients with intraductal carcinoma who were treated by biopsy alone demonstrated two important differences from patients with lobular carcinoma *in situ*: an earlier development of subsequent carcinoma and a tendency for the carcinoma to involve the ipsilateral breast. As shown in Table 10-5, in one series, 39% of such patients developed carcinoma 10 years or less after biopsy. Although many of these series report excision of intraductal cancers that presented as masses, the experience at Memorial Sloan-Kettering Cancer Center comprises a group of patients with intraductal carcinoma identified on later pathologic review (of the same "benign" biopsies obtained between 1940 and 1950 and reported in the paper on lobular carcinoma *in situ* cited above).[62] Thus, these patients did not present with masses caused by malignant disease, and their clinical course might be likened to what could be expected in patients whose intraductal carcinomas are found on mammography today (i.e., presenting with suspicious microcalcifications and no masses) if they were to be followed by excision alone.

Unsuspected breast cancer has been found at the time of autopsy in elderly women dying of causes other than breast cancer. In a series of 70 patients older than 70 years of age, only 4 patients (5.7%) had intraductal cancer; 1 of these patients had microinvasion.[63] These findings contrast with the much higher incidence of unsuspected prostatic cancer found in men at autopsy,[64] suggesting that breast cancer is most likely to express itself as a clinical entity during the patient's lifetime.

Axillary Lymph Node Metastases

It is recognized that clinical assessment of axillary lymph node status is associated with a significant incidence of error. Both false-positive and false-negative impressions

Table 10-5
Combined Results of Follow-up of Patients With Untreated Intraductal Carcinoma*

Source	*No. Cases of Untreated Intraductal Carcinoma*	*Type of Untreated Carcinoma*	*Development of Subsequent Carcinoma No. (%)*	*Interval to Development of Subsequent Carcinoma*
Dean and Geschickter	8	Comedo	6 (75)	≤ 4 yr
Kraus and Neubecker	4	Papillary	2 (50)	10–12 yr
Farrow	25	Unspecified	5 (25)	1–8 yr
Haagensen et al.	11	Papillary	8 (73)	≤ 10 yr
Betsill et al.	25	Papillary	7 (28)	10 mo–24 yr (average of 9.7 yr)
Total	73		28 (39)	

* Untreated in this context means diagnosis by biopsy without further therapy.
(Betsill WL, Rosen PP, Lieberman PH, et al: Intraductal carcinoma. JAMA 238:1863, 1978.)

have been documented by comparison to pathologic examination of axillary nodes. An error in clinical evaluation of approximately one-third is widely accepted.[65]

The pathologic status of the axillary nodes is considered to be the most important prognostic factor for patients with carcinoma of the breast. In a 30-year follow-up of patients undergoing radical mastectomy at Memorial Sloan-Kettering Cancer Center, survival was more closely correlated with axillary node status than with the size of the primary cancers.[22] All patients with negative nodes had a 75% survival rate. Involvement of the lower axillary lymph nodes (level I) was associated with a 40% survival rate, and this survival rate decreased with more advanced axillary nodal disease. However, it is likely that the total number of nodes involved is more important in determining prognosis than is the level of the axilla at which metastases are found.[23] This theory has been confirmed by a recent analysis of patterns of axillary lymph node metastases in over 1200 specimens studied by Rosen and coworkers.[41] A progressive spread from a low axillary level (I) to a high axillary level (II) was noted as the number of positive nodes increased. Only 3% of patients had "skip" metastases (most of which involved level II nodes with negative level I nodes). This figure represents 3% of all patients having axillary metastases, and only 1.6% of all 1228 patients who had axillary dissections. Fifty percent of these metastases were limited to level II; only 0.5% would have had undetected nodal metastases if the dissection had included levels I and II. A close correlation exists between the level of nodal involvement and the total number of involved nodes (Table 10-6). When the highest level of nodal involvement was level I, only 14% of patients had four or more lymph nodes involved. Conversely, if levels II and III were involved, 78% and 98% of patients, respectively, had more than three nodes affected.

One of the controversies in breast cancer management is whether removal of axillary nodal metastases is a therapeutic practice or whether it is merely a staging procedure, allowing identification of patients who are at high risk for recurrence and are, therefore, candidates for adjuvant systemic treatment. Earlier advocates of the latter hypothesis believe that axillary node sampling is adequate, and that little therapeutic or staging benefit is achieved by thorough axillary dissection.[66]

Boova and associates also studied this problem, evaluating 200 consecutive mastectomy specimens from patients who underwent complete axillary dissections.[67] As in the Memorial series cited above, 60% had no axillary metastases. Of the 40% with axillary lymph node involvement, seven patients (8.8%) had metastases to levels II or III, or both, if level I was uninvolved pathologically. This figure represents 5.5% of the entire group, indicating that a level I dissection is an accurate predictor of the entire axilla in 95% of patients.

The difficulty in interpreting these studies is that they are performed in the pathology laboratory on radical or modified radical mastectomy specimens. Although axillary levels are indicated by the placement of tags in the operating room, indistinct boundaries between levels are possible. A study of perhaps greater clinical value is the one by Davies and colleagues which was carried out at Guy's Hospital.[42] They compared findings on clinical examination with those obtained on axillary node biopsy (done in the operating room), those reported on axillary node sampling in the same patients, and those derived from complete axillary dissection. Axillary node biopsy failed to detect metastases in 42% of patients, and axillary node sampling, or excision of nodes in the axillary tail, missed 14% of the patients with axillary metastases. Even if one believes that axillary dissection is only a staging procedure, it is apparent that a significant number of patients with involved nodes would not be detected by some types of axillary sampling.

Axillary lymph nodes are not routinely subjected to serial sections, a tedious and costly undertaking. In studies of patients with negative axillary nodes in whom serial sectioning of nodes was undertaken, Pickren showed that more than 20% of patients with uninvolved axillary nodes

Table 10-6
Distribution of Number of Lymph Nodes With Metastases Related to Highest Axillary Level Involved

Highest Axillary Level Involved	*No. of Positive Lymph Nodes (Percentage of Patients With Metastases at Stated Level)* ≤ 3	4–8	≥ 9
I	86%	12%	2%
II	22%	43%	35%
III	2%	19%	79%

(Rosen PP, Lesser MT, Kinne DW, et al: Discontinuous or "skip" metastases in breast carcinoma. Analysis of 1228 axillary dissections. Ann Surg 197:276, 1983.)

did, indeed, have microscopic metastases in one or more nodes.[68] His findings were later confirmed in another study by Wilkinson and associates.[69] The survival rates for such patients were the same as those for patients with negative nodes. Of importance is the fact that the nodes had been removed, a strong suggestion that these patients benefited from complete axillary dissection.

How many pathologically positive nodes are missed by not clearing the specimen? The clearing process, advocated by Pickren[68] and Haagensen,[70] yields a higher number of nodes, but it is a time-consuming, expensive process. The axillary fat is dissolved over a period of several days, allowing the identification and examination of even very small nodes. In a study by Morrow and associates,[71] axillary nodes removed at the time of mastectomy were examined in the usual manner by pathologists at Memorial Sloan-Kettering Cancer Center, where the average yield is 20 nodes per specimen. Without the knowledge of the pathologists involved, the remainder of the axillary fat was subjected to clearing. Several more nodes were identified in this manner. However, no patient with negative nodes at the first examination was found to have positive nodes in the cleared specimen. Patients initially identified as having involved axillary nodes had further metastatic deposits recovered in the cleared specimen, but this was not judged to be of significant clinical benefit. Therefore, clearing of lymph node dissections is not carried out in our institution.

The biological significance of axillary nodal metastases as predictors of the risk for systemic recurrence is not questioned. However, if not detected (or removed), they do not invariably develop into clinically significant lymphadenopathy. In NSABP trial B-04, which was recently updated with 10-year results,[72] one-third of patients with breast cancer and clinically negative axillae underwent radical mastectomy. Forty percent had pathologically involved nodes. However, one-third of the patients treated by total mastectomy and observation of the axilla developed clinical disease that was histologically confirmed in the axilla in 17.8% of cases. It is assumed that the groups are comparable in this randomized, prospective study, indicating that not all patients with pathologically involved axillary nodes that are left untreated will develop clinically evident disease in the axilla.

Interpretation of Results

Standard parameters for reporting results are local-regional recurrence and survival. Local recurrence after mastectomy is defined as recurrence in either the chest wall or axilla. Regional recurrences are those that affect the ipsilateral supraclavicular or parasternal nodes, reflecting internal mammary nodal involvement. In breast-preserving procedures, local recurrence may affect the breast (whether irradiated or left untreated), and the distinction between persistent and new cancer is sometimes difficult and arbitrary. If, within a few years of primary treatment, the cancer recurs beneath the scar or in the same quadrant and has a similar histologic pattern to that of the primary tumor, it is generally considered to be persistent cancer that was not completely eradicated by the surgical excision or irradiation, or a combination of both. However, a recurrence many years later elsewhere in the breast probably represents a new neoplasm. This distinction is important because ideally, the persistence of cancer may be avoided by adequate excision with clear margins and a boost dose of radiation therapy to the tumor site; the latter, however, will probably develop in a certain percentage of cases with time.

Survival is best defined as disease-free survival, or no evidence of disease (NED). Overall survival figures are also reported and include patients who have had recurrences but who are still alive.

Recurrences, especially those that are local-regional, should be defined according to the site of first recurrence. It is recognized, however, that local recurrence may develop in a patient with distant metastases as a phenomenon associated with reseeding of the chest wall or axilla from other disease.

Although most recurrences after mastectomy occur within 5 years of treatment, a significant number of recurrences appear between 5 and 10 years. In his recent report of NSABP trial B-04, Fisher noted that the trends observed at 5 years were unchanged at 10 years.[72] Although more recurrences were noted in all groups, they were in line with what had been observed at 5 years, lending weight to the interpretation of the 5-year results. However, in that NSABP trial, all patients underwent mastectomy with variations in treatment of the axillae. In ongoing trials of breast preservation with or without irradiation, longer intervals to the development of recurrence may be anticipated, indicating that a follow-up period of longer than 5 years is needed.

Long-Term Results After Mastectomy

Robbins and Berg report 30-year follow-up studies on 1458 patients treated at Memorial Sloan-Kettering Cancer Center with standard radical mastectomy.[73] Thirteen percent of

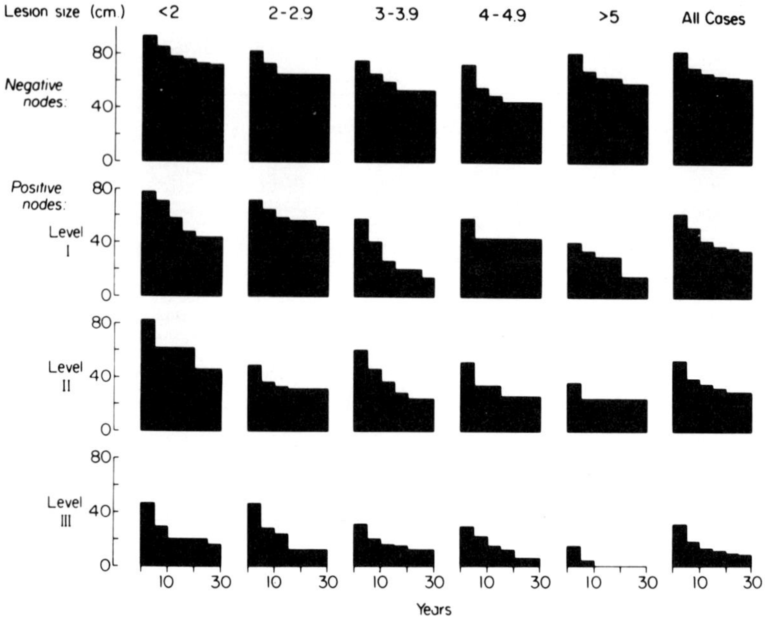

FIGURE 10-17. Data from 30-year Memorial Sloan-Kettering Cancer Center study, showing survival rates of patients in relation to node metastases and tumor size. (Adair et al. Cancer 33:1145, 1974.)

these women survived for 30 years free of cancer; of the remaining 87%, 57% died of breast cancer. Twenty-four percent died of other causes and 7% were lost to follow up. As can be seen from Figure 10-17, axillary nodal status was a more important determinant of prognosis than was the size of the primary tumor. Patients with tumors of less than 2 cm in diameter and involved nodes fared worse than did those with large tumors and negative nodes. Although the majority of patients in this study died of breast cancer, the death rate does not approach the 85% predicted by Mueller from the Syracuse Tumor Registry.[74] A contrary view is supported in a paper by Brinkley and Haybittle.[75] They studied 704 women who were treated surgically for breast cancer between 1947 and 1950 and who underwent follow-up for 22 years. After 21 years, they observed that the survival curve for these patients paralleled the expected survival curve for the normal population. This finding suggested a cure rate of about 18% for all patients with breast cancer and 30% for patients with Stage I or Stage II disease. Twenty-five percent of the survivors had axillary metastases, suggesting that some patients with this unfavorable clinical setting were cured by surgery alone and would not have benefited from systemic therapy. However, the number of patients dying of breast cancer more than 20 years after treatment was 12 times the expected rate in the general population, indicating the long-term risk incurred by patients with this disease.

Rutqvist and co-workers utilized logarithms of survival times in a study of 14,731 women with breast cancer from Norway.[76] With follow-up periods ranging from 5 to 18 years, the cured fractions were estimated to be 54%, 27%, 19%, and 2% for Stages I, II, III, and IV disease, respectively. The authors noted that the lognormal model accounted for both a late excess mortality and a cured fraction of patients.

Haagensen reviewed his 51-year personal experience with 1036 patients treated by radical mastectomy.[77] Results were reported according to the Columbia Clinical Classification system. The local recurrence rate 10 years after radical mastectomy was 3.7% in Stage A patients and 12% in Stage B patients. Pathologically involved nodes were recovered in 31% of Stage A patients, and 28% of Stage B patients had pathologically negative nodes. The overall 10-year disease-free survival rate was 77% for patients with negative nodes and 49% for patients with positive nodes.

The 10-year follow-up of 304 patients treated at Memorial Sloan-Kettering Cancer Center and classified by the TNM system was reported by Schottenfeld and associates.[78] Eighty-five percent of these patients were treated by radical mastectomy, with the remainder being treated by extended radical, modified radical, or total mastectomy. Thirty-six percent of patients with Stage II or III disease received postoperative radiotherapy. Adjuvant systemic therapy was not being administered during this era.

No local recurrence developed in Stage I patients within 10 years, but local recurrence was noted in 6% of Stage II and III patients. These findings are comparable to the local recurrence risk reported by Haagensen,[77] and are summarized in Table 10-7.

Overall 10-year survival rates, according to pathologic TNM stage, were 91% for patients with Stage I disease, 57% for those with Stage II disease, and 34% for patients with Stage III disease. In patients with negative axillary nodes, the 10-year survival risk, according to the size of the primary tumor, was 82% for those with tumors of less than 2 cm in diameter, 65% for those with tumors of 2 cm to 5 cm, and 44% for patients with primary tumors greater than 5 cm in diameter. Overall, patients with negative nodes had a 71% survival rate compared with a 48% survival rate in those with positive nodes. As in the Robbins series, the level of axillary metastases correlated with sur-

Table 10-7
Ten-Year Results in 304 Patients From Memorial Sloan-Kettering Cancer Center

TNM Stage	*% of Patients*	*Observed Survival*	*Local Recurrence (%)*
I	22	90.9	0
II	58	57.1	6 (II and III)
III	20	33.9	

(Schottenfeld D, Nash AG, Robbins GF, et al: Ten-year results of the treatment of primary operable breast carcinoma. A summary of 304 patients evaluated by the TNM system. Cancer 38:1001, 1976.)

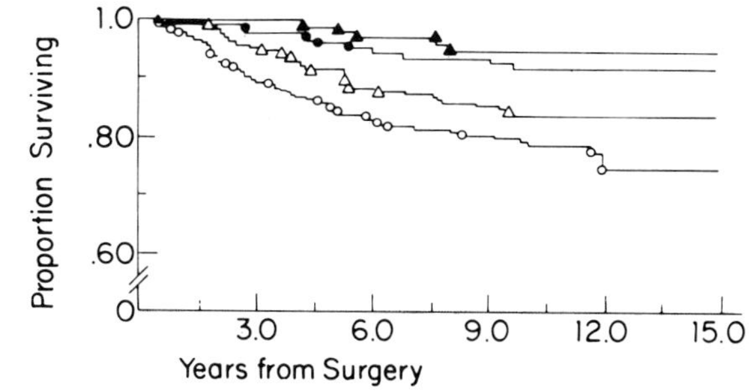

FIGURE 10-18. The estimated distribution of time to recurrence and estimated distribution of survival time for 382 patients with T1N0M0 breast carcinoma. (*Triangles* represent the total proportion of patients surviving; *circles* represent the proportion of the total number of patients who are alive without recurrence; *solid figures* represent results from Group A, whereas *open figures* represent results from Group B.) (Rosen PP, Saigo PE, Braun DW Jr, et al: Predictors of recurrence in Stage I (T1N0M0) breast cancer. Ann Surg 193:15, 1981.)

vival. If the highest axillary node involved was level I, the survival rate was 65%. The survival rate decreased to 30% if levels II and III were involved by metastases. As noted earlier, there is a close correlation between the level of involvement and the total number of nodes harboring metastases.

In a retrospective review of patients with small breast cancers treated at Memorial Sloan-Kettering Cancer Center, Rosen and colleagues showed that patients with pathologic TINOMO (Stage I) disease had a disease-free survival of 84%.[79] As seen in Figure 10-18, it took 12 years before the survival curve flattened, and patients with tumors less than or equal to 1.0 cm in diameter fared better than those whose cancers measured 1.1 cm to 2.0 cm. Thirty-nine percent of those with the larger tumors who had lymphatic tumor emboli developed distant recurrence. This finding approximates the survival rate of patients with pathologically involved nodes, and at this center, is an indication for adjuvant systemic therapy when axillary nodes are uninvolved.

Patients with Stage II lesions and pathologically involved nodes have a poorer prognosis than do patients with T1N0 disease, again indicating that nodal status is a more important prognostic indicator than is tumor size.[80] Interestingly, even if one axillary node is involved with micrometastases (a lesion with a diameter smaller than or equal to 2 mm), the disease-free survival (56%) is the same as in patients with one axillary macrometastasis, and both groups are advised to receive adjuvant systemic therapy (Fig. 10-19). The importance, in terms of survival, of the number of nodes involved is shown in the series reported by Wilson and co-workers, in which 5-year survival curves showed a gradual decrease as the number of nodes increased (Fig. 10-20).[23] The 5-year survival rate was greatest (91.5%) if no nodes were involved; the survival rates decreased to 82.3% if one node was involved, to 77.3% if 2 to 3 nodes were involved, and the rate continued to decrease in stepwise fashion to 38.9% if 21 or more nodes were involved with metastases. These findings emphasize the prognostic significance of axillary lymph node involvement and point to the need for effective systemic therapy to control occult distant metastases in these patients. The latter emphasis, however, has tended to reduce

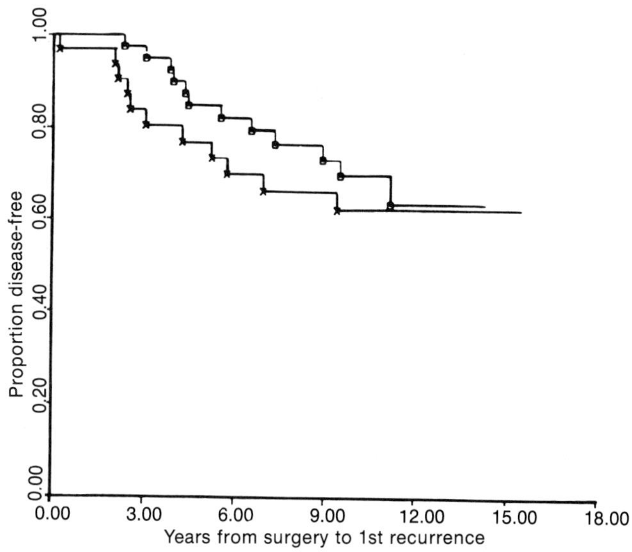

FIGURE 10-19. Disease-free survival curves from T1N1M0-staged patients with a metastasis in a single axillary lymph node. Micrometastasis occurred in 41 patients, and macrometastasis was found in 32 patients. (Rosen PP, Saigo PE, Braun DW Jr, et al: Prognosis in Stage II (T1N1M0) breast cancer. Ann Surg 194:585, 1981.)

the importance ascribed to adequate local-regional control. Recent retrospective reports have reiterated the need for an adequate, thorough surgical approach in patients with Stages II or III breast cancer.[81,82] Also, should patients with these stages of cancer have negative axillary nodes on pathologic examination, their disease-free survival rates are high enough that most oncologists do not consider them to be candidates for systemic treatment. Fracchia and associates showed an overall 10-year survival rate of 75%

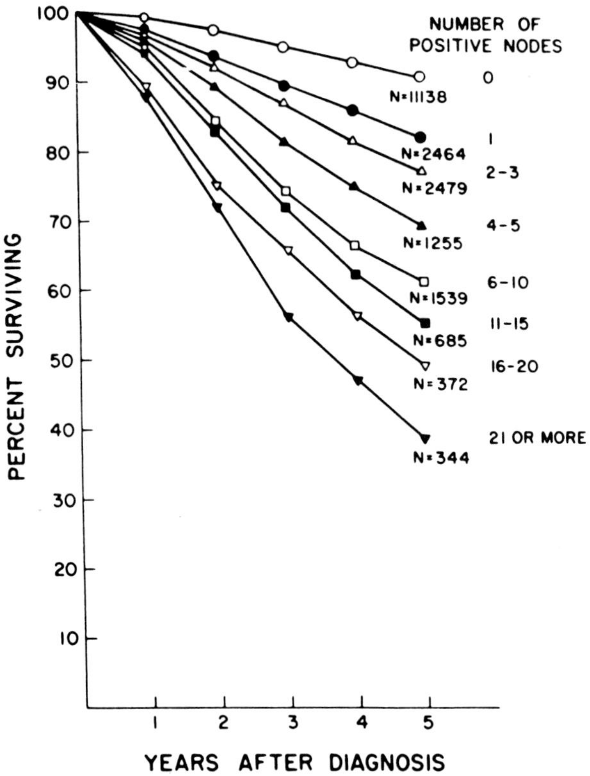

FIGURE 10-20. Actuarial survival of patients with carcinoma of the breast according to the number of positive nodes. (Wilson RE, Donegan WL, Mettlin C, et al: The 1982 survey of carcinoma of the breast in the United States by the American College of Surgeons. Surg Gynecol Obstet 159:309, 1984.)

following radical mastectomy in patients with Stage III disease with no involved axillary nodes.[83]

Surgical Trials

Extended Radical Mastectomy Versus Radical Mastectomy

The rationale for extended radical mastectomy, which includes removal of the internal mammary lymph nodes, is based upon studies showing nodal involvement with metastases, which is most commonly seen in patients with cancers of the central or inner breast quadrant. Turner-Warwick, using injection of dye and colloidal gold into the skin of the breast, showed that 25% of the lymph leaving the breast courses to the internal mammary nodes,[84] and thus may be derived from all quadrants of the breast.

Biopsy of the internal mammary nodes at the time of modified radical mastectomy was done by Handley.[16] Twenty-two percent of his patients had involved nodes, and this percentage increased in patients with tumors of the central or inner breast quadrant, or those with involved axillary lymph nodes. When these patients underwent irradiation of the internal mammary chain, their survival rates did not differ from those in patients undergoing radical mastectomy.

In nonrandomized series, investigators, such as Urban[85] and Deemarski and Seleznev,[86] showed a survival advantage in patients undergoing extended radical mastectomy over those treated by radical mastectomy. Others, such as Dahl-Iversen, could show no difference.[17]

A multicenter, prospective, randomized trial was organized by Lacour and co-workers in 1963 to compare extended radical to radical mastectomy.[87] In this trial, 1453 patients with T1, T2, or T3, N0, or N1M0 breast cancer were studied between 1963 and 1968. In 1976, the 5-year results were reported, showing no difference in relapse-free or overall survival rates in either group.[87] One subgroup of patients, those with T1 and T2 cancer involving the central or inner breast quadrant and positive axillary nodes, showed a survival advantage if treated by extended radical mastectomy. Five-year survival rates of 71% were observed in these patients, compared to a 52% survival rate in patients treated by radical mastectomy ($p = 0.01$). No other subgroups showed differences in survival rates (including those with medial or central T1 and T2 disease with negative axillary nodes, or patients with medial or central T3 cancers with positive axillary nodes). In 1981, Veronesi reported on a subset of patients who underwent 10-year follow-up among a group of 716 patients who were evaluated.[88] No radiotherapy or chemotherapy was given to any group of patients. The two groups showed virtually the same relapse-free survival rate (49.7% and 47.3%) and overall survival rate (60.7% and 57%). No significant difference was noted between the survival rates of patients with negative nodes and survival in those with positive axillary nodes. Subset analyses, based upon the number of nodes involved or the size and location of the primary tumor, showed no differences between the two operations. However, Veronesi recently reported the prognostic importance of internal mammary lymph node metastases, and advised biopsy of the first intercostal space in selected patients.[89]

Extended radical mastectomy is a procedure that is seldom practiced in this country. A recent national survey indicated that it represented 1.1% of breast cancer operations performed in more than 24,000 patients treated in 1976.[23] Should the internal mammary nodes be left untreated? Although postmastectomy irradiation to this lymph node chain and the supraclavicular area (hockey-stick portal) has been carried out for many years and has been shown to result in better local control in patients with positive axillary nodes,[90] no influence on survival has been demonstrated. This subject will be reviewed in detail in the section on postmastectomy radiotherapy, later in this chapter. In NSABP trial B-04, patients with medial or central breast cancers were analyzed in a report published in 1981.[91] In this study, 1665 patients treated in 34 institutions were randomized to undergo either radical mastectomy, total mastectomy with postoperative regional irradiation, or total mastectomy with delayed axillary dissection (in those patients whose nodes became clinically involved). Based on an 82-month median follow-up, no difference in disease-free or overall survival was noted among the three groups. Postoperative radiotherapy did not influence overall survival rates in patients with medial or central lesions when compared to survival rates in patients with lateral lesions. In no subgroup, including patients with positive axillary nodes, could any advantage be shown.

Our current practice is to advise all patients with positive axillary lymph nodes demonstrated on pathologic analysis to undergo systemic therapy. Many of these patients have metastases to the internal mammary nodes which are not recognized or treated either surgically or by radiotherapy, and the hope is that the systemic therapy will control the disease. Long-term follow-up of the subset of patients with central and medial lesions will be undertaken to determine any differences in local (especially parasternal) recurrence and overall survival.

The management of patients with pathologically documented negative axillary nodes and medial or central cancers is more difficult. Perhaps internal mammary lymphoscintigraphy, as advocated by Ege,[92] will become accurate enough to pinpoint the group with involved internal mammary nodes. Based upon Urban's analysis of patients undergoing extended radical mastectomy, 13% of patients with medial or central lesions and negative axillary nodes will have positive internal mammary nodes.[85] A reasonable practice, as advocated by Veronesi,[88] is to attempt to identify this group by extrapleural internal mammary lymph node biopsy (usually practical in interspaces 1 or 2). When metastases are found in these patients, systemic therapy is advised.

Radical Mastectomy Versus Modified Radical Mastectomy

As noted earlier, there was a shift in practice from performing radical mastectomy to performing modified radical mastectomy in the mid 1970s in this country, but this change was not based upon data generated in any prospective randomized trial. The reasons given earlier in this chapter, including the awareness and input on the part of patients, were persuasive enough to force this change. Also, retrospective studies, such as that of Baker and colleagues,[93] showed no significant difference in 5-year survival between patients undergoing radical mastectomy and those undergoing modified radical mastectomy at any stage of disease.

A randomized prospective trial comparing radical mastectomy to modified radical mastectomy in 311 patients has been reported by Maddox and co-workers.[94] This was a surgical and adjunctive chemotherapy trial conducted in the state of Alabama between 1975 and 1978. All patients with pathologically involved axillary lymph nodes received one year of cyclophosphamide (Cytoxan), methotrexate, and 5-fluorouracil (CMF). With a median follow-up of 5.5 years, no significant differences in disease-free or overall survival rates were noted. However, there was a trend toward improved 5-year survival rates in the group having radical mastectomy (84%) over the survival rate in those undergoing modified radical mastectomy (76%) ($p = 0.14$). Also, higher local recurrence rates were noted in patients undergoing modified radical mastectomy than in those having radical mastectomy, although the difference was not statistically significant ($p = 0.09$). Although the sample size for Stage III patients was small (36 patients), local recurrence in this subgroup was highest in patients undergoing modified radical mastectomy (20% recurrence rate versus 6.3% in those undergoing radical mastectomy). A longer follow-up period is needed to evaluate thoroughly the significance of this study.

Another randomized trial, conducted by Turner and colleagues in the United Kingdom, compared 534 patients undergoing either modified radical or radical mastectomy. No Stage III patients were included in this study.[95] Once again, no difference in disease-free or overall survival was noted, but a trend of improved survival at 5 years was observed in the group undergoing radical mastectomy (85%), compared to the 5-year survival rate in those having modified radical mastectomy (78%).

NSABP trial B-04, begun in 1971, did not include a modified radical mastectomy arm, but did randomize patients to undergo a variety of approaches to axillary lymph nodes, and all patients underwent breast removal. If the axillae were clinically negative, patients underwent either radical mastectomy, total mastectomy and irradiation of axillary nodes (perhaps the equivalent of modified radical mastectomy), or total mastectomy with delayed axillary dissection (if the nodes subsequently became clinically involved). Patients with clinically involved nodes at the time of presentation underwent either radical mastectomy or total mastectomy and irradiation to the axilla.

Ten-year results, published recently,[72] demonstrated no significant differences in disease-free survival or overall survival (57%) among the three groups of patients with clinically negative axillae. Similarly, patients with clinically involved nodes showed no survival difference (38% in each group).

In the patients treated with radical mastectomy, 40% of patients with clinically negative axillary nodes proved to have histologically positive nodes. Assuming that the same percentage of patients undergoing total mastectomy had microscopic involvement of these nodes, it is interesting to note that only 18% underwent axillary dissection as a result of the development of clinically positive nodes. This may indicate that not all histologically positive nodes will become biologically active, although the authors admit that another event, such as tumor recurrence elsewhere, death, or microscopic foci of tumor in nodes which never became clinically detectable, might have occurred. Another possible interpretation is that, in patients treated by total mastectomy alone, the untreated positive nodes might have served as a source of further dissemination, leading to a higher rate of distant metastases. Because this did not occur, there is no support in this study for the concept that metastases, by themselves, instigate metastases. Also of importance is the fact that, in the patients receiving irradiation to the axilla, the foci were well controlled, with only 3.1% of affected patients presenting with axillary recurrence. Radiotherapy in patients with clinically positive nodes was less successful, with 12% developing recurrence.

Although it provides interesting answers to the biological behavior of breast cancer, this study provides little guidance in the management of patients today. With increased utilization of breast-sparing approaches and the widespread use of adjuvant systemic therapy for patients with positive axillary nodes, most, if not all, patients with breast cancer are advised to undergo axillary dissection as part of the staging and treatment process. If, prior to treatment, patients are judged not to be candidates for systemic therapy (perhaps owing to advanced age, severe medical illness, or other factors), this study would indicate that either irradiation of the nodes or observation with delayed nodal dissection once clinical involvement occurs is a reasonable option.

Breast Preservation Procedures

As noted in the section on Surgical Procedures (above), the preferred terms and techniques in breast-preserving approaches are wide excision, partial mastectomy, or limited resection, consisting of excision of the tumor with grossly normal margins. The terms lumpectomy, tumorectomy, and segmental mastectomy are imprecise.

Partial mastectomy alone, with no radiotherapy, has been carried out in many institutions. As can be seen in Table 10-8, the relapse rate in the ipsilateral breast ranged from 25% to 37% within 5 years or less for the stages of infiltrating breast cancers treated by this method. This finding is comparable to the local recurrence rate reported by Hermann and associates in the Cleveland Clinic experience.[96] In a group of carefully selected patients with small, peripheral, unicentric tumors, constituting 18% of the entire Cleveland Clinic breast cancer experience, partial mastectomy alone was performed. With a 15-year follow-up period, local recurrence developed in 23% of patients (16% had recurrence at the excision site, whereas 7% had recurrence at another site in the breast). Another group developed axillary lymph node metastases. Even though many of these patients were cured after so-called salvage mastectomy, these recurrence rates have led most oncologists to prefer other approaches.

Table 10-8
Results of Partial Mastectomy Alone as Treatment for Early Breast Cancer

Institution	Stage	Breast Relapse Rate (%)	Follow-up (Yr)
Princess Margaret	T1–T2,N0	25	5
Royal Marsden	T1–T2,N0	33	5
Suffolk	T1–T2,N0 or N1	37	3
McGill	T1–T2,N0	28	5
Children's Hospital, San Francisco	T1–T2,N0 or N1	28	2

Many prospective randomized studies comparing mastectomy to breast-preserving approaches, with or without irradiation, have been conducted and will be reviewed in detail in the section on radiotherapy (below). However, some aspects of these trials deserve emphasis in this surgical discussion.

In the two trials conducted at Guy's Hospital,[97,98] overall interpretation is limited by the fact that inadequate doses of radiotherapy were administered to the two groups. During a period of 3 weeks, patients underwent either radical mastectomy plus 3000 cGy to axillary, internal mammary, and supraclavicular fields, or wide excision plus 3800 cGy to the breast and, for a period of 2 weeks, 3000 cGy to axillary and supraclavicular fields. The second series repeated these treatments except, unlike the first series, it included patients younger than 50 years of age and was limited to those with clinically negative axillary nodes. In the first series, no differences in survival rates in patients with Stage I disease was noted, but an advantage for mastectomy-treated patients in the second series was apparent. This was interpreted as an improved survival in the mastectomy group between the first and second series (Fig. 10-21). Hayward attributes this difference to the lower local recurrence in the second series compared to that in the first (8% and 14%, respectively), attributable, perhaps, to a more careful surgical approach in the second series.[98] In the first series, procedures were carried out by junior surgeons in training; in the second, full-time surgeons working in a breast unit did the procedures.

In the Milan trial, patients with small primary tumors (clinically staged as T1N0 disease) underwent either quadrantectomy, axillary dissection, and radiation therapy (QUART), or radical mastectomy.[99] Good local control was observed in the QUART arm of the study, with the development of 12 recurrent or new cancers in the ipsilateral breast of 352 patients followed for 10 years.[100] This wide excision may have encompassed most multifocal disease, as suggested in the pathologic analysis of mastectomy specimens by Holland and associates,[60] and may explain the good local control rate despite the lack of a boost dose to the tumor site. This finding emphasizes the impression that an inverse relationship exists between surgical and radiotherapeutic approaches to achieve optimal local control in the breast—that is, the wider the surgical excision, the lesser is the need for boost radiotherapy, and vice versa.

Several important points will be discussed later in this chapter in the analysis of the NSABP B0-6 trial.[101] In this study, patients with clinical Stage I and II breast cancer with lesions measuring less than or equal to 4 cm in diameter were randomized to undergo either total mastectomy, segmental mastectomy, or segmental mastectomy with radiotherapy to the remaining breast. All groups underwent axillary dissection and all patients with pathologically involved nodes received adjuvant chemotherapy. In the study design, all patients shown to have involved margins on histologic analysis at the time of segmental mastectomy (10% of patients) underwent total mastectomy

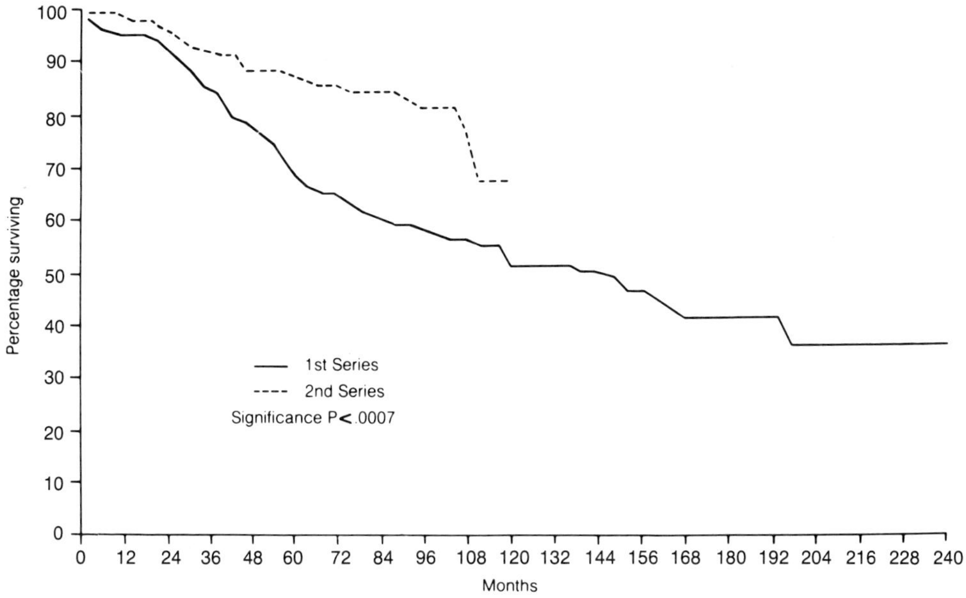

FIGURE 10-21. Comparison of survival rates in patients with Stage I disease who underwent radical mastectomy in the first and second Guy's Hospital series. The better results in the second series are attributed to more careful, thorough dissection. (Harris JR, Hellman S, Silen W: Conservative Management of Breast Cancer, Philadelphia, JB Lippincott, 1983)

and were kept in their respective trial groups. Although this eliminated the risk of possible breast recurrence (which one would surmise would be a high risk owing to the positive margins), this subgroup had larger primary tumors and more involved axillary nodes than did the other groups, placing them at higher risk for the development of distant metastases.

The high rate of breast recurrence in the group undergoing segmental mastectomy (28% at 5 years) is in keeping with prior nonrandomized studies (see Table 10-8) and cannot be considered surprising. Determination of the percentage of these patients who are able to undergo salvage mastectomy and the results of long-term follow-up will be important aspects of this study. Although Fisher points out that 5-year follow-up in NSABP trial B-04 predicted the 10-year results (which makes a case for ascribing increased importance to 5-year results in breast cancer studies), there are important differences in the two studies. Principally, the breast preservation approaches in trial B-06 will require longer follow-up owing to possible delayed recurrence (or development of new cancer) in the breasts preserved, whether irradiated or not. The risk for this development and the results of treatment in these subgroups will require a longer follow-up period.

Salvage Mastectomy

Salvage mastectomy is carried out in patients in whom recurrent (or new) breast cancer develops following breast preservation approaches. If the axilla was treated initially (either by surgical dissection or irradiation), the procedure is a total mastectomy. In our experience, wound healing has not been a problem when salvage mastectomy was carried out in a previously irradiated breast.

Results of this treatment approach have varied. In some series, survival in the subgroup undergoing salvage mastectomy equalled or was better than the survival in patients undergoing breast preservation initially, with or without irradiation.[96] However, Amalric and co-workers described pathologic findings in salvage mastectomy specimens.[102] The procedure was carried out in 32% of patients followed for 10 years after primary breast irradiation. Active residual (or new) carcinoma was found in 56% of patients. The remainder had no residual disease, radionecrosis, or tumor of uncertain viability.

These findings have led other groups to report salvage mastectomy survival rates in patients with documented viable cancer in the mastectomy specimens. Osborne and colleagues, reporting 20-year results after performing breast preservation procedures with irradiation, found that 5-year results after salvage mastectomy correlated with the original axillary status.[103] The survival rate was 42% for patients with a clinically negative axilla, and zero if the axilla was clinically positive initially. Local excision resulted in a decreased survival rate, and another subgroup of patients was considered to be inoperable as a result of the local extent of disease or distant metastases.

Harris and co-workers analyzed long-term risk for recurrence and results of salvage mastectomy.[104] Two series in France and one in Canada, in which the pathology of the specimens could be confirmed and survival assessed, were combined in this study. The risk of developing recurrence persisted for 14 years, although it was greatest during the first 5 years after treatment. In 22% of the patients included in the study, breast cancer developed in the irradiated breast. Salvage mastectomy resulted in a survival rate of 50%.

Other Considerations

As will be discussed in the section on radiotherapy (below), several retrospective and prospective randomized studies show that breast preservation approaches in selected patients with breast cancer offer disease-free and overall survival rates that approach those achieved by mastectomy. This represents an advance in therapy that offers patients an important option. However, it is appropriate to point out that it does not represent an advance in terms of an increased survival rate or less extensive treatment. Both of these misinterpretations have been presented in lay press analyses, and may mislead patients and physicians alike. The hope is that more patients with earlier stages of disease will present for screening and diagnosis because they understand that mastectomy is no longer a uniform approach to treatment. This, in itself, may lead to improved survival following adequate therapy.

Psychological and cosmetic results are also important, and these will be reviewed in other sections of this book. It is apparent that patients undergoing breast preservation procedures have significant physical and psychological problems[105,106] that, in some studies, are comparable to those in patients treated by mastectomy. Cosmetic results are likely to improve in breast-sparing operations with improved selection of patients, pre-treatment cooperation between surgeons and radiotherapists, and improved surgical and radiotherapy techniques. How these results will compare to those achieved in mastectomy patients undergoing reconstruction must await further analyses.

REFERENCES

1. Breasted JH: The Edwin Smith Surgical Papyrus, Vols. 1 and 22. Breasted JH (trans): Chicago, University of Chicago Oriental Institute Publications, 1930
2. Robbins GF (ed): Silvergirl's Surgery: The Breast, pp 7–13. Austin, Texas, Silvergirl, Inc., 1984
3. Banks WM: A brief history of the operations practiced for cancer of the breast. Br Med J 1:5, 1902
4. Cooper WA: The history of the radical mastectomy. Ann Med Hist 3:36, 1941
5. Lewison EF: Breast Cancer and Its Diagnosis and Treatment, pp 1–27. Baltimore, Williams and Wilkins, 1955
6. Power, Sir D'A: The history of the amputation of the breast to 1904. Liverpool Med Chir J 42:29, 1934
7. Degenshein GA, Ceccarelli F: The history of breast cancer surgery. Part 1. Early beginnings to Halsted. Breast 3:28, 1977
8. Paget J: On disease of the mammary areola preceding cancer of the mammary gland. Rep St. Bartholomew's Hosp 10:87, 1874
9. Robbins GF (ed): Silvergirl's Surgery: The Breast, pp 33–127. Austin, Texas, Silvergirl, Inc., 1984
10. Halsted WS: The treatment of wounds with especial reference to the value of the blood clot in the management of dead space. Johns Hopkins Hosp Rep 2:255, 1890–1891
11. Halsted WS: The results of operations for the cure of cancer of the breast performed at the Johns Hopkins Hospital from June, 1889 to January, 1894. Johns Hopkins Hosp Bull 4:297, 1894–1895
12. Meyer W: An improved method of the radical operation for carcinoma of the breast. Med Rec 46:746, 1894
13. Haagensen CD: Diseases of the Breast, 3rd ed, pp 864–871. Philadelphia, WB Saunders, 1986
14. Halsted WS: The results of radical operations for the cure of carcinoma of the breast. Ann Surg 46:1, 1907
15. Handley WS: Parasternal invasion of the thorax in breast cancer and its suppression by the use of radium tubes as an operative precaution. Surg Gynecol Obstet 45:721, 1927
16. Handley RS, Thackray AC: Invasion of the internal mammary lymph nodes. Br Med J 1:61, 1954
17. Dahl-Iversen E: Recherches sur les metastases microscopique des ganglions lymphatiques parasternaux dans le cancer du sein. Int J Chir 11:492, 1951
18. Margottini M: Recent developments in the surgical treatment of breast carcinoma. Acta Un Int Cancer 8:176, 1952
19. Urban JA, Baker HW: Radical mastectomy in continuity with en bloc resection of the internal mammary lymph node chain. Cancer 5:992, 1952
20. Wangensteen OH: Remarks on extension of the Halsted operation for cancer of the breast. Ann Surg 130:315, 1949
21. Haagensen CD: Diseases of the Breast, 3rd ed, pp 872–938. Philadelphia, WB Saunders, 1986
22. Adair F, Berg J, Joubert L, et al: Long-term follow-up of breast cancer patients: The 30-year report. Cancer 33:1145, 1974
23. Wilson RE, Donegan WL, Mettlin C, et al: The 1982 survey of carcinoma of the breast in the United States by the American College of Surgeons. Surg Gynecol Obstet 159:309, 1984
24. Gazet J-C, Rainsbury RM, Ford HT, et al: Survey of treatment of primary breast cancer in Great Britain. Br Med J 290:1793, 1985
25. Patey DH, Dyson WH: The prognosis of carcinoma of the breast in relation to the type of operation performed. Br J Cancer 2:7, 1948
26. Kinne DW, DeCosse JJ: Modified radical mastectomy for carcinoma of the breast. Am Surg 48:543, 1982
27. Moosman DA: Anatomy of the pectoral nerves and their preservation in modified mastectomy. Am J Surg 139:883, 1980
28. Cody HS III, Egeli RA, Urban JA: Rotter's node metastases: Therapeutic and prognostic considerations in early breast carcinoma. Ann Surg 199:266, 1984
29. Durkin K, Haagensen CD: An improved technique for the study of lymph nodes in surgical specimens. Ann Surg 191:419, 1980
30. Kay S: Evaluation of Rotter's lymph nodes in radical mastectomy specimens as a guide to prognosis. Cancer 18:1441, 1965
31. Handley R, Thackray A: Conservative radical mastectomy (Patey's operation). Ann Surg 170:880, 1969
32. Maier WP, Leber D, Rosemond GP, et al: The technique of modified radical mastectomy. Surg Gynecol Obstet 145:69, 1977
33. Croce EJ: A neoclassical radical mastectomy. Surg Gynecol Obstet 147:921, 1978
34. Roses DF, Harris MN, Gumport SL: Total mastectomy with axillary dissection. Am J Surg 134:674, 1977
35. Auchincloss H: Significance of location and number of axillary metastases in carcinoma of the breast. A justification for a conservative operation. Ann Surg 158:37, 1963
36. Madden JL, Kandalaft S, Bourque R: Modified radical mastectomy. Ann Surg 175:624, 1972
37. Urban JA: Carcinoma of the breast. In Cooper P (ed): The Craft of Surgery. Boston, Little, Brown & Co, 1964
38. Haagensen CD: Diseases of the Breast. 3rd ed, p 872. Philadelphia, WB Saunders, 1986
39. Harris JR, Hellman S, Kinne DW: Limited surgery and radiotherapy for early breast cancer. N Engl J Med 313:1365, 1985
40. Saphir O, Amromin GD: Obscure axillary lymph-node metastasis in carcinoma of the breast. Cancer 1:238, 1948
41. Rosen PP, Lesser MT, Kinne DW, et al: Discontinuous or "skip" metastases in breast carcinoma. Analysis of 1228 axillary dissections. Ann Surg 197:276, 1983
42. Davies GC, Millis RR, Hayward JL: Assessment of axillary lymph node status. Ann Surg 192:148, 1980

43. Pigott J, Nichols R, Maddox WA, et al: Metastases to the upper levels of the axillary nodes in carcinoma of the breast and its implications for nodal sampling procedures. Surg Gynecol Obstet 158:255, 1984
44. Schnitt SJ, Connolly JL, Harris JR, et al: Pathologic predictors of early local recurrence in stage I and II breast cancer treated by primary radiation therapy. Cancer 53:1049, 1984
45. Fisher B: Reappraisal of breast biopsy prompted by the use of lumpectomy. Surgical strategy. JAMA 253:3585, 1985
46. Assa J: The intercostobrachial nerve in radical mastectomy. J Surg Oncol 6:123, 1974
47. Aitken DR, Minton JP: Complications associated with mastectomy. Surg Clin North Am 63:1331, 1983
48. Say CC, Donegan W: A biostatistical evaluation of complications from mastectomy. Surg Gynecol Obstet 138:370, 1974
49. Beatty JD, Robinson GV, Zaia JA, et al: A prospective analysis of nosocomial wound infection after mastectomy. Arch Surg 118:1421, 1983
50. Budd DC, Cochran RC, Sturtz OC, et al: Surgical morbidity after mastectomy operations. Am J Surg 135:218, 1978
51. Lotze UT, Duncan MA, Gerber LH, et al: Early versus delayed shoulder motion following axillary dissection. Ann Surg 193:288, 1981
52. Aitken DR, Hunsaker R, James AG: Prevention of seromas following mastectomy and axillary dissection. Surg Gynecol Obstet 158:327, 1984
53. Haagensen CD: Diseases of the Breast, 3rd ed, p 915. Philadelphia, WB Saunders, 1986
54. Wood KM: Intercostobrachial nerve entrapment syndrome. South Med J 71:662, 1978
55. Lagios MD, Westdahl PR, Rose MR: The concept and implications of multicentricity in breast carcinoma. In Sommers SG, Rosen PP (eds): Pathology Annual, pp 83–102. New York, Appleton-Century-Crofts, 1981
56. Rosen PP, Fracchia AA, Urban JA, et al: "Residual" mammary carcinoma following simulated partial mastectomy. Cancer 35:739, 1975
57. Schwartz GF, Patchesky AS, Feig SA, et al: Multicentricity of nonpalpable breast cancer. Cancer 45:2913, 1980
58. Rosen PP, Braun DW, Kinne DW: The clinical significance of preinvasive breast carcinoma. Cancer 46:919, 1980
59. Lagios MD, Richards VE, Rose ME, et al: Segmental mastectomy without radiotherapy. Cancer 52:2173, 1983
60. Holland R, Solke HJV, Mravunac M, et al: Histologic multifocality of Tis, T1-2 breast carcinomas. Cancer 56:979, 1985
61. Rosen PP, Lieberman PH, Braun DW, et al: Lobular carcinoma in situ of the breast. Am J Surg Pathol 2:225, 1978
62. Betsill WL, Rosen PP, Lieberman PH, et al: Intraductal carcinoma. JAMA 239:1863, 1978
63. Kramer WM, Rush BF Jr: Mammary duct proliferation in the elderly. Cancer 31:130, 1973
64. Franks LM: Latent carcinoma of the prostate. J Pathol Bacteriol 68:603, 1954
65. Haagensen CD: Diseases of the Breast, 3rd ed, pp 851–863. Philadelphia, WB Saunders, 1986
66. Fisher B, Wolmark N, Bauer M, et al: The accuracy of clinical nodal staging and of limited axillary dissection as a determinant of histologic nodal status in carcinoma of the breast. Surg Gynecol Obstet 152:765, 1981
67. Boora RS, Bonanni R, Rosato FE: Patterns of axillary nodal involvement in breast cancer. Predictability of level one dissection. Ann Surg 196:642, 1982
68. Pickren JW: Significance of occult metastases—A study of breast cancer. Cancer 14:1266, 1961
69. Wilkinson EJ, Hause LL, Hoffman RG, et al: Occult axillary lymph node metastases in invasive breast carcinoma: Characteristics of the primary tumor and significance of the metastases. Pathol Annu 17 (Pt 2):67, 1982
70. Haagensen CD: Diseases of the Breast, 3rd ed, pp 658–663. Philadelphia, WB Saunders, 1986
71. Morrow M, Evans J, Rosen PP, et al: Does clearing of the axillary lymph nodes contribute to accurate staging of breast carcinoma? Cancer 53:1329, 1984
72. Fisher B, Redmund C, Fisher ER, et al: Ten-year results of a randomized clinical trial comparing radical mastectomy and total mastectomy with or without radiation. N Engl J Med 312:674, 1985
73. Robbins GF, Berg J: Curability of patients with invasive breast carcinoma based on a 30-year study. World J Surg 1:284, 1977
74. Mueller CB, Ames F, Anderson GD: Breast cancer in 3558 women: Age as a significant determinant in the rate of dying and causes of death. Surgery 83:123, 1978
75. Brinkley D, Haybittle JL: The curability of breast cancer. Lancet 2:95, 1975
76. Rutqvist LE, Wallgren A, Nilsson B: Is breast cancer a curable disease? A study of 14,731 women with breast cancer from the cancer registry of Norway. Cancer 53:1793, 1984
77. Haagensen CD, Bodian C: A personal experience with Halsted's radical mastectomy. Ann Surg 199:143, 1984
78. Schottenfeld D, Nash AG, Robbins GF, et al: Ten-year results of the treatment of primary operable breast carcinoma. A summary of 304 patients evaluated by the TNM system. Cancer 38:1001, 1976
79. Rosen PP, Saigo PE, Braun DW Jr, et al: Predictors of recurrence in stage I (T1N0M0) breast cancer. Ann Surg 193:15, 1981
80. Rosen PP, Saigo PE, Braun DW Jr, et al: Prognosis in Stage II (T1N1M0) breast cancer. Ann Surg 194:576, 1981
81. Fracchia AA, Cody HS III, Eisenberg BL, et al: Stage II carcinoma of the breast: The importance of adequate local therapy. Breast 9:23, 1983
82. Cody HS III, Bretsky S, Urban JA: The continuing importance of adequate surgery for operable breast cancer. Breast 32:242, 1982
83. Fracchia AA, Evans JF, Eisenberg BL: Stage III carcinoma of the breast. Ann Surg 192:705, 1980
84. Turner-Warwick RT: The lymphatics of the breast. Br J Surg 46:574, 1959
85. Urban JA: Management of operable breast cancer. The surgeon's view. Cancer 42:2066, 1978
86. Deemarski LY, Seleznev IK: Extended radical operations on breast cancer of medial or central location. Surgery 96:73, 1984
87. Lacour J, Bucalossi P, Cacers E, et al: Radical mastectomy versus radical mastectomy plus internal mammary dissection. Five-year results of an international cooperative study. Cancer 37:206, 1976
88. Veronesi U, Valagussa P: Inefficacy of internal mammary nodes dissection in breast cancer surgery. Cancer 47:170, 1981
89. Veronesi U, Cascinelli N, Greco M, et al: Prognosis of breast cancer patients after mastectomy and dissection of internal mammary nodes. Ann Surg 202:702, 1985
90. Host H, Brennhovd IO: The effect of post-operative radiotherapy in breast cancer. Int J Radiol Oncol Biol Phys 2:1061, 1977
91. Fisher B. Wolmark N, Redmond C, et al: Findings from NSABP Protocol No. B-04: Comparison of radical mastectomy with alternative treatments. II. The clinical and biological significance of medial-central breast cancers. Cancer 48:1863, 1981
92. Ege GN, Clark RM: Internal mammary lymphoscintigraphy

in the conservative management of breast carcinoma: An update and recommendations for a new TNM staging. Clin Radiol 36:469, 1985
93. Baker RR, Montague ACW, Childs JN: A comparison of modified radical mastectomy to radical mastectomy in the treatment of operable breast cancer. Ann Surg 189:553, 1979
94. Maddox WA, Carpenter JT, Laws HL, et al: A randomized prospective trial of radical (Halsted) mastectomy versus modified radical mastectomy in 311 breast cancer patients. Ann Surg 198:207, 1983
95. Turner L, Swindell R, Bell WGT: Radical versus modified radical mastectomy for breast cancer. Ann R Coll Surg Engl 63:239, 1981
96. Hermann RE, Esselstyn CB Jr, Crile G Jr, et al: Results of conservative operations for breast cancer. Arch Surg 120:746, 1985
97. Atkins H, Hayward JL, Klugman DJ, et al: Treatment of early breast cancer—a report after ten years of a clinical trial. Br Med J 2:423, 1972
98. Hayward JL: The Guy's Hospital trials on breast conservation. In Harris JR, Hellman S, Silen W (eds): Conservative Management of Breast Cancer, pp 77–90. Philadelphia, JB Lippincott, 1983
99. Veronesi U, Saccozzi R, Del Vecchio M, et al: Comparing radical mastectomy with quadrantectomy, axillary dissection, and radiotherapy in patients with small cancers of the breast. N Engl J Med 305:6, 1981
100. Veronesi U, Del Vecchio M, Greco M, et al: Results of quadrantectomy, axillary dissection, and radiotherapy (QUART) in T1N0 patients. In Harris JR, Hellman S, Silen W (eds): Conservative Management of Breast Cancer, pp 91–99. Philadelphia, JB Lippincott, 1983
101. Fisher B, Bauer M, Margolese R, et al: Five year results of a randomized clinical trial comparing total mastectomy and segmental mastectomy with or without radiation in the treatment of breast cancer. N Engl J Med 312:665, 1985
102. Amalric R, Santamaria F, Robert F, et al: Radiation therapy with or without primary limited surgery for operable breast cancer: A 20-year experience at the Marseilles Cancer Institute. Cancer 49:30, 1982
103. Osborne MP, Ormiston N, Harmer C, et al: Breast conservation in the treatment of early breast cancer. A 20-year follow-up. Cancer 53:349, 1984
104. Harris JR, Recht A, Amalric R, et al: Time course and prognosis of local recurrence following primary radiation therapy for early breast cancer. J Clin Oncol 2:37, 1984
105. Sanger CK, Reznikoff M: A comparison of the psychological effects of breast-saving procedures and modified radical mastectomy. Cancer 48:2341, 1981
106. Schain W, Edwards BK, Gorrell CR, et al: Psychosocial and physical outcomes of primary breast cancer therapy: Mastectomy vs excision biopsy and irradiation. Breast Cancer Res Treat 3:377, 1983

Adjuvant Radiotherapy

Jay R Harris and Samuel Hellman

Radiotherapy has been used in the primary treatment of early breast cancer as an adjuvant treatment following mastectomy and as definitive treatment following biopsy of the tumor. This section summarizes and evaluates the available data on the use of adjuvant radiotherapy. Definitive radiotherapy is discussed in the following section.

HISTORY

In 1895, Wilhelm Roentgen, using a primitive cathode ray tube, discovered a new form of radiation that was able to penetrate various materials and darken photographic plates. To distinguish this new form of radiation from others, he chose to call it x-ray radiation. Within the next year, Henri Becquerel demonstrated that some naturally occurring materials in uranium crystals emit a form of radiation resembling x-rays. Three years later, Marie and Pierre Curie reported their discovery of a new radioactive substance found in pitchblende, which they named radium. These physicists provided the basic tools to be used in the treatment of cancer by radiotherapy—x-rays, created by the bombardment of accelerated electrons on a target, and gamma rays, emitted by radium and other radioactive materials.

It was with remarkable speed that these tools were used in the treatment of cancer. Within a year after Roentgen reported his discovery, patients with cancer were being treated with x-rays. One of these early practitioners was Francis Henry Williams, a physician at Boston City Hospital, Harvard Medical School, who built improved x-ray machines and treated patients with cancer as early as 1896. By 1905, over 2000 patients had been irradiated at City Hospital, and in 1906, Williams published an article in the Boston Medical Journal entitled "A further note on a method of using the Roentgen rays; the consideration of primary treatment of some early cases of breast cancer by these rays." He wrote:

> I have found this method helpful in treating cancer of the breast. In one case of schirrus carcinoma involving about two-thirds of the breast, the microscopic examination made after death (from other causes) showed that the diseased cells had disappeared. Further consideration to their use as a primary means of treatment in early growths of the breast should be given based on its efficiency in recurrent cases and the possibility of avoiding metastases by early treatment.[1]

These early practitioners demonstrated the ability of x-rays to shrink and, in some cases, to eliminate completely cancerous growths. They were limited, however, by the rudimentary equipment available at that time and by the absence of a technique and treatment schedule able to deliver radiotherapy to the tumor while sparing normal tissues. The energy of x-ray machines available prior to 1920 was in the range of 120 to 135 kVp, compared to the greater than 4000 kVp (4 MV) typically used today. These older x-ray machines delivered their maximal dose at the skin surface with a rapid fall-off into deeper tissues. They typically delivered only 16% of their maximal dose at a depth of 5 cm, whereas modern equipment delivers 80% or more at that depth. Because of the poor penetration of these low-energy x-rays, doses were limited to what the skin could tolerate, and tumors situated at deeper levels were thus spared. X-ray machines with energies of greater than 1 MV (commonly referred to as supervoltage) were not commercially available in large numbers until the 1960s. The two major forms of supervoltage machine used are cobalt-60 irradiators and linear accelerators.

It was quickly recognized that the safe use of radiotherapy depended on extending the course of treatment over time. Massive single exposures to radiation resulted in significant and progressive adverse effects on normal tissues. During the early part of the 20th century, Henri Coutard in Paris used radiotherapy to treat tumors of the head and neck and, by careful observation, determined that best results were achieved by delivering relatively small doses of radiation daily over an extended period of time. This fractionation and protraction of treatment allowed for greater recovery of normal tissues and still killed tumor cells. Worldwide experience has since determined that daily doses in the range of 180 to 200 cGy yield optimal results when treatment is administered once a day.

The development of improved methods for delivering radiotherapy externally (external beam radiotherapy) was paralleled by the development of methods for delivering radiotherapy internally (brachytherapy). Such internal radiotherapy could be delivered either by direct insertion into the tissues (interstitial) or by insertion into body cavities (intracavitary). From 1900 to 1910, Abbe in the United States and Finzi in England explored the therapeutic applications of radium. Between 1910 and 1930 at the Institut du Radium of Paris and the Fondation Curie, Regaud and Lacassagne developed more convenient and stable forms of radium, as well as guidelines for its use. In the 1930s, Patterson, at the Holt Radium Institute in Manchester, England, developed standardized rules for radium application. He devised dosage tables based on these standardized rules and thus established a practical method for ensuring accurate dosimetry of treatment. After World War II, researchers devoted much effort to developing newer and more convenient radioactive sources, such as iridium-192 seeds, and a system of dosimetry consistent with their use. Considerable credit for this development should be given to Bernard Pierquin.

THE RESPONSE OF BREAST CANCER TO IRRADIATION

The ability of a given radiotherapy program to eradicate tumors can only be judged by long-term follow-up of patients thus treated. In situations in which clinically detectable cancer is present, one can also determine rates of complete response. Ultimately, however, the critical endpoint is permanent eradication of the tumor, defined as the absence of tumor regrowth, over time, in the treated area. When all clinically detectable cancer has been surgically removed, one cannot determine complete response rates and must instead compare the rate of recurrence in treated patients to that in untreated patients with similar tumors.

Among the first to document the dose required to sterilize subclinical deposits of breast cancer was Fletcher from the M.D. Anderson Hospital.[2] He examined the incidence of supraclavicular node relapse in patients with positive axillary nodes treated with radical mastectomy. Prior retrospective reports from Christie Hospital in Manchester and Memorial Hospital in New York City had indicated a relapse rate of 20% to 25% when no postoperative radiation was given. Fletcher found that when 3000 to 3500 cGy in 4 weeks was given postoperatively to the supraclavicular region, relapse was confined to 6 of 89 patients or 7%; when 4000 cGy in 4 weeks was administered, supraclavicular relapse occurred in 4 of 121 patients or 3%; and when 5000 to 5500 cGy in 4 weeks was used, supraclavicular relapse was noted in only 4 of 273 patients or 1.5%. These inferential data provide support for 4500 to 5000 cGy in 4 1/2 to 5 weeks being adequate for the eradication of subclinical deposits of breast cancer in a high percentage of cases. Similar but less convincing results were obtained in attempts to eradicate subclinical disease in the chest wall. Of 70 patients with positive axillary nodes treated with radical mastectomy and postoperative radiation, chest wall recurrence was seen in only 7, or 10%. Forty-six of these 70 patients (66%) had more than 50% of their nodes involved, and most of the remainder had grave signs. Fletcher estimated that local recurrence in this group, if left untreated, would have been at least 30%.

Fletcher's observations regarding the dose required to eradicate subclinical deposits of breast cancer have been confirmed in the 10-year results of a trial conducted by the NSABP.[3] The results of this trial will be discussed in detail below. In this trial (B-04), 1074 patients with clinically negative axillary nodes were randomized for treatment with either radical mastectomy, total mastectomy with no axillary treatment, or total mastectomy and postoperative radiation delivered to the chest wall and draining lymph node areas, including the axilla. Among the patients actually treated with total mastectomy without axillary treatment, 21% subsequently developed axillary relapse and underwent delayed axillary dissection. In comparison, only 3% of the patients treated with total mastectomy and radiotherapy to the axilla had axillary relapse. These patients received a total of 5000 cGy in 5 weeks to the axilla. This appears to have eradicated subclinical axillary disease and reduced the risk of axillary recurrence in approximately 86% of patients (18%/21%).

MASTECTOMY AND ADJUNCTIVE RADIOTHERAPY

Postoperative Radiotherapy

Historically, the first major use of radiotherapy in the primary management of patients with breast cancer was not as definitive treatment, but rather as adjuvant therapy following mastectomy. The experience gained from postoperative radiotherapy has provided important lessons on the natural history of the disease and guidelines for the optimal use of radiation in treating breast cancer without mastectomy.

There were two rationales for the use of prophylactic postoperative radiotherapy. The first was that prophylactic radiotherapy reduced the risk of local-regional tumor recurrence by eradicating residual microscopic disease that had spread beyond the margin of surgical resection. It was also argued that once local-regional recurrences were manifested clinically, they could be treated effectively in approximately 50% of patients.[4–6] In addition, these recurrences were often very distressing for afflicted patients. As a result, postoperative radiation has been used in high-risk patients simply to prevent local recurrence. The second rationale for postoperative radiotherapy was to improve survival. According to this view, residual local-regional disease after mastectomy may be the only site of persistent cancer and a source of subsequent distant metastases. Patients without residual local-regional disease, or those who already have distant metastases, will fail to show any improvement in survival with this form of adjuvant therapy.

The usefulness of postoperative radiation therapy in reducing local recurrence after mastectomy has been well documented. In the absence of postoperative radiation therapy, there is a significant risk of local recurrence (Table 10-9). This risk is related to axillary nodal involvement. If axillary nodes are involved, local recurrence is seen in 25% to 27% of patients, whereas if axillary nodes are uninvolved, local recurrence is seen in only 4% to 8% of patients.[7,8]

The addition of postoperative radiotherapy to treatment with radical mastectomy has resulted in a marked decrease in the risk of local-regional recurrence. The benefits of such treatment have been shown through experience at the Joint Center for Radiation Therapy (JCRT).[9] Between July of 1968 and December of 1972, 352 patients with Union Internationale Contre le Cancer (UICC) Stages I through III operable breast cancer were treated with supervoltage radiotherapy following mastectomy. Seventy-one percent of these patients had pathologically positive axillary lymph nodes. The chest wall recurrence rate for all patients was 5.1%, and the overall regional recurrence rate was 0.9%. The incidence of chest wall recurrence was 3% for patients with negative nodes, 2% for patients with one to three positive nodes, and 12% for patients with four or more positive nodes. These results compare favorably with those shown in Table 10-9, and demonstrate the value of selective postoperative radiotherapy in reducing local-regional recurrence.

Another series of patients from the M.D. Anderson Hospital also illustrates the benefits derived from the use of postoperative radiotherapy.[10] Between 1963 and 1977, 920 patients underwent postoperative radiation following radical or modified radical mastectomy. None of these patients received adjuvant chemotherapy. Peripheral lymphatic irradiation (to the internal mammary and supraclavicular nodes) was administered to patients with histologically positive axillary lymph nodes and to those with primary tumors of the central or inner breast quadrant, regardless of the status of their axillary nodes. Chest wall irradiation was added when the primary tumor was greater than 5 cm in diameter, when grave signs were present, or when there was significant axillary lymph node involvement. Initially, irradiation of the chest wall was added when more than 50% of the recovered nodes were involved, but later, this irradiation was done when 20% or more of the recovered nodes were involved. The dose to the chest wall was 5500 to 6000 cGy, and the dose to the peripheral lymphatics was ≥ 5000 cGy.

The follow-up period in these patients ranged from 4 to 18 years. The incidence of local-regional recurrence is shown in Table 10-10. Supraclavicular recurrence was minimal in irradiated patients, and chest wall recurrence was significantly less common when compared to the recurrence rate in patients who were not irradiated (see Table 10-9). The results shown in Table 10-10 also suggest that chest wall irradiation is useful in reducing chest wall recurrence, particularly in high-risk patients (those patients with four or more positive nodes). The authors also compared the 10-year rate of distant relapse in this series to the rate obtained in a series of patients treated with radical mastectomy alone. This retrospective comparison suggests that the rate of distant relapse in node-positive patients may be reduced by the use of postoperative radiation.

Although improvement in local-regional control with adjuvant radiation therapy following radical mastectomy was well documented, its effect on survival remained uncertain. The survival value of postoperative radiotherapy ideally would be determined by means of a prospective

Table 10-9
Likelihood and Site of First Relapse 5 to 10 Years After Radical Mastectomy

	Fisher[8] *Axillary nodes*		*Valagussa*[7] *Axillary nodes*	
Site of Relapse	*Involved (%)*	*Not Involved (%)*	*Involved (%)*	*Not Involved (%)*
Local-regional only	18	6	25	4
Distant only	49	20	43	20
Local-regional and distant	9	2		

Table 10-10
Incidence of Local-Regional Recurrence After Radical Mastectomy and Postoperative Radiotherapy (M.D. Anderson Hospital)

Site of Irradiation	No. Positive Axillary Nodes	% Recurrence	
		Chest Wall	Supraclavicular Region
Peripheral lymphatics	0	5	1
	1–3	9	2
	≥4	20	1
Peripheral lymphatics and chest wall	0	2	2
	1–3	8	1
	≥4	11	3

randomized clinical trial. However, there are significant methodologic problems in properly performing such a study. One major problem is that the technical aspects of the radiation therapy must be carefully monitored, since postoperative radiotherapy is effective only if the correct volume is treated with the correct dose. Many of the earlier series used techniques that either did not ensure adequate coverage of all the draining lymph nodes, or did not use a dose sufficient for the eradication of microscopic deposits of breast cancer (approximately 5000 cGy in 5 weeks). Another major problem is the large number of patients required for such a study. As discussed below, the survival benefit from postoperative radiation, if it exists, is likely to be minimal, approximating 5%. To have a 90% chance of detecting a 7% difference at a statistically significant level of $p = 0.05$, for example, 2000 patients are required. Finally, randomization in these trials must be strict. It is tempting for clinicians to avoid radiotherapy in patients with a good prognosis and to administer radiotherapy in patients with a poor prognosis. Since the expected survival benefit, if it exists, is likely to be minimal, such deviations from true randomization could easily obscure a benefit from postoperative radiotherapy. These considerations will be addressed in the discussion of clinical trials on postoperative radiotherapy, below.

Manchester Trial

There are now seven trials in which patients have been randomized after some form of mastectomy (total, modified radical, or radical) to receive either postoperative radiotherapy or no further treatment. The first of these trials was conducted at the Christie Hospital in Manchester, England. The results were first reported in 1959 by Paterson and Russell,[11] later by Easson in 1968,[12] and most recently, by Palmer and Ribeiro in 1985.[13] The study covered the period between January 1949 and June 1955 and included a total of 1461 patients for analysis. All patients underwent radical mastectomy and then received either postoperative radiotherapy or no further treatment. The trial was divided into two series based on two distinctly different methods of postoperative radiotherapy. The first, applied to 720 patients treated between 1948 and 1952, was described as the quadrate technique. This technique was designed to irradiate the chest wall and axilla, using three anterior tangent beams and a fourth posterior beam directed at the upper axilla. This technique did not attempt to treat the internal mammary or supraclavicular nodal regions. The second technique, applied to 741 patients treated from 1953 to 1955, was termed the peripheral technique, and was designed to irradiate the axillary, supraclavicular, and internal mammary lymph node regions. In this technique, the skin flaps were left unirradiated. In both techniques, the radiation was in the orthovoltage range. The dose used in the quadrate technique was between 3500 and 4000 cGy, administered over a period of 3 weeks. The dose used in the peripheral technique was 3250 cGy at the midpoint of the axilla. These treatments produced moist desquamation in many patients, and generally left permanent stigmata. There was a small but definite incidence of necroses, especially noted with the quadrate technique.

The 10-year incidence of local recurrence is shown in Table 10-11. Local recurrence was defined as malignant disease appearing within the skin flap area of the chest wall or in the ipsilateral axillary, supraclavicular, or parasternal areas. The use of prophylactic postoperative radiotherapy reduced the incidence of local recurrence by 40%. The 10-year incidence of local recurrence was not subdivided by technique of radiotherapy, but the 5-year results indicated that, as expected, the peripheral technique primarily reduced nodal recurrence and the quadrate technique primarily reduced chest wall recurrence.[11] When local recurrence was diagnosed in the patients who received no therapy initially (the "watched" group), local radiotherapy was generally administered. When local recurrence was diagnosed in the treated group, no further treatment was given. Table 10-11 also indicates the incidence of local recurrence persisting at death. Uncontrolled local recurrence at the time of death occurred in roughly 15% of the dying patients in each group. Thus, local irradiation after recurrence controlled the disease until death in a similar proportion of cases as did prophylactic postoperative irradiation.

The overall survival curves for up to 30 years for the watched and treated (both quadrate and peripheral)

Table 10-11
Local Tumor Control in the Manchester Trial: Comparison of Radical Mastectomy to Radical Mastectomy and Radiotherapy

		Incidence of Local Recurrence Within 10 years (%)		*Incidence of Local Recurrence Persisting at Death (%)*	
Clinical Stage	*No. of Cases*	*Treated*	*Watched*	*Treated*	*Watched*
I	527	9.5	16.0	5.0	7.5
II	934	25.0	41.5	18.5	21.0
Total	1461	19.0	32.0	14.0	16.0

Easson EC: Post-operative radiotherapy in breast cancer. In Forrest AP, Kunkler PB (eds): Evolution of Post-Operative Radiotherapy, pp 118–127. Edinburgh, E & S Livingstone, 1968.

groups were similar.[13] When the results were analyzed separately for patients with histologically negative and positive axillary nodes, the rate of survival was better in the subgroup of patients with negative nodes who did not receive radiotherapy, but this difference was not statistically significant. When the results were analyzed further by separating the two techniques of radiotherapy, in the subgroup of patients with negative nodes treated with the quadrate technique, survival was significantly better in the watched group ($p = 0.05$) (Fig. 10-22). Overall, the authors concluded that the use of prophylactic postoperative local radiotherapy was not associated with an improved survival rate at 30 years when compared to local radiotherapy used only after local recurrence.

This study contains significant flaws, and caution is required in interpreting its results. First, randomization was not strictly adhered to, and nonrandomized patients were included in the analysis. As a result, there were proportionally more node-negative patients in the watched group than in the treated group. Of the 526 node-negative patients, 283 (or 54%) were watched and 243 (or 46%) were treated. For patients with positive nodes, the number of positive nodes in patients in both the treated and watched groups was not analyzed. It is, therefore, uncertain whether the groups were balanced in regard to prognosis. The technique and doses of radiotherapy used may also be criticized. All patients were treated using orthovoltage radiation, the daily dose of radiotherapy was high by current standards, and the total doses given were lower than the dose needed for the eradication of subclinical disease. The techniques used also did not adequately cover the tumor-bearing volume. Nodes in the supraclavicular and internal mammary regions did not receive a full dose.[14] As a result, the rate of local tumor control was not optimal in the study. Local recurrence was seen in 19% of treated patients in this trial, whereas the anticipated local recurrence rate is 5% to 10% when optimal techniques and doses are used. This early trial fails to indicate a survival benefit from the use of prophylactic radiotherapy, but also illustrates many of the methodologic problems involved in adequately addressing the question. It also raises the possibility that radiotherapy might be harmful in this setting.

NSABP Trial B-02

The second of these trials was conducted by the NSABP (B-02).[15] This trial was begun in 1961, and the 5-year results were published in 1970 by Fisher and colleagues. Patients undergoing conventional radical mastectomy were randomly assigned to a group receiving postoperative radiotherapy or to a control group. This straightforward randomization was complicated by the possibility of further randomization to receive triethylthiophosphamide (TSPA) or a placebo, depending on the woman's nodal and menopausal status, and the discretion of the participating institution. In addition, the results of treatment of 142 patients in a control group included in a separate but simultaneous study designed to test the value of adjuvant oophorectomy were added to the results. In this study, radiotherapy was directed to the axillary apex, internal mammary, and supraclavicular regions. Doses were 3500 Roentgens (R) given over a period of 3 weeks or less or 4500 R given within 5 weeks or less. Approximately 25% of patients were treated using orthovoltage radiation. A total of 1882 patients were entered into the trial, but 41% of these were withheld from analysis either because the patient was declared ineligible after randomization (569 patients) or because complete data were not available (210 patients). As a result, 1103 patients were eligible for analysis, of whom 954 were followed for 18 months or more and 415 were followed for 5 years or more.

The overall results of the NSABP B-02 trial at 5 years, shown in Table 10-12, failed to reveal a significant advantage in relapse-free survival for patients treated with prophylactic postoperative radiotherapy. Patients treated with radiotherapy had fewer regional recurrences than did patients in the control group and proportionally more distant recurrences as a first site of failure. Since radiotherapy was not directed to the chest wall, local recurrence was similar in the two groups. Sixty-four percent of the irradiated patients had positive axillary nodes compared to only 56% of the control group, suggesting a randomization bias that selected patients with more advanced disease for treatment with postoperative irradiation. When the relapse-free survival results were examined according to the

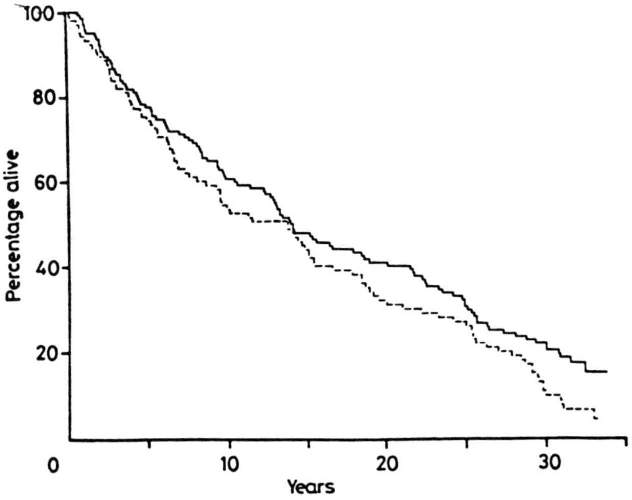

FIGURE 10-22. Survival in the Manchester trial comparing radical mastectomy (*solid line,* n = 142) and radical mastectomy combined with radiotherapy (*broken line,* n = 105) [p = 0.05] in the subgroup of patients with negative nodes treated with the quadrate technique. (Palmer MK, Ribeiro GG: Br Med J 291:1088, 1985.[13])

Table 10-12
5-Year Results of NSABP Trial Testing the Value of Postoperative Radiotherapy*

Site of First Relapse	*Postoperative Radiotherapy*	*Control Group*
Number of patients	91	235
Local recurrence (%)	7.8	10.6
Regional recurrence (%)	0.6	6.0
Distant metastasis (%)	40.0	32.3
Total failed (%)	49.4	49.8

* National Surgical Adjuvant Breast Project.

histologic status of axillary nodes (Table 10-13), a slight, but statistically insignificant, survival advantage was noted for irradiated patients. Overall, the results of the NSABP trial failed to show a survival advantage from the use of prophylactic postoperative radiotherapy. The trial has been criticized, however, for its flaws in study design, poor adherence to randomization, short follow-up time, and deficient radiation technique and doses. In addition, the high percentage of patients who were disqualified from analysis and the inclusion of patients from another study make it difficult to draw firm conclusions from these results.

Despite its flaws, the results of this study do provide some guidelines in determining which patients are likely to benefit from postoperative regional irradiation. Table 10-13 shows the incidence of regional recurrence as the first site of treatment failure for irradiated patients and the control group alike. In approximately 3% of nonirradiated patients with negative axillary nodes or one to three pos-

Table 10-13
5-Year Results of NSABP Trial Testing the Value of Postoperative Radiotherapy*

	No. Patients Followed for 5 years	*Axillary Nodes Negative*	*1–3 Axillary Nodes Positive*	*≥ 4 Axillary Nodes Positive*
		Regional Recurrence (%)		
Postoperative radiotherapy	56	0	0	1.5
Control group	96	2.1	4.5	12.5
		Relapse-Free Survival (%)		
Postoperative radiotherapy		78.6	49.1	28.4
Control group		76.0	47.8	18.0

* National Surgical Adjuvant Breast Project.

itive axillary nodes, regional recurrence represented the first site of treatment failure. This 3% is presumed to represent the maximal possible survival benefit to be gained by adding postoperative regional irradiation, since regional irradiation is of no survival value in patients with distant spread or in patients without residual regional disease. A maximal survival difference of 3% between treated and untreated groups is unlikely to be discerned. For patients with four or more positive nodes, 1.5% of irradiated patients had a regional recurrence as the first site of treatment failure compared to 12.5% of the control group. A similar advantage in relapse-free survival (28.4% versus 18%) was also observed for irradiated patients in this subgroup. In all groups, the majority of failures was attributable to distant spread. The results from this NSABP trial indicate that the percentage of patients likely to benefit from postoperative regional irradiation is small, since treatment failure is primarily due to distant metastases.

Oslo Trial

The third trial testing the value of prophylactic postoperative radiotherapy was conducted at the Norwegian Radium Hospital in Oslo between 1964 and 1972.[16] A total of 1088 patients with operable breast cancer entered the trial. All patients underwent radical mastectomy and ovarian irradiation, and were then randomized to groups receiving postoperative radiotherapy or no further treatment. The trial was divided into two series based on the technique and doses of radiotherapy. In the first series (1964 to 1967), orthovoltage irradiation was used, and the chest wall, axillary, supraclavicular, and internal mammary regions were treated with doses ranging from 1800 to 3600 R over a period of 4 weeks. In the second series (1968-1972), cobalt-60 irradiation was used, and the draining lymph node areas were treated with a single portal to a dose of 5000 cGy in 4 weeks. In this series, the chest wall was not treated.

All patients in this study were followed for at least 11

Table 10-14
10-Year Incidence of Local or Regional Recurrence (Oslo Study)

	No. Patients	Local or Regional Recurrence No.	%
200 kV x-ray irradiation	282	20	7.1
Control group	264	41	15.5
Cobalt-60 irradiation	265	13	4.9
Control group	277	35	12.6

years. The 10-year crude incidence of local or regional recurrence is shown in Table 10-14. Both of the radiotherapy programs significantly reduced local-regional recurrence, although cobalt-60 treatment appeared to be somewhat more effective. Cobalt-60 irradiation reduced the rate of recurrence to 39% of that in the control subjects, whereas orthovoltage treatment reduced the rate of recurrence to 46% of that in the control group. The 10-year relapse-free and overall survival results are shown in Table 10-15.

In this study, Stage I and II refer to pathologic staging. Relapse-free survival was not affected by orthovoltage irradiation relative to the control group in patients with either Stage I or II disease. Patients with Stage I disease who received cobalt-60 irradiation had a relapse-free survival rate that did not differ significantly from that of the control group ($p = 0.12$). Patients with Stage II disease receiving cobalt-60 irradiation had an improved relapse-free survival rate compared to that of the control group ($p=0.04$). Cobalt-60 irradiation was associated with a slightly lower overall survival rate relative to that of the control group in patients with Stage I disease ($p = 0.08$) and no significant difference in survival in those with Stage II disease ($p = 0.15$). In the second series, the cause of death was examined for Stage I patients. There were 32 deaths attributable to breast cancer among the patients treated with cobalt-60 irradiation and 31 deaths due to breast cancer among the control group. There were 27 deaths from other causes among the patients treated with cobalt-60 irradiation and only 17 deaths from other causes among the control subjects. This discrepancy was attributable to an increased incidence of myocardial infarctions in the patients treated with cobalt-60 irradiation. Interestingly, the technique of cobalt-60 irradiation involved a portal 6-cm in width that was directed anteriorly to the internal mammary nodes, thereby delivering a considerable dose to the heart.

The Oslo study may be criticized on a number of points. The routine use of radiation castration makes the results difficult to interpret. The irradiation technique and doses used in the orthovoltage series were clearly inadequate, and in the cobalt-60 series, the chest wall was not treated. Most significantly, the number of patients in the study was small. This is particularly true of the second series, in which a total of only 186 patients with Stage II disease were studied. As a result, the likelihood of detecting a difference in the results of the treatments, if one exists, is small. The results indicate an improvement in relapse-free survival at 10 years ($p = 0.04$) for patients with Stage II disease who received cobalt-60 irradiation postoperatively compared to that for the control group. This benefit, however, must be balanced against the risk of such treatment, which will be discussed further below.

Stockholm Trial

The fourth of the trials examining the value of postoperative radiotherapy is part of a larger study testing the value of both preoperative and postoperative radiotherapy conducted at the Radiumhemmet in Stockholm between 1971 and 1976.[17] In all cases, the diagnosis was confirmed preoperatively by fine needle aspiration cytology. Nine hundred and sixty patients with operable breast cancer were then randomized to groups undergoing either modified radical mastectomy alone (321), preoperative radiotherapy and modified radical mastectomy (316), or modified radical mastectomy and postoperative radiotherapy (323). Radiotherapeutic technique and equipment differed considerably between the preoperative and postoperative arms of the study. The preoperative group was irradiated with cobalt-60 tangential beams to the chest wall encompassing the internal mammary lymph nodes, and a matching direct field to the supraclavicular and axillary nodes. In contrast, the postoperative group was treated with an electron beam field to the chest wall and internal mammary nodes, and cobalt-60 irradiation to the supraclavicular and axillary nodes. The prescribed dose in each radiotherapy arm was 4500 cGy in five-times-weekly fractions of 175 cGy for 5 weeks.

The results of the Radiumhemmet trial with all patients followed to death or to the end of 1984 are shown in Tables 10-16 and 10-17. The follow-up time was 8 to 14 years, with a mean follow-up period of 11 years. Table 10-16 shows the number of patients in the irradiated groups and the nonirradiated group who developed local or distant relapse within 8 years. Preoperative and postoperative irradiation was equally effective in reducing the likelihood of a local-regional recurrence. The likelihood of distant relapse, however, was similar in all three groups. Table 10-17 shows the 5-year rates of relapse-free and overall survival for the three groups. Relapse-free survival was significantly improved by the use of either preoperative or postoperative radiotherapy. The overall relapse-free survival rate at 10 years was 59% for patients treated with preoperative irradiation and 62% for those treated with postoperative irradiation, compared to 47% for patients treated with surgery alone. The difference is statistically significant at the level of $p = 0.05$. However, the overall survival rate at 10 years for patients receiving either form of adjuvant radiotherapy was not statistically superior to the survival rate of patients treated with surgery only.

Table 10-15
10-Year Survival Results (Oslo Study)

	Stage I Disease			Stage II Disease		
	No. of Patients	Relapse-Free Survival (%)	Survival (%)	No. of Patients	Relapse-Free Survival (%)	Survival (%)
200 kv x-ray irradiation	173	75	75	109	45	40
Controls	172	74	76	92	38	44
Cobalt-60 irradiation	170	70	75	95	56	59
Controls	186	76	80	91	43	55

Table 10-16
Crude Incidence of Recurrence from the Stockholm Trial on Adjuvant Radiotherapy

		Site of Recurrence	
	No. of Patients	Local-Regional	Distant
Radiotherapy and surgery	639	44 (7%)	191 (30%)
Surgery only	321	84 (26%)	110 (34%)
		$p < 0.001$	p = NS

Table 10-17
Ten-Year Rates of Relapse-Free and Overall Survival from the Stockholm Trial on Adjuvant Radiotherapy

	Relapse-Free Survival (%)	Overall Survival (%)
Preoperative radiotherapy	59	66
Postoperative radiotherapy	62	65
Surgery only	47	61
	$p < 0.05$	p = NS

The authors also reviewed the cumulative incidence of distant metastases and breast cancer deaths for patients treated with postoperative irradiation and those treated with surgery alone according to their nodal status on pathologic examination. No difference in the incidence of distant metastases was seen for node-negative patients in either group. In node-positive patients, however, there was a lower rate of distant metastases following radiotherapy (47% at 11 years) than in the control group (60% at 11 years, p = 0.01). No difference was noted in the frequency of breast cancer deaths in node-negative patients in either group. In node-positive patients, the use of radiotherapy was associated with a 7% lower rate of breast cancer death (p = 0.09). The results from this study indicate that preoperative and postoperative radiation are equally effective in preventing local recurrence. The data also suggest that there may be a small (4% to 5%) survival advantage for patients treated with adjuvant radiotherapy compared to nonirradiated patients.

Overview of Randomized Trials

Recently, results were collected of an overview of randomized trials of postoperative radiotherapy following modified or radical mastectomy.[18] Included in this study were the results from the Manchester trials (through 1981), the Oslo trial (through 1980), the Stockholm trial (through 1982), and an unpublished small trial from Heidelberg. The results from the NSABP trial B-02 could not be included in this study since further follow-up had not been obtained since the initial report published in 1970. The results of these various trials were combined by the use of a summary logrank statistic (Mantel-Haenzel) obtained by adding together, across trials, the difference between observed and "expected" deaths. No difference was seen in the summary observed-minus-expected deaths comparing patients treated with and without radiotherapy over the first 15 years after surgery. After 15 years, there was a lower rate of survival associated with the use of radiotherapy (p = 0.005). Of note is the fact that the results obtained after 15 years are essentially restricted to the Manchester trials. The cause of death in these trials is not given.

Trials Involving Radiotherapy Following Total Mastectomy

Three additional trials examine the use of radiotherapy after total mastectomy rather than after radical or modified radical mastectomy. Since modified radical mastectomy and radical mastectomy entail an axillary dissection, subsequent axillary recurrence is rare. For this reason, radiotherapy after these procedures is used primarily to treat the chest wall and supraclavicular and internal mammary nodal regions. Total mastectomy does not include an axillary dissection, and postoperative radiotherapy in this setting is therefore used to treat the axilla as well. The use of postoperative radiotherapy after total mastectomy has a bearing on the related issue of the importance of treating the axillary lymph nodes. One other trial from Southampton, England addressed this same issue, but long-term results from this trial are not available at this time.[19]

One of these studies was conducted in the United States by the NSABP (trial B-04) between 1971 and 1974.[3] The relevant portion of this trial relates to treatment of patients with clinically negative axillary nodes. These patients were randomized to groups undergoing either radical mastectomy, total mastectomy with postoperative radiotherapy, or total mastectomy alone. A total of 1159 patients were randomized, of whom 1079 (93%) were eligible for analysis. Supervoltage radiotherapy was used, and the following doses were delivered over a period of 5 weeks: 4500 cGy to the supraclavicular and internal mammary node regions, 5000 cGy to the mid-axilla, and 5000 cGy to the chest wall.

The 10-year rates of local or regional recurrence as a first site of failure are shown in Table 10-18. Of note, 65 patients treated with total mastectomy alone (17.8%) who subsequently were found to have positive nodes requiring an axillary dissection were not considered to have had a treatment failure unless the nodes could not be removed completely.

Since 38.6% of patients treated with radical mastectomy had histologically involved nodes, it is reasonable to assume that a similar percentage of patients treated with total mastectomy also had positive nodes. The results in Table 10-18 indicate that the combination of total mastectomy and radiotherapy provided the best level of local-regional tumor control, although the risk of local or regional recurrence was low in all treatment groups. Figure 10-23 shows the 10-year relapse-free survival curves for the three treatment groups. No significant differences in either relapse-free or overall survival were noted.

The second trial bearing on the issue of total mastectomy and postoperative radiotherapy was conducted by the Cancer Research Campaign (CRC). Between 1970 and 1975, 2800 patients with operable breast cancer were randomized to groups undergoing total mastectomy or total mastectomy and postoperative radiotherapy. Of these, 2243 patients were considered to be eligible for analysis. Either orthovoltage or supervoltage radiotherapy was delivered

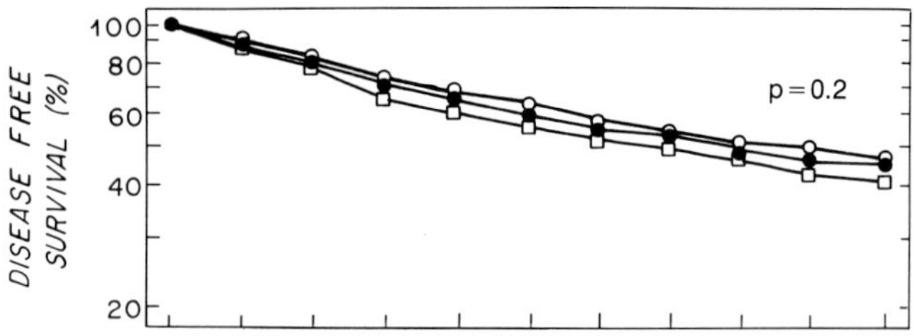

FIGURE 10-23. Disease-free survival in the National Surgical Adjuvant Breast Project trial B-04 was recorded for patients with clinically negative axillary nodes treated with radical mastectomy (*solid circles*), total mastectomy and radiotherapy (*open circles*), or total mastectomy alone (*open squares*). (Fisher B et al: N Engl J Med 312:674, 1985. Reprinted by permission).

to the chest wall, axillary, internal mammary, and supraclavicular regions. Patients treated with orthovoltage received doses in the range of either 2850 cGy in 3 weeks to 4050 cGy in 6 weeks in three fractions per week, or 3250 cGy in 3 weeks to 4600 cGy in 6 weeks in five fractions per week. These figures were multiplied by 1.1 for supervoltage treatment.

The first report of the trial was published in 1976[20] and a follow-up report was published in 1980.[21] By 1980, 1194 patients had been followed for at least 5 years. The results at 5 years are shown in Table 10-19. The use of postoperative radiotherapy significantly reduced the likelihood of local or regional recurrence. An analysis of the specific sites of local-regional recurrence was not provided. No significant differences in the rate of distant metastasis or in survival were noted. The CRC trial is unique among these studies in that it studied a population large enough to permit detection of small differences. The results at 5 years indicate a 3% advantage for patients undergoing postoperative radiotherapy and the 95% confidence limits range from a 1% survival advantage for total mastectomy to a 7% survival advantage for total mastectomy and radiotherapy. The CRC trial may be criticized, however, on the basis of the technique of radiotherapy used. Orthovoltage treatment was used, and the range of doses and fractionation schedules was too broad. As a result, local-regional control with radiotherapy was not

Table 10-18
Local and Regional Recurrence Rates at 10 years in NSABP Trial B-04*

	Radical Mastectomy (%)	*Total Mastectomy and Radiotherapy (%)*	*Total Mastectomy (%)*
Local recurrence	5.8	1.7	8.5
Regional recurrence	2.5	3.7	4.6
Local + regional recurrence	0.8	0	0.8
Total	9.1	5.4	13.9

* National Surgical Adjuvant Breast Project.

Table 10-19
Results of CRC Trial at 5 Years*

	Total Mastectomy (%)	Total Mastectomy and Radiotherapy (%)	p
Local-regional recurrence	29.1	10.9	<0.001
Distant metastasis	35.0	32.8	0.28
Survival	69.6	72.6	0.38

* Cancer Research Campaign.

Table 10-20
Results of the Manchester Trial at 5 and 10 Years

	No. Patients	Local Recurrence (%) 5 yr	10 yr	Alive Without Distant Recurrence (%) 5 yr	10 yr	Survival (%) 5 yr	10 yr
Total mastectomy	359	38	44	62	47	69	55
Total mastectomy and postoperative radiotherapy	355	19	25	71	56	74	62
		$p < 0.0001$		$p = 0.07$		$p = 0.20$	

optimal. The local-regional recurrence rate at 5 years was 11%, whereas the local-regional recurrence rate at 10 years in the NSABP trial was only 5%.

The third trial related to the issue of postoperative radiotherapy after total mastectomy was performed in Manchester, England. The relevant portion of this trial involved randomization of 714 patients with T1 or T2, N0, M0 breast cancer to groups undergoing either total mastectomy or total mastectomy and postoperative radiotherapy. All patients who were premenopausal or perimenopausal were offered castration. Apart from a chest x-ray to exclude pulmonary metastases, staging was accomplished by clinical examination alone. Postoperative radiotherapy was administered by one of two techniques:

Quadrate technique—a combination of five orthovoltage (300 kV) fields designed to irradiate the chest wall and draining lymph node areas (3700 cGy in 3 weeks)

Peripheral and tangential pair technique—a combination of an anterior "hockey-stick" field to the internal mammary, supraclavicular, and axillary nodal areas (4 MV, 4000 cGy in 3 weeks) and a pair of tangential fields to the chest wall (300 kV, 3000 cGy in 3 weeks)

The initial report of this trial was published in 1978, and a subsequent report was published in 1982.[22]

The results at 5 and 10 years are shown in Table 10-20. Local recurrence was significantly reduced with the addition of radiotherapy. There was an improvement in both metastases-free status and survival, but these differences were not significant at a level of $p = 0.05$. The radiotherapy used in this trial was not optimal; local recurrence after total mastectomy and radiotherapy was also greater than that seen in the NSABP B-04 trial. In addition, 24% of patients underwent castration, and the effect of this treatment is difficult to determine. Randomization may not have been strict; 57% of patients assigned to radiotherapy had T2 tumors, whereas only 52% of patients assigned to surgery alone had T2 tumors.

The Value of Axillary Treatment

The NSABP B-04, CRC, and Manchester trials all address the issue of the value of treatment to the axilla, an issue which merits further consideration. Four possible situations may exist when a patient presents with a breast cancer and clinically negative axillary nodes:

1. Cancer is confined only to the breast.
2. Cancer involves the breast and other sites.
3. Cancer is confined to the breast and axilla.
4. Cancer involves the breast and axilla and other sites.

It is important to note that only patients in category 3 will benefit from axillary treatment. Other patients either do not require it or cannot benefit from it because they already have disease at other sites. Since only 30% to 40% of patients with clinically negative nodes are actually found to have axillary involvement on histologic examination, and since the correlation between axillary involvement and involvement at other sites is so high, the percentage of patients in category 3 must be small. For example, if one assumes that 80% of patients with axillary involvement have occult involvement at other sites, and that 35% of patients with clinically negative axillary nodes have histologically positive nodes, then one can estimate that the percentage of patients in category 3 is approximately 7%. (Note: These estimates are based on data presented in Chapter 9.)

This possible survival benefit is even smaller if delayed axillary treatment is curative in some patients. The 10-year results of the NSABP B-04, CRC, and Manchester trials indicate a survival advantage of 4% to 7% for patients who receive axillary treatment. These results are consistent with that predicted above. This improvement in survival is too small, however, to be distinguished with confidence from no improvement at all.

The Value of Postoperative Radiotherapy

The same type of analysis used above to evaluate the use of axillary treatment may also be applied to the use of postoperative radiotherapy in patients treated with modified radical or radical mastectomy. In this analysis, the appropriate possible situations are even more complex. Proponents of postoperative radiotherapy argue that when axillary nodes are involved, other local or regional sites (e.g., the chest wall, internal mammary, or supraclavicular regions) are also frequently involved. It has been well documented that, when axillary nodes are involved, internal mammary nodes are involved in 25% to 40% of patients, and supraclavicular nodes are involved in 15% to 30% of patients. The likelihood of chest wall involvement has not been well documented since biopsy of this region is difficult. Since the lymphatics to the internal mammary nodes course through the chest wall, the likelihood of chest wall involvement is probably as high as that of internal mammary node involvement. The critical issue relating to the survival value of postoperative radiotherapy is the likelihood that breast cancer involves the breast, the axilla, and these other local or regional sites, but not distant sites. As with the value of axillary treatment, discussed above, there are significant subgroups of patients who do not require further local-regional treatment after mastectomy or who cannot benefit from it because they already have disease at other sites. As a result, the actual subgroup that could possibly benefit from such treatment is likely to be extremely small.

The discussion provided above is based on a highly mechanistic view of the disease process. According to this view, the disease is assumed to spread sequentially in most patients, arising in the breast and spreading first to the regional nodes, and only then to distant sites. It also assumes that untreated sites of disease will always progress. As shown above, even in this view, the possible value of treating nodes is small since not all patients have involvement of nodes and since the correlation between nodal involvement and occult involvement at distant sites is high. Devitt, a surgeon in Ottawa, Canada, was one of the first to suggest an alternative view.[23] Devitt retrospectively reviewed the outcome in 922 breast cancer patients treated at his institution between 1946 and 1959. Patients were treated with either radical mastectomy with full axillary dissection or total mastectomy with limited axillary dissection. This decision was based solely on the discretion of the surgeon. Devitt compared the 5- and 10-year survival rates for patients with pathologic Stage II disease treated with these two surgical procedures. He pointed out a potential bias in this comparison. It was possible that, in some patients treated with total mastectomy and a limited axillary dissection, nodal metastases might be missed because of the limited nature of the surgery. If this were true, patients classified as either Stage I or II by limited dissection would have a poorer prognosis as a group than patients classified by full dissection. Despite this bias, patients with either Stage I or II disease who were treated with total mastectomy fared at least as well as those treated with radical mastectomy. This observation suggested to Devitt that removal of the axillary lymph nodes did not improve the rate of long-term survival. Devitt also noted that, although axillary recurrences were more common among patients with Stage I and II breast cancer treated with total mastectomy than among those treated with radical mastectomy, these recurrences did not adversely affect the rate of survival of the group as a whole. Axillary recurrence was often seen many years after primary treatment, and patients with axillary recurrence invariably manifested distant metastases simultaneously or shortly afterward. This suggested to Devitt that axillary node recurrence might be merely the first expression of disseminated disease—an *indicator* of subsequent systemic relapse, not an *instigator* of such relapse. He theorized that breast cancer was systemic in all patients, and that the detection of nodal involvement was merely a manifestation of a deficient host response in the suppression of the disease. Axillary treatment or nodal treatment of any kind was, therefore, of no value and might, in fact, be harmful in suppressing further host defenses. Given the calculations presented above, it is clear that predictions of outcome based on these two different views are too similar to permit a validation of one of these by scientific means.

The available results on the routine use of postoperative radiotherapy are consistent with either a small increase in the likelihood of survival or no improvement at all. It has been suggested that there may be particular subsets of patients for whom radiotherapy may be of value. One subset of possible interest includes patients with primary tumors of the inner or central breast and positive axillary nodes, a group known to be at significant risk (i.e., 40% to 50%) for internal mammary node involvement. In the Oslo trial, patients with positive nodes and inner or central primary tumors who were treated with mastectomy and radiotherapy had a survival advantage at 10 years over patients treated with mastectomy alone, but the number of patients in this subgroup was small, and the difference was not statistically significant (58% versus 40%, $p = 0.08$). In the Stockholm trial, there was a survival advantage for patients receiving adjuvant radiotherapy in whom the internal mammary nodes were adequately treated, but the number of patients in these groups was also small, so that the difference was only of borderline statistical significance. The results of these two studies provide suggestive evidence that postoperative radiotherapy is of value in this subset. The results from the CRC and NSABP trials are not pertinent to this premise since information on axillary histology is not available for patients in these trials. In neither trial, however, was there a significant advantage in the use of radiotherapy for patients with primary tumors of the inner or central breast.

The above discussion has focused on the possible value of adjuvant radiotherapy in improving survival. It is also possible that postoperative radiotherapy is useful in certain situations simply to provide local tumor control. Local recurrence can be a highly distressing event in a patient's life and, as discussed elsewhere in this book, is poorly controlled once it becomes manifest. Many clinicians have argued that patients at high risk for local recurrence should receive postoperative radiotherapy simply to provide local tumor control.

Assessment

At present, it remains undetermined whether there is a subset of patients who would derive a survival benefit from postoperative radiation. Patients in this subset would have to have residual local or regional cancer following mastectomy, but no distant metastases. The likelihood of having residual local or regional cancer after mastectomy is relatively small. Furthermore, if residual cancer is present, there is a high likelihood that the patient will also have occult distant metastases. As a result, this critical subset is certain to be small, perhaps 5% of patients. Of critical importance is the fact that, at present, there are no effective means of identifying this subset. There is suggestive evidence that patients at high risk for local recurrence—those with primary tumors in the medial or central portion of the breast and positive axillary nodes—are more likely to be included in this subset.

The available data from clinical trials are consistent with the view that postoperative radiotherapy confers either a small survival benefit or none at all. It is unlikely that a conclusive study can be performed to answer this question. Given the available facts, however, it does not appear reasonable to recommend postoperative radiation routinely. Furthermore, the whole issue of postoperative radiation needs to be reevaluated in terms of the results now being achieved with adjuvant chemotherapy. For patients not treated with adjuvant chemotherapy, postoperative radiation for patients in high-risk groups is reasonable both for prevention of local recurrence and for its minimal potential survival benefit. The role of postoperative radiation in the treatment of patients receiving adjuvant chemotherapy is discussed later in this section.

Preoperative Radiotherapy

The use of preoperative irradiation has some theoretical advantages not found with postoperative irradiation. One would expect to see an improvement in local-regional control with preoperative irradiation similar to that found with postoperative treatment. In addition, it has been suggested that preoperative irradiation might inactivate cancer cells that are dislodged during the manipulations of mastectomy, thereby decreasing the incidence of distant spread. Despite these theoretical advantages, preoperative radiotherapy has been used infrequently in the treatment of operable breast cancer and has only recently been evaluated in the Stockholm trial described above.

The failure of preoperative radiotherapy to improve survival rate significantly suggests that metastasis is not enhanced by the manipulations of surgery. Preoperative radiotherapy may also increase the risk of complication associated with mastectomy. Alund and co-workers examined the frequency of wound infection and seroma formation in patients included in the Stockholm trial and found that these complications were more common in patients treated with preoperative radiotherapy than in patients not treated with radiotherapy.[24] Preoperative radiation may also interfere with the accurate evaluation of the axillary lymph nodes by eradicating the cancer in positive nodes. In the Stockholm trial, histologic axillary involvement was found in 38% of patients treated with modified radical mastectomy without radiation, compared with only 20% of patients treated with preoperative radiotherapy. At present, the chief guideline for the use of adjuvant chemotherapy is the finding of axillary node metastases. A significant fraction of patients with positive axillary nodes who might benefit from adjuvant chemotherapy would not be identifiable if they were treated with preoperative radiotherapy.

IMPACT OF ADJUVANT CHEMOTHERAPY ON THE USE OF POSTOPERATIVE RADIOTHERAPY

The results presented above on the use of postoperative radiotherapy emphasize the limitations of local-regional treatment (beyond mastectomy) and the importance of systemic involvement in determining curability for most patients. An appreciation of these results has spurred the development of adjuvant systemic therapy—principally, adjuvant chemotherapy. The results available at this time show a significant improvement in relapse-free survival with the use of adjuvant chemotherapy, particularly in premenopausal women. The current status of the use of adjuvant chemotherapy is presented elsewhere in this book. This section will review the influence of adjuvant chemotherapy on local-regional tumor control and examine

Table 10-21
First Treatment Failure in Local-Regional Area Only (Milan Trial Results at 10 Years)

	Control Group	*Group Receiving CMF**
Total entered	26/179 (14.5%)	24/207 (11.6%)
Total relapsed	26/118 (22.0%)	24/111 (21.6%)
Chest wall only	8/179 (4.5%)	6/207 (2.9%)
Supraclavicular nodes only	11/179 (6.1%)	9/207 (4.3%)
Chest wall and supraclavicular nodes	4/179 (2.2%)	4/207 (1.9%)
Internal mammary nodes	3/179 (1.7%)	5/207 (2.4%)

* Cyclophosphamide (Cytoxan), methotrexate, and 5-fluorouracil.

whether there is any possible role for postoperative radiotherapy in conjunction with adjuvant chemotherapy.

The effect of adjuvant chemotherapy on local-regional control has not been fully established. In the Milan trial, which compared the results of adjuvant treatment with CMF in patients undergoing mastectomy to the results obtained in an untreated control group, the 10-year probability of relapse-free survival was 43% for patients receiving CMF and 31% for the control group ($p < 0.01$).[25] The results at 10 years failed to show a significant improvement in local-regional tumor control in the group receiving CMF (Table 10-21). In this group, the 10-year local-regional recurrence rate was 11.6%, compared to a rate of 14.5% in the untreated control group ($p =$ NS).

The trial conducted at the Dana Farber Cancer Institute (DFCI) and JCRT demonstrated similar results.[26] In this trial, patients with one to three positive nodes or with a T3 primary tumor and negative nodes received either CMF or methotrexate and 5-fluorouracil (MF). Patients with four or more positive nodes received Cytoxan/Adriamycin (C/A) for either 5 or 10 cycles. With a median follow-up time of 44 months, the crude incidence of local-regional recurrence was 6% for the patients treated with CMF or MF and 25% for patients treated with C/A. The results from Rush-Presbyterian-St. Luke's Hospital in Chicago were similar.[27] One hundred and four patients with Stage II breast cancer treated with modified or radical mastectomy and multi-agent adjuvant chemotherapy had a local-regional recurrence rate of 19.2% with a median follow-up of 62 months. Local-regional recurrence occurred in 3 of 53 patients (6%) with one to three positive nodes and 12 of 51 patients (24%) with four or more positive nodes. These results indicate that the likelihood of local-regional recurrence is not markedly reduced by the use of adjuvant chemotherapy when compared to that associated with treatment by mastectomy alone.

There are reasons to suspect that adjuvant chemotherapy might be less effective in decreasing local-regional recurrence than in eradicating systemic micrometastases. One reason is that the local-regional tumor burden is likely to be considerable when axillary nodes are positive, particularly if a modified radical mastectomy is performed instead of a radical mastectomy. Modified radical mastectomy, even with complete axillary dissection, is known to leave a significant number of axillary nodes behind in the interpectoral and subclavicular regions that would be removed by a radical mastectomy.[28,29] In fact, many surgeons today do not perform a full axillary dissection as part of a modified radical mastectomy. Histologic slides of clinically uninvolved nodes frequently reveal extensive involvement microscopically. As noted before, even radical mastectomy does not treat disease in the chest wall or the internal mammary or supraclavicular nodal regions—sites likely to be involved when axillary nodes are positive. Based on all of these considerations, it is reasonable to be concerned that the residual local-regional tumor burden is considerable in patients with positive axillary nodes treated with modified radical mastectomy. It is also possible that the surgery itself may alter the blood supply to the region, thus preventing adequate levels of drugs from being delivered to the region.

If these speculations on the relative levels of local-regional and systemic tumor burdens are correct, they form a rationale for the use of postoperative radiotherapy in conjunction with adjuvant systemic therapy. This rationale is based on a concern regarding drug resistance.[30] It is now generally accepted that when the tumor burden exceeds a certain level, drug resistance of tumor cells is observed. If patients with positive axillary nodes treated with mastectomy have a significant residual tumor burden in the untreated supraclavicular and internal mammary nodes, as well as in the operative site, adjuvant chemotherapy appears to be ineffective since local recurrence rates are unchanged. Adjuvant radiotherapy may be critical in reducing the residual local-regional tumor burden sufficiently to avoid the emergence of drug-resistant tumor cells, thereby allowing adjuvant chemotherapy to eradicate systemic micrometastases effectively.

There are practical problems to be addressed in treating patients with both adjuvant chemotherapy and radiotherapy. The question of the integration of modalities is complex. Prompt initiation of postoperative radiotherapy may be favored in order to minimize the absolute number of tumor cells exposed to chemotherapy. This could reduce the likelihood of subsequent drug resistance. On the other hand, some suggest that adjuvant chemotherapy must be administered promptly in order for benefit to be derived. This implies that the operation itself may abet metastases, which may be eliminated by the prompt administration of chemotherapy. There is also concern that initial radiotherapy may inhibit the ability to administer full doses of chemotherapy. This latter issue is controversial, but many institutions, such as the JCRT, have found it feasible to deliver full-dose chemotherapy after radiotherapy.[31–34] Other institutions have indicated that the prior use of postoperative radiotherapy prevents delivery of full doses of chemotherapy.[35,36] Bedwinek pointed out that the studies that have shown interference with drug delivery have used a direct anterior field to treat the internal mammary nodes, whereas studies that have not shown interference have used tangential fields for treatment of internal mammary nodes.[37] Direct anterior internal mammary node fields treat considerably greater volumes of circulating blood and bone marrow than do tangential fields. Also, in delivering chemotherapy after radiotherapy, modification of the drug dose levels should be based on the neutrophil count and not the total white cell count. Radiotherapy is known to reduce the lymphocyte count significantly. This reduction may persist for several months following completion of treatment.

One reasonable approach to the integration of chemotherapy and radiotherapy may be to use postoperative radiotherapy after adjuvant chemotherapy. As part of the DFCI adjuvant chemotherapy trial discussed above,[26] patients completing chemotherapy were randomized to groups receiving either postoperative radiotherapy or no further therapy. Median follow-up was 44 months at the time of analysis. The results of this trial are shown in Table 10-22.

These results indicate that patients with four or more positive nodes have a high rate of local-regional recurrence after chemotherapy alone, but that radiotherapy after chemotherapy may effectively reduce the likelihood of local recurrence, with results comparable to those associated with immediate postoperative radiotherapy. These results suggest that the use of postoperative radiotherapy after adjuvant chemotherapy is effective and does not interfere with drug delivery.

A number of other studies have examined the issue of adding postoperative radiotherapy to adjuvant chemotherapy.[35] One study from the University of Arizona was initially meant to be a prospective trial for patients with Stage II breast cancer who were randomly assigned to groups receiving A/C either with or without postoperative radiotherapy.[38] The randomization was far from strict, with 82 patients being treated with A/C alone and 56 with A/C and postoperative radiotherapy. Of the patients treated with A/C alone, 56 had one to three positive nodes, and 26 had four or more positive nodes. In contrast, of the patients treated with A/C and postoperative radiotherapy, 22 had one to three positive nodes, and 34 had four or more. No improvement in relapse-free survival was seen with the addition of radiotherapy in this study.

Table 10-22
Results of an Adjuvant Chemotherapy (CTX)—Radiotherapy (XRT) Trial (Dana Farber Cancer Institute)

	1 to 3 Positive Nodes		*≥4 Positive Nodes*	
	CTX	*CTX→XRT*	*CTX*	*CTX→XRT*
Number of patients	33	32	51	44
% Local-regional recurrence	6%	6%	25%	7%
			(p = 0.03)	
% Total failure	21%	18%	49%	45%

Another study was performed by the Southeastern Cancer Study Group.[39] In this study, 276 patients with four or more positive nodes were randomized to groups receiving six cycles of CMF, 12 cycles of CMF, or postoperative radiotherapy followed by six cycles of CMF. The results of this study are shown in Table 10-23. The use of postoperative radiotherapy improved local-regional control and relapse-free survival, but the differences were not statistically significant.

At the Mayo Clinic, 313 patients with Stage II breast cancer were randomized to groups receiving phenylalanine mustard (L-pam); Cytoxan, 5-fluorouracil, and prednisone (CFP); or CFP and postoperative radiotherapy. Radiotherapy was given to the internal mammary, supraclavicular, and axillary nodal regions to a total of 5000 cGy. Treatment to the chest wall was administered only in a few patients with more advanced local disease. The results, published in 1984, showed that the use of radiotherapy significantly reduced the rate of local-regional recurrence. The incidence of local-regional recurrence was 10% in patients treated with CFP and radiotherapy, compared to 26% in patients treated with L-pam and 30% in patients treated with CFP alone.[40] Overall disease-free survival at 5 years was improved in patients who received CFP, but was not significantly improved by the use of postoperative radiotherapy. The 5-year relapse-free survival rate was 34% for patients treated with L-pam, 48% in those treated with CFP, and 53% in those treated with combined CFP and radiotherapy. The toxicity associated with the radiotherapy was considerable in this study, as detailed in an earlier report.[41] Edema of the arm was diagnosed in 54% of patients treated with CFP and radiotherapy, compared to 23% of the other patients. Of the patients treated with postoperative radiotherapy, 15% developed radiation pneumonitis, 5% developed radionecrosis, and 3% had brachial plexopathy.

Cooper and colleagues from the Piedmont Oncology Association published a preliminary report on a group of 158 patients with Stage II disease who were randomized to receive L-pam with or without radiotherapy or CMF with or without radiotherapy.[42] The number of patients in each of these subgroups was small (32 to 44 patients). The results at 3 years showed an advantage in relapse-free survival for patients treated with CMF over those treated with L-pam; no advantage was ascribed to postoperative radiotherapy.

Another preliminary study was reported by Buzdar and associates from M.D. Anderson Hospital.[43] In this study, 238 patients with operable breast cancer were treated with adjuvant 5-fluorouracil, adriamycin and Cytoxan (FAC) with or without nonspecific immunotherapy with bacille Calmette Guérin (BCG) vaccine and with or without postoperative radiotherapy. With a median follow-up of 33 months, no advantage in relapse-free survival was seen with the use of radiotherapy or BCG vaccine.

Table 10-23
Results of the SECSG Trial Testing the Value of Adjuvant Chemotherapy and Radiotherapy*

	CMF† × 6 Cycles	*CMF† × 12 Cycles*	*Radiotherapy and CMF† × 6 Cycles*
Local-regional recurrence	12/119 (10%)	6/55 (11%)	4/102 (4%)
Total relapses	60/119 (50%)	31/55 (56%)	39/102 (38%)

* Southeastern Cancer Study Group.
† Cyclophosphamide (Cytoxan), methotrexate, and 5-fluorouracil.
Marcial VA, Velez-Garcia E, Moore M, et al: Radiotherapy related adjuvant chemotherapy initiation delay in breast cancer with positive nodes: Does it affect prognosis? A Southeastern Cancer Study Group report. Proc Am Soc Ther Rad Oncol 11 (suppl 1): 150, 1985

At the present time, the utility of postoperative radiotherapy in conjunction with adjuvant chemotherapy is unproven. There are theoretical reasons to consider its use, but the preliminary results from clinical trials do not indicate a clear advantage in survival over the use of adjuvant chemotherapy alone. If such an approach is to be considered, it should be done in a way that will not interfere with the effective delivery of adjuvant chemotherapy.

REFERENCES

1. Williams FH: A further note on a new method of using the Roentgen rays; consideration of primary treatment of some early cases of breast cancer by these rays. Boston Med J 154:641, 1900
2. Fletcher G: Local results of irradiation in the primary management of localized breast cancer. Cancer 29:545, 1972
3. Fisher B, Redmond C, Fisher ER, et al: Ten-year results of a randomized clinical trial comparing radical mastectomy and total mastectomy with or without radiation. N Engl J Med 312:674, 1985
4. Bedwinek JM, Lee J, Fineberg B, et al: Prognostic indicators in patients with isolated local-regional recurrence of breast cancer. Cancer 47:2232, 1981
5. Aberizk WJ, Silver B, Henderson IC, et al: The use of radiotherapy for treatment of isolated local-regional recurrence of breast cancer after mastectomy. Cancer 58:1214, 1986
6. Chew KK, Montague ED, Oswald MJ: Results of irradiation in the treatment of loco-regional breast cancer recurrence. Cancer 56:1269, 1985
7. Valagussa P, Bonadonna G, Veronesi U: Patterns of relapse and survival following radical mastectomy: Analysis of 716 consecutive patients. Cancer 41:1170, 1978
8. Fisher B, Wolmark N, Bauer M, et al: The accuracy of clinical nodal staging and of limited axillary dissection as a determinant of histologic nodal status in carcinoma of the breast. Surg Gynecol Obstet 152:765, 1981
9. Weichselbaum RR, Marck A, Hellman S: The role of postoperative irradiation in carcinoma of the breast. Cancer 37:2682, 1976
10. Tapley N, Spanos WJ, Fletcher GH, et al: Results in patients with breast cancer treated by radical mastectomy and postoperative irradiation with no adjuvant chemotherapy. Cancer 49:1316, 1982
11. Paterson R, Russell MH: Clinical trials in malignant disease. Part III. Breast cancer: Evaluation of postoperative radiotherapy. J Fac Radiol 10:175, 1959
12. Easson EC: Post-operative radiotherapy in breast cancer. In Forrest AP, Kunkler PB (eds): Evolution of Post-operative Radiotherapy, pp 118–127. Edinburgh, E & S Livingstone, 1968
13. Palmer MK, Ribeiro GG: Thirty-four year follow-up of patients with breast cancer in a clinical trial of postoperative radiotherapy. Br Med J 291:1088, 1985
14. Fletcher G, Montague ED: Does adequate irradiation of the internal mammary chain and supraclavicular nodes improve survival rates? Int J Radiat Oncol Biol Phys 4:481, 1978
15. Fisher B, Slack NH, Cavanaugh PJ, et al: Postoperative radiotherapy in the treatment of breast cancer: Results of the NSABP clinical trial. Ann Surg 172:711, 1970
16. Host H, Brennhoud IO, Loeb, M: Post-operative radiotherapy in breast cancer—Long-term results from the Oslo study. Int J Radiat Oncol Biol Phys 12:727, 1986
17. Wallgren A, Arner O, Bergstrom J, et al: Radiation therapy in operable breast cancer—results from the Stockholm trial in adjuvant radiotherapy. Int J Radiat Oncol Biol Phys (in press)
18. Cuzick J, Stewart H, Peto R, et al: Overview of randomized trials of post-operative adjuvant radiotherapy in breast cancer. Cancer Treat Rep (in press)
19. Turnbull AR, Turner DTL, Chant ADB, et al: Treatment of early breast cancer. Lancet 2:7, 1978
20. Cancer Research Campaign Working Party: Management of early cancer of the breast. Br Med J 1:1035, 1976
21. Cancer Research Campaign Working Party: Cancer research campaign trial for early breast cancer. Lancet 2:55, 1980
22. Lythgoe JP, Palmer MK: Manchester regional breast study—five- and ten-year results. Br J Surg 69(12):693, 1982
23. Devitt JE: The significance of regional node metastases in breast cancer. Can Med Assoc J 93:289, 1965
24. Alund M, Granberg PO, deSchryler A, et al: Surgical complications after radiation therapy for carcinoma of the breast. Surg Gynec Obstet 144:235, 1977
25. Bonadonna G, Valagussa P, Rossi A, et al: Ten-year experience with CMF-based adjuvant chemotherapy in resectable breast cancer. Breast Cancer Res Treat 5:95, 1985
26. Griem K, Henderson IC, Gelman R, et al: The role of radio-

therapy in patients receiving adjuvant chemotherapy after mastectomy: Results of a randomized trial. Proc Am Soc Ther Radiol Oncol. Int J Radiat Oncol Biol Phys II (suppl 1): 151, 1985
27. Rao AR, Murthy AK, Hendrickson FR, et al: Analysis of risk factors for loco-regional failure in stage II (T1N1M0 and T2N1M0) breast carcinoma treated with mastectomy and adjunctive chemotherapy. Proc Am Soc Ther Radiol Oncol. Int J Radiat Oncol Biol Phys 11 (suppl 1): 151, 1985
28. Caceres E, Lingan M, Delgado P: Evaluation of dissection of the axilla in modified radical mastectomy. Surg Gynecol Obstet 143:395, 1976
29. Hultborn A, Hulten L, Roos B, et al: Effectiveness of axillary lymph node dissection in modified radical mastectomy with preservation of pectoral muscles. Ann Surg 179:269, 1974
30. Goldie JH, and Coldman AJ: A mathematic model for relating the drug sensitivity of tumors to their spontaneous mutation rate. Cancer Treat Rep 63:1727, 1979
31. Glick J, Danoff B, Haller D, et al: Integration of full dose adjuvant CMF with definitive radiation for primary breast cancer (abstr). Proc Am Soc Clin Oncol 2:98, 1983
32. Come S, Botnick L, Lange R, et al: Concurrent radiation therapy and chemotherapy in the primary management of pathologic stage II breast cancer (abstr). Proc Am Soc Clin Oncol 2:99, 1983
33. Lippman ME, Lichter AS, Edwards BK, et al: The impact of primary irradiation treatment of localized breast cancer in the ability to administer systemic chemotherapy. J Clin Oncol 2:21, 1984
34. Bonadonna G, Valagussa P, Zucali R, et al: Feasibility of adjuvant chemotherapy plus radiotherapy in operable breast cancer. In Harris JR, Hellman S, Silen W (eds): Conservative Management of Breast Cancer, pp 329–336. Philadelphia, JB Lippincott, 1983
35. Levine JF, Coleman CN, Cox RS, et al: The effect of postoperative and primary radiation therapy on delivered dose of adjuvant chemotherapy in breast cancer (abstr). Proc Am Soc Clin Oncol 1:C-329, 1982
36. Holland JF, Glidewell O, Copper RG: Adverse effect of radiotherapy on adjuvant chemotherapy for carcinoma of the breast. Surg Gynecol Obstet 150:817, 1980
37. Bedwinek J: Adjuvant irradiation for early breast cancer. An ongoing controversy. Cancer 53:729, 1984
38. Jones SE, Salmon SE, Allen H, et al: Adjuvant treatment of node-positive breast cancer with adriamycin-cyclophosphamide with or without radiation therapy: Interim results of an ongoing clinical trial. Recent Results Cancer Res 80:162, 1982
39. Marcial VA, Velez-Garcia E, Moore M, et al: Radiotherapy related adjuvant chemotherapy initiation delay in breast cancer with positive nodes: Does it affect prognosis? A Southeastern Cancer Study Group report. Proc Am Soc Ther Radiol Oncol. Int J Radiat Oncol Biol Phys 11 (suppl 1): 150, 1985
40. Ahmann DL, O'Fallon JR, Scanlon PW, et al: A preliminary assessment of factors associated with recurrent disease in a surgical adjuvant clinical trial for patients with breast cancer with special emphasis on aggressiveness of therapy. Am J Clin Oncol 5:371, 1982
41. Ahmann DL, Payne WS, Scanlon PW, et al: Repeated adjuvant chemotherapy with phenylalanine mustard or 5-fluorouracil, cyclophosphamide, and prednisone with or without radiation, after mastectomy for breast cancer. Lancet 1:893, 1978
42. Cooper MR, Rhyne AL, Muss HB, et al: A randomized comparative trial of chemotherapy and irradiation therapy for stage II breast cancer. Cancer 47:2833, 1981
43. Buzdar AU, Blumenschein GR, Smith TL, et al: Adjuvant chemotherapy with Fluorouracil, Doxorubicin and cyclophosphamide, with or without bacillus Calmette-Guérin and with or without irradiation in operable breast cancer. A prospective randomized trial. Cancer 53:384, 1984

Conservative Surgery and Radiotherapy

Jay R. Harris and Samuel Hellman

The transition from radical mastectomy to modified radical mastectomy (described in the section on surgical management earlier in this chapter) greatly improved cosmetic and functional results for treated patients. Even modified radical mastectomy, however, involves amputation of the breast. Loss of a body part, particularly that of the breast, can be associated with profound psychological distress.[1–3] This observation has provided the impetus for the development of breast-preserving treatment for patients with breast cancer. Experience with postoperative radiotherapy demonstrated the ability of moderate dose radiotherapy to eradicate subclinical deposits of breast cancer. These results suggested the possibility that more conservative surgery, combined with radiotherapy, might be an effective means of obtaining local tumor control with breast preservation. This section summarizes the results obtained with this treatment, and indicates factors to be considered in the use of this approach, including patient selection, the extent of surgical resection required, and the technique of radiotherapy to be employed.

The concept of combining conservative surgery with radiation as a substitute for more radical surgery is not new. Keynes, a surgeon at St. Bartholomew's Hospital in London, began to treat patients with operable carcinoma of the breast in this manner as early as 1924.[4] Because of the rudimentary external beam radiation equipment available at that time, Keynes treated patients with radium needle implantation of the breast and draining lymph node areas (Fig. 10-24). A 10-year retrospective review from St. Bartholomew's Hospital was published in 1953.[5] For patients with disease clinically confined to the breast, the 10-year survival rate was 27% following simple surgery and radium treatment, compared to 26% for patients treated with radical surgery. The incidence of local-regional recurrence was 13% with conservative treatment and 6% with radical surgery. Subsequent experience has shown that implantation of large and complex volumes, such as the breast and draining lymph node areas, cannot provide the radiation dose homogeneity required for optimal local-regional control. Implantation now is reserved for boosts to localized areas, following more homogeneous radiation to the larger volumes using high-energy external beam radiation.

Two early advocates of conservative surgery combined with radiation were Vera Peters and Sakari Mustakallio. Beginning in 1939, Peters, a radiotherapist at the Princess Margaret Hospital in Toronto, treated patients with T1 or T2, N0 breast cancers with excision and radiation.[6] In order to compare her results to those achieved

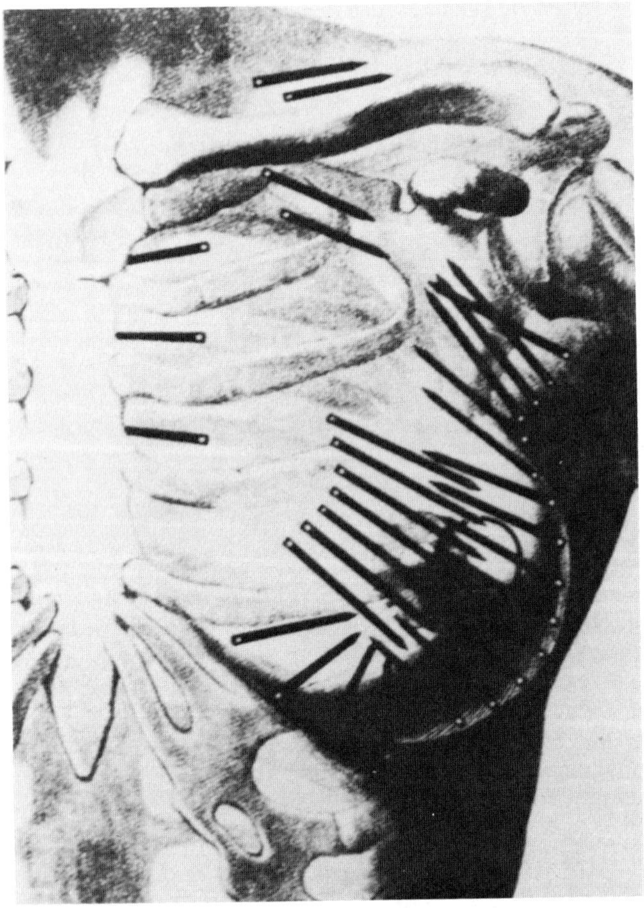

FIGURE 10-24. Distribution of radium needles in patients treated by Sir Geoffrey Keynes. Note needles placed in the axillary, supraclavicular, and internal mammary node regions. (Freeman CR et al: J Can Assoc Radiol 32:125, 1981.[24])

with radical surgery, she performed a matched pair analysis in which each of 184 patients treated with excision and radiation was matched by age, size of primary tumor, and year of treatment to three patients treated with radical mastectomy and radiation. These results, carried out to 30 years, do not show any significant differences in survival.

Similarly, beginning around 1940, Mustakallio in Helsinki used simple excision with radiation to treat patients with clinically negative axillary nodes. The radiation therapy given by Mustakallio is considered inadequate by current standards. Using orthovoltage equipment, he delivered a surface dose of 2100 cGy in six fractions to the breast and lymph node areas. As a result of this technique, 26% of his patients developed local-regional recurrence by 10 years.[7] Despite this high local recurrence rate, a 5-year survival rate of 79% and a 10-year rate of 71% was observed. In a more recent review of Mustakallio's experience, Rissanen and Holsti retrospectively compared the results of local excision and radiation to the results of radical mastectomy and radiation.[8] They found that the 10-year total survival rates were similar for the two treatments in patients with T1 primary tumors, but noted a survival advantage for the more radical surgery in patients with T2 primary tumors. This advantage is, in part, attributable to the selection of older patients for conservative surgery. When the results are analyzed by the age of patients, as well as by T stage, the only subgroup in which the more radical surgery appears to be of benefit is patients 65 years of age or older with T2 primary tumors.

Based on the findings obtained in early retrospective studies, a controlled clinical trial was performed at Guy's Hospital starting in 1961. In this study, patients with T1 or T2, N0 or N1 breast cancers were allocated randomly to groups undergoing either radical mastectomy and postoperative irradiation or wide excision and postoperative irradiation. The first results from this study were reported in 1972,[9] a second report was published in 1977,[10] and the most recent report was published in 1983.[11] In addition, a second series with the same randomization was performed at a later time, but was restricted to patients with clinically negative nodes.

In the first Guy's Hospital trial, patients were treated using an orthovoltage machine. They received 3500 to 3800 cGy over a period of 3 weeks to the breast, and 2500 to 2700 cGy over an 18-day period to the axilla. It is important to point out that the patients treated with wide excision did not undergo axillary dissection. Although the doses delivered to the breast approximated those required for control of microscopic disease, the dose to the axilla was extremely low. This was especially true for the patients with Stage II disease, many of whom had gross axillary disease. As a result, an excess of axillary recurrences was noted in the group treated with wide excision. Of the patients without palpable axillary nodes (N0) treated with wide excision, 33% developed local-regional recurrence. Of the similarly treated patients with enlarged axillary nodes (N1), 63% developed local-regional recurrence. In comparison, only 15% of the N0 patients and 24% of the N1 patients treated with radical mastectomy developed local-regional recurrence. The higher rate of local-regional recurrence noted in the group undergoing wide excision was attributable to an excess of axillary recurrences. As noted above in the section on Adjuvant Radiotherapy, Fletcher had demonstrated that, with adequate radiation doses, recurrences in node-bearing areas were uncommon. Current data indicate that axillary recurrences are rare following doses of 5000 cGy or greater. Of interest is that, with the higher doses used to treat the breast in the Guy's Hospital study, recurrence in the breast was uncommon in patients treated with wide excision.

The results of the Guy's Hospital trial are shown in Table 10-24. For patients with clinically negative nodes, the 15-year rate of freedom from distant relapse was 53% for the group treated with wide excision and 54% for the group treated with radical mastectomy. The 15-year survival rate was 41% for the group undergoing wide excision and 36% for the group undergoing radical mastectomy ($p = NS$). For patients with clinically positive nodes, a survival advantage at 15 years was noted for patients treated with radical mastectomy. However, 36% of patients in the

Table 10-24
Fifteen-Year Results from the Guy's Hospital Trial Comparing Wide Excision and Radiotherapy to Radical Mastectomy and Radiotherapy

	Freedom from Distant Relapse (%)		*Survival (%)*	
	Stage I	*Stage II*	*Stage I*	*Stage II*
Wide excision and radiotherapy	53	36	41	34
Radical mastectomy and radiotherapy	54 (P=NS)	33 (P=NS)	36 (P=NS)	45 (P<0.05)

group treated with wide excision were free of distant relapse, compared to 33% of those who underwent radical mastectomy (p = NS). The results of the first series clearly indicate that adequate doses of radiation are required to prevent recurrences in the axilla. The latest results of this series also show an advantage in long-term survival for patients with clinically positive axillary nodes treated with radical mastectomy rather than wide excision and low-dose radiation.

The latest published results of the second series (N0 patients) indicate an advantage not only in local-regional control, but also in freedom from distant relapse and survival, for the group undergoing radical mastectomy over the group undergoing wide excision. The median follow-up in this series was 8 years. Longer follow-up in this second series will be required to be certain of any difference in the long-term rate of survival between the two groups. Any improvement in survival for patients treated with radical mastectomy would imply that treatment of axillary disease is of importance to long-term survival.

RETROSPECTIVE STUDIES

Over the past 2 decades, there have been reports from a number of centers in Europe on the use of primary radiation therapy to treat patients with early breast cancer. One study from the Institut Curie, reported by Calle and colleagues, describes the long-term results of this treatment, and has a bearing on the use of local excision prior to irradiation.[12] In this study, the records of 606 patients with operable breast cancers treated with primary radiation therapy between 1960 and 1971 were reviewed. All patients had a minimum follow-up of 10 years. The likelihood of survival for the group of patients overall was equivalent to that of a similarly staged group of women treated with radical mastectomy at the Memorial Sloan-Kettering Cancer Center in New York. Two methods of treatment were used. For patients with tumors smaller than 3 cm in diameter, excision of the tumor was combined with external beam irradiation. For patients with tumors larger than 3 cm, only a needle biopsy of the tumor was performed, and external beam irradiation, at a dose of 5000 to 6000 cGy, was administered. Women whose tumors did not show significant regression following treatment underwent immediate mastectomy. The remainder received further irradiation to the tumor region for a total of 8000 cGy, using either electron beam treatment or cobalt-60 irradiation. The dose of 8000 cGy represented an attempt to eradicate residual gross disease.

The results in patients treated with excision were highly satisfactory. One hundred forty-three women underwent excision of the tumor and radiation, and only 20 of these women (14%) experienced treatment failure in the breast or axillary region. In addition, of the 18 women who underwent salvage surgery following such a failure, 13 (72%) were alive and free of disease with a minimum follow-up of 4 years following the surgical procedure. Generally, the cosmetic result was good to excellent; in only 4% of women was it poor. In contrast, the results for the 463 patients treated without excision were less satisfactory. Of these, 163 patients did not show sufficient regression after receiving 5000 to 6000 cGy, and so underwent immediate mastectomy. The remaining 300 patients completed their full course of radiation therapy. Eighty-four (28%) of these 300 women had local or regional recurrences. In addition, the cosmetic results in this group of patients treated with high-dose irradiation without excision were less satisfactory. Fifteen percent of these women had a poor cosmetic result. These results suggest that excision of the tumor is important, both for local tumor control and for achieving a good cosmetic result by allowing lower doses of radiotherapy to be used.

Another large series reported by Pierquin and coworkers from Creteil illustrates the importance of local excision and interstitial implantation as part of primary radiation therapy. Between 1961 and 1977, these researchers treated 408 patients with operable breast cancer using primary radiation therapy.[13,14] Eighteen percent of these women had T3 lesions, 58% had T2 tumors, and 24% had T1 tumors. In general, only patients with T1 tumors underwent excision. Other patients were treated, after undergoing needle biopsy, with their tumors *in situ.* A dose of 4500 cGy was delivered by external beam irradiation to the breast and draining lymph nodes, with an additional 1500 to 2400 cGy being delivered to the lower axilla and internal mammary nodes, depending upon the clinical nodal status of the patient. All patients received additional irradiation to the tumor site by an interstitial implant using iridium-192. The implant dose was 1500 to 2500 cGy following local excision, or 3700 cGy following needle biopsy. The local-regional recurrence rate at 10 years was 8% for patients with T1 lesions, 9% for those with T2 lesions, and 15% for those with T3 lesions. These excellent rates of local tumor control demonstrate the usefulness of interstitial implantation in maximizing local tumor control. Cosmetic results were correlated with the use of local excision and radiation dose. The cosmetic results were considered to be very good in 72% of patients with T1 lesions treated with local excision and lower radiation doses, but this figure declined to only 51% in those with T2 lesions who were treated with needle biopsy and higher radiation doses. Because of the poorer cosmetic results in patients treated without local excision and with higher doses of radiation, excision of the tumor prior to radiation is now recommended for all women.

The experience at the Institut Gustave-Roussy in Villejuif, France was reviewed by Clarke and associates. Between 1970 and 1981, 436 patients with T1 and small T2 breast cancers were treated with conservative surgery and radiotherapy. Mean follow-up time was 5 years. Local-regional control was 93% at 5 years and 90% at 10 years.[15] This study will be reviewed in greater detail in a later section.

More recently, a large number of institutions in this country and Canada have begun to treat patients with breast cancer with conservative surgery and radiotherapy. Montague reported on a group of 291 patients with Stage I and II breast cancer treated with conservative surgery and radiotherapy at the M.D. Anderson Hospital between 1955 and 1980.[16] Prior to 1974, conservative surgery consisted of excision of the gross tumor; the axilla was evaluated on clinical grounds alone. Beginning in 1974, a segmental mastectomy and a dissection of the lateral axilla were routinely performed. Radiotherapy was delivered to the breast in all patients and to nodal areas in selected patients, depending on the findings on axillary dissection. The entire breast received 4500 to 5000 cGy in 5 weeks, and an additional 1000 to 2000 cGy was given to the tumor bed. Local recurrence was detected in eight of 134 patients (6%) with Stage I disease and in eight of 157 patients (5%) with Stage II cancer. The actuarial rate of survival for patients with clinical Stage I disease was 85% at 5 years and 78% at 10 years. The survival rate for those with clinical Stage II disease was 78% at 5 years and 73% at 10 years. These results are comparable to those obtained following treatment with mastectomy at that institution.

As noted above, Peters, from the Princess Margaret Hospital, was an early advocate of breast-preserving procedures. Clark reported on a group of 605 patients with T1 to T3 N0 breast cancer treated with conservative surgery and radiotherapy at that institution between 1958 and 1980.[17] All patients underwent at least excision of the gross tumor. Axillary surgery was not commonly performed. Radiotherapy was delivered to the breast in all patients and to the regional nodes in 253 patients. Patients typically received 4000 cGy in 3 weeks. Twenty-four percent of patients received a boost of 500 cGy to the tumor site. The relapse rate in the breast at 5 years was 9% for patients who received a boost and 13% for patients who did not. At 10 years, the breast relapse rates were 18% and 20%, respectively. The rate of survival for patients with T1N0 cancers was 87% at 5 years, 74% at 10 years, and 60% at 15 years. The rate of survival for patients with T2N0 cancers was 77% at 5 years, 68% at 10 years, and 55% at 15 years.

At the JCRT, 525 patients with Stages I and II breast cancer were treated with conservative surgery and radiation therapy between 1968 and 1980.[18] Eleven patients had contralateral breast cancer treated, making a total of 536 treated breast cancers. Local tumor control was 90% at 5 years for all patients. For patients treated with excisional biopsy, whole breast irradiation, and a boost to the primary site, local tumor control at 5 years was 94% for those with Stage I disease and 92% for those with Stage II disease (Fig. 10-25). The actuarial rate of survival at 5 years was 93% for patients with clinical Stage I breast cancer and 82% for those with clinical Stage II disease.

MODERN PROSPECTIVE TRIALS

Since 1970, there have been four prospective randomized trials—two from Europe and two from North America—with published results that compare conservative surgery and radiotherapy with mastectomy. One of these trials is from the National Cancer Institute of Italy in Milan.[19] From June of 1973 to May of 1980, 701 patients with T1N0 breast cancer who were eligible for evaluation were studied. Of these, 349 were randomized to a group having radical mastectomy and 352 were randomized to undergo conservative surgery and radiotherapy. Conservative surgery consisted of resection of the involved quadrant of the breast and full axillary dissection. Radiotherapy was delivered to the breast through two opposing tangential fields, and a total of 5000 cGy was administered in 5 weeks. An additional 1000 cGy was delivered to the tumor site using orthovoltage radiotherapy. From 1973 to 1975, patients

FIGURE 10-25. Local tumor control by clinical stage, JCRT. (Recht A et al: Semin Oncol [in press][18])

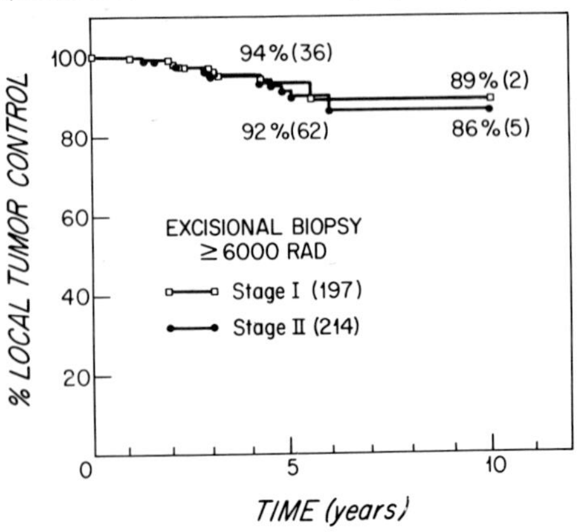

with positive nodes were further randomized to groups receiving radiotherapy to the draining lymph node areas or no further treatment. After 1975, all patients with positive nodes were treated with 12 cycles of CMF. The two arms of the study were well-balanced with regard to age, tumor size, and axillary nodal status. Microscopic evidence of axillary metastases was found in 25% of patients treated with radical mastectomy and in 27% of patients treated with conservative surgery and radiotherapy.

Ten years after the beginning of the trial, five patients in the group undergoing mastectomy and five in the group treated with conservative surgery and radiotherapy had developed a local recurrence. In the group treated conservatively, seven additional patients developed a second primary cancer in the ipsilateral breast. Eighty patients have died since the start of the trial, 41 from the group treated with mastectomy and 39 from the group treated with conservative surgery and radiotherapy. Sixty of these patients died of breast cancer, 30 from each group. Relapse-free survival and overall survival over the 10-year period was similar for the two groups (Fig. 10-26). In the subset of patients with positive axillary nodes, relapse-free survival was better for the patients treated with conservative surgery and radiotherapy than for those undergoing mastectomy (87% versus 72% at 5 years, $p = 0.02$). Adjuvant CMF was administered to 119 patients with positive nodes. CMF was administered simultaneously with radiotherapy without major problems and without the need for significant dose reductions.

In 1976, a randomized trial, begun in the United States by the NSABP, compared mastectomy to segmental mastectomy with and without radiotherapy as local treatment in 1843 patients with Stage I or II cancer with lesions measuring up to 4 cm in diameter. All patients underwent axillary dissection and patients with positive nodes received adjuvant chemotherapy. Segmental mastectomy referred to a resection of the tumor with enough normal tissue removed to ensure that the specimen margins were tumor-free. In 10% of patients assigned to the group undergoing segmental mastectomy, tumor-free margins were not obtained, and a total mastectomy was performed. Radiotherapy was delivered to the breast by opposed tangential fields to a dose of 5000 to 5300 cGy in 5 to 6 weeks. The regional lymph nodes were not treated, and a boost to the tumor site was not used. For the greater part of the study, patients were assigned to treatment by "prerandomization." Using this procedure, patients were randomly assigned to treatment after assessment of their eligibility, but before the protocol was explained or consent was obtained. The published results of the trial are from patients who accepted the assigned therapy.[20] One hundred and seventy-four patients (8%) refused their assigned treatment.

FIGURE 10-26. Probability of relapse-free survival in 701 patients treated with radical mastectomy or conservative surgery and radiotherapy in Milan trial. (Veronesi U in Tobias JS, Peckham MJ (eds): Primary Management of Breast Cancer. London, E. Arnold, 1985)

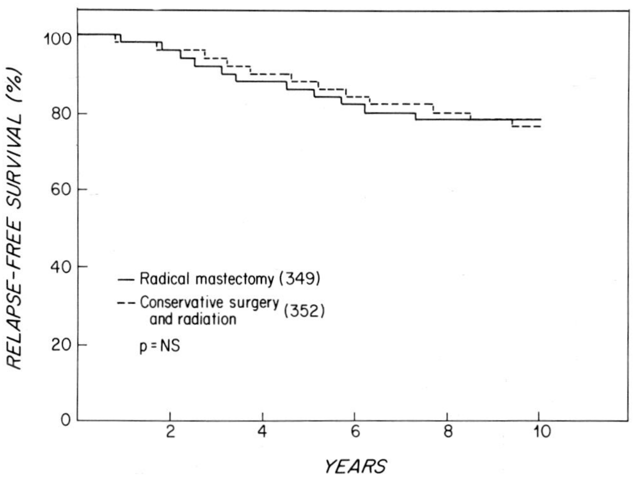

The probability that patients in this series with tumor-free margins who were treated with segmental mastectomy with or without radiotherapy remained free of tumor in the ipsilateral breast was compared. Of patients who received radiotherapy, 7.7% had a recurrence in the treated breast, compared to 28% of patients who did not receive radiotherapy ($p < 0.001$). This benefit for radiotherapy was seen both in patients with negative and positive nodes. In node-negative patients treated with segmental mastectomy alone, the 5-year breast relapse rate was 24%, compared to 10% when radiotherapy was added ($p < 0.001$). In node-positive patients (who were also treated with adjuvant chemotherapy), patients treated with segmental mastectomy alone had a 5-year breast relapse rate of 36%, compared to 2% when radiotherapy was added ($p < 0.001$). These results suggest that chemotherapy is not highly effective in preventing breast recurrence, but that radiotherapy and chemotherapy are additive, if not synergistic, in reducing tumor recurrence in the breast.

The impact of this increased risk of breast recurrence on relapse-free and overall survival in patients treated with segmental mastectomy alone was assessed. Of note was the fact that a recurrence in the treated breast was not scored as an event in the disease-free survival of a patient unless a salvage mastectomy could not be performed. Disease-free survival at 5 years was significantly worse for patients treated with segmental mastectomy than for patients treated with segmental mastectomy and radiotherapy (65% versus 73%, $p = 0.02$). However, overall survival at 5 years was comparable in the two treatment groups. It is conjectural at this point as to whether this difference in disease-free survival (owing to increased distant relapse and unsalvageable local recurrence) will be translated into a difference in survival after 5 years. These results were also analyzed in regard to the histologic status of the axillary lymph nodes (Table 10-25). The results indicate that the benefit in disease-free survival seen with radiotherapy was confined to the subgroup of patients with negative nodes. These patients had improved rates of disease-free survival (81% versus 68%, $p = 0.005$) and distant-disease-free survival (83% versus 73%, $p = 0.02$) at 5 years when radiotherapy was added.

Table 10-25
Comparison of Segmental Mastectomy (SM) with Segmental Mastectomy and Radiotherapy (SM+XRT) according to Nodal Status in Patients with Tumor-Free Margins (NSABP Trial B-06)

Five-Year Results	*Negative Nodes* SM (n=358)	SM+XRT (n=373)	*Positive Nodes* SM (n=207)	SM+XRT (n=193)
Disease-free survival	68% (p=0.005)	81%	57%	61%
Distant disease-free survival	73% (p=0.02)	83%	66%	65%
Survival	90%	91%	74%	79%

The outcome in patients treated with total mastectomy compared to that in patients treated with segmental mastectomy and radiotherapy is shown in Figure 10-27. Disease-free survival and overall survival were better for patients treated with segmental mastectomy and radiotherapy than for those undergoing total mastectomy, but this was only of marginal significance ($p = 0.04$ and $p = 0.01$, respectively). One may safely conclude that no disadvantage was attributed to the use of conservative surgery or radiotherapy.

The NSABP B-06 trial addresses two separate issues. One is the need for radiotherapy in patients treated with segmental mastectomy when margins are tumor-free. The results obtained in this study confirm the results obtained in retrospective studies, which have shown a local recurrence rate of approximately 30% when radiotherapy was not added[21–25] and a local recurrence rate of 5% to 10% when radiotherapy was added. At 5 years, relapse-free survival was worse for patients treated with segmental mastectomy than for those who also received radiotherapy, but overall survival was comparable. Of potential significance is the fact that this difference in disease-free survival was restricted to patients with negative axillary lymph nodes. It should be stressed that patients with negative nodes have a greater potential for cure with local treatment than do patients with positive nodes because their disease is more likely to be local than systemic. In this trial, patients with negative nodes who were treated with segmental mastectomy and radiotherapy had a 10% lower risk of distant relapse than did patients treated with segmental mastectomy alone (see Table 10-25). This observation (if confirmed by a longer follow-up period) will provide a strong impetus for early detection combined with effective local treatment. Early detection will improve the probability of diagnosing breast cancer when nodes are still negative, and effective local treatment in patients with negative nodes appears to improve the chances of freedom from distant relapse. Conversely, patients with positive nodes have a high risk of systemic disease, and effective local treatment is not likely to have a major impact on their likelihood of survival. The second issue addressed by the NSABP trial relates to the relative effectiveness of mastectomy and conservative surgery/radiotherapy as local treatment for patients with early breast cancer. These preliminary results at 5 years indicate a comparable outcome for these two forms of treatment.

The third trial was performed at the Institut Gustave-Roussy in Villejuif, France under the sponsorship of the World Health Organization.[26] The trial, started in 1972, included 179 patients with T1 N0 or N1 M0 breast cancers who were randomized to undergo either modified radical mastectomy or local excision of the tumor, axillary dissection, and radiotherapy. With a median follow-up time of 4 1/2 years, no differences in the rate of local recurrence or survival were observed between the two groups.

The fourth trial was performed at the National Cancer Institute in Bethesda, Maryland starting in 1979.[27] As of September of 1984, 165 patients with T1 or T2, N0 or N1, M0 breast cancer entered the study and were randomized to undergo either modified radical mastectomy or tumor excision, axillary dissection, and radiotherapy. With a median follow-up of 27 months, there were no significant differences in outcome noted between the two groups.

ANALYSIS OF FAILURE

By closely monitoring patterns of failure within the treated breast, the results of future treatment may be able to be improved. An analysis of failure was performed on the 366 Stage I and II breast cancers treated at the JCRT between 1968 and 1979.[28] Local recurrence was defined as any detection of cancer in the treated breast occurring before the development of disseminated disease. In almost all cases, recurrence was documented by a biopsy; however, four patients refused biopsy and were scored as having recurrent disease on the basis of clinical grounds alone. Local recurrence was classified as either: *true recurrence*, occurring within the margins of the boost or at the site of the primary tumor in the absence of a boost; *marginal miss*, occurring near the site of the primary tumor but just outside the border of the boost; or *recurrence elsewhere in the breast*, at a site at least several centimeters from the boosted volume and a substantial distance from the pri-

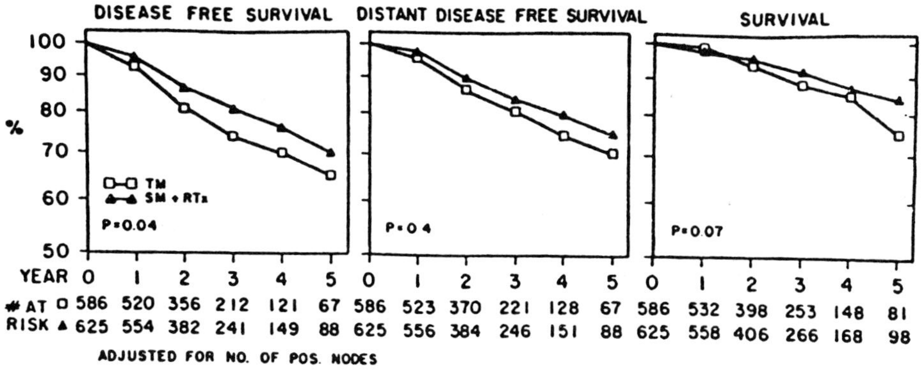

FIGURE 10-27. Life-table analysis showing disease-free survival, distant-disease-free survival, and overall survival of patients treated with total mastectomy (*TM*) or with segmental mastectomy plus radiation (*SM + RTx*). (Data are from the National Surgical Adjuvant Breast Project trial B-06.) (Fisher B et al. New Engl J Med 312:665, 1985. Reprinted by permission)

mary tumor. Either true recurrences or marginal misses were viewed as a recurrence of the original cancer. There were 30 recurrences in the 366 treated breasts, for a crude recurrence rate of 8.2%. The overall 5-year actuarial local recurrence rate was 9%. The actuarial local recurrence rates at 5 years were 4% for clinical Stage I disease and 12% for clinical Stage II tumors ($p = 0.12$). The effect of the type of biopsy on the probability of local recurrence was examined. Among the 342 breasts treated with excisional biopsy, there were 22 local recurrences, yielding a 7% actuarial probability of local recurrence at 5 years. Among the 24 breasts treated with less-than-excisional biopsy, there were eight local recurrences, yielding a 35% actuarial probability at 5 years. This difference was statistically significant ($p < 0.0001$). In those patients treated with excisional biopsy, the recurrences consisted of 11 true recurrences, 8 marginal misses, and 3 recurrences elsewhere in the breast. In the patients treated with less-than-excisional biopsy, there were 6 true recurrences, 2 marginal misses, and no recurrences elsewhere in the breast. Two of the 30 patients also had simultaneous clinical evidence of axillary recurrence, and two had skin nodules over the treated breast at the time of recurrence of the primary tumor. There were no supraclavicular or internal mammary node failures.

The actuarial probabilities of true recurrence, marginal miss, or a recurrence elsewhere in the treated breast were examined for the 342 breast cancers treated with excisional biopsy. The probability of true recurrence with time is shown in Figure 10-28. At 5 years, the actuarial probability of a true recurrence was 4%. No true recurrences were seen after 6 years in the 56 patients followed for longer than that period of time. The likelihood of a true recurrence appeared to be related to the radiation dose delivered to the primary tumor site, but the results did not achieve statistical significance. Eighty-nine patients who received a total dose of less than 6000 cGy had a 7% probability of a true recurrence at 5 years. In comparison, 144 patients who received 6000 to 6999 cGy had a 4% probability of a true recurrence at 5 years, and 109 patients who received 7000 cGy or greater had a 1% probability at 5 years (the difference between the groups receiving the lowest and highest doses, $p = 0.06$).

The probability of a marginal miss with time is shown in Figure 10-28. At 5 years, the actuarial probability of a marginal miss was 4%. No marginal miss occurred more than 7 years after treatment among the 33 patients still available for observation beyond 7 years. The likelihood of a marginal miss was examined in relation to the dose to the primary tumor site and the volume of the boost used (measured by the number of iridium-192 seeds). Marginal miss was not related either to the dose to the primary site or to the volume of the boost used.

For patients treated with excisional biopsy, the overall probability of a recurrence of the primary tumor (either a true recurrence or a marginal miss) was 7% at 5 years. In an attempt to determine the value of a boost in reducing the probability of recurrence of the primary tumor in these patients, results of treatment were compared for the 243 patients boosted to 6000 cGy or greater and the 91 patients who received less than 6000 cGy. This comparison was limited by physician selection. Patients at great risk for local recurrence (i.e., those with large primary tumors or close or microscopically positive margins) were more often selected for a boost. Despite this selection bias, patients who received 6000 cGy or more had a 6% probability of recurrence of the primary tumor at 6 years, compared to a 12% probability for patients receiving less than 6000 cGy ($p = 0.37$).

Three patients, all undergoing excisional biopsy, were scored as having recurrence elsewhere in the breast at 57, 72, and 95 months. This represented an actuarial rate of 1% at 5 years and 3% at 6 years. The probability of the development of a contralateral primary tumor was calculated for comparison. If one assumes that microscopic foci of multicentric breast cancer are equally present in both breasts, this comparison evaluates the usefulness of whole-breast irradiation in eradicating these foci. The probability of a metachronous contralateral primary tumor was 5% at 5 years (15 patients) (see Figure 10-28).

In examining this analysis of failure, it is important to stress that the purpose of breast irradiation following conservative surgery is two-fold: control of the primary tumor and eradication of microscopic foci of multicentric cancer in the ipsilateral breast. It appears reasonable to view a true recurrence or a marginal miss as a failure to control the primary tumor, and a recurrence elsewhere in the breast as a failure to eradicate multicentric cancer. Ninety percent of breast relapses in this series were either true recurrences or marginal misses representing failures to

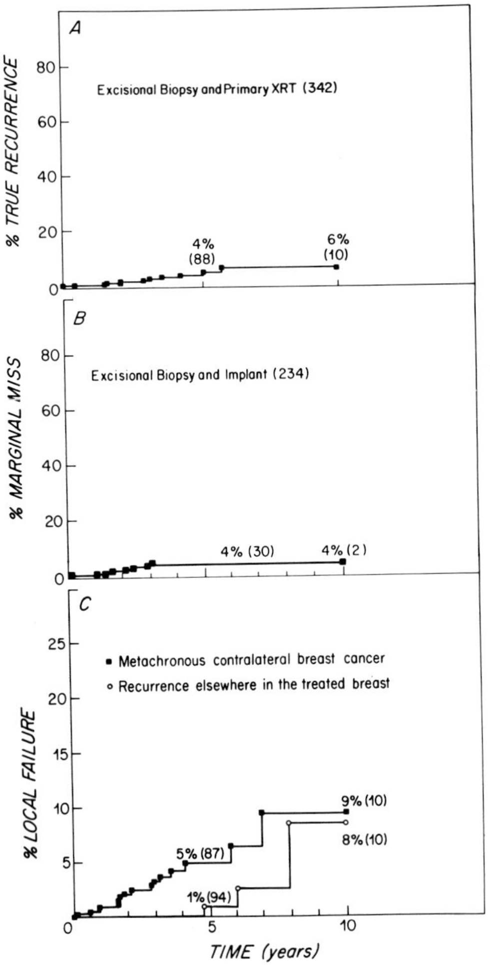

FIGURE 10-28. Actuarial probability of true recurrence (*A*), marginal miss (*B*), or recurrence elsewhere in the breast (*C*) in patients treated with excisional biopsy and radiotherapy at JCRT. For calculation of marginal miss probability, only patients undergoing interstitial implantation were included. (Recht A. Int J Radiat Oncol Biol Phys 11:1271, 1985)

control the primary tumor. The risk of a true recurrence or a marginal miss remained at a fairly constant rate for the first 7 years after treatment. No failures to control the primary lesion were noted after 7 years in the 33 patients followed for longer than that length of time. For true recurrences, a clear (but not statistically significant) dose-response trend was noted, with rare true recurrences seen at levels above 6000 cGy. In analyzing the risk of a marginal miss occurring, a relationship between the volume of the boost and the likelihood of a marginal miss was anticipated, but was not noted. It is possible that the lack of a volume-response relationship in these data is related to a selection bias by physicians who used larger boosts in patients thought to be at higher risk for local recurrence. The risk of recurrence elsewhere in the ipsilateral breast is thought to be related primarily to the incidence of multicentricity of breast cancer (but may be attributable to intralymphatic spread from the primary tumor in some cases). Both the frequency and the significance of multicentric disease in the ipsilateral breast vary from 13% to 74%.[29–31] This large variation is a result of many factors, including the precise definition of multicentricity used and the extent of the pathologic examination. The frequency of multicentric disease in the opposite breast has not been well documented. The frequency of contralateral breast carcinoma (in patients with infiltrating ductal histology) was 15% in one series in which a wide, mirror-image biopsy was done at the time of ipsilateral mastectomy.[32] In another, more recent study, human breasts were examined *in toto* by a subgross sampling technique in 63 cancer-containing breasts, 44 breasts that were contralateral to cancer-containing breasts, and 185 breasts from random autopsies.[33] Additional primary foci of intraductal carcinoma that were unrelated to invasive carcinoma were found in 53% of the cancer-containing breasts, 48% of the contralateral breasts, and only 6% of the breasts from random autopsies. These observations support the view that the frequency of multicentric, predominantly intraductal, breast cancer is equal in both the involved and contralateral breasts. Since, in the majority of cases, multicentric breast cancer represents small foci of cancer, it is anticipated that the use of whole-breast irradiation to a level of 4500 to 5000 cGy will eradicate them. These data provide support for this approach by demonstrating that the likelihood of a recurrence elsewhere in the breast is very low. Further, by using the likelihood of a contralateral breast cancer as a control (representing untreated multicentric disease), these data indicate that the use of whole-breast irradiation appears to eradicate effectively, or at least to suppress, these multicentric foci of breast cancer. However, these data on recurrence elsewhere in the treated breast are still preliminary since it may take a long time to manifest such failures. Additional follow-up will be required to be certain of these results.

COSMETIC RESULTS AFTER CONSERVATIVE SURGERY AND RADIOTHERAPY

The cosmetic results seen after treatment with conservative surgery and radiotherapy have generally been good to excellent.[5,6,34] The results obtained at the JCRT are typical of other reported series and will be presented here in some detail. The JCRT results have been presented in three separate publications. The first report detailed the cosmetic outcome in 29 patients (31 treated breasts) treated between 1968 and 1975.[35] Three principal treatment factors were identified which influenced the cosmetic outcome. The first was the extent and location of the biopsy procedure. Two patients had unsatisfactory cosmetic results solely because of excessively wide resections. In many other patients, the surgical scar was obvious, thus diminishing the overall cosmetic result. The optimal technique for resecting the tumor is discussed in greater detail in the previous section on surgical management. The second factor that influenced the cosmetic result was the time/dose schedule of the radiotherapy. A direct correlation was found between radiation dose (measured in units of rets) and resultant fibrosis and retraction in the treated breast. Increasing doses of external beam radiation were associated with greater degrees of retraction and fibrosis of the treated breast. All six patients who received 6000 cGy to the whole breast had significant retraction and fibrosis, whereas patients who received 5000 cGy rarely showed significant changes. The third factor influencing the cosmetic outcome was the technique of radiotherapy. Skin changes occurred infrequently in these patients as a result of the use of supervoltage equipment and the avoidance of bolus. (Bolus is material placed on the skin during radiotherapy to circumvent the skin-sparing property of supervoltage radiation). Many of the patients in this study underwent interstitial implantation, and two of these patients developed mild skin changes related to this procedure. These skin changes may be minimized by careful positioning of the iridium-192 seeds at a reasonable distance (1 cm) from the skin surface. An additional technical detail concerns the use of wedges as tissue compensators for the tangential fields to the breast. When linear accelerators are used, unwedged fields are typically associated with significant inhomogeneity in radiation dose (> 40% to 50%). This may be corrected easily (to ≤ 15%) by the addition of wedges as compensators. A final technical detail regards the treatment field arrangement. If a third field is directed anteriorly to treat the axillary and supraclavicular node regions, it must be matched to the tangential fields in a way that minimizes overlap between fields. Such overlap can produce an area of fibrosis and skin changes at the match line. This match line effect was seen in some patients who otherwise had excellent results. These technical factors will be reviewed in the section on technique of treatment, below.

The second report on cosmetic results obtained at the JCRT detailed the outcome in 239 patients treated between 1976 and 1980 with conservative surgery and radiotherapy and without chemotherapy.[36] Four patients had bilateral cancer, making a total of 243 breasts available for analysis. Follow-up ranged from 24 to 78 months, with a median of 33 months. Figure 10-29 shows the change in the overall cosmetic results after the completion of primary radiation treatment. At 6 months, 84% of the patients had an excellent result. Over the next 2 years, the percentage of patients scored as excellent decreased, so that at 30 months, 64% of the patients had an excellent result. Thereafter, further deterioration was uncommon. Of the 69 patients who underwent follow-up for longer than 3 years, only 4 (6%) showed a decline from excellent or good results to fair or poor results past the 3-year point. At 60 months, 77% were judged to have had an excellent result. When excellent and good results were combined, a highly satisfactory cosmetic outcome was achieved in 97% of the patients at 6 months, in 91% at 30 months, and in 86% at 60 months. At 60 months, 9% of the patients had a fair result, and 5% had a poor result.

This study also described the frequency and severity of breast edema after primary radiation treatment (Figure 10-30). Breast edema diminished with the duration of follow-up. At 6 months, 35% of patients had breast edema (which was mild in 32% and moderate in 3%); at 60 months, 23% of the patients had breast edema (deemed to be mild). The use of axillary dissection influenced the incidence and degree of breast edema. At 6 months, 75% of the patients not undergoing axillary dissection were free of breast edema, compared with 60% of those undergoing a dissection (p = 0.03). At 30 months, 87% of the patients who did not undergo axillary dissection were free of edema, compared with 78% of those who did have axillary dissection (p = 0.26). At 48 months, the corresponding results were 94% and 83%, respectively (p =

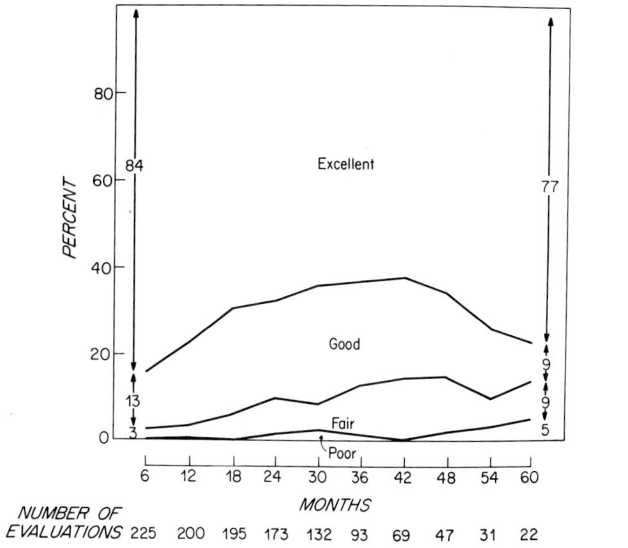

FIGURE 10-29. Overall cosmetic results after completion of primary radiation treatment at the Joint Center for Radiation Therapy. (Beadle GF et al. Cancer 54:2911, 1984)

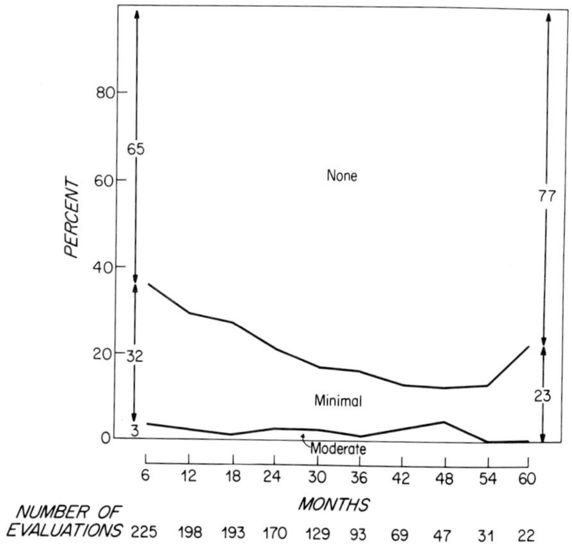

FIGURE 10-30. The frequency and severity of breast edema after completion of primary radiation treatment at the Joint Center for Radiation Therapy. (Beadle GF et al. Cancer 54:2911, 1984)

0.59). When the number of axillary lymph nodes removed at dissection was used as a guide to the extent of surgery, patients having 1 to 10 nodes sampled were noted to have a lower frequency of breast edema at all time-points than patients having 11 or more nodes sampled. The differences were most striking at 6 months, when only 46% of the patients with 11 or more nodes sampled were free of edema, compared with 64% of those who had 1 to 10 nodes sampled ($p = 0.19$). Long-term moderate or severe breast edema was rare in these patients. At 48 months, none of the 16 undissected patients had moderate edema, whereas 2 of 30 patients who underwent axillary dissection had moderate edema ($p = 0.76$). These findings indicate that breast edema after radiotherapy is common when axillary dissection has been performed, that the extent of breast edema is directly related to the extent of axillary dissection, and that breast edema diminishes with time after treatment. These findings are similar to those described by Clarke and colleagues.[37]

This study also indicated that the size of the interstitial implant and the dose delivered by the implant influenced the cosmetic outcome.[36] Patients with small implants tended to have better cosmetic results than did patients with large implants. The size of the implant was measured by the number of seeds used. Implants containing 100 seeds or more were considered to be large. Forty-two percent of patients with large implants had an excellent cosmetic result at 36 months, compared with 59% of patients with small implants ($p = 0.43$). In patients with small implants, the overall cosmetic result appeared to correlate with the implant dose. Eighty-one percent of patients who received less than 1800 cGy using a small implant had an excellent cosmetic result at 42 months, compared with 39% of those receiving 1800 cGy or greater ($p = 0.13$). These observations have been useful in setting guidelines for the use of interstitial implantation, discussed below.

The third publication from the JCRT on the cosmetic result following treatment examined the effect of adjuvant chemotherapy on the cosmetic outcome.[38] Preliminary results indicated a worsening of the cosmetic outcome when chemotherapy was added compared to the outcome when patients were treated with radiotherapy alone. This difference was due primarily to a shift in chemotherapy-treated patients from an excellent to a good overall cosmetic result. Breast retraction was more common in patients treated with adjuvant chemotherapy. Since the median follow-up time for chemotherapy-treated patients was only 34 months, further follow-up is required. These results, however, are similar to the preliminary results obtained by Ray and co-workers.[39]

COMPLICATIONS

The possible complications of radiotherapy include carcinogenesis (cancer of the contralateral breast, leukemia, and soft tissue sarcoma), decreased arm mobility, radiation pneumonitis, brachial plexopathy, radiation-related heart disease, and an increased risk of arm edema. Since the technique used for postoperative radiotherapy is similar to that used for radiotherapy as primary treatment, data on complications after both approaches are relevant to this discussion. Taken together, the various studies presented indicate that significant complications may be seen after radiotherapy for breast cancer, but that the risk of such complications is extremely low when good technique and adequate doses are employed.

Carcinogenesis

One possible complication of radiotherapy is the induction of cancer in the opposite breast. Breast tissue is known to be sensitive to radiation carcinogenesis.[40] The latency period between exposure and the detection of the induced cancer is at least 10 years. As discussed in the section on epidemiology, a number of factors have been identified that influence the likelihood of radiation carcinogenesis of breast tissue. Two critical factors are radiation dose and age at exposure. The influence of dose on the risk of carcinogenesis is illustrated in the study by Baral and associates, which reported the effect of radiation on benign breast conditions in young women.[41] The risk of carcinogenesis increased linearly with doses of up to 1000 cGy. With doses above 1000 cGy, however, there was a bending of the curve and an actual decrease in the risk of carcinogenesis. When doses in the therapeutic range (greater than 4500 cGy) are used, the risk appears to be negligible. To explain this phenomenon, it has been hypothesized that radiation results in two competing processes: carcinogenesis and cell inactivation. Carcinogenesis is viewed as a linear process, whereas cell inactivation is viewed as an exponential process with an initial shoulder region. Based on these relationships, there is a relatively greater risk of carcinogenesis at lower doses. At higher dose levels, though, cell inactivation becomes dominant, and the risk of carcinogenesis decreases. Since the dose to the opposite breast from a course of postoperative or primary radiotherapy is in the range of 100 to 300 cGy,[42] tumor induction in the opposite breast is a matter for potential concern.

Age at exposure to radiation is the other important risk factor for carcinogenesis in human tissue. The highest risk occurs in females exposed before 19 years of age; with increasing age, the risk of carcinogenesis declines. The risk for women over the age of 35 years is not detectable.[43] This factor would mitigate against a significant risk of tumor induction for most breast cancer patients.

Two studies address the issue of contralateral breast cancer after postoperative radiotherapy. In one, the records of patients treated at the Ontario Cancer Treatment and Research Foundation (London Clinic) from 1953 to 1971 were reviewed.[44] Three hundred and sixty-nine patients underwent radical mastectomy, and 1120 underwent radical mastectomy and postoperative radiotherapy. Patients who developed contralateral breast cancer were significantly younger than those who did not develop cancer of the opposite breast. The cumulative probability of contralateral breast cancer, projected to 20 years, was not influenced by the use of postoperative radiotherapy.

The other study, from the M.D. Anderson Hospital, was conducted between 1947 and 1976.[45] Of 2082 patients with Stage I and Stage II breast cancer, 409 were treated with surgery alone, and 1673 were treated with surgery and radiotherapy. Follow-up ranged from 5 to 34 years, with a median of 5.7 years. The median follow-up of the two groups was similar. Of note is the fact that patients in the group receiving radiotherapy were younger and, therefore, more likely to develop contralateral breast cancer. Forty percent of the patients in that group were 50 years of age or younger, compared to only 25% of the patients treated with surgery alone. Despite this fact, 57 of the 1673 patients (3.4%) who received radiotherapy developed contralateral breast cancer, compared to 30 of the 409 patients (7.3%) who were treated with surgery alone. For patients undergoing follow-up for 10 years or more, the rate of contralateral breast cancer was similar in both treatment groups. These data suggest that the risk of cancer of the opposite breast is not significantly increased by the use of postoperative radiotherapy. As noted above, this is perhaps related to the relatively advanced age of patients with breast cancer.

Sarcomas of soft tissue or bone are a rare, but well documented, complication of radiotherapy. In a recent study from Memorial Sloan-Kettering Cancer Center, a total of 42 osteogenic sarcomas were reported between 1921 and 1983 arising in sites of prior radiotherapy given for nonosseous conditions.[46] This represented 3% of all osteogenic sarcomas seen at that institution. Six of these patients had originally been treated for breast cancer. The median latency period from the time of radiotherapy to the detection of the sarcoma was 10.5 years, with a range of 3.5 to 33 years. Since the total number of patients at risk was unknown, it was not possible to calculate an actuarial risk for the condition or its radiation dose response. A total of 20 soft tissue sarcomas arising in irradiated areas were seen over a 50-year period at Memorial Sloan-Kettering Cancer Center.[47] The median latency period was 12 years. Four of these patients had originally been treated for breast cancer. None of the cases of bone or soft tissue sarcoma occurred with doses below 3000 cGy in 3 weeks.

Acute nonlymphatic leukemia (ANLL) is also a well described but rare complication of radiotherapy. The median latency period for the appearance of ANLL is shorter than that for solid tumors, generally 4 to 7 years after exposure.[48] Radiation dose is also a factor in the risk of leukemia. An increased incidence of leukemia has been observed after low-dose radiotherapy (1000 to 2000 cGy) delivered to the pelvis for benign conditions,[49–51] but this increase is not associated with therapeutic levels of radiotherapy (4000 cGy or greater).[52–54] Perhaps because the amount of bone marrow irradiated is small, ANLL is a rare occurrence after treatment for breast cancer when adjuvant chemotherapy is not used. At the JCRT, none of 422 patients treated with primary radiotherapy without adjuvant chemotherapy, with a median follow-up time of 59 months, developed ANLL. The risk of ANLL was also evaluated for patients treated with radiotherapy as part of NSABP trials B-04 and B-06.[55] Four of the 1116 patients eligible for evaluation developed ANLL, yielding a relative risk of 10.3 ($p < 0.01$). Two of the patients who developed ANLL were younger than 50 years of age (with a relative risk of 33, $p < 0.05$), and two were older than 50 years of age (with a relative risk of 6, p = NS). The risk of ANLL after radiotherapy with adjuvant chemotherapy has not been as well documented because the experience with this combination is more limited. In the experience of the JCRT, 103 patients were treated with primary radiotherapy and adjuvant chemotherapy, with a median follow-up time of 59 months. Of these patients, one developed ANLL. This patient underwent 2 years of adjuvant chemotherapy which included the use of an alkylating agent.

Arm Edema

The most frequent complication of radiotherapy for breast cancer is arm edema. The issue of arm edema is discussed in greater detail elsewhere in this book. The etiology of the disorder is poorly understood, but it is probably associated with obliteration of lymphatics in the axilla and scarring secondary to thrombophlebitis and infection. Bretton and Nelson reported on the incidence of arm edema after radical mastectomy from 14 separate series.[56] The incidence of arm edema in patients undergoing radical mastectomy varied from 7% to 63%; the average incidence was 20% to 25%. This incidence was clearly related to the use of postoperative radiotherapy. In patients treated with radiotherapy, the incidence of arm edema ranged from 50% to 85%, whereas in patients treated without radiotherapy the incidence ranged from 8% to 46%. Additional information is available from the Stockholm trial.[57] As part of this trial, precise volumetric measurements of edema were made in patients in each of three treatment groups (those undergoing modified radical mastectomy alone, those treated with modified radical mastectomy and postoperative radiotherapy, and those who underwent preoperative radiotherapy and modified radical mastectomy). In all cases, radiotherapy was delivered to the entire axilla for a total dose of 4500 cGy in 5 weeks. In all three treatment groups, some arm edema was noted; the mean volume of the ipsilateral arm in each group was significantly greater than that of the contralateral arm ($p < 0.01$). Modified radical mastectomy resulted in a 2.2% increase in volume, compared to an increase of 4.5% associated with preoperative radiotherapy and a 4.8% increase associated with postoperative radiotherapy (comparison of radiotherapy versus no radiotherapy, $p < 0.01$). Severe arm edema was uncommon in all treatment groups, occurring in 1% of the patients treated with mastectomy alone, 2% of those undergoing postoperative radiotherapy, and 3% of patients receiving preoperative radiotherapy.

The risk of arm edema was recently reviewed in a group of patients treated with primary radiation therapy at the JCRT.[58] Full axillary irradiation was used in the large majority of patients. The risk of arm edema was found to be related to the use and extent of axillary surgery. The actuarial risk of arm edema at 6 years was 4% for patients treated without axillary surgery and 13% for patients undergoing axillary surgery ($p = 0.006$). Patients treated with full axillary dissection, defined as including a stripping of the axillary vein, had a 37% risk of arm edema at 6 years, whereas patients who underwent a lesser axillary procedure had only a 7% risk of arm edema ($p < 0.001$). Arm edema in this series was either mild or moderate, with no patients having severe edema. An unanswered question at this time is whether the use of a more limited supraclavicular field, which treats the supraclavicular fossa and the axillary apex but spares the dissected portion of the axilla, also increases the risk of arm edema. Available results indicate that both the extent of axillary surgery and the use of axillary irradiation influence the risk of arm edema. If a full dissection has been performed, the use of postoperative radiotherapy, including treatment of the axilla, will significantly increase the risk of arm edema.

Brachial Plexopathy

Another possible complication of treatment to the axillary and supraclavicular region is injury to the brachial plexus. The classic radiation-induced injury is dose-related and very rarely occurs with doses less than 5000 cGy.[59–60] It is characterized by mild discomfort in the shoulder and by paresthesia and weakness in the arm and hand. Typically, there is evidence of soft tissue fibrosis in the supraclavicular and infraclavicular regions. The neurologic deficits are usually permanent and may be progressive. The onset of the syndrome is also related to dose. With doses less than 6000 cGy, the time to onset is generally greater than 1 year, whereas with doses of 6000 cGy or greater, the interval to onset may be shorter than 1 year. Sometimes, it may be difficult to distinguish this syndrome from carcinomatous involvement of the brachial plexus.[61,62] This differential diagnosis will be discussed in Chapter 14 in the section on complications of breast cancer. At the JCRT, 6 of 735 patients with Stage I or II tumors who were treated between 1968 and 1981 developed radiation-induced brachial plexus injury. Reversible brachial plexopathy, one form of radiation-related injury of the brachial plexus seen at the JCRT, occurs at doses less than 5000 cGy. It has a short latency period (a median latency period of 4.5 months), and is characterized by transient paresthesia and weakness. This condition was observed in eight patients with Stage I to III tumors who were treated between 1975 and 1978. They constituted approximately 3% of the total number of patients. Reversible brachial plexopathy has been observed to occur more commonly in patients who also receive adjuvant chemotherapy than in those treated without chemotherapy (4.8% versus 0.4%, $p < 0.01$).[63] The syndrome appears to have been clustered temporally since instances of the syndrome since 1978 have been rare. The temporal clustering and relation to the use of adjuvant chemotherapy suggest an infectious etiology. Similar plexopathies have been noted to occur in clusters without radiotherapy. No recognized therapeutic regimen has been developed for either of these radiation-related brachial plexus injuries.

Soft Tissue and Bone Disorders

The use of postoperative radiotherapy may be associated with alterations of the soft tissues and bones in the treatment volume. Studies from both Sweden[57] and Denmark[64] have shown decreased range of movement in the area of the shoulder joint in patients treated with mastectomy and postoperative radiotherapy compared to that observed in patients treated with mastectomy alone. These effects are generally mild, and are thought to be secondary to fibrosis of the irradiated soft tissue. The relationship of this effect to radiation dose or volume has not been defined. Demineralization of bone may occur after radiotherapy, and may be associated with fracture in some cases. This effect appears to be dose-related, and is increased with the use of orthovoltage treatment, which is associated with a greater absorption of dose by bone. In the experience of Langlands and co-workers, severe osteitis of the shoulder girdle (defined as the presence of prominent, mottled translucencies with gross osteoporosis or dense sclerosis documented on radiographs) occurred in 13% of patients treated with mastectomy and postoperative radiotherapy.[65] Patients were treated with orthovoltage and received 4000 to 4500 cGy over a period of 3 or 4 weeks. Severe osteitis was more likely to occur in patients treated with the more rapid fractionation schedule (3 weeks) than in those treated for the longer period. Only 1 of the 17 patients with severe osteitis suffered a traumatic fracture of the neck of the humerus. At the JCRT, there have been no instances of traumatic fracture of the humerus, although traumatic fractures of the ribs have been seen, particularly early in the series when relatively higher doses of radiotherapy were used. Of the patients treated between 1968 and 1981, 24 patients developed traumatic rib fractures.

Fibrosis of soft tissue in the treated area is a common sequela of treatment. The degree of fibrosis is related to dose. In patients treated with a dose of 4500 to 5000 cGy in 5 weeks, the degree of fibrosis is generally slight. In localized areas to which supplemental radiation has been administered at a higher dose, the degree of fibrosis is increased. Soft tissue necrosis may be a sequela of such treatment. At the JCRT, 1 of 525 patients developed soft tissue necrosis subsequent to localized, high-dose irradiation.

It is important to emphasize that, although significant bone and soft tissue effects are rare following moderate-dose radiotherapy (4500 to 5000 cGy over a period of 5 weeks), their incidence may be increased greatly by increasing the radiation dose or by merely altering the fractionation schedule. Kim and co-workers examined the likelihood of soft tissue effects following postoperative radiotherapy administered using a number of different fractionation schedules.[66] Patients were treated with one of the following regimens: 4900 cGy in 10 fractions over a period of 32 days, 4410 cGy in nine fractions over a period of 30 days, 5000 cGy in 13 fractions over a period of 18 days, or 4600 cGy in 20 fractions over a period of 28 days. There was no difference in the rate of acute reaction or local recurrence among the various fractionation schedules. However, significant subcutaneous fibrosis was seen in 33% of the patients who received 490 cGy × 10, as well as in 17% of those who received 385 cGy × 13 and in 4% of the patients who received 230 cGy × 20. Montague documented the likelihood of soft tissue complications in patients treated using a fractionation schedule of either 200 cGy per day administered five times per week or 333 cGy per day administered three times per weeks.[67] Patients treated only three times per week received the same weekly dose and the same total dose, yet exhibited a marked increase in soft tissue complications. Spanos and associates reported on a group of patients with Stage III breast cancer who were treated with a protracted course of radiotherapy.[68] Of a group of 91 patients who received 8100 cGy or more over a period of 10 weeks, 11 developed severe fibrosis and 13 developed necrosis. Six of the 13 cases of necrosis occurred more than 6 years after treatment. Because of the protracted fractionation, severe acute reactions were not seen. More recently, Ferguson and colleagues from the University of Chicago described similar late soft tissue effects in a group of patients treated with orthovoltage radiotherapy to a median dose of 6000 cGy.[69] These studies emphasize the impact of both total dose and daily dose on the likelihood of soft tissue complications following radiotherapy.

Heart and Lung Injuries

Injury to the heart and lung are possible complications after postoperative radiotherapy, and their likelihood is related to the technique and doses used. Radiation-related pericarditis is a known effect of radiotherapy when the majority of the pericardium is irradiated to a dose exceeding 3500 cGy. Patients with pericarditis typically present 6 to 18 months after treatment with symptoms of effusion and chest pain. Instances of pericarditis have been observed following radiotherapy for Hodgkin's disease, especially in patients in whom large mediastinal masses are present.[70] Radiation-related pericarditis is rare after radiotherapy for breast cancer. At the JCRT, only 1 of the 525 patients with Stage I or II breast cancer developed symptomatic pericarditis after treatment. This patient presented with synchronous bilateral breast cancer and was treated with a direct anterior field to both internal mammary chains, consequently receiving treatment in a significant portion of her pericardium. A detailed study was recently undertaken at the JCRT on the effects of heart and pericardium irradiation as a part of primary radiotherapy for 20 patients with early breast cancer. All patients were irradiated with tangential fields to the breast and internal mammary nodes. A direct anterior field was used in only one patient. Computed tomography (CT) scans of the thorax indicated that approximately 10% of the heart volume was included in the treatment volume using this technique. Electrocardiographic (EKG) changes were common 6 months to 1 year after treatment, and included rightward shift of both frontal plane QRS and T axes, and inversion of one or more leads V2 to V6. These EKG changes all resolved within 2 years. Three patients were found to have transient, asymptomatic, pericardial effusions on echocardiography. A follow-up period of up to 5 years failed to reveal any decrement in left ventricular function, as monitored by exercise EKG or rest and peak radionuclide ventriculography.[71]

The recent report from the Oslo trial on the use of postoperative radiotherapy suggests that patients with Stage I disease who are treated with cobalt-60 have a higher risk of dying from causes other than breast cancer, and that this risk is attributable to an increased risk of myocardial infarction compared to that in patients who are untreated.[72] Radiotherapy has been identified as a factor in the rate of atheromatous formation in large vessels, and has been implicated as a risk factor for myocardial infarction in patients treated for Hodgkin's disease.[73] An increased risk of myocardial infarction after postoperative radiotherapy for breast cancer has not been noted in other series. In the 10-year results of the NSABP B-04 trial, deaths (from all causes) in the absence of breast cancer occurred in 67 of 646 patients (10%) who received radiotherapy and 117 of 1019 patients (11%) who did not receive radiotherapy.[74] In the Oslo trial, the routine use of a 6-cm-wide anterior field to treat the internal mammary nodes was probably a factor in the observed incidence of myocardial infarction.

Postoperative radiotherapy may increase the risk of cardiomyopathy in patients who are also treated with Adriamycin. Loprinzi and co-workers reported on 32 patients with locally advanced breast cancer treated with primary radiotherapy and Adriamycin-containing chemotherapy.[75] Eight of these patients (25%) developed symptomatic cardiac toxicity. Of note is the fact that this complication appeared in 7 of 18 patients with left-sided cancers and only 1 of 14 patients with right-sided cancers ($p < 0.05$). The radiotherapy involved a direct anterior field to treat the IMNs in all cases, and doses were somewhat higher than those used in postoperative radiotherapy. DeLena and associates reported contrasting results.[76] They treated 132 patients with locally advanced breast cancer with Adriamycin-containing chemotherapy, randomizing them to undergo either radical mastectomy or primary radiotherapy. Two cases of cardiomyopathy were seen, both of which occurred in the group undergoing mastectomy. It is difficult to determine the cause of these contrasting results since the technique and doses of radiotherapy employed were similar in the two studies. Both described the use of a direct anterior field. It is likely that the risk of cardiomyopathy would be greatly reduced by the use of tangential fields or electron beams to treat the IMNs.

Radiation pneumonitis is a recognized complication

of thoracic radiotherapy.[77–80] Patients with radiation pneumonitis typically present 6 to 18 months after treatment with a dry cough, shortness of breath, and low-grade fever. The likelihood and severity of this complication are directly related to the volume of the lung irradiated and the dose used. Small segments of lung may be irradiated to 6000 cGy without evidence of symptomatic pneumonitis, whereas 2000 cGy to an entire lung is likely to result in the complication. Symptomatic radiation pneumonitis is an uncommon complication of radiotherapy for breast cancer. At the JCRT, 9 of 735 patients treated for early breast cancer with primary radiotherapy developed symptomatic radiation pneumonitis. In all cases, the symptoms were transient, and no patient developed permanent respiratory problems.

The volume of lung irradiated and the dose depend on the technique of radiotherapy.[81] The use of tangential fields to the breast, which extend medially 3 cm across the midline, treats approximately 25% of the ipsilateral lung, and is rarely associated with symptomatic radiation pneumonitis. This technique, however, adequately covers the IMNs in only 80% of patients.[82] Attempts to cover the IMNs in all patients by the use of a direct anterior field or by the use of deeper tangential fields greatly increase the volume of lung irradiated. Conversely, the use of electron beam to treat the IMNs, or the use of tangential fields to the breast that extend medially to midline and do not regularly include the IMNs, is associated with a considerably smaller volume of lung irradiated.

The use of radiotherapy to treat the supraclavicular and axillary regions is typically associated with subsequent radiographic changes in the irradiated lung. These changes are characterized by fibrosis corresponding to the treated area and pleural thickening, but are rarely associated with symptomatic pneumonitis. These radiographic changes may be confused with evidence of metastatic disease or with lung cancer by physicians unfamiliar with them.

It has been suggested that postoperative radiotherapy may increase the risk of metastases, either by a direct local effect or by a decrease in generalized host defenses. Dao and Kovaric examined the outcome in a group of 354 patients treated with mastectomy, with or without postoperative radiotherapy.[83] Of the patients treated with radical mastectomy alone, 14% developed ipsilateral lung metastases, and 34% developed chest wall recurrence. Of the patients treated with postoperative radiotherapy, 37% developed ipsilateral lung metastases, and 52% developed chest wall recurrence. These two groups of patients were believed to be comparable with regard to both clinical and pathologic features. However, all the relevant randomized trials show a decrease in the rate of local recurrence with the addition of postoperative radiotherapy, suggesting that the findings of Dao and Kovaric are spurious. Dao and Kovaric also reported that, in a small number of irradiated patients, a multitude of skin lesions limited to the irradiated field developed. This observation has occasionally been noted by other clinicians, as well. In 1974, Stjernsward suggested that the use of postoperative irradiation increased mortality by suppressing host immunity.[84] He combined the results of six studies (the two parts of the Manchester study, the NSABP trial B-02, and two studies comparing total mastectomy and postoperative radiotherapy to radical or extended radical mastectomy), and found an increased mortality rate associated with the use of radiotherapy. As discussed above, all of the four more recent studies testing the value of postoperative radiotherapy have demonstrated a small, but not statistically significant, advantage in survival with the use of radiotherapy. The recent report by Palmer and Ribeiro provides some support for this position.[85]

The effect of postoperative radiotherapy on immune response has been studied by a number of investigators.[86–88] This treatment has been clearly shown to decrease the total T-cell population, as well as the responses to various mitogens, but not to produce any significant changes in serum immunoglobulins. The alterations in T-cells are seen during radiotherapy and may persist for years. The significance of these immunologic changes on breast cancer survival is dubious. Baral and colleagues studied the degree of radiation-related immunologic changes in 100 patients with carcinoma of the breast. The degree of suppression in the T-cell population and in mitogen response was not related to patient age or the stage of the tumor.[86] More importantly, prognosis was not correlated with the degree of immunosuppression.

THE TIME COURSE AND PROGNOSIS OF LOCAL RECURRENCE FOLLOWING CONSERVATIVE SURGERY AND RADIOTHERAPY

There are significant differences in the time course and prognosis of local recurrence after treatment with conservative surgery and radiotherapy compared to that observed after mastectomy. The incidence, time course, and significance of recurrence in the chest wall and regional lymph nodes after radical mastectomy for breast cancer have been well documented.[89–94] Such local recurrence is most common during the first 3 years after mastectomy, thereafter decreasing in frequency, and rarely occurring after 10 years. The prognosis for patients with local recurrence following radical mastectomy is poor. Long-term survival is rare even after effective radiation treatment to the area of recurrence.

To determine the time course and implications of local recurrence after conservative surgery and radiotherapy, data were combined from three institutions in which a total of 152 patients (6 with bilateral disease) were treated prior to 1967.[95] All patients diagnosed with local recurrence had pathologically documented evidence of recurrence. Figure 10-31 shows the actuarial rate of local tumor control plotted semi-logarithmically for the 158 breast cancers treated with primary radiation therapy. The risk of a local recurrence was fairly constant (approximately 2% per year) over the first 14 years after treatment. No local recurrences were diagnosed between 14 and 20 years. One patient developed a local recurrence at 21 years and 2 months. There were 35 local recurrences in the 158

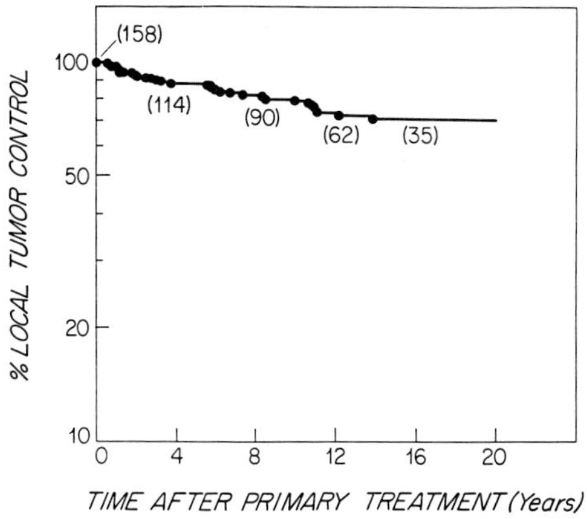

FIGURE 10-31. Actuarial local tumor control in 158 breast cancers treated with primary radiation therapy. The numbers in parentheses indicate the number of breast cancers that are at risk at specified points of time. Data analyzed at the Joint Center for Radiation Therapy. (Harris JR et al. J Clin Oncol 2:37, 1984)

breast cancers treated, for a crude 15-year rate of 22%. Of the 35 local recurrences, 16 were in the breast only (the exact site within the breast was usually not specified), 3 occurred in the ipsilateral axilla only, 7 occurred in both the breast and axilla, and 9 arose in unspecified locations. The overall 15-year actuarial rate of local tumor control was 71%.

Two of the 35 patients who developed local recurrence had simultaneous distant relapse, and 3 patients refused further local treatment. Thirty of the 33 patients who developed an isolated local recurrence underwent secondary surgery (mastectomy in 28 patients) in the hope of cure. The actuarial rate of freedom from distant relapse after this event was 58% at 5 years and 50% at 10 years. The actuarial rate of freedom from distant relapse was examined in relation to the site of local recurrence (breast versus axilla), and to the interval from initial treatment to local recurrence. The value of these comparisons was limited by the small number of patients in each subgroup. However, no statistically significant difference in freedom from distant relapse was noted for the 16 patients who had recurrences only in the breast compared to that in the 10 patients who had recurrences in the axilla (50% versus 33%, $p = 0.31$). There was also no significant difference in distant relapse rates for the 16 patients with local recurrence occurring within 5 years of initial treatment compared to the 14 patients in whom local recurrence arose more than 5 years after initial treatment (43% versus 58%, $p = 0.35$).

The results of this study, which are similar to those from other studies with long-term follow-up, stress two major points. First, unlike with mastectomy, local recurrence after primary radiation therapy is not predominantly confined to the first 3 years after treatment. By the use of actuarial calculations, the risk of local recurrence has been shown to be fairly constant for at least 14 years. The other major point is that approximately 50% of patients with breast cancer in whom isolated local recurrence occurs after primary radiation therapy are apparently cured by secondary surgery. In contrast, patients with isolated local recurrence after undergoing mastectomy are rarely cured by further local treatment. In one study of 215 patients who were initially treated with mastectomy and who subsequently had isolated local recurrence treated with radiation therapy, the 5-year survival rate was 21% and the 10-year rate was 5%.[93] These findings are in contrast to the 58% and 50% rates of freedom from distant relapse at 5 and 10 years, respectively, noted for primary radiation therapy. In addition, the primary radiation therapy data suggest that patients with early and late local recurrences have a similar prognosis following secondary surgery. Taken together, these two points indicate that patients treated with primary radiation therapy require close follow-up for the detection of curable local recurrence, and that this follow-up is required for at least 10 to 15 years after treatment. A more comprehensive review of local recurrence after mastectomy and conservative surgery and radiotherapy is presented in Chapter 14.

Risk Factors for Local Recurrence

Type of Biopsy

Local recurrence appears to be more common among patients who undergo a less-than-excisional biopsy than among those treated with excisional biopsy. At the JCRT, the 5-year local recurrence rate was 7% following excisional biopsy and 31% following less-than-excisional biopsy ($p < 0.0001$). Similarly, Bedwinek and associates observed a local recurrence rate of 5% following excisional biopsy and a 20% rate following less-than-excisional biopsy.[96] All patients received the same radiotherapy, regardless of the type of biopsy. It is possible that increased radiation dose may compensate for a less extensive surgical procedure. Pierquin found that patients with T1 tumors treated with excision and 6900 cGy delivered to the primary site had a similar risk of local recurrence as did patients with T2 tumors who were treated with less-than-excisional biopsy and 8200 cGy delivered to the primary site (8% versus 7% at 10 years).[13] Amalric noted that, for patients with T1 tumors, the local recurrence rate at 10 years was 11.4% after excisional biopsy and 7500 cGy delivered to the primary site and 11.5% after less-than-excisional biopsy and a dose of 8000 cGy to the primary site.[34] However, for patients with T2 tumors, the local recurrence rate at 10 years was 12.7% after excisional biopsy and a dose of 7500 cGy compared to a rate of 35.1% after less-than-excisional biopsy and 8000 cGy.[34]

Tumor Size

Tumor size has not been shown to be a significant risk factor for local recurrence after excisional biopsy and radiotherapy. The results from the JCRT indicate that the 5-year local recurrence rates are similar for all tumor sizes up to 5 cm in diameter. In the NSABP B-06 trial, local recurrence at 5 years is similar for T1 and T2 tumors (6.5% versus 9.6%, respectively, p = NS). Local recurrence rates were also similar in a report from the Institut Gustave-Roussy, but the number of T2 tumors was limited. In the experience at that institution, 20 of 345 T1 tumors (6%) recurred, compared to 1 of 35 T2 tumors (3%).[15]

Axillary Node Status

The pathologic status of the axillary nodes has also not been shown to be an important factor in local recurrence. At the Institut Gustave-Roussy, local-regional recurrence was observed in 4% of patients with negative nodes and 7% of patients with positive nodes (p = NS).[15] These results were obtained in patients who did not receive adjuvant systemic therapy. In the Milan and NSABP B-06 trials, the local recurrence rate was, in fact, lower for node-positive patients treated with radiotherapy and adjuvant chemotherapy than for node-negative patients treated with radiotherapy alone. In the NSABP B-06 trial, the local recurrence rate at 5 years was 10% for patients with negative nodes and 2% for patients with positive nodes. In the Milan trial, the local recurrence rate was 4% for patients with negative nodes and 0% for patients with positive nodes.

Pathologic Features of the Primary Tumor

Investigators at the JCRT have studied the influence of the pathologic features noted in the excision specimen on the subsequent risk of local recurrence.[97,98] During the study period, the extent of surgical resection for the primary tumor was typically limited; in the large majority of patients, the tumor was excised grossly with a small rim of adjacent breast tissue but without regard to the microscopic margins of resection. The most recent report examines the risk of local recurrence in 356 patients with infiltrating duct cancer treated between 1968 and 1980 in whom there was sufficient adjacent breast tissue for pathologic review. Previous results from the same series emphasized that patients with significant intraductal carcinoma present in the tumor and in the adjacent tissue were at high risk for local recurrence. Patients were classified as having significant intraductal carcinoma in the primary tumor ("within +") if 25% or more of the tumor was intraductal. Patients were classified as having intraductal carcinoma in adjacent breast tissue ("adjacent +") if intraductal carcinoma was clearly noted to extend beyond the infiltrating margin of the tumor or if foci of intraductal carcinoma were noted in sections of grossly normal breast tissue.

Figure 10-32 shows the probability of local tumor control based on the presence of these two features. Patients with significant intraductal carcinoma in both the primary tumor and the adjacent breast tissue (considered to have "extensive intraductal involvement") had a 23% risk of local recurrence at 5 years compared to a risk of 0% for patients with significant intraductal carcinoma in the primary tumor alone, 3% for patients with intraductal

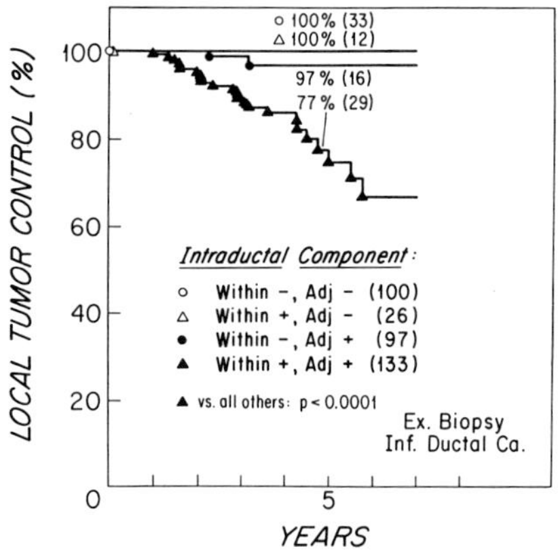

FIGURE 10-32. Data from the Joint Center for Radiation Therapy on local tumor control following excision and radiotherapy, as related to the presence of intraductal carcinoma within the tumor and in the adjacent breast tissue.

carcinoma in the adjacent tissue alone, and 0% for patients with neither feature ($p < 0.0001$). The risk of local recurrence for patients with extensive intraductal involvement was not related to the size of the primary tumor, the clinical or pathologic status of the axillary nodes, the nuclear grade, or the radiation dose delivered to the primary site. Patients with high nuclear grade and extensive intraductal involvement tended to manifest local recurrence sooner after treatment than did patients with low nuclear grade and extensive intraductal involvement. Patients with extensive intraductal involvement who received less than 6000 cGy to the primary site tended to fail directly at the site of the primary tumor, whereas patients who received a supplemental boost to the primary site to greater than 6000 cGy tended to fail at the edge of the boost. Patients with extensive intraductal involvement had the same risk of distant relapse as did patients without extensive intraductal involvement, suggesting that these features do not simply denote a more aggressive form of the disease.

The reason for the association of extensive intraductal involvement with a high risk of local recurrence is not obvious. Intraductal carcinoma in the presence of infiltrating carcinoma may represent either spread of tumor cells through the ductal system or a diffuse, premalignant condition. It is possible that the presence of extensive intraductal carcinoma may define a form of breast cancer that qualitatively responds less favorably to radiation than do the majority of cases. Alternatively, this combination of pathologic features may identify a form of breast cancer that differs quantitatively; that is, tumors with these features may have a greater residual tumor burden following gross excision than do other tumors. The fact that nearly all of the local recurrences in the group with extensive intraductal involvement represented failures to control the primary tumor (classified as either a true recurrence or a marginal miss) rather than the development of a new primary tumor elsewhere in the breast suggests that intraductal carcinoma in the presence of infiltrating carcinoma may represent local spread of the primary tumor. The pattern of failure presented here is consistent with the latter explanation. When patients with extensive intraductal carcinoma did not receive supplemental radiation to the primary site, there was a high rate of true recurrence (a local recurrence arising at the primary site). This implies that the dose delivered to the entire breast in these patients (4500 to 5000 cGy in 5 weeks) was insufficient to control the tumor burden at the primary site. When these patients received a supplemental dose of radiation to the primary site for a total dose of 6000 cGy or greater, true recurrences were virtually eliminated, but there was a high incidence of recurrence at the edge of the supplemental area (marginal miss). This suggests that, although the higher dose of radiation was sufficient to control the increased tumor burden at the primary site, the area of this increased tumor burden may have been greater than anticipated.

These results indicate that the presence of extensive intraductal carcinoma identifies a form of breast cancer that is prone to locally extensive intraductal spread. Since intraductal carcinoma is rarely associated with the fibrotic reaction commonly associated with infiltrating carcinoma, the breast often feels normal to the examining physician or to the operating surgeon, even when intraductal carcinoma is extensive. Thus, large numbers of tumor cells may remain within the ducts without being either visible or palpable after gross excision of the tumor mass.

In a further attempt to explain the increased local recurrence rate observed in patients with extensive intraductal carcinoma treated with gross excision and radiotherapy, an additional clinical and pathologic study was performed at the JCRT.[99] In this study, pathologic material from 72 patients seen between May of 1982 and September of 1984 and treated with gross excision of the primary tumor and a re-excision of the primary site was reviewed. Twenty-seven of these patients underwent re-excision because of extensive intraductal involvement in the excision specimen; the rest underwent re-excision because of close margins of resection. Patients with extensive intraductal involvement in the initial excision specimen were more likely to have residual cancer on re-excision than patients who did not exhibit this initial finding (88% versus 48%, $p = 0.002$). However, the likelihood of residual cancer was high in all groups. The amount of residual infiltrating cancer was similar, on average, for all groups, and was not large. In comparison, the amount of residual intraductal cancer was significantly greater, on average, for patients with extensive intraductal involvement noted in the initial excision specimen than for other patients. In addition, the likelihood of finding a considerable amount of residual intraductal cancer was 44% for patients with extensive intraductal involvement seen initially, compared to a likelihood of only 7% for other patients. For comparison, the 10-year risk of local recurrence was 35% for patients with extensive intraductal involvement treated with excision and radiotherapy and 8% for other patients treated identically. These results indicate that patients with extensive intraductal involvement noted in an initial excision specimen are more likely to have residual cancer on re-excision. They are also more likely to have more extensive residual cancer, which is typically intraductal in nature. These results support the concept that extensive intraductal involvement identifies a group of patients in which cancer spreads along associated ducts, and that the most likely explanation for the high local recurrence rate observed in patients with extensive intraductal involvement treated with gross excision and radiotherapy is their residual tumor burden following a simple gross excision of the tumor.

The importance of associated intraductal carcinoma as a risk factor for local recurrence has been examined in a series of patients from the Institut Gustave-Roussy[15] and in the Milan trial.* In neither series was the risk of local recurrence related to the intraductal component, but it should be noted that the initial surgical procedure was larger than a gross excision in both series. These results suggest that associated intraductal carcinoma is not an important risk factor for local recurrence when a more extensive resection of the primary is performed.

Other Risk Factors

Other pathologic features considered to be risk factors for local recurrence are Bloom grade and lymphatic involvement. At the Institut Gustave-Roussy, the local-regional recurrence rate was greater for patients with Bloom Grade III tumors (8 of 74, or 11%) than for those with Grade II tumors (11 of 170, or 6%) or Grade I tumors (1 of 139, or 1%) ($p < 0.001$).

The importance of involved margins of resection as a risk factor for local recurrence has not been well established. There are practical problems in assessing the importance of this factor. It is essential to ink the margins of resection in order to assess them for involvement. Moreover, there is no clear definition of involved margins; it can imply cancer that is present at an inked surface or cancer that lies within some arbitrary distance from an inked margin. It also depends on the number of sections assessed for involvement. The few studies that have examined this issue have not noted a significantly increased risk of local recurrence for patients with involved margins over that in other patients. In the experience of the Institut Gustave-Roussy, 24% of patients had involved margins and had a local-regional recurrence rate of 9% (8 of 88 patients) compared to a rate of 4% (12 of 274 patients) for those with uninvolved margins. Of note in this series is the fact that all patients received a boost to the primary site to 6000 cGy or greater. Similarly, Alpert and co-workers reported no increase in the risk of local recurrence for patients with involved margins.[100]

The age of patients also has not been clearly established as a risk factor for local recurrence. The experience from the Institut Curie in Paris suggests that patients who are 30 years old or younger have a higher risk of local

*Veronesi, U: personal communication.

recurrence than do older patients.[101] Local recurrence developed in 20% of the 35 patients who were 30 years old or younger but in only 4% of the 294 older patients ($p < 0.01$). This trend was also noted by Durand and co-workers, who found an 11% rate of local recurrence in patients 35 years of age or younger and a 1% rate in older patients.[102] Studies at the University of Pennsylvania and at the Institut Gustave-Roussy have both failed to show an increased risk of local recurrence for younger women.

A number of treatment factors have been studied for their impact on local recurrence. The extent of resection beyond excisional biopsy has not been identified as an important factor. At the Institut Gustave-Roussy, local-regional recurrence was seen in 4 of 47 patients (9%) treated with quadrantectomy compared to 20 of 389 patients (5%) treated with excisional biopsy. Similarly, Chu and colleagues did not find an advantage to quadrantectomy over excisional biopsy for patients treated with radiotherapy, including a boost to the primary site.[103] It is important to note, however, that the crude recurrence rate of 2% (8 of 352 patients) at 9 years observed in patients treated with quadrantectomy in the Milan trial is the best reported result for patients with T1 tumors. As noted above, the results seen at the JCRT suggest that the optimal extent of resection may depend on the extent of associated intraductal carcinoma. Patients without extensive intraductal involvement are adequately treated with excisional biopsy, whereas patients with extensive intraductal involvement require wide resection.

The impact of time-dose factors of radiotherapy on the risk of developing local recurrence has been discussed in a number of studies. Kurtz and co-workers found that local recurrence was greater when a dose of 800 cGy or less per week was administered than when a dose of greater than 800 cGy was given.[104] At the Royal Marsden Hospital, a high rate of local recurrence was also noted to be associated with a weekly dose of 800 cGy or less.[105] At the Institut Gustave-Roussy, local-regional recurrence occurred in 14 of 164 patients (9%) when treatment was protracted compared to 10 of 269 patients (4%) when the treatment period was shorter ($p < 0.05$).

The importance of a boost to the primary site as a risk factor has not clearly been determined. The utility of a boost must be considered in relation to the extent of surgical resection. It is likely that a boost is more important after excisional biopsy than after quadrantectomy. The major impetus for not using a boost as a standard part of treatment lies in the results obtained in the NSABP B-06 trial in which no boost was used. In this trial, a 5-year risk of a breast relapse after excision and radiotherapy of 8% was observed, which is comparable to the results obtained at other institutions when a boost was employed. However, the 3-year median follow-up time in the NSABP trial may not be adequate to assess fully the risk of local recurrence. Furthermore, the absence of tissue compensators in the NSABP trial may have resulted in an increased inhomogeneity of radiation dose and a relatively greater effective dose delivered to the tumor site.

The Role of Surgical and Radiotherapeutic Technique in Assessing the Risk of Local Recurrence

In discussing possible risk factors for local recurrence after conservative surgery and radiotherapy, it is important to interpret results in light of the techniques of surgery and radiotherapy employed. Risk factors for local recurrence seen at one institution may not apply to another institution if significantly different techniques are employed.

Techniques of Radiotherapy at the Joint Center for Radiation Therapy

BREAST AND REGIONAL LYMPH NODES. Any technique used for primary radiation therapy must:

- Minimize the doses given to the lung and heart
- Adequately cover the volume(s) at risk
- Avoid overlapping of fields ("hot spots"), which may cause complications, or underlapping of fields ("cold spots"), which may result in recurrences
- Be reproducible from treatment to treatment
- Deliver a homogeneous dose throughout the target volume

To achieve these goals, the following must be used:

- Table rotation, gantry rotation, and beam blocks to match fields together at the junction of the en face supraclavicular/axillary field and breast tangents and to match the posterior edges of the tangents, thereby minimizing lung dose
- Wedges in the beam to compensate for the contour of the breast
- Radionuclide lymphoscintigraphy to localize the internal mammary lymph nodes (if they are to be treated)
- Inclusion of the lower IMNs in the tangential fields, since the use of a "hockey stick" greatly increases the lung volume and, if left-sided, the heart volume treated. (The upper IMNs are included in the supraclavicular field.)

Since 1977, the JCRT has used the "hanging block" technique to achieve these goals; for more technical descriptions, refer to the report by Svensson and colleagues.[106] The hanging block technique will eventually be replaced by the "corner block" technique,[107] but the geometry of the two techniques is the same. The corner-block technique is shown in Figure 10-33. The match line is set up and checked for accuracy by the use of a beam alignment device described elsewhere.[108]

BREAST TANGENTS. The minimum tumor dose in the tangent fields is prescribed at a point 1.5 cm from the midpoint of the deep intersection of the tangential fields. The dose is normalized to 100% at this point. The maximum dose should be adjusted, with the use of wedges, to below 110% to 115%, while ensuring that the remainder of the volume has as homogeneous a dose as possible.

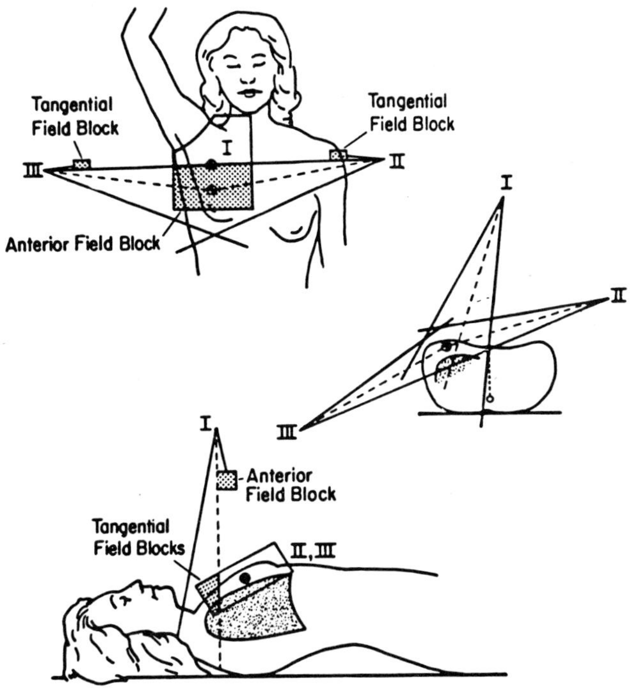

FIGURE 10-33. Set-up geometry of the treatment technique in the coronal, transverse, and sagittal planes. The treatment fields as indicated on the diagram are (I) anterior, (II) medial tangential, and (III) lateral tangential. The half-beam block of the anterior field and the corner blocks of the tangential fields are shown by the labeled, shaded areas in the coronal and sagittal views. (Adapted from Svensson GK et al: Int J Radiat Oncol Biol Phys 6:689, 1980)

Most patients are treated on a 4-MV or 6-MV linear accelerator, although some patients with large breasts are better treated on the 8-MV machine. (In this situation, it may be necessary in some patients to apply bolus to the lumpectomy site intermittently in order to increase skin dose. In general, it is undesirable cosmetically and unneeded in terms of tumor control to give the skin the full dose of radiation.)

The entire breast is ordinarily included in the tangential fields. The borders of the fields are as follows:

Inferior—A 1-cm margin is given inferior to the inframammary fold.

Superior—The margin of the breast is determined by palpation, and is given a 1-cm margin. When a three-field technique is used, the placement of the match line will depend on the location of the primary tumor and breast, but will usually be at about the second intercostal space (usually at the inferior edge of the sternoclavicular junction radiographically).

Lateral—The lateral exit of the tangents is placed in such a way as to include all breast tissue with a 1-cm margin, which usually places it at the mid-axillary line.

Medial—If the internal mammary nodes are *not* to be treated, then the medial exit of the tangents will be at the midline. If the internal mammary nodes *are* to be included, then the medial border is either set by lymphoscintigraphy or placed 3 cm across midline.

Anterior—A 2-cm margin of light is given above the highest point of the breast.

Posterior—The edges of the tangents should be coincident; the medial and lateral borders determine their exact position.

Occasionally, a substantial part of the superior portion of the breast will be in the supraclavicular/axillary field; in such cases, especially with primary tumors of the upper quadrant, careful attention to the adequacy of the match between fields is necessary. It is preferable *not* to place the match line through the primary surgical scar. The use of netting to compress and position the breast in patients with larger breasts is often helpful in reducing the volume of normal tissue that would otherwise be treated and in allowing reproducible set-up and dosimetry.

REGIONAL LYMPH NODES. Treatment of the regional lymph nodes is as follows. In the *full axillary/supraclavicular en face field,* treatment with a daily dose, prescribed at a depth of 5 cm, is used. No bolus is used. The field is angled approximately 10 degrees from the vertical to avoid treating the cervical spinal cord; a small block (running along the outer edges of the pedicles) may also be needed for this field. The borders of the field are as follows:

Inferior—This border is determined by the match line, usually at the second intercostal space (see the description of the borders of the breast tangents, above).

Superior—Radiologically, this is usually the most superior aspect of the first rib. Except in unusual situations, it is preferable not to clear skin (or "flash") in the supraclavicular region.

Lateral—This border is usually two-thirds of the medial to lateral distance through the humeral head; most of the humeral head should be blocked. In some patients with very extensive axillary disease, it may be necessary to clear skin (and also treat AP-PA).

Medial—This set-up is started at the center of the suprasternal notch (the midline), and the gantry is then angled as noted.

The *medial supraclavicular en face field* involves treatment of the axillary apex, upper internal mammary, and supraclavicular lymph nodes (e.g., in the case of a medial primary tumor and adequate, positive, limited, axillary dissection) without treating all of the axillary nodes. The lateral border of the field is stopped at the coracoid process rather than at the humeral head, and the dose is prescribed at a depth of 3 cm. The lower internal mammary lymph nodes will usually be included in the tangential fields when treated, as discussed above. The use of radionuclide lymphoscintigraphy is strongly encouraged to minimize the amount of lung and heart treated, and to ensure adequate coverage of the internal mammary nodes.

BREAST BOOST TECHNIQUES. A boost dose, intended to deliver to the primary site a higher dose than can cosmetically be tolerated by the entire breast, is used to minimize the likelihood of a recurrence at the primary site. This may be done in several ways, depending on the size of the breast, the location and size of the primary tumor, the available equipment, and the personal preference and experience of the radiotherapist. Interstitial implant or electron beam boosts are used in almost all patients. The preoperative description of the lesion, mammography, and operative notes may be helpful in selecting the boost technique.

IMPLANTS. Implants are preferred when the depth to the chest wall from the skin surface in the region to be boosted is greater than 3.5 cm to 4 cm (that is, the depth at which the skin dose from an electron beam becomes excessive). This depth is typically determined by ultrasonography.

A typical implant covers an area 6 cm to 7 cm wide, using two or more planes of needles, with a separation between planes of approximately 1.5 cm. The exact shape will depend on the location of the implant. The needles should encompass the entire target volume in length and width, which ordinarily includes the entire surgical scar. The depth of the implant in the breast and its thickness depend on the original size and depth of the primary tumor and on the size of the breast.

At the JCRT, implants are performed using plastic-coated, platinum-filtered, iridium-192 wire that has been divided into seeds 0.6 cm in length, with a 0.4-cm separation between seeds. Implants should be loaded so that the outermost seed is 0.5 cm to 1.0 cm from the skin surface.

The maximum inhomogeneity of an implant varies with geometry and loading. It is desirable to keep the maximum dose to a level that is less than about twice the minimum target dose; this may sometimes be accomplished by loading the center strands with "colder" sources.

Usually, an implant may be performed using local anesthesia and sedation (usually intravenous diazepam). General anesthesia may be preferable in patients undergoing large-volume implants. An anesthesiologist should be available to administer general anesthesia and intubation if the patient does not tolerate more limited anesthesia.

ELECTRONS. A typical electron beam field is a circle or square that is 6 cm to 8 cm in diameter, defined by lead cut-out or by collimators (with appropriate attention to fall-off at the field edges). Fields may also be rectangular or elliptical. The JCRT technique uses 3-MeV to 11-MeV electrons (depending on thickness), and the dose is prescribed at the 80% isodose depth on the central axis. Energies exceeding 11 MeV will deliver an excessive dose to the skin and may compromise the cosmetic result. The volume covered is, in principle, the same as if an implant were used.

Breast ultrasonography may be helpful in determining whether the patient is a suitable candidate for electron boost, as well as what level of energy to use. This study should be performed with the patient in the proposed treatment position, with the field borders outlined on skin.

It may be helpful to flatten the breast by manipulating its position, exerting pressure from a lead cut-out, or taping. However, care must be taken not to move the target volume out of the field.

Set-up of electron fields is most reproducible when accomplished with the aid of a set-up photograph and a clear film template on which the field borders are drawn and landmarks and tattoos are noted. Once treatment begins, the area may be inked on the skin.

PHOTONS. In some circumstances, an external beam boost (such as an en face or three-field anterior plus wedged pair) may or must be used. One must try, however, to minimize exit dose to the underlying lung (e.g., by angling of an en face field). Also, the breast tissue outside the desired boost area will likely receive a higher dose with external beam boosts than with electron or implant boosts, and this may adversely affect the cosmetic results. A plan that decreases irradiation outside the boost volume should, therefore, be chosen. Occasionally, photons and electrons may be combined, but this practice may be associated with problems of dosimetry and complications of set-up and reproducibility that require careful attention by the radiotherapist and technologist.

AXILLARY BOOST TECHNIQUES. Occasionally, it is necessary to administer a dose exceeding 4600 cGy to the axilla. The en face supraclavicular/axillary field has a relatively high inhomogeneity, and delivers a substantial dose to the pectoralis major muscle. Administering too high a dose through this en face field may result in excessive and symptomatic fibrosis of this muscle and telangiectasia and atrophy of the overlying skin. Hence, an axillary boost technique should be used for a portion of the treatment. (In patients with gross residual adenopathy, or in those in whom homogeneity of dose is of special concern, consideration should be given to using opposed AP-PA fields for the entire treatment.)

EN FACE AXILLARY BOOST. For delivery of an en face axillary boost, the patient is positioned as usual, and the couch, gantry, and collimator are angled to direct the beam from the axilla towards the supraclavicular nodes. The anterior edge of the field should be posterior to the posterior edge of the pectoralis major muscle, documented by palpation and visually. The dose is usually prescribed at a depth of 5 cm, although this may vary from case to case. Either photons or high-energy electrons may be used, although the skin dose delivered is higher with electrons.

POSTERIOR AXILLARY BOOST. Posterior axillary boosts have the disadvantages of traversing a greater area of normal tissue than do en face axillary boosts and of delivering an additional (though limited) dose to the pectoralis major muscle. However, set-up and reproducibility are easier with this method than with the en face axillary boost. The superior border parallels the clavicle, the inferior border is blocked to match the tangents, the medial border is about 2 cm into the lung from the chest wall, and the lateral border is at the middle of the humeral head. The dose is prescribed from the posterior surface to a depth of the separation minus 5 cm.

The axillary/supraclavicular field should not be treated unless one of the following applies:

There is extensive nodal involvement (e.g., > 50% of the number of nodes removed).
Significant extracapsular extension is present.
Axillary sampling is inadequate technically.
Gross residual disease is noted.
Axillary dissection is not performed, and the potential morbidity of treatment is acceptable.

Because of an already substantial risk of arm edema, the guidelines to irradiation of the axilla, presented above, may have to be modified in patients undergoing full axillary dissection. Therefore, it is critical that the radiotherapist be aware of the extent of axillary surgery, particularly whether the axillary vein was stripped, before deciding whether to treat the full axillary field.

TREATMENT OF THE INTERNAL MAMMARY LYMPH NODES. As with treatment of the axilla, the desirability of treating the internal mammary nodes with radiation is controversial, with various positions being strongly upheld at different institutions (e.g., the NSABP approach versus that advocated by those at M.D. Anderson Hospital). There is little evidence that treatment of the internal mammary nodes with extended radical mastectomy or preoperative or postoperative irradiation increases survival, and although parasternal recurrences are by no means unknown, clinically, they occur much less often than one would predict, based on the frequency of pathologic involvement of the internal mammary nodes. However, there might well be small sets of patients in whom control of nodal disease will make the difference between cure and further dissemination of disease. (Patients with positive axillary nodes who are treated only with radical mastectomy, not all of whom succumb to systemic metastases, may belong to this category.) Another argument in favor of treating the internal mammary nodes applies to patients who will undergo adjuvant systemic therapy; the full benefit of adjuvant treatment may only be realized when there is maximum local-regional control.

The main toxic potential of irradiation of the internal mammary nodes (which may be enhanced by chemotherapy) is directed at the heart and lungs. The volume of lung irradiated is increased by the use of the supraclavicular field, and the volume of heart (for left-sided primary tumors only) irradiated is increased by moving the medial border of the tangents further over the midline. In addition, the potential problems arising from the matching of fields must be considered. At present, the risks of irradiation to the internal mammary nodes appear to be small, but there is no consensus regarding the indications for their treatment.

Radionuclide lymphoscintigraphy has not yet been shown to have sufficient resolution and reliability to be used to select patients for internal mammary node irradiation. However, a "positive" finding on lymphoscintigraphy should be among the factors considered in making such a decision. Because of the above considerations, treatment of the internal mammary nodes is never mandatory, but may be advantageous in selected patients. At present, reasonable guidelines dictate that the internal mammary nodes *not* be treated when:

Axillary dissection is negative.
The patient's age or medical condition makes the potential side effects of internal mammary node treatment particularly hazardous.
The volume of lung or heart that would have to be treated is greater than usual.

The internal mammary nodes *may* be treated when:

The axillary nodes are pathologically positive (especially in patients with four or more positive nodes).
The primary tumor is in a medial quadrant (especially when the axillary nodes are positive, but also, in some cases, when they are negative).
Axillary dissection is not performed, and the patient is otherwise suitable for internal mammary node treatment.

When the internal mammary nodes are treated, one should use either a medial supraclavicular or full supraclavicular/axillary field to ensure adequate treatment of the internal mammary nodes in the first and second intercostal spaces, which are usually not fully included in the tangent field. The use of a "hockey stick" is strongly discouraged; if it must be employed, then it is better to use it for only a portion of the entire treatment.

TREATMENT OF THE SUPRACLAVICULAR LYMPH NODES. Even microscopic involvement of the supraclavicular lymph nodes almost certainly reflects a high likelihood of systemic disease; their treatment, therefore, is unlikely to affect survival. Thus, treatment of the supraclavicular lymph nodes is never absolutely indicated. However, in any situation in which the upper internal mammary nodes or full axillary region is to be treated, an en face field will be needed for therapy, and the supraclavicular nodes should be included in this field since no added morbidity is expected.

RECOMMENDED MINIMUM TUMOR DOSES. The following doses are based upon JCRT treatment techniques, and may not be directly equivalent to doses from other institutions. In general, complete information regarding techniques and sample isodose curves and prescription points must be known before such comparisons may be made.

WHOLE-BREAST TREATMENT. The purpose of treating the breast outside the immediate vicinity of the primary region is to destroy subclinical foci of carcinoma. The dose tolerated by the entire breast is compatible with this purpose in the great majority of patients.[35] Whether modestly higher doses (5000 cGy) are desirable in certain settings (e.g., in patients with large postoperative hematomas or infiltrating lobular histology) is not known.

Recommended treatment doses are as follows:

Most patients: 4500 cGy in 25 fractions in 5 weeks or 4600 cGy in 23 fractions in 4.6 weeks
Patients with large breasts or separations: 4500 cGy in 25 fractions in 5 weeks
Patients in whom chemotherapy has been administered or is planned: 4500 cGy in 25 fractions in 5 weeks

BREAST BOOST. As discussed above, the role of the boost is related to the extent of surgical resection. Hence, occasionally, there may be patients in whom the boost dose may be reduced or even eliminated (e.g., in those undergoing quadrantectomy or with extremely wide and histologically negative margins and small primary tumors). However this decision must be carefully weighed against the known effectiveness of doses exceeding 6000 cGy in reducing the incidence of true recurrences as compared to the effectiveness of doses less than 6000 cGy.* Occasionally, it may be desirable to increase the boost dose modestly (e.g., in patients with known positive margins).

Recommended doses for breast boosts are as follows:

Implants: 1800 cGy, usually at 40 cGy to 50 cGy per hour
Electrons: 1600 cGy, at 200 cGy per fraction (prescribed at the 80% isodose depth)
Photons: 1000 cGy to 1600 cGy at 200 cGy per fraction
TOTAL DOSE TO SITE OF THE PRIMARY TUMOR: 6100 cGy to 6300 cGy

INTERNAL MAMMARY NODES. If treated, the internal mammary node should be included in tangent fields with the entire breast (lower nodes) and in the en face supraclavicular/axillary fièld (upper nodes).

AXILLARY LYMPH NODES. If treated, the axillary lymph nodes should receive 4500 cGy to 4600 cGy in 23 to 25 fractions over a period of 4.6 to 5 weeks in most cases. When extracapsular disease is present, axillary nodes should be boosted to a total dose of 5000 cGy to 5400 cGy. For gross residual disease, a boost to a total dose not exceeding 5600 cGy should be used. One could consider using AP-PA fields from the start of treatment.

*Joint Center for Radiation Therapy: unpublished data.

FOLLOW-UP

Physical Examination

Careful examination of both breasts and the regional lymph nodes should be performed at 4- to 6-month intervals. It is preferable for a patient to be followed by all specialists participating in her care. Because the risk of a breast recurrence or a new contralateral primary tumor persists indefinitely, the patient should undergo follow-up for life. Eventually, the initial follow-up schedule may need to be modified because of the patient's desires or logistics. If the patient moves to another area, her follow-up care should be undertaken by physicians who are familiar with both primary radiotherapy and the changes that may result in the treated breast.

Mammography

The optimal interval between follow-up mammographic studies has not been established, although a 12-month interval appears to be reasonable for most patients. The initial post-treatment mammograms should be obtained 4 to 8 months following completion of treatment, by which time acute changes attributable to irradiation will have subsided completely. Because of postradiation changes, the mammograms should preferably be reviewed by a radiologist with a special interest and competence in mammography. Comparison to previous mammograms is also often vital in correct interpretation. Film-screen mammography with modern equipment and good technique is usually preferable to xeromammography.

Laboratory Tests

Routinely ordered laboratory tests (e.g., chest radiographs, complete blood counts, liver chemistries, carcinoembryonic antigen studies, bone scans, or liver scans) are not indicated unless the patient has symptoms or signs suggestive of a potential recurrence. These tests may also be ordered in patients enrolled in a formal protocol requiring such evaluative measures.

Breast Biopsy

Biopsy of the irradiated breast is indicated when physical or mammographic changes are noted which, in the view of an experienced observer, are not clearly secondary to irradiation and surgery. Although changes secondary to irradiation are usually minor, some may be difficult or impossible to distinguish from recurrence without the aid of biopsy. Biopsy of the irradiated breast is not likely to be followed by cosmetic or other complications;[109] hence, when doubt exists, it is usually prudent to perform a biopsy.

Moderately sized open biopsy (1 cc to 20 cc) appears

to be safe and accurate for this purpose. Smaller biopsies and needle biopsies may have a substantial false-negative rate (a rate of 14% at the JCRT), whereas larger biopsies are much more prone to lead to problems of healing, infection, and cosmesis.

WORKSHOP REPORT

Because of the increased use of conservative surgery and radiotherapy (in the face of uncertainty regarding the optimal technique of treatment), a workshop devoted to the technique of conservative surgery and radiotherapy for early breast cancer was held in New York City in June of 1985. The workshop faculty included 24 invited experts. The purpose of the workshop was three-fold:

1. To define more precisely the terms for the various types of surgical procedures used
2. To identify important considerations in the selection of patients for this treatment
3. To identify areas of agreement and disagreement regarding the techniques of surgery and radiotherapy

The report of this workshop was published in 1985.[110] The following sections summarize the content of the workshop and indicate the consensus reached on the issues primarily related to radiotherapy. As such, they may not precisely reflect the views of every faculty member on each of the points discussed. The consensus developed on the surgical aspects of the treatment is presented in the section on surgery at the beginning of this chapter.

Patient Selection

The major criterion for patient selection is the feasibility of adequately resecting the primary tumor without major cosmetic deformity. Patients with two widely separated primary tumors in the same breast, demonstrated either clinically or mammographically, are considered to be poor candidates for breast-conserving treatment. Patients whose mammograms reveal diffuse (i.e., affecting multiple quadrants), clustered microcalcifications that are shown to be malignant on histologic examination also should not be treated with a breast-conserving approach. Furthermore, the treatment of any patient with diffuse, clustered microcalcifications, even if they are not proven to be malignant, is of concern since subsequent mammographic follow-up of these patients may be extremely difficult. High-quality mammograms are essential in the consideration of a patient for conservative surgery and radiotherapy, both in terms of identifying other possible primary lesions in the same breast and in delineating further the extent of the palpable primary tumor.

The question of location as a factor in the selection of patients for conservative surgery and radiation therapy principally centers on patients with tumors directly under the nipple-areolar complex. In such patients, an adequate resection of the primary lesion might entail a resection of the nipple-areolar complex, but this type of resection may be preferable to mastectomy. Furthermore, reconstruction of the nipple-areolar complex may be accomplished following radiotherapy. Similarly, in patients with a primary lesion of the breast associated with Paget's disease, resection of the involved portion of the nipple and areola, in conjunction with resection of the primary tumor and followed by radiotherapy, is considered to be a reasonable treatment approach.

A number of other factors are viewed as relative contraindications to breast-conserving treatment and should be considered jointly by the surgeon and radiotherapist before definitive treatment is initiated. Among these factors are the patient's age, the size of the breast, and the size of the tumor. Treatment with radiotherapy may be more difficult in older patients, in patients with very large or pendulous breasts, and in those with primary tumors that are larger than 4 cm in diameter.

Radiotherapy of the Primary Tumor

The extent of surgery and the radiation dose required for local tumor control are complementary; the more extensive the surgical procedure, the lesser the amount of irradiation that will be required for tumor control. The entire breast should be treated with 180 cGy to 200 cGy per day, up to a total dose of 4500 cGy to 5000 cGy. Doses exceeding 5000 cGy to the entire breast commonly result in an unacceptable degree of fibrosis and retraction and should, therefore, be avoided. Controversy persists regarding the need for supplementary irradiation (a boost dose) to the primary site, and, if used, the preferred technique and dose. Most published series on the use of conservative surgery and radiotherapy have incorporated a boost. The use of a boost should depend on the extent of the initial surgical procedure. In patients treated with a local or wide excision in whom the margins of resection are close, a boost is recommended. In patients treated with wide excision with clearly negative margins, or in those treated with quadrantectomy, the value of a boost is less certain. Since the merit of administering a boost in these patients is somewhat uncertain, it should be stressed that the technique and dose of the boost used should not significantly diminish the cosmetic result.

Radiotherapy of the Regional Lymph Nodes

The radiotherapist should be aware of the extent of the axillary dissection performed, and should plan the radiotherapy treatment accordingly. Because irradiation of the dissected portion of the axilla is associated with a significant risk of arm edema, it should be avoided. In patients with a primary lesion located in the lateral portion of the breast and negative axillary nodes confirmed on dissection, the use of tangential fields to the breast alone is clearly favored. The major area of controversy relates to irradiation of the internal mammary and supraclavicular nodes in patients with positive nodes confirmed on dissection or in those with medial breast lesions. These patients are known to be at significant risk for subclinical involvement in these nodal areas, and some radiotherapists favor irradiation of these areas to prevent tumor recurrence. Significant technical requirements must be met in order to treat these areas without complication. The available information, however, does not indicate that such treatment improves the chances for cure. The results seen in both randomized trials comparing mastectomy to conservative surgery and radiotherapy were achieved using radiotherapy of the breast alone, even in patients with positive nodes. Treatment of the breast alone is acceptable in all situations, but it is reasonable to treat the internal mammary and supraclavicular areas in patients with positive nodes or with medially-placed lesions, provided it can be done safely.

Presently, there are important questions and concerns but little firm data on which to base the practice of integrating adjuvant chemotherapy and radiotherapy in patients with positive nodes. Concerns have been raised regarding both delays in the initiation of either chemotherapy or radiation and the concomitant use of these modalities. Additional studies are required for clarification of these issues.

REFERENCES

1. Bartelink H, Van Dam F, Van Dongen J: Psychological effects of breast-conserving therapy in comparison with radical mastectomy. Int J Radiat Oncol Biol Phys 11:381, 1985
2. Morris T, Greer H, White P: Psychological and social adjustment to mastectomy: A two-year follow-up study. Cancer 40:2381, 1977
3. Jameson K, Wellisch B, Pasnau R; Psychosocial aspects of mastectomy. Am J Psychiatry 135:432, 1978
4. Keynes GL: Conservative treatment of cancer of the breast. Br Med J 2:643, 1937
5. Williams IG, Murley RS, Curwen MD: Carcinoma of the female breast: Conservative surgery and radical surgery. Br Med J, p 787, Oct 10, 1953
6. Peters MV: Cutting the "Gordian knot" in early breast cancer. Ann R Coll Phys Surg Can 8:186, 1975
7. Rissanen PM: A comparison of conservative and radical surgery combined with radiotherapy in the treatment of stage I carcinoma of the breast. Br J Radiol 42:423, 1969
8. Rissanen PM, Holsti P: Vergleich zwischen konservatier und radikaler chirugie, kombiniert mit strahlentherapie bei der behandlung des brustkrebses im stadium I. Strahlentherapie 147:370, 1974
9. Atkins H, Hayward JL, Klugman DJ, et al: Treatment of early breast cancer: A report after 10 years of a clinical trial. Br Med J 2:423, 1972
10. Hayward JL: The Guy's Hospital trials of treatments of "early" breast cancer. World J Surg 1:314, 1977
11. Hayward JL: The Guy's Hospital trials on breast conservation. In Harris JR. Hellman S, Silen W (eds): Conservative Management of Breast Cancer, pp 77–90. Philadelphia, JB Lippincott, 1983
12. Calle R, Vilcoq JR, Pilleron JP, et al: Conservative treatment of operable breast carcinoma by irradiation with or without limited surgery—Ten-year results. In Harris JR, Hellman S, Silen W (eds): Conservative Management of Breast Cancer, pp 3–9. Philadelphia, JB Lippincott, 1983
13. Pierquin B: Conservative treatment for carcinoma of the breast. Experience of Creteil—Ten-year results. In Harris JR, Hellman S, Silen W (eds): Conservative Management of Breast Cancer, pp 11–14. Philadelphia, JB Lippincott, 1983
14. Pierquin B, Owen R, Maylin C, et al: Radical radiation therapy of breast cancer. Int J Radiat Oncol Biol Phys 6:17, 1980
15. Clarke DH, Le MG, Sarrazin D, et al: Analysis of local-regional relapses in patients with early breast cancer treated by excision and radiotherapy: Experience of the Institut Gustave Roussy. Int J Radiat Oncol Biol Phys 11:137, 1985
16. Montague ED, Ames FC, Schell SR, et al: Conservative surgery and irradiation as an alternative to mastectomy in the treatment of clinically favorable breast cancer. Cancer 54:2668, 1984
17. Clark RM: Alternatives to mastectomy—The Princess Margaret Hospital experience. In Harris JR, Hellman S, Silen W (eds): Conservative Management of Breast Cancer, pp 35–46. Philadelphia, JB Lippincott, 1983
18. Recht A, Connolly JL, Schnitt SJ, et al: Conservative surgery and primary radiation therapy for early breast cancer: Results, controversies, and unresolved problems. Semin Oncol (in press)
19. Veronesi U: Randomized trials comparing conservation techniques with conventional surgery: An overview. In Tobias JS, Peckham MJ (eds): Primary Management of Breast Cancer: Alternatives to Mastectomy Management of Malignant Disease Series, pp 131–152. London, E. Arnold, 1985
20. Fisher B, Bauer M, Margolese R, et al: Five-year results of a randomized clinical trial comparing total mastectomy and segmental mastectomy with or without radiation in the treatment of breast cancer. N Engl J Med 312:665, 1985
21. Clark RM, Wilkinson RH, Mahoney LJ, et al: Breast cancer: A 21-year experience with conservative surgery and radiation. Int J Radiat Oncol Biol Phys 8: 967, 1982
22. Montgomery AC, Greening WP, Levene AL: J R Soc Med 71:339, 1978
23. Tagart REB: Partial mastectomy for breast cancer. Br Med J 2:1268, 1978
24. Freeman CR, Belliveau NJ, Kim TH, et al: Limited surgery with or without radiotherapy for early breast carcinoma. J Can Assoc Radiol 32:125, 1981
25. Lagios MD, Richards VE, Rose M, et al: Segmental mastectomy with radiotherapy: Short-term follow-up. Cancer 52:2173, 1983
26. Sarrazin D, Le M, Rouesse J, et al: Conservative treatment versus mastectomy in breast cancer tumors with microscopic diameter of 20 mm or less. Cancer 53:1209, 1984
27. Findlay P, Lippman M, Danforth D, et al: A randomized trial comparing mastectomy to radiotherapy in the treatment of stage I-II breast cancer. Proc Am Soc Clin Oncol 4:60, 1985
28. Recht A, Silver B, Schnitt S, et al: Breast relapse following primary radiation therapy for early breast cancer. I: Classification, frequency, and salvage. Int J Radiat Oncol Biol Phys 11:1271, 1985
29. Fisher ER, Gregorio R, Redmond C, et al: Pathologic findings from the NSABP (Protocol No. 4). Cancer 35:247, 1975
30. Gallagher HS: Multicentricity in breast cancer. In Harris JR, Hellman S, Silen W (eds): Conservative Management of

Breast Cancer, pp 117–122. Philadelphia, JB Lippincott, 1983
31. Rosen PP, Fracchia AA, Urban JA, et al: "Residual" mammary carcinoma following simulated partial mastectomy. Cancer 35:739, 1975
32. Urban JA: Bilaterality of cancer of the breast: Biopsy of the opposite breast. Cancer 20:1867, 1967
33. Alpers CE, Wellings SR: The prevalence of carcinoma in situ in normal and cancer associated breasts. Hum Pathol 16:796, 1985
34. Amalric R, Santamaria F, Robert F, et al: In Harris JR, Hellman S, Silen W (eds): Conservative Management of Breast Cancer, pp 15–22. Philadelphia, JB Lippincott, 1983
35. Harris JR, Levene MB, Svensson G, et al: Analysis of cosmetic results following primary radiation therapy for stages I and II carcinoma of the breast. Int J Radiat Oncol Biol Phys 5:257, 1979
36. Beadle G, Silver B, Botnick L, et al: Cosmetic results following primary radiation therapy for early breast carcinoma. Cancer 54:2911, 1984
37. Clarke D, Martinez A, Cox RS, et al: Breast edema following staging axillary node dissection in patients with breast cancer treated by radical radiotherapy. Cancer 49:2295, 1982
38. Beadle GF, Come S, Henderson IC, et al: The effect of adjuvant chemotherapy on the cosmetic results after primary radiation treatment for early breast cancer: A preliminary analysis. Int J Radiat Oncol Biol Phys 10:2131, 1984
39. Ray GR, Fish VJ, Marmor JB, et al: Impact of adjuvant chemotherapy on cosmesis and complications in stages I and II carcinoma of the breast treated by biopsy and radiation therapy. Int J Radiat Oncol Biol Phys 10:837, 1984
40. Boice JD Jr, Land CE, Shore RE, et al: Risk of breast cancer following low-dose radiation exposure. Radiology 131:589, 1979
41. Baral E, Larsson LE, Mattson B: Breast cancer following irradiation of the breast. Cancer 40:2905, 1977
42. Fraass BA, Roberson PL, Lichter AS: Dose to the contralateral breast due to primary breast irradiation. Int J Radiat Oncol Biol Phys 11:485, 1985
43. Boice JD Jr, Monson RR: Breast cancer in women after repeated fluoroscopic examinations of the chest. J Natl Cancer Instit 59:823, 1977
44. McCredie JA, Inch WR, Alderson M: Consecutive primary carcinomas of the breast. Cancer 35:1472, 1975
45. Schell SR, Montague ED, Spanos WJ, et al: Bilateral breast cancer in patients with initial stage I and II disease. Cancer 50:1191, 1982
46. Huvos AG, Woodard HQ, Cahan WG, et al: Postradiation osteogenic sarcoma of bone and soft tissues. A clinicopathologic study of 66 patients. Cancer 55:1244, 1985
47. Kim JH, Chu FC, Woodard HQ, et al: Radiation-induced soft tissue and bone sarcoma. Radiology 129:501, 1978
48. Smith PG, Dole R: Age and time dependent changes in the rates of radiation-induced cancers in patients with ankylosing spondylitis. In International Atomic Energy Agency: Late Biological Effects of Ionizing Radiation, Vol 1, pp 203–218. Vienna, International Atomic Energy Agency, 1978
49. Alderson MR, Jackson SM: Long-term follow-up of patients with menorrhagia treated by irradiation. Br J Radiol 44:295, 1971
50. Brinkley D, Haybittle JL: The late effects of artificial menopause by x-radiation. Br J Radiol 42:519, 1969
51. Doll R, Smith PG: The long-term effects of x-irradiation in patients treated for metropathia hemorrhagica. Br J Radiol 41:362, 1968
52. Boice JD Jr, Hutchinson GB: Leukemia in women following radiotherapy for cervical cancer: Ten-year follow-up of an international study. J Natl Cancer Instit 65:115, 1980
53. Simon N, Brucer M, Hayes R: Radiation and leukemia in carcinoma of the cervix. Radiology 74:905, 1960
54. Zippin C, Bailer JC, Hohn HI, et al: Radiation therapy for cervical cancer: Late effects on life span and on leukemia incidence. Cancer 28:937, 1971
55. Fisher B, Rockette H, Fisher E, et al: Leukemia in breast cancer patients following adjuvant chemotherapy or postoperative radiation: The NSABP experience. J Clin Oncol 3:1640, 1985
56. Bretton RC, Nelson PA: Causes and treatment of postmastectomy lymphedema of the arm. JAMA 180:95, 1962
57. Swedborg I, Wallgren A: The effect of pre- and post-mastectomy radiotherapy on the degree of edema, shoulder joint mobility, and gripping force. Cancer 47:877, 1981
58. Larson D, Weinstein M, Goldberg I, et al: Edema of the arm as a function of the extent of axillary surgery in patients with stage I and II carcinoma of the breast treated with primary radiotherapy. Int J Radiat Oncol Biol Phys 12(9): 1575, 1986
59. Stoll BA, Andrews JT: Radiation-induced peripheral neuropathy. Br Med J 1:834, 1966
60. Match RM: Radiation-induced brachial plexus paralysis. Arch Surg 110:384, 1975
61. Thomas JE, Colby MY: Radiation-induced or metastatic brachial plexopathy? A diagnosis dilemma. JAMA 222:1392, 1972
62. Bagley FH, Walsh JW, Cady B, et al: Carcinomatous versus radiation-induced brachial plexus neuropathy in breast cancer. Cancer 41:2154, 1978
63. Salner AL, Botnick LE, Herzog AG, et al: Reversible brachial plexopathy following primary radiation therapy for breast cancer. Cancer Treat Rep 65:797, 1981
64. Ryttov N, Blichert-Toft M, Madjen EL, et al: Influence of adjuvant irradiation on shoulder joint function after mastectomy for breast cancer. Acta Radiol Oncol 22:29, 1983
65. Langlands AO, Souter WA, Samuel E, et al: Radiation osteitis following irradiation for breast cancer. Clin Radiol 28:93, 1977
66. Kim JH, Chu FCH, Hilaris B: The influence of dose fractionation on acute and late reactions in patients with postoperative radiotherapy for carcinoma of the breast. Cancer 35:1583, 1975
67. Montague ED: Experience with altered fractionation in radiation therapy of breast cancer. Radiology 90:962, 1968
68. Spanos WJ, Montague ED, Fletcher GH: Late complications of radiation only for advanced breast cancer. Int J Radiat Oncol Biol Phys 6:1473, 1980
69. Ferguson DJ, Sutton HG, Dawson PJ: Late effects of adjuvant radiotherapy for breast cancer. Cancer 54:2319, 1984
70. Kaplan H: Hodgkin's Disease, 2nd ed, pp 427–429. Cambridge, Harvard University Press, 1980
71. Loeffler JS, Goldberg I, Reiser TA, et al: Non-invasive cardiac evaluation after definitive radiation therapy for carcinoma of the breast. Proc Am Soc Ther Radiol Oncol. Int J Rad Oncol Biol Phys 11 (Suppl 1): 103, 1985
72. Host H, Brennhoud IO, Loeb M: Post-operative radiotherapy in breast cancer—Long-term results from the Oslo study. Int J Radiat Oncol Biol Phys 12:727, 1986
73. Kaplan H: Hodgkin's Disease, 2nd ed, pp 429–438. Cambridge, Harvard University Press, 1980
74. Fisher B, Redmond C, Fisher ER, et al: Ten-year results of a randomized clinical trial comparing radical mastectomy and total mastectomy with or without radiation. N Engl J Med 312:674, 1985

75. Loprinzi CL, Carbone PP, Tormey DC, et al: Aggressive combined modality therapy for advanced local-regional breast carcinoma. J Clin Oncol 2(3):157, 1984
76. DeLena M, Varini M, Zucali R, et al: Multimodal treatment for locally advanced breast carcinoma. Cancer Clin Trials 4:229, 1981
77. Crystal RG, Fulmer JD, Roberts WC, et al: Idiopathic pulmonary fibrosis: Clinical, histologic, radiographic, physiologic, scintigraphic, cytologic and biochemical aspects. Ann Intern Med 85:769, 1976
78. Emirgil C, Heinemann HO: Effects of irradiation of chest on pulmonary function in man. J Appl Physiol 16:331, 1961
79. Gross NJ: Pulmonary effects of radiation therapy. Ann Intern Med 86:81, 1977
80. Smith JC: Radiation pneumonitis. Am Rev Respir Dis 87:647, 1963
81. Roberson PL, Lichter AS, Iler V, et al: Dose to lung in primary breast irradiation. Int J Radiat Oncol Biol Phys 9:97, 1983
82. Siddon RL, Kaplan WD, Anderson JW, et al: Three-dimensional internal mammary lymphoscintigraphy: Implication for radiation therapy treatment planning. Proc Am Soc Ther Radiol Oncol. Int J Rad Oncol Biol Phys 11 (Suppl 1): 102, 1985
83. Dao TL, Kovaric J: Incidence of pulmonary and skin metastases in women with breast cancer who received postoperative irradiation. Surgery 52:203, July, 1962
84. Stjernsward J: Decreased survival related to irradiation postoperatively in early operable breast cancer. Lancet 2:1285, 1974
85. Palmer MK, Ribeiro GG: Thirty-four year follow-up of patients with breast cancer in a clinical trial of postoperative radiotherapy. Br Med J 291:1088, 1985
86. Baral E, Blumgren H, Idelstrom K, et al: Prognostic relevance of radiation induced immune suppression in breast carcinoma. ACTA Radiol Oncol 18:313, 1979
87. Toivanen A, Granberg I, Nordman E: Lymphocyte subpopulations in patients with breast cancer after postoperative radiotherapy. Cancer 54:2919, 1984
88. Rotstein S, Blomgren H, Petrini B, et al: Long-term effects on the immune system following local radiation therapy for breast cancer. I. Cellular composition of the peripheral blood lymphocyte population. Int J Radiat Oncol Biol Phys 11:921, 1985
89. Aberizk WJ, Silver B, Henderson IC, et al: The use of radiotherapy for treatment of isolated local-regional recurrence of breast cancer after mastectomy. Cancer 58:1214, 1986
90. Chew KK, Montague ED, Oswald MJ: Results of irradiation in the treatment of loco-regional breast cancer recurrence. Cancer 56:1269, 1985
91. Valagussa P, Bonadonna G, Veronesi U: Patterns of relapse and survival following radical mastectomy: Analysis of 716 consecutive patients. Cancer 41:1170, 1978
92. Fisher B, Wolmark N, Bauer M, et al: The accuracy of clinical nodal staging and of limited axillary dissection as a determinant of histologic nodal status in carcinoma of the breast. Surg Gynecol Obstet 152:765, 1981
93. Chu F, Lin FJ, Kim JH, et al: Locally recurrent carcinoma of the breast. Cancer 37:2677, 1976
94. Haagensen CD: Diseases of the Breast, 2nd ed, pp 706–710. Philadelphia, WB Saunders, 1971
95. Harris JR, Recht A, Amalric R, et al: Time course and prognosis of local recurrence following primary radiation therapy for early breast cancer. J Clin Oncol 2:37, 1984
96. Bedwinek JM, Perez CA, Kramer S, et al: Irradiation as the primary management of stage I and II adenocarcinoma of the breast. Cancer Clin Trials 3:11, 1980
97. Harris JR, Connolly JL, Schnitt SJ, et al: Clinical-pathologic study of early breast cancer treated by primary radiation therapy. J Clin Oncol 1:184, 1983
98. Harris JR, Connolly JL, Schnitt SJ, et al: The use of pathologic features in selecting the extent of surgical resection necessary for breast cancer patients treated by primary radiation therapy. Ann Surg 201:164, 1985
99. Brenner M, Schnitt SJ, Connolly JL, et al: The use of re-excision in primary radiation therapy for stage I and II breast carcinoma. Proc Am Soc Ther Radiol Oncol. Int J Rad Oncol Biol Phys 11 (Suppl 1): 186, 1985
100. Alpert S, Ghossein NA, Stacey P, et al: Primary management of operable breast cancer by minimal surgery and radiotherapy. Cancer 42:2054, 1978
101. Vilcoq JR, Calle R, Stacey P, et al: The outcome of treatment by tumorectomy and radiotherapy of patients with operable breast cancer. Int J Radiat Oncol Biol Phys 7:1327, 1981
102. Durand JC, Piojicak M, LeFranc JP, et al: Wide excision of the tumor, axillary dissection, and postoperative radiotherapy as treatment of small breast cancer. Cancer 53:2439, 1984
103. Chu AM, Cope O, Russo R, et al: Patterns of local-regional recurrence and results in stages I and II breast cancer treated by irradiation following limited surgery. Am J Clin Oncol 7:221, 1984
104. Kurtz JM, Spitalier JM, Amalric R: Late breast recurrence after lumpectomy and irradiation. Int J Radiat Oncol Biol Phys 9: 1191, 1983
105. Osborne MP, Ormiston N, Harmer CL, et al: Breast conservation in the treatment of early breast cancer. Cancer 53:349, 1984
106. Svensson GK, Bjarngard BE, Larsen RD, et al: A modified three-field technique for breast treatment. Int J Radiat Oncol Biol Phys 6:689, 1980
107. Siddon RL, Buck BA, Harris JR, et al: Three-field technique for breast irradiation using tangential field corner blocks. Int J Radiat Oncol Biol Phys 9:583, 1983
108. Buck BA, Siddon RL, Svensson GK: A beam alignment device for matching fields. Int J Radiat Oncol Biol Phys 11:1039, 1985
109. Recht A, Harris JR: Negative breast biopsies after primary radiation therapy: Safety and accuracy. Proc Am Soc Ther Radiol Oncol. Int J Rad Oncol Biol Phys 11 (Suppl 1): 131, 1985
110. Harris JR, Hellman S, Kinne DW: Limited surgery and radiotherapy for early breast cancer. N Engl J Med 313:1365, 1985

Adjuvant Systemic Therapy of Early Breast Cancer

I. Craig Henderson

Most patients relapse and die of breast cancer not because of inadequate therapy but because occult, distant metastases are well established by the time the breast cancer is diagnosed.[1] This conclusion is supported by the observation that improved local control of breast cancer with more extensive surgery (e.g., the Halsted radical mastectomy) or adjuvant radiotherapy has not dramatically improved the life expectancy of breast cancer patients. Mortality from this disease plateaued between 1935 and 1965, a period in which there was continual improvement in our ability to reduce the incidence of local recurrence within the breast, on the chest wall, and in regional lymph nodes.

It is a logical extension of these observations that further progress in the cure of breast cancer will be achieved by either diagnosing the disease at a much earlier time, before metastases have occurred, or treating the distant metastases when the primary cancer is first diagnosed. The latter can be achieved by using systemic therapy before, at the time of, or immediately following the removal of the primary tumor. During this preclinical phase, these distant metastases, or micrometastases, have growth kinetics that make the tumor cell more vulnerable to the cytotoxic effects of chemotherapy. The early use of chemotherapy as an adjuvant to surgical resection in experimental animal tumors may result in the cure of tumors that would be incurable when metastatic disease was clinically apparent.[2] Adjuvant chemotherapy has also been successfully used to cure other human tumor types, especially the pediatric cancers.[3]

There have been four major phases of research on the use of adjuvant therapy for breast cancer, and each has contributed to our understanding of the natural history of the disease and to the development of more effective treatment strategies. The first studies were initiated almost 40 years ago, when premenopausal women were treated with adjuvant oophorectomy. The second generation of clinical trials used short courses of cytotoxic chemotherapy immediately following mastectomy—that is, "perioperative" chemotherapy. These studies were conducted between 1958 and 1970. The promise of success generated by these perioperative trials led to new efforts with prolonged and intense chemotherapy programs that use many newly discovered principles of chemotherapy for the treatment of metastatic disease. These trials were begun about 1970. Research during the past 5 to 10 years has increasingly emphasized the definition of subsets of breast cancer patients who are more likely to benefit from one form of adjuvant therapy rather than another and the use of chemotherapy and endocrine therapies in combination or sequentially.

ADJUVANT OOPHORECTOMY

The first adjuvant oophorectomy trials were begun before chemotherapy had been successfully used to treat any solid tumor. Six separate trials were initiated in the years between 1948 and 1965 (Table 10-26). The early results from these trials were interpreted somewhat differently when they were first published than they are now.

In the oldest of these studies, that of the Christie Hospital in Manchester, England, premenopausal women and postmenopausal women less than 2 years from their last menstrual period were randomized to receive either a radical mastectomy (293 patients) or radical mastectomy plus radiotherapy to the ovaries (305 patients). Two-thirds of the patients had histologically involved nodes. The trial has been reported with 10 and 15 years of follow-up.[4,11] There is a survival advantage for the patients who received ovarian radiation, but this is only marginally statistically significant. At 10 years, 55% of the patients receiving ovarian irradiation were alive, compared with 48% of the control group (p=0.07). At 15 years, 45% and 40%, respectively, were alive. The difference in favor of ovarian radiation was somewhat greater for the node-negative (p=0.06 at 10 years) than for the node-positive patients (p=0.16).

The other trials reported prior to 1970[6,7,12] were all smaller and were reported with shorter follow-up than the study from the Christie. These studies showed even less

Table 10-26
Randomized Trials Comparing Adjuvant Oophorectomy or Ovarian Radiation with Local Therapy Only

Trial Group	*Years of Accrual*	*Number of Patients*	*% Node Positive*	*Years of Follow-up*	*Survival Difference (%)‡*	*p*
Christie*[4]	1948–55	598	67	15	5	NS
Norwegian*[5]	1957–63	169	?	15	4	?
NSABP[6]	1961	357	?	5	2	NS
Boston[7]	—	143	90	5	—	NS
Saskatchewan[8]	1964–73	359	48	10	11	<0.05
Toronto[9]†	1965–72	308	46	15	28	0.02
Toronto*[10]	1965–72	137	87	10	4	0.19

* Ovarian ablation obtained with radiotherapy rather than oophorectomy.
† Premenopausal women > age 45 randomized to ovarian irradiation, ovarian irradiation plus prednisone, or local therapy alone.
‡ The difference between the survival of patients in the treated and control groups at last year of follow-up.
NS, not significant

advantage for adjuvant oophorectomy than the study at the Christie, leading most physicians to abandon the idea of adjuvant oophorectomy.

A retrospective analysis from the University of Minnesota suggested that the advantage of adjuvant oophorectomy, if any, derived from a prolongation of the disease-free survival period—that is, the period from diagnosis to first recurrence—but not from an improvement in overall survival rate.[13] A similar observation was made in the Christie study. Patients who were randomized and treated on study between 1948 and 1952 appeared to benefit from adjuvant ovarian radiotherapy; the 10-year survival rate for the irradiated patients was 56%, that for the control group, 42%. No advantage for adjuvant ovarian irradiation was found for the patients treated between 1953 and 1955. The 10-year survival rate was 54% for the irradiated patients and 52% for the control group. An analysis of differences in the patient groups entered during these two periods showed an increased use of therapeutic oophorectomy for palliation of metastases in the later period.[4] No other major differences were identified.

Two ovarian ablation trials conducted in Canada during the mid-1960s failed to show any advantage for adjuvant treatment during the first 5 years of follow-up. In the Toronto trial, patients were stratified on the basis of age.[9,10] Women younger than 45 were randomized to receive either ovarian ablation with radiotherapy or mastectomy alone. Patients over the age of 45 years, whether pre- or postmenopausal, were randomized to receive one of three treatments: ovarian irradiation, ovarian irradiation plus 7.5 mg prednisone daily for 5 years, or no postmastectomy therapy. There was a prolongation of the disease-free survival of the women younger than 45 treated with ovarian radiotherapy, but at 10 years of follow-up this had not reached statistical significance.[10] There was never a disease-free survival or an overall survival advantage for postmenopausal women treated with either radiation ablation or radiation ablation plus prednisone. However, a highly significant disease-free survival and overall survival advantage has developed for those patients who were premenopausal, who were over the age of 45, and who received both radiation ablation and prednisone. The 15-year disease-free survival rate for this group is 68% compared with 50% in the group treated with mastectomy only. This 18% difference is statistically significant ($p=0.04$). At 15 years, 72% of the patients treated with radiation and prednisone are alive, compared with only 44% of the control group ($p=0.02$).[9]

In the Saskatchewan trial, women were randomized after mastectomy to receive either a surgical oophorectomy or no further therapy.[8] After 5 years of follow-up, there was an 8% disease-free survival advantage for the patients treated with oophorectomy ($p<0.05$), but the difference in survival rate between the two groups was only 4%. This was not statistically significant. By the 10th year the difference in survival rate between the two arms had increased to 11% ($p<0.05$). (Fig. 10-34)[8]

In retrospect, it is not surprising that these trials failed to demonstrate an unequivocal advantage for adjuvant en-

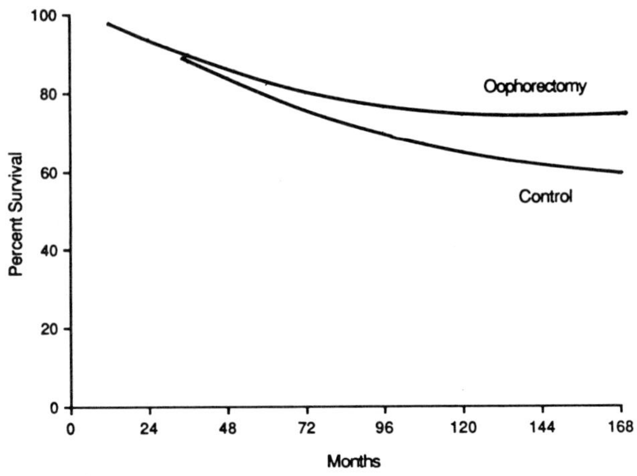

FIGURE 10-34. Survival after mastectomy alone (control; n = 177) or after mastectomy plus oophorectomy (n = 182). (Bryant AJ, Weir JA: Prophylactic oophorectomy in operable instances of carcinoma of the breast. Surg Gyneol Obstet 153:660–664, 1981)

docrine therapy. All of these studies were performed before the discovery of the estrogen receptor protein, and no criteria other than menstrual status were used to select patients. It is unlikely that patients without estrogen receptors will benefit from adjuvant endocrine therapy, but this group constitutes fully one-third to one-half of the patients included in these trials. The power of these studies to detect any beneficial effect is very small indeed. In addition, these studies included both lymph node-negative and node-positive patients. The effect of adjuvant therapy may not be of the same magnitude in these two groups, and longer follow-up will be necessary to detect a benefit in node-negative patients than in node-positive patients. This may explain why differences that eventually emerged in the Saskatchewan and Toronto studies were not apparent during the first 5 years of follow-up.[4]

These studies neither prove nor disprove the value of adjuvant oophorectomy in premenopausal women, but the results do provide rationale for additional controlled studies in which adjuvant oophorectomy is compared with adjuvant chemotherapy. The definition of patients most likely to benefit must be refined in future studies using estrogen receptors and progesterone receptors. Until such studies have been completed, the routine use of adjuvant oophorectomy cannot be recommended.

PERIOPERATIVE CHEMOTHERAPY

The demonstration that tumor cells are readily released into the bloodstream in large numbers at the time of mastectomy led to the idea that perioperative chemotherapy might destroy these cells before they become established as metastatic foci far removed from the breast. These perioperative trials were also conducted with the incorrect notion that a single exposure to a cytotoxic agent could result in destruction of all the cells exposed to the

Table 10-27
Randomized Trials Comparing Adjuvant Perioperative Chemotherapy With Local Therapy Only

Principal Author	*Country*	*Drug*	*Route*	*Schedule*	*Number of Patients*	*Years of Accrual*	*Reported Follow-up (years)*	*Change Disease-Free Survival*	*Survival**
Fisher/NSABP[15]	USA	Thiotepa	IV	In OR and D 1, 2	826	'58–'61	10	↑	↑
Fisher/NSABP[16]	USA	5-FU	IV	D 7–10	657	'61–'67	3	↑	—
Rieche[17]	Germany	Cyclophos	IV	In OR and daily × 1–2 mo	287	'62–'71	5	↑	↑
Garin[17]	USSR	Thiotepa	IV	Daily × 10–14 d	?	?	2.5	↑	—
	—	Cyclophos	?	Daily × 14 d	?	?	2.5	↓	—
Finney[18]	England	Cyclophos	IV	Preop × 4 d, in OR, postop × 4d	83	?	3	↑	↓
Nissen-Meyer[19]	Scandinavia	Cyclophos	IV	Daily × 6 d	1136	'65–'75	17	↑	↑ *
Yoshida[20]	Japan	Cyclophos	PO	D 7–41	351	'74–'76	4	↑	—

Thiotepa, N, N[1], N[11]-triethylenethiophosphoramide; 5-FU, 5-fluorouracil; Cyclophos, cyclophosphamide; IV, intravenous; PO, orally; D or d, day(s), postoperative unless specified; Preop./Postop, before or after surgery; In OR, during surgery; *, statistically significant ($p<0.05$); ↑, improved relative to control group; ↓, treated group fared worse than control group; —, no data available. For many of these studies the statistical significance of observed differences was not reported.

agent—that is, the idea that chemotherapy effects tumor cell kill with zero-order kinetics.

All of the perioperative trials employed regimens of very short duration that were begun at the time of mastectomy or within the first few weeks following mastectomy (Table 10-27). The drugs were usually given intravenously. In several trials, drug dose was administered while the patient was still on the operating room table.[15,17,18] In one study, cyclophosphamide was administered 4 days preoperatively, during the surgery, and for another 4 days postoperatively.[18] (This must be considered the earliest *neo*adjuvant or *proto*adjuvant trial!) In most of these studies, the time to relapse was longer for the treated than for the control group, and in several there was a survival advantage for treatment as well. Except in the largest trials, these differences did not reach levels of statistical significance.

The National Surgical Adjuvant Breast Project (NSABP) initiated its first perioperative trial in 1958. Eight hundred twenty-six patients were randomized and considered evaluable; 417 received thiotepa, and 409 mastectomy only.[16] Patients randomized to the thiotepa arm were given 0.2 to 0.4 mg/kg thiotepa on the day of surgery and 0.2 mg/kg on each of the first 2 postoperative days. No further therapy of any type was administered. At 10 years, there was a 9% survival advantage for the premenopausal women who received thiotepa, and there was a 20% survival advantage for premenopausal women with more than three positive nodes. No benefits were seen for postmenopausal patients treated with thiotepa (Table 10-28).[15] These 10-year differences were not statistically significant. During the first 5 years, the median time to failure in the control group was only 13 months compared with 45 months for the thiotepa group. This difference was statistically significant, as was the 5-year survival advantage for premenopausal women who had more than three histologically involved nodes and who were treated with thiotepa.[21]

The other perioperative chemotherapy study with encouraging results was performed in Scandinavia. Patients were randomized to receive 30 mg/kg of cyclophosphamide intravenously over a 6-day period. In most cases, this chemotherapy was started within a few hours of surgery, but in one hospital, chemotherapy was delayed 2 to 4 weeks while adjuvant radiotherapy was administered. Other forms of adjuvant therapy were not prohibited, including adjuvant oophorectomy or ovarian irradiation, but in retrospect these therapies were equally distributed between the two randomized arms of the study. This study included premenopausal and postmenopausal women, node-positive and node-negative patients.

The Scandinavian study reported more than 15 years of follow-up, and there is a highly significant prolongation of the time to recurrence and a significant increase in overall survival rate (Fig. 10-35). As with the adjuvant oophorectomy trials and in contrast to the NSABP thiotepa trial, no advantage for perioperative chemotherapy was apparent during the first 5 years of follow-up. Since then there has been a steady increase in the difference between the two arms. Most of the patients are now well over age 70, and the survival curves are gradually coming together as increasing numbers of patients die of causes other than breast cancer.[19,22]

Perioperative chemotherapy was abandoned with the recognition that chemotherapy destroys tumor cells by first-order kinetics—that is, chemotherapy kills a fixed percentage of the cells with each dose of drug administered. All subsequent trials have employed at least four to five courses of therapy. However, none of these later trials have follow-up beyond 10 years, and most are not yet 5 years old. The Scandinavian perioperative trial continues to be an important source of convincing evidence that adjuvant chemotherapy is effective in prolonging the survival time of patients with early breast cancer.

Future research on adjuvant chemotherapy must test the hypothesis that longer courses of treatment are more effective than very short perioperative regimens. In a subsequent study, the Scandinavian group randomized node-positive patients to receive either a perioperative course

Table 10-28
Ten-Year Recurrence-Free Survival Rates and Overall Survival Rates Following Perioperative Thiotepa

Patient Group	*Number of Patients*	***Disease-Free Survival (%)*** *Control*	*Thiotepa*
All patients	660	50.5	49.8
Premenopausal	198	46.2	55.4
Postmenopausal	462	52.4	47.7
Premenopausal	97	74.5	72.0
Node negative	43	43.5	40.0
1–3 Positive nodes	58	11.1	31.8
>3 Positive nodes			
		Survival (%)	
All patients	787	45.9	45.8
Premenopausal	206	49.1	58.3
1–3 Positive nodes	45	50.0	47.6
>3 Positive nodes	60	13.5	34.8

Fisher B, Slack N, Katrych D, et al: Ten year follow-up results of patients with carcinoma of the breast in a co-operative clinical trial evaluating surgical adjuvant chemotherapy. Surg Gynecol Obstet 140:528–534, 1975

of cyclophosphamide or 1 year of a combination of cyclophosphamide, methotrexate, and 5-fluorouracil (CMF). Early results from this study suggest that the longer course of treatment is more effective.[19] The Ludwig group in Europe and Australia and the Cancer Research Campaign in Great Britain are conducting trials that may confirm or refute the findings of the Scandinavian group. No preliminary results of these studies have been published. Until they are, perioperative chemotherapy programs should not be routinely employed as a form of adjuvant therapy.

TIMING OF CHEMOTHERAPY INITIATION

Ten hospitals participated in the Scandinavian study, and five contributed most of the patients. All but one of these hospitals observed a beneficial effect from perioperative cyclophosphamide.[23,24] This exception was a radiotherapy institute, and in this hospital there was a delay of 2 to 4 weeks in the initiation of the chemotherapy until after the completion of adjuvant radiotherapy. Radiotherapy was ruled out as a reason for this failure of chemotherapy effect, since the percentage of patients treated with adjuvant radiotherapy was the same in all of the other hospitals. In a multifactorial retrospective analysis, the only factor that seemed to distinguish the use of adjuvant chemotherapy at the radiotherapy institute was this initial delay in the administration of the drug, and this led these investigators to hypothesize that the timing of drug administration may be critical.[23]

Others have been unable to confirm the observation of the Scandinavian group. The M.D. Anderson Hospital performed a retrospective analysis of 460 patients treated with a chemotherapy combination consisting of cyclophosphamide, doxorubicin, and 5-fluorouracil.[25] Patients were separated into groups with intervals between mastectomy and the initiation of chemotherapy of less than 10 weeks, 10 to 13 weeks, 14 to 17 weeks, and more than 18 weeks. No differences in disease-free survival or overall survival rates related to these intervals were observed. However, the shortest postmastectomy interval evaluated in the M.D. Anderson study was 10 weeks. In the Scandinavian study, the longest interval between mastectomy and initiation of chemotherapy was 4 weeks.

The Southwest Oncology Group also performed a retrospective analysis of the relationship between the time that adjuvant L-phenylalanine mustard (L-PAM) or CMF with vincristine and prednisone (CMFVP) was started and failure rate. Patients who began adjuvant therapy less than 14 days, 14 to 28 days or 29 to 42 days postmastectomy had a similar disease-free survival.[26] The Eastern Cooperative Oncology Group (ECOG) found no differences in the treatment failure rate of patients starting therapy within 3 weeks or more than 3 weeks after surgery.[27]

The Ludwig group has begun a prospective randomized trial designed specifically to define the optimal time to begin adjuvant chemotherapy. Two-thirds of the patients are randomized to receive 1 month of CMF beginning on the day of surgery. The other one-third receive no chemotherapy during the first month. All patients are subsequently rerandomized so that eventually one-third of the patients will be treated with only 1 month of CMF, one-third will be treated with 6 months of CMF beginning on the day of surgery, and one-third will be treated with 6 months of CMF after an initial delay of 1 month.

PROLONGED POSTOPERATIVE CHEMOTHERAPY

The third generation of adjuvant chemotherapy trials was built on greater experience in the use of chemotherapy for patients with metastatic disease. The early results from the perioperative chemotherapy trials gave promise that adjuvant chemotherapy was a reasonable approach to the treatment of early breast cancer, and the realization that maximum tumor cell reduction required several courses of chemotherapy led to regimens with durations of 6 months to 2 years. Twenty-five to 30 trials of this type have been conducted, and 18 have been published in either a preliminary or mature form (Table 10-29). Most of these trials were limited to patients with histologically involved lymph nodes, since most investigators were initially hesitant to use a therapy of unknown value and many side effects in a group of patients whose pretreatment prognosis was already quite good. The patients included in these trials fulfilled the usual criteria of "operability." The lesions were not fixed to overlying skin or attached to the chest wall. The lymph nodes, if palpable, were freely movable, and there was no evidence of distant metastases. The similarities between these trials end there. The methods of follow-up are quite variable. Some investigators required follow-up examinations at 3- to 6-month intervals

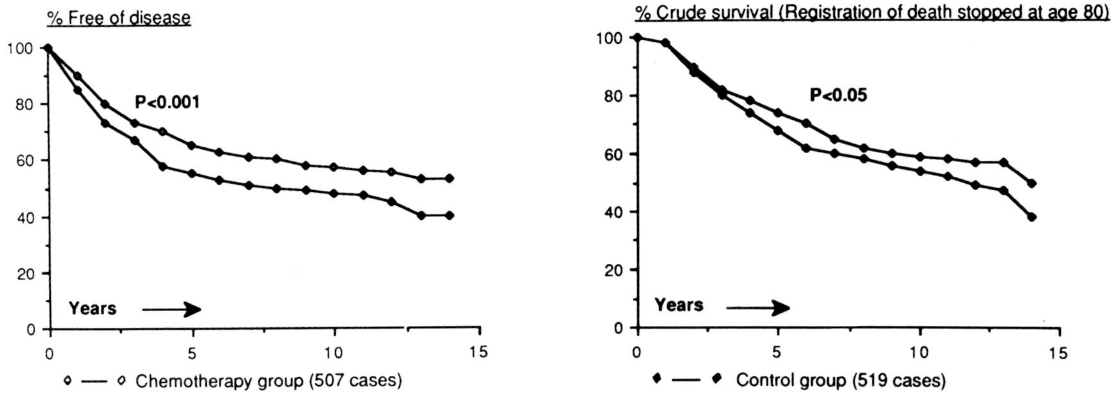

FIGURE 10-35. Survival without recurrence and overall survival of patients randomized to receive a 6-day course of postoperative chemotherapy or local therapy only. (Nissen-Meyer R, Kiellgren K, Manssen R: Adjuvant chemotherapy in breast cancer. Recent Results Cancer Res 80:142–148, 1982)

Table 10-29
Published Studies in Which Patients With Histologically Involved Lymph Nodes Were Randomized to Receive Prolonged Chemotherapy or Local Therapy Alone

Group/Institution	*Years of Accrual*	*Drug(s)*	*Duration of Therapy (Months)*	*Number of Patients Entered*
Japan[28]	1962–76	MMC ± C	9	551‡
Ellis-Fischel[29]	1963–72	Thiotepa	12	167
NSABP[30]	1972–75	L-PAM	24	349
Milan[31]	1973–75	CMF	12	386
Osako (Swiss)[32]	1974–77	LMFP + BCG	6	240‡
English multicenter[33]	1975	CMFV	6	291‡
Guy's/Manchester[34]	1975–79	L-PAM	12	370
Manchester/Guy's[35]	1976–83	CMF	12	327
Heidelberg[36]	1976	LF	24	100
Stockholm/Gottland[37]	1976–82	CMF	12	331‡
W. Midlands[38]	1976–84	CMF-AV	6	462
Glasgow[39]	1976–82	CMF	13	322
Denmark[40]	1977–82	CMF or C	12	1029*
Oxford[41]	1977	L-PAM ± MF	24	273
ECOG[42]	1978–81	CMFP ± T	12	224†
UK/Asia[43]	1978	CMF	18	399
Ludwig[44]	1978–81	CMFPT	12	503†
Vienna[45]	—	CMF, Vlb	36	241

* Only premenopausal patients entered
† Only postmenopausal patients
‡ Some negative-node patients included
Thiotepa, N,N^{1},N^{11}-triethylenethiophosphoramide; F, 5-fluorouracil; C, cyclophosphamide; M, methotrexate; L, chlorambucil; Vlb, vinblastine; P, prednisone; MMC, mitomycin C; T, tamoxifen; L-PAM, L-phenylalanine mustard; A, doxorubicin; V, vincristine

and bone scans at 6- to 12-month intervals. Some reports provide no evidence of systematic follow-up. Some of the trials are quite small, and conclusions based on an analysis of the behavior of subsets within the trial population are tentative at best. In some cases, subsets contain only 15 to 20 patients. The methods of statistical analysis vary, but for many studies there is a paucity of detail in published reports regarding the statistical methods used. For these reasons, each of these trials cannot be given equal weight in reaching conclusions about the efficacy of postoperative chemotherapy for patients with early breast cancer. Two of these trials have been scrutinized more carefully than the others. These are the trials by the NSABP and by the Milan Cancer Institute. These are among the largest of the trials, have the longest duration of reported follow-up, and include both premenopausal and postmenopausal patients with 1 to 3 and more than 3 histologically involved lymph nodes.

The NSABP used L-PAM alone in their first trial of prolonged adjuvant chemotherapy primarily because of its lack of toxicity. This alkylating agent is known to be effective in the treatment of metastatic breast cancer, but a randomized trial has shown that it is less effective than the combination CMF.[46] It may even be less effective than cyclophosphamide as a single agent.[40] Patients accrued to this study between 1972 and 1975, and the first published report appeared in January, 1975.[47] All patients were treated with a radical mastectomy, and none had local radiotherapy. Patients were stratified on the basis of their age (less than 50 or 50 and older) and nodal status (one to three nodes or four plus nodes) and were randomized to receive either L-PAM or a placebo. L-PAM was administered orally, 0.15 mg/kg daily for 5 days every 6 weeks. Seventeen courses of therapy were given in 2 years. Toxicity from L-PAM was limited, and the major toxicity was hematologic. Five percent to 6% of patients had severe nausea and vomiting; one-fourth to one-third had mild nausea. Only 1% to 3% of patients had alopecia; 1% to 4% had stomatitis. Three percent to 4% withdrew because of toxicity, and the percentage of patients withdrawing because of toxicity was about the same among those younger than 50 and older than 50.[48]

The Milan Cancer Institute used a CMF combination as its initial adjuvant program. This regimen was selected in part because of a randomized clinical trial in which patients with metastatic breast cancer were found to have a higher overall response rate to CMF than to L-PAM.[46] Patients entered the Milan study between 1973 and 1975. The basis for patient selection was similar to that used by the NSABP, and stratification was based on age (less than 50 or 50 to 75) and the number of histologically involved lymph nodes (one to three or four plus). Twelve cycles of CMF were given over 1 year. The dose of cyclophosphamide was 100 mg/m^2 administered orally on days 1 to 14 of each 28-day cycle. Methotrexate, 40 mg/m^2, and 5-fluorouracil, 600 mg/m^2, were given intravenously on days 1 and 8.[49] The toxicities were greater with CMF than with L-PAM and included mucositis in 19% of the patients, conjunctivitis in 32%, alopecia in 69% (but only severe enough to require a wig in about 5%), nonhemorrhagic cystitis in 30%, and a complete absence of toxicity in only 2%.[50] Most patients gained weight while on therapy. This averaged 3 kg to 5 kg but was as much as 14 kg in postmenopausal women and 20 kg in premenopausal women.

The 10-year results obtained with these two regimens are remarkably similar, the major difference often being in the p values rather than in the magnitude of the effect (Table 10-30). The difference in the recurrence-free survival rate of treated and control patients is 9% in the L-PAM trial and 12% in the CMF trial. In both trials the disease-free survival advantage for premenopausal women is 17%, and this difference is statistically significant in both studies. There is a small trend in favor of improved disease-free survival rate for postmenopausal women, but this difference is not statistically significant in either study. The greatest benefit is noted in the disease-free survival rate of premenopausal women with one to three positive nodes. Most importantly, treated patients in both trials have a survival advantage of 7% to 8%. For premenopausal women, this survival difference is 14% to 24%. However,

Table 10-30
Ten-Year Results of NSABP and Milan Trials in Which Patients With Histologically Involved Nodes Were Randomized to 1 to 2 Years of Adjuvant Chemotherapy or to Mastectomy Alone

	Recurrence-Free at 10 Years (%)							
	NSABP 30,51				*Milan 31,52*			
Patient Group	*Control*	*L-Pam*	*Diff.*	*p Value*	*Control*	*CMF*	*Diff.*	*p Value*
All patients	29	38	+9	0.06	31	43	+12	0.001
Premenopausal	29	46	+17	0.02	31	48	+17	0.0005
Postmenopausal	28	34	+6	0.49	32	38	+6	0.32
Premenopausal								
1–3 Nodes	41	66	+25	0.02	40	61	+21	0.0002
>3 Nodes	17	22	+5	0.42	15	26	+11	0.03
	Alive at 10 Years (%)							
All Patients	41	48	+7	0.30	47	55	+8	0.10
Premenopausal	37	61	+24	0.02	45	59	+14	<0.02
Postmenopausal	43	41	−2	0.80	50	52	+2	0.89
Premenopausal								
1–3 Nodes	48	81	+33	0.01	51	68	+17	0.025
>3 Nodes	26	35	+9	0.54	30	42	+12	0.29

Table 10-31
Results of Trials in Which Premenopausal Women With Histologically Positive Nodes Were Randomized to Prolonged Chemotherapy or Local Therapy Only

			Survival			
			Disease-Free		*Overall*	
Trial	*Number of Patients*	*Years of Follow-up**	*Trend*	*p Value*	*Trend*	*p Value*
NSABP[51]	120	10	+	0.026	+	0.02
Milan[31]	189	10	+	0.0005	+	0.02
Denmark[40]	1029	6	+	0.001	+	0.2
Osako[53]	60	5	+	0.64	ND	ND
G/M L-PAM[34]	156	5	+	0.14	ND	ND
M/G CMF[35]	168	5	+	0.02	ND	ND
W. Midlands[38]	228	5	+	0.019	ND	ND
Glasgow[39]	ND	4	ND	ND	+	0.5
Oxford[41]	117	5	+	NS	0	NS
Heidelberg[36]	62	1.5	+	0.2	ND	ND

*Date of longest follow-up shown on actuarial disease-free or survival curves for this group of patients.
G/M, M/G, Guy's and Manchester Hospitals; ND, no data; NS, not significant; +, disease-free or overall survival of treated patients superior to control group

the survival curves for treated and control postmenopausal patients are almost superimposable.[30,31] The greatest difference in survival rate is among premenopausal women with a limited number of involved nodes. In the NSABP trial, there is a 33% survival advantage for premenopausal women who have one to three positive nodes and are treated with L-PAM compared with the survival of the control group (p=0.01).

Subsequent randomized trials with a no-treatment control arm confirm the results obtained by the NSABP and Milan in premenopausal, node-positive patients (Table 10-31). In all of these trials there is an improvement in disease-free survival rate, and in five of the trials this trend reaches levels of statistical significance. There is also a consistent survival advantage, but this is not yet statistically significant in any trial except the first two. Since no survival benefit was seen in either the NSABP or the Milan trials during the first 3 to 5 years of follow-up, it is probably too early to anticipate a survival effect in most of these trials.

The largest of these trials is the Danish trial. All patients in this study received local radiotherapy following mastectomy. Patients were subsequently randomized to receive no further therapy, 12 months of cyclophosphamide as a single agent, or the combination CMF. Cyclophosphamide was given orally, 130 mg/m^2, on days one to fourteen of each monthly cycle. The CMF doses used were slightly less than those administered in the Milan trial, but the schedule was unchanged. The dose of cyclophosphamide was 80 mg/m^2, methotrexate 30 mg/m^2, and 5-fluorouracil 500 mg/m^2. Patient selection was similar to that of the Milan and NSABP trials, but randomization to the no-treatment arm was discontinued before the study closed because of early data suggesting a survival advantage for patients on both treatment arms.[54] This overall survival advantage is no longer evident, but there is a significant disease-free survival advantage for patients with either an anaplastic tumor (grade 1) or an estrogen-receptor-negative tumor.[40] Twenty percent of the patients included in this study were perimenopausal (i.e., 1 to 5 years past their last menstrual period), and this may have contributed to the lack of statistical significance in survival trends observed in this study. In addition, the control population in this trial had a statistically significant better survival *after* relapse, compared with patients relapsing following cyclophosphamide and CMF. This is inconsistent with the results of most other adjuvant chemotherapy trials (see below) and may be another reason why no significant survival differences were observed.

Guy's Hospital in London and the South Manchester Hospital in Manchester, England, collaborated in studies designed to confirm or disprove the observations made in the Milan and NSABP trials.[34,35] The doses of L-PAM and CMF used in these studies were about 80% of those used in the earlier trials, but otherwise the trial design was almost identical to that used in the NSABP and the Milan studies. The magnitude of many of the benefits from adjuvant chemotherapy are also quite similar to those obtained in the earlier trials. Disease-free survival differences observed in the L-PAM trial are not statistically significant, but those in the CMF trial are. No survival advantage has emerged, but a strong trend in favor of CMF over mastectomy among premenopausal women suggests that CMF may also impart a survival advantage for this group as well.

The results (or lack of benefit) for postmenopausal women in the NSABP and Milan trials have been confirmed by most other investigators as well (Table 10-32). In most

Table 10-32
Results of Trials in Which Postmenopausal Women With Histologically Positive Nodes Were Randomized to Prolonged Chemotherapy or Local Therapy Only

Trial	Number of Patients	Years of Follow-up	Survival: Disease-Free Trend	Disease-Free p Value	Overall Trend	Overall p Value
NSABP[51]	229	10	+	0.49	+	0.80
Milan[31]	197	10	+	0.32	+	0.89
Stockholm/ Gottland[37]	331	7	−	0.01	−	0.36
Osako[53]	58	5	+	0.57	ND	ND
Ludwig[55]	463	5	+	<0.0001	+	0.76
W. Midlands[38]	234	5	−	0.37	ND	ND
M/G CMF[35]	159	5	+	0.2	ND	ND
G/M L-PAM[34]	214	5	+	0.39	ND	ND
Oxford[41]	156	5	0	NS	0	NS
ECOG[42]	224	4	0	0.09	−	0.82
Heidelberg[36]	21	1.5	+	NS	ND	ND

* Date of longest follow-up shown on actuarial disease-free or survival curves for this group of patients.
G/M, M/G, Guy's and Manchester Hospitals; ND, No data; NS, Not significant, precise *p* value not given; +, disease-free or overall survival of treated group superior to control group

studies there is a trend in favor of better disease-free survival rates for postmenopausal women treated with adjuvant chemotherapy, but this trend reaches statistical significance in only two of the trials. The Ludwig Cooperative Group has conducted the largest trial in postmenopausal women.[55] Node-positive, postmenopausal women, defined by menstrual history or by endocrine testing, were randomized to one of three treatment groups: a combination of CMF with prednisone and tamoxifen, prednisone and tamoxifen alone, or no further treatment. The doses of CMF were identical to those used in the Milan study. Prednisone was administered orally, 7.5 mg per day, continuously throughout the 1-year treatment period. Tamoxifen, 20 mg per day, was also given for 1 year. At the end of 5 years, 39% of the group treated with mastectomy alone were free of recurrence, compared with 56% of the patients treated with prednisone and tamoxifen and 67% of those treated with CMF plus prednisone and tamoxifen ($p<0.0001$).[44] The disease-free survival advantage for patients treated with CMF plus prednisone and tamoxifen was significantly better than that achieved with prednisone and tamoxifen alone ($p=0.02$). An overall survival difference has not yet been reported. Even though adjuvant chemohormonal therapy appeared to be superior to hormonal therapy alone, the added advantage from chemotherapy is small ($p=0.02$).[55]

In several trials, adjuvant chemotherapy had a statistically insignificant but negative effect on the disease-free survival or overall survival rates of postmenopausal women. In the Swedish study, postmenopausal women were randomized to receive 12 months of the Milan CMF regimen, CMF plus tamoxifen, adjuvant radiotherapy alone, or adjuvant radiotherapy plus tamoxifen.[37] Patients on the arms with adjuvant radiotherapy had a much lower local recurrence rate than those given chemotherapy alone or chemotherapy plus tamoxifen. This resulted in a significantly better disease-free survival rate for the patients on the control (i.e., radiotherapy) arms. No difference in overall survival rate was observed.

This analysis of the trials listed in Table 10-29 leads to the conclusions that

1. Adjuvant chemotherapy prolongs the disease-free survival of most treated patients.
2. The magnitude of this benefit is greater in premenopausal women than in postmenopausal women.
3. This disease-free survival advantage may translate into a survival advantage for premenopausal women, but any survival benefit for postmenopausal women is marginal, at best.

IS ADJUVANT CHEMOTHERAPY A CHEMICAL OOPHORECTOMY?

The different effects of adjuvant chemotherapy in premenopausal and postmenopausal women continue to puzzle medical oncologists. Several hypotheses to explain these differences have been suggested:

1. The dose of drug administered to older patients may have been inappropriately reduced, and optimal chemotherapy may not have been delivered.[56]
2. The tumor biology of breast cancer in pre- and postmenopausal women may be different, and either kinetic or other biologic features of premenopausal breast cancer may predispose it to be more sensitive to the cytotoxic effects of chemotherapy.

3. The effect of chemotherapy may be mediated primarily through its impact on the endocrine system, and adjuvant chemotherapy in premenopausal women may actually be a form of "chemical oophorectomy."

There are data to support each of these hypotheses, none of which has been established as an adequate explanation for the differences in the response of pre- and postmenopausal women to adjuvant chemotherapy.

If the effect of adjuvant chemotherapy is mediated primarily through the suppression of ovarian function, one might anticipate that the disease-free survival and overall survival rates of premenopausal women who become permanently amenorrheic would be better than those of patients who do not become amenorrheic. This was not found to be true in the Milan trial.[31] Amenorrhea occurred in 73% of all premenopausal women, in 41% of those younger than 40 years, and in 96% of those older than 40. After the age of 40, amenorrhea was usually permanent; only 4.5% of women in this age-group had a return of menstrual function. Amenorrhea was transient in 39% of the women younger than 40. No correlation could be made between the presence or absence of amenorrhea and the effectiveness of chemotherapy. The disease-free survival rate of women younger than 40 who were treated with mastectomy only (i.e., the control group, n=23) was 17%. The disease-free survival rate of women who had adjuvant CMF and who did *not* develop amenorrhea was 32% (n=19); the disease-free survival rate of those who did develop amenorrhea was 37% (n-13). A similar effect of adjuvant CMF therapy was seen in the subset of premenopausal women with one to three positive nodes: the disease-free survival rate for the control group was 16%, for those without amenorrhea 40%, and for those with amenorrhea 45%. However, permanent amenorrhea may not reflect total ablation of ovarian function, since one-fourth of the women who relapsed after CMF adjuvant chemotherapy had a subsequent response to oophorectomy. This included 6 of 30 patients (20%) who did not develop permanent amenorrhea while on CMF chemotherapy and 6 of 20 (30%) who did.

The findings in the NSABP study were quite similar.[57] Amenorrhea occurred more frequently in women ages 40 to 49 (73%) than in women 39 and younger (22%). Serial measurements of follicle stimulating hormone (FSH), luteinizing hormone (LH), and estradiol (E_2) were performed in 37 premenopausal women on L-PAM. E_2 levels were moderately suppressed both in women older than 40 and in those under 40, but only the older women developed a postmenopausal FSH/LH profile. These findings were correlated with the relative efficacy of L-PAM in improving disease-free survival. The greatest benefit was seen in the women younger than 40. At 4 years, the disease-free survival rate of women under 39 was 32% in the control group and 69% in the group treated with L-PAM (p=0.01). For women ages 40 to 49, the relative disease-free survival rate was 48% and 61%, respectively, in the control and treated population (p=0.09). The patients who appeared to derive the greatest benefit from adjuvant chemotherapy were the younger women, in whom chemotherapy had the fewest endocrine effects. These observations are consistent with those made in the Toronto ovarian ablation study. In that trial, ovarian ablation did not significantly improve the disease-free survival or overall survival rates for women younger than 45, but women older than 45 years had a significant survival benefit from a combination of ovarian ablation and prednisone.[10]

The results from other studies are not all consistent with those obtained in the Milan and NSABP studies. In the Danish trials, amenorrhea occurred in 85% of the patients treated with cyclophosphamide as a single agent and in 80% of the patients treated with CMF.[40] There was a significantly better relapse-free survival rate among the women who developed amenorrhea from cyclophosphamide than those who did not (p=0.0001). However, there was no advantage for those patients who developed amenorrhea while receiving CMF. In the ECOG study comparing CMF, CMFP, and CMFP plus tamoxifen (CMFPT) in premenopausal women, there was a disease-free survival (p=0.006) and an overall survival advantage (p=0.001) among those patients who developed amenorrhea. However, the development of hot flashes on chemotherapy was not associated with an improvement in survival rate.[58] A similar effect of amenorrhea on disease-free survival rate without a noticeable impact on overall survival was seen in the Guy's/Manchester CMF trials.[35]

The Ludwig group randomized premenopausal women to receive either CMF or CMFP.[59] This study was large enough (n = 505 patients) to do an analysis of the effect of therapy in each age-group. As with other studies, the incidence of amenorrhea increased with patient age. About 50% of the women between the ages of 21 and 34 had amenorrhea, compared with 98% of the women between the ages of 40 and 44. At the fourth year of follow-up, the survival rate of women ages 21 to 34 with amenorrhea was twice that of patients without amenorrhea. In contrast, amenorrhea had no effect on the survival rate of women in the 35 to 44 age-group.

Questions about the relative effectiveness of chemotherapy and oophorectomy in premenopausal women can and are being addressed in prospective, randomized trials. In one study, 42 estrogen-receptor-positive, premenopausal women were randomized to receive adjuvant oophorectomy alone or adjuvant oophorectomy plus CMFVP for 1 year. (Both groups were also given adjuvant tamoxifen for 3 years.)[60] If adjuvant chemotherapy has an antitumor effect in addition to its effect on ovarian function, patients treated with both oophorectomy and chemotherapy should have a better disease-free survival or overall survival rate. The 3-year results from this trial show no difference between the two treatment arms. Unfortunately, the number of patients accrued to this study is still too small to permit any meaningful conclusions.

Since chemotherapy does not totally ablate ovarian function (see above), patients treated with chemotherapy plus oophorectomy may have a better survival rate than those treated with chemotherapy alone. A trial of this type has been conducted by the Ludwig group, which randomized 327 premenopausal women with four or more positive nodes to receive 1 year of CMF or CMF plus oophorectomy.[61] At 4 years of follow-up, there was no significant difference in the disease-free survival rates of patients on the two treatment arms ($p = 0.33$).

ADJUVANT CHEMOTHERAPY AND ESTROGEN RECEPTOR STATUS

If the effect of adjuvant chemotherapy is mediated primarily through its endocrine effects, one might anticipate that adjuvant chemotherapy would have a greater impact in patients whose tumors are estrogen receptor positive than in those whose tumors are estrogen receptor negative. Conversely, if the effects of chemotherapy are independent of endocrine function, one might expect chemotherapy effects to be more apparent in patients whose tumors are estrogen receptor negative, since these tumors are likely to have a higher growth fraction and might be expected to be more responsive to chemotherapy.[2,62] Patients with poorly differentiated tumors are more often estrogen receptor negative.[63] Therefore, this is another patient group that might derive added benefit from chemotherapy if its effects are independent of endocrine mechanisms. Unfortunately, the data from clinical trials do not entirely resolve this issue and provide support for both hypotheses.

In the Guy's/Manchester trial comparing adjuvant CMF with mastectomy alone, significant benefits from CMF were observed only in patients who were progesterone receptor positive.[35] The recurrence rate among the progesterone receptor positive patients was 37% in the control group and only 11% in the treated group ($p=0.002$). The recurrence rate among progesterone receptor negative patients was the same in the control and treated groups. In two other studies, the estrogen receptor content did not seem to influence the response to treatment at all,[38,39] and in two studies only the receptor-negative patients appeared to benefit.[27,45] One of these studies was limited to postmenopausal women who were randomized to CMFP, CMFPT, or observation. The CMFP and CMFPT patients had a marginally better disease-free survival rate than the control population ($p=0.09$). However, among the estrogen-receptor-negative patients, those treated with chemotherapy had a significantly better disease-free survival rate ($p=0.01$), and in this group the disease-free survival advantage persisted beyond the first year of observation. A similar advantage for patients treated with chemotherapy was not seen among those who were estrogen receptor positive ($p=0.34$).[27,42] In a Viennese trial, 241 women were randomized to receive either mastectomy plus CMF/vinblastine or mastectomy alone. The 4-year survival rate of the estrogen-receptor-negative patients was 84% with chemotherapy and 37% without ($p<0.05$). The 4-year survival rate of the estrogen-receptor-positive patients was the same with chemotherapy (84%) and without (80%).[45]

In the Viennese study, there was also an excellent correlation between response to chemotherapy and tumor differentiation. Patients with undifferentiated tumors had a 4-year survival of 79% with chemotherapy and 41% without ($p<0.001$), whereas patients with well-differentiated tumors had 4-year survivals of 81% and 85% with and without chemotherapy.[45] Other investigators have observed a similar relationship between the impact of chemotherapy and tumor differentiation. The NSABP found that among those patients with a poor nuclear grade, the 10-year survival of all patients (premenopausal and postmenopausal) was 28% with placebo treatment and 48% with L-PAM treatment ($p=0.007$). Among patients with a good nuclear grade, there was a better survival for the placebo group ($p=0.04$).[64,65] Similar results were observed in the Danish trials.[40]

The question of whether adjuvant chemotherapy is merely a chemical oophorectomy has not been satisfactorily answered. Available data suggest that the benefits of chemotherapy in premenopausal women may, at least in part, be mediated through the effects of chemotherapy on endocrine function, but it seems unlikely that this is the only effect of adjuvant chemotherapy.

DOSE RESPONSE

There is a steep dose-response curve for cytotoxic drugs when they are used in animal models and in the treatment of other tumor types. It is possible that this is an important factor in treating breast cancer as well, but this is not an established principle in the treatment of patients with metastatic breast cancer (see Chapter 13). A retrospective analysis of the Milan trial comparing CMF with mastectomy only suggested that dose might be an important element in the response to adjuvant chemotherapy.[56] Patients were divided into three groups based on the cumulative amount of drug actually given relative to the amount prescribed by the protocol. Patients in group I received 85% or more of the calculated dose, those in group II 65% to 85%, and those in group III less than 65% of the proposed protocol doses. The methodology for calculating cumulative dose was based on the dose per cycle of chemotherapy and adjusted for the number of cycles completed so that patients who relapsed while on therapy did not skew the analysis. Only 20% of patients received level I doses; this included 26% of the premenopausal women but only 14% of the postmenopausal women. Forty-six percent of the patients were treated with level II doses, and 34% with level III doses. There is a highly significant disease-free survival and overall survival advantage for women who received the highest doses. Fifty-six percent of the patients given level I doses but only 39% of those who received level III doses were disease-free at 10 years ($p = 0.006$). Sixty-six percent of those receiving level I doses and 47% with level III doses were alive ($p=0.04$).[31] Although all CMF-treated postmenopausal women did not have significantly better disease-free survival rates than control patients in the Milan study, postmenopausal women treated with level I doses did have a better disease-free survival rate than postmenopausal women treated with lower doses of CMF or postmenopausal patients in the control group (p=0.03).[56] A similar trend has been observed in some of the other trials.[32,35,37] In the Guy's/Manchester trial comparing CMF with mastectomy only, the protocol doses of CMF were 80% of those used in the Milan trials.[35] Nevertheless, only 24% of the patients in this trial received level I doses (i.e., > 85% of the protocol doses, which were 80% of the Milan doses!); 31% received level II, and 45% level III doses. In spite of this, a disease-free survival advantage has emerged for all patients treated in this study, but there is a trend in favor of better disease-free survival for those receiving the highest doses (p=0.19). Unlike the Milan trial, none of these other studies has found that dose effects can explain the differences in the effectiveness of adjuvant therapy in premenopausal and postmenopausal patients.

An equally large number of adjuvant therapy trials have failed to show a dose response.[26,40,66,67] The NSABP has applied several different methodologies of calculating dose response to their data and have shown that it is possible to get a dose response for placebo treatment![68]

No trial specifically designed to evaluate dose response has been published as yet. However, in the Ludwig trial comparing CMF and CMFP, much higher doses of cyclophosphamide, methotrexate, and 5-fluorouracil were given to patients on the CMFP arm than on the CMF arm. An average of 72% of the full CMF dose was given to patients randomized to the CMF arm, compared with 83% for those patients randomized to the CMFP arm. If dose were an important factor, one would anticipate improved disease-free survival or overall survival rates for patients on the CMFP arm. This has not yet been observed. At 4 years, the disease-free survival rate following adjuvant CMF is 77% and after CMFP is 73% (p=0.35).[59]

DEFINING THE OPTIMAL REGIMEN

The original NSABP L-PAM trial was planned as the first in a series of trials with gradual intensification of the chemotherapy program. Experience with other tumor types and with metastatic breast cancer suggested that a combination of chemotherapy should be more effective than a single agent, and an early report from the Milan study that CMF was as effective in postmenopausal women as in premenopausal women[49] encouraged prospective comparisons between a single agent and a combination of drugs. There are now 11 published trials of this type (Tables 10-33 and 10-34).

Many of these trials are small, and the doses of both the single agents and the combination of drugs vary from one study to another. However, there are identifiable trends (Table 10-34). In most studies the disease-free survival and overall survival rates are better when two or three drugs are given rather than a single agent, and this is noted in both pre- and postmenopausal women. Although these disease-free survival trends are statistically significant in a number of studies, there has been a statistically significant survival advantage in only two trials, the Mayo Clinic study[67] and the Southwest Oncology Group trial.[72] The survival advantage observed in the Mayo Clinic trial was limited to premenopausal women. In the Southwest Oncology Group, CMFVP was shown to be superior to L-PAM in both pre- and postmenopausal women. This observation has been published on several prior occasions, but at a recent presentation of the data it was suggested that this observation may, in fact, be an artifact of the methods of analysis.[78] In any case, there are insufficient data to conclude that the survival times of premenopausal or postmenopausal women can be reliably prolonged by the use of multiple drugs rather than a single agent.

Table 10-33
Randomized Trials Comparing a Single Agent With a Combination of Drugs

Study Group	*Trial Design*	*Years of Accrual*	*Number of Patients*	*Follow-up (years)*
Western Group[69]	F vs. CMF	1974–	62	7
Mayo[67]	PAM vs. CFP	1974–80	293	6.5
Northwestern[70]	PAM vs. CFP ± BCG	1975–79	194	4.5
NSABP[71]	PAM vs. PF	1975–76	671	9
SWOG[72]	PAM vs. CMFVp	1975–78	361	8
Fox Chase[73]	PAM vs. CMF	1975–	279	—
Manchester[74]	PAM vs. CMF	1976–81	137	3+
Bowman Gray[75]	PAM vs. CMF	—	158	7+
Alabama[76]	PAM vs. CMF	—	171	4.5
Denmark*[40]	C vs. CMF	1977–82	845	6
Penn State[77]	PAM vs. FAC	—	52	3

PAM, L-phenylalanine mustard; C, cyclophosphamide; M, methotrexate; F, 5-fluorouracil; P, prednisone; V, vincristine; A, Adriamycin; BCG, bacille Calmette-Guerin
* Performed only in premenopausal patients

Table 10-34
Results of Randomized Trials Comparing a Single Agent With a Combination of Drugs

		All Patients				*Premenopausal Patients*				*Postmenopausal Patients*			
		Disease-Free		*Survival*		*Disease-Free*		*Survival*		*Disease-Free*		*Survival*	
		Trend	*p*	*Trend*	*p*	*Trend*	*p*	*Trend*	*p*	*Trend*	*p*	*Trend*	*p*
Western Group	F vs. CMF	+	NS	−	NS	+	<0.05	−	NS	+	NS	−	NS
Mayo	PAM vs. CFP	+	0.088	+	0.221	+	0.016	+	0.011	±	0.560	±	0.738
Northwestern	PAM vs. CFP	±	0.280	ND	ND	ND	ND	ND	ND	ND	ND	ND	ND
NSABP	PAM vs. PF	+	0.31	+	0.36	+	0.62	+	0.81	+	0.45	+	0.32
SWOG	PAM vs. CMFVP	+	0.002	+	0.001	+	0.002	+	0.005	+	0.003	+	0.039
Fox Chase	PAM vs. CMF	+	NS	ND	ND	+	0.056	ND	ND	+	NS	ND	ND
Manchester	PAM vs. CMF	+	0.03	ND	ND	−	NS	ND	ND	+	0.004	ND	ND
Bowman Gray	PAM vs. CMF	±	ND	ND	ND	ND	ND	ND	ND	ND	ND	ND	ND
Alabama	PAM vs. CMF	−	0.30	−	0.026	ND	ND	ND	ND	ND	ND	ND	ND
Denmark	C vs. CMF	ND	ND	ND	ND	−	0.7	±	0.1	ND	ND	ND	ND
Penn State	PAM vs. FAC	−	NS	−	NS	ND	ND	ND	ND	ND	ND	ND	ND

+, Patients treated with multidrug regimen had a better disease-free survival or survival than patients given single drug; −, control patients had a better disease-free survival or survival than treated patients; ND, no data; NS, not statistically significant, precise *p* value not given

Several groups have compared two or three agents with three to five agents, and these studies have also failed to show a clear survival advantage for a larger number of drugs.[58,59,71] The NSABP randomized patients to receive either a combination of L-PAM and 5-fluorouracil (PF) or the same combination with methotrexate (PMF). At 8 years of follow-up, the disease-free survival and overall survival rates of patients given the three-drug regimen of PMF is actually slightly less than that of patients treated with PF, especially among premenopausal women. There is a nonsignificant trend in favor of better survival rates for postmenopausal women who received the three-drug regimen. The Cancer and Acute Leukemia Group B (CALGB) randomized patients to receive either CMF or CMFVP, and there is a trend toward better disease-free survival rates for premenopausal women treated with the five-drug combination ($p = 0.068$). However, this is counterbalanced by a poorer disease-free survival rate for postmenopausal women given CMFVP ($p = 0.72$). No survival advantages of statistical significance have been observed for any group of patients receiving CMFVP. Both the ECOG and the Ludwig group have randomized premenopausal women to receive either CMF or CMFP, and there is a slight trend in favor of CMF in both trials. However, none of the differences in disease-free survival or overall survival rates have reached statistical significance.[58,59]

THE ROLE OF DOXORUBICIN (ADRIAMYCIN)

Doxorubicin is used as an adjuvant relatively infrequently because of its cardiotoxicity. A doxorubicin regimen has been compared with a no-treatment control arm.[38] In this study, patients were randomized to receive doxorubicin and vincristine together at hour 0. Cyclophosphamide and methotrexate were given 6 hours later. 5-Fluorouracil and leucovorin rescue of the methotrexate were given at hour 18. This chemotherapy regimen was repeated every 21 days for eight cycles. The results obtained with this doxorubicin-containing program are similar to those achieved with CMF: There has been a significant decrease in the number of recurrences in the premenopausal group but not in the postmenopausal group. There is no significant difference between the survival rates of treated and control patients.

Three studies have compared a doxorubicin combination with a nondoxorubicin combination or with the single agent L-PAM. In one of these studies, patients were randomized to receive 1 year of CMF using the Milan dose schedule or to receive doxorubicin (Adriamycin), vincristine, cyclophosphamide, and 5-fluorouracil (AVCF).[79] Patients on this combination were given doxorubicin, 30 mg/m^2, on day one; vincristine, 1 mg/m^2, on day two; and a combination of cyclophosphamide, 300 mg/m^2, and 5-fluorouracil, 400 mg/m^2, on days three through six. Two hundred and forty-nine node-positive and node-negative patients have been randomized on this study. At 5 years there is a statistically significant ($p = 0.003$) disease-free survival advantage for premenopausal node-positive patients receiving AVCF rather than CMF, but there is no difference in the effectiveness of the AVCF and CMF regimen among postmenopausal women ($p = 0.62$) or in node-negative patients ($p = 0.58$). A survival trend in favor of AVCF for premenopausal patients has not reached statistical significance. In another very small trial ($n = 52$) patients were randomized to receive either L-PAM or a combination of 5-fluorouracil, doxorubicin, and cyclophosphamide (FAC).[77] There were no differences in the disease-free survival or overall survival rates of patients on these two regimens, and the trend was surprisingly in favor of the use of L-PAM alone.

The NSABP has compared the combination with L-

PAM, 5-fluorouracil, and doxorubicin (PAF). The results of this study have not been published, but the data were presented at the National Consensus Conference on Adjuvant Therapy in September, 1985.[78] At that time both premenopausal and postmenopausal patients treated with the doxorubicin-containing regimen had a significantly better disease-free survival and overall survival rate than patients treated with PF. If this observation is confirmed by others, the introduction of doxorubicin into adjuvant therapy regimens may significantly improve the results achieved with these programs.

Future strategies for adjuvant chemotherapy trials parallel those performed in patients with metastatic breast cancer. One of these is the use of alternating regimens designed to explore the Goldie-Coldman hypothesis.[80] Goldie and Coldman have suggested that resistance to chemotherapy develops after a very few courses of therapy and that the maximum benefit obtained from a regimen is achieved quickly. The use of alternating non–cross-resistant regimens may permit the administration of the maximum dose of each drug in the combination and at the same time expose the tumor to a large number of different drugs before pleiotropic resistance appears. (See the section entitled Chemotherapy of Metastatic Disease in Chapter 13.) An early study using two non–cross-resistant regimens randomized patients to receive either a combination of CMFP for six cycles followed by four cycles of doxorubicin and vincristine (AV) or the same alternating program with delayed escalation of drug dose.[81] No significant difference was seen in the disease-free survival rates of patients on these two regimens. However, a historical comparison of the disease-free survival and overall survival rates of postmenopausal women treated with this regimen and similar patients treated with CMF alone suggested that CMFP alternating with AV might be superior. The CALGB randomized patients to receive either CMFVP for 14 months or CMFVP followed by 6 months of vinblastine, doxorubicin, thiotepa, and Halotestin (VATH).[82] With a median follow-up of almost 2 years, there is a significantly better disease-free survival rate ($p = 0.01$) for patients crossed over to VATH. An ongoing ECOG program involves randomization of patients to either CMFPT or CMFPTH alternating with thiotepa, doxorubicin, vinblastine, tamoxifen, and Halotestin (TAVTH),[83] and an NSABP trial randomizes patients to cyclophosphamide/doxorubicin (CA), CMF, or CA as an induction regimen followed by delayed therapy with CMF after an interval in which no chemotherapy is administered.[30] There are no preliminary results from these trials.

The use of doxorubicin-containing regimens or alternating programs represents exciting possibilities for the future, but there are insufficient data to recommend them for routine use at the present time.

DURATION OF THERAPY

The duration of adjuvant chemotherapy jumped abruptly from several days in the perioperative trials to several years in the second generation of studies, with no intervening steps to define the optimal treatment duration. There are several potential advantages to shorter courses of therapy. First, if the maximum benefit is achieved within several cycles of drug, as suggested by Goldie and Coldman[80] then a demonstration that a short course is as effective as a longer course is a first step to the introduction of alternating regimens. Second, a short course of therapy is, by definition, less toxic than a longer course. If maximum benefit is achieved after several months, the use of shorter regimens will increase the therapeutic index of most adjuvant therapies.

Some of the trials designed to address this issue are outlined in Table 10-35. Duration of therapy in these trials has varied from 15 weeks in the Dana-Farber Cancer Institute trial to 2 years in the Southwest Oncology Group study. All of these trials were limited to patients with histologically involved lymph nodes. The Southwest Oncology Group trial is further limited to node-positive patients who are estrogen receptor negative. Thus far, no one has shown a significant survival advantage for a longer therapy over a shorter period.

The Dana-Farber trial was initiated in 1974.[84] Patients were randomized to receive either 15 weeks or 30 weeks of a combination of cyclophosphamide (500 mg/m^2) and doxorubicin (45 mg/m^2) given on day one of a 3-week cycle. All patients entered into this study had more than four positive nodes or nodes in the highest axillary zone; at the time of this analysis, half the patients had relapsed and one-third were dead. There is no significant difference in the time to recurrence or the overall survival rate of patients randomized to the two arms of the study (Fig. 10-36). However, the probability of a false-negative (a beta, or type II, error) is still considerable. The chance that a disease-free or survival difference of the magnitude observed in the original NSABP L-PAM trial or the Milan CMF trial would not be detected in this study is about 25%. There is a 50% to 60% chance that such differences would not be detected among the premenopausal patients in this trial.

In the Milan trial, patients were randomized to either 6 or 12 months of CMF using the dose schedule employed in the original CMF trial.[31] Almost three times as many premenopausal women were entered into this trial as in the Farber trial, although women with one to three nodes as well as four positive nodes were included in the study. After 8 years, there is a slight trend in favor of 6 cycles over 12 cycles of CMF, but this is not statistically significant. This trend is greatest among postmenopausal women and among those with more than four histologically involved nodes. The shorter treatment appears to be most advantageous in those groups of patients who derived the *least* benefit in the first CMF trial.

In the Southeast Oncology group study, patients were also randomized to either 6 or 12 months of CMF therapy using the Milan dose schedule.[66] Patients with more than four histologically involved nodes were also randomized to a third arm, 6 months of CMF plus adjuvant radiotherapy. This is the only study in which there is an advantage for a longer course of therapy, but this advantage is limited to premenopausal women, especially those with one to three

Table 10-35
Trials Evaluating the Optimal Duration of Adjuvant Chemotherapy

Parameter	*DFCI*[84]	*Milan*[31]	*Trial Group* *SECSG*[66]	*SAAK*[85]	*SWOG*[86]
Regimen	CA	CMF	CMF ± XRT	LMF	CMFVP
Duration	weeks 15 vs 30	months 6 vs 12	months 6 vs 12	months 6 vs 18	years 1 vs 2
Number of patients					
entered	286	466	620	419	391
evaluable	286	459	440	351	312
Premenopausal	113	324	185	—	152
1–3 nodes	10	197	100	—	74
≥ 4 nodes	102	127	85	—	78
Postmenopausal	173	135	255	—	171
1–3 nodes	7	84	123	—	76
≥ 4 nodes	161	51	132	—	95
Length of follow-up					
year initiated	1974	1975	1976	1976	1979
median (years)	5.3	7.9	3.5	5.0+	3.5

C, cyclophosphamide; M, methotrexate; F, 5-fluorouracil; L, chlorambucil; V, vincristine; P, prednisone; XRT, radiotherapy; A, doxorubicin

positive nodes ($p = 0.03$). No differences in overall survival rate have been reported.

In spite of the possibility that longer duration of therapy may prove to be better in one or another subset of patients, the magnitude of any such benefit is likely to be very small. For this reason, short courses of therapy are now becoming standard arms in current randomized trials, and in practice 6 months of CMF may be considered the standard program for premenopausal women with operable breast cancer and histologically involved nodes.

TOXICITY OF ADJUVANT CHEMOTHERAPY

The toxicities associated with adjuvant chemotherapy are identical to those that occur when chemotherapy is used in patients with metastatic disease. Their import, however, is quite different. Patients with metastatic breast cancer are usually symptomatic, and the chemotherapy is likely to improve the quality of life by relieving those symptoms. Patients with early breast cancer are generally asymptomatic except for the anxiety associated with the diagnosis of cancer. For these patients, toxicity without a net prolongation of survival time at least equal to the time during which the patient experiences chemotherapy side effects is likely to result in a net decrease in overall quality of life.

The frequency of side effects and types of toxicities experienced will vary with the regimen used. Combinations of drugs and high drug doses are usually associated with considerably more toxicity. Most of the drugs used will cause myelosuppression and thrombocytopenia. Cyclophosphamide alone will cause moderate alopecia in about 50% of patients. Alopecia is rarely seen in patients treated with L-PAM or chlorambucil alone. Doxorubicin causes total alopecia in all treated patients, as well as cardiotoxicity, a side effect that is unique for that drug. The incidence of congestive heart failure in adjuvant trials in which doxorubicin was combined with 5-fluorouracil and cyclophosphamide (FAC)[87] or with cyclophosphamide alone (CA)[88] is 4% to 7%. In both of these studies, the incidence of congestive heart failure in patients who received a cumulative doxorubicin dose of <300 mg/m^2 is 1%. Vincristine is among the few agents that do not cause much myelotoxicity, and it is frequently used in drug combinations because it does not compromise the dose of myelosuppressive drugs used in the combination. However, vincristine causes neurotoxicity, which frequently limits its use. In most cases this neurotoxicity is limited to paresthesias of the hands and the feet, but on occasion it may be severe enough to cause a paralytic ileus or incapacitating, total paresis. Cyclophosphamide has been reported to cause cystitis in 5% to 30% of patients.[26,50] However, hemorrhagic cystitis or cystitis of any type is rarely a serious problem. Mucositis or stomatitis is most frequently associated with the administration of methotrexate, although many other drugs may cause this as well, and 5-fluorouracil may cause an irritating conjunctivitis.

The incidence of the most common acute side effects associated with the combination chemotherapy regimens CMF, CMFP, and CMFPT are outlined in Table 10-36. The use of prednisone in any drug combination ameliorates the nausea and vomiting and some of the myelosuppression associated with chemotherapy. On the other hand,

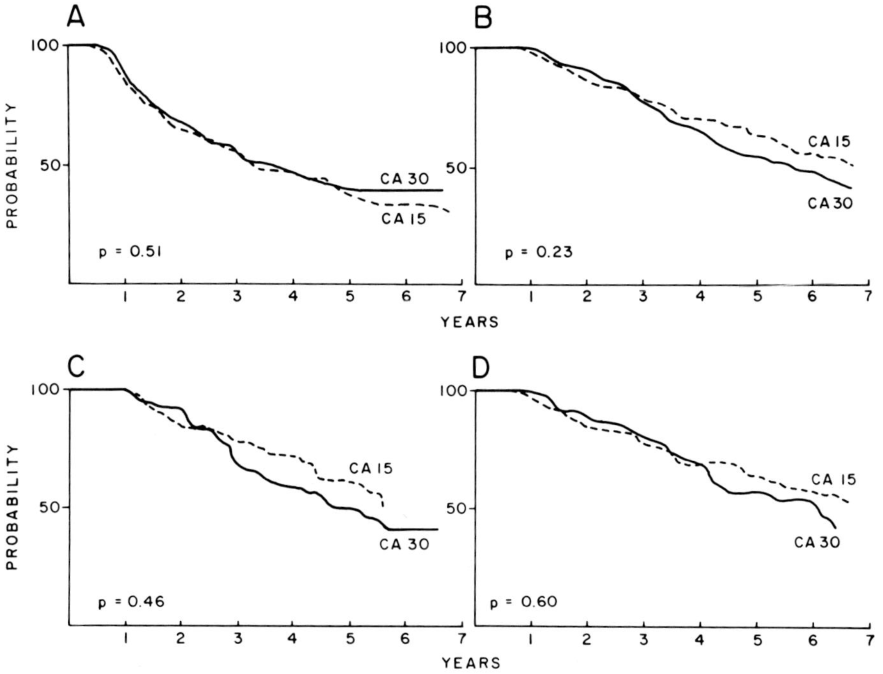

FIGURE 10-36. Disease-free survival and overall survival of patients randomized to receive either 15 or 30 weeks of therapy with cyclophosphamide and adriamycin (CA) on the DFCI trial. *(A)* Time to recurrence (TTR) of all patients, 145 given 15 weeks (median TTR 39 months) and 141 given 30 weeks (median TTR 44 months). *(B)* Survival of all patients, median survival 84 months for 15 week patients and 65 months for the 30 week patients. *(C)* Survival of premenopausal patients, 53 given 15 weeks (median survival 67 months) and 60 given 30 weeks (median survival 61 months). *(D)* Survival of postmenopausal patients, 92 given 15 weeks (median survival 84 months) and 81 given 30 weeks (median survival 73 months). (Henderson IC, Gelman RS, Harris JR, et al: Duration of therapy in adjuvant chemotherapy trials. NCI Monographs 1:95–98, 1986)

Table 10-36
Incidence of Toxicity in Frequently Used Adjuvant Chemotherapy Regimens

	Incidence (%) in				
	Premenopausal Patients			*Postmenopausal Patients*	
Symptom	*CMF*	*CMFP*	*CMFPT*	*CMFP*	*CMFPT*
Nausea/vomiting requiring support	19	5	9	4	6
WBC < 2,000	13	21	20	22	19
PPHS <50,000	3	1	2	7	7
Deep vein thrombophlebitis	0.5	2	3	4	13
Peripheral edema	12	31	38	26	25
Cushingoid changes	0	20	17	22	12
Musculoskeletal pain	8	14	20	18	23
Weight gain > 20%	21	35	43	12	9
Hot flashes	57	58	71	12	18

(Modified from Tormey DC, Taylor SG, Kalish LA, et al.: Adjuvant systemic therapy in premenopausal (CMF, CMFP, CMFPT) and postmenopausal (observation, CMFP, CMFPT) women with node positive breast cancer. In Jones SE, Salmon SE (eds): Adjuvant Therapy of Cancer IV, New York, Grune & Stratton, 1984)

there is increased incidence of deep vein thrombophlebitis, peripheral edema, and weight gain associated with the prednisone.

There are also acute psychological side effects from the administration of chemotherapy.[89,90] These psychological problems may be related to the physical toxicities accompanying chemotherapy, since patients randomized to CMF following mastectomy have been reported to have significantly more anxiety, depression, and overall psychological morbidity than patients randomized to mastectomy and L-PAM or to mastectomy only.[89] In this study, the least psychological toxicity was seen among those patients given L-PAM. In other studies, the patient's prognosis was a more important determinant of psychological morbidity than the treatment given.[91] Some physicians and patients find the psychological morbidity of adjuvant chemotherapy "dose limiting." Psychological toxicity is emphasized more in the European than in the American literature, and there may be an important cultural component to this side effect. In an American study in which patients experienced a variety of psychological complications, 74% stated they would still recommend adjuvant chemotherapy to friends in a similar situation.[92] In some cases, the hope that chemotherapy will improve a poor prognosis may counterbalance many of the discomforts associated with the therapy. The fact that American middle-class women are often more keenly aware of their prognosis as a result of considerable media attention to this disease may provide a partial explanation for the greater acceptance of chemotherapy on this side of the Atlantic.

Long-term toxicities, such as an increased incidence of second malignancies or chronic immunosuppression as a result of adjuvant chemotherapy, are more difficult to measure accurately. These drugs are carcinogens, but some, such as L-PAM and chlorambucil, may be more carcinogenic than the others. As with most carcinogens, there is likely to be a dose response and a latent period for the induction of second tumors with these drugs. An increased incidence of second malignancies must be distinguished from the increased risk of second breast cancers and other malignancies, which already exist in any cohort of breast cancer patients. The potential for inducing second cancers is dramatically illustrated by one report of three cases of acute myelogenous leukemia developing in 13 breast cancer patients treated with more than 4 years of chlorambucil.[93] This underscores the need to use these agents cautiously in any group of patients in which chemotherapy has not yet proved beneficial.

The NSABP is one of the few groups with sufficient numbers of patients and long enough follow-up to perform a meaningful analysis for second malignancies. This group has reported 27 cases of leukemia (0.5%) and 7 cases of myeloproliferative syndrome among 5299 patients treated with L-PAM or L-PAM plus other drugs.[94] All of these leukemias were detected within 5 years of the completion of chemotherapy. At 10 years, the cumulative risk of developing leukemia in patients otherwise free of metastases or a second primary breast tumor was $1.11 \pm 0.30\%$ in the chemotherapy treated patients, $1.37 \pm 0.74\%$ in patients treated with postoperative radiotherapy and no chemotherapy, and $0.06 \pm 0.05\%$ in patients treated with surgery only. This represents an 11-fold ($p<0.01$) increase in the risk of developing leukemia and a 24-fold increase in the risk of developing acute myelogenous leukemia ($p<0.01$) following adjuvant treatment with L-PAM. In spite of this, the benefits of adjuvant therapy far outweigh the risk of leukemia in the NSABP studies. A similar increase in leukemia has not been observed in the Milan CMF studies.[95]

The incidence of other types of malignancies has also been reported to be increased in one study. In a Japanese trial conducted between 1962 and 1976, 262 patients were randomized to receive adjuvant mitomycin C and 255 to a no-treatment control group.[96] The incidence of second malignancies in the control population equaled that of the general population in the regional cancer registry, but the ratio of expected to observed second malignancies in the treated group was 6.22:21. One hundred twenty-seven node-negative patients were included in this study, and 9% developed a second malignancy. In a historical series in the same hospital the 10-year mortality from breast cancer in node negative patients was 15%. Investigators from Scandinavia, Milan, Switzerland, Tucson, and Guy's/Manchester in England collaborated in an analysis of the combined incidence of second tumors in more than 2500 patients included in their trials.[97] With a median follow-up of 8 to 14 years, the incidence of all types of second malignancies was 3.1% in the surgical controls and 2.7% in those treated with adjuvant chemotherapy. This is consistent with several earlier retrospective studies, which found no relationship between exposure to limited doses of thiotepa and second malignancies.[29,98] No increase or decrease in the incidence of second primary breast tumors has been observed in any of these studies.[31,98,99]

ADJUVANT CHEMOTHERAPY IN NODE-NEGATIVE PATIENTS

Most adjuvant chemotherapy trials have limited entry to those patients with histologically involved lymph nodes. Several preliminary reports have appeared on the use of adjuvant chemotherapy in patients without nodal involvement, but most of these failed to demonstrate a clear advantage for chemotherapy.[32,38,79,100–102] The most mature of these trials was conducted in Switzerland, where 122 node-negative patients were randomized to either no treatment or the relatively nontoxic combination of chlorambucil, methotrexate, and 5-fluorouracil (LMF).[32] This was administered monthly for six courses and was used in a randomized trial for node-positive patients as well. Early reports of this trial suggested that there was a significant benefit for adjuvant LMF in node-negative but not in node-positive patients.[103] The most recent report from this trial shows an 8-year survival of 84.2% for node-negative patients treated with LMF (plus BCG) and 69.2% for the patients treated with surgery only ($p=0.07$).[32] In the West Midlands trial, node-negative patients were randomized to receive eight cycles of LMF or surgery only. At a maximum follow-up of 7 years, no statistically significant differences have emerged. Thirty-two of the 226 treated patients and 34 of 241 control patients have recurred ($p=0.531$).[38] An even smaller West German trial using CMF also shows a nonsignificant trend in favor of the patients receiving adjuvant therapy.[100]

In Milan, 89 node-negative patients who were also estrogen receptor negative were randomized to 12 courses (9 months) of a new intravenous CMF regimen or to no further therapy.[102] With a median follow-up of 2 years, all of the treated patients but only 75% of the control patients are alive. These differences are statistically significant.

Ongoing trials are being conducted in node-negative patients by the NSABP, the Ludwig Cooperative Group, and the ECOG. Since the early relapse rate among patients who are node negative will be small, it is not anticipated that definitive results will be available from these trials for 5 years or more. Until then, patients without histologically involved nodes should not be treated with adjuvant chemotherapy.

ADJUVANT HORMONE THERAPY

Several adjuvant hormone therapy trials using diethylstilbestrol (DES) were attempted in postmenopausal women at about the same time that the adjuvant oophorectomy trials, described above, were initiated. None of these trials was very large, and none has been reported with mature results. Presumably this option was not pursued seriously because of the lack of encouraging results from the early adjuvant oophorectomy trials. In addition, the use of estrogens is associated with considerable toxicity. (See Chapter 13 for discussion on the toxicities of endocrine therapy and the mechanisms by which endocrine therapy might prolong patient survival in an adjuvant setting.)

The discovery of tamoxifen, with its almost total lack of toxicity, stimulated renewed interest in adjuvant endocrine therapy, especially for postmenopausal women, who did not seem to derive much benefit from adjuvant chemotherapy. The first tamoxifen trial was begun in Copenhagen in 1975. Premenopausal women were randomized to receive either tamoxifen or no further treatment. Postmenopausal women were randomized to receive DES, tamoxifen, or no further treatment. DES therapy was discontinued before the end of the 2-year treatment period because of toxicity in more than half of the patients randomized to that arm. With more than 8 years of follow-up, no significant advantage was observed for premenopausal women given tamoxifen ($p = 0.31$), but the recurrence-free survival rate of postmenopausal women on tamoxifen was 70% compared with 73% for those given DES and only 44% among those treated with placebo. These differences in recurrence-free survival rate are significant ($p = 0.004$), but no overall survival data are available from this trial.[104]

Most subsequent trials have confirmed this original observation (Table 10-37). One of the largest of these trials was conducted by the Nolvadex Adjuvant Treaty Organization (NATO), in England. Patients entered into this study were randomized to no further therapy after mastectomy or to treatment with tamoxifen, 10 mg twice daily for 2 years. Postoperative radiotherapy was optional for patients in both arms. This study included premenopausal women who were node positive and postmenopausal women who were node positive or node negative. The majority of the patients were postmenopausal (89%), but less than half of all the patients entered into the study had histologically involved nodes. This study has been reported with actuarial analysis through the fifth follow-up year. There is a highly significant ($p = 0.0001$) improvement in event-free survival rate and a significant ($p = 0.0019$) improvement in overall survival rate for all patients entered into the study. The event-free survival and overall survival curves for this study are shown in Figure 10-37. (An event in this study is either a recurrence or death from any cause.) An advantage in event-free survival and overall survival rate was seen for patients who were premenopausal and postmenopausal and for both the node-positive and node-negative group. A Cox analysis showed no interaction between treatment effect and either menopausal or nodal status.[106]

One puzzling observation in the NATO trial is the lack of correlation between tamoxifen effect and estrogen receptor status. As in other studies patients who had a low (or negative) estrogen receptor value had a poorer prognosis than patients with a high value. The estrogen receptor had prognostic importance whether a low receptor value was defined as less than 5 fmol/mg cytosol protein or less than 30 fmol/mg cytosol protein. In this trial, however, unlike other studies, tamoxifen reduced the breast

Table 10-37
Randomized Trials Comparing Adjuvant Tamoxifen With Local Therapy Alone

	Tamoxifen			*Total*		*Percent*	*Effect on*			
Trial Group	*Dose (mg)*	*Duration*	*Time of Accrual*	*Number of Patients*	*Percent Postmenopausal*	*Node Positive*	*DFS§*	*p*	*Survival§*	*p*
Copenhagen[104]	30	2 years	1975–78	343	38	ND	+	0.015	ND	ND
Christie[105]	20	1 year	1976–82	961	61	53	+	0.04	+	0.05‡
Sweden[101]*	40	2 years	1976–82	1028	100	32	+	0.01	+	0.34
NATO[106]	20	2 years	1977–81	1129	89	44	+	0.0001	+	0.0019
Denmark[107]	30	1 year	1977–84	1650	100	83	+	0.003	0	0.53
Ludwig[108]†	20†	1 year	1978–81	629	100	100	+	0.001	+	0.32
ECOG[109]	20	2 years	1978–82	170	100	100	+	0.0004	0	0.56
Toronto[110]	30	2 years	—	366	100	100	+	0.018	ND	ND

* 20% of patients also received adjuvant CMF; equally distributed between treated and control group
† Patients also received 7.5 mg of prednisone per day
‡ For postmenopausal patients $p = 0.24$
§ +, an advantage was observed for the treated patients
DFS, disease-free survival; ND, no data; NS, not significant

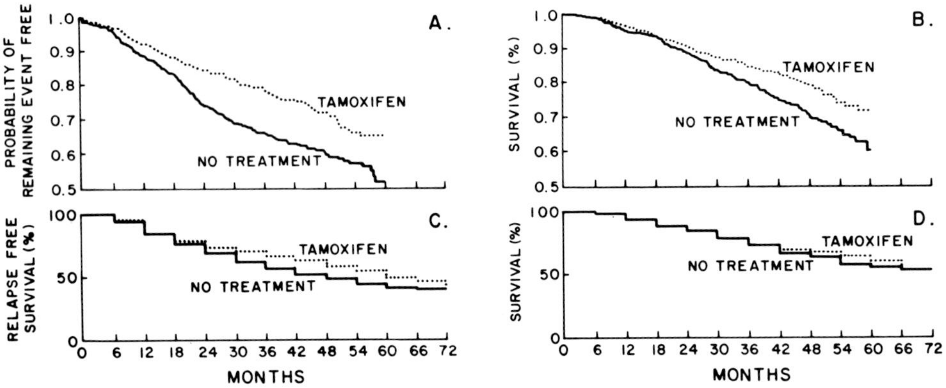

FIGURE 10-37. Effect of adjuvant tamoxifen on disease-free (event-free) survival and overall survival in the NATO and Danish trials. *(A)* Event-free survival, adjuvant tamoxifen for 2 years versus mastectomy ± radiotherapy alone in the NATO trial ($p < 0.0001$) *(B)* Overall survival for patients in the NATO trial ($p = 0.0019$). *(C)* Disease-free survival, adjuvant radiotherapy plus 48 weeks of adjuvant tamoxifen versus adjuvant radiotherapy alone in the Danish trials ($p = 0.003$). *D* Overall survival of patients in the Danish trial ($p = 0.53$). (Baum M, Nolvadex Adjuvant Trial Organization: Controlled trial of tamoxifen as single adjuvant agent in management of early breast cancer: analysis at six years. Lancet 1:836–839, 1985) (Rose C. Mouridsen HT, Thorpe SM, et al: Patients with high risk of recurrence: 72 months of lifetable analysis and steroid hormone receptor status. World J Surg 9: 65– 4, 1985).

cancer mortality of patients with a low (or negative) estrogen receptor level, as well as that of those with a high estrogen receptor (ER) level. The ratio of observed to expected deaths among the tamoxifen-treated patients was 0.63 for those with an ER less than 5 fmol/mg cytosol protein, 0.82 with ER greater than 5 fmol/mg, 0.76 for ER less than 30 fmol/mg, and 0.71 for ER greater than 30 fmol/mg. A Cox analysis showed no difference in the tamoxifen effect within these subgroups.[106]

Only one other trial group has observed a survival advantage for the use of adjuvant tamoxifen.[105] This was the study performed at the Christie Hospital in Manchester. Premenopausal women were randomized to receive either a radiation-induced oophorectomy or adjuvant tamoxifen for 1 year. Postmenopausal women were randomized to receive either no therapy after completion of their mastectomy or mastectomy plus tamoxifen for 1 year. At 7 years, there is a statistically significant improvement in event-free survival rate ($p = 0.04$) and overall survival rate ($p = 0.05$) for all patients. However, when subsets are analyzed, the prolongation of survival time in postmenopausal women does not reach statistical significance.

Many of the differences observed between the trials outlined in Table 10-37 can be accounted for by differences in size or length of follow-up. It is puzzling, however, why the very large Danish trial, with a total of 1650 postmenopausal women, has thus far failed to show results similar to those observed in the NATO study. As with all the other trials, there is a prolongation of disease-free survival, but unlike the NATO trial no benefit in overall survival has been observed (Fig. 10-37).[107] In addition, the improvement in disease-free survival time observed in the Danish trial is limited to patients whose tumors are strongly estrogen-receptor positive, those who have well-differentiated tumors, and those who are in the younger postmenopausal age-group. Women between the ages of 50 and 59 who were treated with tamoxifen had a disease-free survival advantage of 18% ($p = 0.01$). For those older than 70 years, there was only a 5% difference ($p = 0.35$). In an analysis of adjuvant tamoxifen effects in patients with levels of ER less than 10 fmol/mg cytosol protein, 10 to 99 fmol/mg, and greater than 100 fmol/mg, there was a statistically significant advantage for tamoxifen treatment only among those with levels of ER greater than 100 fmol/mg ($p = 0.01$). The disease-free survival rates of tamoxifen-treated patients whose levels of ER were 10 to 99 fmol/mg was actually less than that of the no-treatment control group, but this difference did not reach statistical significance ($p = 0.11$).

In one adjuvant tamoxifen study, entry was limited to patients known to be estrogen-receptor positive or to have an unknown estrogen-receptor status; estrogen-receptor-negative patients were excluded.[109] However, in most of the studies some estrogen-receptor-negative patients were included, but the effects of tamoxifen were seen exclusively in the estrogen-receptor-positive patients.[101,108,110] Thus, the experience of the NATO investigators is inconsistent with that of most other trialists.

The original goals of adjuvant systemic therapy were to eradicate subclinical or micrometastatic foci of disease, to improve overall survival rate, and possibly even to cure some patients who would not be cured with local therapy only. The toxicities associated with cytotoxic chemotherapy are such that any benefit short of this (e.g., a prolongation of disease-free survival without an improvement in overall survival) will be unacceptable to many patients and physicians. However, an improvement in disease-free survival might be considered an important benefit if the therapy is inexpensive and nontoxic. Tamoxifen is certainly nontoxic, and all of the published data indicate that disease-free survival may be reproducibly prolonged, especially in postmenopausal women. The data for premenopausal women are still too limited to draw conclusions about the effectiveness of tamoxifen in this group.

The ability of tamoxifen to significantly prolong overall survival is less clear. The NATO trial stands out as an important exception to the other studies, and the reason for this has not been satisfactorily explained. The magnitude of the benefits observed for tamoxifen in the NATO study are as great as any observed with the use of adjuvant chemotherapy in postmenopausal women, and the results from this trial provide rationale for further research, if not the basis for the routine use of tamoxifen as an adjuvant.

ADJUVANT CHEMOHORMONAL THERAPY

Reasonable arguments can be made that combinations of chemotherapy and endocrine therapy might be additive, synergistic, or antagonistic. In some trials, the response rate to chemohormonal combinations in patients with advanced breast cancer is superior to the response rate obtained with chemotherapy alone. (See the section entitled Chemotherapy for Metastatic Disease in Chapter 13). It has been hypothesized that even a small reduction in overall tumor burden by hormonal therapy early in the course of treatment might substantially increase the percentage of patients whose tumor would be totally eradicated by adjuvant chemotherapy.[111] Endocrine therapy may have no effect on the tumor stem cell,[112] and the total cell kill may be very small. However, this effect could be critical if it reduces the chances of developing chemotherapy-resistant mutants.[111] The current enthusiasm for chemohormonal combinations is more likely related to tamoxifen's lack of toxicity than to theoretical considerations regarding potential synergism between these two modalities. It is assumed that the addition of tamoxifen to a chemotherapy combination may be helpful and is unlikely to be harmful.

However, there are theoretical reasons why endocrine therapy and chemotherapy might actually be antagonistic. Tumor cells that respond to hormone therapy rapidly enter a resting or G_0 phase shortly after the administration of the endocrine therapy.[113] If the chemotherapy and endocrine therapy were directed at the same cell population, this effect of endocrine therapy might make the tumor cell much less sensitive to the cytocidal effect of chemotherapy. This antagonism between tamoxifen and chemotherapy can be demonstrated in tissue culture models, such as MCF-7. When a combination of tamoxifen and either 5-fluorouracil or doxorubicin is placed on growing MCF-7 cells, the cytotoxic effects of the combination are less than the cytotoxic effects obtained with either drug alone.[114] These antagonistic effects of tamoxifen have been observed in both estrogen-receptor-positive cell lines (e.g., MCF-7) and estrogen-receptor-negative lines (e.g., MDA-4668). DES usually stimulates the growth of MCF-7 cells *in vitro* but may be synergistic with melphalan in killing tumor cells.[115] However, melphalan and tamoxifen used together were antagonistic in this system, presumably because tamoxifen-treated cells had decreased uptake of ^{14}C-melphalan compared with cells not previously exposed to tamoxifen. Low concentrations of estrogen will increase the proportion of cells in S-phase. Low concentrations of estrogen and cytosine arabinoside together enhance the cell killing seen with cytosine arabinoside alone.[116] With higher doses of estrogen this enhancement is lost, probably because the higher doses suppress cell proliferation.

Because of, or in spite of, these theoretical considerations, randomized trials have been performed for premenopausal and postmenopausal women comparing the efficacy of tamoxifen plus chemotherapy with chemotherapy alone (Table 10-38). In most of these studies there is a clear improvement in disease-free survival rates for patients given chemohormonal therapy. However, overall survival time has been improved in only three studies, and these small survival trends are not statistically significant.[43,101,119]

The study showing the greatest benefit for chemohormonal therapy is the largest of these studies.[119] This is the NSABP study, in which both pre- and postmenopausal women were randomized to receive either 2 years of L-PAM and 5-fluorouracil (PF) or these two drugs plus tamoxifen (PFT). At 5 years, 52% of the patients treated with tamoxifen and chemotherapy are alive and free of recurrence, compared with only 47% of the patients receiving PF alone ($p = 0.001$). However, the survival rates of patients in the two treatment groups are identical (Table 10-39). There is a consistent pattern of marked improvement in disease-free survival rate and a strong trend for better overall survival rate for all groups of postmenopausal women treated with PFT. The converse is true for younger women, in whom an overall survival advantage was found for patients in the control group (i.e., for patients given PF without tamoxifen).[119] In some subsets, especially those who are estrogen-receptor or progesterone-receptor negative, these differences are marginally significant ($p = 0.06$ and 0.07)(Table 10-39).

The lack of efficacy of chemohormonal therapy in premenopausal women observed by the NSABP has not been noted by other investigators, who have found that the addition of tamoxifen to chemotherapy has had no effect[58] or beneficial effect[121] in premenopausal patients. Contradictory results of this type often arise when the effects of treatment are very small, and very large trials with long follow-up may be needed to obtain a reliable estimate of the effect of tamoxifen added to chemotherapy in premenopausal patients. Until then, adjuvant tamoxifen should not be used for premenopausal patients outside the context of a clinical trial.

Most of the emphasis in recent studies has been on comparisons of chemohormonal therapy with chemother-

Table 10-38
Randomized Trials Comparing Chemotherapy Alone with Chemotherapy and Tamoxifen Combinations

Trial Group	Menstrual Status	Regimen: Chemotherapy Combination	Tamoxifen Dose (mg)	Tamoxifen Duration	Time of Accrual	Years of Follow-up	Number of Patients	Effect on: DFS	p	Surv	p
Case Western[117,118]	1	CMF	40	1 year	1974–79	8–9	312	+	0.04	–	0.3
England/Asia[43]	1	CMF	40	2 years	1978–	2.5	399	+	ND	+	ND
Sweden[101]	2	CMF	40	2 years	1976–82	5	173	+	NS	+	NS
NSABP[119,120]	2	PF	20	2 years	1977–80	5	1082	+	0.001	+	0.27
ECOG[27]	2	CMFP	20	1 year	1978–81	3	142	+	0.31	0	0.91
SWOG[86]	2	CMFVP	20	1 year	1979–	—	194	ND	ND	ND	ND
NSABP[119,120]	3	PF	20	2 years	1977–80	5	779	+	0.98	–	0.27
ECOG[58]	3	CMFP	20	1 year	1978–82	4	369	0	0.53	0	0.53
Mayo/NCCTG[121]	3	CFP	20	1 year	—	—	370	+	0.01	ND	NS

Menstrual Status: 1, mixed pre- and postmenopausal; 2, postmenopausal only; 3, premenopausal only.
DFS, disease-free survival; surv, survival; ND, no data; NS, not statistically significant; + denotes better DFS or survival for the group given chemohormonal therapy; – denotes better survival for group given chemotherapy without tamoxifen

Table 10-39
Disease-Free Survival and Overall Survival Rates in Patients Randomized to Receive Chemotherapy or Chemohormonal Therapy, Subdivided by Age and Receptor Status

	Percent Disease-Free at 5 Years: PAM/FU	PAM/FU/T	p Value	Percent Alive at 5 Years: PAM/FU	PAM/FU/T	p Value
All Patients	47	52	0.002	67	67	0.8
Age < 50	49	50	0.98	67	64	0.27
ER– PR–	41	38	0.4	56	44	0.06
ER– PR+	55	43	0.4	65	66	0.9
ER+ PR–	55	41	0.08	70	56	0.07
ER+ PR+	51	60	0.1	69	75	0.4
Age ≥ 50	44	54	0.001	67	70	0.27
ER– PR–	29	39	0.4	44	46	0.9
ER– PR+	45	48	0.9	58	59	0.7
ER+ PR–	52	48	0.6	75	67	0.3
ER+ PR+	45	56	0.002	76	74	0.9

ER– includes patients with estrogen receptor value 0–9 fmol/mg cytosol protein.
ER+ includes all values ≥ 10 fmol/mg.
PR– includes patients with progesterone receptor values 0–9 fmol/mg.
PR+ includes all values ≥ 10 fmol/mg.
(Fisher B, Redmond C, Brown A, et al: Adjuvant chemotherapy with and without tamoxifen: Five-year results from the National Surgical Adjuvant Breast and Bowel Project Trial. J Clin Oncol 4:459–471, 1986)

apy. Because of the demonstrated efficacy of adjuvant tamoxifen alone in postmenopausal women, further trials are likely to emphasize comparisons between chemohormonal therapy and hormonal therapy. The ideal trial might be a three-way randomization between chemotherapy, endocrine therapy, and chemohormonal therapy. The Ludwig group randomized postmenopausal patients to receive a combination of daily prednisone and tamoxifen (pT), CMF + pT, or observation only. Patients treated with chemohormonal therapy had a significantly better disease-free survival rates than patients given chemotherapy alone ($p = 0.02$).[55] Preliminary results are available from a similar randomized comparison of CMFVP plus tamoxifen and tamoxifen alone in 94 postmenopausal women. Forty-two premenopausal women in this trial were treated with oophorectomy as well.[60] At 3 years, the disease-free survival rate was significantly higher for postmenopausal women given CMFVP plus tamoxifen ($p = 0.05$). There was no difference in the overall survival rates of the two groups of premenopausal patients. Both of these trials suggest that chemotherapy does have an antitumor effect in addition to or synergistic with the effect of endocrine therapy.

OVERVIEW ANALYSES

Most of the adjuvant therapy trials described in this chapter are relatively small. The adjuvant chemotherapy trials with a no-treatment control arm all have less than 500 patients (250 per treatment arm), with the exception of the Danish trials. Those comparing adjuvant tamoxifen with no treatment all have less than 1200 (600 patients per treatment arm). In order to reliably detect survival differences of 10% or 15% between the two treatments for early breast cancer, a study should include at least 1200 patients.[122,123] Most physicians would consider an increase from a 60% to a 70% 10-year survival rate for all patients with breast cancer an important clinical advance. An improvement of this magnitude would also be scientifically important, since it would prove the hypothesis that patients die of metastatic breast cancer because metastases are well established before the initial diagnosis of breast cancer. Acceptance of this principle is an important first step in the development of more effective treatment programs.

One approach to this problem of size is the development of even larger randomized trials. The most recent NSABP trial, the NATO trial, and the Danish Cooperative Breast Group Trials are all examples of such herculean efforts. It is tempting to add up or "pool" the data from several randomized trials in an effort to amplify the results. However, this process negates the value of randomization and is apt to be as misleading as historical comparisons were in previous generations.[1] For example, survival data for patients given adjuvant chemotherapy in London in 1979 might be pooled and compared with the survival data for a cohort of untreated patients in New York in 1974. There are many reasons, other than the treatment itself, why the survival rates of these two groups of patients might be different, and a comparison that assumes that they differ only in the fact that one was treated with adjuvant therapy is apt to be misleading.

Methods of combining data and analyzing the overall effect of treatment were described by Mantel and Haenszel,[124] and these methods have been accepted as valid by most statisticians. Using this methodology, patients treated on one arm of a study are always compared with patients randomized to the other treatment arms of the study and never compared directly with patients treated in another trial. It is assumed from the null hypothesis that if there is no treatment effect, total deaths in the trial will be distributed among the treatment arms in the same proportion as patients were randomized to each of these treatments. In this way, the expected (E) number of deaths on each treatment arm is calculated. The actual number of treatment deaths observed (O) in each arm is then noted, and the number of expected deaths is subtracted from the number of observed deaths ($O - E$) in each treatment arm. If the treatment had no effect, $O - E$ should be zero or differ from zero randomly. On the other hand, if there is a beneficial effect, the number of expected deaths should be larger than the number of observed deaths (i.e., $O - E$ should be a negative value). In performing an overview analysis, the $O - E$ and the variance are determined for *each* trial in a series of trials that have a similar experimental design. For example, an analysis of this type might involve a series of trials that differ only in the use of adjuvant tamoxifen in one of the two treatment arms. The $O - E$ values and the variance from each of the trials is then summed. Levels of statistical significance are determined by the relationship between the summed $O - E$ and the variance. (See Chapter 17, Interpreting Clinical Data.)

This methodology has previously been applied successfully to an analysis of the effect of β-blockers on mortality due to myocardial infarction.[125] Sixteen trials testing the effect of long-term administration of β-blockers were performed. Thirteen of the studies were published, and only two demonstrated a statistically significant benefit. The others had shown no benefit or a nonsignificant disadvantage for the patients treated with β-blockers. However, when an $O - E$ was calculated for all of the studies, it was found that the acute mortality resulting from myocardial infarction was reduced from 10% to 8% ($p<0.0001$). Although this difference of 2% appears quite small, it represents a 20% reduction in the number of *deaths* that might otherwise have occurred. (This is roughly equivalent to saying that the short-term probability of dying of a myocardial infarction or the odds of death have been reduced by 20%.) In light of the worldwide mortality due to myocardial infarction, this represents a large number of lives saved.

A similar analysis has been performed using the data from the many adjuvant chemotherapy and adjuvant tamoxifen trials. This overview analysis has not yet been published as a full report, but it was presented at the National Institutes of Health Consensus Conference held in Bethesda, Maryland, in September, 1985, and influenced the recommendations of the Consensus panel (see below). In fact, it would be difficult to justify the conclusions reached by that panel with only the published literature and no information at all from the overview analysis.

The overview analysis of adjuvant therapy trials was performed by Richard Peto and his colleagues at Oxford University. Data were provided by investigators from every country where such trials have been conducted. Many of the individual trials from which these data were derived are still going on have not yet been published, and this is a major obstacle to publication of the overview.

More than 16,000 patients randomized on tamoxifen trials and more than 14,000 patients randomized on chemotherapy trials were included in this analysis. Entry into the analysis was not restricted to studies with a no-treatment arm. The tamoxifen trials included patients randomized to receive chemotherapy plus tamoxifen versus chemotherapy alone, as well as trials in which patients were randomized to tamoxifen versus mastectomy. In a similar fashion, chemotherapy trials included patients who were randomized to chemotherapy plus tamoxifen versus tamoxifen alone, as well as trials in which patients were randomized to chemotherapy versus mastectomy. All studies were included in which there was only one difference between the two treatment arms: the addition of tamoxifen to one arm of the tamoxifen studies or the addition of chemotherapy to one arm of the chemotherapy studies. The effects analyzed are short-term effects. Many of the studies have a median follow-up of only a couple of years, and no results can be projected beyond the first 5 years at the present time.

It was concluded from this overview that *both* adjuvant tamoxifen and adjuvant chemotherapy could significantly reduce short-term mortality from breast cancer ($p = 0.0001$ or less). The greatest reduction in mortality rate was observed when chemotherapy was given to premenopausal women. The estimated reduction in the odds of death for a premenopausal woman treated with any adjuvant chemotherapy was 25%, and CMF-type regimens (i.e., CMF, CMFP, CMFVP, and so on) might reduce the odds of death by more than one-third. The effects of adjuvant therapy in postmenopausal women were more limited. Tamoxifen might reduce the odds of death in this group by 18%. Chemotherapy of any type might reduce the odds of death for postmenopausal women by 8%. CMF-type regimens might reduce the odds of death for postmenopausal women by 17%. There were insufficient data on the use of tamoxifen in premenopausal women to draw even preliminary conclusions.

Peto estimated that the magnitude of the survival benefit at 5 years would vary with treatment and age-group from 3% to 9%. The 5-year survival rate of the control patients in the tamoxifen trials was 70%. These were the patients who had mastectomy alone, mastectomy plus radiotherapy, or mastectomy plus chemotherapy. With the addition of tamoxifen, the estimated 5-year survival rate was increased to 73%. For women older than 50 years, the estimated 5-year survival rate without tamoxifen was 67% and with tamoxifen was 72%. For all women randomized on trials that involved a CMF-type regimen, the 5-year survival rate with mastectomy only or mastectomy plus tamoxifen was 65%. With the addition of chemotherapy, the estimated 5-year survival rate was increased to 70%. For women younger than 50, chemotherapy increased the estimated 5-year survival rate from 64% to 73%. In the women over the age of 50, chemotherapy increased the estimated 5-year survival rate from 65% to 68%. Although these figures have been widely quoted in the public press and have been discussed in lectures and workshops worldwide, it is important to recognize that the analysis has not yet been published with full details. This is a large task that requires the cooperation of many investigators, careful checking of all data items, and prior publication of at least the methods of each individual study. It is highly unlikely that the broad conclusions derived from this overview analysis are likely to change, but the precise magnitude of the effects may be different in future publications.

The overview analysis presented in September of 1985 was the culmination of work begun 1½ to 2 years earlier by the Oxford group. The first analysis of these data was presented to the trialists involved in October of 1984 at a meeting held at London Heathrow. This first analysis is summarized in a very rudimentary form in a meeting report published in the Lancet, November 24th, 1984.[126]

The use of an overview analysis permits the detection of potentially large and important differences (e.g., a 25% reduction in mortality) that are still too small to detect in most individual trials. This is its major advantage. However, an overview analysis is more closely related to a literature review than to a randomized trial and cannot substitute for a large, well-designed, well-conducted trial, nor can it detect subtle differences between treatment effects that might be observed in an individual study. For example, there may have been very poor compliance in the administration of drug in a large percentage of the trials included in an overview analysis. Presumably there would be no treatment effect in those trials in which the drug was not given! However, if these trials were given the same weight in an overview, they would dilute any real treatment effect that might have been observed in those trials where there was good compliance. In the overview process, there is rigorous quality control of the individual trials to ascertain that the process of randomization resulted in equal distribution of known prognostic and predictive factors such as the number of involved lymph nodes, the size of the tumor, the age of the patients, and the receptor status (when known). However, the overview process cannot control the many variables that do not appear on a data flow sheet.

COST-BENEFIT ANALYSIS OF ADJUVANT THERAPY

A demonstration that therapy improves survival rates or is otherwise beneficial is not in itself sufficient to recommend the therapy as standard treatment. Ideally the magnitude of a benefit should be defined precisely so that it can be weighed against any cost related to the therapy, especially toxic costs. Further, a cost-benefit rato should ideally be expressed in a common unit of measurement. For example, months of life gained as a result of treatment might be balanced against months of quality of life lost because of toxicity.

Traditionally, the end point of primary therapy has been "cure." There are many reasonable definitions of the term "cure,"[127] but they all involve survival without recurrent disease. Primary therapy has usually been viewed as an all-or-nothing event. A mastectomy or local-regional radiotherapy administered before distant metastases occur is likely to eradicate the tumor forever. Patients thus treated might reasonably expect to be cured. Conversely, the use of mastectomy or local-regional radiotherapy in a patient who already has metastatic disease will not prolong survival time. The original goals of adjuvant chemotherapy and adjuvant hormonal therapy were to "cure" patients

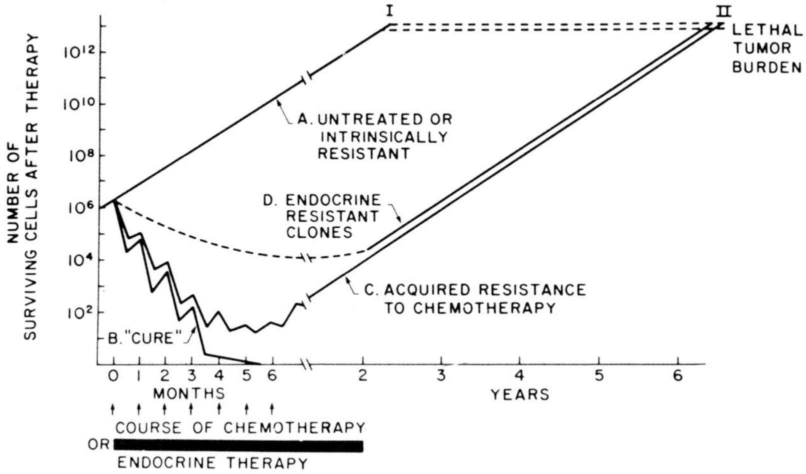

FIGURE 10-38. Theoretical effects of adjuvant therapy on tumor cells. *(A)* Tumor growth in untreated patients or patients with cells intrinsically resistant to chemotherapy and/or endocrine therapy. Lethal burden of tumor mass reached at point I. *(B)* Tumor regression in patient with total elimination of tumor burden and presumably "cured." *(C)* Tumor regression and regrowth in patient with initial sensitivity and subsequent acquired resistance to chemotherapy. *(D)* Tumor regression in patient with endocrine-sensitive clones of cells and subsequent outgrowth of endocrine-resistant clones. Lethal tumor burden reached at point II for patients responding on curves C and D.

using similar definitions. It was hoped that such treatment would eradicate the cancer stem cell. Anything short of total eradication of tumor in at least some patients was not seriously considered as a reasonable end point.

This all-or-none approach to primary therapy may obcure real survival benefits from adjuvant therapy that are short of cure. This is illustrated in Figure 10-38. With each course of chemotherapy, there is a reduction of the total cell burden (curves B and C). Since chemotherapy destroys tumor cells by first-order kinetics, one would not expect drugs to eradicate the last cancer cell, but it is plausible that the reduction in tumor burden might be sufficient to allow normal defense mechanisms to destroy the few remaining cells and result in cure (curve B). Untreated tumors or tumors with instrinsic resistance to therapy would continue to grow, and the patient would die when the total body burden of cells reached approximately 10^{12}. This is shown as curve A on Figure 10-38, and the point at which the patient would die is shown as point I. There are several other possible effects of therapy. Patients might have an incomplete response to chemotherapy and acquire resistance to the drugs being used. If the therapy were not changed, these tumors would eventually begin to regrow. However, the time from initial diagnosis to the point at which the total tumor burden reached a fatal level might be delayed. This is shown as line C on Figure 10-38, and death would occur at point II. Endocrine therapy might have a similar effect, causing either a reduction in tumor cell mass or a static inhibition of growth long enough to delay death until point II on Figure 10-38 (curve D). If the interval between point I and point II on Figure 10-38 is long enough to counterbalance any inconvenience or toxicity associated with the therapy, this would represent a rather important effect short of cure.

Although it is likely that the effect of therapy on each patient will be in the same direction—that is, most patients will either benefit, have no change in survival, or have a shortened survival as a result of therapy—the magnitude of this effect may vary considerably from one patient to the next. For example, one patient may live 10 years longer as a result of treatment, another patient only 6 months longer, and another patient may have a slight reduction in survival as a result of treatment. It is also possible that the benefit of therapy will differ between subsets of patients. For example, it is possible that the average survival benefit observed in patients with one to three nodes will be either greater or less than the average and range of survival benefits observed in patients with four or more nodes.

If it were possible to use each patient as her own control, the average effect of therapy could be determined by calculating either the mean or the median in the differences between expected survival without treatment and observed survival time with treatment. This is illustrated in Figure 10-39, where two hypothetical cohorts are shown and the hypothetical effect of therapy on the survival of each patient is estimated. Those patients with positive numbers had a survival advantage of the magnitude shown. Those patients with negative values had a slightly shorter survival as a result of treatment. Under these circumstances, the mean or median impact of therapy on survival can be easily calculated for the entire group or for each cohort. In this example, all patients treated with the adjuvant therapy lived an average of 40 (mean) or 42 (median) months longer than if they had had no therapy; the range of survival change was −6 to +120. The greatest effect was seen in those patients with one to three nodes, where the mean and median survival differences were 56 and 52 months, respectively. The patients with more than four nodes had a more modest survival benefit, with a mean of 17 and a median of 12 months, of improvement. Of course, patients cannot literally serve as their own controls, and this is the reason randomized trials are performed.

The results of randomized trials are usually interpreted by (1) visual inspection of the difference between the survival curve of the treated and the control patients (Fig. 10-40*A*), (2) calculation of the difference in the percentage survival rates at the end of those two curves (14.2% in Fig. 10-40*A*), or (3) determination of the level

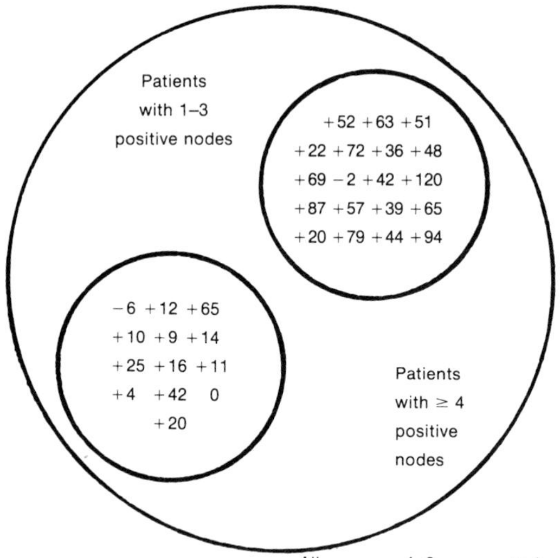

Change in Survival (Months)	All Patients	1–3 Nodes	≥ 4 Nodes
Mean	40	56	17
Median	42	52	12
Range	−6, +120	−6, +120	−6, +65

FIGURE 10-39. Schematic representation of the change in survival which might be observed in two cohorts of patients if each could serve as her own control. One cohort represents premenopausal patients with 1–3 involved lymph nodes; the other premenopausal women with four or more involved nodes. Means and medians have been calculated for each cohort and for the entire "study" population.

of statistical significance for the differences observed. It is tempting to draw the *erroneous* conclusion that the only patients who benefit from treatment are those who lie between the two curves. This conclusion is based on the incorrect assumption that patients who relapse following therapy have had no benefit. This assumption leaves a very small subset of patients who might be considered the beneficiaries of treating all patients—in this case, the 14.2% of patients between the ends of the two curves.

There are other, more appropriate methods of calculating the average survival benefit using data from randomized trials. For example, the mean difference in the survival times of the two patient groups could be calculated by subtracting the area under the survival curve of the control patients from the area under the survival curve of the treated. Alternatively, the median survival time of the control group could be subtracted from the median survival time of the treated group. This is illustrated in Figure 10-40*B*, where the difference in the horizontal distances at the 60th percentile point has been calculated for the premenopausal patients entered into the original Milan CMF trial. The calculations in Figure 10-40*B* suggest that 1 year of CMF will prolong survival time by an average of 3.5 years. Some patients will derive greater benefit, and an equal proportion less. This figure also illustrates one of the more important limitations of these methods. A difference in the medians cannot be determined until the median follow-up of the group with the longest survival time exceeds the median survival time of that group. The mean difference in survival time of the two groups cannot be calculated until all or most of the patients are dead. Therefore, this type of analysis is never suitable for early data and is never better than the assumptions that must be made regarding the future survival times of patients in a trial who have not died by the time the analysis is performed.

An analysis of this type can be used to express the relative cost and benefits of therapy. In spite of the evidence that there may be some long-term adverse effects from adjuvant therapy (see toxicity section, above), most of the toxicity is seen early on, while the chemotherapy is still being administered. There is a large subjective component in measurements of toxicity, and "severe" to one patient or one physician may be "mild or moderate" to another. However, there are few who would consider 6 months of CMF "quality survival." However, this loss of quality survival might be considered worthwhile if the average gain in survival time is 3.5 years, as in Figure 10-40*B*. A more modest benefit (e.g., 9 to 12 months) would be acceptable to some patients, but not to others, and the most important advantage of an analysis in which the cost and benefits are expressed in months of quality life gained or lost is that the patient can readily understand this ratio and herself decide whether this is an appropriate trade-off for her.

A similar approach has been proposed by Gelber and colleagues in the Ludwig group.[128] They have calculated the average *T*ime spent *W*ithout *S*ymptoms of disease and *S*ubjective *T*oxicity (TWiST) for postmenopausal women randomized in the Ludwig trial to receive CMFpT, p+T, or observation. The percentage of patients with 5 years of TWiST is 58% ± 4 for the CMFpT group, 46% ± 4 for the p+T group, and 35% ± 4 for the observation group. These differences are statistically significant. This can also be expressed as the amount of TWiST gained as a result of therapy. This was 569 months per 100 patients treated with CMFpT and 343 months per 100 patients in the p+T group.

THE NIH CONSENSUS STATEMENT ON ADJUVANT CHEMOTHERAPY FOR BREAST CANCER, SEPTEMBER, 1985

The National Institutes of Health (NIH) has sponsored a series of conferences designed to evaluate the usefulness of biomedical technology and to produce a consensus statement that will be useful to both health professionals and the public at large. The panels selected to develop these consensus statements are usually broad based and include physicians from a number of different specialities as well as other health professionals and lay persons. There have been several such panels to evaluate the status of adjuvant chemotherapy.[129,130] The most recent of these was conducted in September of 1985, and the recommendations are outlined in Table 10-40. These positions are

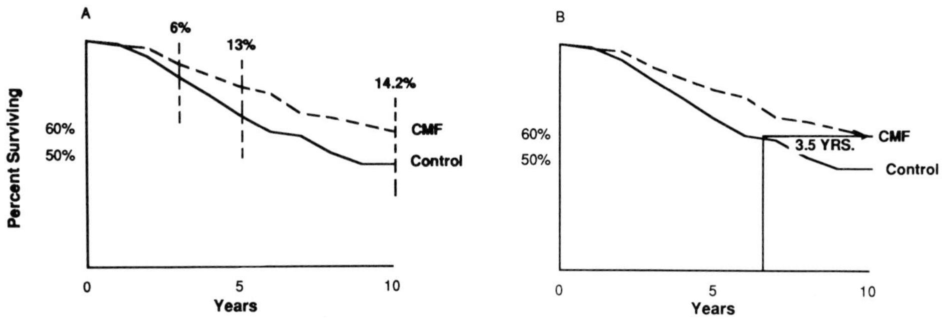

FIGURE 10-40. Ten-year survival of all premenopausal patients treated in the Milan CMF trial. *(A)* The usual way of interpreting survival curves by calculating the vertical difference between the curves at various time points following entry onto study. *(B)* Estimating the average survival benefit by calculating the difference in the medians of the two curves. Since the median has not yet been reached for the treated group in this study, a horizontal at the 60th percentile has been used. (Bonadonna G, Valagussa P, Rossi A, et al: Ten-year experience with CMF-based adjuvant chemotherapy in resectable breast cancer. Breast Cancer Res Treat 5:95–115, 1985)

Table 10-40
NIH Consensus Statement on Adjuvant Chemotherapy of Breast Cancer, September, 1985

Optimal adjuvant therapy is unknown for any patient group. Participation in a clinical trial is the treatment of choice for all *breast cancer patients.*

For treatment outside of a clinical trial:

Patient Group	*Recommended Therapy*
Premenopausal	
Node positive	Chemotherapy, optimal regimen unknown
Node negative	None
Postmenopausal	
Node positive Receptor positive	Tamoxifen
Node positive Receptor negative	None
Node negative	None

somewhat different from those of the consensus panel 5 years earlier.[129] The 1985 panel concluded that adjuvant chemotherapy and adjuvant hormonal therapy effectively prolong survival time of all node-positive breast cancer patients. However, they also concluded that it is not yet possible to define the optimal treatment for any subset of patients. Although the panel reviewed data on a variety of different chemotherapy and tamoxifen regimens given for varying lengths of time, they could not reach a conclusion that one drug or drug combination, duration, or dose is clearly superior to all others. For this reason, the panel emphasized that all patients should continue to participate in a controlled clinical trial whenever possible.

The panel also recognized that the majority of patients will continue to be treated outside of a clinical trial. In this setting, they felt there was justification for treating only two groups of patients: premenopausal women with histologically involved nodes and postmenopausal women with positive nodes who are also estrogen-receptor positive. Adjuvant chemotherapy, rather than tamoxifen, should be used in premenopausal patients. The panel recognized that both chemotherapy and tamoxifen have improved the survival rates of postmenopausal patients. However, tamoxifen can do this with very little toxicity, and for this reason it is the treatment of choice for this group. The panel did not feel there are sufficient data to recommend tamoxifen for postmenopausal, node-positive, estrogen-receptor-negative patients. Adjuvant chemotherapy was not recommended for either premenopausal or postmenopausal women who are node negative, although the panel thought that in cases where the tumor is large, estrogen receptors are negative, and there is a high degree of anaplasia, individual patients and physicians might want to consider this option.

CONCLUSIONS

The evidence that the natural history of breast cancer can be perturbed by the use of adjuvant systemic therapy is substantial, and it is fair to conclude that during the past decade we have moved away from the question "Does adjuvant therapy work?" to a new generation of questions:

1. In which clinical situations can adjuvant therapy be reliably applied?
2. Can the therapeutic index be increased by decreasing the toxicity of adjuvant therapy?
3. In what ways can the efficacy of adjuvant therapy be increased, and at what cost?

One of the greatest dangers of premature acceptance of clinical results is a premature closure of ongoing trials and further research. Although adjuvant therapy may improve the survival rates of all patients by 3% to 5% and of some groups of patients by as much as 10%, it is unlikely that the current regimens will decrease the overall mortality from breast cancer to a figure below 50%. It would be sad if the medical community were to accept this as satisfactory for future years.

At the same time, it is clear that most patients will not go on to a clinical trial, either because the patient is not eligible or does not wish to participate in the trial. Under these circumstances, we concur with the recommendations of the NIH consensus panel and suggest that 6 months of CMF is the program of choice for premenopausal women. In spite of the demonstrated benefit of chemotherapy in postmenopausal women, the small gain is more than counterbalanced by the large cost in toxicity. The tamoxifen trials have shorter follow-up than the adjuvant chemotherapy trials, and the maximum potential of adjuvant endocrine therapy to eradicate all tumor and cure any group of patients may be quite small. However, the very limited toxicity of tamoxifen, the unequivocal improvement in disease-free survival rates for treated postmenopausal women, and the possibility that survival may be improved by tamoxifen as well justify the routine use of this agent for 2 years following mastectomy in postmenopausal node-positive women who are estrogen-receptor positive. In our estimation, no other patient should be treated with any regimen outside the context of a controlled clinical trial.

REFERENCES

1. Henderson IC, Canellos GP: Cancer of the breast: The past decade. N Engl J Med 302:17–30, 78–90, 1980
2. Skipper HE: Kinetics of mammary tumor cell growth and implications for therapy. Cancer 28:1479–1499, 1971
3. Frei III E: Selected considerations regarding chemotherapy as adjuvant in cancer treatment. Cancer Chemother Rep 50:1–8, 1966
4. Cole MP: A clinical trial of an artificial menopause in carcinoma of the breast. Inserm 55:143–150, 1975
5. Nissen-Meyer R: Adjuvant cytostatic and endocrine therapy: Increased cure rate or delayed manifest disease. In Bulbrook RD, Taylor DJ (eds): Commentaries on Research in Breast Disease, Vol 1, pp 95–109. New York, Alan R. Liss, 1979
6. Ravdin RG, Lewison EF, Slack NH, et al: Results of a clinical trial concerning the worth of prophylactic oophorectomy for breast carcinoma. Surg Gynecol Obstet 31:1055–1064, 1970
7. Nevinny HB, Nevinny D, Rosoff CB, et al: Prophylactic oophorectomy in breast cancer therapy: A preliminary report. Am J Surg 117:531–536, 1969
8. Bryant AJ, Weir JA: Prophylactic oophorectomy in operable instances of carcinoma of the breast. Surg Gynecol Obstet 153:660–664, 1981
9. Meakin JW, Allt WEC, Beale FA, et al: Ovarian irradiation and prednisone following surgery and radiotherapy for carcinoma of the breast. Breast Cancer Res Treat (suppl) 3:45–48, 1983
10. Meakin JW, Allt WEC, Beale FA, et al: Ovarian irradiation and prednisone therapy following surgery and radiotherapy for carcinoma of the breast. Can Med Assoc J 120:1221–1228, 1979
11. Cole MP: Prophylactic compared with therapeutic x-ray artificial menopause. In Joslin CAF, Gleave EN (eds): The Clinical Management of Advanced Breast Cancer, 2nd Tenovus Workshop, pp 2–11. Cardiff, Wales, Alpha Omega Alpha Publishing, 1970
12. Nissen-Meyer R: Suppression of ovarian function in primary breast cancer. In Forrest APM, Kunkler PB (eds): Prognostic Factors in Breast Cancer, pp 139–145. Edinburgh E&S Livingston, 1968
13. Kennedy BJ, Mielke PW Jr, Fortuny IE: Therapeutic castration versus prophylactic castration in breast cancer. Surg Gynecol Obstet 118:524–540, 1964
14. Henderson IC: Adjuvant endocrine therapy. In Allegro JC (ed): The Management of Breast Cancer through Endocrine Therapies, pp 38–57. Lawrenceville, NJ, Excerpta Medica, 1984
15. Fisher B, Slack N, Katrych D, et al: Ten year follow-up results of patients with carcinoma of the breast in a co-operative clinical trial evaluating surgical adjuvant chemotherapy. Surg Gynecol Obstet 140:528–534, 1975
16. Fisher B, Ravdin RG, Ausman RK, et al: Surgical adjuvant chemotherapy in cancer of the breast: Results of a decade of cooperative investigation. Ann Surg 168:337–356, 1968
17. Tormey DC: Combined chemotherapy and surgery in breast cancer: A review. Cancer 36:881–892, 1975
18. Finney R: Adjuvant chemotherapy in the radical treatment of carcinoma of the breast—a clinical trial. Am J Roentgenol 111:137–141, 1971
19. Nissen-Meyer R, Host H, Kjellgren K, et al: Scandinavian trials with one single postoperative course vs 12 courses. Recent Results Cancer Res 96:48–54, 1984
20. Yoshida M, Murai H, Miura S: Chemotherapy with mitomycin-C and cyclophosphamide adjuvant to surgery for breast cancer. Jpn J Clin Oncol 9:27–34, 1979
21. Fisher B: Adjuvant chemotherapy in breast cancer. Int J Radiat Oncol Biol Phys 4:295–298, 1978
22. Nissen-Meyer R, Host H, Kjellgren K, et al: Perioperative adjuvant chemotherapy of breast cancer: The Scandinavian experience. Recent Results Cancer Res (in Press) 1986
23. Nissen-Meyer R, Kjellgren K, Malmio K, et al: Surgical adjuvant chemotherapy. Cancer 41:2088–2098, 1978
24. Nissen-Meyer R, Kjellgren K, Mansson B: Adjuvant chemotherapy in breast cancer. Recent Results Cancer Res 80:142–148, 1982
25. Buzdar AU, Smith TL, Powell KD, et al: Effect of timing of initiation of adjuvant chemotherapy on disease-free survival in breast cancer. Breast Cancer Res Treat 2:163–169, 1982
26. Glucksberg H, Rivkin SE, Rasmussen S, et al: Combination chemotherapy (CMFVP) versus L-phenylalanine mustard (L-PAM) for operable breast cancer with positive axillary nodes: A Southwest Oncology Group Study. Cancer 50:423–434, 1982
27. Taylor SG, Kalish LA, Olson JE, et al: Adjuvant CMFP versus CMFP plus tamoxifen versus observation alone in postmenopausal, node-positive breast cancer patients: Three-year results of an Eastern Cooperative Oncology Group study. J Clin Oncol 3:144–154, 1985
28. Koyama H, Wada T, Takahashi Y, et al: Surgical adjuvant chemotherapy with mitomycin C and cyclophosphamide in

Japanese patients with breast cancer. Cancer 46:2373–2379, 1980
29. Kardinal CG, Donegan WL: Second cancers after prolonged adjuvant thiotepa for operable carcinoma of the breast. Cancer 45:2042–2046, 1980
30. Wolmark N, Fisher B: Adjuvant chemotherapy in stage II breast cancer: A brief overview of the NSABP clinical trials. World J Surg 9:699–706, 1985
31. Bonadonna G, Valagussa P, Rossi A, et al: Ten-year experience with CMF-based adjuvant chemotherapy in resectable breast cancer. Breast Cancer Res Treat 5:95–115, 1985
32. Senn HJ, Jungi WF, Amgwerd R, et al: Adjuvant chemoimmunotherapy with LMF + BCG in node-negative and node-positive breast cancer: 8 year results. In Senn H (ed): Recent Results in Cancer Research. Adjuvant Chemotherapy of Breast Cancer, pp 90–101. New York, Springer-Verlag, 1984
33. Wheeler TK, Edelstyn GA, Bates TS, et al: Four drug combination chemotherapy following surgery for breast cancer. In Jones SE, Salmon SE (eds): Adjuvant Therapy of Cancer II, pp 269–276. New York, Grune & Stratton, 1979
34. Rubens RD, Knight RK, Fentiman IS, et al: Controlled trial of adjuvant chemotherapy with melphalan for breast cancer. Lancet 1:839–843, 1983
35. Howell A, Bush H, George WD, et al: A controlled trial of adjuvant chemotherapy with cyclophosphamide, methotrexate and fluorouracil for breast cancer. Lancet 2:307–311, 1984
36. Kaufmann M, Fournier DV, Sievers H, et al: Adjuvant chemotherapy with chlorambucil and 5-fluorouracil in primary breast cancer (Cooperative Study Heidelberg). In Mouridsen HT, Palshof T (eds): Breast Cancer—Experimental and Clinical Aspects, pp 157–160. Elmsford, NY, Pergamon Press, 1980
37. Wallgren A, Baral E, Beling U, et al: Tamoxifen and combination chemotherapy as adjuvant treatment in postmenopausal women with breast cancer. In Senn HJ (ed): Recent Results in Cancer Research. Adjuvant Chemotherapy of Breast Cancer, pp 197–203. New York, Springer-Verlag, 1984
38. Morrison JM, Howell A, Grieve RJ, et al: The West Midlands Oncology Association trials of adjuvant chemotherapy for operable breast cancer. In Jones SE, Salmon SE (eds): Adjuvant Therapy of Cancer IV, pp 253–259. New York, Grune & Stratton, 1984
39. Smith DC, Crawford C, Dykes EH, et al: Adjuvant radiotherapy and chemotherapy in breast cancer. In Jones SE, Salmon SE (eds): Adjuvant Therapy of Cancer IV, pp. 283–289. New York, Grune & Stratton, 1984
40. Brincker H, Mouridsen HT, Rank F, et al: Evidence of a castration-mediated effect of adjuvant chemotherapy (CT) in a randomized trial of cyclophosphamide monotherapy versus CMF in premenopausal stage II breast cancer. Proc Am Soc Clin Oncol 4:56, 1985
41. Gough MH, Durrant KR, Giraud-Saunders AM, et al: A randomized controlled trial of prophylactic cytotoxic chemotherapy in potentially curable breast cancer. Br J Surg 72:182–185, 1985
42. Taylor IV SG, Olsen JE, Cummings FJ, et al: Observation compared to adjuvant chemo-hormonotherapy in postmenopausal breast cancer: The ECOG trial. Proc Am Soc Clin Oncol 4:61, 1985
43. Senanayake F: Adjuvant hormonal chemotherapy in early breast cancer: Early results from a controlled trial. Lancet 2:1148–1149, 1984
44. Goldhirsch A, The Ludwig Breast Cancer Study Group: Randomized trial of chemo-endocrine therapy, endocrine therapy, and mastectomy alone in postmenopausal patients with operable breast cancer and axillary node metastasis. Lancet 1:1256–1260, 1984
45. Jakesz R, Kolb R, Reiner G, et al: Effect of adjuvant chemotherapy in stage I and II breast cancer is dependent on tumor differentiation and estrogen receptor status. Proc Am Soc Clin Oncol 4:69, 1985
46. Canellos GP, Pocock S, Taylor S, et al: Combination chemotherapy for metastatic breast carcinoma. Cancer 38:1882–1886, 1976
47. Fisher B, Carbone P, Economou S, et al: L-phenylalanine mustard (L-PAM) in the management of primary breast cancer. N Engl J Med 292:117–121, 1975
48. Glass A, Wieand S, Fisher B, et al: Acute toxicity during adjuvant chemotherapy for breast cancer: The National Surgical Adjuvant Breast and Bowel Project (NSABP) experience from 1717 patients receiving single and multiple agents. Cancer Treat Rep 65:363–376, 1981
49. Bonadonna G, Brusamolino E, Valagussa P, et al: Combination chemotherapy as an adjuvant treatment in operable breast cancer. N Engl J Med 294:405–410, 1976
50. Bonadonna G, Rossi A, Valagussa P, et al: The CMF program for operable breast cancer with positive axillary nodes: Updated analysis on the disease-free interval, site of relapse and drug tolerance. Cancer 39:2904–2915, 1977
51. National Surgical Adjuvant Project of Breast and Bowel Cancers: Progress report. Twenty-eighth semi-annual meeting. National Surgical Adjuvant Breast Project. Pittsburgh, 1986
52. Bonadonna G, Rossi A, Valagussa P: Adjuvant CMF chemotherapy in operable breast cancer. Ten years later. World J Surg 9:707–713, 1985
53. Senn H, Jungi WF, Amgwerd R: Chemo(immuno)therapy with LMF+BCG in node-negative and node-positive breast cancer. In Salmon SE, Jones SE (eds): Adjuvant Therapy of Cancer III, pp 385–393. New York, Grune and Stratton, 1981
54. Brincker H, Mouridsen HT, Andersen KW: Adjuvant chemotherapy with cyclophosphamide or CMF in premenopausal women with stage II breast cancer. Breast Cancer Res Treat 3:91–95, 1983
55. Ludwig Breast Cancer Study Group: Adjuvant therapy for postmenopausal women with operable breast cancer. Part I—a randomized trial of chemo-endocrine versus endocrine therapy versus mastectomy alone. In Salmon SE, Jones SE (eds): Adjuvant Therapy of Cancer IV, pp 379–391. New York, Grune & Stratton, 1984
56. Bonadonna G, Valagussa P: Dose-response effect of adjuvant chemotherapy in breast cancer. N Engl J Med 304:10–15, 1981
57. Fisher B, Sherman B, Rockette H, et al: L-phenylalanine mustard (L-PAM) in the management of premenopausal patients with primary breast cancer. Cancer 44:847–857, 1979
58. Tormey DC: Clinical results III: Experience of randomized trials without surgical controls. In Senn HJ (ed): Recent Results in Cancer Research. Adjuvant Chemotherapy of Breast Cancer, pp 155–165. New York, Springer-Verlag, 1984
59. Ludwig Breast Cancer Study Group: A randomized trial of adjuvant combination chemotherapy with or without prednisone in premenopausal breast cancer patients with metastases in one to three axillary lymph nodes. Cancer Res 45:4454–4459, 1985
60. Hubay CA, Pearson OH, McGuire WL: Randomized trial of endocrine versus endocrine plus cytotoxic chemotherapy in women with stage II, estrogen receptor positive breast cancer. Proc Am Soc Clin Oncol 5:324, 1986
61. Ludwig Breast Cancer Study Group: Chemotherapy with or

without oophorectomy in high-risk premenopausal patients with operable breast cancer. J Clin Oncol 3:1059–1067, 1985
62. Meyer JS, McDivitt RW, Stone KR, et al: Practical breast carcinoma cell kinetics: Review and update. Breast Cancer Res Treat 4:79–88, 1984
63. Fisher ER, Osborne CK, McGuire WL, et al: Correlation of primary breast cancer histopathology and estrogen receptor content. Breast Cancer Res Treat 1:37–41, 1981
64. Fisher B, Fisher E, Redmond C: Long term survival with adjuvant chemotherapy related to tumor differentiation: The NSABP experience. Proc Am Soc Clin Oncol 4:65, 1985
65. Fisher B, Fisher ER, Redmond C: Ten year results from the NSABP clinical trial evaluating the use of L-phenylalanine mustard (L-PAM) in the management of primary breast cancer. J Clin Oncol 4:929–941, 1986
66. Velez-Garcia E, Moore M, Vogel CL, et al: Postsurgical adjuvant chemotherapy in women with breast cancer and positive axillary nodes: The Southeastern Cancer Study Group (SECSG) experience. In Salmon SE, Jones SE (eds): Adjuvant Therapy of Cancer IV, pp 273–282. New York, Grune & Stratton, 1984
67. Ahmann D, O'Fallon J, Scanlon P, et al: A preliminary assessment of factors associated with recurrent disease in a surgical adjuvant clinical trial for patients with breast cancer with special emphasis on the aggressiveness of therapy. Am J Clin Oncol 5:371–381, 1982
68. Redmond C, Fisher B, Wieand HS: The methodologic dilemma in retrospectively correlating the amount of chemotherapy received in adjuvant therapy protocols with disease-free survival. Cancer Treat Rep 67:519–526, 1983
69. Chlebowski R, Weiner J, Luce J, et al: Significance of relapse after adjuvant treatment with combination chemotherapy or 5-fluorouracil alone in high-risk breast cancer. Cancer Res 41:4399–4403, 1981
70. Cohen E, Scanlon EF, Caprini JA, et al: Follow-up adjuvant chemotherapy and chemoimmunotherapy for stage II and III carcinoma of the breast. Cancer 49:1754–1761, 1982
71. Fisher B, Redmond C, Fisher ER: A summary of findings from NSABP trials of adjuvant therapy. In Salmon SE, Jones SE (eds): Adjuvant Therapy of Cancer IV, pp 185–194. New York, Grune & Stratton, 1984
72. Rivkin SE, Glucksberg H, Foulkes M: Adjuvant therapy of breast cancer: A Southwest Oncology Group Experience. In Senn HJ (ed): Recent Results in Cancer Research. Adjuvant Chemotherapy of Breast Cancer, pp 166–174. New York, Springer-Verlag, 1984
73. Creech RH, Dayal H, Alberts R, et al: A comparison of L-PAM and low dose CMF as adjuvant therapy for breast cancer patients with nodal metastases. Proc Am Assoc Cancer Res 24:148, 1983
74. Howat JMT, Hughes R, Durning P, et al: A controlled clinical trial of adjuvant chemotherapy in operable cancer of the breast. In Salmon SE, Jones SE (eds): Adjuvant Therapy of Cancer III, pp 371–376. New York, Grune & Stratton, 1981
75. Cooper R, Muss H, Ferree C, et al: A six and one-half year follow-up of a randomized adjuvant study of chemotherapy (CT) with and without radiation therapy (RT) for stage II breast cancer. Breast Cancer Res Treat 6:169, 1985
76. Carpenter JT, Maddox WA, Laws HL, et al: Favorable factors in the adjuvant therapy of breast cancer. Cancer 50:18–22, 1982
77. Simmonds MA, Lipton A, Harvey HA, et al: FAC vs. L-PAM chemotherapy for adjuvant treatment of breast cancer in postmenopausal women. Proc Am Soc Clin Oncol 22:438, 1981
78. National Consensus Conference on Adjuvant Therapy, Bethesda, Md., September 1985
79. Misset JL, De Vassal F, Jasmis C, et al: Five year results of the French adjuvant trial for breast cancer comparing CMF to a combination of Adriamycin (ADM), vincristine (VCR), cyclophosphamide (CPM), and 5-fluorouracil (5-FU). In Salmon SE, Jones SE (eds): Adjuvant Therapy of Cancer IV, pp 243–251. New York, Grune & Stratton, 1984
80. Goldie JH, Coldman AJ, Gudauskas GA: Rationale for the use of alternating non-cross-resistant chemotherapy. Cancer Treat Rep 66:439–449, 1982
81. Brambilla C, Rossi A, Valagussa P, et al: Adjuvant chemotherapy in postmenopausal women: Results of sequential non-cross-resistant regimens. World J Surg 9:728–737, 1985
82. Perloff M, Norton L, Korzun A, et al: Advantage of an Adriamycin (A) combination plus Halotestin (H) after initial cyclophosphamide, methotrexate, 5-fluorouracil, vincristine and prednisone (CMFVP) for adjuvant therapy of node-positive stage II breast cancer. Proc Am Soc Clin Oncol 5:xxx, 1986
83. Carbone PP: Multiple trials of adjuvant chemohormonal therapy in the treatment of breast cancer: Preliminary results—the ECOG experience. Breast Cancer Res Treat 3:35–38, 1983
84. Henderson IC, Gelman RS, Harris JR, et al: Duration of therapy in adjuvant chemotherapy trials. NCI Monographs 1:95–98
85. Jungi WF, Alberto P, Brunner KW, et al: Short- or long-term chemotherapy for node-positive breast cancer: LMF 6 versus 18 cycles. SAKK study 27/76. In Senn HJ (ed): Recent Results in Cancer Research. Adjuvant Chemotherapy of Breast Cancer, pp 175–177. New York, Springer-Verlag, 1984
86. Rivkin SE, Knight WAI, McDivitt R, et al: Adjuvant therapy for breast cancer with positive axillary nodes designed according to estrogen receptor status. World J Surg 9:723–727, 1985
87. Buzdar AU, Marcus C, Smith TL, et al: Early and delayed clinical cardiotoxicity of doxorubicin. Cancer 55:2761–2765, 1985
88. Henderson IC: Personal Experience.
89. Maguire GP, Tait A, Brooke M, et al: Psychiatric morbidity and physical toxicity associated with adjuvant chemotherapy after mastectomy. Br Med J 281:1179–1180, 1980
90. McArdle CS, Cooper AF, Morran C, et al: The emotional and social implications of adjuvant chemotherapy in breast cancer. In Salmon SE, Jones SE (eds): Adjuvant Therapy of Cancer II, pp. 319–325. New York, Grune & Stratton, 1979
91. Taylor SE, Lichtman RR, Wood JV, et al: Illness-related and treatment-related factors in psychological adjustment to breast cancer. Cancer 55:2506–2513, 1985
92. Meyerowitz BE, Sparks FC, Spears IK: Adjuvant chemotherapy for breast carcinoma: Psychosocial implications. Cancer 43:1614–1618, 1979
93. Lerner HJ: Acute myelogenous leukemia in patients receiving chlorambucil as long-term adjuvant chemotherapy for stage II breast cancer. Cancer Treat Rep 62:1135–1138, 1978
94. Fisher B, Rockette H, Fisher ER, et al: Leukemia in breast cancer patients following adjuvant chemotherapy or postoperative radiation: The NSABP experience. J Clin Oncol 3:1640–1658, 1985
95. Valagussa P, Tancini G, Bonadonna G: CMF adjuvant program for breast cancer: A 10-year report on second malignancies. Proc Am Soc Clin Oncol 6:75, 1986
96. Wada T: Second cancers following postoperative adjuvant

trol but also decreased the likelihood of distant metastases.[11,12] This provides direct evidence for the correlation between local control and distant metastases, emphasizing that tumors inadequately treated locally can give rise to distant disease.

These recent studies provide data supporting a renewed emphasis on the importance of local control, but they do not imply that local treatment is the only consideration. Even in groups in which the earliest clinically detectable tumors are well treated locally, there are a significant number of patients who develop occult metastases, presumably from occult micrometastases present at the time of initial treatment. Stage I cancers are those 2 cm or less in diameter without axillary lymph node metastases. Radical treatment of such tumors results in a very high probability of local control; however, about one-quarter of these patients will succumb to disseminated distant metastases. This likelihood increases with increasing tumor size, lymph node involvement, and histologic grade.[10] Various adjuvant hormonal and chemotherapeutic treatments are therefore being added to local therapy in groups of patients thought to have a high risk of occult metastases. The results of such studies have been interpreted in a variety of ways. There appears to be no doubt that such treatment regimens influence survival rates. How they do so and the implications of such survival curve changes have been the subject of disagreement and controversy. Some believe such treatments result in more cured patients, whereas others believe that the treatment only transiently delays the appearance of metastases. Some believe such treatment is effective for many patients, is important, and is therefore worth administering to an even larger group of patients. Others believe that the results apply to a small number of patients, are of minor consequence, and thus adjuvant therapy should not be administered to large numbers of patients. For proponents of adjuvant therapy, the results of recent studies are promising, suggesting the development of even more potent and, therefore, potentially toxic therapies and that these be administered to many patients in order to gain maximum benefit of such adjuvant effects. For the more skeptical, the search should be for further demonstration of efficacy of adjuvant therapy, less toxic therapy, and better delineation of patient groups appropriate for treatment. A synthesis of both of these opinions seems likely. The analysis of a large number of trials confirms that adjuvant therapy has a real therapeutic effect.[13] The next step is to understand the nature and magnitude of this effect. To do this, one must consider the nature of survival curves and the changes predicted by the experimental manipulation.

In general, the presentation of survival curves has one of several purposes: to determine the natural history of the disease, to identify factors influencing outcome, and to assess the results of some therapeutic maneuver. Survival curves are usually constructed according to an actuarial method, with both the abscissa and the ordinate displayed linearly. When comparisons are made with a control group receiving a standard therapy, the curves are compared using nonparametric techniques, and if a statistically significant difference is noted, the data are assumed to indicate an improvement in the level of cure. Such differences in survival curves do not necessarily imply differences in curability but rather may indicate delay in metastases or a decreasing force of mortality. Such curves are made more difficult to evaluate when plotted in linear fashion. Such linear curves often give the impression that a tail is emerging, suggesting a cured population (Fig. 10-41). When this is viewed with a semilogarithmic plot, it is often determined that patients are dying at a constant rate.[14] The slope of such a semilogarithmically plotted survival curve may be considered as the force of mortality of the disease. For breast cancer, it appears as though the curve is even more complicated. Figure 10-42 shows the semilogarithmic plot of two series of patients[15,16] for whom long follow-up is available. The curves are exponential, but an inflection point is noted at 10 years. This marks a change in the force of mortality from a constant force of approximately 10% per year for 10 years to approximately 2% to 3% per year. Such biphasic survival curves have been explained by suggestions that rather than being a homogeneous group of patients, the patients studied are a mixture of two populations, one with an aggressive disease having the 10% force of mortality and the other having a more indolent disease. By back-extrapolation of the survival curve, one can determine that this more indolent force of mortality applies to approximately 60% of the original population. This secondary force of mortality is still greater than that for the age-adjusted peer population, suggesting there is still an excess mortality

FIGURE 10-41. A comparison of patient survival plotted *(A)* linearly and *(B)* semilogarithmically. In both curves, patient survival is decreased 25% each year. The use of a semilog plot more accurately depicts this constant force of mortality. (Harris JR, Hellman S: Observations on survival curve analysis with particular reference to breast cancer. Cancer 57:925–928, 1986)

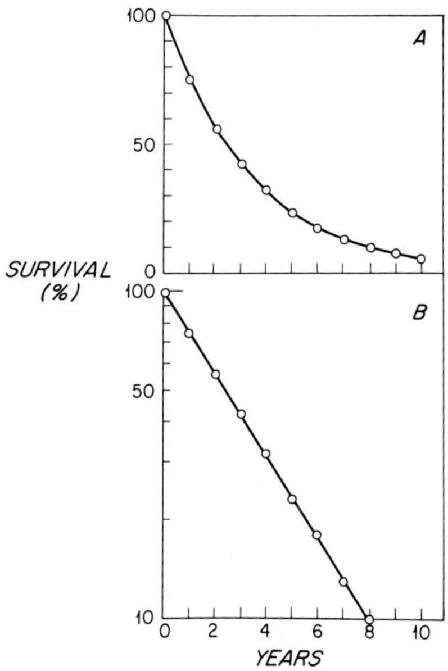

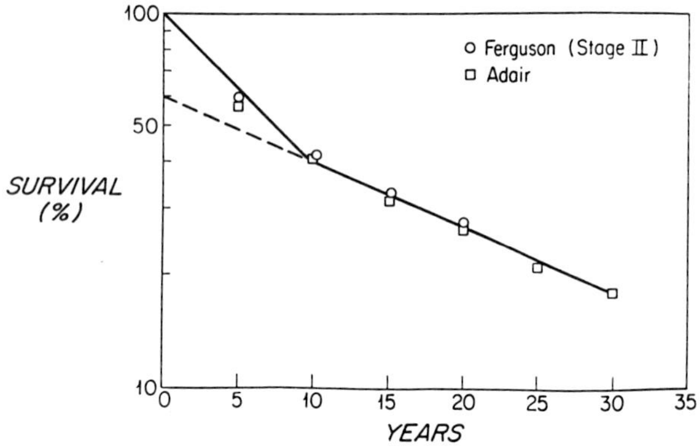

FIGURE 10-42. Semilog plot of survival for breast cancer patients treated by mastectomy (Stage II). Notice change in slope at 10 years (inflection point). (Harris JR, Hellman S: Observations on survival curve analysis with particular reference to breast cancer. Cancer 57:925–928, 1986)

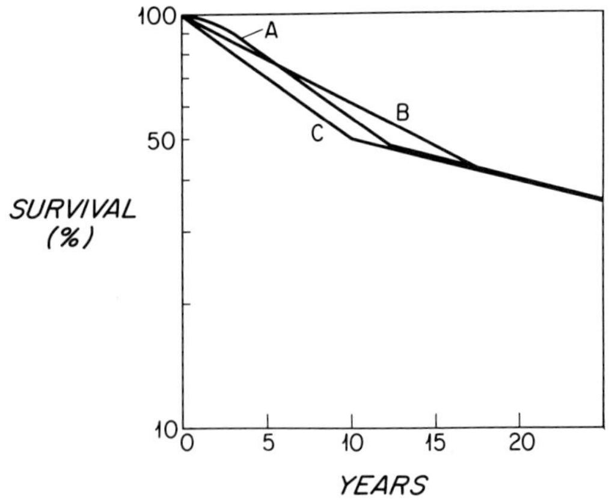

FIGURE 10-43. A comparison of survival curves after three hypothetical treatments for breast cancer. Curve C, control group; curve A, delayed force of mortality for 3 years; curve B, decreased force of mortality for 10 years. Notice that despite early survival advantages for groups A and B, long-term survival is identical. (Harris JR, Hellman S: Observations on survival curve analysis with particular reference to breast cancer. Cancer 57:925–928, 1986)

even in this group. In fact, some have questioned whether breast cancer is ever cured.[17,18] Recent studies suggest that there is clearly a cured population and that this secondary force of mortality disappears but not until after at least 25 years.[19,20] Cure in the statistical sense can only be determined when the curve becomes parallel to that of the age-adjusted peer population. If this occurs and there is still an excess mortality due to the cancer, then there must be a compensatory decrease in mortality due to other causes. This presumably is an unlikely event.

Figure 10-43 gives examples of survival curve alterations induced by different therapies. Curve C represents a survival curve for a control group treated by surgery alone. In this example, the initial force of mortality is 8%, the inflection point is at 10 years, and the secondary force of mortality of 2.5% then obtains. Curve A represents the results of a therapy that produces delay in mortality, but following such delay both the initial and secondary forces of mortality are unchanged, as is the proportion of patients in each group. Early analysis of such survival curves will indicate a marked advantage to treatment A. In fact, for those therapies that cause delay, differences between the groups are greatest during the early years. Curve B is the result of a therapy that decreases the initial force of mortality but does not change the secondary force of mortality nor the proportion of patients in each group. For such a treatment, initial analysis will show only small differences; however, differences will increase, reaching a maximum at the inflection point in curve C and then diminishing. Thus, progressively spreading curves, which may give the impression of increased effectiveness, may not be representative of eventual differences in cure. Differences in cure can only be determined when the study has been followed past the control group inflection point. For adjuvant therapy, this has been seen in the randomized control study reported by Meakin and colleagues.[21] The results of this study demonstrate a decrease in the initial force of mortality and a decrease in the proportion of patients for whom this force of mortality applies. Ten-year analysis of the Milan adjuvant chemotherapy studies appears to begin to identify a similar effect for those premenopausal patients with only one to three positive nodes. However, sufficient time has not elapsed past the inflection point for definite determination of this. The effects of therapy with cyclophosphamide, methotrexate, and 5-fluorouracil (CMF) primarily appear to be a delay in the force of mortality. This does not mean that this is not important nor that a change in the inflection point will not occur. It does mean, however, that long-term follow-up is necessary in order to determine whether this is occurring.

The situation may be further complicated if the therapy has differing effects on the various subpopulations treated. For example, it is possible that a new therapy may be curative for one group within the treated population but deleterious for a different group. Figure 10-44 demonstrates the results of such a treatment. In this example, curve C represents conventional therapy and curve A such an alternative form. Curve A results in an increase in the initial force of mortality but an overall improved cure rate. Early analysis would have erroneously concluded that treatment A is inferior to treatment C. Thus, early analysis may be not only premature but frankly misleading. This early detrimental effect associated with increased cure is shown in the results of any therapy that detrimentally affects those patients not cured by it. A good example of this is the adverse effects of surgery when the patient's tumor cannot be removed. The patient then suffers the consequences of the surgical procedure itself and the resulting mortality and morbidity without deriving benefit. Another example is the use of inadequate radiation applied to patients unlikely to benefit. This has resulted in impaired survival.[22] The use of bone marrow transplanta-

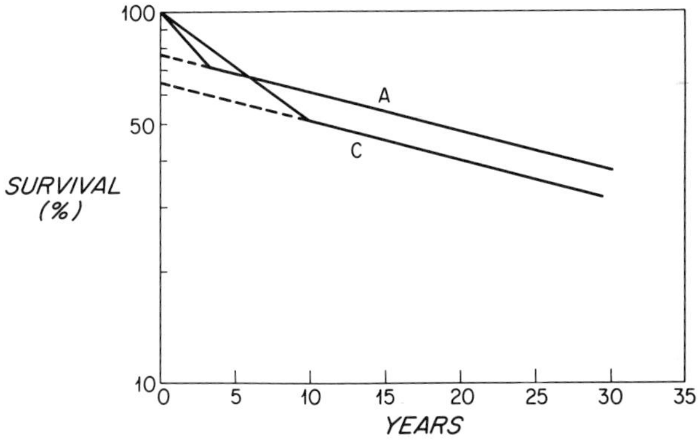

FIGURE 10-44. A comparison of survival curves after two hypothetical treatments for breast cancer. Curve C, control group; curve A, increased force of mortality initially but long-term survival improved. Notice that at 3 years, treatment A appears inferior to treatment C. (Harris JR, Hellman S: Observations on survival curve analysis with particular reference to breast cancer. Cancer 57:925–928, 1986)

tion to treat a disease ameliorated but less frequently cured by conventional chemotherapy is a graphic illustration of this effect. Such bone marrow transplantation is associated with a high morbidity and mortality and, therefore, would be detrimental for those not cured, but it would result in cure for patients not successfully treatable by other means. One might even interpret the most recent results of the Milan trial comparing 6 and 12 months of treatment with adjuvant CMF chemotherapy for breast cancer in this light. These results suggest that patients treated with 12 months of CMF are not improved and in fact, may be adversely affected. When these results are analyzed by the degree of node involvement, patients with one to three positive nodes had similar survival rates after either 6 or 12 months of treatment. The patients with four or more positive nodes treated for 12 months had a survival rate inferior to those treated for 6 months. Perhaps these results are due to two opposing effects of the chemotherapy—the first, an improvement in survival rate associated with tumor kill, and the second, a decrease in survival rate associated with the deleterious effects of such treatment on the host. Patients treated with the longer treatment program obviously are exposed to such deleterious effects for a longer period. When the tumor burden is small (patients with one to three positive nodes), the beneficial effect outweighs the deleterious one, and thus no difference is seen in the two groups differing in treatment duration. With patients with a larger tumor burden (four or more positive nodes), there appears to be little to be gained from such adjuvant chemotherapy, and thus the deleterious effects predominate for the patients treated for a longer period.

This interpretation illustrates the complex evaluation required when considering the initial portions of the survival curve when the population studied is not homogeneous and the treatment applied has both beneficial and deleterious effects. Such observations underscore the frustrations of clinical cancer research, particularly in breast cancer, which has such a long natural history. To assess accurately new forms of therapy, long follow-up is required. The prediction of the effect of such treatments allows one to anticipate the types of survival curve differences that should be seen and are necessary if we are to interpret early information properly. For clinicians caring for patients with breast cancer, there is a strong desire to improve the results of treatment. This has led to the common practice of reporting early results. This is necessary if we are to apply new information as soon as possible, but great care must be used in analysis lest erroneous conclusions be drawn.

What appears to emerge from these considerations of systemic adjuvant therapy is the importance of the identification of the risk of occult metastases in the individual patient. When the risk is high, then aggressive adjuvant treatment seems appropriate. As the toxicity of such treatment decreases, then the population of patients for whom it might be applied increases. Conversely, when the therapy is only modestly effective, its greatest application may be only for those with a very small tumor burden rather than for those with a large tumor burden. As treatment efficacy increases, then it becomes more applicable to those with larger tumor burdens. This emphasizes the importance of studying such aggressive therapies in patients in whom the tumor burden is high. This group appears to gain less from conventional adjuvant therapy, thus making them candidates for such experiments. Therapies that delay the progress of disease without increasing cure may still be of value if the delay is significant, the therapy is relatively nontoxic, and the population of patients is older. Such may be the case with adjuvant tamoxifen therapy in the postmenopausal woman. Those therapies that increase cure are, of course, especially desirable in the younger patient.

These treatment considerations offer many opportunities for influencing the natural history of breast cancer. Optimism should prevail, since even with the current state of knowledge, it appears that much can be done. Early diagnosis can significantly reduce mortality. This can be implemented by active screening programs, breast self-examination, and the opportunity for patients to seek medical attention at the earliest possible moment. Techniques that assure adequate local therapy appear to decrease the possibility for distant metastases. Such effective local therapies appear to be at hand. As the form of local treatment becomes more acceptable, patients will be less fearful and may seek treatment earlier. Adjuvant hormonal therapy and chemotherapy appear to offer real reduction in the probability of dying of breast cancer. How much of this is delay in appearance of metastases, reduced force of mortality, or actual improvement in cure remains to be seen. However, that there is a significant meaningful effect appears certain. We need to understand what the nature of this effect is and for whom such adjuvant therapies are appropriate. Although analysis of early results is risky, it is necessary if we are to advance in our treatment of breast cancer. In advocating such advances, we must be tentative and willing to change. Our current therapies—surgery, radiation therapy, and chemotherapy—are often toxic and may have only modest effects on outcome. Where this is the case, we should look for and expect changes. Until we devise a simple, effective, nonmorbid therapy, we should remain open to all potential therapeutic advances.

REFERENCES

1. Breasted JH: The Edwin Smith Surgical Papyrus, Vol. 1, p 363, 463, Chicago, University of Chicago Press, 1930
2. Meyer W: An improved method of the radical operation for carcinoma of the breast. Med Rec 46:746, 1894
3. Halsted WS: The results of operations for the care of cancer of the breast performed at the Johns Hopkins Hospital from June 1889 to January 1894. Johns Hopkins Hosp Bull 4:297, 1894–5
4. Halsted WS: The results of radical operations for the cure of carcinoma of the breast. Ann Surg 46:1, 1907
5. Urban JA: Breast cancer 1985: What have we learned? Cancer 57:636–643, 1986
6. McWhirter R: The value of simple mastectomy and radiotherapy in the treatment of breast cancer. Br J Radiol 21:599, 1948
7. Bonadonna G, Valagussa P, Rossi A: Ten year experience with CMF-based adjuvant chemotherapy in resectable breast cancer. Breast Cancer Res Treat 5:95–115, 1985
8. Shapiro S, Vemet WL, Strax P, et al: Ten to fourteen year effects of breast cancer screening on mortality. J Natl Cancer Inst 69:349–353, 1982
9. Tabar L, Gad A, Holmberg LH, et al: Reduction in mortality from breast cancer after mass screening with mammography. Lancet 1:829–832, 1985
10. Koscielny S, Tubiana M, Le MG, et al: Breast Cancer: Relationship between the size of the primary tumour and the probability of metastatic dissemination. Br J Cancer 49:709–715, 1984
11. Fisher B, Bauer M, Margolese R, et al: Five year results of a randomized clinical trial comparing mastectomy and segmental mastectomy with or without radiation in the treatment of breast cancer. N Engl J Med 312:665–673, 1985
12. Harris JR, Hellman S: Affecting the natural history of breast cancer. (in press)
13. Peto R: Review of mortality results in randomized trials in early breast cancer. Lancet 11:1205, 1984
14. Harris JR, Hellman S: Observations on survival curve analysis with particular reference to breast cancer. Cancer 57:925–928, 1986
15. Adair F, Berg J, Voubert L, et al: Long-term follow-up of breast cancer patients: The 30 year report. Cancer 33:1145–1150, 1974
16. Ferguson DV, Meier P, Karrison T, et al: Staging of breast cancer and survival rates: An assessment based on 50 years of experience with radical mastectomy. JAMA 248:1337–1341, 1982
17. Park WW, Lees VC: The absolute curability of cancer of the breast. Surg Gynecol Obstet 93:129–157, 1951
18. Fox MS: On the diagnosis and treatment of breast cancer. JAMA 241:489–494, 1979
19. Brinkley D, Haybittle JL: The curability of breast cancer. Lancet 2:95–97, 1975
20. Rutqvist LE, Wallgren A, Nilsson B: Is breast cancer a curable disease? A study of 14,731 women with breast cancer from the Cancer Registry of Norway. Cancer 53:1793–1800, 1984
21. Meakin JW, Allt WEC, Beale FA, et al: Ovarian irradiation and prednisone following surgery and radiotherapy for carcinoma of the breast. Breast Cancer Res Treat (suppl 1) 3:45–48, 1983
22. Palmer MK, Ribeiro GG: Thirty-four year follow-up of patients with breast cancer in a clinical trial of postoperative radiotherapy. Br Med J 291:1088–1091, 1985

In Situ Cancers

11

Frank E. Gump

The concept of *in situ* cancer was introduced into American medicine in 1932 by Broders[1] in an effort to better define the transition between benign and malignant epithelium. The basic concept stresses abnormal cells that remain confined to their original boundaries, and *in situ* cancers have been studied in a variety of organs. An important corollary is the absence of clinical findings; diagnosis is by microscopic examination.

The term was formally applied to the breast by Foote and Stewart in 1941 in their description of lobular carcinoma *in situ*.[2] This description was consistent with the original concept of *in situ* lesions, which were thought to represent an intermediate point in the progression to overtly invasive, malignant disease. *In situ* lesions were not considered static or capable of regression; rather, inevitable progression was postulated. Such a straightforward relationship posed no problem for the clinician. If a lesion will inevitably progress to invasive cancer, aggressive treatment is obviously called for.

Recent studies have forced a re-evaluation of the *in situ* concept as far as the breast is concerned. *In situ* ductal and lobular lesions continue to be recognized and reported in increasing numbers by pathologists. However, the malignant potential of these lesions is no longer considered a simple, straightforward problem, and therapeutic recommendations have become increasingly controversial.

This chapter examines the diagnosis, prevalence, and natural history of the two types of *in situ* breast cancers. The two types will be contrasted and related to both benign proliferation and invasive cancer. Therapeutic recommendations will be based on these data, recognizing that limited information makes specific treatment recommendations difficult.

LOBULAR VERSUS INTRADUCTAL CARCINOMA *IN SITU*

The diagnosis of carcinoma depends on histologic evidence of cells no longer confined by their natural boundaries. For that reason, the term *in situ* carcinoma has always been somewhat contradictory. The original descriptions of *in situ* lesions were in association with invasive cancer. Cells that clearly resembled those of the invading tumor were seen within adjacent ducts and lobules but were labeled *in situ* because they were still confined to the normal breast structures. Two separate diagnoses evolved. The first, involving breast lobules, was identified as lobular carcinoma *in situ* (LCIS); the second related to the small terminal ducts and was referred to as intraductal carcinoma *in situ* (DCIS). LCIS has a distinctive histologic appearance. Epithelial cells proliferate and completely fill the acinar lumens. As the acini are filled by this new population of cells, the affected lobules become larger and more prominent. It is thought that the new strain of cells evolves from the normal epithelium of both acini and terminal ducts. As a rule, duct involvement from LCIS can readily be distinguished from *in situ* intraductal carcinoma, so the two types of lesions are not usually confused.[3]

A diagnostic problem does exist as far as DCIS is concerned. Pathologists have focused on the various histologic patterns such as solid, comedo, cribriform, cartwheel, cobweb, or papillary, and when the cells are confined within ducts the term DCIS has been applied. These lesions were usually detected as a clinically palpable mass or possibly as Paget's disease of the nipple. This variant of breast cancer was extremely rare, as exemplified by a 1978 American College of Surgeons national survey of breast carcinoma, showing that intraductal carcinoma *in situ* constituted 0.84% of 24,000 new breast cancers recorded that year.[4] A different perspective on DCIS lesions comes from the report of the Breast Cancer Detection Demonstration Project because this massive screening effort relied heavily on mammography.[5] A total of 3557 cancers was detected, and they were classified into four types. The first category was noninfiltrating or *in situ* lesions, category two consisted of invasive lesions less than 1 cm in diameter, category three comprised lesions greater than 1 cm, and a fourth category existed because size was not stated in some instances. There were 782 cancers recorded in the noninfiltrating group, and this constituted 22% of the total number of cancers detected. Although this sizable percentage of *in situ* cancers is consistent with any mammographic screening effort, many of these lesions were actually palpable. Biopsies were performed solely because of an abnormality seen on mammography in 461 patients (59%), whereas in 258 patients (33%) the tumor was both palpable and evident on x-ray. In an additional 43 patients (6%) with *in situ* carcinoma, the lesion was detectable only on physical examination.

When DCIS is defined in this fashion, it does not conform to the original *in situ* concept (a microscopic lesion that cannot be detected clinically), but the histologic similarity to purely microscopic intraductal lesions resulted in the application of the common term DCIS. This semantic problem was of little concern until the widespread use of mammography brought large numbers of patients with the microscopic lesion to our attention. At this point, the term DCIS can mean anything from a 5-cm clinically obvious lesion (with or without axillary metastases) to a minute focus of occult calcification on a mammogram. Clinicians must distinguish between patients with clinical (palpable) lesions and those with the microscopic lesions (usually diagnosed following biopsy for microcalcifications). When mammographic screening is employed, the number of DCIS patients will be dramatically increased. This can readily be appreciated when one contrasts the extremely low incidence reported by the American College of Surgeons Survey in 1978 with the figure from the Breast Cancer Demonstration Project.

The section on DCIS will emphasize the differences between the grossly obvious and the microscopic forms of the disease but will focus on the latter because it is more consistent with the *in situ* concept.

LOBULAR CARCINOMA *IN SITU*

LCIS was first identified as a specific entity in 1941.[2] This is somewhat surprising, given that the lesion is easily recognized microscopically and that the breast was extensively studied by generations of pathologists up to that time. It is worth remembering that the original paper by Foote and Stewart is subtitled *A Rare Form of Mammary Cancer.* These authors reviewed 300 mastectomies and found two patients with the pure *in situ* lesion. In another 12 patients, the lesion was accompanied by conventional infiltrating lobular carcinoma. Foote and Stewart recognized that the lobular lesion had special characteristics when seen alone. Most importantly, it was a microscopic and not a gross diagnosis, and it did not metastasize. However, the concept promulgated in the paper was that both the lobular and invasive forms constituted a single disease that represented a rare form of breast cancer. Although this concept was widely accepted, increasing evidence has been presented that the microscopic lesion described by Foote and Stewart has characteristics very unlike those of carcinoma.

The true incidence of the lesion is not known, since it does not form a palpable tumor and therefore cannot be identified clinically or grossly. The available information comes from biopsy studies, mastectomy specimens, and autopsy studies. The studies of breast biopsies involve selected patient populations, since a clinical problem would have led to the biopsy. Furthermore, since the lesion that necessitated the biopsy is not LCIS, the incidence depends on the amount of adjacent tissue excised and the care with which it is examined. Finally, biopsy material allows examination of only a small portion of the breast.

Autopsy and mastectomy studies avoid the biases of tissue selection, but mastectomy specimens usually come from patients with cancer. Autopsy studies of patients dying without breast disease represent the best approach, but examination of all the breast tissue constitutes an enormous effort and for that reason it has been accomplished only in a small number of breasts. In summary, biopsy studies are available in large numbers but suffer from patient and tissue selection; autopsy studies have been limited but probably provide a better guide to prevalence in the general population.

One of the most extensive and thorough reviews of biopsy material was carried out by Haagensen from the files of the Surgical Pathology Laboratory at Columbia's College of Physicians and Surgeons.[6] Specimens from more than 5000 patients who underwent a biopsy between 1930 and 1972 for what was reported as benign disease were reviewed, and 211 cases of lobular neoplasia—Haagensen's term for LCIS—were identified. This study revealed that lobular neoplasia constituted 3.6% of all benign epithelial breast lesions. A lower figure was reported by Wheeler and associates, who reviewed 3570 benign lesions. These authors found LCIS in 0.8% of their biopsies,[7] whereas Andersen found it in 1.5% of his series of 3299 benign lesions.[8]

Every review of this condition has stressed the fact that it is primarily found in premenopausal women. Haagensen noted that 88% of his patients were premenopausal and 12% were postmenopausal.[9] Rosen reported 22 premenopausal patients and 8 menopausal women.[10] Only 9 of his patients were postmenopausal. This suggests that LCIS regresses after menopause, but the nature of biopsy material forces one to be cautious. The overwhelming number of benign epithelial lesions that require biopsy appear during the reproductive years, and since the diagnosis of LCIS is made as a result of these biopsies, it is obvious that all such reviews would reflect this age distribution. It has been shown that there is normally some degree of involution of the lobular elements of the breast with advancing age. It may be that LCIS follows this pattern and that the decrease in lesions is real. Regardless of this fact, the risk of cancer, which will be discussed subsequently, certainly does not decrease after menopause.

Autopsy studies are better suited to examine age distribution, but they are also subject to limitations. LCIS probably does not represent a static process. Any effort to better understand the natural history of the lesion would have to focus on the initiation and possible regression of the process, and such information cannot come from an autopsy study. Some degree of selection is also present in that most studies are skewed toward elderly patients and the small numbers usually make it impossible to dissect out risk factors relating to breast cancer.

One of the earliest and most extensive autopsy reports was carried out by Frantz and associates.[11] Although the incidence of cystic disease was under investigation, it is of note that no cases of LCIS were found in 225 autopsies. Frantz's paper appeared 10 years after the report of Foote and Stewart, and she was well aware of the lesion described by these authors. A wide age range (13 to 88) was covered, and the median was 45 years.

Another autopsy series presented a very different picture in that an appreciable number of neoplastic lesions were found.[12] This Danish study is of interest in that it comes from a country with both a high autopsy rate and one of the highest rates of breast cancer. The material came from 83 consecutive unselected autopsies of women over the age of 20. However, the age of the study group was not further specified. A thorough investigation of glandular tissue was carried out, as evidenced by the fact that 57 to 166 blocks were reviewed from each breast. Six patients were known to have breast cancer, and three of them actually died of metastatic disease. A total of 14 *in situ* cancers were detected; 3 of these were pure LCIS, another 3 were in association with DCIS. The remainder were ductal lesions. The authors noted that their frequency of *in situ* cancers was higher than previous reports but attributed this to the completeness of their histologic search.

A recent study by Alpers and Wellings failed to substantiate these findings despite extensive investigation of 185 randomly selected breasts from autopsies of 101 patients.[13] The sampling technique was exhaustive and permitted the identification of essentially the entire breast epithelium.[14] No instances of LCIS were found. This may in part reflect the age of the patients, since 70% of them were 50 years or older at the time of death. The age factor was even more marked in another autopsy study, reported by Kramer and Rush,[15] of women dying without known breast disease. These authors found no instances of LCIS in 140 breasts, but their study group was confined to women over 70 years of age.

Alpers and Wellings also studied breasts with cancer and contralateral to cancer. In 59 breasts with a clinically identified primary tumor, they found 8 (13.6%) with LCIS. In 44 breasts contralateral to a breast with invasive cancer, 6 such lesions were identified. This suggests that LCIS, although a rare lesion in the general population, may be a significant marker for clinical carcinoma.

The malignant potential of LCIS, and hence the proper treatment, remains a subject of controversy. Information regarding the natural history of LCIS comes entirely from patients treated by biopsy alone and then followed for a suitable interval. Although all authors stress that they are studying LCIS occurring alone—in other words, in the absence of invasive cancer—there has been no agreement on the inclusion of patients with prior invasive cancer in the other breast. Haagensen includes patients in whom true carcinoma had occurred in one breast prior to the diagnosis of lobular neoplasia occurring alone in the other breast.[16] Such cases were excluded in the reports of Hutter and Foote[17] and Wheeler and associates.[7] Since the question of malignant potential relates to cancer developing in the ipsi- or contralateral breast, the time sequence—that is, whether the carcinoma was identified prior to or subsequent to the point when a biopsy turned up LCIS in one breast—should be of secondary importance. This view is certainly consistent with Haagensen's view that lobular neoplasia represents a marker of risk rather than a lesion that will transform itself into an invasive cancer.

Haagensen reported on 297 patients who underwent a biopsy between 1930 and 1977.[9] All but four patients were observed for 5 or more years, and 208 of them from 11 to 47 years. The average follow-up was 16.3 years, and only two were lost. Breast cancer developed in 63 patients, or 21% of the total series. If the 10 patients whose LCIS was diagnosed after an invasive cancer of the opposite side were excluded, the percentage would fall to 18% (53 of 287). Table 11-1 contrasts the four series available for review.

The Memorial Hospital series, recently updated by Rosen,[18] has the longest period of follow-up but the most patients lost. This series also has the highest percentage of patients that went on to develop invasive cancer. The fact that 16% of the patients could not be traced raises a question about the 37% figure. Patients are easier to trace if they come to mastectomy, and if the patients that were lost remained disease free, the figure would fall to 31%, which more closely approximates the results reported by other authors (see Table 11-1).

Wheeler and associates reported on 35 patients, 6 of whom developed invasive cancer.[7] Andersen studied 52 patients with a long period of follow-up. Fifteen of them developed cancer.[8]

The simple percentage of patients developing subsequent carcinoma is probably not the best way to compare these reports because it is too dependent on the length of follow-up. An actuarial analysis could be used, but the ratio of observed to expected cases is probably preferable because this method of analysis not only takes into account the years of follow-up but also the ages and calendar years at which the patients were expected to develop carcinoma.

Haagensen used the state of Connecticut incidence rates for breast cancer by 10-year and 5-year age-groups to determine that 8.93 of his patients would have been

Table 11-1
Lobular Carcinoma in Situ (LCIS)

Study	*Number of Patients*	*Patients Lost to Follow-up*	*Mean Length of Follow-up*	*Cancer in Biopsied Breast (No Mastectomy)*	*Cancer in Other Breast*	*Total Number of Patients Developing Cancer*
Wheeler et al, 1974[7]	35	0	15.7	1/25 (4%)	5/34 (15%)	6/35 (17.1%)
Andersen, 1974[8]	52	0	15	9/46 (20%)	9/52 (17.3%)	15/52 (28.8%)
Rosen et al, 1978[18]	99	15	24	18/83 (22%)	17/83 (20%)	31/84 (36.9%)
Haagensen et al, 1981[16]	268	2	14.7	27/257 (10.5%)	27/258 (10.5%)	48/266 (18%)

expected to develop breast cancer. The greater number of observed cases resulted in a ratio of observed to expected cases of 6.9 to 1. Rosen and associates presented similar data also using the Connecticut Tumor Registry data. Their ratio was 9:1 when calculated on the basis of 77 of the 99 patients for whom all necessary information was available. Andersen also reported the ratio of observed to expected carcinomas in his series of patients. He excluded five patients in whom invasive cancer was diagnosed prior to the appearance of LCIS in the opposite breast. In the remaining 44 patients, the ratio of observed to expected cancers was 12:1. The ratios in the two large series (Columbia and Memorial) are similar, which is reassuring since these two reports provide our best guide to the natural history of this lesion when treated by biopsy alone.

It is important to note that all series agree that patients developing cancer do so with equal frequency in the biopsied and the opposite breast. Despite this fact, it has not always been possible to document that the actual lesion is bilateral. Tissue was available from both breasts in 73 of the patients in the Columbia series, and only 19 patients (26%) were found to have bilateral LCIS. This may reflect the spotty distribution of the lesion as well as the fact that a biopsy provides limited material for examination.

Mirror-image biopsies done in patients with LCIS provide additional information regarding the bilaterality of the lesion. Newman reported on 26 such patients subjected to mirror-image biopsies, and LCIS was found in 6 of them.[19] Urban's larger series of 159 mirror-image biopsies included 26 patients with LCIS. Nine patients were found to have LCIS in the contralateral breast.[20] Therefore, the incidence of LCIS in the opposite breast varies from 23% (Newman) to 35% (Urban), with Haagensen's figure of 26% falling in between. These percentages are based on biopsy specimens, and if all of the contralateral breast could be examined the percentages would undoubtedly be higher. As noted before, the low incidence of histologically documented bilaterality in patients with LCIS should not obscure the fact that invasive cancers appear with equal frequency in both breasts.

There is uncertainty on how to view the malignant potential of the actual lesion in the breast. Are the small round cells with pale cytoplasm that fill the acini truly malignant cells, or is this simply a proliferative process that serves to mark a patient as being at increased risk of developing breast cancer? Cancers that develop in patients with LCIS are usually invasive ductal rather than lobular on histologic examination.[6,7] Haagensen reported on the microscopic type of 51 of the 54 carcinomas that developed in his series. Thirteen were invasive lobular and could conceivably have come from the lobular lesion diagnosed previously. However, the remaining lesions were primarily infiltrating ductal, the most common histologic type in any series of invasive breast cancers. At this time, the processes relating LCIS to invasive carcinoma are not known. Many efforts have been made both by light[21] and electron microscopy[22] to identify features that might be useful in distinguishing patients at greater or lesser risk of developing invasive cancer, but no reliable guides have been developed.[23]

The available information makes it clear that a patient diagnosed as having LCIS has three options available: (1) to do no surgery and rely on close observation, a course first advocated by Haagensen; (2) an ipsilateral mastectomy with biopsy of the opposite breast and contralateral mastectomy if LCIS is found, and finally, (3) bilateral mastectomy. The role of radiation in the treatment of LCIS has yet to be defined.

Haagensen felt that observation was justified given the fact that the ratio between observed and expected cases of breast cancer was 6.9:1.[9] A similar risk ratio exists for women with mothers who have bilateral breast cancer, and, although there is obviously concern in this situation, mastectomy is not recommended. For that reason it was Haagensen's policy to offer close observation to patients with LCIS. This approach has been continued to the present day. Patients are carefully instructed, and an abstract of Table 11-1 is presented to the patient and her family. Follow-up visits take place every 4 to 6 months, and an annual mammogram is mandatory. Research studies involving blood, cyst fluid, and tissue markers are under way in an effort to identify patients with the greatest likelihood of developing cancer, but clear guidelines have not yet emerged.

Haagensen and Bodian examined the effect of other risk factors acting on patients with LCIS.[16] In patients with LCIS, no family history of breast carcinoma, and no gross cystic disease, the ratio of observed to expected carcinoma was 5.9:1. When there was cystic disease but no family history, the ratio was 5.6:1. In patients with LCIS and a mother or sister with breast cancer, the risk was 8.5:1, indicating a cumulative predisposition to breast cancer when the risk factors of lobular neoplasia and family history are combined.

When the policy of observation was introduced, it was Haagensen's hope that close follow-up would result in early detection so that mastectomy would be curative. The program has been effective in that patients developing cancer while under observation have had clinical Stage I disease. However, lymph node metastases were noted in 23% of the patients after axillary clearing, and this figure is little different from the 28% recorded for all Stage I patients presenting to the Columbia-Presbyterian Breast Service. More recent concepts concerning the natural history of breast cancer require a re-evaluation of the efficacy of early detection, so the risks have to be carefully reviewed with the patient.

Mastectomy on the involved side with contralateral biopsy has long been advocated by the Memorial Hospital Breast Service.[24] As noted previously, contralateral biopsies would be expected to show LCIS in approximately 25% of the patients, but the remaining 75% whose biopsies were negative would still be exposed to the same risk that led to mastectomy on the side of the original biopsy. It is for this reason that bilateral mastectomy would appear to be a more logical approach in patients who elect surgery as opposed to observation.

Patients will obviously be involved in the choice between close follow-up and bilateral mastectomy. The emotional impact of such surgery has to be balanced against the patient's anxiety about breast cancer. Clearly this is a personal decision. We have continued to follow Haagensen's view that LCIS (or his preferred name, lobular neoplasia) is a powerful marker for invasive carcinoma without direct participation in the process of malignant transformation. Similar views have been expressed by others[13,25] and have encouraged us to continue to offer close observation as the standard method of treatment. The controversy surrounding this lesion is discussed openly, and patients are encouraged to participate in the final decision.

INTRADUCTAL CARCINOMA *IN SITU*

Pathologists tend to consider *in situ* carcinoma as a midpoint in the process of epithelial unrest that starts with proliferation and atypia and ends with invasive cancer. Certainly pathologists will at times experience difficulty in separating *in situ* carcinoma from severe atypia, as well as *in situ* carcinoma from microscopic invasion. There has even been a tendency to regard the two *in situ* cancers as alternative morphological manifestations of epithelial proliferation in the breast. The clinician, however, is faced with the need to treat patients identified at different points along this presumed pathway, and certain guidelines are necessary. The discussion of LCIS makes it clear that the relationship between *in situ* and invasive cancer is complex. The following section illustrates that similar problems exist when intraductal lesions are considered, and even more importantly, the two *in situ* cancers have differences that will affect decisions regarding treatment.

Most autopsy studies show DCIS to be the more common of the two *in situ* lesions, but Andersen has recently expressed the opposite view.[23] Since true *in situ* lesions do not make a clinically palpable mass, the exact incidence of both lesions remains unknown. The selection and especially the age of the study group will play a major role in the incidence of the two lesions. However, autopsy studies make it clear the DCIS is still an uncommon finding in the general population. The thought that the breast might resemble the prostate in harboring large numbers of microscopic, clinically undetected carcinomas has not been borne out. Kramer and Rush, in a study mentioned previously, put this question to the test.[15] They studied 140 breasts from women who died after the age of 70 but found only 4 instances of DCIS. Alpers and Welling, whose detailed autopsy study was also mentioned previously, found nine patients, for an incidence of 5.9%.[13] Sandison found 6 patients with DCIS in 766 randomly selected patients without clinical evidence of breast cancer.[26] The Danish study by Nielsen and colleagues stands out as it did in the LCIS section because of its high incidence of *in situ* cancer.[12] The figure of 16% should be regarded cautiously, since it is a small, generally uncharacterized sample and the paper presented no illustrations of the ductal lesions listed as DCIS.

The frequency of DCIS in biopsy material is very dependent on the time period under review. In the large retrospective slide reviews done at Memorial[18] and Vanderbilt,[27] the study periods were 1940–1950 and 1950–1968, respectively. This was prior to the large-scale use of mammography, and, even though approximately 10,000 biopsies were reviewed at both institutions, very few intraductal carcinomas were found. The Memorial study reported 30 women,[24] and the Vanderbilt group found 28 patients.[27] Patients with Paget's disease were excluded, and these were true microscopic lesions. These reviews would indicate that DCIS is less common than LCIS. The Memorial review identified 99 patients with the lobular lesion, or about 3 times the number of *in situ* ductal cancers. However, the picture has changed dramatically since the advent of routine mammographic screening. The tendency for intraductal lesions to precipitate calcium into the lumen of the abnormal duct has resulted in a large-scale increase in the number of DCIS patients.

An abnormal mammogram may necessitate a biopsy in the absence of a palpable mass for a number of reasons. However, microcalcifications represent the specific indication associated with intraductal carcinoma *in situ*. It is important to point out that large, invasive, and easily palpable carcinomas may also be associated with microcalcifications. The mammogram will usually show a density or some parenchymal distortion. If true *in situ* cancer is involved, the microcalcifications represent the only abnormality and the surgeon will recognize no gross abnormality when the breast tissue is cut.[28] When x-ray calcifications represent the only indication for biopsy, between

50% and 75% of the cancers will be *in situ* lesions,[29,30] and the vast majority of those will be ductal rather than lobular.[31] When the histopathology is reviewed, the calcium is usually in the necrotic centers of malignant ducts. When LCIS is the only finding, the calcium is in adjacent tissue rather than involved acini. This would explain the high incidence of ductal lesions when biopsies are done for microcalcifications.[32] The association between DCIS and calcium deposition appears to be specific, although the distribution of the microcalcifications and the histologic lesions in the breast do not necessarily correspond.[33]

Although DCIS was long thought to be a straightforward, malignant lesion, a few publications in the early 1970s questioned this concept.[34,35] However, the first definitive study detailing the natural history of this lesion when treated by biopsy alone appeared in 1978 when Betsill and colleagues reported on 25 women.[36] These patients were identified in the review of almost 10,000 biopsies done at Memorial Hospital for benign disease between 1940 and 1950. The 99 patients found to have LCIS were discussed previously. Clinical records were available for 15 of the 25 women with DCIS, including 10 with long-term follow up. The follow-up period in this later group averaged 21.6 years, and seven of the ten patients developed cancer after an average interval of 9.7 years. Is this an incidence of 70% (7 of 10) or 28% (7 of 25)? An earlier paper by Farrow did not address this problem specifically, but in a general discussion of *in situ* cancers, he included 25 patients with DCIS treated by local excision only.[37] Six patients (24%) developed invasive cancer, but the total number of patients observed was not reported. Reports by Haagensen,[38] Dean and Geschickter,[39] and Kraus and Neubecker[40] are not relevant because these were often large and always clinically obvious lesions. The present discussion of DCIS remains focused on microscopic lesions that would not be detected clinically (except possibly on mammogram).

The only other study that examined such patients was recently reported by Page and associates.[27] It resembles the Memorial Study in that 28 women with DCIS were found in reviewing a large number of breast biopsies. These women were treated by biopsy only, since the original diagnosis given to the surgeon was "benign." Follow-up information was obtained on all 28 patients, and 7 developed invasive cancer, suggesting a 25% incidence. However, three patients were followed for less than 3 years, and two died of unrelated causes within 2 years of biopsy. Another had bilateral mastectomies shortly after the biopsy. The remaining 18 women who did not develop carcinoma were observed from 8 to 27 years (average 16 years). The information presented above suggests that approximately 20% to 30% of patients with DCIS will go on to invasive carcinoma. However, it is conceivable that all of the *in situ* cancer was removed by the biopsy in some patients. In patients whose DCIS is treated by mastectomy, residual DCIS was found in 60% in one series[41] and 66% in another.[42] Therefore, no additional lesions could be demonstrated in about one-third of the patients. If we accept 30% as the risk of developing invasive cancer after a biopsy showing DCIS and 60% of the patients have residual disease in the breast, the risk of the ductal lesion progressing to invasive cancer would be about 50%. Such assumptions regarding residual DCIS may have validity, because when additional DCIS is found in the breast the lesions are usually in the same quadrant as the biopsy.[43] Table 11-2 lists and compares the various DCIS reports discussed above.

Although the percentage of patients who go on to invasive carcinoma is roughly similar in DCIS and LCIS, this should not obscure the fact that important differences exist (Table 11-3). The major one relates to the site of invasive cancer when it appears following DCIS treated by biopsy only. These cancers are inevitably on the side of the biopsy and usually at the site of the biopsy wound.[27] This implies that progression of the actual intraductal lesion took place in those patients and constitutes the major justification for a different approach to the two *in situ* lesions.

Table 11-2
Ductal Carcinoma in Situ (DCIS)

Study	Number of Patients	Type of DCIS Gross	Micro	Mean Follow-up (Years)	Patients with Breast Cancer: Number	Percent of Total	Percent of Patients Followed	Interval to Breast Cancer (Years)
Dean & Geschickter[39]	8	8	0	7	6	75	75	1–4
Kraus & Neubecker[40]	4	4	0	10	2	50	50	10–12
Farrow[37]	25	?25	? 0	not stated	5	20	20	1–8
Haagensen[38]	11	11	0	13.5	8	73	73	Av. 4.7
Betsill et al[36]	25	0	25	21.6	7	28	70	Av. 9.7
Page et al[27]	28	0	28	15	7	25	28	Av. 6.1

Table 11-3
Comparison of Lobular Carcinoma in Situ and Ductal Carcinoma in Situ

	Lobular Carcinoma in Situ	*Ductal Carcinoma in Situ*
Age	Primarily premenopausal	Pre- and postmenopausal
Physical findings	None	None with micro form Mass with gross form
Metastases	None	None with micro form Possible with gross form
Malignant potential	Bilateral risk	Risk in biopsied breast, usually in biopsy area
Mammogram	No specific findings	Microcalcifications

The traditional recommendation has been ipsilateral total mastectomy. Although lymph node metastases have been reported in patients with DCIS,[42] these have always been in patients with clinically obvious lesions and not the truly microscopic lesions. Mastectomy constitutes effective therapy, with a cure rate that approaches 100%.[24] However, it comes at a high price, especially to women who have been promised that early detection will allow them to preserve their breast.

Radiation therapy and wide local excision have both been employed, although experience with these alternatives remains limited. A recent report by Montague included 345 patients treated with conservation therapy and irradiation.[44] Fifty-four were classified as "minimal cancer," an unfortunate term that combines the two *in situ* lesions with small invasive cancers. The author did state that 34 patients had noninvasive intraductal carcinomas and only 1 of the total group of 54 had a local recurrence. This was in an untreated axilla and may well have been from the invasive group. The 10-year disease-free survival rate was 92%, but this means very little since the *in situ* and small invasive cancers were considered together.

Findlay and Goodman were the first to present specific information regarding the results of radiotherapy in the treatment of DCIS.[45] From 1979 to 1981, these authors treated 14 patients. Two of the 14 required mastectomy for recurrence 19 and 36 months following initial treatment. Careful reading of their paper makes it clear that these patients had gross and not microscopic disease. These patients have recently been incorporated into a larger group of DCIS patients reported by Recht and coworkers.[46] The combined group totaled 40 patients treated between 1976 and 1983. Patients having predominantly or exclusively LCIS were excluded, as were patients with clinical Paget's disease. Clinical features that led to the diagnosis of DCIS were listed, and most of the patients had gross disease. A palpable mass was present in 27, and an additional 4 patients had bloody nipple discharge. The remaining nine patients underwent biopsy solely because of a positive mammogram; in three of them, the mammogram showed a mass, and three others were "positive" but details were not available. The final three patients underwent biopsy with microcalcifications as the only indication. The median follow-up was 44 months, and four local recurrences were recorded. At the time of recurrence, three of the four patients had mammograms, and the recurrence was detected only on mammography in these three patients. The mammographic findings were microcalcifications. These findings are consistent with a recent case report involving a patient whose purely microscopic DCIS was treated by irradiation.[47] The patient again developed microcalcifications 3 years later, and, when biopsied, the tissue was grossly normal but microscopic DCIS was present once again.

Recht and co-workers noted that three of the four local recurrences were in patients who presented with nipple discharge and a central primary tumor. This was obviously the gross rather than the purely microscopic form of DCIS and could be related to incomplete excision of the tumor. The same authors had previously reported a series of patients with invasive cancers and noted that extensive intraductal disease within the tumor and in the adjacent grossly normal breast tissue appears to result in a much higher rate of recurrence within the irradiated breast.[48] When *in situ* tumor was present in tissue adjacent to the invasive tumor, a 17% failure rate was noted at 5 years. It is not clear if this reflects a problem related to complete excision or radiation resistance of DCIS. Since the breast epithelium is not sterilized by irradiation, the continued presence of breast tissue may give rise to additional foci of DCIS.

Additional information regarding radiotherapy in the treatment of DCIS comes from the National Surgical Adjuvant Breast Project (Protocol 6).[49] When pathologists reviewed the slides of the 2072 patients in the trial, they found 78 that fit their criteria for DCIS. Fifty-one of these patients had been treated by lumpectomy; 29 received radiation afterward and the remaining 22 were observed. Seven local recurrences were recorded during the average follow-up period of 39 months—five in the lumpectomy alone group but only two in the lumpectomy group that received radiation. Unfortunately, this series represents almost entirely gross DCIS in that there was only one patient biopsied because of an abnormal mammogram. All the others presented with a palpable tumor, and the average size was 2.2 cm. Clearly, this study does not deal with a microscopic lesion that cannot be detected grossly.

The material presented in Table 11-2 as well as the above discussion suggests a need to re-examine the definition of DCIS. At this time, the diagnosis encompasses everything from large breast tumors with or without axillary and systemic involvement to a minute focus of abnormal cells lining a single duct in grossly normal breast tissue. We have recently reviewed all patients with the diagnosis of DCIS seen at the Columbia Presbyterian Medical Center between 1983 and 1985 in an effort to better define this lesion.[50] During this 3-year period, a total of 70 patients with a variety of breast problems were listed as having DCIS as their major diagnosis. An effort was made to separate this group into the gross and microscopic form of DCIS using a number of criteria. A patient who had a palpable mass that was clearly neoplastic on biopsy or presented with nipple discharge or an ulcerated nipple was considered to have the gross form of DCIS. If the biopsy specimen had the appearance of normal breast tissue, the lesion was categorized as the microscopic form of DCIS.

Forty-eight of the 70 patients had a palpable mass or nipple discharge or both, and an additional 4 patients had Paget's disease of the nipple. Purely microscopic DCIS was diagnosed in 16 patients; 13 of these were biopsied with mammographic microcalcifications as the only indication, and in the remaining 3 patients microscopic DCIS constituted an incidental finding in the course of surgery for benign lesions. In one patient, the DCIS was adjacent to fibroadenoma, in another a cyst led to the biopsy, and in the third of these patients DCIS was found in a mastectomy specimen removed for LCIS. The DCIS in these last three patients would be equivalent to that reported in the two large retrospective reviews discussed previously, except that the diagnosis of DCIS was made at the time of the original biopsy.

Two patients require special mention in that they presented with microcalcifications on mammography and had no abnormal physical findings. Although such a presentation would be regarded as an occult carcinoma, at the time of biopsy they were found to have a grossly obvious lesion that was clearly recognized as such by both the surgeon and the pathologist. For that reason, these patients were placed in the gross rather than the microscopic DCIS category.

Sixty-one of the patients were treated by total mastectomy, and in 58 this was accompanied by an axillary dissection. Six patients, all of them in the gross DCIS category, were treated with lumpectomy followed by irradiation. Two patients from the microscopic group were treated by wide excision, and one patient failed to return after her biopsy.

Pathologic findings in the patients with gross DCIS subjected to mastectomy were much like those seen in invasive cancers, but there was a lesser incidence of axillary node involvement. Twelve of the 16 patients with the microscopic form of DCIS had an axillary dissection, but all nodes were negative for metastatic tumor. Residual disease was found in 5 of the 16 patients with microscopic DCIS when they were subjected to additional surgery. In one of these patients the residual disease was limited to the biopsy area, but in the other four it was also found elsewhere in the breast.

Our review of 70 recent DCIS patients suggests that categorization into gross and microscopic forms is not only feasible but absolutely necessary in order to rationalize treatment. The limited malignant potential of DCIS evidenced in the reviews by Betsill and Page reflects only the microscopic form. DCIS appearing in conjunction with mammographic microcalcifications is probably similar, but its natural history has yet to be evaluated. The gross form of DCIS should be treated as if it were invasive cancer, even though it probably has a somewhat better prognosis.[9] Treatment of the microscopic form is a more difficult issue. Mastectomy and radiotherapy have been discussed, but radiotherapists have yet to single out the microscopic form for special consideration. It is clear that the reported series deal primarily with the gross form of the disease.

Wide local excision represents the third treatment option for DCIS. Most of the previous reports also involve gross disease, such as discussed by Millis and Thynne.[51] These authors reported a long-term follow-up study of patients with DCIS treated by a variety of surgical approaches. From a review of 85 patients, 26 were considered acceptable for detailed study. Eight patients were treated by wide local excision, and 2 recurred locally. However, all of the patients had clinically obvious lesions when first diagnosed. A more encouraging view of wide local excision was reported by Ashikari and colleagues.[52] These authors reported on *in situ* lesions in 18 patients, none of whom developed recurrence during an average 4-year follow-up period. Unfortunately 13 of the 18 had LCIS, and only 5 had DCIS.

The reviews by Betsill and Page make it clear that not all patients with microscopic DCIS will go on to develop invasive cancer. For that reason, a policy of close observation can be considered. It is not clear what wide excision will add if this approach is elected, since excision of a microscopic lesion that may or may not correlate with the mammographic microcalcifications is a difficult task. Furthermore our small series indicated that four of the five patients with residual tumor had DCIS away from as well as within the biopsy site.

A summary of the treatment recommendations set forth above would be as follows:

1. The gross form of DCIS can be treated by mastectomy and axillary dissection or by lumpectomy, axillary dissection, and radiotherapy. Wide excision alone for gross DCIS appears to be associated with a high rate of local recurrence, judging from the NSABP Protocol 6.[49]
2. Microscopic DCIS has traditionally been treated by total mastectomy. However, the fact that progression to invasive cancer is not inevitable when the disease constitutes an incidental finding means that observation with or without re-excision can be considered. This might be especially applicable in elderly women, given the long time interval between biopsy and invasive cancer when progression does take place. Microscopic DCIS found as the result of microcalcifications may well have a natural history similar to that found incidentally, but this relationship has yet to be established with certainty.

Radiotherapy has also been applied in the treatment of microscopic DCIS, but the reported studies deal almost solely with gross disease, making evaluation difficult.

SUMMARY

In situ cancers of the breast are being recognized with increasing frequency because of mammography and more painstaking examination of biopsy specimens. LCIS is histologically well defined, and pathologists and clinicians agree that it is a completely microscopic lesion. There is no clinical abnormality, and even though biopsy of microcalcifications may at times yield the diagnosis, the relationship is probably not specific. The malignant potential is low and is not related to the biopsy site or even the breast that yielded the biopsy. LCIS can best be considered a marker of increased risk. Treatment remains controversial, the alternatives being close observation, unilateral mastectomy with contralateral biopsy, or bilateral mastectomy.

DCIS is a lesion currently in transition but with important differences from LCIS. Until recently it was an infrequently documented form of breast cancer, representing 1% to 2% of all new cases. It usually presented as a mass or Paget's disease, which is not consistent with the *in situ* concept set forth in this chapter—a microscopic lesion that cannot be recognized clinically. Mammography has added a new diagnostic dimension, because microcalcifications may alert the clinician to the presence of the lesion despite the fact that it cannot be detected grossly. Efforts to understand the natural history of this lesion require careful distinction between patients with the microscopic form of the disease and patients with tumors of varying size whose histology remains intraductal. Many reports fail to differentiate between gross and microscopic versions, because pathologists have applied the term DCIS to both. The distinction is critical to clinicians attempting to evaluate the significance of this lesion. The malignant potential of the lesion, when microcalcifications are the sole indication for biopsy, has yet to be studied. However, the Betsill and Page studies provide important information. This is because both groups reviewed large numbers of "benign" biopsies and in the process of this herculean effort found a number of patients whose DCIS had been overlooked. These biopsies were done at a time when mammography was in its infancy, but the microscopic lesions uncovered by these investigators are similar in appearance to those found in many patients who underwent biopsy on the basis of microcalcifications.

The incidence of invasive cancer in these two reports on DCIS is only slightly higher than that reported for LCIS. However, concern about the malignant potential of the ductal lesion is far greater, because when invasive cancer develops it is inevitably in the breast that was biopsied and usually in close proximity to the scar. Treatment options for microscopic DCIS include observation with or without wide excision, but total mastectomy has been the usual recommendation. Patients often find it difficult to accept the need for a mastectomy when their disease is diagnosed at such an early stage. On the other hand, aggressive local treatment may be justified when one encounters breast cancer at a time when the possibility of systemic involvement is remote.

REFERENCES

1. Broders AC: Carcinoma in situ contrasted with benign penetrating epithelium. JAMA 99:1670–1674, 1932
2. Foote FW, Stewart FW: Lobular carcinoma in situ: A rare form of mammary cancer. Am J Pathol 17:491–496, 1941
3. Carter D: Interpretation of Breast Biopsies, p 76. New York, Raven Press, 1984
4. Rosner D, Bedwani RN, Vana J, et al: Non-invasive breast carcinoma: Results of a national survey by the American College of Surgeons. Ann Surg 192:139–147, 1980
5. Baker LH: Breast Cancer Detection Project: Five-year summary report. CA 32:194–225, 1982
6. Haagensen CD, Lane N, Lattes R, et al: Lobular neoplasia (so-called lobular carcinoma in situ) of the breast. Cancer 42:737–769, 1978
7. Wheeler JE, Enterline HT, Roseman JM, et al: Lobular carcinoma in situ of the breast: Long-term follow-up. Cancer 34:554–560, 1974
8. Andersen JA: Lobular carcinoma in situ: A long-term follow-up in 52 cases. Acta Pathol Microbiol Scand. (A) 82:519–525, 1974
9. Haagensen CD: Diseases of the Breast, 3rd ed. Philadelphia, WB Saunders, 1986
10. Rosen PP, Senie RT, Farr GH, et al: Epidemiology of breast carcinoma: Age, menstrual status, and exogenous hormone usage in patients with lobular carcinoma in situ. Surgery 85:219–228, 1979
11. Frantz VK, Pickren JW, Melcher GW, et al: Incidence of chronic cystic disease in so-called normal breasts. A study based on 225 postmortem examinations. Cancer 4:762–783, 1951
12. Nielsen M, Jensen J, Andersen J: Precancerous and cancerous breast lesions during lifetime and at autopsy. Cancer 54:612–615, 1984
13. Alpers CE, Wellings SR: The prevalence of carcinoma in situ in normal and cancer-associated breasts. Hum Pathol 16:796–807, 1985
14. Wellings SR, Jensen HM, Marcum RG: An atlas of subgross pathology of the human breast with special reference to possible precancerous lesions. J Natl Cancer Inst 55:231–240, 1975
15. Kramer WM, and Rush BF Jr: Mammary duct proliferation in the elderly. Cancer 31:130–137, 1973
16. Haagensen CD, Bodian C, Haagensen DE Jr: Breast Carcinoma, Risk and Detection, p 238. Philadelphia, WB Saunders, 1981
17. Hutter PVP, Foote FW: Lobular carcinoma in situ: Long-term follow-up. Cancer 24:1080, 1969
18. Rosen PP, Lieberman PH, Braun DW, et al: Lobular carcinoma in situ of the breast. Am J Surg Pathol 2:225–251, 1978
19. Newman W: In situ lobular carcinoma of the breast: Report of 26 women with 32 cancers. Ann Surg 157:591–599, 1963
20. Urban JA: Bilaterality of cancer of the breast: Biopsy of the opposite breast. Cancer 20:1867–1870, 1967
21. Giodano JM, Klopp CT: Lobular carcinoma in situ: Incidence and treatment. Cancer 31:105–109, 1973
22. Nesland JM, Johannessen JV: Malignant breast lesions. J Submicrosc Cytol 14:553–575, 1982
23. Andersen JA, Schiodt T: On the concept of carcinoma in situ of the breast. Pathol Res Pract 166:407–414, 1980
24. Rosen PP, Braun DW, Kinne DE: The clinical significance of pre-invasive breast carcinoma. Cancer 46:919–925, 1980
25. Andersen JA: Lobular carcinoma in situ of the breasts: An approach to rational treatment. Cancer 39:2597–2602, 1977
26. Sandison AT: An autopsy study of the adult human breast.

Washington DC: US Dept of Health, Education and Welfare, National Cancer Institute, Monograph No 8, pp 44–51, 1962
27. Page DL, Dupont WD, Rogers LW, et al: Intraductal carcinoma of the breast. Cancer 49:751–758, 1982
28. Millis RR, Davis R, Stacey AJ: The detection and significance of calcifications in the breast. Br J Radiol 49:12–26, 1976
29. Rosen PP, Schneider RE: Non-palpable breast lesions detected by mammography and confirmed by specimen radiography. Breast 3:13–16, 1977
30. Schwartz GE, Patchesfsky AS, Feig SA, et al: Multicentricity of non-palpable breast cancer. Cancer 45:2913–2916, 1980
31. Powell RW, McSweeney MB, Wilson C: X-ray calcifications as the only basis for breast biopsy. Ann Surg 197:555–559, 1983
32. Egan RL, McSweeney MB, Sewell CW: Intramammary calcifications without an associated mass in benign and malignant diseases. Radiology 137:1–7, 1980
33. Lagios MD, Westdahl PR, Margolin FR, et al: Duct carcinoma in situ. Cancer 50:1309–1314, 1982
34. Silverberg SG, Chitale AR: Assessment of significance of proportions of intraductal and infiltrating tumor growth in ductal carcinoma of the breast. Cancer 32:830–837, 1973
35. Westbrook KC, Gallager HS: Intraductal carcinoma of the breast: A comparative study. Am J Surg 130:667–670, 1975
36. Betsill WL, Rosen PP, Lieberman PH, et al: Intraductal carcinoma: Long-term follow-up after treatment by biopsy alone. JAMA 239:1863–1867, 1978
37. Farrow JH: Current concepts in the detection and treatment of the earliest of the early breast cancers. Cancer 25:468–477, 1970
38. Haagensen CD: Diseases of the Breast, ed 2. pp 528–544. Philadelphia, WB Saunders, 1971
39. Dean L, Geschickter CF: Comedo carcinoma of the breast. Arch Surg 36:225–234, 1938
40. Kraus FT, Neubecker RD: The differential diagnosis of papillary tumors of the breast. Cancer 15:444–455, 1962
41. Rosen PP, Senie R, Schottenfeld D, et al: Non-invasive breast carcinoma. Frequency of unsuspected invasion and implications for treatment. Ann Surg 189:337–382, 1979
42. Carter D, Smith RRL: Carcinoma in situ of the breast. Cancer 40:1189–1193, 1977
43. Shah JP, Rosen PP, Robbins GF: Pitfalls of local excision in the treatment of carcinoma of the breast. Surg Gynecol Obstet 136:721–725, 1973
44. Montague ED: Conservative surgery and radiation therapy in the treatment of operable breast cancer. Cancer 53:700–704, 1984
45. Findlay P, Goodman R: Radiation therapy for treatment of intraductal carcinoma of the breast. Am J Clin Oncol 6:281–285, 1983
46. Recht A, Danoff BS, Solin LJ, et al: Intraductal carcinoma of the breast: Results of treatment with excisional biopsy and irradiation. J Clin Oncol 3:1339–1343, 1985
47. Wecksell A, Attkiss MD, Shahamatpour M: Recurrent intraductal breast carcinoma following radiation therapy: A case report. Breast 8:13–15, 1982
48. Harris JR, Connolly JL, Schnitt SJ, et al: The use of pathologic features in selecting the extent of surgical resection necessary for breast cancer patients treated by primary radiation therapy. Ann Surg 201:164–169, 1985
49. Fisher ER, Sass R, Fisher B, et al: Pathologic findings from the National Surgical Adjuvant Breast Project (Protocol 6) 1. Intraductal carcinoma (DCIS). Cancer 57:197–208, 1986
50. Jicha DL, Gump FE, Ozzello L: Ductal carcinoma in situ (DCIS); a revised concept. (in press)
51. Millis RR, Thynne GSJ: In situ intraductal carcinoma of the breast: A long-term follow-up study. Br J Surg 62:957–962, 1975
52. Ashikari R, Huvos AG, Snyder RE: Prospective study of non-infiltrating carcinoma of the breast. Cancer 39:435–439, 1977

Recurrent Disease

12

Ian E. Smith

Approximately 50% of all patients with breast cancer relapse within 10 years of diagnosis,[1–3] and the risk of relapse appears to continue thereafter, even with 30 years of follow-up.[4] Metastatic breast cancer is at present incurable, and so, nearly always, is local recurrence after mastectomy. But the diversity of relapse patterns and their range of natural history are unique in cancer medicine, and they present a major challenge in clinical management. This chapter discusses these patterns of recurrence, their prognostic significance, and the role of currently available techniques for their detection.

LOCAL-REGIONAL AND DISTANT METASTATIC RELAPSE PATTERNS

Breast cancer can recur both locally and at distant metastatic sites. Table 12-1 compares the incidence of local-regional and distant metastatic recurrence in patients treated by radical mastectomy, without postoperative radiotherapy or adjuvant systemic treatment. Even after radical surgery, local-regional relapse occurs first in 15% to 30% of all patients who are going to relapse.[1,3,5–12] This figure is not insignificant, but in terms of treatment strategy it has often wrongly been allowed to overshadow the main problem in breast cancer: The considerable majority of patients who relapse do so initially in distant metastatic sites (around 70% to 80%), and that is why they die.

Intrinsic biologic factors do not appear to influence this relative pattern of local-regional and metastatic recurrence to any great extent. Axillary node involvement remains the single most important adverse prognostic factor in breast cancer, and patients with involved nodes have a very much higher incidence of both local-regional and distant metastatic relapse than those without.[1,3,6,10,11] However, the presence or absence of axillary node involvement appears to have no significant influence on the *relative* incidence of relapse (Table 12-1).[3,10]

The time at which relapse occurs after primary treatment (tumor-free interval) also has little influence on relative relapse patterns. In serial analyses of the same group of patients, the relative incidences of relapse were 17% (local-regional) and 83% (metastatic) at a median follow-up of 14 months[13] and 22% (local-regional) and 78% (metastatic) after 10 years.[11] Likewise, relapse patterns in the studies outlined in Table 12-1 appear similar whether follow-up is short (2 years)[8] or long (10 years).[1,3] Finally, in a large retrospective analysis, the time course to relapse followed an identical exponential curve for 150 patients developing local recurrence and 215 patients developing distant metastases.[14]

Distant Metastases

Sites

Data on the first sites of distant metastatic relapse after mastectomy are listed in Table 12-2. Reporting methods vary for different studies, particularly with regard to analyzing multiple site recurrence, and detailed comparisons are difficult. Nevertheless, bone is the most common first site of relapse in all studies and is frequently involved initially in more than 50% of patients when multiple first sites are included.[1,3,5,8,10,12,14–16]

The second most common site of first relapse is lung or pleura, occurring alone in around 15% to 30% of patients. Most studies fail to differentiate between these two sites, but where this has been done, lung is the more common site for initial relapse, with a rate of 15% to 25% compared with 8% to 9% for pleura.[10,12] Isolated first relapse in liver (3% to 9%) is surprisingly uncommon, considering the high incidence of liver metastases at autopsy (Table 12-3). As a rule for clinical management, therefore, hepatic abnormalities in the absence of metastatic disease elsewhere should be fully investigated and not assumed without question to represent metastatic dis-

Table 12-1

Relative Rates (%) of Local-Regional and Distant Metastatic Relapse in Patients Treated With Radical Mastectomy Alone Without Adjuvant Therapy or Radiotherapy

Study	*Number of Relapse Patients*	*Relative Relapse Rate (%)* Local-Regional Alone	Metastatic
Haagensen[1]	193	22	78
Valagussa et al[3]	94 N− *	26	74 (19)†
	290 N+	26	74 (13)†
Fisher et al[6]	402	18	78 (5)†
Bonadonna et al[11]	118	22	78
Strender et al[7]	124	26	74
PTBCSG[8]	78	28	72
Lee[10]	36 N− *	17	83 (14)†
	69 N+	19	81 (23)
Fisher et al[5]	117	33	67

* N−/+ Axillary node involvement
† Both distant and local-regional relapse

ease. First presentation with central nervous system (CNS) metastases is rare, but does occur in 1% to 7% of patients and should be borne in mind when an otherwise well patient develops neurologic abnormalities.

Few intrinsic factors appear to influence the site of first distant metastasis. Some studies have suggested that axillary node-negative patients may have a higher relative incidence of lung and pleural metastases than those with involved nodes,[1,10] but others have found the opposite.[3] Conflicting data have likewise been reported for the relationship between node status and the incidence of bone metastases,[1,3,10] and cumulative evidence suggests no significant association between node status and sites of first metastatic spread. The same appears true for tumor-free interval.[3,10,14]

Time to recurrence after mastectomy does not influence the site of first metastasis,[14] and this is borne out by comparing data from studies with short (2-year)[8] and long (10-year) follow-up (Table 12-2)[1] and from a study reanalyzing data from the same group of patients at 3 years and 10 years.[16] Estrogen receptor (ER) status is reported as having no influence on site of first relapse,[17] although one report suggests without data that ER-positive patients have a higher incidence of bone relapse.[10]

Irrespective of initial clinical sites of metastases, the number of detectable metastatic sites increases inexorably during the course of disease, and postmortem studies reveal the protean nature of metastatic spread (Table 12-3). Particular attention is drawn to the high incidence of adrenal metastases (around 30% to 40%), which are nearly always undetected clinically, but there are few organs in which metastases have not been recorded. It is one of the curiosities of breast cancer that its initial metastatic pattern should be so varied and yet its final outcome so uniform.

Time to First Metastases

Breast cancer is unique in the potential length of its natural history (Chapter 9), and patients can relapse clinically more than 25 years after initial diagnosis.[1,12] Although they are of biologic interest, these late relapses are rare, and the majority of patients who are going to develop recurrence do so early, within 2 years of diagnosis. Table 12-4 summarizes the cumulative incidence of relapse per year in patients developing metastases after radical local treatment (usually radical mastectomy) without adjuvant systemic therapy. The data show that 50% to 75% of patients who are going to relapse do so within 2 years and 65% to 85% within 3 years.[5,14,23–25] The time to metastatic relapse has been shown to follow an exponential curve, indicating a constant risk of recurrence,[14] and this is confirmed in other studies when time to relapse has also been plotted graphically.[5,24]

A close relationship between tumor size at presentation and time to first metastasis has been shown in a large retrospective analysis of 2648 patients.[26] At extremes, median time to relapse after initial treatment for all relapsing patients with tumors less than 2.5 cm in diameter was 42 months, compared with only 4 months for those with tumors greater than 8.5 cm.

Likewise, axillary node status, although not significantly affecting patterns of recurrence (see above), may influence time to first metastasis. In one study, 70% of patients with node involvement who were going to relapse did so within 3 years, compared with only 55% of node-negative patients.[25] For patients with one to three nodes involved, the relapse rate was 61% compared with 78% for those with four or more nodes. In contrast, time to onset of metastases does not appear to be influenced by age, menopausal status, or the site of first metastases.[14,23]

Survival After First Metastasis

Once metastases occur, the prognosis is poor, and Haagensen rightly described distant metastases as "the sword of Damocles that hangs over the patient who has had a locally successful radical mastectomy."[1] Median survival from the time of first metastatic relapse ranges from 11 to 24 months, 3-year survival from 12% to 36%, and 5-year survival from 5% to 18% (Table 12-5).[9,14,15,23,24,27–29] However, a small number of patients live for more than 10 years after detection of metastases,[15,24,27] and one study reported 5% of patients still alive 15 years later (all initially presenting with clinical stage N_0 disease).[27]

Prognostic Factors Influencing Survival

Several intrinsic biologic factors appear to influence prognosis after metastatic relapse.

SITE. In studies published both before and since the beginning of the current era of combination chemotherapy for metastatic disease, patients who first present with bone metastases have a better prognosis than those with

Table 12-2
Initial Sites of Distant Metastatic Relapse (% Incidence)

		Site (s) of Initial Relapse						
Study	*Patients*	*Bone*	*Lung/ Pleura*	*Liver*	*Soft Tissue*	*CNS*	*Other*	*Multiple*
Donegan[15]	922*	29	19	4	12	2	4	32*
Haagensen[1]	297	33	31	8	10	7	7	—
Fisher et al[5]	37	46	35	—	—	3	27	—
Valagussa et al[16]	66	42	23	3	—	2	5	26
PTBCSG[8]	56	39	14	5	—	2	14	25
Karabali-Dalamaga et al[14]	215	32	13	9	—	—	—	25
Lee[10]	146	43	32	5	7	3	10	—
Smith[12]	329	38	24	8	10	1	4	15

* Includes local-regional recurrence

Table 12-3
Percentage of Metastatic Involvement at Different Sites at Autopsy

Site of Involvement	*Vidaria et al*[18] (n=647)	Warren & Witman[19] (n=160)	Saphillo & Parker[20] (n=43)	Haagensen[21] (n=100)	Coombes et al[22] (n=50)
Bone	70	44	—	71	74
Lungs	66	59	65	69	58
Pleura	—	37	23	51	46
Liver	61	58	56	65	70
Nodes	56	72	—	76	—
Skin	—	34	7	30	20
CNS	25	—	9	22	18
Peritoneum	25	12	9	13	14
Adrenals	38	31	41	49	26
Thyroid	20	—	—	24	< 10
Pituitary	20	—	—	—	< 10
Ovary	15	9	16	20	10
Kidney	13	—	14	17	10
Pancreas	12	—	11	17	—
Intestine	10	—	—	18	—
Uterus	13	—	—	15	—
Spleen	—	14	23	17	< 10
Heart	—	—	—	11	< 10
Pericardium	—	5	21	19	10

visceral metastases,[9,15,28] and this has been our own experience. In our unit, over the past 10 years, patients presenting with bone metastases had a better median survival after relapse (34 months) than those with metastases in other sites, including pleura, 28 months (NSD); lung, 17 months ($p < 0.01$); and liver, 12 months ($p < 0.01$) (Fig. 12-1). Similarly, survival after combination chemotherapy is better for patients with bone than with visceral metastases, although the response rate is no better.[30]

Further data on survival after specific sites of relapse from both comparative and noncomparative studies are listed in Table 12-6. Pleura as a single site of relapse carries a good prognosis,[12,31] but in one study median survival was reduced from 48 to 12 months in the presence of multiple-site relapse.[31] Brain relapse usually carries a poor prognosis,[32–38] but again median survival was much longer (15 versus 4 months) when this was the sole initial site of relapse.[33] Occasional 3- to 4-year survivors have been reported,[32,33] and for otherwise fit patients, active treatment is therefore worthwhile. The same is true for leptomeningeal relapse; median survival is around 2 to 6 months,[39–42] but with active intrathecal treatment, occasional patients survive 2 years or more.[43]

Multiple sites of concurrent relapse carry a worse

Table 12-4
Cumulative Percentage Relapse Per Year After Diagnosis in Patients Developing Metastatic Breast Cancer After Radical Local Treatment Without Adjuvant Chemotherapy

Study	Number of Patients	Cumulative Percentage Relapse				Maximum Length of Follow-up (Years)
		1 Year	2 Years	3 Years	5 Years	
Romsdahl et al[23]	177	29	59	72	—*	13 years
Karabali-Dalamaga et al[14]	215	50	75	85	95	9 years
Powles et al[24]	51	20	50	75	85	11 years
Valagussa et al[25]	92 N−			55	77	
	287 N+			70	86	10 years
Fisher et al[5]		30	60	80	100	5 years

* 97% relapsed at 12 years
Maximum length of follow-up, which influences cumulative relapse, is given for each study

Table 12-5
Survival From Time of First Metastases in Patients Developing Metastatic Breast Cancer

Study	Patients With Metastases	Survival			
		Median (Months)	3-Year	5-Year	Long-Term
Fey et al[9]	359	20	25%	12%	Longest 8 years
Karabali-Dalamaga et al[14]	215	12	16%	4%	Longest 7 Years
Romsdahl et al[23]	177	18	24%	8%	4% 8 years
Powles et al[24]	158	16	25%	18%	2% 10 years
Donegan[15]	1091	11	12%	5%	2% 10 years
Clark et al[27]	94	16	20%	12%	5% 15 years*
Cutler et al[28]	888	14	18%	7%	—
Paterson et al[29]	719	19	28%	10%	Longest 8 years

* Clinically staged N0 at presentation

prognosis than single sites. In one study, median survival from relapse for patients with two or more sites of involvement was 17 to 19 months, compared with 23 months for visceral metastases and 27 months for bone metastases.[9] In another, survival decreased with each additional metastatic site; with one site, median survival was 19 months; with two, 13 months; with three, 10 months; and with four, 6 months. Three-year survival similarly decreased from around 25% for one site to less than 3% for four sites.[28] Survival after chemotherapy is likewise worse for patients with multiple relapse sites and a large total tumor burden.[30]

DISEASE-FREE INTERVAL. Several centers have shown that the shorter the disease-free interval (DFI) between initial diagnosis and metastatic relapse, the worse is the prognosis after relapse.[9,12,28] At extremes, a DFI of less than 1 year is associated with a median survival after relapse of 7 to 18 months, compared with 25 to 36 months for a DFI of greater than 5 years. However, patients who have metastatic disease at presentation do rather better than those with a short DFI (median survival 12 months versus 7 months),[28] illustrating that the extent of disease at presentation does not necessarily reflect its tempo.

AXILLARY NODE STATUS. Despite the powerful adverse prognostic significance of involved axillary nodes on overall survival, this parameter appears to have little or no influence on survival from first metastasis.[17,29,44–46] The survival consequences of axillary node involvement are instead largely mediated through the disease-free interval between initial diagnosis and relapse.

TUMOR SIZE AND STAGE AT PRESENTATION. These parameters also have a major influence on overall prognosis,[47,48] but once again neither tumor size[43] nor clinical

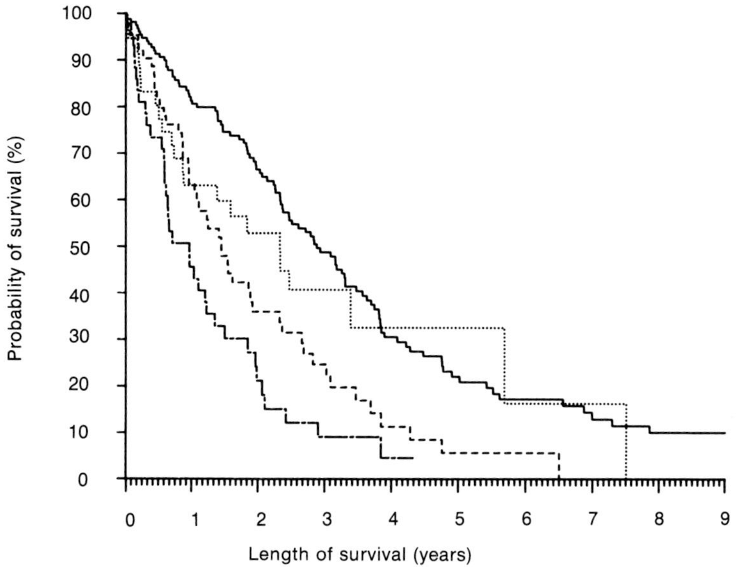

FIGURE 12-1. Survival (years) by site from date of first relapse. Bone (——), pleura (. . . .), lung (– – –), liver (– · –).

Table 12-6
Survival of Patients Developing Metastatic Breast Cancer Related to Specific Sites of First Relapse

	Survival from First Relapse		
Site of First Relapse	*Median (Months)*	*3 Years*	*Reference*
Pleura	28–48*	40%	12, 28, 31
	9–12†	—	28, 31
Bone	14–34	45%	9, 12, 15, 28
Lung	17–20	20%	12, 28
Liver	6–12	<10%	12, 15, 28
Brain	1–8 † 15*	Occasional	28, 32–42
Meninges	2–6	0%	39–43
Marrow	> 8 ‡	—	177

* Single site relapse
† Multiple site relapse
‡ Median time to disease progression

Table 12-7
Survival (in Months) After First Recurrence Related to Positive or Negative Cytoplasmic Estrogen (ER) and Progesterone (PR) Receptors

	Survival (Months)			
Study	*ER+*	*ER−*	*PR+*	*PR−*
Hahnel et al[17]	39	14		
Moseley et al[49]	38	22		
Paterson et al[29]	15	10		
Howell et al[45]	42	14	44	14
Stewart et al[44]	36	12		
Howat et al[46]	48	19	62	20

stage[29] has any effect on survival after relapse, implying that their main influence is likewise on the disease-free interval between diagnosis and first metastasis.

ESTROGEN AND PROGESTOGEN RECEPTOR STATUS. There is a general consensus that patients whose tumors contain estrogen or progestogen receptors have a better prognosis than those without (Chapter 9). In contrast to axillary node status and tumor size, the influence of receptors on survival appears to relate almost entirely to survival after first relapse. Several studies have shown that the time to first relapse is unaffected by the presence or absence of ERs, whereas median survival after recurrence for ER-positive patients is longer than for ER-negative patients by 5 to 29 months (Table 12-7).[17,29,44–46, 49] The same is true for progestogen receptors, and prolongation in survival here may be even greater (30 to 42 months) for receptor-positive patients.[45,46] Patients who are both ER negative and progestogen-receptor negative do particularly badly; one study found a median survival from starting treatment of only 4 months compared with around 20 months when one or more receptors were positive,[50] and another found that median survival was 37 months less than for patients in whom both receptors were positive.[46] This may not simply reflect intrinsic biologic differences between receptor-positive and -negative tumors but may indicate a survival benefit achieved by response to endocrine therapy. In one study, only ER-positive patients who responded to endocrine therapy achieved significant survival prolongation; nonresponding positive patients had the same survival as nonresponding receptor-negative patients.[45]

Local-Regional Recurrence After Mastectomy

Local-regional recurrence in the chest wall or in regional nodes as first site of relapse occurs in about 10% to 20%

of patients after mastectomy.[1,3,5–7, 10,14,51–54] It is usually an ominous event with a poor prognosis.

The majority of recurrences (about 55% to 90%) are in the chest wall, and usually within the central scar or under a skin graft, where one has been used;[1,5,10,50,51,54–57] only a minority occur in the axilla or the supraclavicular fossa. In most studies, the incidence of local recurrence is very significantly increased in patients presenting with clinical[6] or histologic axillary node involvement[1,3,51,52,54] and rises to 40% in some series with multiple-node (8 or more) involvement.[1,51,54] In contrast, the incidence in histologically node-negative patients is 3% to 10%,[1,3,51,52] and 10% where nodes are clinically negative.[16] The incidence also increases with increasing tumor size at presentation[51,52] and with skin infiltration or edema.[51,52]

Time to Recurrence

As with distant metastases, the majority of local recurrences occur within 2 years of diagnosis (about 55% to 80%), and about 90% have occurred within 5 years.[1,5,6,14,51–55,58] However, again as with distant relapse, occasional chest wall recurrences have been reported 10 years or more after primary treatment.[54–56, 58,59] The pattern of time to onset of first recurrence for local-regional and for distant relapse is almost identical where this has been compared[9,14,54] and follows an exponential curve indicating constant risk of relapse.[14]

Prognostic Significance and Survival

There is compelling evidence to suggest that local-regional recurrence is a first manifestation of systemic relapse in the great majority of patients. Distant metastases are reported as following local recurrence in 81%,[60] 89%,[55] 94%,[3] 96%,[61] 97%[54] and 100%[56] of patients, and nearly always within 2 years (although once 16 years later).[56]

Median survival is significantly longer from first local relapse than from first systemic relapse,[9,12,14,61] but prognosis is nevertheless poor, with a median survival of around 2 to 3 years and a 5-year survival of 12% to 36% (Table 12-8).[9,12,14,55,56,58,60,62]

Despite this generally poor prognosis, it must be noted that some studies report a small number of long-term survivors, with a 10-year survival of 5% to 22%[56,58,62] and with one patient dying 23 years after local relapse.[56] Prognosis is best for patients developing single rather than multiple recurrences,[55,56,60] and in one series the 10-year survival rate after solitary chest wall recurrence was 22%.[58] This appears to relate to whether further surgery with or without radiotherapy can eradicate recurrent disease.[56,58,62] Other good prognostic factors include solitary lesions of less than 1 cm,[60] a DFI of more than 2 years from diagnosis,[55,56,60,62] and histologic grade 1 and 2 tumors.[58] Factors that do not appear to have prognostic significance include age,[14] menopausal status,[14,56,58,60,62] site of recurrence on chest wall or in nodes,[60,62] and, as with distant metastases, axillary node status at presentation.[56,60] Clinical stage at presentation is reported as having prognostic significance in one study[62] but not in two others.[56,60]

Recurrence After Breast Conservation

With current renewed interest in breast conservation, it is important to note that local recurrence in the conserved breast does not carry the same ominous prognosis as chest wall recurrence.

The reported incidence varies from 1.4% to 21.5%,[27,59,63–70] depending on patient selection, stage, type of conservative treatment, and duration of follow-up. Breast recurrence, in contrast to chest wall recurrence, is associated with distant metastatic disease in only a minority of patients and salvage surgery is usually possible with a good subsequent prognosis. The overall 10-year survival of patients undergoing salvage surgery is reported as 69% to 81% and is as good as overall survival in patients who have not had a recurrence in the breast.[27,63,64,71] This topic is dealt with in more detail elsewhere.

STAGING FOR DISTANT METASTASES

Bone

Bone is the most common site of first metastatic spread (Table 12-2) and has an eventual autopsy incidence of around 70% (Table 12-3). Pain is the most common presenting symptom and occurs in around 65% of patients, although local tenderness is uncommon.[70]

Biochemical Investigations

Biochemical investigations are of only moderate value. Serum alkaline phosphatase is elevated in 50% to 93% of patients with established skeletal metastases,[72–75] but in two studies it antedated clinical and radiologic evidence of recurrence in only 25% to 29% of patients.[75,76] The urinary excretion of hydroxyproline (OHP) or the OHP:creatinine ratio is elevated in 93% of patients with bone metastases,[73,75,77–79] but in only 38% at first evidence of bone involvement.[77] Elevated levels are found in a minority of patients with early breast cancer at presentation,[74,75,78–81] and these have a significant correlation with early bone recurrence.[75,80,81] However, in all studies, there is a high incidence of false-negative results and lead-time interval is short (6 to 9 months median).[76,78,80,81] The overall predictive value for the development of bone metastases is therefore considered poor.[75,76,81]

X-rays and Radionuclide Scans

X-rays and radionuclide scans are the two principle investigations currently available for the detection of bone metastases. Radionuclide scintiscanning usually employs ^{99m}Tc-labeled phosphate as a label, although the less sensitive 18F was used in many early studies.[82,83]

Table 12-8
Survival After First Local-Regional Recurrence, in Patients Initially Treated With Mastectomy

Study	*Patients Initially Relapsing Local-Regionally*	*Survival*		
		Median (Months)	*5-Year*	*Long-Term*
Bedwinek et al[60]	129	34	36%	
Gilliland et al[56]	60*	>24	18%	5% 10 years
Chu et al[55]	215	30	21%	5% 10 years
Karabali-Dalamaga et al[14]	150	24	26%	8% 7 years
Fey et al[9]	146	22	12%	0% 10 years
Fentiman et al[58]	73†	34	30%	13% 10 years
Beck et al[62]	121	38	37%	22% 10 years
Smith[12]	201	34	28%	10% 9 years

* Four patients no mastectomy
† Only patients with skin recurrence

There have been many reports comparing scintiscans with x-rays for sensitivity (number of positive tests/number of patients with disease), specificity (number of negative tests/number of patients without disease) and accuracy (correct tests/total number of patients).[72,84–94] From these, a general conclusion can be drawn; scintiscans are more sensitive than x-rays (around 80% compared with around 50%) but have a lower specificity. This is because abnormal radionuclide uptake can occur in many benign conditions.[94,95] In contrast, the characteristic osteolytic and osteoblastic lesions seen on x-rays are usually diagnostic of metastases but tend to occur late, and it has been estimated that at least 50% bone destruction must occur before a metastasis is seen radiologically.[96]

On balance, most studies conclude that scintiscanning is more accurate than x-rays in investigating patients with suspected metastases, but this has recently been challenged in a detailed study comparing both incidence and sites of involvement using both techniques.[97] Scintiscanning without recourse to x-ray verification had a very high false-positive rate and a poor detection rate at certain sites, including skull and pelvis (60%) and femurs (35%). The authors concluded that a five-plate limited radiologic skeletal survey alone had a 92% accuracy in detecting metastatic disease and was superior to scintigraphy.

There is controversy over the value of scintiscan screening at presentation to detect early occult bone metastases in asymptomatic patients. In an influential study, 12/50 early stage patients (24%) had abnormal 18F-scintiscans at presentation and developed bone metastases within 5 years, compared with only 26% of patients whose initial scintiscan was negative.[98] Although these findings have had some support,[99,100] other studies have in general found a much lower incidence of positive scans in early stage patients at diagnosis (around 2% to 10%),[101–113] with a variability of 1.9% to 20.2% between different centers in one.[101] In addition, although positive scans in these studies did in general carry a worse prognosis, this was much more marginal than that originally suggested,[98] with a relapse rate of only 10% to 50% over follow-up intervals of 18 months to 9 years.[97,102,103,114] These authors and others[105,115] concluded that such data do not justify routine scintiscanning as an initial staging investigation in the asymptomatic patient, except in the context of a research trial.

Scintiscanning and x-rays have been evaluated in women with asymptomatic minimal (less than 0.5 cm palpable mass) or occult (detected only on mammography) breast cancer detected at screening clinics.[116] Both investigations were always normal, and the authors concluded that they were unnecessary here. This is a useful finding, given the increasing number of patients with early breast cancer detected at screening.

A final argument for routine scintiscanning at presentation would be to provide a baseline for subsequent scans. Several groups have studied the "conversion" of an originally negative scan to a positive one at follow-up.[99,103,106,111,117] These report a conversion rate of 6% to 30% over periods ranging from 11 months to 9 years. As might be expected, such conversion is a bad prognostic sign and usually implies bone metastases, with a median survival from time of conversion in one study of only 17.5 months.[103] However, lead-time over radiologic detection was usually short or nonexistent, and such information probably has little value in planning clinical management with currently available therapies.

Computed Tomography

Computed tomographic (CT) scanning has recently been used to investigate 20 patients with abnormal radionuclide scans but with normal skeletal x-rays.[118] In 11 patients, this technique demonstrated 13 metastases, all of which were subsequently confirmed clinically or radiographically; in addition, benign diseases were identified in three patients and no abnormalities in six, all of whom remained disease free. CT scanning would therefore appear to be significantly superior to conventional radiology for correctly diagnosing scintiscan abnormalities. At present, cost and time rule this out as a standard staging procedure, but the technique may have a useful role to play in the further investigation of lesions that are clinically suspicious on scintigraphy when conventional x-rays are unhelpful.

Liver

Liver is an uncommon site of solitary first metastases (Table 12-2), but liver metastases are eventually found in about 55% to 75% of autopsies (Table 12-3).

Clinical

Although clinical evaluation of the liver is an essential first step in the investigation of possible metastases, its potential is limited in that 50% of livers with gross metastatic involvement remain clinically impalpable.[117] Likewise, clinical examination fared badly against other techniques in a comparative study, detecting only 33% of patients with subsequently proven metastases.[119]

Biochemistry

Biochemical liver function tests (LFTs) have a low specificity in detecting liver metastases,[120–123] given the many other causes of liver dysfunction. Nevertheless, LFTs and in particular alkaline phosphatase are reasonably sensitive in detecting breast cancer metastases. In one study, 78% of patients with pathologically proven liver metastases had a raised alkaline phosphatase, including 37/39 patients (95%) with a positive radionuclide scan.[124] Others have reported abnormal LFTs (usually alkaline phosphatase) in 100% of patients with proven liver metastases,[125] and one group found liver radionuclide scans or ultrasonography to be abnormal only in patients with an elevated alkaline phosphatase.[126] These various authors therefore recommend scans or ultrasonography only in patients with abnormal LFTs.

Radionuclide Scanning and Ultrasonography

Radionuclide scans are usually carried out with technetium 99m tagged to sulphur colloid,[127,128] which is uniformly taken up by the Kupffer cells of the reticuloendothelial system, leaving metastases as "cold" areas of decreased or absent uptake. This limits detectability to lesions of approximately 2 cm for superficial sites and larger than this for deeper lesions.[129–131] Gray-scale ultrasonography distinguishes echo-density differences between tissues[132] and can detect lesions of 0.5 to 1.0 cm under favorable conditions.[129,133] The technique can often differentiate between malignant and benign lesions, including cysts, and has the additional advantages over scintiscanning of providing precise anatomical location of lesions and of allowing the biliary tree and porta hepatis to be examined.[134] However, the accuracy of ultrasonography is operator dependent,[135,136] and the limits of detection are reduced if metastases are echo poor[129,133] or if there is excess bowel gas or the patient is obese.[129,135]

The two techniques therefore offer a trade-off between sensitivity, which is higher for isotope scanning, and specificity, which is higher for ultrasonography. The overall accuracy of both techniques in patients suspected of having liver metastases is very similar, at around 75% to 90%, as assessed by subsequent biopsy, autopsy, or the development of unequivocal clinical features,[119,128,130,137–145] and at present there is therefore little to choose between the two techniques. A sensible suggestion has been that isotope scanning should be used as the initial approach on the basis of a higher sensitivity, using ultrasonography as a follow-up investigation on the basis of its increased specificity to clarify the nature of suspicious lesions.[129,131] Ultrasonography is likewise indicated if the biliary tree and porta hepatis require assessment.

Computed Tomography

CT scanning is a more recent addition to diagnostic imaging techniques for liver metastases. It is based on the detection of tissue differences in radiodensity,[146] and its limits of detection with or without iodinated dye for contrast enhancement are lesions of around 1.5 cm.[131] Its accuracy, like that of scintiscanning and ultrasonography, is around 75% to 90%[136,143,147–149] and may even be a little higher on the basis of comparative studies.[135,150] Whether these marginal benefits of CT scan are enough to justify the extra cost on a routine basis is arguable.

Screening for Liver Metastases at Presentation

Attempts to detect occult liver metastases at presentation have proved disappointing. Clinical assessment for malignant hepatomegaly has a very low yield; in one series this was found in only one of 138 patients.[72] The estimation of serum liver function tests may be moderately helpful. In a series of 91 patients, 24 who had raised alkaline phosphatase at presentation had a median survival of only 20 months compared with 4 years for those with normal levels.[124] However, 44% of patients with normal LFTs also developed liver metastases within 5 years.

Routine liver scanning at presentation is unrewarding and has been reported as abnormal in 0%,[102] 1%,[125] and

13%[117] of patients. In the last study, only 24% of patients with initially abnormal scans developed liver metastases within 5 years, compared with 14% with initially normal scans. In the same study, ultrasonography was initially abnormal in only 7% of patients and the incidence of subsequent liver metastases was identical to that for patients with normal ultrasonography. Scans or ultrasonography at presentation should therefore be reserved for patients with clinical or biochemical abnormalities suggestive of liver involvement.

Lungs

The lung is the second most common site for first presentation of metastatic disease (Table 12-2), and the autopsy incidence of pulmonary metastases is around 60% to 70% (Table 12-3).

Standard chest radiography is a mandatory staging investigation in a newly presenting patient with breast carcinoma, before any treatment decision is made. In a consecutive series of 296 patients, chest radiography at presentation demonstrated metastatic disease in 18 (6%), and this represented the highest yield of any single screening test.[117] Chest radiography is also a simple and valuable follow-up investigation. In the same study, 47% of patients who subsequently developed metastatic disease within a 5-year period had metastases detected on chest radiography, and again this represented the highest yield of any single investigation.

Radionuclide scintigraphy is no more accurate than conventional chest radiography in detecting nodular pulmonary metastases.[151] Whole-lung tomography is more sensitive than chest radiography,[152–154] and CT scanning is more sensitive than either, with an ability to detect lesions of 2 mm to 3 mm in lung parenchyma.[155,156] However, at present there seems no good therapeutic justification for the routine use of CT scanning in the follow-up of asymptomatic patients with normal findings on chest radiography.

Carcinomatous lymphangitis can be a difficult diagnostic problem. This is reported as occurring in 8% to 25% of patients, often as a late or terminal event,[157,158] and autopsy studies suggest a higher incidence of around 40%.[158] The diagnostic problem arises because around 25% to 30% of patients have a normal chest radiograph,[158,159] and as many as 40% more may have nonspecific interstitial changes without characteristic metastatic nodules.[159] ^{99m}Tc-scintiscanning can show multiple irregular perfusion defects,[158] but the definitive diagnostic investigation is transbronchial biopsy, with a reported accuracy of 70% to 100%.[160,161]

In this context, it should be noted that breast carcinoma is associated with an unusually high incidence of endobronchial metastases. In one study, these were confirmed at fiber-optic bronchoscopy and biopsy in 35% of patients with unexplained pulmonary symptoms or nonspecific x-ray changes,[162] and an autopsy series reported an incidence of 37%, although the lesions were nearly always microscopic.[163]

Central Nervous System

The incidence of CNS metastases at presentation is very low (Table 12-2), and there is no current justification for routine CNS screening at this stage. One study investigated the role of CT scan screening of patients with breast cancer at presentation and failed to detect any intracranial lesions.[164] Despite an eventual autopsy incidence of around 20% (Table 12-3) and as much as 30% in some series,[32,165,166] the clinical incidence remains low, at around 10% for brain metastases[32,33] and 5% for leptomeningeal disease,[39] and does not justify routine screening in the absence of a specific clinical indication.

CT scanning can detect lesions of 6 mm to 10 mm and is currently the best investigation for detecting intracranial metastases.[167–169] It is significantly superior to radionuclide scanning, in terms of both sensitivity and specificity.[169–172] It is also more effective at demonstrating multiple lesions and infratentorial lesions and can produce information on cerebral herniation, ventricular displacement, and obstructive hydrocephalus.[168] Cerebrospinal fluid (CSF) analysis is not usually helpful in detecting intracranial metastases unless there is associated meningeal involvement.[32,173]

Leptomeningeal disease should be suspected in any patient with signs suggesting multifocal CNS disease. The diagnosis is established by the demonstration of tumor cells in cytologic examination of CSF. CSF protein is usually raised, and CSF glucose is frequently low.[39,174] One study has suggested that a presenting CSF glucose of 10 mg/ml or less is the single most important adverse prognostic factor for patients with meningeal involvement.[39] CSF carcinoembryonic antigen (CEA) levels are frequently elevated in patients with meningeal disease,[173,175] and it has been reported that alterations in CEA levels during therapy may assist in determining response to intrathecal treatment.[175] However, false-positive elevations of CSF CEA have also been reported in patients with extensive dorsolumbar spinal involvement but without meningeal disease.[173]

Bone Marrow

With conventional aspiration cytology techniques, the incidence of bone marrow infiltration in patients with suspected or proven metastatic disease ranges from 13% to 45%.[117,176–179] The great majority of these patients also have evidence of bone metastases, and in one study only 6% of patients with marrow infiltration did not have associated bone involvement.[176] In terms of clinical management, if it is felt necessary to investigate bone marrow at all, then it would seem reasonable to restrict marrow aspirates to patients with established bone metastases, in the absence of other specific indications.

At initial presentation the incidence of marrow metastases is very low, and bone marrow examination is quite unrewarding.[115,117,180,181] In one series, metastases were detected in only 1/254 patients (0.4%),[117] and this patient also had metastatic disease elsewhere. The routine use of conventional marrow aspirates as a staging investigation therefore is not recommended. However, it is of interest that an immunocytochemical technique using a polyclonal antibody that recognizes an epithelial membrane antigen (anti-EMA)[182] increases the detection rate of marrow metastases in patients without skeletal recurrence.[183] The same technique has been used to demonstrate tumor cells in multiple marrow aspirates from 31 of 110 patients (28%) presenting with early stage disease; none of these patients had any evidence of marrow infiltration on conventional aspirate cytology.[184] The eventual prognostic significance of this finding must await long-term follow-up.

TUMOR MARKERS

Many different tumor-derived and tumor-associated products including oncofetal proteins, hormones, enzymes, nucleosides, polyamines, and acute-phase proteins have been studied as possible tumor markers in the detection and monitoring of breast cancer. Initially, their potential has been investigated in metastatic disease. However, the principal value of any such tumor marker would lie in its ability to detect minimal residual cancer at a time when appropriate therapy might significantly alter the outcome.

Markers in Association With Overt Metastases

The most widely studied tumor marker in breast cancer has been the oncofetal protein CEA. Many studies have shown this to be elevated in 70% to 80% of patients with overt metastases,[74,185–189] and in one, CEA levels of greater than 10 ng/ml were associated with metastatic disease in 100% of patients.[180] Abnormal levels correlate in particular with bone and liver metastases and with multiple sites of disease.[187,188] However, CEA has a low specificity, and moderately raised levels may occur in many other conditions.

Details of other marker substances commonly raised in metastatic disease are listed in Table 12-9. These include ferritin in 68%[191] to 88%[74] of patients, C-reactive protein (CRP) in around 80%,[74] α-glycoprotein (AGP) in around 75%,[74, 192] sialyl transferase in around 60%,[74,193] alkaline phosphatase in around 65%,[74] β-oncofetal antigen in around 55%,[194] and the nucleoside dimethylguanosine in around 65%.[194,195] Recently, attention has also focused on antigens that might be recognized by antibodies raised against breast cancer and breast tissue products. Two of these, Thomsen-Friedenreich (T) antigen and human tissue polypeptide antigen (TPA), are elevated in the great majority of patients with metastatic breast cancer.[196–198] However TPA is also elevated in more than 25% of patients with benign breast disease.[198]

Many other markers have also been reported as elevated, but in a minority of metastatic breast cancer patients.[194] These include calcitonin[74,199,200] and β-HCG[74,195]

Despite this plethora of available markers, many are redundant in that they are no more effective than readily available conventional investigations for detecting metastases. It has been shown that their sensitivity can be increased by selecting only a few key markers in combination. Thus, all of a series of 17 patients with metastases had abnormalities in at least three out of ten tumor markers, and several combinations of only two markers also detected 100% of patients, including CEA and ferritin, CRP and ferritin, CEA and AGP, and ferritin and AGP.[74] Another group likewise detected 97% of metastatic patients measuring a combination of plasma CEA, β-HCG, and urinary dimethylguanosine.[195]

Table 12-9
Tumor Markers Commonly Found Elevated in Patients With Metastatic Breast Cancer

Markers	*Incidence (%)*	*Reference*
Oncofetal products		
CEA	70–80	74, 185–189
Oncofetal antigen (OFA)	55	194
Ferritin	68–88	74, 191
Proteins		
C-reactive protein	80	74
Pregnancy-associated macroglobulin (PAM)	35	194
α-Acid glycoprotein (AGP)	75	74, 192
β_2-microglobulin	50	207
Gross cystic disease fluid protein (GCDFP)	40–50	206
Enzymes		
Sialyl transferase	60	74, 193
Alkaline phosphatase	65	194
5-nucleotide phosphodiesterase	55	208
Nucleosides		
Dimethylguanosine	65	194, 195
Pseudouridine	50	194
Methylinosine	46	194
Antigens		
Thomsen-Friedenreich (T) antigen	100	196
Tissue polypeptide antigen (TPA)	80	197, 198

Markers in Association with "Early" or Occult Disease

Despite some clear-cut correlations between raised tumor markers and the prediction of occult metastatic disease, no marker or combination of markers has shown the extreme sensitivity required to make early and accurate predictions of minimal occult disease.

In patients with early stage disease presenting for surgery, preoperative CEA levels of more than 3 ng/ml were associated with an increased incidence of a recurrence.[201] Likewise, in three studies persistently elevated postmastectomy levels were shown to correlate with significantly increased recurrence rates and poor prognosis.[201–203] However, another study found CEA levels to be raised in only 12% of patients with early stage disease, and no correlation emerged between initially elevated CEA and subsequent relapse.[194]

In a very detailed marker study, the same group[194] investigated a total of 26 tumor markers in patients presenting with early breast cancer. As with CEA, other markers were elevated only in a minority of patients (e.g., sialyl transferase in 16%, calcitonin in 25%, and CRP in 4%), whereas many putative markers were normal in all patients. With follow-up on patients who subsequently relapsed, no difference emerged in relapsers between those with or without abnormal markers at initial presentation. In a different study, only 67% of patients with positive nodes (and therefore a presumed poor prognosis) had one or more abnormalities in CEA, HCG, or dimethylguanosine.[195]

Studies have also been carried out to determine whether tumor marker substances can be used as early predictors of metastatic recurrence. Serially rising plasma CEA levels in postmastectomy patients anticipated metastatic relapse in 48 of 65 (74%), with a mean lead time over standard investigations of 4.8 months (range 1 to 12 months).[190] Rapid rates of rise indicated liver or bone metastases. A French group found that 11 of 27 patients (41%) who developed relapse had elevated CEA levels preceding clinical signs by a median 6 months; in 12 patients (44%) CEA never rose.[204] In a detailed study, CEA, γ-glutamyltranspeptidase (γ-GT), hydroxyproline, alkaline phosphatase, ferritin, CRP, α-AGP, erythrocyte sedimentation rates, dimethylguanosine, and pregnancy-associated macroglobulin were serially measured in postmastectomy patients at three-month intervals.[194] A rising CEA antedated clinical recurrence in 8 of 23 patients (35%), alkaline phosphatase in 4 of 23 (17%), γ-GT in 2 of 16 (13%), and three others (CRP, α-AGP, and hydroxyproline) in one patient each. Overall, even with all markers, only 13 of 23 (57%) patients had antecedent rises. These had a short lead interval, averaging 3 months (range 1 to 15 months). The authors concluded that the use of only three markers (CEA, alkaline phosphatase, and γ-GT) in association with chest radiography and clinical examination would have been as effective in the detection of metastatic disease.

These meticulous and painstaking studies demonstrate that tumor markers for breast cancer are so far not sensitive enough to detect minimal residual disease reliably or to influence plans for adjuvant treatment.

RECOMMENDATIONS FOR STAGING AND FOLLOW-UP

In recent years there has been an increasing tendency to overinvestigate patients with breast cancer, and this has been correctly criticized.[115,181] The more sophisticated investigative techniques have their main value in sorting out diagnostic problems; when used routinely in asymptomatic patients, they can become a costly extravagance, making no useful contribution to patient management. The recommendations listed below are therefore suggested for routine clinical practice. A more elaborate approach should be reserved for appropriate research studies.

Staging at Presentation

The key investigations at first presentation should be detailed clinical assessment, mammography, peripheral full blood count, biochemical liver function tests including in particular alkaline phosphatase, and a standard chest x-ray. As discussed above, other more elaborate investigations on a routine basis have an extremely low yield or produce positive results of uncertain significance and do not help in clinical management. In particular, liver scintiscans, ultrasonography, and bone marrow aspirates are unnecessary in the absence of specific clinical or biochemical abnormalities. Despite some persisting controversy, the weight of evidence suggests that the same is true for bone scintiscans.

Follow-up

Several studies have shown that with routine follow-up (clinical examination and biochemical liver tests every 3 to 6 months with annual chest radiography, and scintiscans only for specific indications) the great majority of those who relapse (86% to 97%) are first detected clinically, through symptoms or signs.[115,181,205] In one study in which 254 patients were observed routinely, only 8 out of 98 who relapsed (8%) were detected through investigations, at a total cost in x-rays, blood tests, and scans of around $90,000 at pre-1980 prices.[181]

Even with a much more elaborate series of follow-up investigations in a research study (10 tumor markers assayed every 3 months, chest x-ray, skeletal x-rays, bone and liver scintiscanning, and bone marrow aspirate every 6 months) 40% of patients who relapsed were still first detected clinically, and a median lead interval of only 3 months was achieved in those detected by tumor marker abnormalities.[76] Of all patients who relapsed, 98% would have been detected using a simple screen of clinical assessment; serum alkaline phosphatase, γ-GT, and CEA; and chest radiography.

Our policy is therefore to use this basic screen for routine follow-up, with a strong emphasis on clinical assessment and with more elaborate investigations reserved for patients in whom abnormalities are detected. We recommend three-month follow-up intervals during the first 2 years, when risk of relapse is greatest, and six-month intervals thereafter, with patients instructed to return early if symptoms develop between visits. Breast conservation is an indication for more frequent follow-up to detect local recurrence. Current treatment for metastatic disease has a very limited potential, and on this basis reassurance for the asymptomatic patient makes more sense than a sophisticated search for early recurrence.

REFERENCES

1. Haagensen CD: The surgical treatment of mammary carcinoma. In Haagensen CD: Diseases of the Breast, pp 669–773. Philadelphia, WB Saunders, 1971
2. Fisher B, Slack N, Katrych D, et al: Ten-year follow-up results for patients with carcinoma of the breast in a cooperative trial evaluating surgical adjuvant chemotherapy. Surg Gynecol Obstet 140:528–534, 1975
3. Valagussa P, Bonadonna G, Veronesi U: Patterns of relapse and survival following radical mastectomy: Analysis of 716 consecutive patients. Cancer 41:1170–1178, 1978
4. Brinkley D, Haybittle JL: Long term survival of women with breast cancer. Lancet 1:1118, 1984
5. Fisher B, Slack NH, Cavanaugh PJ, et al: Post-operative radiotherapy in the treatment of breast cancer: Results of the NSABP clinical trial. Ann Surg 172:711–730, 1970
6. Fisher B, Redmond C, Fisher ER, et al: Ten-year results of a randomized clinical trial comparing radical mastectomy and total mastectomy with or without radiation. N Engl J Med 312:674–681, 1985
7. Strender L, Wallgren A, Arndt J, et al: Adjuvant radiotherapy in operable breast cancer: Correlation between dose in internal mammary nodes and prognosis. Int J Rad Oncol Biol Phys 7:1319–1325, 1981
8. Primary Therapy of Breast Cancer Study Group (PTBCSG): Identification of breast cancer patients with high risk of early recurrence after radical mastectomy. II: Clinical and pathological correlations. Cancer 42:2809–2826, 1978
9. Fey MF, Brunner KW, Sonntag RW: Prognostic factors in metastatic breast cancer. Cancer Clin Trials 4:237–247, 1981
10. Lee Y-TN: Breast carcinoma: Pattern of recurrence and metastasis after mastectomy. Am J Clin Oncol 7:443–449, 1984
11. Bonadonna G, Valagussa P, Rossi A, et al: Ten-year experience with CMF-based adjuvant chemotherapy in resectable breast cancer. Breast Cancer Res Treat 5:95–115, 1985
12. Smith IE: Unpublished data
13. Bonadonna G, Brusamolino E, Valagussa P, et al: Combination chemotherapy as an adjuvant treatment in operable breast cancer. N Engl J Med 294:405–410, 1976
14. Karabali-Dalamaga S, Souhami RL, O'Higgins NJ, et al: Natural history and prognosis of recurrent breast cancer. Br Med J 2:730–733, 1978
15. Donegan WL: Patterns and prognosis of advanced breast carcinoma. Missouri Med 67:853–858, 1970
16. Valagussa P, Tesoro Tess JD, Rossi A, et al: Adjuvant CMF: Effect on site of first recurrence, and appropriate follow-up intervals, in operable breast cancer with positive axillary nodes. Breast Cancer Res Treat 1:349–356, 1982
17. Hahnel R, Woodings T, Vivian AB: Prognostic value of oestrogen receptors in primary breast cancer. Cancer 44:671–676, 1979
18. Viadaria E, Cotter R, Pickren JW, et al: An autopsy study of metastatic sites of breast cancer. Cancer Res 33:179, 1973
19. Warren S, Witman EM: Studies on tumour metastases: The distribution of metastases in cancer of the breast. Surg Gynecol Obstet 57:81–94, 1937
20. Saphillo O, Parker ML: Metastases of primary carcinoma of the breast with special reference to spleen, adrenal glands and ovaries. Arch Surg 42:1003–1034, 1941
21. Haagensen CD: Diseases of the breast, p 426. Philadelphia, WB Saunders, 1971
22. Coombes RC, Powles TJ, Ford HT, et al (eds): Breast Cancer Management, p 206. New York, Grune & Stratton, 1981
23. Romsdahl MM, Sears ME, Eckles NE: Post-treatment evaluation of breast cancer. In Breast Cancer Early and Late, pp 291–299, 13th Annual Clinical Conference on Cancer, 1968 at the University of Texas, MD Anderson Hospital and Tumour Institute. Chicago, Year Book Medical Publishers, 1970
24. Powles TJ, Smith IE, Ford HT, et al: Failure of chemotherapy to prolong survival in a group of patients with metastatic breast cancer. Lancet 1:580–582, 1980
25. Valagussa P, Bonadonna G, Veronesi U: Patterns of relapse and survival in operable breast carcinoma with positive and negative axillary nodes. Tumori 64:241–258, 1978
26. Koscielny S, Tubiana M, Le MG, et al: Breast cancer: Relationship between the size of the primary tumour and the probability of metastatic dissemination. Br J Cancer 49:709–715, 1984
27. Clark RM, Wilkinson RH, Mahoney LJ, et al: Breast cancer: A 21 year experience with conservative surgery and radiation. Int J Radiat Oncol Biol Phys 8:967–975, 1982
28. Cutler SJ, Asire AJ, Taylor III SG: Classification of patients with disseminated cancer of the breast. Cancer 24:861–869, 1969
29. Paterson AHG, Zuck VP, Szafran O, et al: Influence and significance of certain prognostic factors on survival in breast cancer. Eur J Cancer Clin Oncol 18:937–943, 1982
30. Swenerton KD, Legha SS, Smith T, et al: Prognostic factors in metastatic breast cancer treated with combination chemotherapy. Cancer Res 39:1552–1562, 1979
31. Poe RH, Qazi R, Israel RH, et al: Survival of patients with pleural involvement by breast carcinoma. Am J Clin Oncol 6:523–527, 1983
32. Tsukada Y, Fouad A, Pickren JW, et al: Central nervous system metastasis from breast carcinoma. An autopsy study. Cancer 52:2349–2354, 1983
33. DiStefano A, Yap HY, Hortobagyi GN, et al: The natural history of breast cancer patients with brain metastases. Cancer 44:1913–1918, 1979
34. Hendrickson FR: The optimum schedule for palliative radiotherapy for metastatic brain cancer. Int J Radiat Oncol Biol Phys 2:165, 1977
35. Horton J, Baxter DH, Olson KB: The management of metastases to the brain by irradiation and corticosteroids. Am J Roentgenol 3:334–336, 1971
36. Lang EF, Slater J: Metastatic brain tumour: Results of surgical and non-surgical treatment. Surg Clin North Am 44:865, 1964
37. Nisce LZ, Hilaris BS, Chu FC: A review of experience with irradiation of brain metastases. Am J Roentgenol 3:329–340, 1971
38. Order SE, Hellman S, Von Essen CF, et al: Improved quality of survival following whole-brain irradiation for brain metastases. Radiology 91:149, 1968
39. Yap HY, Yap BS, Rasmussen S, et al: Treatment for meningeal carcinomatosis in breast cancer. Cancer 49:219–222, 1982
40. Little JR, Okajaki H: Meningeal carcinomatosis. Arch Neurol 30:138–143, 1974
41. McKelvey EM: Meningeal involvement with metastatic carcinoma of the breast treated with intrathecal methotrexate. Cancer 22:576–580, 1968
42. Shapiro WR, Posner JB, Ushio Y, et al: Treatment of meningeal neoplasia. Cancer Treat Rep 61(4):733–743, 1977
43. Bramlet D, Gilberti J, Bender J: Meningeal carcinomatosis: Case report and review of the literature. Neurology 26:287–290, 1976
44. Stewart JF, King RJB, Sexton SA, et al: Oestrogen receptors, sites of metastatic disease and survival in current breast cancer. Eur J Cancer 17:449–453, 1981
45. Howell A, Harland RNL, Bramwell VHC, et al: Steroid hor-

mone receptors and survival after first relapse in breast cancer. Lancet 1:588–591, 1984
46. Howat JMT, Harris M, Swindell R, et al: The effect of oestrogen and progesterone receptors on recurrence and survival in patients with carcinoma of the breast. Br J Cancer 51:263–270, 1985
47. Duncan W, Kerr GR: The curability of breast cancer. Br Med J 2:781–783, 1976
48. Fisher B, Slack NH, Bross DJ: Cancer of the breast: Size of neoplasm and prognosis. Cancer 24:1071–1080, 1969
49. Moseley HS, Peetz ME, Keenan EJ, et al: Endocrine ablation for metastatic breast cancer: A reappraisal of hormone receptors. Am J Surg 140:164–172, 1980
50. Stewart J, King R, Hayward J, et al: Estrogen and progesterone receptors: Correlation of response rates, site and timing of receptor analysis. Breast Cancer Res Treat 2:243–250, 1982
51. Donegan WL, Pevez-Masa CM, Watson RF: A biostatistical study of locally recurrent breast carcinoma. Surg Gynecol Obstet 122:529–540, 1966
52. Zimmerman KW, Montague ED, Fletcher GH: Frequency, anatomical distribution and management of local recurrences after definitive therapy for breast cancer. Cancer 19:1967–1974, 1966
53. Auchinloss H: The nature of local recurrence following radical mastectomy. Cancer 11:611–619, 1958
54. Spratt JS: Locally recurrent cancer after radical mastectomy. Cancer 20:1051–1053, 1967
55. Chu FCH, Lin FJ, Kim JH, et al: Locally recurrent carcinoma of the breast. Cancer 37:2677–2681, 1976
56. Gilliland MD, Barton RM, Copeland EM: The implication of local recurrence of breast cancer. Ann Surg 197:284–287, 1983
57. Tough ICK: The significance of recurrence in breast cancer. Br J Surg 53:877–900, 1966
58. Fentiman IS, Matthews PN, Davidson OW, et al: Survival following local skin recurrence after mastectomy. Br J Surg 72:14–16, 1985
59. Montague ED: Conservation surgery and radiation therapy in the treatment of operable breast cancer. Cancer 53:700–704, 1984
60. Bedwinek JM, Lee J, Fineberg B, et al: Prognostic indicators in patients with isolated local-regional recurrence of breast cancer. Cancer 47:2232–2235, 1981
61. Marshall KA, Redfern A, Cady B: Local recurrence of carcinoma of the breast. Surg Gynecol Obstet 139:406–408, 1974
62. Beck TM, Hart NE, Woodward DA, et al: Local or regionally recurrent carcinoma of the breast: Results of therapy in 121 patients. J Clin Oncol 1:400–405, 1983
63. Clarke DH, Le MG, Sarrazin D, et al: Analysis of local-regional relapses in patients with early breast cancers treated by excision and radiotherapy: Experience of the Institut Gustave-Roussy. Int J Radiat Oncol Biol Phys 11:137–145, 1985
64. Kurtz JM, Spitalier JM, Amalric R: Late breast recurrence after lumpectomy and irradiation. Int J Radiat Oncol Biol Phys 9:1191–1194, 1983
65. Vilcoq JR, Calle R, Stacey P, et al: The outcome of treatment by tumorectomy and radiotherapy of patients with operable breast cancer. Int J Radiat Oncol Biol Phys 7:1327–1332, 1981
66. Calle R, Pilleron JP, Schlienger P, et al: Conservative management of operable breast cancer: Ten years experience at the Foundation Curie. Cancer 42:2045–2053, 1978
67. Veronesi U, Saccozzi R, Del Vecchio M, et al: Comparing radical mastectomy with quadrantectomy, axillary dissection and radiotherapy in patients with small cancers of the breast. N Engl J Med 305:6–11, 1981
68. Fisher B, Bauer M, Margolese R, et al: Five-year results of a randomized clinical trial comparing total mastectomy and segmental mastectomy with or without radiation in the treatment of breast cancer. N Engl J Med 312:667–673, 1985
69. Pierquin B, Owen R, Maylin C, et al: Radical radiation therapy of breast cancer. Int J Radiat Oncol Biol Phys 6:17–24, 1980
70. Hellman S, Harris JR, Levene MB: Radiation therapy of early carcinoma of the breast without mastectomy. Cancer 46 (4:suppl):988–994, 1980
71. Amalric R, Santamaria F, Robert F, et al: Radiation therapy with or without primary limited surgery for operable breast cancer. Cancer 49:30–34, 1982
72. Galasko CSB: Skeletal metastases and mammary cancer. Ann Roy Coll Surg Engl 50:3, 1972
73. Cushieri A: Urinary hydroxyproline excretion in early and advanced breast cancer—a sequential study. Br J Surg 60:800–806, 1973
74. Coombes RC, Powles TJ, Gazet JC, et al: A biochemical approach to the staging of human breast cancer. Cancer 40:937–944, 1977
75. Gielen F, Dequeker J, Wildiers J, et al: Relevance of hydroxyproline excretion in bone metastasis in breast cancer. Br J Cancer 34:279–285, 1976
76. Coombes RC, Powles TJ, Gazet JC, et al: Biochemical markers in human breast cancer. Lancet 1:132–135, 1980
77. Coombes RC, Dearnaley DP, Buckman R, et al: Detection of bone metastases in patients with breast cancer. Invasion Metastasis 2:177–184, 1982
78. Guzzo CE, Pachas WN, Pinals RS, et al: Urinary hydroxyproline excretion in patients with cancer. Cancer 24:382–387, 1969
79. Roberts JG, Williams M, Henk JM, et al: The hypronosticon test in breast cancer. Clin Oncol 1:33–43, 1975
80. Cuschieri A: Urinary hydroxyproline excretion and survival in cancer of the breast. Clin Oncol 1:127–130, 1975
81. Grant CS, Hoare SA, Millis RR, et al: Urinary hydroxyproline and prognosis in human breast cancer. Br J Surg 71:105–108, 1984
82. Barrett JJ, Smith PHS: Bone imaging with ^{99m}Tc polyphosphate: A comparison with 18F and skeletal radiography. Br J Radiol 47:387–392, 1974
83. Fogelman I: Diphosphonate bone scanning agents—current concepts. Eur J Nucl Med 7:506–509, 1982
84. Simpson WJ, Orange RP: Total body scanning with 85Sr in the diagnosis of metastatic bone disease. Canad Med Assoc J 93:1237, 1965
85. Briggs RC: Detection of osseous metastases. Evaluation of bone scanning with 85Sr. Cancer 20:392, 1967
86. French RJ, McCready VR: The use of 18F for bone scanning. Br J Radiol 40:655, 1967
87. Harmer CL, Burns JE, Sams A, et al: The value of Fluorine-18 for scanning bone tumours. Clin Radiol 20:204, 1969
88. Milner TH, Maynard CD, Cowan RJ: Evaluation of 85Sr bone scans and roentgenograms in 100 patients. Arch Surg 103:371, 1971
89. Gnekow WC, Denards GL, Poole GJ, et al: Review of a 5-year experience with the radiostrontium bone scintiscan. Calif Med 117:1, 1972
90. Pistenma DA, McDougall IR, Kriss JP: Screening for bone metastases. JAMA 231:46–50, 1975
91. Citrin DL, Bessent RG, Grieg WR: A comparison of the sensitivity and accuracy of the ^{99m}Tc phosphate bone scan and skeletal radiograph in the diagnosis of bone metastases. Clin Radiol 28:107–117, 1977
92. Parthasarathy KL, Landsberg R, Bakshi SP, et al: Detection of bone metastases in urogenital malignancies utilizing Tc

99m-labelled phosphate compounds. Urology 2:99–102, 1978
93. Brady LW, Croll MN: The role of bone scanning in the cancer patient. Skeletal Radiol 3:217–222, 1979
94. Lentle BC, Russell AD, Percy JS, et al: Bone scintiscanning updated. Ann Intern Med 84:297–303, 1976
95. Corcoran RJ, Thrall JH, Kyle RW, et al: Solitary abnormalities in bone scans of patients with extraosseous malignancies. Radiology 121:663–667, 1976
96. Edelstyn GA, Gillespie PJ, Grebbell FS: The radiological demonstration of osseous metastases. Clin Radiol 18:158, 1967
97. Perez DJ, Milan J, Ford HT, et al: Detection of breast carcinoma metastases in bone: Relative merits of x-rays and skeletal scintigraphy. Lancet 2:613–616, 1983
98. Galasko CSB: The value of scintigraphy in malignant disease. Cancer Treat Rev 2:225–272, 1975
99. Citrin DL, Bessent RG, Greig WR, et al: The application of ^{99m}Tc phosphate bone scan to the study of breast cancer. Br J Surg 62:201–204, 1975
100. Kirkman S, Henk JM: The value of bone scanning in the staging of breast cancer. Clin Radiol 30:11–14, 1979
101. British Breast Group: Bone scanning in breast cancer. Br Med J 2:180–181, 1978
102. Nomura Y, Kondo H, Yamagata J, et al: Evaluation of liver and bone scanning in patients with early breast cancer, based on results obtained from more advanced cancer patients. Eur J Cancer 14:1129–1136, 1978
103. Kunkler IH, Merrick MV, Rodger A: Bone scintigraphy in breast cancer: A nine-year follow-up. Clin Radiol 36:279–282, 1985
104. Rossing N, Munck O, Pors Nielsen S, et al: What do early bone scans tell about breast cancer patients? Eur J Cancer Clin Oncol 18:629–636, 1982
105. Khandekar JD, Burkett FE, Scanlon EF: Sensitivity, specificity and predictive value of bone scans in breast cancer. Proc Am Assoc Cancer Res 19:379, 1978
106. Gerber FH, Goodreau JJ, Kirchner PT, et al: Efficacy of pre-operative and post-operative bone scanning in the management of the breast carcinoma. N Engl J Med 297:300–303, 1977
107. Baker RR, Holmes ER, Alderson PO, et al: An evaluation of bone scans as screening procedures for occult metastases in primary breast cancer. Ann Surg 186:363–368, 1977
108. Taaning E, Nielsen J, Rossing N, et al: Skeletal metastases in operable cancer of the breast. Ugeskr Laeger 141:994–997, 1979
109. Hahn P, Vikterlof KJ, Rjdman H, et al: The value of whole body bone scan in the pre-operative assessment in carcinoma of the breast. Eur J Nucl Med 4:207–210, 1979
110. Kirkman S, Henk JM: The value of bone scanning in the staging of breast cancer. Radiology 30:11–14, 1979
111. McKillop JH, Blumgurt LH, Wood CB, et al: The prognostic and therapeutic implications of the positive radionuclide bone scan in clinically early breast cancer. Br J Surg 65:649–652, 1978
112. Elston CW, Blamey RW: Staging breast cancer: Role of bone scanning. Br Med J 2:603–605, 1977
113. Butzelaar MJM, Van Dongen JA, Van Der Schott JB, et al: Evaluation of routine pre-operative bone scintigraphy in patients with breast cancer. Eur J Cancer 13:19–21, 1977
114. Roberts MM, Hayward JL: Bone scanning and early breast cancer: Five-year follow-up. Lancet 1:997–998, 1983
115. Winchester DP, Sener SF, Khandekar JD, et al: Symptomatology as an indicator of recurrent or metastatic breast cancer. Cancer 43:956–960, 1979
116. Schaffer DL, Kalisher L: Incidence of bone metastases in women with minimal and occult breast carcinoma. Radiology 124:675–680, 1977
117. Coombes RC: The staging of human breast cancer: Physical staging techniques. In Coombes RC, Powles TJ, Ford HT, et al (eds): Breast Cancer Management, pp 77–96. New York, Grune & Stratton, 1981
118. Muindi J, Coombes RC, Golding S, et al: The role of computed tomography in the detection of bone metastases in breast cancer patients. Br J Radiol 56:233–236, 1983
119. Smith IE, Taylor KJW, McCready VR, et al: A comparison of grey-scale ultrasound with other methods for the detection of liver metastases from breast carcinoma. Clin Oncol 2:47–53, 1976
120. Schaefer J, Schiff L: Liver function tests in metastatic tumor of the liver: Study of 100 cases. Gastroenterology 49:360–363, 1965
121. Baden H, Anderson B, Augustenborg G, et al: Diagnostic value of gamma-glutamyltranspeptidase and alkaline phosphatase in liver metastases. Surg Gynecol Obstet 133:769, 1971
122. Kim NY, Yasmineh WG, Frier EF, et al: Value of alkaline phosphatase, 5-nucleotidase, gamma-glutamate dehydrogenase activity measurements (single and combined) in serum in diagnosis of metastases to the liver. Clin Chem 23:2034, 1977
123. Irvin TT, Edwards JP, Goligher JC: The value of plasma gamma-glutamyltranspeptidase in the detection of hepatic metastases. Br J Surg 60:347, 1973
124. White DR, Maloney III JJ, Muss HB, et al: Serum alkaline phosphatase determination. JAMA 242:1147–1149, 1973
125. Wiener SN, Sachs SH: An assessment of routine liver scanning in patients with breast cancer. Arch Surg 113:126–127, 1978
126. De Ribas L, Coombes RC, Gazet JC, et al: Tests for liver metastases in breast cancer. Evaluation of liver scan and liver ultrasound. Clin Oncol 6:225, 1980
127. Harper PV, Lathrop KA, Jimenez F, et al: Technetium 99m as a scanning agent. Radiology 85:101–109, 1965
128. McAfee JG, Ause RG, Wagner HN Jr: Diagnostic value of scintillation scanning of the liver. Arch Intern Med 116:95, 1965
129. Cosgrove DO, McCready VR: Diagnosis of liver metastases using ultrasound and isotope scanning techniques. J R Soc Med 71:652–657, 1978
130. Ostfeld DA, Meyer JE: Liver scanning in patients with short interval autopsy correlation. Radiology 138:671–673, 1981
131. Clouse ME: Roentgenographic techniques for the diagnosis and management of liver tumours. Semin Oncol 10:159–175, 1983
132. Taylor KJW, Carpenter DA, McCready VR: Grey-scale echography in the diagnosis of intrahepatic disease. J Clin Ultrasound 1:284–289, 1973
133. Khan O, Slack N, Cosgrove D: Ultrasound imaging in staging and monitoring. In Stoll BA (ed): Screening and Monitoring of Cancer, pp 79–95. New York, John Wiley & Sons, 1985
134. Taylor KJW, Sullivan D, Rosenfield T, et al: Grey-scale ultrasound and isotope scanning: Complementary techniques for imaging the liver. Am J Roentgenol 128:277–281, 1977
135. Snow JH Jr, Goldstein HM, Wallace S: Comparison of scintigraphy, sonography and computed tomography in the evaluation of hepatic neoplasms. Am J Roentgenol 132:915–918, 1979
136. Grossman ZD, Wistow BW, Bryan BJ, et al: Radionuclide imaging, computed tomography and grey scale ultrasonography of the liver: A comparative study. J Nucl Med 18:327–332, 1977

137. Nagler W, Bender MA, Blau M: Radioisotope photoscanning of the liver. Gastroenterology 44:36–45, 1963
138. Ariel IM, Molander D, Galey D: Hepatic gamma scanning. An aid in determining treatment policies for cancer involving the liver. Am J Surg 118:5–13, 1969
139. Ferrier FL, Hatcher CR Jr, Achard JL, et al: The value of liver scanning for detection of metastatic cancer. Am J Surg 35:112, 1969
140. Poulose KP, Reba RC, DeLand FH, et al: Role of liver scanning in the preoperative evaluation of patients with cancer. Br Med J 4:585, 1969
141. Castagna J, Benfield JR, Yamada H, et al: The reliability of liver scans and function tests in detecting metastases. Surg Gynecol Obstet 134:463, 1972
142. Lunia S, Parthasarathy KL, Bakshi S, et al: An evaluation of ^{99m}Tc-sulfur colloid liver scintiscans and their usefulness in metastatic workup. A review of 1,424 studies. J Nucl Med 16:62, 1975
143. Alfidi RJ, Haaga JR, Havrilla TR, et al: Computed tomography of the liver. Am J Roentgenol 127:69–74, 1976
144. Vicary FR, Shirley I: Ultrasound and hepatic metastases. Br J Radiol 51:596–598, 1978
145. Galli G, Maini CL, Salvation M, et al: The diagnostic application of radiocolloid liver scintigraphy in breast carcinoma. Nucl Med 21:140–144, 1982
146. Scherer U, Rothe R, Eisenburg J, et al: Diagnostic accuracy of CT in circumscript liver disease. Am J Roentgenol 130:711–714, 1978
147. Yeh HC, Rabinowitz JG: Ultrasound and computed tomography of the liver. Radiol Clin North Am 18:321–338, 1980
148. Levitt RG, Sogel SS, Stanely RJ, et al: Accuracy of computed tomography of the liver and biliary tract. Radiol 124:123–128, 1977
149. MacCarthy RL, Stephens DH, Hattery RR, et al: Hepatic imaging by computed tomography. A comparison with ^{99m}Tc-sulfur colloid, ultrasonography and angiography. Radiol Clin North Am 17:137–155, 1979
150. Djang WT, Young SW, Castelline RA, et al: Computed tomography of the liver: Evaluating focal defects on radionuclide liver-spleen scans. Am J Roentgenol 141:937–940, 1984
151. Ali MK, Hare CD, Miller JM: Regional pulmonary function in metastatic carcinoma to the lung studied with Xenon-133. Cancer 27:460–466, 1971
152. Polga JP, Watnick M: Whole lung tomography in metastatic disease. Clin Radiol 27:53–56, 1976
153. Neilfeld JP, Michaelis LL, Doppman JL: Suspected pulmonary metastases. Correlation of chest x-ray, whole lung tomograms and operative findings. Cancer 39:383–387, 1977
154. Sindelar WF, Bagley DH, Felix EL, et al: Lung tomography in cancer patients. Full lung tomograms in screening for pulmonary metastases. JAMA 240:2060–2063, 1978
155. Chang AE, Schaner EG, Conkle DM, et al: Evaluation of CT in the detection of pulmonary metastases. Cancer 43:913–916, 1979
156. Husband J, Grimer DP: Staging testicular tumours: Role of CT scanning. J R Soc Med 78(b):25–31, 1985
157. Goldsmith HS, Bailey HD, Callahan EL, et al: Pulmonary lymphangitic metastases from breast carcinoma. Arch Surg 94:483–494, 1967
158. Green N, Kern W, Levis R, et al: Lymphangitic carcinomatosis of the lung: Pathologic diagnostic and therapeutic considerations. Int J Radiat Oncol Biol Phys 2:149–153, 1977
159. Janover ML, Blennerharsett JB: Lymphangitic spread of metastatic cancer to the lung. Radiology 101:267–273, 1971
160. Joyner LR, Schienhorn DJ: Transbronchial forceps lung biopsy through the fiberoptic bronchoscope. Chest 67:532–535, 1975
161. Aranda C, Sidhu G, Sasso LA, et al: Transbronchial lung biopsy in the diagnosis of lymphangitic carcinomatosis. Cancer 42:1995–1998, 1978
162. Morris AJR, O'Sullivan JP, Millard FJC, et al: Fibreoptic bronchoscopy as an aid to diagnosis of respiratory symptoms in breast cancer patients. Br J Cancer 48:731–734, 1983
163. Rosenblatt MB, Lisa JR, Trinidad S: Pitfalls in the clinical and histologic diagnosis of bronchogenic carcinoma. Dis Chest 49:396–404, 1966
164. Lewi HJ, Roberts MM, Donaldson AA, et al: The use of computer assisted tomography as a staging investigation of patients with carcinomas of the breast and melanoma. Surg Gynecol Obstet 151:385-386, 1980
165. Willis RA: Pathology of Tumours, 4th ed, pp 174–175. Scarborough, Ont, Butterworth & Co, 1967
166. Cifuentes N, Pickren JW: Metastases from carcinoma of mammary gland: An autopsy study. J Surg Oncol 11:193–205, 1979
167. Black P: Metastatic tumours of the central nervous system: Cerebral metastases. In Abeloff MD (ed): Complications of Cancer, pp 283–312. Baltimore, Johns Hopkins Press, 1979
168. Weisberg LA: Computerized tomography in intracranial metastases. Arch Neurol 36:630–634, 1979
169. Dearnaley DP, Kingsley DPE, Husband JE, et al: The role of computed tomography of the brain in the investigation of breast cancer patients with suspected intracranial metastases. Clin Radiol 32:375–382, 1981
170. Deck MDF, Messina AV, Sackett JF: Computed tomography in metastatic disease of the brain. Radiology 119:115–120, 1976
171. Bardfeld PA, Passalaqua AM, Braunstein P, et al: A comparison of radionuclide scanning and computed tomography in metastatic lesions of the brain. J Comput Assist Tomogr 1:315–318, 1977
172. Buell V, Niendorf HP, Kazner E, et al: Computerized transaxial tomography and cerebral serial scintigraphy in intracranial tumours—rates of detection and tumour-type identification. J Nucl Med 19:476–479, 1978
173. Dearnaley DP, Patel S, Powles TJ, et al: Carcinoembryonic antigen estimation in cerebrospinal fluid in patients with metastatic breast cancer. Oncodev Biol Med 2:305–311, 1981
174. Sondak V, Deckers PJ, Feller JH, et al: Leptomeningeal spread of breast cancer: Report of case and review of the literature. Cancer 48:395–399, 1981
175. Yap BS, Yap HY, Fritsche HA, et al: CSF carcinoembryonic antigen in meningeal carcinomatosis from breast cancer. JAMA 244:1601–1603, 1980
176. DiStefano A, Tashima CK, Yap HY, et al: Bone marrow metastases without cortical bone involvement in breast cancer patients. Cancer 44:196–198, 1979
177. Ingle JN, Tormey DC, Bull JM, et al: Bone marrow involvement in breast cancer. Cancer 39:104–111, 1977
178. Thrupkaew AK, Henkin RE, Quinn JL: False negative bone scans in disseminated metastatic disease. Radiology 113:383–386, 1974
179. O'Mara RE: Bone scanning in osseous metastatic disease. JAMA 229:1915–1917, 1974
180. Ingle JN, Tormey DC, Tan HK: The bone marrow examination in breast cancer. Cancer 41:670–674, 1978
181. Scanlon EF, Oviedo MA, Cunningham MP, et al: Preoperative and follow-up procedures on patients with breast cancer. Cancer 46:977–979, 1980
182. Heyderman E, Steele K, Ormerod MG: A new antigen on the epithelial membrane: Its immunoperoxidase localisation in normal and neoplastic tissue. J Clin Pathol 32:35–39, 1979
183. Dearnaley DP, Sloane JP, Ormerod MG, et al: Increased detection of mammary carcinoma cells in marrow smears using antisera to epithelial membrane antigen. Br J Cancer 44:85–90, 1981

184. Redding WH, Monaghan P, Imrie SF, et al: Detection of micrometastases in patients with primary breast cancer. Lancet 2:1271–1274, 1983
185. Laurence DJR, Stevens U, Bettelheim R, et al: Role of plasma carcinoembryonic antigen in diagnosis of gastrointestinal, mammary and bronchial carcinoma. Br Med J 3:605–609, 1972
186. Steward AM, Nixon D, Zamcheck N, et al: Carcinoembryonic antigen in breast cancer patients—serum levels and disease progress. Cancer 33:1246–1252, 1974
187. Tormey DC, Waalkes TP, Snyder JJ, et al: Biological markers in breast carcinoma. III. Clinical correlations with carcinoembryonic antigen. Cancer 39:2397–2404, 1977
188. Chu TM, Nemoto T: Evaluation of carcinoembryonic antigen in human mammary carcinoma. J Natl Cancer Inst 51:1119–1122, 1973
189. Myers RE, Sutherland DJA, Kellen JA, et al: CEA in breast cancer. Cancer 42:1520–1526, 1978
190. Staab HJ, Ahlemann LM, Koch HL, et al: Serial carcinoembryonic antigen (CEA) determinations in the management of patients with breast cancer. Oncodevel Biol Med 1:151–160, 1980
191. Marcus DM, Zinberg N: Measurement of serum ferritin by radioimmunoassay results in normal individuals and patients with breast cancer. J Natl Cancer Inst 55:791–795, 1975
192. Roberts JG, Keyser JW, Baum M: Serum alpha l-acid glycoprotein as an index of dissemination in breast cancer. Br J Surg 62:816–819, 1975
193. Kessel J, Allen J: Elevated plasma sialyltransferase in the cancer patient. Cancer Res 35:670–672, 1975
194. Coombes RC: Biochemical markers in breast cancer. In Coombes RC, Powles TJ, Ford HT, et al (eds): Breast Cancer Management, pp 153–169. New York, Grune & Stratton, 1981
195. Tormey DC, Waalkes TP, Ahmann D, et al: Biological markers in breast carcinoma. I. Incidence of abnormalities of CEA, HCG, three polyamines, and three minor nucleosides. Cancer 35:1095–1100, 1975
196. Springer GF, Murthy MS, Desai PR, et al: Breast cancer patients cell-mediated immune response to Thomsen-Friedenreich (T) antigen. Cancer 45:2949–2954, 1980
197. Luthgens M, Scwegel G: Follow-up by tissue polypeptide antigen and CEA in radio-oncologic surveillance and therapy. Tumour Diag 2:179–188, 1981
198. Nemoto T, Constantine R, Chu TM: Human tissue polypeptide antigen in breast cancer. J Natl Cancer Inst 63:1347–1350, 1979
199. Coombes RC, Easty GC, Detre SI, et al: Secretion of immunoreactive calcitonin by human breast carcinomas. Br Med J 4:197–199, 1975
200. Silva OL, Chisholm RC, Becker KL: Hypercalcitonemia in cancer of the breast. Clin Res 35:596A, 1975
201. Haagensen DE, Kister SJ, Vandervoord JP, et al: Evaluation of carcinoembryonic antigen as a plasma monitor for human breast carcinoma. Cancer 42:1512–1519, 1978
202. Wang DY, Bulbrook RD, Hayward JC, et al: Relationship between plasma carcinoembryonic antigen and prognosis in women with breast cancer. Eur J Cancer 2:615–618, 1975
203. Myers RE, Sutherland DJ, Meakin JW, et al: Carcinoembryonic antigen in breast cancer. Cancer 42:1520–1526, 1978
204. Chatall JF, Chupin F, Ricolleau G, et al: Use of serial CEA assays in detecting relapses in breast cancer involving high risk of metastases. Eur J Cancer 17:233–238, 1981
205. Cantwell B, Fennelly JJ, Jones M: Evaluation of follow-up methods to detect relapse after mastectomy in breast cancer patients. Ir J Med Sci 151:1–5, 1982
206. Haagensen DE, Barry WF, McCook TA, et al: The value of serial plasma levels of CEA and gross cystic disease fluid protein in patients with breast cancer and osseous metastases. Ann Surg 191:599–603, 1980
207. Papaioannou D, Geggie P, Klassen J: Study of serum beta-2 microglobulin levels in breast cancer patients. Clin Chim Acta 99:37–41, 1979
208. Buckman R, Coombes RC, Dearnaley M, et al: Some clinical uses of biological markers. In Bonadonna G (ed): Breast Cancer Diagnosis and Management. Vol 1: Cancer Investigation and Management, pp 109–126. New York, John Wiley & Sons, 1984

Treatment of Metastases

13

Selection of Therapy

George P. Canellos

PROGNOSTIC FACTORS IN METASTATIC DISEASE

Metastatic breast cancer may appear at any time following primary therapy, with the risk of metastatic disease remaining present for up to 30 years following the initial diagnosis. The incidence of metastases, if they are to occur, is dependent on a number of factors, including the size of the primary mass, the histologic appearance of the tumor, and the extent of axillary and internal mammary lymph node involvement. Metastatic breast cancer may be manifested in several ways: (1) it may be present at the time of initial diagnosis of the primary disease; (2) it may occur as a local-regional recurrence in skin or soft tissue contiguous to the primary resection site, or in contiguous lymph nodes in the axilla, internal mammary chain, and supraclavicular area (affecting approximately 15% of all patients); (3) it may arise as distant metastases to bone, viscera, soft tissue, or the central nervous system (which occurs in approximately 60% of patients); or (4) it may involve both local-regional and distant metastases (in about 25% of patients). In recent years, an increasing number of patients have undergone some form of adjuvant systemic therapy, but most studies show that this therapy does not alter the pattern of dissemination. Among the possible metastatic sites, bone is the most common site (40% to 60% of patients), followed by lung (15% to 22% of patients), pleura (10% to 14% of patients), soft tissue (7% to 15% of patients), and liver (5% to 15% of patients).[1,2]

The prognosis for any metastatic tumor is determined by the intrinsic biologic characteristics of the tumor, which influence its proliferative rate and invasiveness, as well as the organ systems with the predominant burden of tumor at the time of diagnosis of metastatic disease. Clinical factors assessed at the time of diagnosis may also be helpful in determining prognosis. These factors identified by retrospective analysis include historical, clinical, hematologic, and biochemical characteristics. Univariate analyses of prognostic factors from various series have defined a large number of variables that significantly influence not only response to therapy, but also duration of survival. These factors are delineated in Table 13-1.[3–6] Multivariate analyses utilizing the proportional hazard model of Cox have also been performed, incorporating into the model those factors that were significant on univariate analysis. This technique has produced a number of models into which most patients may be grouped.[7]

The M.D. Anderson study resulted in a classification of all patients according to four levels of hazard ratio. The six variables utilized to construct these prognostic groups, including serum lactic dehydrogenase (LDH) levels, performance status, lung involvement, prior radiotherapy, serum alkaline phosphatase levels, and extent of disease, provided the best fit in a regression model to predict survival. The median survival for each of the four groups was 172, 104, 83, and 53 weeks, respectively. The wide variability in median survival emphasizes the importance of this type of analysis in the interpretation of treatment data and in the prospective design of clinical trials. However, since most clinicians do not have the facilities to perform such analyses, attempts have been made to sort patients into prognostic groups according to the pattern of metastatic disease. One series from the Southeastern Cancer Study Group divided all patients into five clinical prognostic groups: those with early, widespread dissemination to all major organs (with a median survival of 4 months); those with either nodular or lymphangitic pulmonary involvement (with a median survival of 18 months); those with osseous involvement (with a median survival of 29 months); patients with pleural involvement

Table 13-1
Variables Influencing Response to and Survival Following Chemotherapy in Patients With Breast Cancer

	M. D. Anderson[3] (n-619)	*SEG*[4] (n-304)		*SWOG*[5] (n-281)	*Arizona*[6] (n-138)
Chemotherapeutic regimen	5-Fluorouracil, Adriamycin, and cyclophosphamide (FAC)	FAC	Cyclophosphamide, methotrexate, 5-fluorouracil, vincristine, and prednisone (CMFVP)	Adriamycin, CMFVP	Adriamycin, cyclophosphamide
Variables influencing response	Performance status; prior therapy; weight loss; hemoglobin and platelet count; LDH, alkaline phosphatase, and albumin levels; extent of metastases; % of dose	Prior therapy, absence of bone and pleural involvement, lymphocytosis	Absence of visceral metastases, performance status of > 70%	Disease free interval (DFI), performance status, liver involvement	Number of metastases, patient's age, liver involvement
Variables influencing duration of response	———	Lymphocytosis, absence of pleural metastases, performance status of > 70%, postmenopausal with a bone dominant pattern	Absence of pleural metastases or lymphangitic involvement	———	Absence of lung involvement, patient's age, quality of response
Variables influencing survival	Prior therapy, response to hormones, performance status, weight loss, complete blood count, results of liver function test, extent of disease	Lymphocytosis, performance status of > 70%, bone dominant pattern	Absence of lymphangitic or pleural involvement, performance status of > 70%	———	Number of metastatic sites, performance status, patient's age, DFI

SEG, Southeastern Oncology Group; SWOG, Southwestern Oncology Group.

and ipsilateral effusion (with a median survival of 44 months); and those with local skin and nodal involvement with occasional bone metastases (with a median survival of 27+ months).[4] Another series analysis simplified the grouping to three categories: pure local and pure osseous dissemination (associated with a median survival of 27 months); pure visceral involvement (with a median survival of 23 months); and mixed dissemination patterns with metastasis in at least two or more organ sites (associated with a median survival of 17 to 19 months).[8] The minor differences in this sort of grouping limit its usefulness in the selection of therapy.

Primary tumor characteristics, such as the size of the primary tumor, the number of axillary nodes involved, and the type of primary therapy, have no effect on prognosis following appearance of metastases. Similarly, certain characteristics, such as the age of patients (in most series), their menstrual status, or a family history of breast cancer, are unrelated to prognosis of metastatic disease. Some biologic characteristics of the metastatic tumor may be assessed at diagnosis, including duration of disease-free interval from the time of primary treatment; estrogen and progesterone receptor content of the primary tumor and possibly, the metastatic tumor; response to prior endocrine therapy; and whether relapse has occurred during administration of adjuvant endocrine or cytotoxic therapy. In addition, an assessment of the extent of involvement may be made through clinical studies that determine the presence of disease in lungs, liver, abdomen, and bone. The M.D. Anderson group, in its analysis of prognostic factors, scored metastatic sites according to a strong suspicion of involvement or minimal, moderate, or extensive involvement.[3] This weighting of extent of involvement was used in the prognostic analysis. The impact of the extent of metastatic disease on the host may be assessed by performance status, peripheral blood counts, liver function studies, serum calcium levels, and serum LDH levels, which may reflect the tumor mass. Other markers, such as carcinoembryonic antigen (CEA), have not generally been useful in measuring the extent of disease. Although CEA studies have limited usefulness in quantifying volume of tumor, the CEA level is elevated in only 44% to 69% of patients with metastatic disease. This elevation occurs with greatest frequency in patients with liver metastases.[9] The combined assessment of CEA, alkaline phosphatase, and γ-glutamyl transpeptidase levels provides a serum marker profile that, when persistently elevated in serial measurement, may anticipate overt clinical metastases by only 3 months.[10] Patients with elevated CEA levels that persist following mastectomy may have a higher recurrence rate than do similar patients with CEA levels in the normal range. Measures of proliferative activity, such as tritiated thymidine labeling of the primary tumor mass, have been shown to correlate with disease-free interval; the higher the labeling index, the greater the likelihood of early relapse.[11] Estrogen receptor-positive tumors tend to have lower labeling indices than do receptor-negative tumors.[12]

THERAPEUTIC APPROACHES TO PATIENTS WITH METASTATIC DISEASE: THE DECISION TO TREAT

The choice of systemic therapy and the indications for instituting such therapy are often based on the experience and bias of the physician who is faced with the decision. Since, in almost all instances, systemic therapy for metastatic disease is palliative, the decision to offer therapy should ideally be based on an assessment of the extent of metastatic disease, the rate of disease progression (if possible to determine), the biologic features of the tumor (such as hormone receptors), the presence of symptoms, and the likelihood that the patient will tolerate the treatment without undue toxicity. The latter point cannot be overemphasized, as a vast number of women facing therapy for metastatic disease have preconceived notions about the toxicity of therapy, especially cytotoxic chemotherapy. In the recent past, these notions included fear of the toxicity of additive sex steroid hormones or ablative endocrine surgery.

Undoubtedly, systemic therapy may relieve most, if not all, symptoms in patients with metastatic disease. It is unclear, however, whether systemic therapy significantly prolongs overall survival, despite relief of symptoms. In certain patients, such treatment certainly can temporarily reverse an imminently fatal progression of systemic disease, such as extensive liver involvement, but in the totality of metastatic breast cancer, such patients are difficult to identify. Retrospective analysis of the M.D. Anderson experience suggests that survival rates have improved since the advent of systemic chemotherapy.

As a general rule, patients with symptoms related to the metastatic tumor should receive a trial course of the appropriate systemic therapy, whether it be hormonal or cytotoxic. However, there is no body of evidence that dictates that immediate systemic therapy for early, asymptomatic, metastatic disease will influence the duration of the patient's survival. However, such patients are often treated prematurely, usually because of the anxiety of the patient and the reluctance of the clinician to follow the disease without offering treatment. In these days of informed patients, it is becoming more difficult to withhold therapy from patients whose metastatic disease may be detected earlier than in the past as a result of more frequent examinations and the greater technical sophistication of radiographic techniques. In asymptomatic patients, assessment of the extent of metastases and the rate of progression through close follow-up is a reasonable, but perhaps emotionally difficult, approach. Slowly progressive, asymptomatic pulmonary nodules or bone lesions in non–weight-bearing sites may easily be followed with appropriate radiographic studies and do not require immediate treatment. Therapy is usually offered to symptomatic patients with metastatic lesions in sites that are likely to produce symptoms in the near future. The latter group includes those with destructive bone metastases in weight-bearing bone; diffuse lymphangitic pulmonary metastases; extensive hepatic involvement with functional impairment; asymptomatic brain metastases; or extensive bone marrow replacement with low-grade anemia, leukoerythroblastosis, or thrombocytopenia. Isolated bone lesions and brain metastases may be treated with radiation therapy delivered to the critical areas and close follow-up without systemic therapy. Femoral, humeral, and acetabular metastases may be associated with pain and pathologic fracture; the risk of this occurring is 13% to 30% in patients with radiographic evidence of femoral metastases. This incidence has prompted many orthopedic surgeons to adopt the viewpoint that fracture is inevitable if an osteolytic lesion is greater than 2.5 cm in diameter and involves the cortex. Many recommend prophylactic internal fixation in such high-risk groups.[13] This recommendation has been questioned by others who have demonstrated that only 5% of such high-risk patients sustain femoral fractures while receiving radiation therapy or while involved in subsequent follow-up.[14] Generalized bone pain from multiple metastases, hepatic pain, functional deterioration with jaundice secondary to rapid expansion of liver metastases, dyspnea secondary to lymphangitic spread in the lung, and symptomatic recurrent effusions may all be reversed by prompt administration of systemic therapy.

THERAPEUTIC APPROACHES TO PATIENTS WITH CHEST WALL RECURRENCE AND LOCALLY EXTENSIVE DISEASE

The same principles of treatment may be applied to patients with isolated chest wall recurrences, but in these instances, the lesion(s) may be carefully followed without specific therapy as there is usually no immediate morbidity from such local recurrences, especially if they occur late in the course of the disease. However, in most circumstances, localized radiation therapy is offered, since it is impossible to predict the natural history of each local recurrence. The clinical setting of a local recurrence may influence prognosis, and thus, the relative urgency for local therapy. For example, a patient with a single recurrence measuring less than 1 cm and with a disease-free interval of longer than 24 months has a median survival of 5.25 years, compared to a survival of 1.4 years in those without these features.[15] If restaging of the patient demonstrates extensive distant metastases as well as a local recurrence, then systemic therapy alone, with frequent assessment of the local recurrence, may constitute initial therapy. Radiation therapy may be deferred until there is evidence of a lack of response or escape from systemic therapy. Some patients with locally advanced (Stage III) disease may be treatable by surgery, especially in the absence of clinical extension to the axillary nodes and chest wall fixation. A high 5-year survival rate has been observed in the absence of histologic involvement of axillary nodes, even in the presence of edema or skin involvement.[16] Surgery is usually contraindicated in inflammatory carcinoma since historically, it is associated with a poor 5-year survival rate. This rate has recently improved owing to the use of cytotoxic chemotherapy as initial treatment, followed by local therapy, usually involving irradiation.[17] It is unclear whether both irradiation and surgery, in addition to systemic therapy, are required for optimal therapy of locally advanced tumor. In a patient with an isolated distant metastasis for whom systemic therapy is also planned, local "debulking" therapy with surgery or radiation therapy has not been shown to improve survival, and thus is not generally recommended. Patients whose symptoms may be related to the presence of metastasis and who may require immediate relief, such as those with obstruction of a viscus or vessels, or extradural compression of the spinal cord, represent an exception to this rule.

HORMONAL THERAPY FOR METASTATIC DISEASE

Since hormonal therapy is less toxic than cytotoxic chemotherapy, it is usually selected as the first modality in patients with metastatic disease. The indications for systemic hormonal therapy are, however, the same as for chemotherapy—namely, symptomatic disease with bone pain; serous effusions; symptomatic soft tissue or lymph node masses on the chest wall, axilla, groin, or abdomen; and hypercalcemia. The choice of endocrine therapy is usually based on demonstration of estrogen receptor in the primary tumor or, when the estrogen receptor is unknown, the pattern of metastases and the disease-free interval. In general, late-appearing metastases (those arising more than 2 years after mastectomy) that are confined to bone, pleura, or soft tissue have a greater likelihood of responding to endocrine therapy. If a falsely negative estrogen receptor assay has been obtained, a therapeutic trial of endocrine therapy is warranted when the clinical presentation indicates a slowly progressing tumor with the above characteristics.[18] The fact that metastatic disease occurred while adjunctive endocrine therapy was being administered should not preclude a trial of another hormonal agent since such a recurrence does not necessarily imply total refractoriness to other endocrine treatment in estrogen receptor-positive tumors. The choice of endocrine therapy is usually determined by the patient's menstrual status at the time of metastases. At present, oophorectomy remains the standard approach in premenopausal or perimenopausal patients, but recent trials have shown tamoxifen to have a comparable effect in premenopausal women. Moreover, patients who are refractory to tamoxifen may subsequently respond to oophorectomy. Antiestrogens are the standard treatment in postmenopausal patients. Other agents, such as megestrol acetate, diethylstilbestrol, androgens, or aminoglutethimide hydrocortisone, may be considered for treatment of postmenopausal patients with estrogen receptor-positive tumor who relapse on adjuvant tamoxifen (Figs. 13-1 and 13-2).

COMBINATION CHEMOTHERAPY IN THE TREATMENT OF METASTATIC DISEASE

Patients with metastatic disease that is refractory to hormonal therapy, or those with known hormone receptor-negative metastases are potential candidates for cytotoxic chemotherapy. It should be emphasized, however, that asymptomatic, hormone-refractory disease does not necessarily require the immediate institution of combination chemotherapy. The same principles described earlier should apply to the urgency of systemic therapy in a given case. As a general rule, cytotoxic chemotherapy is the systemic treatment of choice when symptomatic progression occurs after a trial of hormonal therapy, and when rapid reversal of metastatic disease is required owing to rapid progression of metastatic tumor with inflammatory changes in the liver, lung, or chest wall.

When systemic therapy is required, the addition of hormonal agents to cytotoxic chemotherapy does not increase the response rate over chemotherapy alone. However, the converse may be true—namely, combined cytotoxic and hormonal therapy may yield a higher response rate than hormonal therapy alone. In general, these treatment modalities are better used in sequence, with their administration guided by the nature and pace of the metastatic disease. Chemotherapy added to hormonal therapy does not improve overall survival but may prolong the interval between initiation of treatment and treatment failure.[19]

When systemic chemotherapy is required, combination chemotherapy produces a higher response rate per unit of time than do single agents. The choice of cytotoxic combination chemotherapy is not crucial, as all of the commonly used regimens have similar response rates for all metastatic sites and have no differences in survival. Treatment regimens containing Adriamycin differ very little in terms of response benefit from the standard non-Adriamycin programs, such as CMF, CMFP, or CMFVP.* When comparing CMF or CMFP to Adriamycin, the initial

*C, cyclophosphamide; M, methotrexate; F, fluorouracil; P, prednisone; V, vincristine.

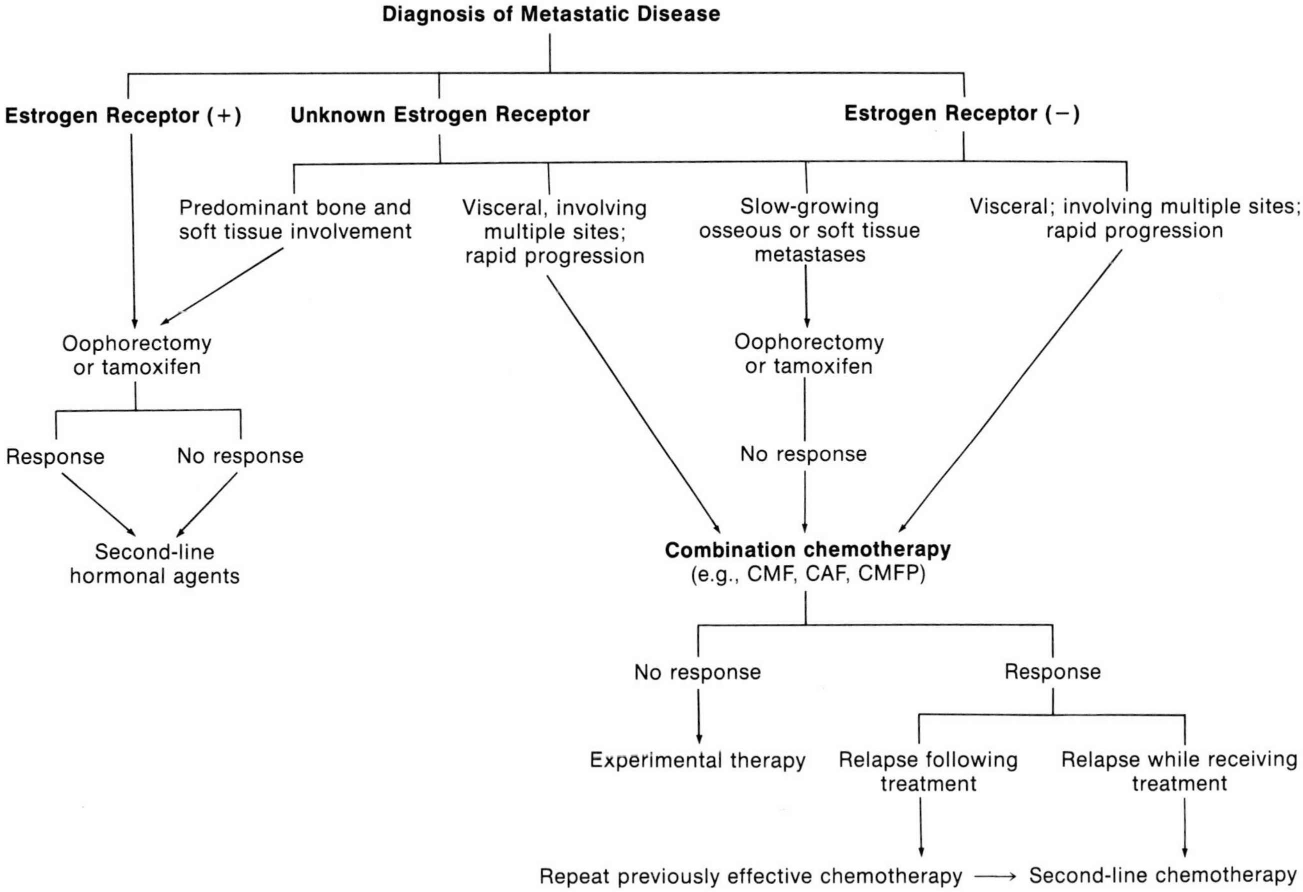

FIGURE 13-1. Selection of therapy for metastatic breast cancer in premenopausal women.

regimen does not influence the likelihood of response to the alternative program when used as "crossover" treatment.[20] Likewise, a relapse while off adjuvant therapy does not preclude a response to the same regimen used to treat distant metastases. The survival of patients is usually not influenced by the particular regimen.

In most circumstances, the diagnosis of metastatic disease is not a medical emergency. Since regimens of combination chemotherapy or endocrine therapy for metastases are palliative, new agents showing some promise in the treatment of breast cancer might better be investigated early in the natural history of metastatic disease. Extensively pretreated patients rarely respond to third-line chemotherapy.

When the clinical picture suggests rapidly progressive metastases, especially in multiple visceral sites such as the liver or lung, combination chemotherapy using standard regimens with demonstrated efficacy is the treatment of choice as it offers the opportunity for the most rapid reversal of tumor in these sites. A recent analysis of 381 patients demonstrated that duration of survival from the time of the first distant metastasis is not significantly influenced by whether a complete or partial response is achieved. This similarity in survival, regardless of response, occurred whether the patient received hormonal or cytotoxic chemotherapy as the initial systemic treatment.[21]

Patients presenting with extensive bone marrow involvement resulting in compromise of peripheral blood counts are treatable and may respond to systemic chemotherapy, but myelosuppression is likely to be severe. In such circumstances, and in the absence of estrogen receptor data, an initial hormonal treatment approach is preferred. The skeleton is the most common site of metastasis in patients with advanced breast cancer; eventually, such metastases are detected in the majority of patients. About 25% of those who present with metastases will have disease that is initially confined to bone. The initial therapeutic modality is usually hormonal, but eventually, cytotoxic chemotherapy is used. Objective radiographic evidence of tumor regression and bone healing may be obscure, but symptomatic improvement may be expected in a large percentage of patients.[22]

The average duration of response (or time interval to

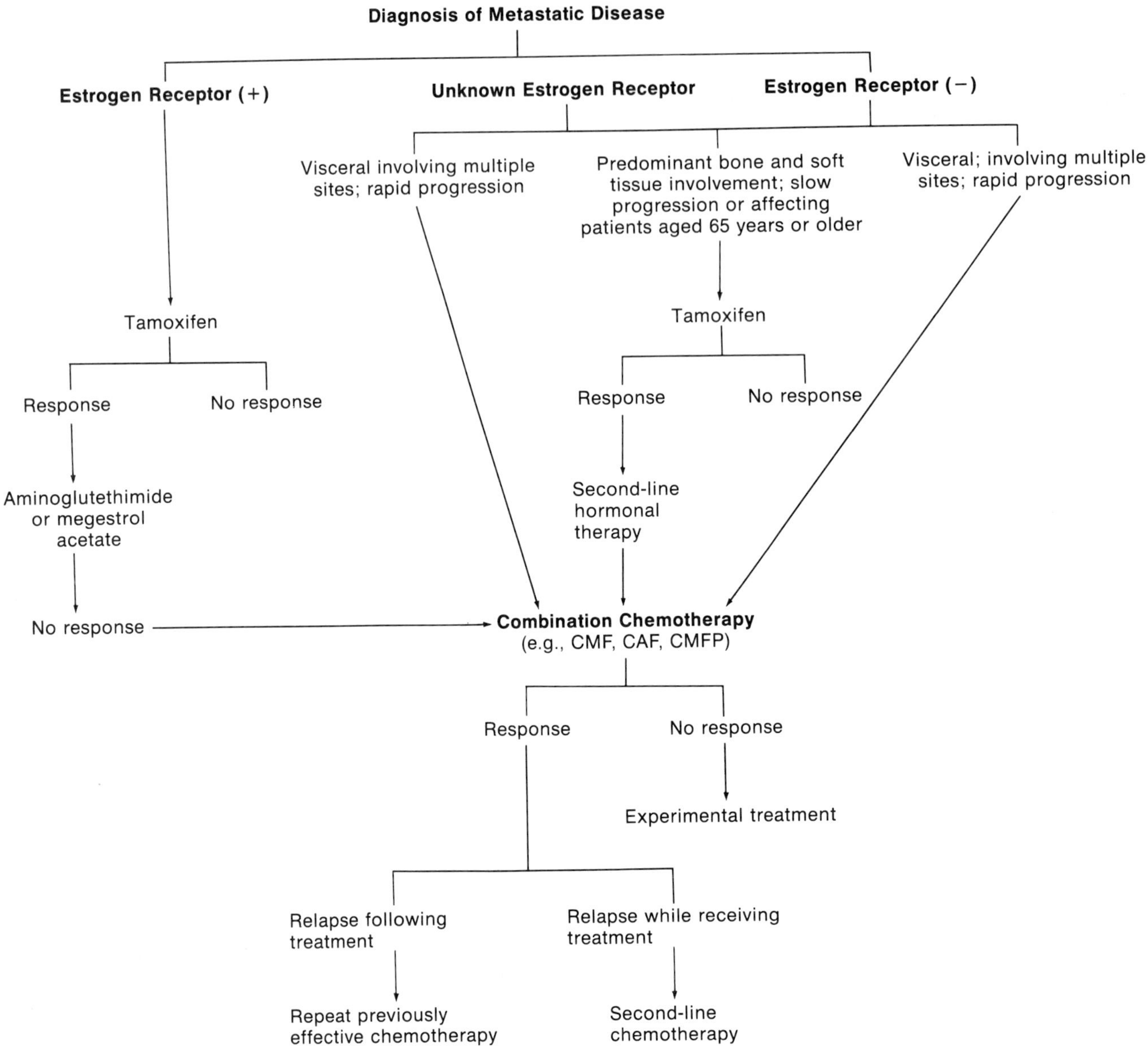

FIGURE 13-2. Selection of therapy for perimenopausal and postmenopausal women with metastatic breast cancer.

disease progression) following chemotherapy is usually quite short, averaging 6 to 8 months. The tendency of most physicians is to continue chemotherapy relentlessly until disease progression is evident since most patients achieve only a partial regression of their tumor. Few studies have addressed the issue of response duration in patients achieving a rare complete or good partial response. It is possible that a shorter duration of therapy in patients who respond well may permit the readministration of a previously effective treatment regimen. Since chemotherapy is palliative in patients with advanced disease, optimal use of therapeutic programs currently known to be effective may be achieved through shorter courses of therapy. It is difficult to assess the impact of dose itself on the benefits of combination chemotherapy. Analysis of the dose rate from multiple trials suggests that the likelihood of response is proportional to the use of full doses. Whether survival is similarly prolonged is less certain.[23] Clearly, in the case of adjuvant therapy, maximal-dose chemotherapy is desirable. However, the extent to which patients with metastatic disease should be treated is unclear since there is a level of toxicity at which many patients will refuse further treatment or at which they may be placed at risk of drug-related lethality.

REFERENCES

1. Bruce SJ, Carter DC, Fraser J: Patterns of recurrent disease in breast cancer. Lancet 1:433, 1970
2. Lee YN: Breast carcinoma: Pattern of recurrence and metastasis after mastectomy. Am J Clin Oncol 7:443, 1984
3. Swenerton KD, Legha SS, Smith T, et al: Prognostic factors in metastatic breast cancer treated with combination chemotherapy. Cancer Res 39:1552, 1979
4. Smalley RV, Lefante J, Bartolucci A, et al: A comparison of cyclophosphamide, Adriamycin, and 5-fluorouracil (CAF) and cyclophosphamide, methotrexate, 5-fluorouracil, vincristine, and prednisone (CMFVP) in patients with advanced breast cancer. Breast Cancer Res Treat 3:209, 1983
5. George SL, Hoogstraten B: Prognostic factors in the initial response to therapy by patients with advanced breast cancer. J Natl Cancer Inst 60:731, 1978
6. Nash CH III, Jones SE, Moon TE, et al: Prediction of outcome in metastatic breast cancer treated with Adriamycin combination chemotherapy. Cancer 46:2380, 1980
7. Hortobagyi GN, Smith TL, Legha SS, et al: Multivariate analysis of prognostic factors in metastatic breast cancer. J Clin Oncol 1:776, 1983
8. Fey MF, Brunner KW, Sonntag RW: Prognostic factors in metastatic breast cancer. Cancer Clin Trials 4:237, 1981
9. Wang DY, Bulbrook RD, Hayward JL, et al: Relationship between plasma carcinoembryonic antigen and prognosis in women with breast cancer. Eur J Cancer 11:615, 1975
10. Coombes RC, Powles TJ, Gazet JC, et al: Assessment of biochemical tests to screen for metastases in patients with breast cancer. Lancet 1:296, 1980
11. Silvestrini R, Daidone MG, Gasparini G: Cell kinetics as a prognostic marker in node-negative breast cancer. Cancer 56:1982, 1985
12. Moran RE, Black MM, Alpert L, et al: Correlation of cell-cycle kinetics, hormone receptors, histopathology, and nodal status in human breast cancer. Cancer 54:1586, 1984
13. Beals RK, Lawton GD, Snell WE: Prophylactic internal fixation of the femur in metastatic breast cancer. Cancer 28:1350, 1971
14. Cheung DS, Seitz CB, Eyre HJ: Nonoperative management of femoral, humeral, and acetabular metastases in patients with breast cancer. Cancer 45:1533, 1980
15. Bedwinek JM, Lee J, Fineburg B, et al: Prognostic indicators in patients with isolated loco-regional recurrence of breast cancer. Cancer 47:2232, 1981
16. Fracchia AA, Evans JF, Eisenberg BL: Stage III carcinoma of the breast—A detailed analysis. Ann Surg 192:705, 1980
17. Sherry MM, Johnson DH, Page DL, et al: Inflammatory carcinoma of the breast—Clinical review and summary of the Vanderbilt experience with multi-modality therapy. Am J Med 79:355, 1985
18. Henderson IC, Canellos GP: Cancer of the breast—The past decade. N Engl J Med 302:17–30, 78–90, 1980
19. Viladiu P, Alonso MC, Avella A, et al: Chemotherapy versus chemotherapy plus hormonotherapy in postmenopausal advanced breast cancer patients—A randomized trial. Cancer 56:2745, 1985
20. Tormey DC, Gelman R, Band PR, et al: Comparison of induction chemotherapies for metastatic breast cancer—An Eastern Cooperative Oncology Group trial. Cancer 50:1235, 1982
21. Paterson AHG, Szafran O, Hanson J, et al: Response to treatment and its influence on survival in metastatic breast cancer. Am J Clin Oncol 8:283, 1985
22. Smalley RV, Scogna DM, Malmud LS: Advanced breast cancer with bone-only metastases—A chemotherapeutically responsive pattern of metastases. Am J Clin Oncol 5:161, 1982
23. Hryniuk W, Bush H: The importance of dose intensity in chemotherapy of metastatic breast cancer. J Clin Oncol 2:1281, 1984

Surgery for Metastatic Disease

Jeanne A. Petrek

BIOPSIES OF LOCAL RECURRENCES

Patients with local recurrences after mastectomy often undergo biopsy—especially if that is their first sign of recurrence—both to confirm the existence of the recurrence and to obtain tissue for various studies. The tumor volume requirements of the various tests should be considered carefully when planning which lesion is selected for analysis and which method of biopsy is used. In addition to hormone receptor assays, the tissue may be used for electron microscopy, tissue culture, antigen typing, or other tests. Different fixatives are required for various tests; indeed, if formalin is used consistently in all tissue samples, the opportunity for performing valuable diagnostic tests may be lost.

Repeat surgery on tight skin flaps or in areas of previous irradiation is often difficult. After the suspect tissue is removed, the surrounding skin may not be adequate or pliable enough to bring the edges together. Tension in a previously irradiated area (because of the decreased blood supply) will often lead to necrosis and the formation of a long-standing, open wound. Conversely, thin skin flaps often will not tolerate undermining to any useful degree. Although a small, split-thickness, skin graft would be an ideal option in other areas and may occasionally be used in postmastectomy patients, one must remember that such skin grafts do not fare well with irradiation, and an open, nonhealing wound may still result.

In light of these factors, one must be mindful both of the indications for biopsy and the kind of biopsy undertaken if a local recurrence is not to be made worse. For example, if a subcutaneous nodule is incompletely excised and closed under tension so as to prevent complete incisional healing, a malignant ulceration may result. If left alone (perhaps with biopsy of a more advantageous area being undertaken), the subcutaneous nodule may remain subcutaneous, or a longer period of time may elapse before it invades and disrupts the skin.

A variety of techniques exist for acquiring tissue, depending on the location of the tissue and the amount of tissue required.

ASPIRATION BIOPSY. Aspiration biopsy involves the aspiration of cells and tissue fragments through a needle that has been inserted into the suspect tissue. Usually, an 18- or 20-gauge needle is used. Some tumor growth patterns, often the "softer" tumors, are more amenable to the withdrawal of a sufficient sample of loose cells. It is probably important not to aspirate material as the needle is being withdrawn through the skin in order to keep all the collected tumor cells within the needle shaft, thus preventing their implantation in the skin. Cytologic analysis of these cells may provide a diagnosis of malignant disease, depending upon the experience of the cytologist involved. However, keloids and inflammatory or benign reparative changes—especially in patients who have undergone previous irradiation—may be confusing to the cytologist. It is important to provide the cytologist with maximal information about such factors; in many cases, only a histologic diagnosis will suffice.

CORE NEEDLE BIOPSY. Core needle biopsy involves biopsy with a special needle that will yield sufficient tissue for histologic analysis. Typically, a core of tissue that is 1mm to 2 mm in width and 2 cm long is obtained. A sheath or carrier needle is advanced over the core specimen (to hold it inside the needle) before being withdrawn from the tumor. The sheath contains the tumor cells, thereby preventing the skin's exposure to them and thus, the possible risk of implantation as the needle is being withdrawn.

A core needle biopsy is advantageous because only a single needle puncture site is required. The technique is useful in the biopsy of a large area, such as a breast, but its usefulness declines in postmastectomy local recurrences. In the latter cases, the suspect tissue has to be adequately large and sufficiently raised off the chest wall so that the 2-cm (or more) needle tract can be placed parallel to the body. As with aspiration biopsy, it is possible to miss the malignant tissue entirely, with resultant collection of benign cells.

INCISIONAL BIOPSY. Incisional biopsy refers to the removal of a small wedge of tissue from a larger tumor mass. Such biopsies are often used for the diagnosis of large masses that would require a major surgical procedure even for local excision. The disadvantage of using an incisional biopsy in a patient with a local recurrence is that there is a very real possibility of creating an oozing and ulcerated area. However, an incisional biopsy is sometimes useful, especially in cases in which performing a larger excisional biopsy would open and contaminate new tissue planes. For example, if a major resection of the local recurrence were being planned, a small incisional biopsy (to obtain a definitive histologic diagnosis) would initially be best. As part of this procedure, needle tracts or incisions should be aligned carefully so that they may conveniently be removed as part of the subsequent procedure.

EXCISIONAL BIOPSY. Excisional biopsy is the procedure of choice for most local recurrences. This technique removes the entire suspect tissue with some margin of surrounding normal tissue. It is not uncommon to biopsy several suspected lesions at one time. Care should be taken not to use instruments or gloves that may have come into contact with tumor when obtaining tissue from a potentially noncontaminated area.

OVERVIEW OF OPERATIVE TECHNIQUES FOR ENDOCRINE ABLATION

OOPHORECTOMY. Oophorectomy can usually be performed in a half hour or so, either by a general surgeon or a gynecologist. The ovaries are not deep visceral organs, and are loosely attached by the fallopian tubes and the ovarian pedicle. In patients without significant obesity, previous pelvic operations, or pelvic disease, such as endometriosis, the ovaries can easily be brought to the surface of the abdomen. Ligatures are then placed around the fallopian tubes and ovarian pedicle (which contains the ovarian artery), and the ovary is excised. The uterus and almost all of the fallopian tubes are left in place. The postoperative period of hospitalization is about 3 to 5 days, and usually depends on the degree of ileus caused by handling the intestines in an attempt to evaluate possible liver metastases.

Even though oophorectomy is a simple surgical procedure, it still involves general anesthesia and a hospitalization. A patient must be in acceptable medical condition for this procedure, and problems, such as pulmonary or hepatic metastases with a significant decrease in lung or liver function, should not be present.

ADRENALECTOMY. Adrenalectomy is a much more difficult procedure than oophorectomy, requiring significant expertise in retroperitoneal surgery. If the patient is thin, both the adrenals and ovaries may be approached through a single, long, midline incision. Since the adrenals lie in the area that is farthest back in the retroperitoneum, abdominal obesity may be a significant hindrance to the success of such an operation.

Excision of the adrenals through the bed of the resected 11th or 12th ribs, with the patient lying prone, is an ideal approach since the adrenals are easily reached and the incision and operative area are small. Because the intestines are not exposed, ileus is avoided. The postoperative stay averages about 5 days. Because of these advantages, many surgeons prefer to use the flank approach (with the patient prone) even if an oophorectomy is planned; they then reposition the anesthetized patient into a supine position for a standard pelvic incision.

Meticulous postoperative care is crucial after bilateral adrenal removal. Because it is difficult to determine how much corticosteroid should be administered owing to the stress of the operation and postoperative period, patients are usually "overtreated" with steroids in order to avoid a hypoadrenal state. In view of this excess dosage during the postoperative period, metabolic changes, including sodium conservation and potassium excretion, should be anticipated and corrected. After the immediate postoperative period, mineral corticoids are replaced, usually by α-fluorohydrocortisone. Corticosteroid replacement therapy must be continued forever, and the dosage must be increased whenever there is an increased need as a result of intercurrent injury or illness.

HYPOPHYSECTOMY. Hypophysectomy has appealing endocrine aspects of both a theoretical and practical nature. In addition to altering the trophic stimulation of the ovaries and adrenals, pituitary ablation may decrease tumor growth by removing prolactin and growth hormone. However, the same response rates derived from adrenalectomy or hypophysectomy suggest similar mechanisms of action.[1,2] The choice between hypophysectomy and adrenalectomy depends largely on the physician involved and on whichever specialized technique is best developed in a particular community.

Pituitary destruction has been performed by transcranial resection and with the recently popular transsphenoidal resection. Selective destruction by a radioactive implant has also been used in some centers. In addition, cryosurgery may be performed with the patient under local anesthesia, using stereotactic placement of freezing probes. Hypophysectomy by any approach is associated with a milder postoperative recovery than adrenalectomy. However, the effects of total pituitary destruction, the complicated postoperative maintenance therapy required, and the small but definite risk of a cerebrospinal fistula and diabetes insipidus detract from the advantages of hypophysectomy.

BONE BIOPSY

Since modern medical, surgical, and radiation therapy is both specific and complex, as well as associated with risk, tissue diagnosis of suspected bone metastases is often necessary. Open surgical biopsy has greater morbidity, takes longer to perform, may delay therapy, and is more expensive than other procedures. Accordingly, closed or percutaneous bone biopsy, performed by invasive radiologists or surgeons, has become popular. The most common areas for biopsy are the spine, pelvis, and long bones, in that order.[3]

Since 1930, when the first series of successful aspiration biopsies at Memorial Hospital in New York City was reported,[4] more than 8000 percutaneous needle aspirations have been reported in the English-language literature.[3] In 1945, the Memorial Hospital group summarized 12 years' experience with 567 aspirations, yielding an 82% accuracy rate.[5] One group reported 7165 cases in 33 years, with an overall accuracy of 74%.[6] In almost all subsequent series, the accuracy rate was similar—75% or higher.[3]

Modern bone trephine or core techniques date to 1947, when the drill biopsy method was introduced as a modification of aspiration biopsy.[7] The first needle was simple, squared at the tip, and sharpened. It was attached to a drill, a technique that provided a core of tissue. In 1956, Ackermann described a biopsy set that could routinely recover a tissue core that was 1.5 mm in diameter.[8] He reported more than 200 uncomplicated, semi-random biopsies, some of which documented the presence of cancer in radiologically normal bones.[9]

The other core needle biopsy set in frequent use today was first reported by Craig in 1956.[10] Its main feature is the 3.5-mm diameter tissue core that is obtainable. Recently, the Tru-Cut biopsy needle, so useful in soft tissue procedures, has been utilized to a small extent for the nonosseous component of skeletal tumors.[11]

During the past 5 decades, other techniques have been developed that support aspiration and trephine biopsy. Many of these are radiologic: image-intensified fluoroscopy, biplane fluoroscopy, high-resolution television chains, radionuclide bone scintigraphy, and computed tomography. Simultaneously, histopathologic and cytopathologic diagnostic capabilities have become more sophisticated.

The patient must be evaluated carefully to determine whether another procedure with less risk or potential morbidity would yield the desired diagnosis. Because of the rare complications encountered, percutaneous biopsies are not performed if the results would not change the treatment and affect management. With the aid of combined imaging procedures (radiography, scintigraphy, and computed tomography), the most accessible skeletal lesion and the proper anatomic approach should be chosen for biopsy.

The patient must be comfortable and the part to be sampled must be stable. The needle chosen should be optimal for the particular biopsy, a decision governed by the location and character of the lesion. The optimal approach may always be to combine aspiration and trephine biopsies.

In the past, the bone core has been regarded as the prime biopsy specimen and the osseous blood obtainable through the biopsy trocar has sometimes been ignored. However, more recently, in cases in which both bone cores and osseous blood were available, the osseous blood showed better malignant morphologic structure and was better diagnostic material than the bone core in almost all cases.[12] In some patients in whom insertion of a large biopsy trocar was considered to be dangerous, only needle puncture and aspiration of osseous blood were performed. Needles as small as 20-gauge have been used.

Handling Bone Biopsy Specimens

Tissue aspirates of marrow may be handled in various ways. Most commonly, they are collected and embedded in paraffin for routine histologic sections. However, they may also be processed for cytologic examination. The choice should depend on the preference of the pathology department responsible for the evaluation.

Trephine cores are usually placed in formalin, decalcified, embedded in paraffin, sectioned, and stained. The common problem of crushing artifact may be minimized by using needles with a large internal diameter and by exercising care in handling the specimen once it has been removed from the patient, especially when pushing the trephine core from the cutting needle. Specimen-to-finger contact should be avoided.

Touch preparations, if desired by the pathologist, may be prepared prior to placing the specimen in formalin. However, this practice increases the likelihood of crush artifacts.

Imaging Procedures Before Bone Biopsy

Fluoroscopic guidance, particularly biplane and image-intensified fluoroscopy, is the most common modality used in bone biopsies. In the future, however, computed tomography (CT) may become increasingly utilized. CT scanning may influence the choice of biopsy site, needle type, and needle position, and may help to plan fluoroscopically-guided skeletal biopsies.[13] The imaging techniques are often necessary for open (surgical) incisional biopsy, as well as for percutaneous biopsy.

If the bone lesion is imaged only on bone scan, techniques involving injection of the periosteum with methylene blue-lidocaine or the embedding of a spring hookwire into the suspect tissue have been used prior to open incisional biopsy.[14]

Complications

A review of the literature indicates that there have been approximately 20 complications from percutaneous bone biopsies that have been considered important enough to report.[3] Although this is undoubtedly an underestimation, it does provide some measure of risk. There have been nine pneumothoraces reported from performing rib or thoracic spine biopsies, many of which did not require placement of a chest tube. However, there are also rare serious complications, such as transient or permanent paraplegia and peripheral nerve injuries with resultant footdrop. Five spinal cord injuries have been recorded, including one case of meningitis and two that resulted in death. Therefore, serious neurologic injury occurred in 0.08% of the procedures reported, and resultant death occurred in 0.02%.[3]

There are no absolute contraindications for percutaneous bone biopsy. The risk of a particular biopsy should always be measured against the risk of alternative diagnostic methods or of not obtaining a specific diagnosis, but biopsies should not be performed if the results would not affect treatment or management.

Percutaneous skeletal biopsy for suspected bone metastases has many advantages and very few disadvantages. It can be done rapidly, safely, economically, and nearly painlessly with only local anesthesia. Sometimes, open incisional biopsy will be required. Accuracy depends upon careful technical performance and an insistence upon specimen adequacy.

REFERENCES

1. Fracchia AA, Farrow JH, Miller TR, et al: Hypophysectomy as compared with adrenalectomy in the treatment of advanced carcinoma of the breast. Surg Gynecol Obstet 140:528, 1975
2. Wilson RE, Piro AS, Aliapoulos MA, et al: Evaluation of adrenalectomy and hypophysectomy in treatment of metastatic cancer of the breast. Cancer 24:1322, 1969
3. Murphy WA, Destouet JM, Gilula LA: Percutaneous skeletal biopsy 1981: A procedure for radiologists—Results, review, and recommendations. Radiology 139:545, 1981
4. Martin HE, Ellis EB: Biopsy by needle puncture and aspiration. Ann Surg 92:169, 1930
5. Synder RE, Coley BL: Further studies on the diagnosis of bone tumors by aspiration biopsy. Surg Gynecol Obstet 80:517, 1945
6. Schajowicz F, Hokama J: Aspiration (puncture or needle) biopsy in bone lesions. Recent Results Cancer Res 54:139, 1976
7. Ellis F: Needle biopsy in clinical diagnosis of tumours. Br J Surg 34:240, 1947
8. Ackermann W: Vertebral trephine biopsy. Ann Surg 143:373, 1956
9. Ackermann W: Application of the trephine for bone biopsy. JAMA 184:133, 1963
10. Craig FS: Vertebral-body biopsy. J Bone Joint Surg 38:93, 1956
11. deSantos LA, Lukeman JM, Wallace S, et al: Percutaneous needle biopsy of bone in the cancer patient. AJR 130:641, 1978
12. Hewes RC, Vigorita VJ, Freiberger RH: Percutaneous bone biopsy: The importance of aspirated osseous blood. Radiology 148:69, 1983
13. Hardy DC, Murphy WA, Gilula LA: Computed tomography in planning percutaneous bone biopsy. Radiology 134:447, 1980
14. Froelich JW, McKusick KA, Strauss HW, et al: Localization of bone lesions for open biopsy. Radiology 146:549, 1983

Radiotherapy

Beryl McCormick

The role of radiation therapy in the treatment of breast metastases has remained unchallenged throughout the recent and continuing controversy surrounding primary breast cancer therapy. Radiation remains the most effective means of local control for symptomatic breast metastases.

Breast cancer is well recognized as a tumor of moderate radiosensitivity. In the curative setting, 4500 to 5000 cGy in 5 weeks is an established dose for the sterilization or "cure" of subclinical breast cancer; higher doses are indicated for bulky disease. Precise treatment planning is necessary to ensure delivery of that dose to a relatively "tight" target volume containing the tissues at risk for breast cancer, thereby avoiding or sparing as much of the surrounding normal tissue as possible.

Radiation treatment of metastases has many similarities to and some marked differences from radiation treatment for cure. First and foremost, the concept of ensuring a therapeutic gain remains. Irradiation must be accomplished in such a way as to ensure that the benefits to the patients outweigh the complications or the side effects from the treatment. Although this statement seems so obvious that it barely warrants saying, in actuality, it is a complex guideline to adhere to in patients with metastatic disease. Although the risk/benefit ratio has been clearly established for curative treatment, in patients with metastases, the radiation oncologist must weigh many factors that vary greatly from case to case in determining the optimal treatment approach.

Fortunately, the organs most likely to be involved by breast cancer metastases—the bones, lung, pleura, soft tissue, and skin—are quite tolerant of irradiation and usually can be treated by this modality.[1] The potential benefits to a patient with symptomatic metastases are clear: the symptoms disappear or decrease markedly. In the case of an impending fracture in a weight-bearing bone, even if symptoms are not present, the benefits again are clear. The bone begins to recalcify and a fixation procedure may be able to be avoided. However, the risks may not be so clear. In the curative setting, great emphasis is placed, and rightly so, on potential complications involving the tissue in the path length of the beam, which is especially important since long-term survival is anticipated. In the palliative setting, these potential complications must be calculated in the same way, but must also be considered in light of the patient's anticipated life span. For example, in a patient whose life span is measured in weeks, a treatment associated with daily nausea for 3 to 4 weeks would be unacceptable. In the same patient, the risk of a lens cataract or skin telangiectasia occurring several years post-treatment would constitute an acceptable and anticipated side effect risk. For each metastatic consultation, the radiation oncologist must weigh similar factors, risks, and benefits in terms of the symptoms and of the overall condition of the patient.

TREATMENT PLANNING

Once the decision to treat has been made, careful treatment planning is indicated. All diagnostic studies documenting the metastases are reviewed. In patients with bone metastases, these studies should include a recent bone scan as it is a more sensitive test than is an x-ray study. Physical examination and the patient's own account of the location of bone pain or similar symptoms are equally important in treatment planning. As a rule, and in contrast to the approach in primary treatment planning, every effort is made to include involved sites adjacent to the symptomatic metastases whenever feasible; this practice is in anticipation of those adjacent sites becoming symptomatic in the near future. In patients with bone metastases, this would mean treating the entire segment of the bone involved, including adjacent, nonsymptomatic "hot spots" demonstrated on a bone scan. In patients with brain metastases, this guideline translates to the inclusion of the whole brain in the radiation treatment portal. Such planning avoids the development of symptoms in areas close to the metastasis in question that would otherwise be difficult to treat because of overlap with a previous field.

Simulation should be scheduled as part of the treatment planning process whenever possible. In certain emergency situations, when anatomic land marks must be relied upon for the placement of the portal, high-quality "beam films" verifying that the site of interest is included in the beams as planned are equally acceptable.

Permanent documentation of the site treated, usually accomplished by means of tattoos on the skin, is necessary once the portals have been finalized. Patients with breast cancer frequently have relatively long life spans, with many subsequent episodes of symptomatic metastases. The radiation oncologist must be able to pinpoint previously treated portals, thus avoiding overlap of those with subsequent treatment portals.

TECHNIQUE

Selection of a therapy unit and treatment technique depends on two factors: the facilities available in the department and the location of the symptomatic metastases. For most bone, brain, and thoracic metastases, and for those similarly located deep within uninvolved tissue, parallel opposing fields using the photon beam from a linear accelerator or a cobalt unit provide acceptable dosimetry. Electron beam therapy, using an energy level and penetration appropriate to the clinical situation, is indicated for fairly superficial soft tissue or cutaneous lesions and for rib metastases. If these beams are not available, skillful use of a cobalt beam using "glancing" or tangential techniques will provide useful palliation in many clinical situations. For metastases in an extremity, rib, or cutaneous location, a 250-kV unit may also provide acceptable dosimetry.

The appropriate dose for the palliation of breast metastases should be selected on the basis of both the site to be treated and the life expectancy of the patient. At one end of the spectrum is a lesion that represents the first and only failure in a patient who has had a long disease-free interval from her initial treatment. For example, in the case of a chest wall failure in such a patient, 4500 to 5000 cGy, fractionated at 200 cGy per day, 5 days per week, to the entire chest wall region is needed. A boost dose might even be indicated in this situation if the recurrence site was not surgically excised prior to therapy.[2] A similar course of 4000 cGy in 4 weeks, in 250-cGy fractions, would also be appropriate for the first and only bone metastasis in a patient.

In the more common clinical situation, the area to be treated is the most symptomatic of multiple metastatic sites, and the life expectancy of the patient is measured in weeks to months. Several studies have reviewed various dose/fraction schemes for such patients in an effort to identify a rapid and effective, yet safe, radiation prescription. Doses ranging from 1000 cGy delivered in two treatments to 4000 cGy administered in 20 treatments over a 4-week period in one study,[3] and from 1500 cGy given in five fractions in 1 week to 3000 cGy administered in 10 fractions over a period of 2 weeks in a second study[4] yielded equally effective relief from bone pain. A similar study of dose/fractionation schemes for brain metastases from the Radiation Therapy Oncology Group again showed similar results, with doses ranging from 2000 cGy given in five fractions in 1 week to 4000 cGy given in 20 treatments.[5] Thus, the range of appropriate doses is wide. In prescribing treatment, the volume and sensitivity of uninvolved organs in the beam's path length must be considered. Short treatment courses are quite safe for bone lesions of the extremities since skin and connective tissue are relatively radiotolerant organs. Slower courses are better suited for large pelvic bone metastases in which small and large bowel tolerance is limited and complications may be acute. Between these extremes lie most clinical situations. The dose-fractionation scheme we use most frequently for bone metastases is 3000 cGy delivered in 10 fractions over 2 weeks' time. Clinical judgment is the last word in each situation.

ANTICIPATED RESPONSE

The most common metastases treated by radiation therapists are bone metastases. Some degree of pain relief over a period of 12 months was noted in 91% of patients with bone metastases in a study from Memorial Hospital that included only patients with breast cancer.[6] In a study at the Swedish Hospital in Seattle, complete and permanent pain relief was observed in 82% to 86% of patients with bone metastases from breast cancer. In this study patients received either 1000 cGy in two fractions or 4000 cGy in 20 fractions; there was no difference in the palliation achieved with these two dose-schedules.[3] Both the Memorial and Swedish Hospital studies relied on patients' subjective evaluations of pain relief. In addition to pain relief, radiographic bone healing and prevention of pathologic fractures are measures of the response of bone metastases to a palliative course of radiation. The Memorial study also assessed the postradiation improvement of the treated bone lesions on x-ray studies and found a radiologic improvement within 3 months of the completion of radiation in 78% of the patients treated.[6] A second study, conducted by Cheng and colleagues from the University of Utah, reviewed 59 patients with bone metastases from breast cancer who would routinely be considered for surgical fixation. These patients had lesions that were large and lytic or that had destroyed more than half of the cortex of a weight-bearing bone. Treatment of these patients consisted of a dose of 3000 cGy delivered in 10 fractions. Only 6% of the femoral lesions and none of the acetabular or humeral lesions sustained a fracture following initiation of radiation. Of course, should fracture occur, surgical fixation is indicated, followed by a course of palliative irradiation if it has not already been administered in that area.[7]

Response rates for other metastases from breast cancer are also quite high following palliative irradiation. A Memorial Hospital study that reviewed cases of brachial plexus metastases noted a 75% response rate.[8] A study from the Massachusetts General Hospital reported a treatment response in 6 of 7 patients with ureteral metastasis from breast cancer.[9] In the Radiation Therapy Oncology Group's study of fractionation in patients with brain metastases from breast cancer only, an 85% response rate was noted.[5] Similar response rates may be expected for most other symptomatic metastases, as noted in the following chapter.

SPECIAL TECHNIQUES

Hemi-body Irradiation

On occasion, widespread symptomatic breast cancer metastases are encountered in patients whose disease is refractory to any systemic chemotherapy. For some of these patients, single-exposure, hemi-body irradiation may be appropriate, and may provide rapid relief of symptoms. This technique, developed at the Princess Margaret Hospital in Toronto for palliative purposes,[10] has been further utilized by others—most notably, the group at the University of Rochester.[11] The patient is theoretically divided in half at the level of the umbilicus or at the iliac crest, and the most symptomatic half of the body is treated with a large field and a single dose of between 600 cGy and 800 cGy. Following such treatment, pain relief is rapid, occurring within 48 hours in 80% of the patients treated for a variety of primary lesions at the University of Rochester.[11]

Patients must be hospitalized for this procedure. For those undergoing upper-body irradiation, side effects, including hypotension, tachycardia, mild fever, nausea, and vomiting, are encountered within the first 24 hours after treatment. For those receiving lower-body treatments, acute side effects are minimal. In both upper- and lower-body treatments, the bone marrow exhibits a marked tolerance to the treatment, and blood counts usually return to pretreatment levels within a period of 3 to 5 weeks.[10] After that time, the nonirradiated half of the body may be treated if widespread symptoms also affect that portion, and if the response to the first half-body treatment has been good.

Subtotal Skin Electron Beam Therapy

Inflammatory breast cancer may recur in the skin of patients following initial therapy, and may spread to encompass wide areas of the chest, back, upper abdomen, arms, and opposite breast. The regions involved are frequently too large to include in conventional electron beam portals. In such cases, subtotal skin electron beam therapy should be considered. This technique was developed for widespread, cutaneous, malignant diseases, such as mycosis fungoides, and has been adapted by Nisce and colleagues at Memorial Hospital for widespread inflammatory breast cancer recurrences.[12] A factor affecting the efficacy of the technique is the thickness of the lesions. Generally, dosimetry is developed for just one electron beam energy for this technique. At Memorial Hospital, this beam will penetrate to 7 mm below the skin surface. In patients with lesions that do not exceed this thickness, treatment is administered on a once-weekly schedule using special shields to block those portions of the patient's skin that are clearly uninvolved by the disease. Doses of 400 cGy weekly for 6 weeks are prescribed, with boost doses sometimes being administered locally, as needed, for small areas of bulky or resistant disease.

Nisce noted a complete response in 17 of 22 patients treated, and a partial response in an additional 3 patients. The mean duration of that response was 8.3 months. Although this technique is not widely available, it should be considered in special situations, such as in patients with wide-spread skin metastases from recurrent inflammatory breast carcinoma.

Treatment of Ocular Metastases

The most common tumor presenting in the eye is a metastatic lesion, and the breast is the most common site of the primary lesion in such cases.[13–15] This is discussed in detail in the next chapter. A complaint of blurred vision or decreased activity is associated with disease of the choroid, and proptosis, ptosis, or visual loss is associated with extrabulbar soft tissue involvement.[14] CT scanning is of great value in diagnosis and treatment planning in patients with extrabulbar metastases. A careful ophthalmic examination will usually reveal choroid lesions.

Choroid lesions are best treated with a lateral field that is well collimated and positioned with the anterior border entering the eye just posterior to the lens. The field is angled a few degrees posterior to the lens in order to avoid an exit dose through the lens of the contralateral eye. A dose of 3000 cGy, delivered in 10 fractions over 2 weeks, is appropriate, and has been noted to produce a response in 89% of patients.[15]

For extrabulbar lesions, the treatment technique depends on the size and location of the lesion. A CT scan should be utilized in the planning process. In patients with retrobulbar lesions, the radiation dose should be delivered to this entire anatomic region, even if the disease appears to involve only one muscle. An electron beam with an eye shield, a lateral photon field, or a wedged pair of fields is appropriate. In patients with anterior extrabulbar lesions, which occur rarely, treatment planning will vary with each case. In all cases, the lens and the lacrimal gland should be protected whenever possible.

Radiation Castration

Irradiation may also play an indirect role in the management of breast metastases when it is directed at the ovaries to induce a therapeutic castration. This technique is no longer used as widely as it was in the past, but it remains an alternative to surgical castration when indicated.

Reviews of some of the earlier reports of this technique are remarkable for the low doses prescribed[16,17] (i.e., 450 cGy to 900 cGy), as well as the difficulty encountered in assessing the dosimetry used.[18,19] The menstrual cycle may be interrupted with low doses of irradiation, but much higher doses are necessary to induce a true castration. Recent reports suggest that doses of between 1500 cGy and 3000 cGy are needed for castration,[20–23] with the higher doses being universally recommended for young women, and the lower doses being recommended for those who are perimenopausal or menopausal. With conventional fractions of 200 cGy per day, doses of at least 2000 cGy for older women and at least 2500 cGy for younger patients are recommended.

The time interval between the cessation of radiation therapy and the reduction in ovarian hormone production is slightly longer than that following surgical ablation. Although Nathanson reported the onset of hot flashes and night sweats just 2 to 3 weeks following the last radiation treatment,[24] most studies suggest that 6 weeks to 2 months is the usual time interval.[20,23,25] Two months after treatment, Lalanne and colleagues documented similar levels of urinary gonadotropin in two groups of patients, one of which had been castrated by irradiation and one of which had undergone surgical castration.[20]

RETREATMENT

As is mentioned many times throughout this book, breast cancer, even after it metastasizes, may have a long natural history. Occasionally, the radiation oncologist is called in consultation to consider retreating a previously irradiated area that has become symptomatic. Commonly, further surgery and chemotherapy are no longer options, and the radiotherapist is faced with the decision to do nothing or to treat the patient again, knowingly exceeding the normal tissue tolerance in the area of concern.

Each patient and the possible complications must be evaluated individually and with great care. The normal tissue tolerances that are generally learned and quoted are associated with a small but predictable complication rate for that organ at that dose; higher doses increase the chances of that complication occurring. If a decision is made to re-treat the patient, both the patient and her family should be advised of the increased possibility of late effects. Also, to maximize the normal tissue tolerance that remains, the daily fractionation in any retreatment regimen must be kept low—that is, between 180 and 200 cGy per day. Using these guidelines, successful palliation may again be achieved in a patient whose only other option is an increase in analgesia.

REFERENCES

1. Haagensen CD: Diseases of the Breast, p 716. Philadelphia, WB Saunders, 1971
2. Bedwinek J, Fineberg B, Lee J, et al: Analysis of failures following local treatment of isolated local regional recurrence of breast cancer. Int J Radiat Oncol Biol Phys 7:581, 1981
3. Allen K, Johnson W, Hibbs G: Effective bone palliation as related to various treatment regimens. Cancer 37:984, 1976
4. Tong D, Gillick L, Hendrickson F: The palliation of symptomatic osseous metastases. Cancer 50:893, 1982
5. Gelber R, Larson M, Borgelt B, et al: Equivalence of radiation schedules for the palliative treatment of brain metastases in patients with favorable prognosis. Cancer 48:1749, 1981
6. Garmatis C, Chu F: The effectiveness of radiation therapy in

the treatment of bone metastases from breast cancer. Radiology 126:235, 1978
7. Cheng DS, Seitz CB, Eyre HJ: Nonoperative management of femoral, humeral, and acetabular metastases in patients with breast carcinoma. Cancer 45:1533, 1980
8. Nisce L, Chu F: Radiation therapy of brachial plexus syndrome from breast cancer. Radiology 126:235, 1978
9. Kopelson G, Munzenrider J, Kelley R, et al: Radiation therapy for ureteral metastases from breast carcinoma. Cancer 47:1976, 1981
10. Fitzpatrick P, Rider WD: Half-body radiotherapy of advanced cancer. Can Assoc Radiol 27:75, 1976
11. Salazar O, Rubin P, Keller B, et al: Systemic (half-body) radiation therapy: Response and toxicity. Int J Radiat Oncol Biol Phys 4:937, 1978
12. Nisce L, Poussin-Rosillo H, Kim JH, et al: Subtotal skin electron beam therapy once a week for inflammatory breast carcinoma. Radiology 130:761, 1979
13. Glassburn JR, Klionsky M, Brady LW: Radiation therapy for metastatic disease involving the orbit. Am J Clin Oncol 7:145, 1984
14. Reddy S, Saxena VS, Hendrickson F, et al: Malignant metastatic disease of the eye: Management of an uncommon complication. Cancer 47:810, 1981
15. Maor M, Chan RC, Young SE: Radiotherapy of choroidal metastases. Breast cancer as primary site. Cancer 40:2081, 1977
16. Cole MP: The place of radiotherapy in the management of early breast cancer: A report of two clinical trials. Br J Surg 51:216, 1964
17. Treves N: An evaluation of prophylactic castration in the treatment of mammary carcinoma. An analysis of 152 patients. Cancer 10:393, 1957
18. Taylor GW: Ovarian sterilization for breast cancer. Surg Gynecol Obstet 68:452, 1939
19. Adair FE, Treves N, Farrow JH, et al: Clinical effects of surgical and x-ray castration in mammary cancer. JAMA 128:161, 1945
20. Lalanne CM, Juret P, Hourtoule F, et al: La Castration dans le Cancer du Sein: Chirurgie ou Radiations, pp 323–334. Villejuif, Seine, France, Institut Gustave-Roussy, 1965
21. Farrow JH: The management of metastatic breast cancer by hormone manipulation. Bull NY Acad Med 38:151, 1962
22. Fracchia AA, Farrow JH, DePalo AJ, et al: Castration for primary inoperable or recurrent breast carcinoma. Surgery 128:1226, 1969
23. Stein JJ: Surgical or irradiation castration for patients with advanced breast cancer. Cancer 24:1350, 1969
24. Nathanson IT, Rice C, Meigs JV: Hormonal studies in artificial menopause produced by roentgen rays. Am J Obstet Gynecol 40:936, 1940
25. Stoll BA: Hormonal management of advanced breast cancer. Br Med J 2:293, 1969

Endocrine Therapy in Metastatic Breast Cancer

I. Craig Henderson

Endocrine therapy for breast cancer probably represents the oldest form of systemic therapy for any type of cancer.[1] Breast cancer is one of a very small group of tumors which regress following manipulation of the endocrine system. Not all patients with breast cancer respond to endocrine therapy. Clinical and laboratory research over the past 4 decades has led to a relatively precise delineation of those patients who are likely to benefit from endocrine therapy, but it is still uncertain how endocrine therapy works.

The clinical use of endocrine therapy is based primarily on the empirical observation that approximately one-third of patients with metastatic breast cancer will respond to endocrine manipulation. For most clinical situations, there is little evidence that one form of endocrine therapy is more effective than another (Table 13-2). However, there are exceptions to this rule. Oophorectomy, for example, is effective only in women who are actively menstruating or who are within 1 year of their last menstrual period, and aminoglutethimide and estrogens are effective only in postmenopausal women. Androgens are associated with a slightly lower response rate than other forms of treatment. Beyond these few exceptions, though, the selection of one endocrine therapy over another is usually based on the relative toxicity of the therapeutic regimens being considered. (Note: Throughout this section, menopause is defined in terms of the menstrual status of the patient at the time treatment is initiated, not the patient's menstrual status at the time of diagnosis.)

Patients who respond to endocrine therapy are those with the most indolent forms of the disease. The relatively recent discovery of the estrogen receptor and progesterone receptor proteins has simplified the task of selecting the patients who are most likely to benefit from endocrine therapy. An important predictive factor in response to endocrine therapy is a previous response to another type of endocrine therapy. Conversely, patients who fail to respond to initial endocrine therapy are unlikely to benefit from further attempts at either ablation of the endocrine organs or the addition of any form of endocrine therapy. The median duration of response to endocrine therapy is usually in the range of 12 to 18 months, but rarely, patients will have sustained responses for as long as 3 to 10 years.

Table 13-2
Response Rates of Unselected Patients to Various Forms of Endocrine Therapy

Therapy	*No. of Patients*	*Response Rate (%)*	*Range (%)*	*Reference No.*
Tamoxifen*	1269	32	16–52	2
Oophorectomy†	1674	33	21–41	3
Progestins*	2174	31	9–67	(See Table 13-9)
Aminoglutethimide‡	1153	31	16–43	4
Estrogens*	1683	26	15–38	3
Androgens*	2250	21	10–38	3
Adrenalectomy*	3739	32	23–46	3
Hypophysectomy*	1174	36	22–58	3

* Primarily postmenopausal patients.
† Exclusively premenopausal patients or patients who were within 1 year of their last menstrual period.
‡ Exclusively postmenopausal patients.

In addition, the sequential use of various forms of endocrine therapy may easily result in a cumulative response duration in excess of 2 to 3 years.

POSSIBLE MECHANISMS UNDERLYING ENDOCRINE THERAPEUTIC EFFECTS

Endocrine therapy may cause regression of breast cancers by removing or blocking an important tumor growth factor. This is a particularly attractive hypothesis for explaining endocrine effects because it is supported by clinical, as well as laboratory, observations. Oophorectomy, adrenalectomy, and hypophysectomy are all followed by a prompt decline in the circulating levels of a number of hormones, especially estrogens. Many patients experience relief from breast cancer symptoms concomitant with this change in estrogen level. The thymidine-labeling index, a measure of the percentage of cells synthesizing deoxyribonucleic acid (DNA), decreases abruptly within 1 week in patients responding to either oophorectomy or antiestrogens.[5] Epidemiologic evidence strongly suggests that estrogens either induce breast cancer or promote its growth. (See Chapter 4.) There is little more than anecdotal evidence that the administration of any dose of estrogen will actually stimulate the growth of measurable foci of metastatic breast cancer. However, physiologic doses of estradiol and progesterone, administered intramuscularly and concomitantly, caused an increase in the labeling index (LI) in 7 of 10 tumors. This effect was seen within 3 days of the treatment and occurred in four estrogen receptor-negative tumors, as well as in three estrogen receptor-positive tumors.[6] These observations are consistent with the concept that the growth of breast cancer is maintained or stimulated by estrogens, and that tumor regression occurs as a direct result of removing this stimulus.

Experimental evidence from studies of animal tumors and tissue culture systems supports the hypothesis that estrogens are a growth factor for mammary cancer. 7, 12-Dimethylbenzanthracene (DMBA) will induce mammary cancer in female rats, and many of these tumors will be hormone-dependent. Ovariectomy will cause tumor regression in many, but not all, of these DMBA-induced tumors. If estrogens are administered any time after the ovariectomy, the tumor will again begin to grow.[7] MCF-7 is an established cell line originally derived from a pleural effusion in a patient with metastatic breast cancer. This cell grows slowly in the absence of estrogen. The addition of physiologic concentrations of estradiol will stimulate the incorporation of tritiated thymidine and inorganic phosphate into DNA. Enzymatic activities associated with nucleic acid synthesis are increased, and the number of cells per Petri dish is greater in cultures with 5×10^{-9} mol per liter of estradiol than in cultures with 2.5% charcoal-treated calf serum and no added estradiol.[8]

On the basis of these experiments, it might be anticipated that the removal of estrogens would force the cells into a resting state—i.e., into G_0—but would not necessarily result in cell death. Histologic evaluation of regressing DMBA tumors in rats suggests that this is not the case. Loss of tumor volume in cancers responding to ovariectomy cannot be accounted for by shrinkage of tumor cells or by a decrease in the supporting stroma.[9] An initial event in the involution of these tumors is an increase in intracellular lysosomal enzyme activity, suggesting that the regression of DMBA tumors results from autophagocytosis. Since there is no evidence of lymphocytic invasion, changes in blood supply to the tumor, or other alterations of the supporting stroma, this autophagocytosis must represent a direct effect on the tumor cell of estrogen withdrawal.[10]

The growth-sustaining or growth-promoting effects of estrogens may be mediated through autocrine growth factors. Estrogen-sensitive mammary tumor cells that will not usually grow in male rats will grow when inoculated as a mixture with estrogen-independent cells. The estrogen-independent cells seem to secrete growth factors that support the growth of the estrogen-sensitive cell to the same extent that estrogen supports its growth.[11] *In vitro* studies have shown that conditioned medium from human breast cancer cells will stimulate the proliferation of other breast cancer cell cultures.[12] Established human cell lines secrete a variety of growth factors. The basal secretory levels of some of these autocrine growth factors have been shown to be much lower in estrogen receptor-positive cells than in estrogen receptor-negative cells, but estrogen may selectively stimulate the receptor-positive cells to secrete at a higher level. These experiments are all consistent with the hypothesis that autonomous (hormone-independent) cancer cells differ from hormone-dependent cells in their ability to synthesize growth factors critical to the maintenance of tumor growth.[12]

Despite the evidence that estrogens promote and sustain the growth of endocrine-sensitive cells, all endocrine effects may not be mediated through estrogens. Androgens may inhibit tumor growth by exerting an indirect effect on the supporting tissues surrounding the tumor, rather than on the tumor itself.[13] The ability of estrogens to reactivate growth of a regressing DMBA mammary cancer in rats requires a functional pituitary gland. The inhibitory effects of androgens or estrogens on the DMBA tumor may be overcome by the concomitant administration of high doses of prolactin. Although there is a competitive interaction between estrogens and the antiestrogen tamoxifen, the latter also has a direct cytotoxic effect on MCF-7 cells in tissue culture, affects the secretion of a number of other hormones *in vivo,* and has a weak estrogenic effect on some tissues.

It is puzzling that a single patient may experience tumor regression when estrogens are first administered, subsequently experience another tumor regression at a later time when estrogen therapy is discontinued, and respond yet a third time following more complete estrogen ablation by adrenalectomy or hypophysectomy.[14] Similar observations have been made in laboratory models. High doses of estrogen will inhibit the growth of DMBA-induced mammary cancers in rats.[7] However, the DMBA model and human breast cancer differ in their response to physiologic or moderate doses of estrogens. There are very few data that estrogens promote the growth of human breast cancer at any dose.[15] Sequential responses to the addition and removal of estrogens may reflect the growth and inhibition of clones of tumor cells with different sensitivities to estrogen. Although the growth of MCF-7 cells is usually stimulated by physiologic concentrations of estradiol, a clone that is inhibited by the same concentration of estradiol has been isolated. Four to 5 days after the addition of estradiol, these cells appear to undergo autophagocytosis. Removal of the estradiol at that time does not rescue the cells.[16] Clones of MCF-7 cells that are resistant to the inhibitory effects of diethylstilbestrol (DES) have been isolated. Some of these clones have an increased sensitivity to the cytotoxic effects of tamoxifen.[17] Two estrogen receptor-positive human breast tumors grown in nude mice were shown to have opposite reactions to estradiol: the growth of one tumor was stimulated, whereas the growth of the other was inhibited.[18] Although these experiments provide excellent evidence that clones of cells with similar receptor status and histologic appearance may have different responses to estrogens, they also illustrate the risks involved in basing clinical decisions on the behavior of one animal or tissue culture tumor model.

Animal and tissue culture models are excellent tools for developing hypotheses that can be tested in clinical trials, but each case of human breast cancer is characterized by multiple clones of tumor cells. It is likely that each clone has unique sensitivities to estrogens and other hormones. The net growth or regression of a tumor mass may depend upon the relative growth and regression of dozens of clones within the tumor mass. This concept is schematically illustrated in Figure 13-3.[19] The tumors that are most sensitive to endocrine therapy are characterized by a well-differentiated histologic appearance.[20–22] It is likely that these hormone-sensitive end cells have evolved from stem cells that are more undifferentiated. There may be a variable sensitivity to hormone therapy among those end cells with an estrogen receptor and those without, and possibly, even among different receptor-positive clones. The estrogen-binding detected with immunocytochemical techniques is not a true measure of the estrogen receptor detected by conventional estrogen receptor bioassay, but these techniques are another measure of tumor sensitivity to endocrine therapy, providing information on the percentage of cells that might be receptor-positive.[23] Estrogen-binding is only rarely observed on all cells within a tumor specimen. In one study, 25% of the tumors had no cells with indirect immunofluorescence, 4% of the tumors were characterized by estrogen-binding on all of the cells, and 71% of the tumors had varying numbers of cells with evidence of estradiol-binding.[24] The intensity of immunofluorescent staining varied within each specimen, which may reflect different receptor types or other differences in the way separate clones of tumor process estrogen.

If the stem cell model shown in Figure 13-3 is correct, endocrine therapy would not be expected to destroy the undifferentiated stem cell. This premise has been studied using DMBA rat mammary carcinoma. Fragments were removed from tumors regressing after ovariectomy and from tumors growing in untreated rats. These fragments were transplanted into new hosts and grew equally well. After some time, it was impossible to distinguish in the new host between tumors started from regressing cancers and those started from growing cancers.[9] The stem cell model and these experiments suggest that the potential for endocrine therapy to eradicate breast cancer totally in any patient is limited.

OVARIAN ABLATION

Oophorectomy is the oldest form of endocrine therapy. The overall response rate to such therapy among premenopausal women is 32%. The response rate among

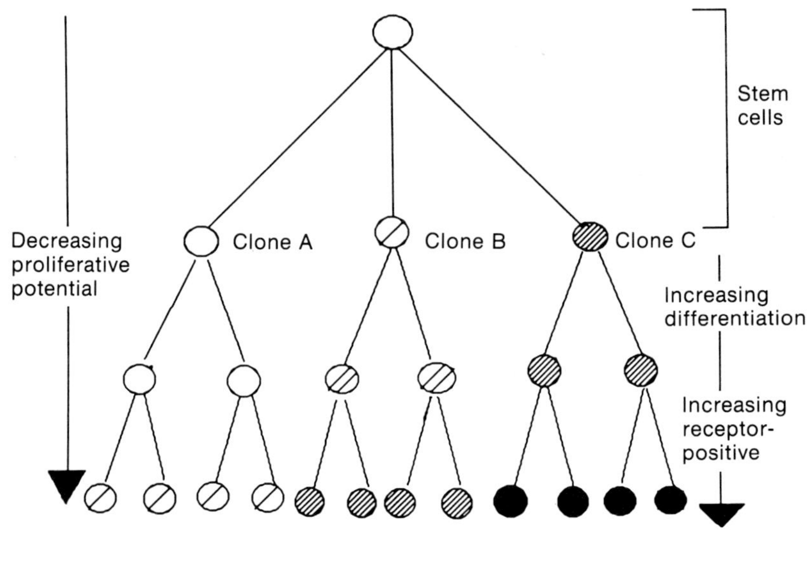

FIGURE 13-3. A model for clonal evolution from breast cancer stem cells. ●, cells that are very sensitive to endocrine therapy; ◍, cells that are moderately sensitive to endocrine therapy; ⊘, cells that are weakly sensitive to endocrine therapy; and ○, cells that are insensitive to endocrine therapy. (Modified from Figures 1 and 3 of Selby P, Bizzar J-P, Buick RN: Therapeutic implications of a stem cell model for human breast cancer: A hypothesis. Cancer Treat Rep 67:659, 1983.)

women younger than 35 years of age is frequently in the range of 15% to 25%.[25,26] In one series of 550 patients, the response rate for these young women was 18%.[27]

It is logical to assume that women who are no longer actively menstruating are unlikely to benefit from oopho rectomy. However, after an initial decline in circulating estrogen levels during the years following the onset of menopause, a gradual increase occurs until levels are reached that are at the lower end of the normal range for reproductive women.[28] There is a surprisingly high vaginal smear cytology maturation index in postmenopausal women, even 20 years after the last menstrual period, and at least one study suggests that this index is higher in patients with breast cancer than in age-matched control subjects.[29] For these reasons, it is not entirely unreasonable to believe that postmenopausal women might respond to oophorectomy as well as premenopausal women do. Indeed, there is a rare study that demonstrates benefit from oophorectomy in postmenopausal women.[30] However, the response rate has usually been disappointingly low in most trials. In the large series from Memorial Hospital, only 3.5% of postmenopausal women had objective evidence of response to therapy.[26] At the Milan Cancer Institute, the response rate was 6% in women who were more than 1 year beyond their last menstrual period.[27] In most cases, the highest reported response rates are less than 20%.[25,31] Following oophorectomy, the estradiol production rate in premenopausal women changes dramatically; similar evaluations of the endocrine profiles of postmenopausal women show no similar changes following oophorectomy.[32]

Ovarian ablation may be achieved with either surgery or radiotherapy. There are no randomized trials comparing these two approaches, and most comparisons of these two methods must be interpreted cautiously because of the bias introduced by selection factors. In the Memorial series, the overall response rate to ovarian ablation was only 16%, compared to a 35% response rate to oophorectomy in menstruating patients. However, most of the patients who were selected for ovarian irradiation in that series were considered to be poor operative risks. A few patients who failed to respond to radiation ablation were subsequently treated with surgical oophorectomy, and none responded.[26] In another retrospective analysis, the response rate to oophorectomy in 97 patients was 30% and the response to radiation ablation in 61 patients was 21%.[33] However, the group undergoing radiation ablation included a much larger proportion of perimenopausal and postmenopausal women than did the group undergoing oophorectomy. Only 36% of the actively menstruating patients included in this series were treated with radiation ablation. Following treatment, there was a delay of 2 to 8 weeks in response to radiation ablation. The response to oophorectomy was described as being more immediate. However, there was a subjective response to irradiation which preceded the objective response in most patients. The duration of response to the two modalities was the same.

In several recent radiation ablation series, patients have achieved response rates similar to those usually associated with surgical oophorectomy. For example, the response rate in sites distant from the radiation field was 32% in 28 patients treated with 1000 cGy at a single exposure; the response rate in women who were actively menstruating was 41%.[31] The percentage of patients still alive and in continuing response 6 months after initiation of therapy was the same whether the patient was treated with radiation ablation or oophorectomy.[34]

The operative mortality rate associated with oophorectomy is minimal, but it may range between 2.5% and 4.5%, depending on the general health of the patients selected for therapy.[26,34] Patients with rapidly progressive disease and extensive visceral involvement often are not good candidates for surgical oophorectomy because they are likely to have a higher operative mortality rate than other patients. This group of patients is also less likely to benefit from endocrine therapy, and it is doubtful whether they should be considered for radiation ablation.

In summary, surgical oophorectomy and ovarian irradiation appear to be equally effective when undertaken in appropriate patients who are actively menstruating, especially in premenopausal women older than 35 years of age. In an otherwise healthy patient who is symptomatic—e.g., from widespread bone metastases—oophorectomy might be preferred over irradiation because of the rapidity of response. In a patient with relatively few symptoms, radiation ablation may be the treatment of choice because hospitalization is not required and there are no postoperative complications. Many premenopausal patients inadvertently receive ovarian irradiation when palliative radiotherapy is administered to painful bony metastases in the lumbar spine or pelvis. Further systemic therapy should not be given to these patients until there is objective evidence of progression in nonirradiated sites. In most cases, 2 to 3 months should elapse after cessation of menses before it is concluded that the radiation therapy has been ineffective.

ADRENALECTOMY AND HYPOPHYSECTOMY

A generation ago, many physicians considered ablative surgery of the adrenal and pituitary glands to be the endocrine therapy of choice in postmenopausal women. The overall response rate to this treatment was equal to that associated with other forms of endocrine therapy available at that time (see Table 13-2). The remissions obtained were notably durable, and chronic toxicity was considered to be less objectionable than the nausea, vomiting, masculinization, and fluid retention associated with the standard additive endocrine therapies of that time—estrogens and androgens. However, the operative morbidity and mortality from adrenalectomy and hypophysectomy were prohibitive at facilities that did not perform large numbers of these procedures (Table 13-3). Overall operative mortality was usually less than 5% but ranged as high as 25%. This is the major reason why neither adrenalectomy nor hypophysectomy are used with any frequency today.

Table 13-3
Mortality Associated With Major Ablative Therapy

	No. of Patients	*Mortality Rate (%)*	*Range (%)*
Adrenalectomy	2000	5.5	0.8–25.0
Transfrontal hypophysectomy	617	4.7	1.2–17.0
Transsphenoidal hypophysectomy	625	4.0	0.0– 7.1
Yttrium-90 implantation	662	1.5	0.2– 5.0

(Robin PE, Dalton, GA: The role of major endocrine ablation. In Stoll BA (ed). Breast Cancer—Early and Late, pp 147–156. Chicago, Yearbook Medical Publishers, 1977.)

Adrenalectomy and hypophysectomy are thought to affect breast cancer by ablating all adrenal function, thus removing the last remaining source of androgens that can be converted to estrogen in postmenopausal women. (See the section on aminoglutethimide, below.)

In one randomized trial, hypophysectomy was shown to be more effective than adrenalectomy.[35] The percentage of patients who responded to hypophysectomy was greater, and the survival of all patients treated with hypophysectomy was longer than that of patients treated with adrenalectomy. However, the mean survival difference was only 8 months for all patients and 9 months for responders. It is not easy to explain these results. The removal of prolactin with the hypophysectomy may have contributed to its added effectiveness, but this cannot be accepted uncritically since there is no other evidence that prolactin is an important factor in either the etiology or the treatment of human breast cancer. In fact, prolactin levels may actually rise in some responsive patients following hypophysectomy, presumably because the hypophysectomy is incomplete.[36]

Hypophysectomy may be performed by surgical extirpation through either a transsphenoidal or a transfrontal approach. There is no evidence that one of these approaches is more effective than the other in inducing response, but the morbidity rate and the complexity of the medical facilities necessary for the transfrontal approach are somewhat greater than that associated with the transsphenoidal approach.[35,37] Hypophysectomy has also been performed with yttrium-90 implantation, and this method is probably as effective as the surgical approaches.[38] However, yttrium-90 implantation has never been widely used because it was first evaluated only a few years prior to the introduction of newer, less toxic forms of endocrine therapy.

In addition to the acute surgical mortality associated with these two forms of ablation, there are chronic, long-term side effects as well. The most important of these side effects is recurrent addisonian crisis. Such crises have been reported to occur in as many as 17% of patients undergoing follow-up for more than 6 weeks postadrenalectomy.[39] Progressive involvement of the visceral organs, infections, and the stress associated with chemotherapy are all apt to increase the frequency and severity of addisonian crises during the final phases of the illness. Hypophysectomy may also be associated with transient diabetes insipidus, and up to 50% of patients may have anosmia. Meningitis may develop in 5% of patients following transsphenoidal hypophysectomy.

ESTROGEN AND ANDROGEN THERAPY

Postmenopausal women respond to estrogen therapy with about the same frequency as they do to major ablative procedures (see Table 13-2). Until tamoxifen, the newer progestins, and aminoglutethimide were introduced, estrogen therapy was generally considered to be the treatment of choice for postmenopausal women. Estrogens are ineffective, even at very high doses, in premenopausal women.[40] As with other forms of endocrine therapy, the best responses are reported among postmenopausal women who are at least 5 years beyond their last menstrual period.[41]

A number of different estrogen preparations and dosages have been used, but the optimal dosage of estrogen is not well established. The most commonly used regimens are DES, 5 mg three times per day (t.i.d.); ethinyl estradiol, 1 mg t.i.d.; or Premarin, 2.5 mg t.i.d.[41,42] Dose-response was evaluated in a randomized trial in which 523 postmenopausal women were treated with either 1.5, 15, 150, or 1500 mg of estrogen per day.[15] Statistically significant higher response rates were associated with the highest dosages: 21% in those patients receiving 1500 mg of estrogen per day, 17% in those receiving 150 mg per day, 15% in those receiving 15 mg per day, and 10% in those receiving 1.5 mg per day. However, the administration of higher doses was also associated with more severe side effects, especially nausea, vomiting, and anorexia. Even though the high response rate associated with the highest dosage may have been statistically significant, it was not necessarily clinically significant. Another important observation from this study is that lower dosages of estrogen do not accelerate tumor growth. For this reason, the estrogen dose may be titrated in an individual patient to the highest tolerated dose rather than to a predetermined optimal level.

Between 25% and 35% of patients who respond to estrogens will have a secondary response if the estrogens are withdrawn at the time of further tumor progression.[43–48] Because of this, many clinical trials require a month or more of observation between the completion of one therapeutic regimen and the initiation of another, especially when another form of endocrine therapy is planned. The incidence of rebound regression in patients who initially fail to respond to estrogen or any other form of endocrine therapy is extremely low; under these circumstances, an interval between treatments is probably not justified.

Androgens have also been shown to be effective in

treating metastatic breast cancer. In randomized trials comparing the efficacy of androgens and estrogens, the response rate to androgens was significantly lower than that achieved with estrogen therapy.[49] Sixteen percent of 218 women randomized to receive DES responded, whereas 10% of the 221 women receiving testosterone responded. This difference in response was statistically significant. No subgroup of patients was found to derive a clear benefit from androgen therapy in comparison to estrogen therapy, although there has traditionally been a tendency to utilize androgens rather than estrogens as second-line therapy in premenopausal patients who have previously responded to oophorectomy.

A variety of androgens have been evaluated in phase II trials, including testosterone propionate, testolactone, calusterone, and fluoxymesterone. Despite considerable effort, an effective androgen that is without masculinizing side effects has not yet been developed.[50–53] Fluoxymesterone (Halotestin), 10 mg p.o., b.i.d., is as effective and nontoxic as any of the other preparations.

Estrogen therapy is associated with a variety of side effects (Table 13-4). Ethinyl estradiol and Premarin may produce fewer side effects—especially, less nausea and vomiting—than diethylstilbestrol. These symptoms may become less severe or may disappear with continued administration of estrogen, and in some cases, nausea and vomiting may be avoided altogether by initiating therapy at a lower dosage (e.g., 0.5 mg of ethinyl estradiol instead of 1.0 mg t.i.d.). Up to one-third of the patients treated with estrogens may withdraw from therapy because of toxicity. The most important side effect is persistent and severe nausea with frequent vomiting. Fluid retention may also be severe in a few cases and may be associated with congestive heart failure. Urinary incontinence and a variety of mild gynecologic symptoms also occur with considerable frequency and should be mentioned to the patient before estrogen therapy is initiated (see Table 13-4).

Androgens are associated with relatively mild symptoms, except for masculinization, which is extremely disturbing to many patients. In some cases, this effect is counterbalanced by a slight euphoria or increased sense of well-being which many patients experience when first starting androgen therapy. Flare and hypercalcemia have been more frequently reported with androgens than with any other form of endocrine therapy.

ANTIESTROGEN THERAPY: TAMOXIFEN

Antiestrogens were initially developed as antifertility drugs. Instead, they actually induce ovulation in infertile women. More importantly, this group of drugs may cause regression of breast cancer, and one of this group—tamoxifen—has become the endocrine therapy of choice for most clinical situations in which palliation of the symptoms of metastatic breast cancer is required. In addition, tamoxifen has become an important form of systemic therapy for the treatment of early breast cancer, and it may significantly prolong survival in some groups of patients. (See Chapter 10.)

Tamoxifen inhibits tritiated thymidine incorporation, suppresses DNA polymerase activity, and reduces total DNA content and total cell numbers when applied to MCF-7 cells growing in tissue culture. There is a reduction in the number of cells in S-phase and an increase in the number of cells in G_1.[54,55] Most of these *in vitro* tamoxifen effects may be prevented or reversed by the addition of estradiol in concentrations equal to 1/1000 of the molar

Table 13-4
Common Side Effects Associated With Administration of Estrogens or Androgens in the Treatment of Metastatic Breast Cancer

Estrogen Symptoms	*Incidence (%)*	*Androgen Symptoms*	*Incidence (%)*
Gynecologic		***Masculinizing***	
Nipple pigmentation	80	Hoarseness	61
Breast engorgement	20	Hirsutism	52
Breast tenderness	16	Hair loss	22
Vaginal bleeding	33	Acne	30
		Increase in libido	37
Gastrointestinal		***Gastrointestinal***	
Anorexia	57	Nausea	18
Nausea	58	Vomiting	11
Vomiting	32	Weight increase	71
Diarrhea	5		
Other		***Other***	
Edema	34	Edema	16
Urinary incontinence	28	Hypercalcemia	10
Congestive heart failure	9		

(Kennedy BJ, Nathanson IT: Effects of intensive sex steroid hormone therapy in advanced breast cancer. JAMA 152:1135, 1953. Copyright 1953, American Medical Association)

concentration of tamoxifen. However, if the tamoxifen remains in the culture media for 3 days prior to the addition of estrogen, the tamoxifen effects are no longer reversible.[56] At very high doses (in the range of 10 μM), cell death occurs within 48 hours.[54] Tamoxifen is associated with a number of other effects as well, but these may not be seen with every tissue culture cell line. For example, tamoxifen inhibits progesterone synthesis in the MCF-7 line but not in the ZR-751 line, a cell line that is normally as estrogen-sensitive as MCF-7. In general, tamoxifen effects are seen exclusively in cell lines with an estrogen receptor protein, but there have been reports of inhibition of the growth of estrogen receptor-negative cell lines as well.[54,55]

In the DMBA rat model, tamoxifen reduces circulating gonadotropin, estrogen, and prolactin levels. Tamoxifen will reduce or prevent the appearance of tumors if antiestrogen therapy is started before the first evidence of tumor growth, but it must be administered continuously in order for this effect to be sustained.[57]

In women, especially in those who are premenopausal, tamoxifen may stimulate ovarian estrogen secretion,[58] suppress pituitary gonadotropins, or exert an estrogenic effect inducing maturation of the vaginal mucosa.[59] Endometrial biopsies taken during the luteal phase of the menstrual cycle of a patient receiving tamoxifen show no evidence of progestational effect.[58] This suggests that tamoxifen may have antiprogestational, as well as antiestrogenic, activity.

A large number of phase II trials of tamoxifen have been performed. The overall response rate is about equal to that seen with estrogens, oophorectomy, and major ablative procedures (see Table 13-2).[2] The range of responses in these studies varies between 15% and 47%. The mean response rate is 34%. The mean and median duration of response has ranged from 5.8 to 20 months, and this, too, is similar to that associated with earlier modes of endocrine therapy.[60]

Two other antiestrogens have also been tested in the clinic: clomiphene and nafoxidine. The response rate achieved with these two agents is similar to that of tamoxifen, and the side effects are quite limited as well.[61] Nafoxidine has been reported to cause cutaneous photosensitivity, and there were isolated reports of bilateral cataracts, also. In some cases, partial hair loss and dryness of skin were problems.[61–63] Clomiphene may have even fewer side effects.[64,65] A few other antiestrogens, such as trioxifene mesylate, have received even more limited evaluation.[66] Tamoxifen has become established as the antiestrogen of choice without demonstrated superiority to the other antiestrogens in controlled trials. It is possible, however, that tamoxifen is slightly less toxic than other antiestrogens.

Tamoxifen has been compared in randomized trials with almost every major form of conventional endocrine therapy (Table 13-5). Four separate trials have failed to show any significant differences in the relative efficacy of estrogens and tamoxifen. The largest of these trials found no difference in the time to treatment failure, duration of response, or survival in patients randomized to receive either DES or tamoxifen (Fig. 13-4).[48] However, there was a statistically significant higher incidence of toxicity in the patients receiving DES. DES caused more than twice the incidence of nausea and vomiting, four times the incidence of edema and heart failure, and three times the incidence of phlebitis associated with tamoxifen. The only side effects that were observed more frequently among the patients treated with tamoxifen than among those treated with DES were hot flashes and leukopenia.

Tamoxifen has been shown to be more effective than fluoxymesterone.[53] Patients treated with tamoxifen had a time to treatment failure ($p = 0.003$) and a survival rate

Table 13-5
Randomized Trials Comparing Tamoxifen Therapy With More Conventional Endocrine Therapy in Postmenopausal Women With Metastatic Breast Cancer

Therapeutic Regimen	*No. of Patients*	*Response Rate (%)*			*Median Duration of Response (mos)*			*Reference No.*
		TAM	*OET*	*p*	*TAM*	*OET*	*p*	
DES, 15 mg	56	31	22		9.5	8.1		67
DES, 3 mg	92	28	31	NS	24.0	24.0	NS	70
DES, 15 mg	143	33	41	0.37	7.9	13.1	0.46	48
DES, 15 mg	27	19	36	NS				69
Ethinyl estradiol, 3 mg	59	33	31	NS	11.0	11.0	>0.10	68
Ethinyl estradiol, 3 mg	43	53	25					71
Fluoxymesterone, 20 mg	79	30	19					53
Hypophysectomy	26	71	67	NS	13.0	12.5	NS	72
Adrenalectomy	51	35	52	>0.1	14+	18+	NS	73

The dosage of tamoxifen was 10 mg twice daily, except in one trial[67] in which a dosage of 10 mg three times daily was used, and three trials[53, 68, 72] in which 20 mg of tamoxifen was administered twice daily. Doses of other drugs reflect the cumulative daily dose. (TAM, tamoxifen; OET, other endocrine therapy; NS, not statistically significant.)

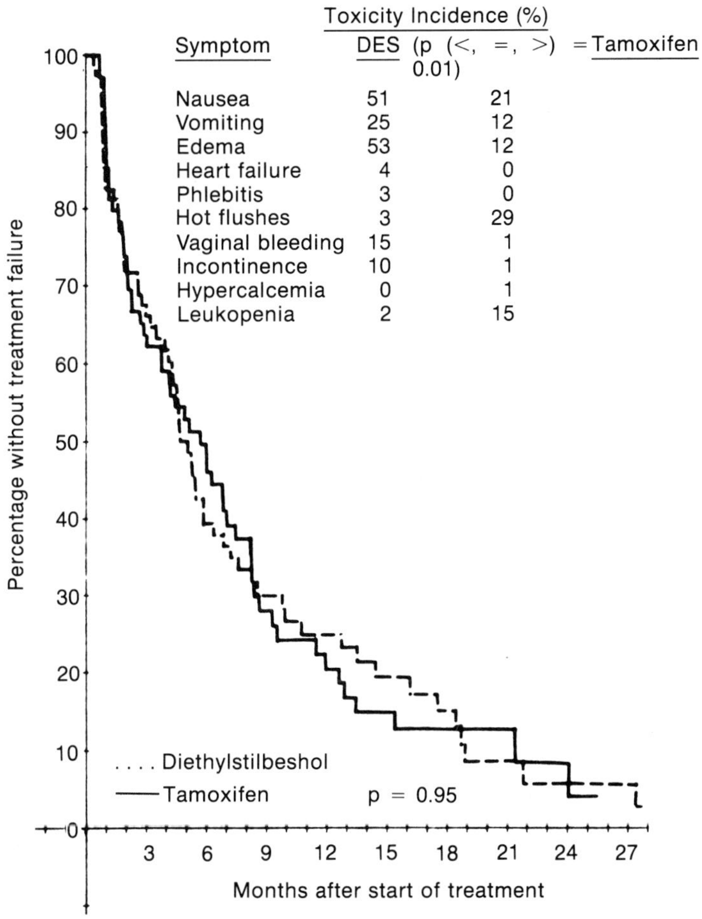

FIGURE 13-4. Time interval to treatment failure in postmenopausal patients with metastatic breast cancer who were randomized to receive either diethylstilbestrol (DES) or tamoxifen. (Ingle JN, Ahmann D, Green SJ, et al: Randomized clinical trial of diethylstilbestrol versus tamoxifen in postmenopausal women with advanced breast cancer. N Engl J Med 304:16, 1981. Reprinted by permission of the New England Journal of Medicine.)

($p = 0.05$) that were significantly greater than those achieved with fluoxymesterone. This observation is in keeping with the results of an earlier generation of studies in which estrogens were shown to be more effective than androgens. The incidence of toxicity was higher and the side effects were more unacceptable with the use of fluoxymesterone than with the use of tamoxifen. Thirty-one of 42 patients treated with fluoxymesterone experienced hirsutism, 5 had abnormal liver enzymes, and therapy was discontinued in 3 patients because of toxicity. Tamoxifen was discontinued in 3 patients because of toxicity, primarily as a result of hypercalcemia. The incidence of hot flashes in patients receiving tamoxifen was much greater than that seen with androgen therapy. Hot flashes occurred in 19 of 37 patients receiving tamoxifen and in none of those receiving fluoxymesterone.

Small trials have been undertaken comparing tamoxifen with major ablative procedures, including hypophysectomy[72] and adrenalectomy.[73] No advantage was demonstrated for hypophysectomy over tamoxifen, and the increased response rate observed for treatment with adrenalectomy in comparison to tamoxifen did not reach a level of statistical significance, nor did it translate into a survival advantage.[73]

Use of Tamoxifen in Premenopausal Women

The initial experience with tamoxifen was limited predominantly to postmenopausal women, in part because oophorectomy is both effective and relatively nontoxic for premenopausal women. Reports from small, uncontrolled trials of tamoxifen in premenopausal women suggest that the frequency of response (72 of 231 patients, or 31%) and the median duration of response (13 to 23 months) are as great as that usually achieved with oophorectomy.[74–79] Also, an initial response to tamoxifen appears to predict a secondary response to oophorectomy at the time the patient has evidence of further progression of her disease. In this series of phase II trials, the response to oophorectomy after a tamoxifen response was 40% (17 of 42 patients). Conversely, the response to oophorectomy in patients who failed to respond to tamoxifen was only 13% (7 of 52 patients). Most of the responders to oophorectomy among the nonresponders to tamoxifen are from a single trial.[74] In this study, none of the 14 patients who responded to tamoxifen had a secondary response to oophorectomy, whereas 5 of 22 patients who failed to respond to tamoxifen had a response to oophorectomy. In another study, a response to tamoxifen was found to be a more powerful predictor of subsequent response to oophorectomy than was the estrogen receptor protein.[76] Thirteen of 15 patients who did not respond to tamoxifen and who were treated secondarily with oophorectomy progressed following oophorectomy; the condition of two of these patients stabilized. Five of the 13 patients who progressed were both estrogen receptor- and progesterone receptor-positive. In this study, the predictive value of a tamoxifen response for subsequent response to oophorectomy was highly significant ($p < 0.004$). There are other case reports of patients responding to oophorectomy despite a failure to respond to tamoxifen,[80] and it is reasonable to recommend oophorectomy following tamoxifen failure in the rare patient who is otherwise an excellent candidate for endocrine therapy and who has no urgent need for response.

Two randomized trials comparing the results of treatment with tamoxifen and with oophorectomy in premenopausal women have recently been reported (Table 13-6).[81,82] Overall, there appears to be no statistically significant differences in response rate, time to treatment failure, duration of response, or survival of patients treated with either of these modes of therapy. The response rate to oophorectomy was higher in one of the trials,[81] and the duration of response was marginally greater following ta-

Table 13-6
Randomized Trials Comparing Tamoxifen and Oophorectomy in Premenopausal Women With Metastatic Breast Cancer

Therapeutic Regimen	*Oophorectomy Arm*	*Tamoxifen Arm*	*p*
Tamoxifen, 10 mg b.i.d[81]			
No. of patients	27	26	
Response rate	37%	27%	0.045
Median TTF	4.8 mo	5.3 mo	0.74
Median response duration	15.9 mo	15.1 mo	NS
Median survival	18.3 mo	30.0 mo	0.44
Secondary response on crossover	5/15 patients (33%)	2/18 patients (11%)	
Prior responders	2/5 patients (40%)	1/6 patients (17%)	
Prior nonresponders	2/10 patients (20%)	1/12 patients (8%)	
Tamoxifen, 20 mg b.i.d.[82]			
No. of patients	52	55	
Response rate	21%	24%	NS
Median response duration	7 mo	20 mo	0.056
Median survival	25 mo	15 mo	0.18

TTF, time to treatment failure for all patients entered into the trial, regardless of their response; b.i.d., twice daily; NS, not statistically significant.)

moxifen treatment in the other,[82] but these differences were of borderline significance. In one of these trials, there appeared to be an advantage for oophorectomy among patients with predominantly visceral disease.[81] None of the 14 patients with predominantly visceral disease who were randomized to receive tamoxifen responded, whereas 8 of the 16 patients who were randomized to undergo oophorectomy had a response. This observation was not confirmed in the other trial.[82]

Premenopausal women treated with tamoxifen experience a variety of menstrual irregularities.[75–79] The incidence of amenorrhea varies from 16% to 39%, and increases with longer duration of tamoxifen therapy.[75,79,83] Patients who respond to tamoxifen are more likely to continue the drug for a long period of time. However, no other association between either amenorrhea or other menstrual abnormalities and a response to tamoxifen has been established. An early onset of oligomenorrhea or amenorrhea is not a predictive factor for subsequent response or failure to respond to tamoxifen.

Dose Schedule for Tamoxifen

Tamoxifen often induces a marked rise in serum estrogen levels in premenopausal women.[58,78] This has led some investigators to utilize a higher-than-usual dose of tamoxifen in patients failing to respond to conventional doses. However, there is no reproducible evidence that these higher doses result in either more frequent suppression of the menstrual cycle[78] or a greater probability of response. In a nonrandomized trial, the response rate among 11 patients treated with 10 mg of tamoxifen twice daily was 27%; in 33 patients treated with 10 mg of tamoxifen three times daily, the response rate was also 27%. All of the complete responses occurred in the group treated with 30 mg per day, but this observation is of questionable statistical or clinical significance.[75]

Several anecdotal reports suggest that higher doses of tamoxifen may be effective in postmenopausal patients who prove to be refractory to lower doses of the drug. An 80-year-old patient who had had stable disease for 6 months while receiving 10 mg of tamoxifen twice daily had an objective response when the dosage was escalated to 20 mg twice daily.[84] In another report, 4 of 12 patients who failed to respond to a dosage of 40 mg of tamoxifen per day subsequently responded to a dosage of 80 mg per day,[85] yet another report found that 1 of 19 patients who were refractory to a dosage of 30 mg per day responded to a dosage of 90 mg per day.[2] Larger studies using higher dosages in patients proven to be refractory to lower dosages of tamoxifen failed to confirm these early observations.[86,87]

Because of these anecdotal observations, randomized trials have been conducted to determine the optimal dosage of tamoxifen. Dosages have ranged from 8 mg to 200 mg/m^2 per day (Table 13-7). None of these trials has shown a significant advantage for the use of a higher dose of tamoxifen. In a National Cancer Institute study, 108 patients were randomized to receive 4, 8, 16, 32, 50, 60, 80, and 100 mg/m^2 of tamoxifen twice daily.[89] Patients within each of these groups were also randomized to receive either tamoxifen alone or tamoxifen plus fluoxymesterone. Dose-response was analyzed by dividing the patients into three dosage groups: less than 12 mg, 12 mg to 32 mg, and greater than 32 mg/m^2 per day. Overall, the response rate

Table 13-7
Randomized Trials Comparing Two Dosages of Tamoxifen in Postmenopausal Patients With Metastatic Breast Cancer

		Response Rate (%)			Median Duration (mos)		
Dosages (mg/day)	No. of Patients	Low Dose	Intermediate Dose	High Dose	Low Dose	High Dose	Reference No.
20 vs 40	68	61		77			88
< 12 vs 12–32 vs > 32	108	41	31	46			89
30 vs 90	143	37		35	13+	11+	85
20 vs 40	237	34		31	18	12	90

was as great in the group of patients receiving the lowest dose (41%) as it was in the group receiving the highest dose (46%). There was a nonsignificant trend toward dose-response among the patients receiving tamoxifen without fluoxymesterone, with response rates of 11%, 10%, and 33% in the groups treated with less than 12 mg, 12 mg to 32 mg, and greater than 32 mg/m^2, respectively. The median time to treatment failure was not significantly different among the three groups. No advantage for higher dosages of tamoxifen was established. A dosage of 20 mg to 40 mg per day is adequate in all situations. In the United States, the standard therapy is 10 mg of tamoxifen twice daily. In Europe, it is usually 20 mg of tamoxifen twice daily.

The use of a twice-daily schedule for tamoxifen is arbitrary. The half-life of tamoxifen is 9 to 12 hours after the initial dose, and 7 days with chronic dosage. When the starting dosage is 10 mg twice daily, a steady-state serum tamoxifen level is reached after 16 weeks of therapy. Tamoxifen is still detectable in the blood 6 weeks after therapy is discontinued.[91] This observation may be important in deciding when to repeat a biopsy for estrogen receptors. Patients may have a false-negative estrogen receptor assay if the tumor tissue is obtained while the patient is being treated with tamoxifen. A waiting period of at least 6 weeks following cessation of tamoxifen therapy may decrease the risk of a false-negative result.

It has been suggested that a loading dosage of 40 mg/m^2 of tamoxifen twice daily for 7 days, followed by chronic dosages of 20 mg/m^2 of the drug once daily thereafter, is most consistent with the known pharmacology of the drug.[91] However, the lack of a dose-response in the randomized trials described above suggests that it is unlikely that an increased response rate, duration of response, or survival would result from this approach. In one study, serum tamoxifen concentrations were greater with dosages of 20 mg twice daily than they were with dosages of 10 mg twice daily, but there was no difference in the mean serum tamoxifen concentrations among responders and nonresponders.[90] Higher doses of tamoxifen have not been found to shorten the interval to first response. The median interval to treatment response in the dosage study conducted by the National Cancer Institute was 41, 69, and 56 days for patients receiving the lowest, intermediate, and highest doses.[89] In a Danish study, patients were randomized to receive either 30 mg or 90 mg of tamoxifen per day. The interval to treatment response was 2.5 and 3.2 months, respectively, which did not constitute a significant difference.[85] Although the usual dose schedule of 10 mg to 20 mg twice daily may not be the simplest dose schedule compatible with an excellent therapeutic result, there is no reason to expect that any other dose schedule would be superior. The long half-life of this drug means that patients may occasionally omit doses of tamoxifen without lowering circulating tamoxifen levels or compromising response, and this may, in fact, be another reason why the drug has proven to be so effective.

Isolated instances of rebound regression have been observed, but such regression has not been studied as carefully as has rebound regression following estrogen therapy. When estrogens were the treatment of choice, there were fewer acceptable alternatives once estrogens failed. When patients fail with tamoxifen therapy, other treatment options are commonly available and are usually employed. In addition, the long half-life of tamoxifen means that an observation period of 4 to 6 weeks, which is the usual observation period for judging an estrogen withdrawal response, may be too short for a tamoxifen withdrawal response to be manifested.

Tamoxifen Toxicity

Few drugs available for the treatment of any disease have less overall toxicity than tamoxifen. However, there is a long list of side effects that occur infrequently with its use (Table 13-8). The most frequent side effect is mild nausea; vomiting is rarely seen. The nausea will usually disappear after a few weeks of therapy, and it may be alleviated by instructing the patient to take the tamoxifen after meals. Hot flashes occur in a substantial proportion of patients, but these are rarely severe enough to require discontinuation of the drug. Nonspecific central nervous system (CNS) symptoms (headache and dizziness) occasionally occur. Transient thrombocytopenia and, less frequently, leukopenia have been observed during the first weeks of therapy, but these conditions do not dictate cessation of tamoxifen therapy. Since thrombocytopenia and leuko-

Table 13-8
Major Side Effects Associated With Tamoxifen Therapy in Postmenopausal Patients With Metastatic Breast Cancer

Symptom	*Incidence (%)*
Gastrointestinal	
Nausea or vomiting	9.5
Anorexia	< 0.5
Weight gain	1.0
Gynecologic	
Hot flashes	8.4
Vaginal discharge	1.0
Vaginal bleeding	< 1.0
Pruritus vulvae	< 1.0
Dermal	
Rash	1.2
Skin dryness	< 0.5
Alopecia	< 0.5
Neurologic	
Headache	1.4
Dizziness	< 1.0
Light-headedness	< 0.5
Depression	< 0.1
Vascular	
Thrombophlebitis	1.0
Pulmonary emboli	< 0.5
Congestive heart failure	< 0.1
General	
Fatigue	1.8
Malaise	1.0
Edema	1.1
Polydipsia	< 0.5
Flare*	5.9
Hypercalcemia*	4.3
Laboratory Abnomalities	
Thrombocytopenia	4.6
Leukopenia	1.6
Abnormal liver function	< 1.0

* See Table 13-17.
(Mouridsen H, Palshof T, Patterson J, et al: Tamoxifen in advanced breast cancer. Cancer Treat Rev 5:131, 1978; Heel C, Brogden RN, Speight TM, et al: Tamoxifen: A review of its pharmacological properties and therapeutic use in the treatment of breast cancer. Int J Curr Ther Appl Pharmacol Rev 16:1, 1978.)

penia have not had serious consequences, most physicians do not routinely monitor the white blood count or the platelet count. Flare, defined as a transient and diffuse increase in bone pain, an increased size in skin lesions or erythema surrounding skin lesions, or hypercalcemia following initiation of tamoxifen therapy, occurs in 4% to 6% of patients.

Retinopathy has been described in four patients who underwent more than 12 months of therapy at dosages between 60 mg and 100 mg/m^2 twice daily.[92] In these four patients, the cumulative dose of tamoxifen exceeded 108 g. Three of the four patients experienced decreased visual acuity which was thought to be irreversible. Changes in the macula included edema and small cysts, along with small, white, refractile opacities. In all four patients, there were punctate areas of depigmentation on the retina, and three of the four patients had whorl-like, superficial, corneal opacities. Psychophysical testing showed bilateral foveal dysfunction, as measured by cone thresholds and abnormalities in color perception. In a follow-up study based on this report, 19 patients underwent careful ocular examinations 3 to 48 months after the initiation of therapy.[93] All of the patients had received conventional doses of therapy, and no abnormalities were found.

As with estrogen therapy, patients receiving tamoxifen have been found to have a slightly increased incidence of thrombophlebitis and various other clotting abnormalities. This affects between 1% and 3% of patients in various studies.[94] It is possible that these clotting abnormalities are related to a depression of the functional antithrombin III levels. These levels were low in 42% of 24 patients being treated with tamoxifen, but were abnormal in only 1 of 11 patients (9%) with breast cancer who were receiving other forms of anticancer treatment. The immunologic antithrombin III levels were normal in 23 of the patients receiving tamoxifen and were elevated in one of those patients.[95]

One observer found a fourfold increase in the incidence of endometrial cancer among patients receiving tamoxifen therapy.[96] This observation has not yet been confirmed and is not considered to be a contraindication to the use of tamoxifen, particularly when it is employed as palliative therapy in symptomatic patients with metastatic disease. The possible development of endometrial cancer is of greater concern when tamoxifen is used for prolonged periods as an adjuvant therapy in postmenopausal women. In any patient receiving a long-term course of tamoxifen, the possibility of endometrial carcinoma should be considered.

PROGESTINS

Early studies of the use of progestins were generally negative and until recently these hormones were thought to be ineffective for palliating the symptoms of metastatic breast cancer. It was not until the introduction of new synthetic progestins in the late 1960s and early 1970s that results began to change.[97] Medroxyprogesterone acetate has been evaluated in more than 19 separate phase II trials, most of which have been conducted in Europe (Table 13-9).[98–105] Much of the impetus for this research came from the observation in a few early trials that high dosages (more than 500 mg per day) appeared to be more effective than lower dosages. A total of 1175 patients who received a variety of doses of medroxyprogesterone acetate were evaluated. The overall response rate was 33%, with the response rate ranging from 10% to 67%. In these trials, 315 patients received dosages of less than 500 mg per day; the response rate among these patients was only 18%. Among the 860 patients receiving more than 500 mg of medroxyprogesterone per day, the overall response rate was 39%, providing further evidence that the differences

Table 13-9
Response Rates of Unselected Patients to Different Progestins

Progestin	*No. of Patients*	*Response Rate (%)*	*Range (%)*	*Reference No.*
Medroxyprogesterone acetate	1175	33	10–67	98–105
Megestrol acetate	810	29	14–43	106–110
Norethistrone	149	39	25–42	98
Hydroxyprogesterone caproate	40	10		98

Table 13-10
*Randomized Trials Comparing Progestins to Other Hormones in the Treatment of Postmenopausal Women With Metastatic Breast Cancer**

Hormone	*No. of Patients*	*Response Rate (%)*		*Time to Treatment Failure (1) or Median Duration of Response (2) (mo)*		*Reference No.*
		Progestin	*OET*	*Progestin*	*OET*	
MA vs TAM	54	14	26	(1) 2.2	1.9	112
MA vs TAM	110	29	31	(1) 8.1	7.6	110
MA vs TAM	120	31	37	(1) 11.5	13.0	109
MA vs TAM	94	30	35			113
HD MPA vs TAM	41	43	25	(2) 5+	13+	114
HD MPA vs TAM	58	54	47			115
HD MPA vs Mepitiostane	87	40	35	(2) 11.3	9.8	103

* Observed differences are not statistically significant.
Abbreviations used : (MA, megestrol acetate; TAM, tamoxifen; HD MPA, high-dose medroxyprogesterone acetate; OET, other endocrine (nonprogestin) therapy.)

between the results of earlier and more recent trials may be related to the dosage of drug used.

Megestrol acetate has also been evaluated extensively, primarily in the United States. Among a total of 810 patients who were evaluated in phase II trials, the overall response rate was 29%, with a range of 14% to 43%.[106–111] Less widely tested, but effective, progestational agents include norethistrone and hydroxyprogesterone caproate.[98]

Progestins, either megestrol acetate or high-dose medroxyprogesterone acetate, have been demonstrated to be as effective as tamoxifen in randomized trials (Table 13-10). None of the differences in response rate reached levels of statistical significance, and no significant survival advantage was observed for either tamoxifen or progestin therapy. However, in one trial, there was a statistically significant survival advantage for perimenopausal women treated with megestrol acetate after an adjustment for stratification factors.[112] In another trial, patients with visceral disease had a significantly greater response rate (37%) if treated with tamoxifen than if treated with megestrol acetate (0%) ($p = 0.003$).[110] However, this observation was not confirmed by other studies.

One of the earliest randomized trials that evaluated progestins is not shown in Table 13-10. This study involved the randomization of patients to groups receiving either stilbestrol (5 mg, three times a day), methyltestosterone (5 mg, three times a day) and Durabolin (50 mg intramuscularly weekly), or hydroxyprogesterone caproate (250 mg intramuscularly, three times a week). The response rate for those receiving the progestin was only 18%, whereas the response rate for those treated with stilbestrol was 47%. Those who received both methyltestosterone and Durabolin had a response rate of 48%.[116]

Dose Schedule for Progestins

The importance of the dose of medroxyprogesterone acetate has been evaluated in four randomized trials (Table 13-11). There was no significant difference in the response rate, the duration of response, or the survival in three of the four trials. However, in the largest of these studies, 93 patients were randomized to receive 500 mg of medroxyprogesterone twice weekly or 1000 mg of the drug, administered intramuscularly daily. In this study, the response rate to the lower, twice-weekly dosage was only

Table 13-11
Randomized Trials Evaluating Dose-Response to Medroxyprogesterone Acetate

Study	*Doses (mg)*	*No. of Patients*	*Response Rate (%)*	*Duration of Response (Mo)*
Robustelli Della Curran et al.[101]	500 vs.	50	44	8
	1000	51	41	9
Pannuti et al.[117]	500 vs.	46	44	6+
	1500	46	46	6+
Cortes Funes et al.[101]	500 vs.	46	28	
	1000	43	35	
Cavalli et al.[102]	500* vs.	93	14	12.7
	1000	91	33†	11.5

* In all cases, the drug was administered daily, intramuscularly, except in one arm of the Cavalli study in which a low dose was given twice weekly, intramuscularly. Differences are not statistically significant except as indicated.
† p = 0.004

14%, compared to a response rate of 33% in the women receiving the higher daily dose. This large and statistically significant difference did not translate into a survival difference.[102]

Higher doses of medroxyprogesterone acetate are associated with an increased incidence of side effects.[117] In one study that compared daily intramuscular dosages of 1500 mg and 500 mg, gluteal abscess occurred in 15% and 2% of patients, facies lunaris occurred in 11% and 4%, increased sweating was noted in 6% and 2%, fine tremors were observed in 19% and 2%, and leg cramps occurred in 19% and 2% of patients, respectively. The increased incidence of abscesses in patients receiving high doses of intramuscular medroxyprogesterone acetate has also been observed by others.[118]

The use of megestrol acetate has been studied, with dosages ranging from 80 mg q.i.d. to 200 mg q.i.d.[119] Only five patients were treated at each of these dosage levels. Since 3 of 5 patients responded to the lowest dosage, and 4 of 5 patients responded to the highest dosage, it is difficult to draw many conclusions about dose-response to megestrol acetate. No unusual side effects were noted when the highest dose of this drug was administered. The major side effects have been a 10% or greater increase in body weight in 15 of 25 patients, and nausea (in 12 of 25 patients). Peak levels of megestrol acetate are achieved 2 hours after administration of an oral dose, and the half-life of the drug is 4 hours. After a single oral dose of 200 mg of megestrol acetate, plasma levels were detectable for 24 hours. Once-daily dosing at high levels resulted in an accumulation phenomenon.[119]

Both megestrol acetate and norethistrone are administered orally. Medroxyprogesterone acetate may be administered either orally or intramuscularly. Pharmacology studies indicate that there is a marked variation in medroxyprogesterone plasma levels among patients, especially when the drug is given by the oral route.[120,121] The peak dose is higher following oral administration than when it is administered intramuscularly, but accumulation of the drug occurs when it is given by the intramuscular route. Over relatively short periods (less than 168 hours), the plasma concentration × time is essentially the same for the two modes of administration.[120] Peak plasma levels are reached 2 to 7 hours following the initial administration of an oral dose of medroxyprogesterone acetate.[120] With the oral route, a steady state is rapidly achieved, whereas with the intramuscular route, a steady state is achieved only after 6 months of therapy.[121] There are no randomized trials that compare the relative efficacy of the oral and the intramuscular routes, but there is no reason to conclude from the available data that one of these routes is more efficacious than the other.

No controversy surrounds the standard dosage of megestrol acetate, which is 40 mg q.i.d. In light of the increased toxicity and lack of unequivocal benefit from higher doses of medroxyprogesterone acetate, it seems reasonable to limit the dosage of this drug to 400 mg per day. This dose has been shown to be effective in two recent trials.[99,104]

Toxicity of Progestins

Although the list of potential side effects associated with the progestins is long (Table 13-12), most of them occur only rarely. These drugs are tolerated almost as well as is tamoxifen. The most important side effect is weight gain, which occurs in 20% to 50% of patients. This weight gain may be dose-related. In one study of medroxyprogesterone acetate, 50% of the patients receiving the drug experienced a weight gain of between 0 and 10 pounds, 20% had a gain of between 11 and 20 pounds, 15% gained

Table 13-12
Toxicity Associated With the Administration of Progestins to Postmenopausal Women With Metastatic Breast Cancer

Symptom	*Incidence (%)* *		
	Megestrol Acetate	*Medroxyprogesterone Acetate*	
		High Dose	*Low Dose*
Gynecologic			
Vaginal bleeding	5		8
Vaginal discharge	Rare		
Hot flashes	<10		<10
Amenorrhea			37
Endocrinologic			
Cushingoid facies	Rare		12
Fluid retention	5	<10	19
Hypertension	Rare		Occurs
Hypertrichosis		< 5	< 5
Acne		Occurs	Infrequent
Diabetes	Rare		Infrequent
Gastrointestinal			
Weight gain	18		<50
Increased appetite			Frequent
Constipation	Rare	Occurs	<10
Nausea/vomiting	11	Infrequent	< 5
Neurologic			
Tremor			16
Depression	Occurs		
Euphoria	Rare		
Nervousness			Infrequent
Other psychiatric symptoms			Infrequent
Headache	Occurs		Infrequent
Insomnia			Infrequent
Dermal/Musculoskeletal			
Rash	4		
Abcesses			17
Infiltration			9
Pruritus	Occurs		
Muscle cramps			16
Slight alopecia			Infrequent
Vascular			
Thrombophlebitis	0		2
Pulmonary embolus			Infrequent
Congestive heart failure			Infrequent
General			
Mild fatigue			Occurs
Increased sweating			17
Drug fever	Rare		
Hypercalcemia	5	Infrequent	<10
Laboratory Abnormalities			
Mild leukopenia (3000–4000)	Occurs		
Mild thrombocytopenia	Rare		

* "Rare" means that one instance was reported, "infrequent" reflects several reports, and "occurs" means that the incidence was difficult to establish, but may exceed 5% to 10%.
(Based on data from references 98, 103, 104, 109–112, and 122–124,)

between 21 and 30 pounds, and 12% gained more than 30 pounds. However, weight increases of more than 20 pounds occurred only in those patients who received more than 800 mg of medroxyprogesterone per day.[104] This weight increase appears to be related to both a marked increase in appetite and fluid retention, which occurred in 37% of the patients. Nine percent of patients experienced mild fluid retention; in 10%, fluid retention was severe. Vaginal bleeding, either while the patient was receiving progestins or at the time treatment was discontinued, occurred in 5% to 10% of patients. Hot flashes may also occur. Neurologic symptoms occur infrequently, except for the fine tremor that is associated with high doses of medroxyprogesterone acetate.

Although hypercalcemia and flare have not been described as frequently with the use of progestins as with the use of tamoxifen, both of these phenomena may appear following initiation of progestational therapy.[99,109] As with tamoxifen, leukopenia and thrombocytopenia occur infrequently and do not require special monitoring.

AMINOGLUTETHIMIDE

Aminoglutethimide, a derivative of glutethimide (Doriden), was first approved for use as an anticonvulsant 20 years ago. It was later found to suppress corticosteroid synthesis as well. For this reason, it was taken off the market as an anticonvulsant in the 1960s and reintroduced as an anticancer agent in the 1970s.

At first, aminoglutethimide was thought to effect a medical adrenalectomy. The major source of estrogen in the postmenopausal woman is indirectly from the adrenal gland, which produces androstenedione. Androstenedione is then converted, via an aromatase reaction in peripheral tissues, to estrone and estradiol (Fig. 13-5).[125] Aminoglutethimide blocks a number of steroid hydroxylations and cleavage enzymes. It is capable of inhibiting the conversion of cholesterol to Δ-5-pregnenolone, thus blocking all adrenal steroid synthesis. Aminoglutethimide may also inhibit the aromatase reaction that is responsible for conversion of androstenedione to estrone in peripheral tissue.

Blocking the cholesterol side chain cleavage reaction may not be necessary in effecting regression of breast cancer with aminoglutethimide. The aromatase reaction is inhibited with much smaller molar concentrations of aminoglutethimide than is the cholesterol side chain cleavage (Fig. 13-6). This may account for the fact that a patient responding to aminoglutethimide may have a hormone profile of increased androstenedione levels with a concomitant decrease in estrone and estradiol levels (Fig. 13-7). Both estrogen and androstenedione levels are suppressed following surgical adrenalectomy.

Adrenal suppression with aminoglutethimide results in negative feedback to the pituitary gland, increased levels of adrenocorticotropic hormone (ACTH), and further stimulation of the adrenal gland to overcome the block. For these reasons, as well as in an attempt to prevent addisonian symptoms, patients who are treated with aminoglutethimide usually receive glucocorticoid replacement therapy also. Dexamethasone was the glucocorticoid selected to prevent reflex increases in ACTH in the first studies in which aminoglutethimide was used as an anticancer drug. Subsequently, aminoglutethimide was found to accelerate its own metabolism, as well as that of dexamethasone.[126] Aminoglutethimide does not affect the metabolism of hydrocortisone, and this glucocorticoid is now recommended as the steroid replacement therapy of choice. The standard dosage of aminoglutethimide is 250 mg q.i.d., administered with 40 mg of hydrocortisone per day. The hydrocortisone may be given in a divided dose (20 mg b.i.d.), or according to a physiologic schedule of 10 mg in the morning, 10 mg in the late afternoon, and 20 mg before bedtime.

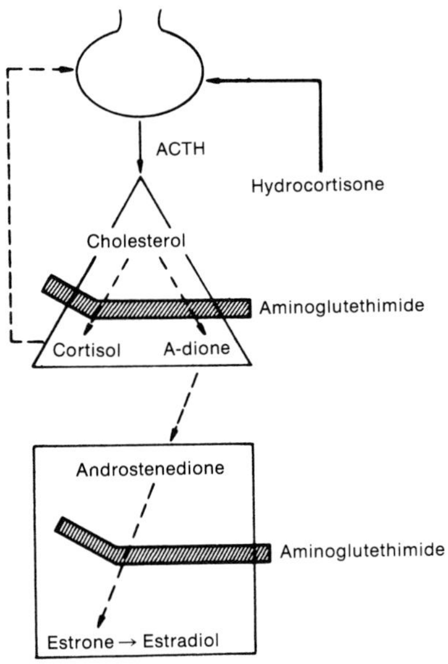

FIGURE 13-5. Sources of estrogen in postmenopausal women and possible sites of aminoglutethimide action. (ACTH, adrenocorticotropic hormone; A-DIONE, androstenedione.) (Santen RJ, Samojlik E, Worgul TJ: Aminoglutethimide. In Santen RJ, Henderson IC (eds): A Comprehensive Guide to the Therapeutic Use of Aminoglutethimide, pp 101–160. Basel, S Karger, 1982.)

Role of Glucocorticoids

Most of the trials evaluating aminoglutethimide have incorporated a glucocorticoid, so it is possible that some of the antitumor effect observed may result from the glucocorticoid itself. Recent trials in which patients have been randomized to receive either tamoxifen or oophorectomy, each with or without prednisolone, have shown a significantly higher response rate when prednisolone was added.[127] There were also a large number of earlier trials in which cortisone, prednisone, dexamethasone, hydrocortisone, or fluorometholone were used as single agents. Only two of these trials were conducted during the past 2

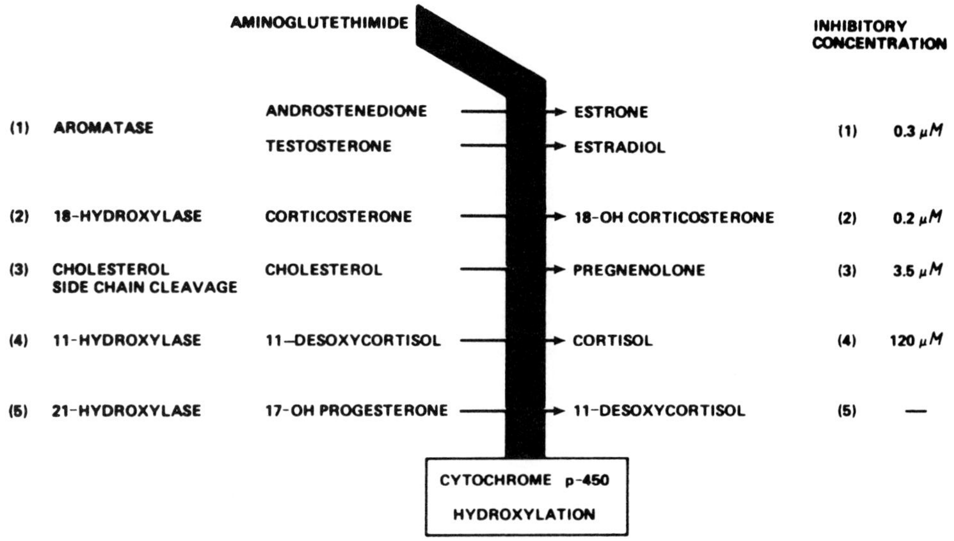

FIGURE 13-6. Enzymatic reactions blocked by aminoglutethimide and inhibitory concentrations of aminoglutethimide necessary to block each reaction. (Santen RJ, Samojlik E, Worgul TJ: Aminoglutethimide. In Santen RJ, Henderson IC (eds): A Comprehensive Guide to the Therapeutic Use of Aminoglutethimide, pp 101–160. Basel, S Karger, 1982.)

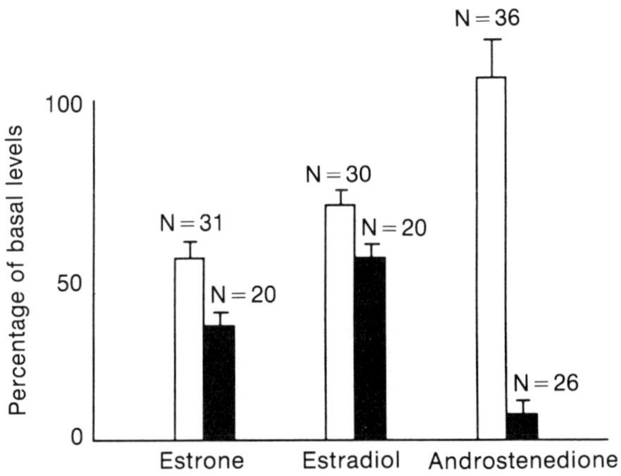

FIGURE 13-7. Hormonal levels following treatment with aminoglutethimide (□) or adrenalectomy (■), expressed as a percentage of pretreatment (basal) levels, ± the standard error of mean. The figure above the bars represents the number of patients studied ($p < 0.01$). (Santen RJ, Worgul TJ: A randomized trial comparing surgical adrenalectomy with aminoglutethimide plus hydrocortisone in women with advanced breast cancer. N Engl J Med 305:545, 1981. Reprinted by permission of the New England Journal of Medicine.)

decades. The overall response rate to glucocorticoid alone was 25% in these trials, and the response rates ranged from 0% in several of the trials to 62% in one trial involving 29 patients.[4]

Aminoglutethimide is also effective without glucocorticoid. (This is discussed in greater detail below.) There are no randomized comparisons of glucocorticoid alone, aminoglutethimide alone, or a combination of both agents, but the combination seems to be the most effective and least toxic method of administering these agents.

Effectiveness of Aminoglutethimide and Hydrocortisone

Aminoglutethimide is as effective as any other form of endocrine therapy in postmenopausal women (see Table 13-2).[4] The response rate to this drug in 19 phase II trials was 31%, with response rates ranging from 16% to 43%. However, aminoglutethimide is ineffective in premenopausal women. There is no evidence that estrogen production is blocked in the ovary, and no responses were seen in 18 premenopausal women treated with aminoglutethimide.[126]

Aminoglutethimide has been compared to major ablative surgery and to tamoxifen in randomized trials (Table 13-13). None of the differences in response rate or duration of response are statistically significant. Analysis of the randomized trials comparing aminoglutethimide with hypophysectomy[128] and with adrenalectomy[129] was confounded by imbalances resulting from patients being too sick to undergo adrenalectomy[129] or patients who refused surgery.[128,129] This fact indicates that surgical ablation is the more toxic of the two modalities. Since it is unlikely that larger trials or better compliance on the part of patients would demonstrate a greater effectiveness for surgical ablation than for aminoglutethimide, the latter has emerged as the preferred treatment.

Aminoglutethimide and tamoxifen are equally effective in most patients. However, two independent investigators have observed that aminoglutethimide is more likely than tamoxifen to induce a response in sites of bone metastases. In one study, 9 of 27 patients (33%) with bone metastases responded to aminoglutethimide, whereas only 4 of 27 patients (15%) had an objective response to tamoxifen ($p = 0.10$).[130] In the other study, 11 of 31 patients (35%) with bone lesions responded to aminoglutethimide, whereas only 5 of 29 patients (17%) responded to tamoxifen.[131] There were no differences in the survival of pa-

Table 13-13
Randomized Trials Comparing the Efficacy of Aminoglutethimide to That of Other Forms of Endocrine Therapy

Treatment Regimen	No. of Patients	Response Rate (%) AG	OET	Median Duration of Response (mo) AG	OET	Reference No.
Hypophysectomy	35	48	21	11.5	4.6	128
Adrenalectomy	69	53	45	17.2	17.1	129
Tamoxifen	75	36	38	10+	9+	130
Tamoxifen	117	30	30	16	20	131
Tamoxifen	220	41	30			132

(AG, aminoglutethimide; OET, other endocrine therapy.)

tients treated with aminoglutethimide or tamoxifen in any of these randomized trials.[130–132]

Dose Schedule for Aminoglutethimide

Since it is possible that the most important mechanism of action for aminoglutethimide is the inhibition of the sensitive aromatase that is responsible for conversion of androstenedione to estrone in peripheral tissues, it is reasonable to ask whether very low doses of aminoglutethimide may be as effective as higher doses of the drug. Two studies have revealed that aminoglutethimide, administered in a dosage of 250 to 500 mg per day with hydrocortisone, will suppress circulating estrogens to the same level as will full doses.[133–135] In one of these studies, patients were initially treated with 62.5 mg of aminoglutethimide twice daily, and the dose was then doubled every month thereafter.[135] Hydrocortisone was not administered. Maximal estrogen suppression was achieved only with dosages of greater than 250 mg per day.

In a phase II trial utilizing 250 mg of aminoglutethimide per day without cortisone, 7 of 30 patients (23%) responded. Only 1 of 7 patients who failed to respond to these low doses subsequently responded to conventional doses. However, the toxicity of aminoglutethimide was not markedly reduced with administration of the lower dose. Thirty-one percent of the patients treated with the low doses experienced lethargy; 12% had nausea. However, 54% experienced no side effects at all.[135]

Other investigators have not found low doses of aminoglutethimide without hydrocortisone to be either as effective or as safe as higher doses of the drug.[136] In one study, 11 of 57 patients (19%) responded to 125 mg of aminoglutethimide administered twice daily; 4 of 17 patients who failed to respond to the low dose subsequently responded at full doses. In this study, three patients died unexpectedly, one of whom had hypotension and a clinical picture that was compatible with an addisonian crisis. A fourth patient had documented low levels of cortisone and hyponatremia while receiving the low dose, but she was asymptomatic. Side effects were only minimally reduced at this dose. Sixteen percent of the patients developed a rash, and one had severe exfoliative dermatitis.

Full doses of aminoglutethimide without glucocorticoid replacement were administered safely to a group of eight patients. One gram of aminoglutethimide per day suppressed plasma estrogens to very low levels without markedly affecting plasma cortisol levels. Plasma levels of testosterone, androstenedione, and 17-hydroxyprogesterone were increased,[137] which probably explains why addisonian crises and other signs of adrenal insufficiency are so rare in patients receiving aminoglutethimide at any dose.

At present, the use of low dosages of aminoglutethimide (less than 500 mg per day) and of aminoglutethimide without hydrocortisone should be restricted to centers that are conducting studies of this drug.

Toxicity of Aminoglutethimide

Aminoglutethimide is a more toxic agent than either tamoxifen or the progestins, but it is generally better tolerated than estrogens or androgens (Table 13-14). As might be expected in a drug that is closely related to Doriden, the major side effects are neurologic. In most reported series, one-third or more of the patients being treated experienced lethargy, but this side effect may be partially circumvented by initiating treatment with 250 mg of aminoglutethimide twice daily together with full replacement doses of hydrocortisone. Full doses of aminoglutethimide may be started after the first month of therapy, and the patient is unlikely to experience toxicity of any kind thereafter. As a result of this treatment approach, patients may experience symptoms of excess glucocorticoid, such as euphoria and insomnia, rather than lethargy. In many patients, the initial treatment with excess glucocorticoid replacement will also result in a dramatic remission of many of the secondary symptoms of metastatic breast cancer. Aminoglutethimide frequently causes a macular-papular, erythemic rash during the first month of ther-

Table 13-14
Side Effects Associated With Administration of Aminoglutethimide to Postmenopausal Women With Metastatic Breast Cancer

Symptoms/Signs	*Incidence (%)*
Neurologic	
Lethargy	36
Dizziness	16
Ataxia	9
Depression	1
Insomnia	< 1
Hallucinations	Rare
Confusion	Rare
Visual disturbances	Rare
Headache	Rare
Endocrinologic	
Cushingoid symptoms	2.8
Hypotension	< 1
Hot flashes	< 1
Hypertension	< 1
Edema	< 1
Inappropriate ADH secretion	Rare
Gastrointestinal	
Nausea/vomiting	14
Weight gain or loss	< 1
Anorexia	Rare
Diarrhea	Rare
Dermal	
Rash	22
Stevens-Johnson syndrome	Rare
General	
Fever	1
Increased sweating	< 1
Leg cramps	1
Weakness	Rare
Laboratory Abnormalities	
All hematologic abnormalities	0.9
Thrombocytopenia	0.8
Leukopenia	0.3
Electrolyte imbalance	Rare
Elevated levels of TSH	Rare

(ADH, antidiuretic hormone; TSH, thyroid-stimulating hormone)
(Messeih AA, Lipton A, Santen RJ, et al: Aminoglutethimide and induced hematologic toxicity: Worldwide experience. Cancer Treat Rep 69:1003, 1985; Stuart-Harris RC, Smith IE: Aminoglutethimide in the treatment of advanced breast cancer. Cancer Treat Rep 11:189, 1984.)

apy. This is usually pruritic and appears about 7 to 10 days after initiation of therapy. Aminoglutethimide should not be discontinued; the pruritus may easily be alleviated by doubling the dose of hydrocortisone for a period of a few days to a week or more. Cushingoid symptoms, which occur rarely with the long-term administration of aminoglutethimide and hydrocortisone, can usually be controlled by slight adjustments in the daily dose of hydrocortisone.

The side effects of aminoglutethimide are usually transient. In one trial, almost 50% of the patients experienced lethargy, and one-third of them developed a rash during the first 6 weeks (Table 13-15).[129] After the first 6 weeks of therapy, only 10% of the patients experienced lethargy, 12% experienced orthostatic dizziness, and none of the patients had a rash. The CNS symptoms associated with aminoglutethimide may occur more frequently in the elderly, so this drug should be used cautiously in this group of patients.

Pancytopenia occurs rarely with aminoglutethimide therapy, but has resulted in a fatal bout of sepsis on a few occasions.[138–142] A retrospective review of the worldwide literature on aminoglutethimide indicates that the incidence of leukopenia or thrombocytopenia is no more than 1.6%.[138] Recently, investigators who use this drug frequently collaborated in a retrospective analysis of their individual cases. They found only 12 of 133 patients (0.9%) had had evidence of hematologic abnormalities.[143] The most frequently observed abnormalities were thrombocytopenia (0.8% of patients) and leukopenia (0.3% of patients). All instances of leukopenia and thrombocytopenia were observed between the second and seventh weeks of therapy. For this reason, it seems prudent to monitor the patient's white blood count and platelet count during the first few months of therapy. These blood tests may be obtained as a baseline and at weeks 4, 8, and 12.[143] The precise mechanisms underlying the leukopenia and thrombocytopenia are not known. Bone marrow biopsies obtained in patients with leukopenia have been normal, suggesting that this side effect occurs primarily as a result of peripheral destruction of the white cells and platelets.

OTHER FORMS OF "MEDICAL ADRENALECTOMY"

Several other aromatase inhibitors have undergone limited clinical evaluation. None has yet shown greater prom-

Table 13-15
Acute and Chronic Side Effects Associated With Aminoglutethimide

	Incidence (%)	
Side Effect	*Within First 6 Weeks*	*After 6 Weeks*
Lethargy	48	10
Rash	33	0
Orthostatic dizziness	20	12
Ataxia	10	2.5
Drug fever	2.5	0
Blood pressure > 140/90	5	2.5

(Santen RJ, Worgul TJ, Samojlik E, et al: A randomized trial comparing surgical adrenalectomy with aminoglutethimide plus hydrocortisone in women with advanced breast cancer. N Engl J Med 305:545, 1981. Reprinted by permission of the New England Journal of Medicine.)

ise than aminoglutethimide. Hydroxyandrostenedione induced regression of metastatic breast cancer in 4 of 11 postmenopausal patients.[144] Almost no toxicity was observed. Unfortunately, the drug must be administered parenterally. In this study, it was given as an intramuscular injection weekly. Trilostane is not an aromatase inhibitor, but it inhibits the 3β-hydroxysteroid dehydrogenase system. As a result, trilostane inhibits the conversion of pregnenolone to progesterone, of 17α-hydroxypregnenolone to 17α-hydroxyprogesterone, and dehydroepiandrosterone (DHEA) to androstenedione. This form of medical adrenalectomy has been evaluated more extensively, but with limited success. In one study, only 1 of 6 patients responded.[145] In another study, 10 of 31 patients (32%) responded, but therapy had to be discontinued in 18% of the patients because of toxicity.[146] In the largest study, 10 of 56 patients (18%) responded.[147]

INHIBITORS OF PITUITARY FUNCTION

There are a number of reasons to anticipate that a drug that affects pituitary function might also affect the growth of breast cancer. The effectiveness of hypophysectomy in the palliative treatment of metastatic breast cancer is well established. In the DMBA rat model, either an increase or decrease in prolactin levels may inhibit the induction of mammary tumors. Once the tumors are established, increases in serum prolactin will enhance tumor growth.[148] However, the role of prolactin in either the induction or promotion of human breast cancer remains tentative, at best.[148–151] In fact, it has been shown that human breast cancer regression following hypophysectomy may actually be associated with increased prolactin levels![152]

Several recent reports have suggested that elevated serum prolactin levels may signify a tumor with a poor prognosis and may predict a low probability of response to either endocrine therapy or chemotherapy.[151,153] Serum prolactin levels were measured in 135 postmenopausal women treated with either tamoxifen alone, tamoxifen plus aminoglutethimide, or tamoxifen combined with both aminoglutethimide and danazol.[151] The mean pretreatment prolactin levels were significantly higher among those 53 patients who responded or had stable disease after treatment with one of these three endocrine agents than among the 82 patients who had progressive disease while receiving therapy ($p = 0.02$). The survival rate of the 15 patients who failed to respond and who had prolactin levels which were greater than 500 mIU/liter was significantly worse than the survival rate of the 66 nonresponders with prolactin levels of less than 500 mIU/liter ($p = 0.006$).

Levodopa is known to suppress prolactin levels, and this drug will relieve bone pain in some patients with metastatic breast cancer. These observations led to the use of a levodopa response as a selection criteria for patients who might benefit from endocrine ablation. Levodopa was administered in divided doses for 4 days. Patients who experienced marked relief of pain were considered to be good candidates for major endocrine ablation.[154] These patients were more likely to have a cytoplasmic estrogen receptor as well.[155]

There have been scattered reports of responses to antiprolactin drugs. In one study, patients were treated with tamoxifen in combination with either levodopa, carbidopa, or bromocriptine. The response rates to these tamoxifen/antiprolactin combinations in patients who had previously been shown to be refractory to tamoxifen varied between 23% and 42%.[156]

Danazol is a synthetic steroid with multiple potential sites of action. Its primary effect is to inhibit pituitary function, but it has also been described as antiestrogenic without being estrogenic and antiprogestational without being progestational. It has some androgenic effects.[157] Danazol binds to androgen and progesterone receptors, as well as to sex hormone-binding globulin and corticosteroid-binding globulin.[158] It has been used to treat endometriosis, and in double-blind, randomized trials, it has been shown to relieve the pain and tenderness of cyclic mastopathy.[159] Danazol, 100 mg to 200 mg three times per day, was administered to 37 postmenopausal and 4 premenopausal patients with metastatic breast cancer.[160] There were seven responses (17%), all among the postmenopausal women. The side effects were described as mild and included lethargy, mild peripheral edema, and hot flashes. Two patients required diuretics for treatment of fluid retention. Danazol has also been used in combination with tamoxifen and aminoglutethimide. The overall response rates to the three-hormone combination was better than the response to tamoxifen alone ($p = 0.05$), but there was no improvement in either the duration of response or survival.[161]

Recent research has focused on the use of luteinizing hormone-releasing hormone (LHRH) analogues, including leuprolide and buserelin. Buserelin was first given intravenously and intranasally to four premenopausal women; two of the four experienced a dramatic improvement.[162] There were no significant side effects. The effects on endocrine function were variable, but plasma gonadotropin levels eventually fell below pretreatment values in all patients. Within 7 weeks, all patients had postmenopausal estradiol concentrations and experienced hot flashes. However, these low estradiol levels were transient in two of the patients. Buserelin was given in combination with tamoxifen to five premenopausal patients.[163] Two of the five responded. As with buserelin alone, there were variable effects on endocrine function. In one patient, there was evidence of ovarian stimulation; multiple follicles and a ruptured follicle were found at oophorectomy following treatment with tamoxifen plus buserelin. However, there was no evidence that tumor growth had been stimulated. Leuprolide was administered to 31 postmenopausal women who had been heavily pretreated with endocrine therapy and other treatments.[164] Twelve of these patients responded (39%). No side effects were noted. Subsequently, leuprolide was administered to 25 premenopausal women, and 11 responded (44%).[165] The median duration of response was 39 weeks. Toxicity was mild and included hot flashes, nausea, and headache. Amenorrhea appeared in all premenopausal patients who stayed on the study for more than 10 weeks. Plasma estrone and estradiol levels fell to postmenopausal levels, but serum follicle stimulating hormone (FSH) and luteinizing hormone (LH) were also suppressed.

THYROID HORMONE

Subclinical hypothyroidism has frequently been noted in patients with advanced breast cancer, and this observation provided the rationale for using triiodothyronine, either alone or in combination with other hormonal therapy or chemotherapy.[166,167] Triiodothyronine was shown in a controlled trial to have no therapeutic effect when used alone.[167] Thyroid substance plus oophorectomy was no more effective than oophorectomy alone,[168] but triiodothyronine plus hydrocortisone was more effective than hydrocortisone alone in postmenopausal women.[166] Triiodothyronine has also been used in combination with cytotoxic chemotherapy, but its contribution, if any, to the effectiveness of the combination has not been assessed.[169] There is currently no role for thyroid hormones in the treatment of breast cancer.

COMBINATION ENDOCRINE THERAPY

There are several potential advantages to combining two or even three endocrine therapies. First, the effect of one endocrine agent, such as tamoxifen, which appears to work via the estrogen receptor, might be potentiated by another agent, such aminoglutethimide, which lowers the levels of circulating estrogens that compete for binding sites on the receptor. A therapy that stimulates the synthesis of new hormone receptors might also prove to be synergistic with an agent that requires the presence of the estrogen receptor to be effective. Different endocrine treatments may affect tumor growth through different mechanisms, and an agent that decreases estrogen might affect the cancer cell quite differently from a progestin. The use of combinations of endocrine therapy might permit further elucidation of the mystery surrounding sequential responses to additive and ablative hormone therapies, and this sequential effect might be manipulated to achieve a more durable and more complete remission.[170,171]

It is equally possible that combinations of hormones will have an antagonistic interaction. For example, aminoglutethimide may decrease circulating levels of medroxyprogesterone acetate when these two hormones are administered together.[172] Combinations of aminoglutethimide and danazol result in the same level of estrogen suppression as achieved with aminoglutethimide alone. However, sex hormone-binding globulin is also decreased as a result of danazol administration, and there is a net increase in circulating free estrogen.[173]

Huggins and colleagues were the first to use several hormones together, combining estrogens and progestins.[174] This combination has also been used recently.[175] Ethinyl estradiol and medroxyprogesterone were administered to 19 previously treated patients, 31% of whom responded. This recent experiment differed from Huggins' original experiments in that the estrogens and medroxyprogesterone were given alternately, with ethinyl estradiol being administered on days 1 and 2 and medroxyprogesterone acetate (600 mg per day) being administered on days 3 through 9.

Combination endocrine therapy has been evaluated in numerous randomized clinical trials (Table 13-16). In some trials, the combination therapy resulted in a higher response rate, but with the exception of the trial in which postmenopausal women were randomized to tamoxifen versus tamoxifen plus prednisolone,[176] there was no survival advantage or even response duration advantage for the combination regimen. One of the earliest of these trials evaluated a combination of DES and testosterone.[177] The combination did not appear to be better than DES alone, but it was significantly better than testosterone alone. Diethylstilbestrol was shown, in this trial as in previous trials, to be superior to the androgen in its ability to induce tumor regression. Tamoxifen has also been used in combination with an androgen, fluoxymesterone, and this combination appeared to induce a significantly higher response rate.[89] The response rate to tamoxifen in this trial was unusually low, which might explain the lack of a survival advantage for the combination regimen. The addition of fluoxymesterone increased the toxicity of the drug regimen, especially the incidence of masculinization, which occurred in 39% of the patients receiving combination therapy and in none of the patients receiving tamoxifen alone.

Tamoxifen was combined with DES in one trial,[178] with aminoglutethimide in two trials,[179,180] and with medroxyprogesterone acetate in one trial.[181] In each of these trials, the increased toxicity from the combination regimen outweighed any advantage that might have been gained. Side effects were observed in 28 of 57 patients treated with both tamoxifen and DES, compared to only 8 of 65 patients treated with tamoxifen alone.[178] Only 1 of 45 patients treated with tamoxifen alone discontinued therapy, whereas 10 of 51 patients discontinued treatment because of toxicity from a combination of tamoxifen and aminoglutethimide.[180]

The one endocrine therapy combination that may be superior to a single hormone is prednisolone plus tamoxifen in postmenopausal women. In a large trial, the response rate with this combination was 36%; with tamoxifen alone, the response rate was only 13% ($p > 0.01$). The unusually low response rate to tamoxifen led the authors of the study to repeat the trial.[127] Preliminary results from the second trial confirmed the significant difference in response rates observed in the first trial. In the second trial, premenopausal women were randomized to oophorectomy or oophorectomy plus prednisolone; postmenopausal women were randomized to receive either tamoxifen alone or tamoxifen plus prednisolone. The response

Table 13-16
Randomized Clinical Trials Evaluating the Efficacy of Combination (Two or More) Endocrine Therapy

Therapy	*No. of Patients*	*Response Rate (%)*	*p*	*Response of Duration (mo)*	*p*	*Survival (mo)*	*p*	*Reference No.*
DES vs	22	46	0.05	8.5+		11+		
Testosterone vs	22	14	0.09	10 +	NS	11+	NS	177
DES + Testosterone	12	41		10 +		12+		
TAM vs	52	15	0.0025	7.6	NS	11.0	0.17	89
TAM + Fluoxymesterone	56	38		7.1		12.7		
TAM vs	65	39	> 0.7	11+				178
TAM + DES	57	37		9+				
TAM vs	9	33	NS				NS	179
TAM + AG	11	36						
TAM vs	49	43	0.54			21.9	0.29	180
TAM + AG	51	49				22.6		
TAM vs	45	44	>0.2	10	NS			181
TAM + MPA	55	25		9				
TAM vs	99	31	0.05	22.8	>0.1		NS	161
TAM + AG + danazol	99	43		18.3				
OOPHOR-X vs	19	21	NS		NS	19	NS	176
OOPHOR-X + PRED	16	44				18		
TAM vs	72	13	<0.01		NS	12	<0.025	176
TAM + PRED	73	36				21		
OOPHOR-X or TAM vs	97	36	<0.05					127
OOPHOR-X or TAM + PRED		54						

(DES, diethylstilbestrol; TAM, tamoxifen; AG, aminoglutethimide; MPA, medroxyprogesterone acetate; OOPHOR-X, radiation ovarian ablation; PRED, prednisolone.)

rate to tamoxifen alone among premenopausal and postmenopausal patients was 36%. The response rate to the combination therapy was 54% ($p < 0.05$).[127]

Sequential administration of tamoxifen and medroxyprogesterone is more effective than either agent alone in causing regression of DMBA rat mammary tumors.[182] Sequential use of these two drugs is now being evaluated in the clinic, as well.[183] Tamoxifen is administered for the first 15 days of therapy, and medroxyprogesterone is administered for the next 15 days. The response rate among patients randomized to receive tamoxifen alone is 48%; among those treated with the alternating regimens, the response rate is 60%. The mean duration of response for those receiving tamoxifen alone is 9.5 months, whereas the response duration in those receiving the alternating regimen is 25 months. There are no survival differences.

Combination endocrine therapy cannot be recommended outside of a clinical trial. Although the response rates may be higher, there is no survival advantage associated with combination regimens. This may be because patients responding to a single endocrine agent subsequently respond to other endocrine agents that are administered in sequence. Patients who are treated with combination hormonal therapy may lose their ability to respond to sequential therapy. The added toxicity observed in some of these trials also outweighs any marginal gain.

FLARE FOLLOWING ENDOCRINE THERAPY

Flare is a poorly defined phenomenon that has been described in many endocrine trials over the last 35 years. The most frequent manifestation of flare is an abrupt, diffuse onset of musculoskeletal pain, beginning hours to as long as several weeks after the initiation of endocrine therapy. Multiple other manifestations of flare have been described, including erythema around skin lesions, increased size of skin lesions which eventually regress,[184] transient changes in liver function studies, transient increases in the intensity of bone scan lesions, fever, and transient elevations in CEA concentrations.[185] The most serious manifestation of flare is hypercalcemia, which commonly occurs spontaneously in patients with breast cancer that is metastatic to bone. The precise relationship between the endocrine therapy and the hypercalcemia is sometimes difficult to document. Occasionally, patients have been challenged repeatedly with the same endocrine therapy and have had repeated elevations of serum calcium within hours to a week or more following initiation of the endocrine therapy.

By definition, flare occurs within the first month of therapy. It has frequently been thought to represent an exacerbation of the patient's disease,[186] and has sometimes been described as a good prognostic sign—or at least, a sign of a hormone-sensitive tumor. However, there is little evidence that tumor growth rates actually increase during a flare. A single case report in which the tumor-doubling time of pulmonary lesions was documented before, during, and after tamoxifen therapy provides a rare clinical documentation of tumor exacerbation.[187] In this instance, the tumor-doubling time was 140 days prior to treatment and 52 days following treatment; the tumor regressed for more than 6 months following discontinuation of the tamoxifen treatment. In other case reports, the presumed exacerbation could have been explained by a continual growth of the tumor lesion(s) without a change in growth rate. Alternatively, the flare phenomenon may reflect normal tissue response as the first sign of tumor regression. The evidence that flare is a reflection of tumor stimulation is not well substantiated.[188]

Flare has been observed with every known endocrine therapy, including the major ablative treatments.[189] Androgens, estrogens, and tamoxifen have most frequently been associated with flare. In recent randomized trials that included tamoxifen studies, the incidence of flare in the tamoxifen treated patients was the same as that in patients treated with estrogens and progestins but was higher than that in patients treated with aminoglutethimide or a combination of hormones (Table 13-17). The lack of flare, manifested either by hypercalcemia or bone pain, was particularly noticeable in the randomized trial that compared tamoxifen therapy alone with a combined regimen of tamoxifen plus prednisolone.[176]

It was once claimed that flare occurred primarily in endocrine-sensitive tumors, and that it was a valuable predictive factor for subsequent response to endocrine therapy.[190] This claim has not been substantiated by most other observers. The probability of a response following a flare reaction is at least as great as that observed in patients without flare, and it is reasonable to continue tamoxifen or other endocrine therapy despite these symptoms as long as the symptoms are not life-threatening. In patients with hypercalcemia, tamoxifen therapy may be continued as long as the serum calcium level is less than 14 mg/dl. However, the patient should be carefully monitored and given adequate fluids, diuretics, and other treatment to control the calcium levels until the patient begins to experience tumor regression.[191]

SELECTION OF PATIENTS FOR ENDOCRINE THERAPY

Long before the discovery of the estrogen receptor protein, clinicians who were experienced in the treatment of metastatic breast cancer were able to identify, on the basis of clinical characteristics, those patients who were most likely to benefit from endocrine therapy. These clinical factors include a long interval between diagnosis and the first evidence of recurrence, a late premenopausal or late postmenopausal status, and disease that is limited to sites

Table 13-17
Incidence of Flare in Randomized Trials Evaluating Two Hormones or Combination Hormonal Therapy

Mode of Therapy	*No. of Patients*	*Incidence of Flare (%)* Hypercalcemia TAM	Hypercalcemia OET	Bone Pain/Skin Lesions* TAM	Bone Pain/Skin Lesions* OET	*Reference No.*
Tamoxifen vs						
DES	141	3	0	3	4	48
Stilbestrol	111	5	7			67
Ethinyl Estradiol	59	7	3	13	7	68
Ethinyl Estradiol	71	3	0			71
Aminoglutethimide	91	4	0			130
Megestrol Acetate	131	6	9			109
Fluoxymesterone	79	5	0			53
Tamoxifen + DES	122			3	0	178
Tamoxifen + Fluoxymesterone	39	0	0	17	14	184
Tamoxifen + Prednisolone	145	7	0	6	0	176

* The patient experienced a transient increase in bone pain, increased growth of measurable skin lesions, or developed erythema with or without other changes around the skin lesions.
(TAM, tamoxifen; OET, other endocrine therapy; DES, diethylstilbestrol.)

Table 13-18
Clinical Characteristics of the Ideal Candidate for Endocrine Therapy

Clinical Characteristic	*Mode of Therapy*	*No. of Patients*	*Response Rate (%)*	*Reference No.*
Long disease-free interval				
Zero	Adrenalectomy	366	38	3
< 2 Yr		953	30	
> 2 Yr		1030	42	
> 5 Yr		237	56	
Age in premenopausal women				
< 35 Yr	Oophorectomy	117	20	25, 26
> 35 Yr		849	33	193
Years postmenopausal in postmenopausal women				
< 5 Yr after LMP	Tamoxifen	157	23	2, 113
> 5 Yr after LMP		275	33	
< 5 Yr after LMP	Megestrol acetate	124	15	108, 113
> 5 Yr after LMP		240	37	122
Disease limited to sites other than the liver				
Liver metastasis	Various	30	23	194
Lung metastasis		73	41	
Nonvisceral metastasis		253	34	

(LMP, last menstrual period.)

outside of the viscera, especially outside of the liver. Moreover, patients who previously responded to an endocrine therapy are more likely to respond again.

The response rates relative to these clinical characteristics are shown for a number of different endocrine therapies in Table 13-18. A disease-free interval of longer than 2 years has arbitrarily been accepted as "long," but the longer the interval, the more likely the patient is to respond to any form of endocrine therapy. The example presented here is from a large retrospective analysis of patients treated with adrenalectomy.[3] Disease-free interval probably reflects the intrinsic pace and biology of the cancer, since patients who have a long disease-free interval usually have a long interval from the diagnosis of metastases to death.[192] This premise is consistent with the general principle that those patients who are most likely to respond to endocrine therapy are those with the most indolent disease. However, patients with a zero disease-free interval—that is, patients who present with metastatic disease at the time of their initial diagnosis—have a higher probability of responding to endocrine therapy than do patients who have metastatic disease several months to a year or so after the initial diagnosis. Presumably, this is because patients who present with metastases at diagnosis represent a mixture of those individuals with very aggressive disease who have sought immediate attention for their breast cancer and those with indolent disease that the patient was able to ignore for long periods of time.

The response rate to oophorectomy among younger premenopausal women, (those younger than 35 years of age) has been consistently lower than the response rate to oophorectomy in older premenopausal women. Whether this will be an important factor in predicting the response of premenopausal women to tamoxifen therapy is not yet clear. There are a few reports of responses to tamoxifen among women younger than 35 years of age,[79,83] but the total number of patients treated is still too small to draw firm conclusions.

Women in the perimenopausal years have the lowest responses of all to every form of endocrine therapy, including both additive and ablative therapy. The overall response rate to tamoxifen in women whose last menstrual period was less than 5 years ago is 23%, compared to a response rate of 33% in women who are more than 5 years into menopause. A similar difference in response rate relative to postmenopausal status is seen with megestrol acetate (see Table 13-18). The response rate to oophorectomy in patients who are more than a year beyond their last menstrual period has been reported to be as low as 6%,[27] and the preponderance of data suggests that estrogens, androgens, aminoglutethimide, and adrenalectomy are all relatively less effective during this period of time than they are 5 years or more after the last menstrual period. In most reports, the response rate continues to increase as the patient ages, and the highest response rates are seen in women who are in their 60s and 70s, and who are 10 to 15 years or more into menopause.

Visceral involvement with metastatic breast cancer is not an absolute contraindication to the use of endocrine therapy, and there are well-documented cases of partial and complete responses of liver metastases following treatment with every known form of endocrine therapy. However, in large series of patients, the response rate to hormones or ablation is usually decreased when the liver is involved, especially when there is extensive replacement of the liver. It has not been well documented that the interval to response following the initiation of endocrine therapy is any longer than the interval to response to chemotherapy. However, if this widely held impression is correct, it may be that patients with short life expectancies, such as those in whom the liver has been replaced extensively by tumor, may not have adequate life expectancy to experience any benefit from endocrine therapy.

The median duration of response to single endocrine therapy is between 1 and 2 years. This, too, is independent of the type of endocrine therapy used. However, the total duration of response to a series of endocrine agents is much longer, and one of the most important principles regarding the use of this modality is that patients who respond to one endocrine therapy and experience subsequent relapse have a greater-than-average probability of responding to another type of endocrine therapy. In most cases, the duration of the second response will be shorter.[195] Many patients respond a third time, and a small number will respond up to 5 times in sequence. In one institution, 69 of 242 patients with metastatic breast cancer were treated with more than one form of endocrine therapy. The successive response rates in these 69 patients were 45/69 (65%) to the first endocrine therapy, 30/69 (43%) to the second treatment regimen, 9/30 (30%) to the third regimen, 1/6 (16%) to the fourth regimen, and 0/1 (0%) to the fifth treatment regimen.[196]

The predictive value of a response to one endocrine treatment regimen for a subsequent response to a second regimen appears to be independent of the type of endocrine therapy used (Table 13-19). The lack of an initial response does not clearly rule out a subsequent response, but with rare exceptions, the probability of a response is two to three times greater if the patient has had a previous response. For example, the response rate to oophorectomy among premenopausal women who have previously failed to respond to tamoxifen is only 15%. In contrast, the response rate is 40% among those patients who have responded initially and then progressed. The response to aminoglutethimide after treatment with tamoxifen shows an even greater differential: only 22% of the nonresponders to tamoxifen but 63% of the responders to tamoxifen subsequently responded to aminoglutethimide therapy.

The development of the estrogen receptor protein has simplified the process of selecting appropriate patients for endocrine therapy. More precisely, the estrogen receptor protein helps to exclude patients who are not likely to benefit from endocrine therapy (Table 13-20). The receptor is predictive of response, regardless of the type of endocrine therapy used. The probability of responding to endocrine therapy in unselected patients is about one in three (33%). The response rate in estrogen receptor-positive patients is doubled, and is usually in the range of 50% to 60%. For those patients who are estrogen receptor protein (ERP)-negative, the response rate is consistently less than 10%. Data on the correlation between estrogen receptor positivity and treatment with progestins, shown in Table 13-20, must be interpreted cautiously. Since widespread use of progestins began at about the time it was recognized that estrogen receptor-negative patients were unlikely to benefit from endocrine therapy, the number of

Table 13-19
Predictive Value of a Response to Endocrine Therapy for Subsequent Response(s) to Further Endocrine Therapy

Therapy Sequence		*No. of Patients* R	*No. of Patients* NR	*Response Rate (%)* *After* R	*Response Rate (%)* *Prior* NR	*Therapy Sequence*		*No. of Patients* R	*No. of Patients* NR	*Response Rate (%)* *After* R	*Response Rate (%)* *Prior* NR	*Reference No.*
Various	→ tamoxifen	46	34	67	15							2
Various	→ progestins	81	70	38	10							102, 104
Various	→ AG	61	205	54	25							126
Tamoxifen	→ oophorectomy	47	62	40	15	Oophorectomy	→ tamoxifen	6	12	17	8	74, 76, 78, 79, 197
						Oophorectomy	→ AG	13	23	69	35	126
Tamoxifen	→ progestins	33	50	30	8	Progestins	→ tamoxifen	8	23	25	13	110, 112, 113
Tamoxifen	→ AG	30	102	63	22	AG	→ tamoxifen	28	83	7	7	126, 130, 131
Tamoxifen	→ estrogens	19	30	37	23	Estrogens	→ tamoxifen	20	54	75	32	48, 67, 71, 198
						Estrogens	→ AG	5	28	0	25	126
Tamoxifen	→ androgens	27	30	41	23	Androgens	→ tamoxifen	26	25	69	36	53, 198, 199
						Androgens	→ Ag	10	35	50	29	126
Tamoxifen	→ ablation*	29	28	59	29	Ablation*	→ tamoxifen	11	13	27	31	72, 199, 200
						Ablation*	→ Ag	3	7	67	29	126

*Ablation, Adrenalectomy or hypophysectomy.
(R, patients who responded to the first therapeutic regimen in the sequence and subsequently progressed; NR, patients who failed to respond to the first therapeutic regimen; AG, aminoglutethimide.

Table 13-20

Response Rates to Endocrine Therapy Among Patients With (ERP+) or Without (ERP−) an Estrogen Receptor

Endocrine Therapy	*Response Rate (%)* in Unselected Patients*	*No. of Patients*		*Response Rate (%) in Patients*		*Reference No.*
		ERP+	*ERP−*	*ERP+*	*ERP−*	
Tamoxifen	32	224	74	54	9	60, 201
Oophorectomy	33	68	83	62	6	194, 202
Progestins	31	279	74	35	8	99, 103, 104, 107, 109–111, 113
Aminoglutethimide	31	96	27	54	6	126, 203–206
Estrogens	26	61	58	57	9	194
Androgens	21	28	26	43	8	194
Adrenalectomy	32	137	60	46	10	194, 202

* Response rates taken from Table 13-2.
(ERP, estrogen receptor protein)

ERP-negative patients included in these studies was very small. In addition, progestins have been used primarily as second-line therapy following a trial with another form of endocrine therapy, especially tamoxifen, and the response to progestins after previous treatment with tamoxifen may be somewhat lower than if the progestin were used as the primary treatment agent.

The development of the estrogen receptor and the progesterone receptor (see Chapter 9) has not completely eliminated the need to heed clinical characteristics. Logistic regression analysis of estrogen receptor values, visceral sites, disease-free intervals, and prior response to therapy demonstrates that the estrogen receptor is easily the most important of these factors, but each of the variables has predictive value.[194] For example, among ERP-positive patients, the probability of a response to endocrine therapy was predicted to be 57% if the disease-free interval was greater than 10 months, and 39% if the interval was less than 10 months. The observed differences were 60% and 25%, respectively. The estrogen receptor is a more powerful predictor of response to endocrine therapy than is prior response to therapy. However, the additional knowledge of prior response to endocrine therapy strengthens the prediction. Fifty percent of all patients who were ERP-positive and who regressed after the first course of endocrine therapy also regressed after a second endocrine treatment regimen. Only 30% of the patients who were ERP-positive and who failed the first course of endocrine therapy responded to subsequent therapy. These differences were statistically significant.

These observations on the relative value of the ERP and the patient's clinical characteristics in predicting response to endocrine therapy suggest that all available data should be used in each therapeutic decision. A very young woman presenting with a short disease-free interval and extensive liver involvement might reasonably be treated initially with chemotherapy, rather than endocrine therapy, even if she were ERP-positive. A premenopausal woman in her 40s presenting with disease limited to the soft tissue and bone, a 3-year, disease-free interval, and a strongly positive ERP might be treated with oophorectomy even if she had not responded to an initial course of tamoxifen. A woman in her 70s or 80s presenting with mildly symptomatic disease affecting the chest wall and several bones might be considered for a trial of tamoxifen even if her ERP was negative or borderline.

OPTIMAL SEQUENCES FOR ENDOCRINE THERAPY

In most situations, there is little difference in the probability of response to one endocrine therapy or another, so the selection of endocrine therapy for an individual patient must be based on other criteria, usually the relative toxicity of the treatment regimen being considered. For this reason, the therapy of choice is usually tamoxifen, oophorectomy, or a progestin (Fig. 13-8). In premenopausal women, the relative toxicity of surgical or irradiation-induced ablation of ovarian function and tamoxifen is subjective. There is no reason why the patient's attitude toward these two approaches should not be considered. Among postmenopausal women, tamoxifen is clearly the treatment of choice. Preliminary data from randomized trials suggest that conventional doses of medroxyprogesterone acetate or megestrol acetate will eventually prove to be as effective as tamoxifen, with a similar level of toxicity. In postmenopausal patients who respond to initial endocrine therapy with tamoxifen or a progestin, the next treatment of choice is aminoglutethimide. Aminoglutethimide is also a reasonable option for premenopausal women who have previously been treated with oophorectomy. In patients with painful bony metastases, aminoglutethimide as a first endocrine therapy may be the treatment of choice. A new problem which has not been systematically studied is the initial endocrine therapy of choice for patients who re-

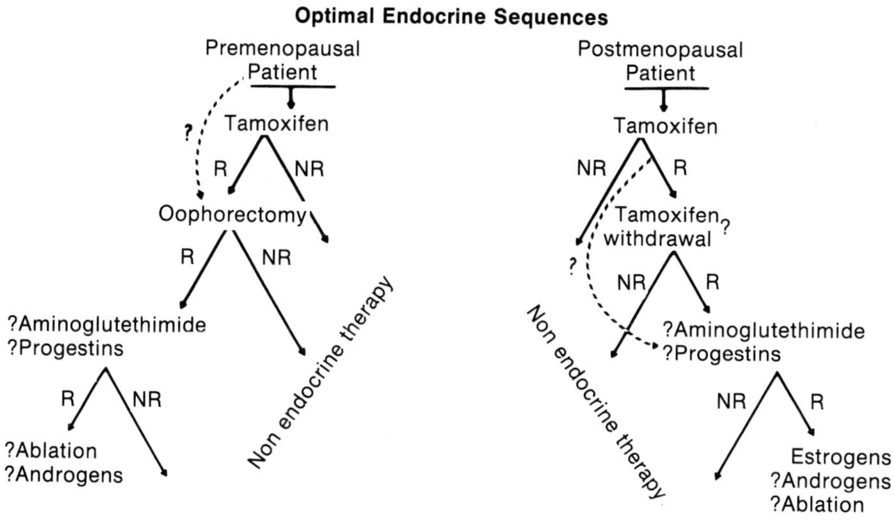

FIGURE 13-8. Optimal sequence for administering different endocrine treatment regimens based on relative toxicities and efficacy in premenopausal and postmenopausal women. (R, response; NR, no response.)

lapse following adjuvant endocrine therapy or adjuvant chemohormonal therapy. The clinical research trials conducted thus far have concentrated predominantly on choosing between two endocrine treatment regimens rather than on defining a complete sequence of therapy. Perusal of the sequential responses in Table 13-19 suggests that the best responses might be obtained by alternating additive-type hormones, such as tamoxifen and the progestins, with ablative approaches, such as oophorectomy and aminoglutethimide, each time there is evidence of disease progression. At the present time, however, there is insufficient evidence to consider this an established principle, and a certain amount of trial and error at each decision point will continue to be necessary until more data from controlled trials are available.

REFERENCES

1. Beatson GW: On the treatment of inoperable cases of carcinoma of the mamma: Suggestions for a new method of treatment with illustrative cases. Lancet 2:104, 1896
2. Mouridsen H, Palshof T, Patterson J, et al: Tamoxifen in advanced breast cancer. Cancer Treat Rev 5:131, 1978
3. Henderson IC, Canellos GP: Cancer of the breast: The past decade. N Engl J Med 302:17–30; 78–90, 1980
4. Stuart-Harris RC, Smith IE: Aminoglutethimide in the treatment of advanced breast cancer. Cancer Treat Rev 11:189, 1984
5. Nordenskjold B, Lowhagen T, Westerberg H, et al: 3H-thymidine incorporation into mammary carcinoma cells obtained by needle aspiration before and during endocrine therapy. Acta Cytol 20:137, 1976
6. Dao TL, Sinha DK, Nemoto T, et al: Effect of estrogen and progesterone on cellular replication of human breast tumors. Cancer Res 42:359, 1982
7. Welsch CW: Host factors affecting the growth in carcinogen-induced rat mammary carcinomas: A review and tribute to Charles Brenton Huggins. Cancer Res 45:3415, 1985
8. Aitken SC, Lippman ME: Effect of estrogens and antiestrogens on growth-regulatory enzymes in human breast cancer cells in tissue culture. Cancer Res 45:1611, 1985
9. Gullino PM, Grantham FH, Losonczy I, et al: Mammary tumor regression. I. Physiopathologic characteristics of hormone-dependent tissue. J Natl Cancer Inst 49:1333, 1972
10. Gullino PM, Lanzerotti RH: Mammary tumor regression. II. Autophagy of neoplastic cells. J Natl Cancer Inst 49:1349, 1972
11. Danielpour D, Sirbasku DA: The role of autocrine growth factors in estrogen-responsive and estrogen-autonomous rat mammary tumor cell growth in vivo. Proc Am Assoc Cancer Res 25:214, 1984
12. Lippman ME, Dickson R, Kasid A, et al: Autocrine and paracrine growth regulation of human breast cancer. J Steroid Biochem, 24:147, 1986
13. Durnberger H, Heuberger B, Schwartz P, et al: Mesenchyme-mediated effect of testosterone on embryonic mammary epithelium. Cancer Res 38:4066, 1978
14. Singhakowinta A, Henderson MD, Vaitkevicius VK: Bilateral adrenalectomy in selected patients with carcinoma of the breast. Surg Gynecol Obstet 138:689, 1974
15. Carter AC, Sedransk N, Kelley RM, et al: Diethystilbestrol: Recommended dosages for different categories of breast cancer patients—Report of the Cooperative Breast Cancer Group. JAMA 237:2079, 1977
16. Bronzert DA, Triche TJ, Gleason P, et al: Isolation and characterization of an estrogen-inhibited variant derived from the MCF-7 breast cancer cell line. Cancer Res 44:3942, 1984
17. Brandes LJ, Hermonat MW: Receptor status and subsequent sensitivity of subclones of MCF-7 human breast cancer cells surviving exposure to diethylstilbestrol. Cancer Res 43:2831, 1983
18. Poulsen HS, Brunner N, Rytter L, et al: Steroid receptor profile of two estrogen-positive human breast tumors grown in nude mice. Proc Am Assoc Cancer Res 25:206, 1984
19. Selby P, Bizzari JP, Buick RN: Therapeutic implications of a stem cell model for human breast cancer: A hypothesis. Cancer Treat Rep 67:659, 1983
20. Fiusgher ER, Osborne CK, McGuire WL, et al: Correlation of primary breast cancer histopathology and estrogen receptor content. Breast Cancer Res Treat 1:37, 1981
21. Silfversward C, Gustafsson J, Gustafsson SA, et al: Estrogen

receptor concentrations in 269 cases of histologically classified human breast cancer. Cancer 45:2001, 1980
22. McCarty KS Jr, Barton TK, Fetter BF, et al: Correlation of estrogen and progesterone receptors with histologic differentiation in mammary carcinoma. Cancer 46:2851, 1980
23. Pertschuk LP, Eisenberg KB, Carter AC, et al: Heterogeneity of estrogen binding sites in breast cancer: Morphologic demonstration and relationship to endocrine response. Breast Cancer Res Treat 5:137, 1985
24. Mercer WD, Lippman ME, Wahl TM, et al: The use of immunocytochemical techniques for the detection of steroid hormones in breast cancer cells. Cancer 46:2859, 1980
25. Dao TL: Ablation therapy for hormone-dependent tumors. Annu Rev Med 23:1, 1972
26. Fracchia AA, Farrow JH, DePalo AJ, et al: Castration for primary inoperable or recurrent breast carcinoma. Surg Gynecol Obstet 128:1226, 1969
27. Veronesi U, Pizzocaro G, Rossi A: Oophorectomy for advanced carcinoma of the breast. Surg Gynecol Obstet 141:569, 1975
28. Chakravarti S, Collins WP, Forcast JD, et al: Hormonal profiles after the menopause. Br Med J 2:784, 1976
29. Senie RT, Lobenthal SW, Rosen PP: Association of vaginal smear cytology with menstrual status in breast cancer. Breast Cancer Res Treat 5:301, 1985
30. Peetzs ME, Awrich AE, Moseley HS, et al: Results of oophorectomy by menstrual and estrogen receptor status in patients with metastatic breast cancer. Am J Surg 141:554, 1981
31. Fitzpatrick PJ, Garrett PG: Metastatic breast cancer: Ovarian ablation with lower half-body irradiation. Int J Radiat Oncol Biol Phys 7:1523, 1981
32. Barlow JJ, Emerson K Jr, Saxena BN: Estradiol production after ovariectomy for carcinoma of the breast: Relevance to the treatment of menopausal women. N Engl J Med 280:633, 1969
33. Lees AW, Giuffre C, Burns PE, et al: Oophorectomy versus radiation ablation of ovarian function in patients with metastatic carcinoma of the breast. Surg Gynecol Obstet 151:721, 1980
34. Lee YTN: Therapeutic castration for advanced breast cancer. Am J Surg 122:42, 1971
35. Hayward JL, Atkins HJB, Falconer MA, et al: Clinical trials comparing transfrontal hypophysectomy with adrenalectomy and with transethmoidal hypophysectomy. In Joslin CAF, Gleave EN (eds): The Clinical Management of Advanced Breast Cancer, pp 50–53. Cardiff, Wales, Alpha Omega Alpha Publishing, 1970
36. McMillin JM, Seal US, Theologides A: Prolactin dynamics following transsphenoidal hypophysectomy for metastatic carcinoma of the breast. Cancer 39:2254, 1977
37. Pearson OH, Brodkey JS, Manni A: Hypophysectomy for stage IV breast cancer. Surg Clin North Am 58:809, 1978
38. Roberts MM: A comparison of transethmoidal hypophysectomy, yttrium 90 implant and adrenalectomy. In Joslin CAF, Gleave EN (eds): The Clinical Management of Advanced Breast Cancer, pp 54–62. Cardiff, Wales, Alpha Omega Alpha Publishing, 1970
39. Santen RJ, Worgul TJ, Lipton A, et al: Aminoglutethimide as treatment of postmenopausal women with advanced breast carcinoma. Ann Intern Med 96:94, 1982
40. Kennedy BJ: Massive estrogen administration in premenopausal women with metastatic breast cancer. Cancer 15:641, 1962
41. Stoll BA: Palliation by castration or by hormone administration. In Stoll BA (ed): Breast Cancer—Early and Late, pp 133–146. Chicago, Year Book Medical Publishers, 1977
42. Smith IE, Ford HT, Gazet JC, et al: Premarin in the management of metastatic breast carcinoma in post-menopausal patients. Clin Oncol 5:159, 1979
43. Kaufman RJ, Escher GC: Rebound regression in advanced mammary carcinoma. Surg Gynecol Obstet 113:635, 1961
44. Nesto RW, Cady B, Oberfield RA, et al: Rebound response after estrogen therapy for metastatic breast cancer. Cancer 38:1834, 1976
45. Cortes EP, Lipshutz MD: Hormonal therapy of breast cancer. Ann Intern Med 88:844, 1978
46. Baker LH, Vaitkevicius VK: Reevaluation of rebound regression in disseminated carcinoma of the breast. Cancer 29:1268, 1972
47. Huseby RA: The use of estrogen in the treatment of advanced human breast cancer. In Segaloff A (ed): Breast Cancer—The Second Biennial Louisiana Cancer Conference, pp 206–216. St Louis, CV Mosby, 1958
48. Ingle JN, Ahmann DL, Green SJ, et al: Randomized clinical trial of diethylstilbestrol versus tamoxifen in postmenopausal women with advanced breast cancer. N Engl J Med 304:16, 1981
49. Cooperative Breast Cancer Group: Results of studies of the Cooperative Breast Cancer Group—1961–63. Cancer Chemother Rep 41:1, 1964
50. Brodkin R, Cooper MR: Calusterone. Ann Intern Med 89:945, 1978
51. Manni A, Arafah BM, Pearson OH: Androgen-induced remissions after antiestrogen and hypophysectomy in stage IV breast cancer. Cancer 48:2507, 1981
52. Goldenberg IS, Waters MN, Ravdin RS, et al: Androgenic therapy for advanced breast cancer in women. JAMA 223:1267, 1973
53. Westerberg H: Tamoxifen and fluoxymesterone in advanced breast cancer: A controlled clinical trial. Cancer Treat Rep 64:117, 1980
54. Jordan VC: Biochemical pharmacology of antiestrogen action. Pharm Rev 36:245, 1984
55. Sutherland RL, Reddel RR, Green MD: Effects of oestrogens on cell proliferation and cell cycle kinetics. A hypothesis on the cell cycle effects of antioestrogens. Eur J Cancer Clin Oncol 19:307, 1983
56. Lippman M, Bolan G, Huff K: Interactions of antiestrogens with human breast cancer in long-term tissue culture. Cancer Treat Rep 60:1421, 1976
57. Jordan VC, Allen KE, Dix CJ: Pharmacology of tamoxifen in laboratory animals. Cancer Treat Rep 64:745, 1980
58. Sherman BM, Chapler FK, Crickard K, et al: Endocrine consequences of continuous antiestrogen therapy with tamoxifen in premenopausal women. J Clin Invest 64:398, 1979
59. Fiorentino P: Clinical experience with antihormone therapy. In Ward HWC (ed): Proceedings of the Symposium on The Hormonal Control of Breast Cancer, p 56. Cheshire, Imperial Chemical Industries, 1975
60. Rose C, Mouridsen HT: Treatment of advanced breast cancer with tamoxifen. Recent Results Cancer Res 91:230, 1984
61. Legha SS, Carter SK: Antiestrogens in the treatment of breast cancer. Cancer Treat Rev 3:205, 1976
62. Bloom HJG, Boesen E: Antiestrogens in treatment of breast cancer: Value of nafoxidine in 52 advanced cases. Br Med J 2:7, 1974
63. Steinbaum FL, DeJager RL, Krakoff IH: Clinical trial of nafoxidine in advanced breast cancer. Med Pediatr Oncol 4:123, 1978
64. Hecker E, Vegh I, Levy CM, et al: Clinical trial of clomiphene in advanced breast cancer. Eur J Cancer 10:747, 1974

65. Haskell CM, Herrmann C Jr, Marsh GG: Clomiphene-induced neurological dysfunction. Lancet 2:1227, 1977
66. Buzdar AU, Powell KC, Legha SS, et al: A phase I-II evaluation of trioxifene mesylate in the treatment of advanced breast cancer. Proc Am Soc Clin Oncol 22:448, 1981
67. Stewart HJ, Forrest APM, Gunn JM, et al: The tamoxifen trial—a double-blind comparison with stilboestrol in postmenopausal women with advanced breast cancer. In Mouridsen HT, Palshof T (eds): Breast Cancer—Experimental and Clinical Aspects, pp 83–87. Elmsford, Pergamon Press, 1980
68. Beex L, Pieters G, Smals A, et al: Tamoxifen versus ethinyl estradiol in the treatment of postmenopausal women with advanced breast cancer. Cancer Treat Rep 65:179, 1981
69. Paschold EH, Slatkoff ML, Muss HB, et al: Hormonal therapy of advanced breast cancer: Efficacy and toxicity of diethylstilbestrol (DES) vs. tamoxifen (TAM). Proc Am Soc Clin Oncol 22:380, 1981
70. Ribeiro GG: A clinical trial to compare the use of tamoxifen vs stilboestrol in the treatment of post-menopausal women with advanced breast cancer. In: Reviews on Endocrine-Related Cancer, Suppl 9, pp 409–414. Wilmington, Delaware, Stuart Pharmaceuticals, 1980
71. Matelski H, Huberman M, Zipoli T, et al: Randomized trial of estrogen vs. tamoxifen therapy for advanced breast cancer. Am J Clin Oncol 8:128, 1985
72. Kiang DT, Frenning DH, Vosika GJ, et al: Comparison of tamoxifen and hypophysectomy in breast cancer treatment. Cancer 45:1322, 1980
73. Nemoto T, Patel J, Rosner D, et al: Tamoxifen (Nolvadex) versus adrenalectomy in metastatic breast cancer. Cancer 53:1333, 1984
74. Hoogstraten B, Fletcher WS, Gad-el-Mawla N, et al: Tamoxifen and oophorectomy in the treatment of recurrent breast cancer. Cancer Res 42:4788, 1982
75. Margreiter R, Wiegele J: Tamoxifen (Nolvadex) for premenopausal patients with advanced breast cancer. Breast Cancer Res Treat 4:45, 1984
76. Pritchard K, Meakin JW, Sawka C, et al: The role and mechanism of action of tamoxifen in premenopausal women with metastatic carcinoma of the breast: An update. Proc Am Soc Clin Oncol 4:54, 1985
77. Wada T, Koyama H, Terasawa T: Effect of tamoxifen in premenopausal Japanese women with advanced breast cancer. Cancer Treat Rep 65:728, 1981
78. Manni A, Pearson OH: Antiestrogen-induced remissions in premenopausal women with stage IV breast cancer: Effects on ovarian function. Cancer Treat Rep 64:779, 1980
79. Planting AST, Alexieva-Figusch J, Blonk-v.d.Wijst J, et al: Tamoxifen therapy in premenopausal women with metastatic breast cancer. Cancer Treat Rep 69:363, 1985
80. Kalman AM, Thompson T, Vogel CL: Response to oophorectomy after tamoxifen failure in a premenopausal patient. Cancer Treat Rep, 66:1867, 1982
81. Ingle JN, Krook JE, Green SJ, et al: Randomized trial of bilateral oophorectomy versus tamoxifen in premenopausal women with metastatic breast cancer. J Clin Oncol 4:178, 1986
82. Buchanan RB, Williams CJ, Hall V, et al: Tamoxifen versus surgical oophorectomy in premenopausal women with advanced breast cancer. Proc Am Soc Clin Oncol 4:59, 1985
83. Pritchard KI, Thomson DB, Myers RE, et al: Tamoxifen therapy in premenopausal patients with metastatic breast cancer. Cancer Treat Rep 64:787, 1980
84. Manni A, Arafah BM: Tamoxifen-induced remission in breast cancer by escalating the dose to 40 mg daily after progression on 20 mg daily. Cancer 48:873, 1981
85. Rose C, Theilade K, Boesen E, et al: Treatment of advanced breast cancer with tamoxifen. Breast Cancer Res Treat 2:395, 1982
86. Goldhirsch A, Joss RA, Leuenberger U, et al: An evaluation of tamoxifen dose escalation in advanced breast cancer. Am J Clin Oncol 5:501, 1982
87. Stewart JF, Minton MJ, Rubens RD: Trial of tamoxifen at a dose of 40 mg daily after disease progression during tamoxifen therapy at a dose of 20 mg daily. Cancer Treat Rep 66:1445, 1982
88. Ward HWC: Anti-oestrogen therapy for breast cancer: A trial of tamoxifen at two dose levels. Br Med J 1:13, 1973
89. Tormey DC, Lippman ME, Edwards BK, et al: Evaluation of tamoxifen doses with and without fluoxymesterone in advanced breast cancer. Ann Intern Med 98:139, 1983
90. Bratherton DG, Brown CH, Buchanan R, et al: A comparison of two doses of tamoxifen (Nolvadex) in postmenopausal women with advanced breast cancer: 10 mg bd versus 20 mg bd. Br J Cancer 50:199, 1984
91. Fabian C, Sternson L, El-Serafi M, et al: Clinical pharmacology of tamoxifen in patients with breast cancer: Correlation with clinical data. Cancer 48:876, 1981
92. Kaiser-Kupfer MI, Lippman ME: Tamoxifen retinopathy. Cancer Treat Rep 62:315, 1978
93. Beck M, Mills PV: Ocular assessment of patients treated with tamoxifen. Cancer Treat Rep 63:1833, 1979
94. Lipton A, Harvey HA, Hamilton RW: Venous thrombosis as a side effect of tamoxifen treatment. Cancer Treat Rep 68:887, 1984
95. Enck RE, Rios CN: Tamoxifen treatment of metastatic breast cancer and antithrombin III levels. Cancer 53:2607, 1984
96. Killackey MA, Hakes TB, Pierce VK: Endometrial adenocarcinoma in breast cancer patients receiving antiestrogens. Cancer Treat Rep 69:237, 1985
97. Hayward J: Corticosteroids and progestogens. In Hayward J (ed): Hormones and Human Cancer, An Account of 15 Years Study, pp 93–98. New York, Springer-Verlag, 1970
98. Lober J, Rose C, Salimtschik M, et al: Treatment of advanced breast cancer with progestins. Acta Obstet Gynecol Scand (Suppl) 101:39, 1981
99. Nemoto T, Patel J, Rosner D, et al: Oral medroxyprogesterone acetate (NSC-26386) in metastatic breast cancer. Proc Am Assoc Cancer Res 24:320, 1983
100. Muggia FM, Cassileth PA, Ochoa M, et al: Treatment of breast cancer with medroxyprogesterone acetate. Ann Intern Med 68:328, 1968
101. Mattsson W: Current status of high dose progestin treatment in advanced breast cancer. Breast Cancer Res Treat 3:231, 1983
102. Cavalli F, Goldhirsch A, Jungi F, et al: Randomized trial of low- versus high-dose medroxyprogesterone acetate in the induction treatment of postmenopausal patients with advanced breast cancer. J Clin Oncol 2:414, 1984
103. Izuo M, Yoshida M, Tominaga T, et al: A phase III trial of oral high-dose medroxyprogesterone acetate (MPA) versus mepitiostane in advanced postmenopausal breast cancer. Cancer 56:2576, 1985
104. Hortobagyi GN, Buzdar AU, Frye D, et al: Oral medroxyprogesterone acetate in the treatment of metastatic breast cancer. Breast Cancer Res Treat 5:321, 1985
105. Davila E, Thompson TT, Riordan D, et al: High-dose oral medroxyprogesterone acetate (HDO-MPA) for advanced breast cancer (BC). Proc Am Soc Clin Oncol 1:76, 1982
106. Canetta R, Florentine S, Hunter H, et al: Megestrol acetate. Cancer Treat Rev 10:141, 1983
107. Johnson PA, Bonomi PD, Wolter JM, et al: Megestrol acetate

versus tamoxifen in advanced breast cancer: A retrospective study. Proc Am Assoc Cancer Res 24:172, 1983
108. Ansfield FJ, Kallas GJ, Singson JP: Clinical results with megestrol acetate in patients with advanced carcinoma of the breast. Surg Gynecol Obstet 155:888, 1982
109. Keller J, Browder H, White JM, et al: Megestrol acetate (MA) compared to tamoxifen (T) in postmenopausal women with advanced breast cancer: Preliminary results. Proc Am Soc Clin Oncol 4:62, 1985
110. Muss HB, Paschold EH, Black WR, et al: Megestrol acetate vs. tamoxifen in advanced breast cancer: A phase III trial of the Piedmont Oncology Association (POA). Semin Oncol 12:55, 1985
111. Gregory EJ, Cohen SC, Oines DW, et al: Megestrol acetate therapy for advanced breast cancer. J Clin Oncol 3:155, 1985
112. Ingle JN, Ahmann DL, Green SJ, et al: Randomized clinical trial of megestrol acetate versus tamoxifen in paramenopausal or castrated women with advanced breast cancer. Am J Clin Oncol 5:155, 1982
113. Morgan LR: Megestrol acetate vs. tamoxifen in advanced breast cancer in postmenopausal patients. Semin Oncol 12:43, 1985
114. Pannuti F, Martoni A, Fruet F, et al: Hormone therapy in advanced breast cancer: High-dose medroxyprogesterone acetate (MPA) vs. tamoxifen (TMX). Preliminary results. In Mouridsen HT, Palshof T (eds): Breast Cancer—Experimental and Clinical Aspects, pp 93–98. Oxford, Pergamon Press, 1980
115. Mattsson W: A phase III trial of treatment with tamoxifen versus treatment with high dose medroxyprogesterone-acetate in advanced postmenopausal breast cancer. In Iacobelli S, DiMarco A (eds): Role of Medroxyprogesterone in Endocrine-Related Tumors, pp 65–71. New York, Raven Press, 1980
116. Jones V: A prospective trial of oestrogens, androgens and progestogens for the treatment of advanced carcinoma of the breast. In Joslin CAF, Gleave EN (eds): The Clinical Management of Advanced Breast Cancer, pp 24–28. Cardiff, Wales, Alpha Omega Alpha Publishers, 1970
117. Pannuti F, Martoni A, Di Marco AR, et al: Prospective, randomized clinical trial of two different high dosages of medroxyprogesterone acetate (MPA) in the treatment of metastatic breast cancer. Eur J Cancer 15:593, 1979
118. De Lena M, Brambilla C, Valagussa P, et al: High-dose medroxyprogesterone acetate in breast cancer resistant to endocrine and cytotoxic therapy. Cancer Chemother Pharmacol 2:175, 1979
119. Morgan LR, Donley PJ, Savage J: High dose megestrol acetate (MA) in advanced breast cancer: Bioavailability, toxicity and response. Proc Am Assoc Cancer Res 24:134, 1983
120. Lober J, Mouridsen HT, Salimtschik M, et al: Pharmacokinetics of medroxyprogesterone acetate administered by oral and intramuscular route. Acta Obstet Gynecol Scand 101:71, 1981
121. Hesselius I, Johansson EDB: Medroxyprogesterone acetate (MPA) plasma levels after oral and intramuscular administration in a long-term study. Acta Obstet Gynecol Scand 101:65, 1981
122. Alexieva-Figusch J, van Gilse HA, Jop WCJ, et al: Progestin therapy in advanced breast cancer: Megestrol acetate—An evaluation of 160 treated cases. Cancer 46:2369, 1980
123. Bonomi P, Johnson P, Anderson K, et al: Primary hormonal therapy of advanced breast cancer with megestrol acetate: Predictive value of estrogen receptor and progesterone receptor levels. Semin Oncol 12:48, 1985
124. Ross MB, Buzdar AU, Blumenschein GR: Treatment of advanced breast cancer with megestrol acetate after therapy with tamoxifen. Cancer 49:413, 1982
125. Santen RJ, Samojlik E, Worgul TJ: Aminoglutethimide. In Santen RJ, Henderson IC (eds): A Comprehensive Guide to the Therapeutic Use of Aminoglutethimide, pp 101–160. Basel, S Karger, 1982
126. Santen RJ: Suppression of estrogens with aminoglutethimide and hydrocortisone (medical adrenalectomy) as treatment of advanced breast carcinoma: A review. Breast Cancer Res Treat 1:183, 1981
127. Rubens RD, Knight RK: The contribution of prednisolone (P) to primary endocrine therapy (PET) in advanced breast cancer. Proc Am Soc Clin Oncol 4:53, 1985
128. Harvey HA, Santen RJ, Osterman J, et al: A comparative trial of transsphenoidal hypophysectomy and estrogen suppression with aminoglutethimide in advanced breast cancer. Cancer 43:2207, 1979
129. Santen RJ, Worgul TJ, Samojlik E, et al: A randomized trial comparing surgical adrenalectomy with aminoglutethimide plus hydrocortisone in women with advanced breast cancer. N Engl J Med 305:545, 1981
130. Lipton A, Harvey HA, Santen RJ, et al: Randomized trial of aminoglutethimide versus tamoxifen in metastatic breast cancer. Cancer Res 42:3434s, 1982
131. Smith IE, Harris AL, Morgan M, et al: Tamoxifen versus aminoglutethimide versus combined tamoxifen and aminoglutethimide in the treatment of advanced breast carcinoma. Cancer Res 42:3430s, 1982
132. Gale KE, Gelman R, Tormey D, et al: Hormonotherapy for metastatic breast cancer. Proc Am Soc Clin Oncol 2:105, 1983
133. Santen RJ, Lipton A, Harvey H, et al: Dose response effects of aminoglutethimide on estrogen levels in women with breast cancer: Validity of low dose regimen. Proc Am Soc Clin Oncol 3:123, 1984
134. Santen RJ, Lipton A, Harvey H, et al: Pharmacologic mechanism of estrogen suppression with aminoglutethimide in women with breast cancer. Proc 13th Int Congr Chemother (Vienna) 218:21, 1983
135. Stuart-Harris R, Bozek T, Gazet JC, et al: Low-dose aminoglutethimide in treatment of advanced breast cancer. Lancet 2:604, 1984
136. Murray R, Pitt P: Low-dose aminoglutethimide without steroid replacement in the treatment of postmenopausal women with advanced breast cancer. Eur J Cancer Clin Oncol 21:19, 1985
137. Vermeulen A: Effects of aminoglutethimide on plasma sex hormone levels in postmenopausal women. In Paesi FJA (ed): Aminoglutethimide: Mechanism of Action and Clinical Results in Breast Cancer, pp 47–58. Basle, CIBA-Geigy, 1982
138. Young JA, Newcomer LN, Keller AM: Aminoglutethimide-induced bone marrow injury: Report of a case and review of the literature. Cancer 54:1731, 1984
139. Kampel LJ, Kurman MR: Severe leukopenia induced by aminoglutethimide. Cancer Treat Rep 68:1277, 1984
140. Vincent MD, Clink HM, Coombes RC, et al: Aminoglutethimide (with hydrocortisone) induced agranulocytosis in primary breast cancer. Br Med J 291:105, 1985
141. Kissin MW, Kark AE: Irreversible thrombocytopenia following aminoglutethimide. Cancer Treat Rep 67:849, 1983
142. Austerlitz J: Leukopenia associated with aminoglutethimide therapy: A case report. Cancer Treat Rep 66:1879, 1982
143. Messeih AA, Lipton A, Santen RJ, et al: Aminoglutethimide-induced hematologic toxicity: Worldwide experience. Cancer Treat Rep 69:1003, 1985

144. Coombes RC, Dowsett M, Goss P, et al: 4-Hydroxyandrostenedione in treatment of postmenopausal patients with advanced breast cancer. Lancet 1:1237, 1984
145. Coombes RC, Powles TJ, Muindi J, et al: Trilostane therapy for advanced breast cancer. Cancer Treat Rep 69:351, 1985
146. Wilkinson PM, Hindley AC, Beardwell CG, et al: Trilostane (T) a new hormonal agent in the treatment of metastatic breast cancer (MBC). Proc Am Soc Clin Oncol 3:113, 1984
147. Williams CJ: Trilostane: A phase II study of a new hormonal agent in postmenopausal women with recurrent breast cancer. Proc Am Assoc Cancer Res 25:212, 1984
148. Smithline F, Sherman L, Kolodny HD: Prolactin and breast carcinoma. N Engl J Med 292:784, 1975
149. Nagasawa H: Prolactin and human breast cancer: A review. Eur J Cancer 15:267, 1979
150. Welsch CW, Nagasawa H: Prolactin and murine mammary tumorigenesis: A review. Cancer Res 37:951, 1977
151. Dowsett M, McGarrick GE, Harris AL, et al: Prognostic significance of serum prolactin levels in advanced breast cancer. Br J Cancer 47:763, 1983
152. Turkington RW, Underwood LE, Van Wyk JJ: Elevated serum prolactin levels after pituitary-stalk section in man. N Engl J Med 285:707, 1971
153. Holtkamp W, Nagel GA, Wander HE: Hyperprolactinemia: A marker of progressive disease and poor prognosis in advanced breast cancer. Proc Am Soc Clin Oncol 3:112, 1984
154. Minton JP: Precise selection of breast cancer patients with bone metastasis for endocrine ablation. Surgery 80:513, 1976
155. Sasaki GH, Leung BS, Fletcher WS: Levodopa test and estrogen receptor assay in prognosticating responses of patients with advanced cancer of the breast to endocrine therapy. Ann Surg 183:392, 1976
156. Ward HWC: Combined anti-prolactin and anti-oestrogen therapy for breast carcinoma. Clin Oncol 3:91, 1977
157. Potts GO, Schane HP, Edelson J: Pharmacology and pharmacokinetics of danazol. Drugs 19:321, 1980
158. Ingle JN: Additive hormonal therapy in women with advanced breast cancer. Cancer 53:766, 1984
159. Dhont M, Van Eyck J, Delbeke L, et al: Danazol treatment of chronic cystic mastopathy: A clinical and hormonal evaluation. Postgrad Med J 55:66, 1979
160. Coombes RC, Dearnaley D, Humphreys J, et al: Danazol treatment of advanced breast cancer. Cancer Treat Rep 64:1073, 1980
161. Powles TJ, Ford HT, Nash AG, et al: Treatment of disseminated breast cancer with tamoxifen, aminoglutethimide, hydrocortisone, and danazol, used in combination or sequentially. Lancet 1:1369, 1984
162. Klijn JGM, deJong FH: Treatment with a luteinizing-hormone-releasing-hormone analogue. Lancet 1:1213, 1982
163. Klijn JGM, deJong FH, Blankenstein MA, et al: Anti-tumor and endocrine effects of chronic LHRH agonist treatment (buserelin) with or without tamoxifen in premenopausal metastatic breast cancer. Breast Cancer Res Treat 4:209, 1984
164. Harvey HA, Lipton A, Santen RJ, et al: Phase II study of a gonadotropin-releasing hormone analogue (leuprolide) in postmenopausal advanced breast cancer patients. Proc Am Soc Clin Oncol 22:444, 1981
165. Harvey HA, Lipton A, Max DT, et al: Medical castration produced by the GNRH analogue leuprolide to treat metastatic breast cancer. J Clin Oncol 3:1068, 1985
166. Davis HL: Hormonal manipulation in the treatment of cancer of the female breast. In Rose DP (ed): Endocrinology of Cancer, Vol 1, pp 61–92. Boca Raton, CRC Press, 1979
167. Hayward J: Pituitary and thyroid hormones. In Hayward J (ed): Hormones and Human Cancer, An Account of 15 Years Study, pp 138–146. New York, Springer-Verlag, 1970
168. O'Bryan RM, Gordon GS, Kelley RM, et al: Does thyroid substance improve response of breast cancer to surgical castration? Cancer 33:1082, 1974
169. Chlebowski R, Irwin LE, Pugh RP, et al: Survival of patients with metastatic breast cancer treated with either combination or sequential chemotherapy. Cancer Res 39:4503, 1979
170. Dowsett M, Harris AL, Smith IE, et al: Endocrine and clinical consequences of combination tamoxifen-aminoglutethimide in postmenopausal breast cancer. Br J Cancer 50:357, 1984
171. Stoll BA: Combination endocrine therapy in breast cancer. Eur J Cancer Clin Oncol 21:413, 1985
172. Van Deijk WA, Blijham GH, Mellink WAM, et al: Influence of aminoglutethimide on plasma levels of medroxyprogesterone acetate: Its correlation with serum cortisol. Cancer Treat Rep 69:85, 1985
173. Dowsett M, Murray RML, Pitt P, et al: Antagonism of aminoglutethimide and danazol in the suppression of serum free oestradiol in breast cancer patients. Eur J Cancer Clin Oncol 21:1063, 1985
174. Landau RL, Ehrlich EN, Huggins C: Estradiol benzoate and progesterone in advanced human breast cancer. JAMA 182:632, 1962
175. Pellegrini A, Massidda B, Mascia V, et al: Ethinyl estradiol and medroxyprogesterone treatment in advanced breast cancer: A pilot study. Cancer Treat Rep 65:135, 1981
176. Stewart JF, Rubens RD, King RJB, et al: Contribution of prednisolone to the primary endocrine treatment of advanced breast cancer. Eur J Cancer Clin Oncol 18:1307, 1982
177. Kennedy BJ, Brown JH: Combined estrogenic and androgenic hormone therapy in advanced breast cancer. Cancer 18:431, 1965
178. Mouridsen HT, Salimtschik M, Dombernowsky P, et al: Therapeutic effect of tamoxifen versus combined tamoxifen and diethylstilboestrol in advanced breast cancer in postmenopausal women. In Mouridsen HT, Palshof T (eds): Breast Cancer—Experimental and Clinical Aspects, pp 107–110. Elmsford, Pergamon Press, 1980
179. Corkery J, Leonard RCF, Henderson IC, et al: Tamoxifen and aminoglutethimide in advanced breast cancer. Cancer Res 42:3409s, 1982
180. Ingle JN, Green SJ, Ahmann DL, et al: Randomized trial of tamoxifen (TAM) alone or combined with aminoglutethimide (AG) and hydrocortisone (HC) in postmenopausal women with metastatic breast cancer. Proc Am Soc Clin Oncol 4:53, 1985
181. Mouridsen HT, Palshof T, Rose C: Therapeutic effect of tamoxifen alone versus tamoxifen in combination with gestagen and oestrogen in advanced breast cancer. In Henningsen B, Linder F, Steichele C (eds): Endocrine Treatment of Breast Cancer—A New Approach, pp 169–177. New York, Springer-Verlag, 1980
182. Boccardo F, Pino G, Zanardi S, et al: Therapeutic synergism of sequential administration of tamoxifen (TMX) and medroxyprogesterone acetate (MPA) in DMBA-induced rat mammary carcinoma. Proc Am Soc Clin Oncol 3:20, 1984
183. Garcia-Giralt E, Jouve M, Palangie T, et al: Sequential administration of tamoxifen and medroxyprogesterone acetate in disseminated breast cancer. Results of a controlled trial. Proc Am Soc Clin Oncol 3:129, 1984
184. Tormey DC, Simon RM, Lippman ME, et al: Evaluation of

tamoxifen dose in advanced breast cancer: A progress report. Cancer Treat Rep 60:1451, 1976
185. Plotkin D, Lechner JJ, Jung WE, et al: Tamoxifen flare in advanced breast cancer. JAMA 240:2644, 1978
186. Clarysse A: Hormone-induced tumor flare. Eur J Cancer 21:545, 1985
187. Legault-Poisson S, Jolivet J, Poisson R, et al: Tamoxifen-induced tumor stimulation and withdrawal response. Cancer Treat Rep 63:1839, 1979
188. Stoll BA: The significance of tumour "stimulation" by tamoxifen. In Henningsen B, Linder F, Steichele C (eds): Endocrine Treatment of Breast Cancer: A New Approach, pp 149–150. New York, Springer-Verlag, 1980
189. Wilson RE, Jessiman AG, Moore FD: Severe exacerbation of cancer of the breast after oophorectomy and adrenalectomy—Report of four cases. N Engl J Med 258:312, 1958
190. Hall TC, Dederick MM, Nevinny HB: Prognostic value of hormonally induced hypercalcemia in breast cancer. Cancer Chemother Rep 30:21, 1963
191. Henderson IC: Hypercalcemia of malignant disease. In Brain MC, Carbone PP (eds): Current Therapy in Hematology-Oncology 1985–86, pp 254–257. Philadelphia, BC Decker, 1985
192. Devitt JE: The enigmatic behavior of breast cancer. Cancer 27:12, 1971
193. Taylor SG III: Endocrine ablation in disseminated mammary carcinoma. Surg Gynecol Obstet 115 (4):443, 1962
194. Byar D, Sears M, McGuire W: Relationship between estrogen receptor values and clinical data in predicting the response to endocrine therapy for patients with advanced breast cancer. Eur J Cancer 15:299, 1979
195. Wilson AJ: Response in breast cancer to a second hormonal therapy. Rev Endocrine-Related Cancer 14:5, 1983
196. Kostraba N, Kiang D, Frenning D, et al: Multiple endocrine therapy (RX) in the management of advanced breast cancer. Am Assoc Cancer Res 21:147, 1980
197. Ingle JN, Krook JE, Green SJ, et al: Randomized trial of bilateral oophorectomy (OX) versus tamoxifen (TAM) in premenopausal women with metastatic breast cancer. Proc Am Assoc Cancer Res 26:163, 1985
198. Ward HWC, Arthur K, Banks AJ, et al: Anti-oestrogen therapy for breast cancer—A report on 300 patients treated with tamoxifen. Clin Oncol 4:11–17, 1978
199. Manni A, Pearson OH, Marshall JS, et al: Sequential endocrine therapy and chemotherapy in metastatic breast cancer: Effects on survival. Breast Cancer Res Treat 1:97, 1981
200. Bruce J, Carter DC, Fraser J: Patterns of recurrent disease in breast cancer. Lancet 1:433, 1970
201. Heel RC, Brogden RN, Speight TM, et al: Tamoxifen: A review of its pharmacological properties and therapeutic use in the treatment of breast cancer. Int J Current Ther Appl Pharmacol Rev 16:1, 1978
202. Dao TL, Nemoto T: Steroid receptors and response to endocrine ablations in women with metastatic cancer of the breast. Cancer 46:2779, 1980
203. Lawrence BV, Lipton A, Harvey HA, et al: Influence of estrogen receptor status on response of metastatic breast cancer to aminoglutethimide therapy. Cancer 45:786, 1980
204. Horsley JS III, Newsome HH, Brown PW, et al: Medical adrenalectomy in patients with advanced breast cancer. Cancer 49:1145, 1982
205. Buzdar AU, Powell KC, Blumenschein GR: Aminoglutethimide after tamoxifen therapy in advanced breast cancer: M.D. Anderson Hospital experience. Cancer Res 42:3448s, 1982
206. Troner MB: Aminoglutethimide in the treatment of metastatic breast cancer. Cancer Res 42:3402s, 1982

Chemotherapy for Advanced Disease

I. Craig Henderson

CHEMOTHERAPY FOR METASTATIC DISEASE

The percentage of patients who have metastatic breast cancer and who respond to cytotoxic chemotherapy is almost twice as large as the percentage who respond to endocrine therapy. Although chemotherapy has many more side effects than endocrine therapy, the palliative value of response outweighs the toxic cost of therapy in symptomatic patients. It is likely that most patients with metastatic breast cancer live longer after successful treatment with endocrine therapy or chemotherapy, but it is very difficult to determine precisely how much additional survival time is gained. A few patients may gain a year or more of additional life, but most appear to gain only a few months. For this reason, the major emphasis in choosing therapy for a patient with metastatic breast cancer must be relief of symptoms at the lowest cost in toxicity.

More than 80 cytotoxic drugs have been tested in patients with metastatic breast cancer during the past three decades. Twenty-five of these agents are active, and ten are used routinely to treat patients with breast cancer. No other solid tumor is responsive to such a wide array of cytotoxic agents in addition to multiple types of endocrine therapy. The response rate to combinations of drugs, and possibly to combinations of endocrine therapy and cytotoxic agents, is higher than the response rate to a single agent. For this reason, combinations are commonly used in practice. However, a single agent may be as effective as a combination in patients who have received extensive prior therapy with hormones, radiation, and drugs, and a single agent may palliate a patient unable or unwilling to tolerate the additional toxicity associated with a combination.

The principles of medical oncology used in treating other types of human malignancies are also applied in the use of chemotherapy for patients with metastatic breast cancer. However, it has not been established in randomized trials that some of these principles, such as dose response, are as important in treating breast cancer as they are in treating the hematologic malignancies. As a result, some investigators are now testing very high doses of drugs with autologous marrow transplant, and others are exploring new approaches such as continuous infusion therapy, drug sequencing, and drug-hormone sequencing.

Definitions of the patients most likely to respond to endocrine therapy are well established. No similar definitions exist to distinguish the patients most likely to benefit from chemotherapy, and tests such as the estrogen receptor assay and the clonogenic (stem-cell) assay have not yet been shown to be helpful. As a result, the selection of patients for treatment with cytostatic drugs continues to be a process of elimination. Symptomatic patients who are

Table 13-21
*Response to and Survival Following Treatment With Commonly Used Drug Combinations for Metastatic Breast Cancer**

Percentage of patients with a partial or complete response	43–82%
Percentage with a complete response	4–27%
Time to Response: Median	7–14 weeks
Maximum	72 weeks
Duration of response: Median	5.3–13 months
Maximum	180+ months
Survival of responders: Median	14.8–33 months
Maximum	180+ months

* Based on data from references 1–26.

not good candidates for endocrine therapy but who have multiple sites of disease should be treated with chemotherapy.

About two-thirds of all patients will have an objective response to chemotherapy (Table 13-21). The objective response rate or overall response rate in these studies is defined as the sum of the partial response rate and the complete response rate. In most cases, a partial response is at least a 50% reduction in tumor volume at one or more sites of metastatic disease without evidence of progression at other sites. A complete response is usually defined as disappearance of all evidence of active disease in every known metastatic site. In most studies, the complete response rate is less than 20% and ranges between 5% and 25% in studies with a large number of patients. The median time to evidence of response is between 2 and 3 months, but a patient may have stable disease and go on to have a true partial or complete response more than a year after starting chemotherapy.[19] Patients who have a complete response may live with unmaintained remissions for 5 to 15 years following the completion of their chemotherapy,[22,24–26] but the survival of most responders will be less than 3 years. In spite of this prolonged survival in a small group of patients, there is no evidence that any patient with metastatic breast cancer has been cured with chemotherapy.

MECHANISMS OF DRUG ACTION

Most cytotoxic drugs kill cells by affecting DNA synthesis or function. In general these drugs are ineffective against cells in a resting state unless the cells divide soon after exposure.[27] Endocrine therapy may be most effective against a well-differentiated cell (i.e., an "end" cell) and is effective because of the unique interaction between the endocrine therapy and a differentiated function of the cell. For example, endocrine therapy is most likely to be effective against a cell with an estrogen receptor, a protein that appears predominately in a differentiated or specialized cell. (See the section on Enodcrine Therapy earlier in this chapter.) In contrast, chemotherapy is effective primarily against the cells that are dividing rapidly, and these are most likely to be the least differentiated cells, or stem cells.[28] Since the stem cell is a progenitor for the differentiated end cell, it might be assumed that chemotherapy has greater potential than endocrine therapy to cure or to prolong the survival time of patients with breast cancer. These observations also provide a rationale for the use of chemotherapy and endocrine therapy together. If there is little or no overlap in the cell populations against which each of these modalities are effective, the two forms of therapy should be additive if not synergistic.

The kinetics of drug cytotoxicity have been studied in animal models and in the treatment of hematologic malignancies. Chemotherapy is thought to destroy cells in a logarithmic fashion, or by first-order kinetics. This means that "a given dose of a given drug will kill the same fraction, not the same number, of different-sized tumor stem cell populations as long as their growth fraction and phenotypic heterogeneity ae the same."[29] This is illustrated by curves *A, B,* and *C* in Figure 13-9. The cell kill with each dose of treatment *A* is about two logs, or 90% of the tumor cell population remaining at the beginning of the treatment interval. Between drug doses, tumor regrowth occurs at the same rate or faster than in the untreated or unresponsive tumor, curve *D* (see below). The tumor cell kill achieved with treatment *B* is less than that achieved with treatment *A,* presumably because the drug was less effective, the drug dose was smaller, or the tumor kinetics were less favorable for response to the drug dose schedule chosen for treatment *B.* Nevertheless, the fraction of cells killed with each course of treatment *B* is constant. Although the initial response of tumor to treatment *C* is identical to treatment *B,* the tumor response decreases with time either because of acquired resistance or decreasing drug dose. Decrease in the size of the clinically measurable mass lags behind the destruction of tumor cells (curve *E*). This more gradual decrease in the size of the tumor mass is the net result of the dynamic tumor cell destruction and regrowth within the mass and reflects the fact that the necrotic debris must be removed by the host before a response is evident. If tumor cells are destroyed by first-order kinetics, chemotherapy will never destroy the "last cell." Presumably the last cells are destroyed by host defense mechanisms in patients cured by chemotherapy. Because of limitations in normal tissue tolerance to cytotoxic drugs, maximum tumor cell kill must be achieved with a series of drug doses rather than one very large dose. However, as illustrated in Figure 13-9, maximal tumor cell kill is achieved only when each drug dose is maximal and the interval between drug doses is short enough to prevent regrowth of the tumor to its original size during this interval.[28]

A number of other principles for the use of chemotherapy have also been established using animal tumor models. For most drugs, there is a steep dose-response curve. A small increment in drug dose may result in a several log increase in cell kill. Conversely, a 20% reduction in drug dose may result in a 50% reduction in tumor cure.[27] Chemotherapy is also thought to be most effective

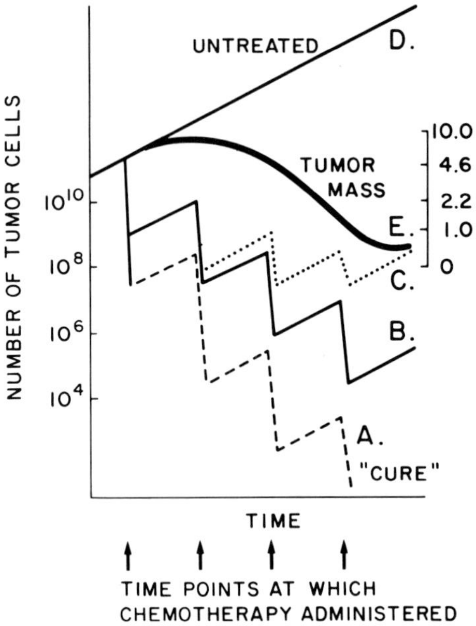

FIGURE 13-9. Schematic illustration of the relationship between clinically observed reduction in tumor mass and kinetics of tumor cell kill following administration of chemotherapy. The tumor cell kill with treatment A is considerably greater than that observed with treatment B or C. Tumor cell increase in the untreated or unresponsive tumor is reflected in curve D. Changes in the size of the tumor mass (curve E) lag behind the changes in the size of the tumor cell population.

if given as early as possible, when tumor masses are small.[30] Tumor growth in micrometastases and in the smallest clinical metastatic deposits is thought to be logarithmic, as illustrated in curve *D* of Figure 13-9. Most or all of the cells are dividing, and the tumor may be very responsive to an effective chemotherapy agent. At the time that tumor masses can easily be detected in x-rays and on physical examination (i.e., at about 1 cm in diameter), tumor growth plateaus, and an increasingly large part of the entire tumor mass is composed of "resting" or nondividing cells. (A growth pattern that results in a plateau in tumor growth rate as the tumor gets larger is referred to as gompertzian growth.) These cells are less responsive to chemotherapy. In addition, many areas of these larger tumor masses are poorly vascularized, and it is difficult to deliver adequate cytotoxic doses of drug to these areas.

In addition to kinetic resistance related to the size of the tumor mass, the tumor cell may have an intrinsic resistance to one or several drugs. Drug-resistant mutant clones appear early in the natural history of tumors, and this is one reason why combinations of drugs are usually more effective than a single agent.[27] New resistant clones also develop quite rapidly after the initiation of therapy.[31] The use of alternating regimens that are non–cross-resistant should be more effective, since maximal doses of each drug regimen could be given and the early introduction of a second regimen might eradicate the new drug-resistant mutants. The observation that resistant mutations occur early and become dominant as the sensitive tumor cells are destroyed means that it is unlikely that prolonged courses of chemotherapy will be more effective than short courses. Although the tumor cannot be eradicated with a single course of therapy, maximal cell reduction will probably be achieved with four to six courses. Resistance to one drug may result in cross-resistance to other drugs of an unrelated class. Pleiotropic drug resistance of this type might be induced by the use of low doses of drug inadequate to fully eradicate the tumor cell burden, and this is one reason why chemotherapy should not be used in situations or in dose schedules of questionable efficacy.[32]

The application of these principles will result in the cure of some tumor types. In general, these tumors are characterized by an undifferentiated morphology, a rapid growth rate, a high growth fraction, and responsiveness regardless of tumor size. Breast cancer does not fulfill these critera. It is only partially differentiated; it has a fairly slow growth rate and a low growth fraction; and response is very dependent on tumor size. For these reasons, breast cancer has been classified as "subcurable."[28] It should not be assumed that these principles do not apply to the treatment of breast cancer, but the best results that can be achieved by the diligent application of these principles may be somewhat less than can be achieved when the principles are applied to tumor models and other human cancers. For example, there is almost certainly a dose-response curve for human breast cancer, but this curve may be too shallow to have a significant effect on survival or even to result in the cure of patients with clinically evident metastases.

THE MEANING OF A RESPONSE TO CHEMOTHERAPY

The efficacy or relative efficacy of a systemic therapy for metastatic disease is usually expressed as the response rate or the duration of response to therapy. These observations made in therapeutic trials emphasize objective end points that can be measured, averaged, and compared. Most studies provide little information on the subjective response of the patients treated, even though the patient's personal goal in accepting therapy is usually palliation of symptoms. What is the correlation between the objective and the subjective response rates to therapy?

The little evidence available suggests that the subjective response rate to chemotherapy exceeds the objective response rate. In one series of trials, it was possible to correlate the percentage of patients who had a decrease in tumor-related pain, an improvement in performance status, or an increase in weight with the objective response rate (Table 13-22).[5] All of these patients had been entered into randomized clinical trials evaluating various combinations of cyclophosphamide, methotrexate, 5-fluorouracil, vincristine, and prednisone. With each combination, the percentage of patients who experienced a decrease in

Table 13-22
Relationship Between Objective Response Rates to Chemotherapy and Relief of Breast Cancer Symptoms

		Percent of Patients With		
Treatment Program†	*Objective Response Rate (CR + PR)**	*Decreased Pain*	*Improved Performance Status*	*Increased Weight*
CM-V	33%	51%	21%	21%
CM-P	44%	64%	37%	43%
CMF-VP	49%	55%	30%	32%
All Regimens	Progressive Disease	33%	10%	17%

* CR, complete response, PR, partial response
† C, cyclophosphamide; M, methotrexate; V, vinblastine; F, 5-fluorouracil; P, prednisone
(Modified from Brunner KW, Sonntag RW, Martz G, et al: Controlled Study in the Use of Combined Drug Therapy for Metastatic Breast Cancer. Cancer 36:1208–1219, 1975.)

pain exceeded the percentage of patients with a complete or partial response. Even patients who had no objective evidence of response had some decrease in pain. This might represent a placebo effect of the therapy, but it is also possible that the reduction in tumor cell burden as a result of therapy was sufficient to relieve symptoms but not large enough to cause a measurable decrease in the size of the tumor mass. It has been shown with animal models that a tumor cell kill in excess of five logs may be insufficient to induce a 50% decrease in the size of a palpable tumor mass.[28] A large part of the breast cancer tumor mass may be supporting stroma, and in some cases total eradication of tumor cells within this stroma may not have a measurable effect on the size of the tumor.[33] Changes in tumor size may also require both eradication of tumor cells and healing. This is true of bone metastases, for which response is usually scored only when there is sclerosis of a previously lytic lesion. A response in the liver cannot be observed until the filling defects on a liver scan have been replaced with normal liver cells.

The relief of symptoms as a result of chemotherapy may persist long after the chemotherapy has been discontinued. Nineteen of 21 patients with metastatic disease to the bone were evaluable for a subjective response after treatment with combination chemotherapy. All 19 experienced initial relief of pain. Sixteen of these patients were observed for variable times without progression of disease after completion of the chemotherapy, and six of the patients remained stable and free of symptoms for periods of 2 years or more after the completion of chemotherapy.[34]

The side effects experienced with chemotherapy are variable from one patient to another, and measurements of the severity of nausea and vomiting, stomatitis, and fatigue are also subjective. It is conceivable that these toxicities might outweigh any benefit resulting from relief of symptoms and cause a net reduction in the quality of life of many or most treated patients. This possibility was evaluated among a group of patients randomized to receive either relatively nontoxic endocrine therapy or combination chemotherapy.[35,36] All patients in this study were asked to complete a linear analogue self-assessment form designed to measure patient responses in four broad categories: symptoms and side effects, anxiety and depression, personal relations, and physical performance.[37] Prior to initiating therapy and periodically following the start of therapy, patients were asked to indicate their response in ten categories (Fig. 13-10). By drawing a vertical line somewhere along a horizontal line with extremes of feeling at each end, the patient could indicate her relative feelings and performance level. For example, the patient could indicate that she was very depressed, very cheerful, or somewhere between those two extremes. Each category was scored by assuming that the left end of the horizontal line represented 1 and the right end 100. As might be expected, patients treated with combination chemotherapy had a significantly greater incidence of alopecia, nausea, and vomiting. However, patients treated with chemotherapy also had a significant increase in sense of well-being ($p<0.05$ at week 11).

The greatest differences in linear analogue self-assessment scores were seen in the comparison between responders and nonresponders to chemotherapy (Fig. 13-11). There were no differences noted during the first 3 weeks of therapy, but thereafter the difference in the incidence of depression grew and was statistically significant at weeks 11 and 15 ($p<0.01$). Other areas in which there was a statistically significant difference in the experience of responders and nonresponders included pain; the frequency of dyspnea; anorexia; the frequency of insomnia; the degree to which the patients had a sense of well-being; the ability to do housework, shopping, and other chores; and the patient's sense of ease in socializing.[37] This suggests (but does not prove) that chemotherapy, even with its attendant side effects, may improve the quality of life for patients symptomatic from breast cancer metastases. An objective response to therapy in this group of patients might reasonably be taken as a reflection or even an underestimation of subjective benefit.

Feel Lousy	Feel Great
Very Depressed	Very Cheerful
Doing Nothing	Very Active
Much Pain	No Pain
Very Nauseous	No Nausea
Poor Appetite	Great Appetite
Unable to perform the work	Able to do as much as desired
Little social activity	Very Active
Very Anxious	Calm
Not At All	Greatly

FIGURE 13-10. Format for performing linear analogue self-assessment (LASA). Patients are asked to place a vertical mark along the horizontal line at the point that best approximates the patient's feeling between the two extremes expressed at the end of each line. The test is scored by measuring the distance between the left end of the line (value 1) and the right end of the line (value 100). (Baum M, Priestman T, West RR, et al: A comparison of subjective responses in a trial comparing endocrine with cytotoxic treatment in advanced carcinoma of the breast. In Mouridsen HT, Palshof T (eds): Breast Cancer—Experimental and Clinical Aspects, pp 223–226. Elmsford, New York, Pergamon Press, 1980.)

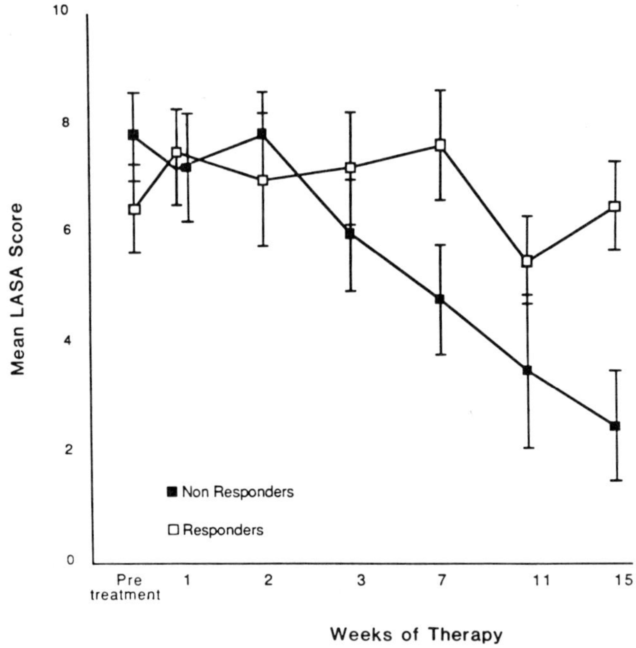

FIGURE 13-11. Mean LASA scores (± se) (see Fig. 13-10) for depression at time point following initiation of therapy for patients responding to (0-0) and patients failing chemotherapy. Difference statistically significant ($p < 0.01$) at weeks 11 and 15. (Baum M, Priestman T, West RR, et al: A comparison of subjective responses in a trial comparing endocrine with cytotoxic treatment in advanced carcinoma of the breast. In Mouridsen HT, Palshof T (eds): Breast Cancer—Experimental and Clinical Aspects, pp 223–226. Elmsford, New York, Pergamon Press, 1980.)

ACTIVITY OF INDIVIDUAL DRUGS

No other solid tumor is as sensitive to such a large array of different drugs and drug groups as breast cancer. However, defining the relative activity of each of these drugs is difficult. Evidence of an objective response must be based on a decrease in the size of measurable lesions, but many of the common sites of breast cancer metastases are not easily measurable. Metastases to bone may form lytic or blastic lesions. The blastic lesions may never show evidence of change. The lytic lesions usually do not decrease in size linearly with response to the drug, but lytic lesions may become sclerotic (i.e., may take on the appearance of a blastic lesion), and this is thought to reflect healing. Pleural effusions are not only difficult to measure but frequently disappear after thoracentesis in spite of evidence of disease progression elsewhere. Conversely, pleural effusions may increase or remain stable in spite of shrinkage of other lesions. Measurement of response to breast cancer therapy is most often based on changes in the size of skin recurrences, lymphadenopathy, or untreated primary breast tumors. Changes in these lesions may also be difficult to interpret since most of them consist of a mixture of breast cancer cells and a reactive stroma. A biopsy specimen of skin lesions after partial response may show very few or no cancer cells and many fibroblasts organizing into a scar.[33,38] Scoring responses to therapy for metastatic breast cancer has a large subjective component, and this is one reason why response rates vary between investigators (and between countries).

A second limitation to comparisons of the relative efficacy of individual drugs or drug programs is differing criteria for a partial or complete response. As a result of recent work by international committees, standard definitions have been formulated and accepted by most trial organzations in the United States and by the UICC worldwide.[38] (A detailed description of these definitions is given in Chapter 17). For most sites of disease, an objective response is defined as a reduction of 50% or more in the sum of the product of the longest perpendicular diameters of measurable sites of disease without evidence of progression at any other sites. A complete response requires disappearance of evidence of active disease at all known sites of metastases without evidence of new metastatic growths. Progression is defined as a greater than 25% increase in the size of measurable lesions. Although these definitions of response were first proposed almost 10 years ago, there is considerable variation in the interpretation of these general rules by individual investigators. These criteria were not used in most of the phase II trials performed in the 1950s and 1960s, when the standard agents for the treatment of metastatic breast cancer were first tested. For this reason, comparisons of the results from these early trials and trials performed after 1975 may be very misleading.[39] The calculated response rate to cyclophosphamide is more than 50% when any patient with an "objective response" is included. The calculated response rate to cyclophosphamide is only 26% when studies that used response criteria other than those recommended by the UICC were excluded (Table 13-23).

The selection of patients for new drug trials has also changed with the development of effective chemotherapy combinations for the treatment of metastatic breast cancer. The extent of the patient's prior therapy, especially the patient's prior chemotherapy, is the single most important predictive factor for a response to subsequent chemotherapy (see below). In phase II trials evaluating 5-fluorouracil, cyclophosphamide, and many of the other standard drugs, most patients had been previously treated with hormone therapy but no chemotherapy. At most, patients in these trials would have had prior exposure to short courses of one or two other single agents. More than half of the phase II trial reports from that era provide no information about prior exposure to chemotherapy, presumably because prior chemotherapy was not seen as an important predictive factor for response or because so few of the patients had had prior chemotherapy. Phase II trials performed in the early 1970s, when doxorubicin was introduced, included many patients who had had only one prior combination chemotherapy regimen. Phase II trials performed today usually include only those patients who have had prior exposure to doxorubicin. Most patients in these studies have had adjuvant combination chemotherapy and one regimen for metastatic disease, and many patients have had three or more combination chemotherapy programs before they are treated with a new drug.

Table 13-23
Definition of Tumor Response: Effect on Response Rates to Chemotherapeutic Agents Used in the Treatment of Metastatic Breast Cancer

	Response Rates (%)	
Drug	*Response if defined as <50% reduction in tumor size or not specified*	*Response if defined as reduction of ≥50% in tumor size**
Cyclophosphamide	52	26
Methotrexate	30	20
5-Fluorouracil	43	22
Vincristine	16	14

* Objective response defined as a reduction of 50% or more in the sum of the product of the longest perpendicular diameters of measurable sites without progression elsewhere. Denominator for response includes all patients started on therapy.

(Hoogstraten B, Fabian C: A reappraisal of single drugs in advanced breast cancer. Cancer Clin Trials 2:101–109, 1979.)

This evolution in the way that new drugs are tested in the clinic makes comparisons between the response rates of single agents tested in different decades meaningless. In an attempt to circumvent this problem, the response rates for single agents in previously untreated patients has been determined whenever possible (see Tables 13-24, 13-26, and 13-31). For the standard agents described in Table 13-24, the overall response rate is close to the response rate obtained in patients without prior exposure to chemotherapy. This is because most of the patients were previously untreated. The difference in response rates between patients with prior therapy or with no prior therapy is most evident for the drugs outlined in Table 13-26. These are promising agents that have been extensively evaluated but have not yet been accepted as standard drugs for the treatment of metastatic breast cancer. The response rate is 50% to 100% greater in patients without prior chemotherapy than in patients who had prior chemotherapy for metastatic breast cancer.

The Standard Drugs

Four drugs, used alone or in combination, constitute the core of almost every cytotoxic program used to treat metastatic breast cancer. These are cyclophosphamide (C), 5-fluorouracil (F), methotrexate (M), and doxorubicin (A). In phase II trials, these four drugs have the highest single-agent activity among all patients studied and among those patients with no prior chemotherapy (Table 13-24). There is only limited cross-resistance between these agents. Cyclophosphamide and 5-fluorouracil were evaluated as single agents in previously untreated patients using a randomized trial with a crossover design. Seven of 32 (22%) of the patients initially randomized to cyclophosphamide and 11 of 30 (37%) of the patients given 5-fluorouracil initially responded. On crossover, 7 of 30 (23%) secondarily treated wth cyclophosphamide and 4 of 32 (13%) secondarily treated with 5-fluorouracil responded.[45] Methotrexate was introduced for the treatment of metastatic breast cancer after the acceptance of cyclophosphamide and 5-fluorouracil, and most of the responses in previously treated patients were in patients with prior exposure to one or both of these drugs (Table 13-24). Doxorubicin was evaluated in a randomized crossover trial with the combination CMF.[3] Although in this study doxorubicin was combined with vincristine (V), vincristine probably contributed little to the responses observed (see below). Before crossover, 56% of patients responded to CMF and 52% to AV. After crossover for progressive disease, 8 of 23 (35%) responded secondarily to AV and 3 of 15 (20%) responded to CMF.

Four of the drugs listed in Table 13-24 are alkylating

Table 13-24
Single-Agent Activity of the Drugs Most Often Used Alone or in Combination to Treat Metastatic Breast Cancer

		Response Rates							
		All Patients			With Prior Chemotherapy*		No Prior Chemotherapy*		
Drug Name	**Years of Publications**	*N**	*%*	*Range*	*N**	*%*	*N**	*%*	**References**
Chlorambucil	1959–68	58	17	0–19	—	—	—	—	40, 41
Cyclophosphamide	1961–79	887	33	11–59	135	22	594	36	42–57
Doxorubicin	1974–85	1122	32	0–87	940	29	182	43	13, 23, 58–79
5-Fluorouracil	1961–81	1921	27	0–68	116	15	667	28	10, 42, 45, 47, 48, 51–53, 80–97
L-Phenylalanine mustard	1965–82	222	20	0–23	45	4	91	25	79, 96, 98–100
Methotrexate	1952–81	547	28	4–54	134	17	76	26	16, 40, 47, 48, 79, 85, 101–109
Mitomycin C	1976–85	307	22	5–35	307	22	0	—	65, 110–114
Thiotepa	1959–68	266	29	8–37	1	—	139	25	40, 52, 57, 96, 97, 115
Vinblastine	1962–72	119	21	0–45	8	0	—	—	79, 116–120
Vincristine	1964–76	251	19	0–40	20	10	12	8	48, 51, 79, 96, 121–123

* N, number of patients evaluated. "Prior Chemotherapy" or "No Prior Chemotherapy" administered for metastatic breast cancer.

agents. It has not been demonstrated in controlled trials that any one of these agents is more effective than the others. In uncontrolled trials, the response rates obtained with cyclophosphamide have consistently been higher than with the other agents. Cyclophosphamide is equally effective whether administered orally or intravenously.[79] In a retrospective analysis of a series of uncontrolled trials, 37 of 106 (35%) patients responded when cyclophosphamide was given as a daily oral dose and 137 of 395 (35%) when it was given intravenously as a loading dose followed by daily oral administration. Only 5 of 25 (20%) patients responded when cyclophosphamide was given by an intermittent intravenous dose schedule. In experimental systems, there is a steep dose-response curve to cyclophosphamide.[124] There are no controlled studies of cyclophosphamide dose in the treatment of metastatic breast cancer, but a retrospective analysis suggested that the dose was not a critical factor.[78] Cyclophosphamide is used in combination with other drugs, both parenterally and orally. It is also one of the only agents that is frequently used alone, rather than in combination, to treat patients with metastatic breast cancer. As a single agent, it has very mild toxicities, and 50 mg to 100 mg daily may be used as an alternative to more intensive combinations in patients, such as the elderly, for whom toxicity is a critical issue. At this dose, chronic myelosuppression will occur, and the drug dose may be titrated to maintain a total white count between 2000 and 3000/μ.

Thiotepa, L- phenylalanine mustard (L-PAM), and chlorambucil cause less acute toxicity, especially less nausea and vomiting, than cyclophosphamide. These drugs have not been used frequently in the treatment of metastatic breast cancer because they are considered less effective than cyclophosphamide, but all of them have been used in one or more adjuvant chemotherapy programs because they are less toxic (see Chapter 10). They have not been used as secondary agents after failure to respond to cyclophosphamide because the alkylating agents have traditionally been thought to be cross-resistant with each other. Recent studies indicate this may not be true, and under some circumstances these agents may even be synergistic.[125]

5-Fluorouracil was one of the first cytotoxic agents to be extensively tested in patients with metastatic breast cancer. This drug is usually administered intravenously, but it is also active when given by the oral route. In a randomized trial, 6 of 25 (24%) patients responded to oral administration and 7 of 24 (29%) to intravenous administration.[82] Pharmacologic studies show that the uptake of 5-fluorouracil following oral administration is erratic,[126] and it is for this reason that this drug is preferentially given intravenously. Four different dose schedules of 5-fluorouracil administration have been evaluated in a randomized trial. None proved superior to the others.[84] 5-Fluorouracil is rarely used as a single agent today, but it is effective when administered weekly in a dose of 500 mg intravenously or orally. More frequently it is used as part of the CMF regimen, in which it is administered on days 1 and 8 of a monthly cycle (see below).

The single-agent activity of methotrexate is equal to that of 5-fluorouracil. In early phase II trials, the use of a single daily dose, continuous infusion, or divided doses of methotrexate resulted in response rates of 38% to 44%. In contrast, the response rate to monthly loading doses was considerably less, 23%.[79] An optimal dose schedule for methotrexate administration has not been determined in controlled trials. As a single agent, methotrexate may be given either weekly or twice weekly, although with frequent administration there may be severe stomatitis. In combination, methotrexate is more frequently given on the same schedule as 5-fluorouracil or in sequence with 5-fluorouracil (see below). Methotrexate is the drug most frequently used for meningeal carcinomatosis from breast cancer.[127] In this setting, the drug is often administered intrathecally, but it may be more effective if given through an Ommaya reservoir. Methotrexate has been administered in doses as high as 7.5 g/m^2, but at doses in this range rescue with leucovorin is required. Eight of 27 patients previously treated with chemotherapy responded to high-dose methotrexate; 9 of these 27 patients had previously been treated with standard doses of methotrexate.[101] High-dose methotrexate has also been used in combination chemotherapy,[16] but there are no controlled trials that demonstrate that such high doses are more effective than conventional doses of methotrexate. The use of leucovorin rescue decreases the myelosuppressive toxicity from methotrexate, and as a result rescued methotrexate used in a combination may permit administration of higher doses of the other drugs included in the combination. Methotrexate doses of 3g/m^2 or more result in therapeutic levels of methotrexate in the cerebrospinal fluid (CSF), and there are reports of other solid tumors metastatic to the brain responding to high doses of methotrexate given intravenously.[128] There are no similar studies demonstrating that high-dose methotrexate will result in an objective decrease in the size of central nervous system metastases from breast cancer, but a few patients have had relief from the symptoms of central nervous system metastases using weekly high-dose methotrexate with leucovorin rescue.[129] High-dose methotrexate does not prevent the appearance of central nervous system metastases, however.[16]

Doxorubicin is the single most active agent in the treatment of metastatic breast cancer. In experimental systems, there is a steep dose response to doxorubicin,[130] but the duration of exposure to the drug is also a critical factor, especially when doxorubicin is added to plateau phase cells (i.e., resting cells) in *in vitro* systems.[131] The dose-response curve is less steep in plateau phase cells, and this observation may be relevant to the treatment of a tumor, such as breast cancer, with a low growth fraction. Uncontrolled clinical trials suggest that doses of 90 to 135 mg/m^2 are more effective than doses of 75 mg/m^2 or less.[63] Only one controlled trial comparing several doxorubicin doses in patients with metastatic breast cancer has been conducted, but 75 mg/m^2 was the highest dose employed in this study.[59] There were no significant differences in response rate among patients considered to be in a "good risk" category who were treated with doses between 45 and 75 mg/m^2. "Poor-risk" patients were randomized to receive either 25 mg/m^2 or 50 mg/m^2, and the response rates to these two doses were 6% and 24%, respectively, suggesting that there may be a dose below which doxorubicin is ineffective or less effective. Doxorubicin is frequently used as a single agent, since it has been shown in randomized trials to be as effective as CFP[75] or CMFVP.[23] When used as a single agent, 60 to 75 mg/m^2 may be administered on a three weekly schedule. This drug is cardiotoxic, and the incidence of congestive heart failure increases sharply after a cumulative dose of 450 mg/m^2 has been given. Weekly doses of methotrexate are less cardiotoxic[132,133] and are probably as effective. Patients with metastatic breast cancer and no prior chemotherapy were randomized to receive a combination of mitomycin C and doxorubicin given on either a weekly or monthly schedule.[134] Eleven of the 26 (42%) patients on the weekly schedule and 14 of the 31 (45%) on the monthly schedule responded. Although the weekly regimen is less cardiotoxic and may be associated with less gastrointestinal toxicity, it does require more frequent visits to the clinic, and there is increased risk of extravasation and subsequent ulceration. There are advantages and disadvantages to each of these doxorubicin schedules, and the selection of one rather than the other will depend on the clinical setting.

The vinca alkaloids, vincristine and vinblastine, are attractive agents for the treatment of any cancer because their mechanism of action is different from the antibiotics and the alkylating agents, and it is probable that they are non–cross-resistant with many of the other standard drugs. Vincristine has been used most extensively. It is not myelosuppressive and may be used in a combination of drugs without compromising the dose of any of the other drugs. The response rate to vincristine is less than that of the other drugs described thus far. In uncontrolled phase II trials, there seemed to be a dose response to this drug. At 12.5 μg/kg, no responses were observed. At 75 μg/kg the response rate was 33%.[79] This was observed in two separate studies, but the toxicity was also noted to increase proportionately. For example, in one study the incidence of severe neurotoxicity was 12% when 34 μg/kg vincristine was administered.[121] Although it has been suggested that vincristine may be synergistic with mitomycin C and doxorubicin,[135] there is very little evidence that this drug adds anything except neurotoxicity to most standard combinations (see below). Since vincristine has very limited activity as a single agent, its role, if any, in the treatment of breast cancer is poorly defined.

Unlike vincristine, vinblastine induces considerable myelosuppression, and there are fewer data on its efficacy when used as a single agent and administered as a bolus. However, because of the possibility that vinblastine is not cross-resistant with other standard agents, it has been used in combination, especially with mitomycin C, as a second-line regimen for the treatment of patients refractory to CMF and doxorubicin.[136–139] None of these studies has established that the combination of mitomycin C and vinblastine together is better than mitomycin C alone. Vinblastine has also been used as a continuous infusion (see below).

Mitomycin C is the newest of the standard agents for the treatment of metastatic breast cancer. When used as a single agent in patients refractory to doxorubicin, response rates have ranged from 12% to 28%.[111,113,114] Mitomycin C has only rarely been used in combination chemotherapy regimens for patients without previous treatment, but in one study a combination of doxorubicin and mitomycin C was used in previously untreated pa-

Table 13-25
Drugs Commonly Used to Treat Breast Cancer:
Recommended Dose Schedule for Use as Single Agents and the Most Important Toxicities

	Single Agent			*Incidence of Toxicities*			
Drug Name	*Dose (mg/m²)*	*Route*	*Schedule*	*Myelo-Suppression*	*Nausea/ Vomiting*	*Alopecia*[145]	*Other Toxicities*
Chlorambucil	1–3	P O	q d	Moderate	Mild	Rare	Leukemia
Cyclophosphamide	400	I V	q d × 5*	Marked	Moderate	4–48%	Cystitis, water retention
	100	P O	q d × 14*	Moderate	Mild		
Doxorubicin	75	I V	q 3 wk	Marked	Moderate	100%	Cardiomyopathy, vesicant
	20	I V	Weekly	Moderate	Moderate	100%	Less cardiomyopathy, stomatitis
5-Fluorouracil	500	I V	Weekly	Moderate	Mild	20–57%	Cerebellar ataxia, stomatitis, conjunctivitis
L-Phenylalanine mustard	6	P O	q d × 5†	Moderate	Mild	Rare	Leukemia
Methotrexate	25	I V	Twice weekly	Moderate	Mild	0–6%	Stomatitis
	12§	I T	q 4 d	Mild	None		Fever, motor dysfunction
	1000–3000	I V with rescue	Weekly[16]	Mild	Mild		Renal failure, seizure, hepatic dysfunction
Mitomycin C	12	I V	q 3 wk[143]	Marked	Mild	Rare	Renal, cardiotoxicity, vesicant
	20	I V	q 6 wk[113]	Marked	Mild		Pulmonary toxicity
Thiotepa	0.2 mg/kg	I V	q d × 5[115, 144]	Moderate	Mild	None	
Vinblastine	4	I V	Weekly	Marked	Mild	3–15%	Mucositis, vesicant
Vincristine	1‡	I V	Weekly	Mild	Mild	22–51%	Neuropathy, Inappropriate ADH, vesicant

* Cycle usually repeated monthly
† Dose schedule used in NSABP trials[142]
‡ Maximum recommended total dose is 2 mg
§ Total dose rather than mg/m²
q, every; d, day; PO, orally; IV, intravenous; intrathecal, (Modified from Chabner BA, Myers CE: Clinical pharmacology of cancer chemotherapy. In DeVita VT Jr, Hellman S, Rosenberg SA: Cancer: Principles and Practice of Oncology, 2nd ed, pp 287–328. Philadelphia, JB Lippincott, 1985)

tients.[140] Twenty-one of 35 (60%) patients responded, but only 1 of 5 patients responded secondarily to CMF after treatment with the doxorubicin/mitomycin regimen. The incidence of cardiopulmonary insufficiency among these patients treated with doxorubicin/mitomycin C was 14%, and two patients died of congestive heart failure. Other programs using mitomycin C as a first-line agent in combination with doxorubicin plus or minus other drugs have failed to show any evidence of increased benefit from the use of mitomycin C, but none of these has been randomized trials in which the use of mitomycin C was a variable.[134,135,141] Mitomycin C is an important drug for the treatment of breast cancer, but at present it should be reserved for use as a single agent in patients who are refractory to treatment with the other standard agents (see below).

All of the standard cytotoxic agents are associated with some nausea and vomiting, but the gastrointestinal toxicities are mild when these drugs are used as single agents (Table 13-25). In combinaton regimens, these symptoms are usually more severe. Most of these drugs—including cyclophosphamide, the vinca alkaloids, and 5-fluorouracil—cause partial alopecia in less than half the patients. Only doxorubicin predictably causes total alopecia in every treated patient. Several of the drugs, especially the alkylating agents, have a potential for inducing leukemia. All but vincristine cause variable degrees of myelosuppression, and both the white count and platelet count should be monitored regularly when these drugs are used. In general, these drugs should be administered under the supervision of a specialist with experience in their use. When used appropriately, these drugs may have minimal side effects and result in significant palliation of symptoms, even in elderly and debilitated patients.

Drugs With Questionable Activity in Metastatic Breast Cancer

Nitrogen mustard and 5-fluoro-2′-deoxyuridine (FUdR) are active drugs in the treatment of metastatic breast cancer. Neither has been used in combinations or has found an established role, primarily because they have no demonstrable advantage over other alkylating agents or 5-fluorouracil in the treatment of breast cancer. Ifosfamide (I) is another very active alkylating agent, and it has been

Table 13-26
Drugs With Variable Single-Agent Activity but No Established Role in the Treatment of Metastatic Breast Cancer

		Response Rates (%)							
		All Patients			With Prior Chemotherapy*		No Prior Chemotherapy*		
Drug Name	**Years of Publications**	N*	%	Range	N*	%	N*	%	**References**
BCNU	1972–73	155	16	7–29	—	—	5	—	39
Bisantrene	1983–85	306	15	5–23	306	15	0	—	71, 147–152
CCNU	1973–81	108	9	0–14	87	9	21	10	13, 153–156
Cisplation	1978–82	119	8	0–14	119	8	0	—	198–202
4′-Demethoxydaunorubicin	1985–86	121	26	11–50	64	17	57	37	70, 157–159
4′-Deoxydoxorubicin	1985–86	56	11	0–21	33	6	23	17	70, 160, 161
Elliptinium	1982–85	228	27	0–33	162	22	66	37	162–166
4′- Epidoxorubicin	1983–86	210	34	16–62	180	27	30	73	67–70, 167–169
Estracyt	1982	97	20	5–39	—	—	12	—	170
5-Fluoro-2′ -deoxyuridine	1963–73	152	35	12–48	—	—	7	—	85, 171–175
Hexamethylmelamine	1969–79	151	11	0–32	151	11	0	—	176–181
Ifosfamide	1974–76	48	27	15–40	28	32	20	20	182, 183
Mitolactol	1976–84	142	17	0–44	142	17	0	—	184–188
Mitoxantrone	1981–85	694	20	3–31	491	18	203	27	71–73, 189–197
Nitrogen mustard	1960–61	95	18	8–25	—	—	39	8	52, 115
Prednimustine	1980–83	166	26	22–40	131	21	35	46	203, 204
Vindesine	1979–82	195	23	4–31	171	21	24	39	205–212

* N, Number of patients evaluated. "Prior Chemotherapy" or "No Prior Chemotherapy" administered for metastatic breast cancer.

combined with doxorubicin and 5-fluorouracil as a first-line regimen to treat patients without prior chemotherapy.[146] Thirty-two of 49 (55%) of the patients responded to this program. This response rate, the duration of response, and the survival time of these patients was not different from that of patients treated at the same institution with a combination of FAC, but the hematuria, nausea, and vomiting observed with FAI was considerably greater. These investigators concluded that ifosfamide was not more effective but was more toxic than cyclophosphamide.

When used as single agents, the nitrosoureas have very limited activity in the treatment of metastatic breast cancer (Table 13-26). BCNU and CCNU appear to be the most promising of these agents in phase II studies (Tables 13-26 and 13-31). These two drugs have been used in combination regimens to determine whether they might be synergistic with any of the other standard agents. The response rate to a combination of doxorubicin and either CCNU, BCNU, or methyl-CCNU varied between 16% and 22% in three studies[213–215] and was 44% in a fourth study.[216] All of these studies were performed with patients who had previously received chemotherapy. The studies were uncontrolled, but the doxorubicin/nitrosourea combination did not appear to be more effective than doxorubicin. BCNU was combined with 5-fluorouracil, imidazole carboxamide, vincristine, and prednisone, and this regimen induced a response in 36 of 92 (39%) patients previously treated with chemotherapy.[217] A similar combination using mitomycin C instead of 5-fluorouracil and imidazole carboxamide induced a 10% response.[218] In the only randomized trial evaluating the efficacy of a nitrosourea in previously untreated patients, the response rate to CAMP (CCNU, L-PAM, methotrexate, and prednisone) was 20%, significantly less than the 50% response rate to CMF.[219]

The response rate to hexamethylmelamine in early phase II trials was 25%.[220] This is a synthetic agent similar to triethylenemelamine, but it may have a mechanism of action different from other alkylating agents. For this reason, hexamethylmelamine has been studied extensively as a single agent (Table 13-26) and more recently in combinations.[179,221–223] One of these was a randomized trial comparing hexamethylmelamine as a single agent with a combination of mitomycin C, hexamethylmelamine, and vincristine.[179] None of the 15 patients treated with hexamethylmelamine alone but 5 of the 27 patients treated with the combination responded. The toxicity associated with hexamethylmelamine is significant. In one study, nausea and vomiting were severe in 67% of the patients and were dose limiting in 14%. Hexamethylmelamine causes neurotoxicity, which was severe in 10 of 19 patients in one study.[180] Hexamethylmelamine has some limited activity in metastatic breast cancer, but the excessive toxicity associated with this drug seems to preclude any future role.

Mitolactol (dibromodulcitol) is related to the alkylating agents but may not be cross-resistant with cyclophosphamide.[187] It is active as a single agent, but its activity in patients previously treated with doxorubicin is limited. In

Table 13-27
Randomized Trials Evaluating the Efficacy of Mitolactol (D) in Combination With Other Drugs

Agents	Authors	Prior Chemotherapy	Number of Patients	Response Rate (%)	Median TTF (Months)	Median Survival (Months)
A vs. DA	Ingle et al[224]	Yes No A	74 77	30 26	3.7 3.2	7.7 7.5
AV vs. DAV	Cummings et al[225]	Yes No A	92 94	27 23	3.8 2.9	8.3 7.1
CAF vs. DAV-CMF	Tormey et al[9]	None	46 48	63 71	NS	NS
MiT vs. DAT	Falkson et al[226]	Limited No A	53 60	28 38	2.9 3.7	7.6 9.7
MiT vs. DAT	Chang et al[227]	Limited No A	12 11	17 45	2.8 3.8	10.0 6.7

None of the observed differences reached statistical significance. A, doxorubicin; V, vincristine; D, mitolactol; Mi, mitomycin C; T, tamoxifen; F, 5-fluorouracil; M, methotrexate; NS, not significantly different; TTF, time to failure.

an early phase II trial (before doxorubicin), 12 of 30 patients (40%) responded to single-agent mitolactol.[188] In more recent trials performed with patients previously treated with doxorubicin, responses were seen in 0 of 22[184] and 1 of 38 patients.[185] Mitolactol has been evaluated in controlled trials with previously treated and untreated patients (Table 13-27). In all of these trials, mitolactol has been combined with doxorubicin in an attempt to develop a combination program that is non–cross-resistant with CMF. However, the combination mitolactol and doxorubicin (DA) was no more effective than doxorubicin alone,[224] and the combination of mitolactol, doxorubicin, and vincristine (DAV) was no more effective than AV alone in previously treated patients.[225] A combination of mitolactol, doxorubicin, and tamoxifen (DAT) was compared with a combination of mitomycin C and tamoxifen (MiT) in two groups of patients with limited prior chemotherapy.[226,227] The mitolactol-containing regimen was significantly better in both of these trials, and the toxicity associated with DAV was significantly greater. The patients treated with DAV had more nausea and vomiting ($p=0.0001$), more alopecia ($p<0.0001$), and more severe leukopenia ($p=0.02$) than the patients on MiT. The mitomycin C regimen caused more thrombocytopenia ($p=0.03$).[226] The potentially non–cross-resistant regimens of DAV and CMF were alternated every three cycles and compared in a randomized study with CAF alone.[9] There was no improvement in response rate, time to treatment failure, or survival for patients on the alternating cycle. Mitolactol is a drug that has activity in breast cancer, has reasonable toxicity, but has no demonstrated advantage over standard agents or synergism with doxorubicin.

Cisplatin has been studied extensively in breast cancer, primarily because of its great activity in other tumor types. Most of these studies have been performed in patients with extensive previous treatment. In one trial, a high dose of cisplatin, 3 mg/kg, induced a response in 4 of 19 (21%) of patients, whereas a dose of 1.5 mg/kg resulted in no responses among 18 treated patients.[199] This was not confirmed by others evaluating a similar dose range.[201] Cisplatin has been evaluated as part of a drug combination in two randomized trials. In both of these trials, a combination of cyclophosphamide, doxorubicin, and cisplatin was compared with either CMFVP[228] or CFP.[229] The first study was performed in patients without prior chemotherapy, and the response rate was 27 of 36 (75%) to CAP and 16 of 36 (44%) to CMFVP ($p<0.01$).[228] The complete response rate and the median duration of response were also longer for the patients treated with CAP. Survival data are still unavailable. In contrast, the second study was performed in patients with prior therapy, and the response rate to CAP was 22 of 45 (49%) and to CFP 19 of 41 (46%). There was no significant difference in the time to treatment failure or survival time. There are insufficient data to conclude that cisplatin has more than very limited activity in the treatment of metastatic breast cancer.

Newer Drugs

Elliptinium is a plant alkaloid that was developed at the Institut Gustave Roussy in Villejuif, France. Experience with this drug outside of France is still limited.[162–164] One of the major advantages of this agent is its lack of bone marrow toxicity. Its major disadvantage is hemolysis, which may be dose limiting. Coombs'-positive reactions have been observed in up to 21% of patients,[166] but hemolysis is usually limited to less than 7% of patients. Severe vomiting may occur in 30% of patients, and administration of the drug requires a central catheter because of associated phlebitis.[163] Patients may experience chills. Antielliptinium antibodies can be detected. Patients may have mild azotemia or other evidence of renal abnormalities, but proximal tubular enzyme markers have not been found to be elevated.[164] The drug is active, and the response rate in previously untreated patients is as high as 37%. This drug has not been used in combination chemotherapy regimens.

Vindesine, new anthracycline analogues, anthracene derivatives, and chemotherapy-hormone esters all represent new drugs or groups of drugs characterized by less toxicity without increased efficacy. Vindesine is a semisynthetic vinca alkaloid that was designed to be less neurotoxic than vincristine and less myelosuppressive than vinblastine. This goal appears to have been achieved. In a randomized comparison of vindesine plus doxorubicin and vincristine plus doxorubicin, 7 of 29 patients treated with the vincristine combination developed paresthesias or constipation; this was dose limiting in 6 of the patients. Seven of the 26 patients treated with the vindesine combination had mild neurotoxicity, and it was dose limiting in only 2 (8%). There was no difference in the marrow toxicity observed with the two programs.[230] Vindesine is as effective as or more effective than the other alkylating agents. It has been evaluated in a randomized comparison with vinblastine and vincristine. None of the patients treated with vincristine as a single agent responded, whereas 30% and 31% responded to vinblastine and vindesine, respectively (Table 13-28).[211] In a randomized trial in which vincristine and vindesine were each combined with doxorubicin, no significant differences in response rate were observed.[230] From these studies, vindesine appears to be as active as vinblastine and more active than vincristine. However, it has not been established that vindesine (or any other vinca alkaloid) contributes in any important way to the overall activity of combinations in which they are included. Vindesine has been combined with cisplatin[231] and mitomycin C,[137] but these regimens were evaluated in uncontrolled trials. In phase II trials of vindesine for the treatment of leukemia, some patients who responded to a 48-hour continuous infusion were refractory to bolus infusions of vindesine.[232] For this reason, both bolus and continuous infusion schedules of vindesine have been evaluated in patients with metastatic breast cancer,[209] and there is very little difference in the response rate to these two schedules. Vindesine may not be cross-resistant with the other vinca alkaloids. In one trial, half of the patients had had vincristine prior to entry into the study. The overall response rate was 19% among these 31 previously treated ptients, and there was no difference in the response rate of patients with or without prior vincristine exposure.[210]

The efficacy of doxorubicin has stimulated a search for another anthracycline that is as effective (or more effective) without the cardiotoxicity associated with doxorubicin. Three promising agents with activity in metastatic breast cancer have been developed. 4′-Epidoxorubicin was synthesized by epimerization of the hydroxyl group at position four of the sugar moiety. 4′-Demethoxydaunorubicin (idarubicin) has a hydrogen substituted for the methyl group at position four in the D ring of daunorubicin. 4′-Deoxydoxorubicin (esorubicin) was synthesized by removing the hydroxyl group at position four of the amino sugar of doxorubicin. Although all three of these drugs are active, 4′-epidoxorubicin has been studied more extensively than the other two (Table 13-29). No significant differences in response rate have been observed in multiple randomized trials comparing doxorubicin and 4′-epidoxorubicin.[68,69,233,234] The acute gastrointestinal toxicity associated with 4′-epidoxorubicin is considerably less than that observed following doxorubicin therapy, but the

Table 13-28
Randomized Trials Evaluating Efficacy of Vindesine

*Drugs**	*Dose Schedule†*	*Number of Patients*	*Response Rate (%)*	*Authors*
Vindesine vs.	1.2 mg/m^2 bolus, days 1–5	16	31	
Vinblastine vs.	1.7 mg/m^2 bolus, days 1–5	13	30	Yap et al[211]
Vincristine	0.4 mg/m^2 bolus, days 1–5	15	0	
A + Vincristine vs.	2 mg bolus, days 1 and 8	29	59	Smith et al[230]
A + Vindesine	5 mg bolus, days 1 and 8	26	62	
Vindesine vs.	1–1.2 mg/m^2 bolus, days 1 and 5	25	24	Fleishman et al[209]
Vindesine	1–1.2 mg/m^2 continuous, days 1–5	26	31	

*A, doxorubicin, 40 mg/M^2 on days 1 and 8.
† Dose of vinca alkaloid; cycle length 4 weeks, [230] 3 weeks, [209] and 3 weeks for vindesine and vinblastine, 2 weeks for vincristine.[211]

Table 13-29
Randomized Trials Evaluating the Efficacy of 4′-Epidoxorubicin

*Drugs**	*Dose Schedule†*	*Number of Patients‡*	*Response Rate (%)§*	*Median (Months) Duration§*	*Authors*
Doxorubicin vs.	75 mg/m²	21(8)	52	13	Brambilla et al[233]
4′-epidoxorubicin	75 mg/m²	21(11)	62	11	
Doxorubicin vs.	60 mg/m² continuous	16(0)	25	5	
4′-epidoxorubicin vs.	90 mg/m² continuous	24(0)	25	8	Hortobagyi et al[234]
4′-epidoxorubicin	90 mg/m² bolus	18(0)	17	7	
Doxorubicin vs.	60 mg/m²	28(0)	25	7	Jain et al[68]
4′-epidoxorubicin	85 mg/m²	24(0)	25	12	
Doxorubicin vs.	75 mg/m²	33(0)	30	—	Van Oosterom et al[69]
4′-epidoxorubicin	90 mg/m²	31(0)	32	—	
Carminomycin vs.	18 mg/m²	29(3)	3	3	Rozencweig et al[235]
4′-epidoxorubicin	90 mg/m²	34(3)	27	7	
FAC vs.	50 mg/m²	77(77)	43	6	Armand et al[236]
FEC*	50 mg/m²	82(82)	45	5	

* F, 5-fluorouracil; A, doxorubicin; C, cyclophosphamide; E, 4′-epidoxorubicin.
† Dose of doxorubicin or 4′-epidoxorubicin, injected every 3 weeks as a bolus except as indicated where 4′-epidoxorubicin or doxorubicin given continuously over 48 hours.
‡ Numbers in parentheses are the number of patients without prior chemotherapy for metastatic disease.
§ Differences not statistically significant except for the comparison of carminomycin with 4′-epidoxorubicin, where $p<0.02$.

severity and frequency of alopecia induced by the two drugs are the same.[70] Cardiotoxicity has been observed with 4′-epidoxorubicin, but both preclinical and clinical studies indicate that 4′-epidoxorubicin is less cardiotoxic than doxorubicin.[237] The median cumulative dose to the appearance of cardiotoxicity with 4′-epidoxorubicin is about half the median cumulative dose at which cardiotoxicity occurs with doxorubicin. However, when identical doses of 4′-epidoxorubicin and doxorubicin are used, less myelosuppression occurs with 4′-epidoxorubicin, and it is possible that 4′-epidoxorubicin is less effective in destroying tumor cells as well. To test this possibility, several trials have used a higher dose of 4′-epidoxorubicin. If the therapeutic index of 4′-epidoxorubicin is truly better than that of doxorubicin, the higher doses of 4′-epidoxorubicin might induce a higher response rate without a proportionate increase in toxicity. In these trials, the response rates to doxorubicin and 4′-epidoxorubicin were still the same, but some of the differences in gastrointestinal toxicity were no longer evident when equimyelosuppressive doses of the two drugs are used.[69,234] 4′-epidoxorubicin has also been used in combination with 5-fluorouracil and cyclophosphamide (FEC), and this regimen has been compared in a randomized trial with FAC.[236] The doses of 4′-epidoxorubicin and doxorubicin were the same, 50 mg/m², and no differences in response rate were observed. However, the FEC regimen was associated with less toxicity. 4′-Epidoxorubicin is clearly an effective agent in the treatment of breast cancer. It may be as effective as doxorubicin, but it remains to be seen whether its therapeutic index is greater than that of doxorubicin.

The anthracene derivatives constitute a new class of drugs that include bisantrene and mitoxantrone. These are the first totally synthetic DNA intercalating agents to be tested in the clinic. Bisantrene differs from mitoxantrone in the nature of the substitutions in the tricycline ring and in the structure of the side chains. The chemical structures of these two compounds are very different, but the clinical spectrum of activity is similar. Because the anthracenes and the anthracyclines are both ring structures, it is often assumed that the anthracenes are anthracycline derivatives. They are not. The fact that they are often compared in randomized trials further confuses this issue. Mitoxantrone has been studied more extensively than bisantrene (Table 13-30). In three separate trials, previously treated patients were randomized to receive either single-agent doxorubicin or mitoxantrone. In each study, the response rate to mitoxantrone was about 10% less than the response rate to doxorubicin.[72,73,240] These differences did not reach levels of statistical significance, and both the durability of response and the survival of patients treated with these two drugs were identical. Alopecia requiring a wig occurred in less than 10% of the mitoxantrone patients compared with almost all of the doxorubicin patients ($p<0.001$). Severe nausea and vomiting, stomatitis, and anorexia occurred significantly less frequently with mitoxantrone. The incidence of congestive heart failure, reduced left-ventricular ejection fractions, and abnormal cardiac biopsy scores was also significantly less following mitoxantrone therapy compared with doxorubicin. In one of the trials, the incidence of congestive heart failure with mitoxantrone was 4% and with doxorubicin 12%.[240] Although the mean endomyocardial biopsy grade increased with increasing doses of mitoxantrone, the severity of

Table 13-30
Randomized Trials Evaluating the Efficacy of Mitoxantrone

*Drugs**	*Dose†*	*Number of Patients‡*	*Response Rate (%) §*	*Median Duration (Months)§*	*Authors*
Doxorubicin vs.	60 mg/m²	39 (3)	33	3	Neidhart et al[73]
Mitoxantrone	12 mg/m²	40 (1)	23	4	
Doxorubicin vs.	75 mg/m²	123 (56)	35	5	Henderson et al[72]
Mitoxantrone	14 mg/m²	126 (59)	25	5	
Doxorubicin vs.	60 mg/m²	59 (0	27	—	
Mitoxantrone vs.	14 mg/m²	60 (0)	15	—	Osborne et al[71]
Bisantrene	320 mg/m²	61 (0)	18	—	
CAF vs.	50 mg/m²	101 (101)	47	6	Vogel et al[238]
CNF	10 mg/m²	103 (103)	41	6	
CAF vs.	50 mg/m²	44 (44)	ND	ND	Stewart et al[239]
CNF	10 mg/m²		ND	ND	

* C, cyclophosphamide; A, doxorubicin; F, 5-fluorouracil; N, mitoxantrone.
† Dose of doxorubicin or mitoxantrone administered intravenously every 3 weeks.
‡ Number in parentheses are the number of patients without prior chemotherapy for metastatic disease.
§ Observed differences are not statistically significant.
ND, No data yet available.

these changes and the doses at which they occurred were less than in patients treated with doxorubicin.[241] Mitoxantrone has been used in combination with cyclophosphamide and 5-fluorouracil. In spite of the addition of two other drugs, the reduced toxicity of mitoxantrone compared with doxorubicin was still evident.[238,239] Response data are available from only one of these trials, and the combination of cyclophosphamide, mitoxantrone, and 5-fluorouracil (CNF) is not significantly different from CAF.[238] Mitoxantrone is an effective new drug with very limited toxicity. It must be concluded from these trials that mitoxantrone is not as effective as doxorubicin, and it should not be used as a substitute for doxorubicin. However, it may be a valuable therapeutic alternative when toxicity is of paramount importance.

Prednimustine is an ester of prednisolone and chlorambucil. This drug has been studied more extensively in Europe than in the United States, and its major advantage is also its lack of toxicity. However, a leukocyte count below 1000 was observed in 7 and a platelet count below 50,000 in 8 of 35 patients. Hematologic toxicity may occur late in the course.[203] Nausea and vomiting also occur, and this may be dose related. Forty-two percent of patients treated on an intermittent schedule but only 21.5% given a continuous daily dose of prednimustine had gastrointestinal toxicity. Alopecia was observed in only two patients.[204] Prednimustine appears to be more effective than chlorambucil and prednisolone given as a combination regimen. Patients randomized to one of two dose schedules of prednimustine had a 22% to 23% response rate. The response rate to chlorambucil and prednisolone was 11% ($p<0.02$). The responses to prednimustine were also more durable. Prednimustine has been used in a combination regimen with methotrexate, 5-fluorouracil, and tamoxifen, but this was an uncontrolled trial. As a result, the contribution of prednimustine to the combination cannot be assessed.[242] Prednimustine may also have a role as a nontoxic therapeutic alternative for patients in whom toxicity is a major consideration.

INACTIVE DRUGS

More than 50 additional drugs have been studied in one or more trials and have been found to have little or no activity in metastatic breast cancer (Table 13-31). Most of these trials were small, and the most recent ones were performed in patients who were heavily pretreated. In some cases, there may be justification for further evaluation. In others, such as with amsacrine, the probability that the drug might prove to be active in metastatic breast cancer is very small. Carminomycin was compared with 4′-epidoxorubicin in a randomized trial, and the response rate was only 3% compared with 27% for the 4-epidoxorubicin (see Table 13-29).[235] Peptichemio is a multipeptide complex of L-PAM, and it has been compared in a randomized trial with the parent drug.[99] None of the 28 patients treated with single-agent L-PAM responded, and 7 of 28 (25%) responded to peptichemio. There were no crossover responses. This agent has also been used in combinations.[299–301] A combination of peptichemio, doxorubicin, and cyclophosphamide was evaluated in patients with limited prior therapy.[300] Fifty-four percent of the patients responded, but this was considered inferior to other doxorubicin-containing regimens commonly used for induction of response. (Etoposide-16) has also been studied

Table 13-31
Inactive Drugs Tested As Single Agents in Phase II Trials

Drug Name	Years of Publications	Number of Patients Studied		Response Rate (%)		References
		Total	Untreated*	Average	Range	
Aclacinomycin-A	1983	32	0	3	—	147
Aclarubicin	1983–85	47	0	0	0– 0	243, 244
Actinomycin-D	1959–65	59	—	8	0–20	40, 245
Amsacrine	1978–83	235	1	5	3–15	246–250
Anquidine	1979–84	27	0	4	0–14	251, 252
Azacytidine	1974	27	6	7	—	155
Aziridinylbenzoquinone (AZQ)	1982–84	81	0	2	0– 7	253–255
Azotomycin	1968	16	—	6	—	39
Bleomycin	1972–81	39	3	3	0– 5	154, 256, 257
Bruceantin	1982	15	0	0	—	258
Carboplatin	1985	14	0	0	—	259
Carminomycin	1979–84	87	3	14	3–29	235, 260, 261
Chlorozotocin	1981–82	43	0	0	0	262, 263
Chromomycin A3	1978	48	0	4	—	264
Cyclocytidine	1978	36	—	3	—	265
Cytembena	1976	15	0	0	—	266
Cytosine arabinoside	1969–70	64	—	9	0–15	79
10-Deaza-aminopterin	1983	29	0	3	—	267
Dianhydrogalactitol	1977–78	41	0	2	0– 4	268, 269
DL-metasarcolysin	1968	35	—	29	—	39
Estradiol mustard	1978	17	—	6	—	270
Ftoratur	1972–79	29	—	17	—	17
Guanazole	1975	5	—	0	—	39
Hydroxyurea	1964	21	—	19	13–14	79
ICRF-159	1977–79	51	0	4	0– 5	268, 271
Imidazole carboxamide	1970–76	51	—	10	0–14	272
Maytansine	1978–81	69	0	1	0– 3	273–275
6-Mercaptopurine	1968	44	—	6	14	276
Methyl-CCNU	1974	61	22	3	3– 3	13, 277
Methyl-GAG	1981	26	0	8	—	278
Mithramycin	1960–63	48	—	13	0–19	39, 245
Neocarcinostatin	1981	13	—	0	0– 0	279
PALA	1982	49	1	8	5–10	280, 281
PCNU	1982–83	43	0	2	0– 4	282, 283
Peptichemio	1980–82	84	0	18	14–25	18, 99
Piperazinedione	1977	42	0	7	—	284
Porfiromycin	1975	6	—	17	—	39
Procarbazine	1972	21	—	5	—	79
Puromycin	1959	6	5	0	—	40
Pyrazofurin	1978	17	0	0	0	285
Rubidazone	1979	32	0	0	0– 0	60, 286
Spirogermanium	1982–84	75	0	4	0–11	287–289
Streptonigrin	1976	21	—	19	—	39
Streptozotocin	1974–81	24	0	0	0– 0	154, 290
Thioquanine	1980	23	0	4	—	291
TIC-mustard	1973	20	20	10	—	153
Tilorone	1981	25	0	0	—	154
TMCA	1967	6	—	17	—	39
Triazinate (Baker's Antifol)	1977–81	59	0	3	0– 8	154, 285, 292
Tubercidin	1975	3	—	33	—	39
VM-26	1984	20	0	5	—	293
VP-16	1975–1981	213	0	<1	0–13	266, 294–298
Yoshi-864	1979	16	—	0	—	39

* No prior chemotherapy administered for treatment of metastatic disease.

extensively. In a randomized trial among previously treated patients without prior exposure to doxorubicin, the response rate to VP-16 alone was 10.5% and to the combination of doxorubicin/vincristine (AV) 20%.[295] No patients responded on crossover from AV to VP-16, but 2 of 15 patients (13%) responded on crossover from VP-16 to AV. VP-16 has been combined with doxorubicin and cyclophosphamide as an induction regimen. In a randomized trial, the overall response rate and the complete response rate to VP-16, doxorubicin, and cyclophosphamide were the same as obtained with more conventional FAC.[302] In a randomized comparison of doxorubicin alone and doxorubicin plus VP-16, there was no difference in the complete response rate or the duration of response.[66] VP-16 does not appear to hold much promise of ever being particularly useful in the treatment of metastatic breast cancer.

THE USE OF DRUG COMBINATIONS

Dr. Ezra Greenspan is often credited with the first report of a combination chemotherapy regimen used to treat metastatic breast cancer.[303] He used thiotepa and methotrexate together and achieved an overall response rate of 60%, with a complete response rate of 25%. This appeared to be superior to the response rates obtained with single agents. Six years later, Dr. Richard Cooper of Buffalo, New York, reported an 88% complete response rate using the combination of cyclophosphamide, methotrexate, 5-fluorouracil, vincristine, and prednisone.[304] This exciting result stimulated widespread interest in the use of combination chemotherapy and established the "Cooper regimen" as a standard with which subsequent combination chemotherapy programs would be compared. No one has duplicated the results initially reported by Cooper, although many have attempted (Table 13-32). The average response rate in subsequent studies was between 50% and 60%, and the complete response rate was usually less than 20%.[23,48,50,305–310] The median duration of response was between 9 and 10 months, and the median duration of the survival of patients treated with this as an initial program was slightly more than a year. Although many physicians still use the original CMFVP program, multiple variations have used slightly less intense combinations of these five drugs or intermittent schedules of CMF or CMFP (Table 13-33).

Cyclophosphamide is probably the only drug in this combination that is absolutely critical for its efficacy. Some single-agent studies have found that cyclophosphamide alone will obtain the same response rate as a combination of four or five of these drugs (see below). On the other hand, vincristine almost certainly adds nothing except neurotoxicity. Five randomized trials were performed in which the only difference between the two arms was the addition of vincristine (Table 13-34).[316–320] Three of these trials used the "Cooper drugs," and two used doxorubicin alone or with CCNU. The patients treated with vincristine had no significant advantage in any of these trials. In fact, in most of the trials patients on the arm in which vincristine was added did slightly worse.

The role of prednisone in the original Cooper regimen is also unclear. Two randomized trials have found that patients treated with a combination of CMFVP or CMFP have a higher response rate than patients treated with CMFV or CMFP.[2,305] In the trial comparing CMFVP and

Table 13-32
Results of Trials Employing Some or All of the Drugs in the Original Cooper Regimen

Regimen	Study	Group	Number of Patients	Response Rate (%) PR + CR	Response Rate (%) CR	Median Duration of Response (Months)	Median Duration of Survival (Months)
CMFVP	Original Cooper[304]	S	60	—	88	10	—
CMFVP	COG[305]	G*	48	63	—	—	13
CMFVP	Bowman-Gray[306]	S*	34	50	3	6	—
CMFVP	Copenhagen[50]	S*	28	63	19	—	—
CMFVP	SEG[48]	G*	35	46	11	9	12
CMFVP	SWOG[23]	G*	106	59	18	8	14
CMFVP	CALGB[307]	G*	86	50	9	9	16
CMFP	NCI[7]	S	40	68	8	8	—
CMFP	ECOG[308]	G*	76	53	5	6	16
CMF	Milan[3,309]	S*	53	53	11	11	17
CMF	ECOG[98]	G*	93	53	15	6	12
CMF	Bowman-Gray[306]	S	38	34	3	6	—
CMF	CALGB[310]	G*	99	37	10	7	14
CMF	Fox Chase[12]	S	46	46	13	—	—

G, Study performed by a co-operative group; S, Single-institution study.
* One arm of a randomized trial.

Table 13-33
Combination Chemotherapy Regimens Commonly Used to Treat Metastatic Breast Cancer

Regimen	*Dose*	*Route*	*Frequency*	*Cycle Length*
"Cooper":* CMFVP[304]				
Cyclophosphamide	2.5 mg/kg	P O	Daily	
Methotrexate	25–50 mg	I V	Weekly	
5-Fluorouracil	12 mg/kg	I V	Daily × 4 then	
	500 mg	I V	Weekly	8 Weeks Induction
Vincristine	35 μg/kg	I V	Weekly	
Prednisone	0.75 mg/kg	P O	Daily, then taper	
CALGB CMFVP[311]				
Induction Phase				
Cyclophosphamide	80 mg/m^2	P O	Daily	
Methotrexate	30–40 mg/m^2	I V	Weekly	
5-Fluorouracil	500 mg/m^2	I V	Weekly	5 Weeks Induction
Vincristine	1 mg/m^2 (max = 1.5 mg)	I V	Weekly	
Prednisone	40 mg/m^2	P O	Daily × 21 then taper	
Maintenance				
Cyclophosphamide	100 mg/m^2	P O	Days 1–14	
Methotrexate	30–40 mg/m^2	I V	Weekly	
5-Fluorouracil	500 mg/m^2	I V	Weekly	4 Weeks
Vincristine	1 mg/m^2 (max = 1.5 mg)	I V	Days 1 + 8	
Prednisone	40 mg/m^2	P O	Days 1–14	
CMF (P)[312, 98]				
Cyclophosphamide	100 mg/m^2	P O	Days 1–14	
Methotrexate	40–60 mg/m^2	I V	Days 1 + 8	4 Weeks
5-Fluorouracil	600–700 mg/m^2	I V	Days 1 + 8	
Prednisone	40 mg/m^2	P O	Days 1–14	
IV CMF[313]				
Cyclophosphamide	600 mg/m^2	I V	Day 1	
Methotrexate	40 mg/m^2	I V	Day 1	3 Weeks
5-Fluorouracil	600 mg/m^2	I V	Day 1	
AV[3]				
Adriamycin	75 mg/m^2	I V	Day 1	3 Weeks
Vincristine	1.4 mg/m^2	I V	Days 1 + 8	
CA[314]				
Cyclophosphamide	200 mg/m^2	P O	Days 3–6	3–4 Weeks
Adriamycin	40 mg/m^2	I V	Day 1	
CAF[6, 20, 315]				
Cyclophosphamide	400–500 mg/m^2	I V	Day 1	
Adriamycin	40–50 mg/m^2	I V	Day 1	3 Weeks
5-Fluorouracil	400–500 mg/m^2	I V	Day 1 + 8	

* This is the original Cooper induction regimen. Doses were reduced by unspecified amounts after the induction period.

CMFV, the response rate to CMFVP was 63%, to CMFV 44%, and the difference only marginally significant ($p = 0.075$).[305] There were no differences in the survival or duration of response following treatment with either of these programs. In an Eastern Cooperative Oncology (ECOG) trial, the response to CMFP (63%) was only slightly larger than the response to CMF (57%), and the difference was not statistically significant ($p > 0.10$).[2] However, the duration of response to CMFP was significantly longer than the duration of response to CMF, the medians being 8.4 and 4.5 months, respectively ($p = 0.05$). The survival of CMFP patients was also significantly longer than the survival of those treated with CMF, the medians being 16.4 and 14.5 months ($p = 0.03$). Patients treated with CMFP had significantly more infections, but the addition of prednisone decreased the incidence of vomiting and was associated with higher white count nadirs. As a result, the average dose of cyclophosphamide, methotrexate, and 5-

Table 13-34
Contribution of Vincristine to Combination Regimens: Randomized Trials in Patients With Metastatic Disease

			Additional Benefit Observed With Vincristine Combination					
			Response		*Duration*		*Survival*	
Study Design	*Study*	*Number of Patients*	*Rate (%)*	*(p)*	*(Mos)*	*(p)*	*(Mos)*	*(p)*
CMFP ± V	CBCG[316]	427	+ 7	(0.72)			0	(0.86)
CF ± V	SWOG[317]	74	− 26	—				
CFP ± V	MAYO[318]	90	− 13	(NS)	− 1	(NS)	− 12	(NS)
A/CCNU ± V	WCSG[319]	35	− 7	(NS)			− 2	(NS)
A ± V	Guys[320]	109	− 5	—	0		+ 4	(0.112)

V, vincristine; C, cyclophosphamide; M, methotrexate; F, 5-fluorouracil; P, prednisone; A, doxorubicin, NS, not significant.

fluorouracil administered with the CMFP regimen was greater than that given in the CMF regimen. For example, during the first three cycles of CMF, the median cyclophosphamide dose administered relative to the dose prescribed in the protocol was 91%, 76%, and 65%. The corresponding doses of cyclophosphamide given to patients treated with CMFP were 94%, 88%, and 88%. These differences were statistically significant. The increased response rate seen with CMFP may reflect the higher doses of CMF given rather than a cytotoxic effect of prednisone. The precise role of prednisone in combination chemotherapy must be sorted out in future trials. The response frequency, response duration, and survival advantages for prednisone-containing combinations is small, and these differences should not be the major consideration in deciding whether this drug is added to any combination. Some patients will find the use of combination chemotherapy much more tolerable if prednisone is added, and in a few patients this may be the only way to continue administration of drug. In others, the side effects—especially cushingoid side effects, which occur uncommonly—may be unacceptable; this is most likely the reaction from patients who are able to tolerate CMF with minimal gastrointestinal toxicity.

The relative efficacy of CMFVP and CMF has been evaluated in only one randomized trial.[306] The CMFVP program used in this trial was not the same as the original Cooper regimen. The response rate to CMF was 34% and to CMFVP 50%. This difference is not statistically significant.

CMF is well tolerated and easy to administer. Cyclophosphamide is usually given orally for the first 14 days of each 28-day cycle, and methotrexate and 5-fluorouracil are given intravenously on day 1 and day 8. The incidence of nausea and vomiting with CMF is about 20%. The incidence of nausea and vomiting with CMFP is about 4% to 6%. (See the section on Adjuvant Systemic Therapy of Early Breast Cancer in Chapter 10.) The reported incidence of alopecia varies considerably from one trial to another, but alopecia usually occurs gradually, beginning about 1 month after the initiation of therapy. Less than half of all patients treated with CMF for 6 months or less will have severe alopecia requiring a wig.

Recently investigators have attempted to increase the efficacy of CMF by sequencing methotrexate and 5-fluorouracil. Preclinical studies in animals performed more than a decade ago suggested that methotrexate and 5-fluorouracil might be antagonistic in some systems.[321] Subsequent *in vitro* studies reached the opposite conclusion and demonstrated synergism if the drugs were appropriately sequenced.[322] With better understanding of the biochemistry and pharmacology of these two drugs, a number of mechanisms have been proposed to explain these interactions.[323] The first clinical trial sequencing methotrexate and 5-fluorouracil was performed in patients with breast cancer.[324] This study included seven patients without prior chemotherapy for metastatic breast cancer and seven patients who had been previously treated with drug combinations that included both methotrexate and 5-fluorouracil. The patients were given 200 mg/m^2 of methotrexate followed 1 hour later by 600 mg/m^2 of 5-fluorouracil. The toxicity with this combination was minimal. The response rates in the initial pilot were impressive. Fifty-three percent of the treated patients responded, including 85% of the patients without prior chemotherapy and 50% of the patients who had had previous treatment with methotrexate and 5-fluorouracil. Unfortunately, no one has been able to duplicate precisely the original results (Table 13-35). Even in patients with no or limited prior chemotherapy, the response rate to sequential MF has been only 21% to 28%.[326,329] A sequence of MF has also been used in combination with cyclophosphamide or cyclophosphamide and prednisone. The overall response rate and duration of response in these uncontrolled trials is similar to what would be expected with CMF or CMFP administered in a conventional fashion.[330,331] Randomized comparisons of sequential and bolus MF have been made in patients with head and neck cancers, and these studies have not substantiated the superiority of the sequential program. This sequential regimen is relatively nontoxic, which may be an advantage when used in adjuvant programs. However, additional clinic visits are required if the

13-35
The Efficacy of Sequencing Methotrexate and 5-Fluorouracil in the Treatment of Metastatic Breast Cancer

	Drug Dose* (mg/m²)			Number of Patients					
Regimen*	MTx	5-FU	Interval* Between MF	Total	Without Prior Chemo.	With Prior MF	Response Rate (%)	Median Duration (Months)	Author
MF	200	600	1 hr	14	7	7	53	—	Gerwitz et al[324]
MF	1500	1500	1 hr	13	0	5	23	> 3	Tisman et al[325]
MF	100–200	600	?	18	18	0	28	—	Plotkin et al[326]
MF	200	600	1 hr	25	0	22	8	> 4	Perrault et al[327]
MF	300	900	7 hr	43	0	Most	28	4.5	Herrmann et al[328]
MF	50	600	6 hr	29	28	5	21	—	Kaye et al[329]
CMF	30	500	24 hr	41	39	0	78	> 8–15	Chang et al[330]
CMFP	200	600	1 hr	37	37	0	43	—	Cadman et al[331]

M or MTx, methotrexate; F or 5-FU, 5-fluorouracil; C, cyclophosphamide; P, prednisone; ?, data unclear.
* Methotrexate and 5-FU sequenced in each study using the indicated doses with 5-FU following methotrexate by the indicated interval.

interval between the two drugs is increased to 8 to 24 hours. There are insufficient data to recommend the routine use of sequential methotrexate and 5-fluorouracil in the clinic at the present time.

Doxorubicin Combinations

Doxorubicin is the most active single drug for the treatment of metastatic breast cancer and lacks cross-resistance with the older Cooper drugs. Doxorubicin alone (or doxorubicin with vincristine, which is probably equal to doxorubicin alone—see Table 13-34) has been shown in randomized trials to be as active as CMFVP, CFP, or CMF (Table 13-36). In some of these studies, the duration of response to doxorubicin as a single agent was significantly shorter than to the combination,[23,76] but the survival of patients treated with doxorubicin alone was not significantly different. Crossover studies in which doxorubicin is used in one arm are difficult to design and interpret, since the congestive heart failure associated with prolonged administration of doxorubicin limits the cumulative safe dose to 450 mg/m². As a result, patients are usually crossed over from the doxorubicin arm to the nondoxorubicin arm before there is evidence of disease progression, creating a bias in the selection of patients for the crossover component of the study. Nevertheless, the secondary response to doxorubicin has not been significantly different from the secondary response to the Cooper drugs. In two of five studies, the secondary response to doxorubicin or a doxorubicin combination was as high as or higher than that achieved with the CMF-type program.[23,75]

In spite of its high single-agent activity, doxorubicin combinations induce even higher response rates. Doxorubicin is often combined with cyclophosphamide and 5-fluorouracil, usually in a 3-week schedule in which all the drugs are administered on day 1 and a second dose of 5-fluorouracil is administered on day 8 (see Table 13-33). Two randomized trials have failed to show any advantage for the addition of 5-fluorouracil to the combination of cyclophosphamide and doxorubicin (CA). In one of these studies, the response rate to CAF (25%) was actually lower than the response rate to CA (42%).[333] This difference was not statistically significant, however. In a larger group study, the response rate to CA was 44% and to CAF was 48%.[21] The survival time of patients randomized to these two treatment arms was identical, but the response duration to CAF was more durable. The median duration of response to CAF was 52 weeks and to CA 29 weeks (p=0.06). Combinations of doxorubicin and 5-fluorouracil (AF); doxorubicin, 5-fluorouracil, and cyclophosphamide (AFC); and these three drugs plus methotrexate (AFCM) have been compared in a randomized study, and no significant differences in response rate, response duration, or survival were observed.[20] Patients randomized to receive vincristine and prednisone in addition to CAF (CAFVP) had a shorter survival time than patients given only CAF.[310] There was no difference in the response rates obtained with these two combinations.

The relative value of doxorubicin and methotrexate in combination regimens has been tested in six randomized trials (Table 13-37). In every one of these studies, there was a trend toward a higher response rate, a more durable response, or even a longer survival time with the doxorubicin-containing program. However, only one group of investigators has repeatedly found a statistically significant survival advantage for treatment with a doxorubicin-containing regimen.[307,310]

Doxorubicin-containing regimens are undeniably more effective in inducing and maintaining a response than non–doxorubicin-containing regimens. However, these advantages are purchased at considerable toxic cost. Alopecia will occur dramatically within 2 weeks of the first dose of doxorubicin in 100% of patients treated. The nausea and vomiting associated with doxorubicin administration may be mild to moderate when doxorubicin is used

Table 13-36
Studies Demonstrating Relative Effectiveness and Lack of Cross-Resistance Between Doxorubicin (A) and the Cooper Drugs

		Pre Crossover		Post Crossover	
Regimen	**Study**	*Number of Patients*	*Response Rate (%)*	*Number of Patients*	*Response Rate (%)*
A vs.	SWOG[23]	283	39	97	36
CMFVP			50*		20
A vs.	Mayo[75]	48	50	20	27
CFP (± V)			46		11
A vs.	ECOG[10]	42	34	—	—
CMF			19		—
AV vs.	Milan[3]	105	52	38	20
CMF			57		35
AV	ECOG[2]	331	56	103	35
CMF (± P)			60		37
AM vs.	Mayo[332]	46	38	32	32
CFP (± V)			59		20

* Difference statistically significant, $p < 0.05$. The observed differences were not noted to be significant.

Table 13-37
The Relative Effectiveness of Doxorubicin and Methotrexate in Combination Programs: Results of Randomized Trials

			Additional Benefit Observed With Doxorubicin Combination					
			Response		Duration		Survival	
Study Design	**Study**	**Number of Patients**	*Rate (%)*	*(p)*	*(Months)*	*(p)*	*(Months)*	*(p)*
CMF vs. CAF	NCI[58]	78	+20	(0.10)	+3	(NS)	+10	(0.13)
	CALGB[310]	181	+18	(0.01)	+4	(0.05)	+11	(0.08)
CMFP vs. CAF	ECOG[308]	155	0	(−)	+5	(0.33)	+ 3	(0.86)
CMFVP vs. CAFVP	Bowman-Gray[8]	175	+ 1	(NS)	+2	(0.47)	—	—
	*CALGB[307]	193	+31	(0.003)	+5	(0.07)	+ 3	(0.24)
	*CALGB[307]	216	+31	(0.002)	+7	(<0.01)	+ 6	(0.01)
CMFVP vs. CAF	SEG[334]	265	+15	(0.01)	0	(−)	+ 3	(<0.1)

* Two arms of a three-arm study comparing CAFVP with a continuous or intermittent schedule of CMFVP.

as a single agent, but a combination of cyclophosphamide and doxorubicin together is frequently associated with 2 to 3 days of protracted vomiting. The major goal of therapy for patients with metastatic breast cancer is to maximize palliation of symptoms at the least cost for the longest period of time. Simple comparisons of response rates and response durations are insufficient to judge which of several regimens is most likely to achieve this goal. The relative toxicities of the two therapies are not factored into the efficacy comparisons, and only one segment of the patient's entire course is considered. Since the Cooper drugs and doxorubicin are non–cross-resistant, sequential use of these agents permits more than one response in 20% to 30% of patients. For this reason, the use of doxorubicin alone followed by CMF at the time of disease progression (or the reverse sequence) may provide the greatest palliation at the least toxic cost for the longest cumulative interval between the first symptom of metastatic disease and the death of the patient.

"Salvage" Chemotherapy

The medical literature is filled with reports of trials in which a limited number of patients "refractory to prior chemotherapy" are treated with one or another combination. Results of these pilot studies are then compared with five to ten similar trials in the literature, most of which have a lower response rate, a shorter duration of response, or shorter median survival time. Most of these studies provide only rudimentary information regarding the patient's prior treatment, and it is rarely possible to correlate response to therapy with the number of prior chemotherapy combinations to which the patient has been exposed. This is unfortunate, since the number of combinations or the number of months of prior therapy may be the most important single factor in determining the patient's response to therapy. On the other hand, most of the studies do provide information on prior exposure to doxorubicin, and these studies of secondary or "salvage" regimens can be conveniently grouped into those in which all or almost all of the patients have had prior doxorubicin treatment and those in which none or almost none have had this exposure (Table 13-38). Since many patients are treated initially with a CMF or Cooper combination, those without prior doxorubicin exposure have usually had only one prior chemotherapy program. The studies performed in patients with prior doxorubicin exposure are somewhat more heterogeneous, since these patients may have had doxorubicin as part of their initial treatment or they may have had a CMF-like program followed by doxorubicin secondarily and the experimental regimen as a tertiary program. It is for this reason that the studies performed in patients with prior doxorubicin exposure generally have a lower overall response rate, a shorter median duration of response, and a shorter survival time.

The secondary or tertiary programs for patients without prior exposure to doxorubicin almost always include this drug. The important question that cannot be adequately answered by a perusal of Table 13-38 is whether these patients are better served by the doxorubicin combinations than by doxorubicin used as a single agent. The only randomized trial addressing this issue compared doxorubicin with a combination of doxorubicin and mitolactol, and the addition of mitolactol did not significantly increase the response rate, response duration, or survival time.[224] Doxorubicin/vincristine (AV) has been compared with AV plus mitolactol, and again, there was no significant advantage for the mitolactol combination.[225]

One of the most active regimens in patients with limited or no prior exposure to doxorubicin appears to be a combination of doxorubicin, vinblastine, thiotepa, and fluoxymesterone (VATH) (see Table 13-38).[338,339] In two separate reports by the same investigators, the response to this program in patients with prior treatment was 45% to 53%, the median duration of response was 11 to 12 months, and the median duration of survival 13 to 16 months. The activity of VATH in these previously treated patients is similar to the activity of CMF or CAF in patients without prior chemotherapy. This program has not been evaluated in a randomized controlled trial, but the results of the pilot suggest that this regimen deserves more careful investigation.

Mitomycin C, vinblastine either as a bolus or continuous infusion, or these two drugs together are the backbone of most combinations used in patients who have failed doxorubicin. Response rates with these tertiary programs vary between 7% and 40%, and the median survival time in all of the studies is less than 6 months (see Table 13-38). It has not been shown in a controlled trial that a patient is better served by a mitomycin C or a vinblastine combination rather than either of these drugs used as a single agent. However, the highest response rate reported from an uncontrolled trial was 40%, and this study involving 30 patients previously exposed to doxorubicin used both of these drugs in combination.[345] Mitomycin C, 20 mg/m^2, was administered intravenously on day 1, and vinblastine, 0.5 mg/kg, was given intravenously on days 1 and 21. The course was repeated at 6- to 8-week intervals. This is a toxic program that may cause severe myelosuppression, neurologic complications (obstipation, hypotension, diplopia), and pulmonary toxicity. Platelet nadirs below 25,000 were observed, and the white blood count may nadir twice during a 6-week course. The first nadir occurs between days 8 and 14 and the second between days 28 and 35.

It is usually assumed that patients who progress after treatment with CMF will never again respond to any of the Cooper drugs, but several reports suggest that this may not be so. Patients failing adjuvant CMF have been reported to have a secondary response to CMF for metastatic disease equal to that of patients who have had no adjuvant chemotherapy.[348–351] This is particularly true of patients who relapse more than 12 months after completion of the adjuvant CMF.[348] Other investigators have found that patients who had relapsed from adjuvant therapy were less responsive.[352–354] Patients with metastatic disease may have a secondary response to CMF by a minor change in dose or schedule of these drugs.[355] Patients have been reported to respond to CMFVP after a failure on CMF,[306] and one study concluded that patients progressing after an initial response to CFP were better served by re-treatment with CFP plus methotrexate and vincristine than by the use of methotrexate and vincristine alone.[356,357] In this study, patients were initially randomized to treatment with either CF or CFP, and the response rates were 54% and 60%, respectively. Seventy-eight of these patients went on to receive CFP-MV at the time of relapse, and 46% responded with a median duration of 8 months. In comparison, only 12% of patients responded to MV alone and 11% to MVP.

An important question that cannot be answered by these studies is whether a patient relapsing from a first-line program would be adversely affected by a trial of a new agent rather than one of the salvage regimens. Neither the individual patient nor future patients are well served by the use of new drugs or new combinations just prior to the patient's death. At that point in the patient's course, pleiotropic resistance is likely to prohibit any type of response, and patients with a 2- to 3-month life expectancy are not likely to express a response. The survival benefit, if any, of the first program used for the treatment of metastatic breast cancer is questionable (see below). In this context, the survival benefit that may be derived from the use of the programs outlined in Table 13-38 is even less certain. At all junctures in a patient's course, the goals of

Table 13-38
Regimens Used in Patients Who Have Failed One or Two Prior Chemotherapy Programs

Drugs		Authors	Number of Patients	Response Rate (%)	Median Duration of Response (Months)	Median Duration of Survival (Months)
Patients *Without* Prior Doxorubicin Exposure:						
Mitomycin C	+ TAM*	Falkson et al[226]	53	28	4.1	7.6
	+ TAM*	Chang et al[227]	12	17	—	10.0
Doxorubicin alone*		Ingle et al[224]	74	30	6.2	7.7
+ Vincristine		Harris et al[335]	50	32	7.0	9.7
+ Vincristine*		Cummings et al[225]	92	27	—	8.3
+ Vinblastine (CI)		Tannir et al[336]	42	43	10.0	—
+ Vinblastine (CI)		Yap et al[337]	23	26	4.5	—
+ Vinblastine + thiotepa + Halo (VATH)		Perloff et al[338]	19	53	11.5	16.0
+ Vinblastine + thiotepa + Halo (VATH)		Hart et al[339]	29	45	11.0	13.0
+ Mitomycin C		Harris et al[335]	24	25	9.6	11.1
+ Mitomycin C		Creech et al[340]	71	51	—	—
+ Mitomycin C + vincristine		Oster et al[341]	15	73	8.0	—
+ Mitomycin C + vincristine + 5-FU (FOAM)		Friedman et al[135]	82	35	6.8	9.4
+ Mitomycin C + vinblastine		Luikart et al[139]	27	33	3.9	—
+ Mitomycin C + mitolactol		Pinnamaneni et al[342]	26	54	10.0	—
+ Mitolactol*		Ingle et al[224]	77	26	5.9	7.5
+ Mitolactol		Tormey et al[187]	50	40	5.1	—
+ Mitolactol	+ Tam *	Falkson et al[226]	60	38	7.7	9.7
+ Mitolactol	+ Tam *	Chang et al[227]	11	45	—	6.7
+ Mitolactol + vincristine*		Cummings et al[225]	94	23	—	7.1
+ VP-16		Vaughn et al[343]	28	36	6.5	—
+ VP-16		Konits et al[344]	30	40	4.9	—
Patients *With* Prior Doxorubicin Exposure:						
Mitomycin C	+ Tam*	Chang et al[227]	8	40	—	4.0
	+ Tam*	Falkson et al[226]	35	23	—	4.6
	+ Tam + Halo*	Falkson et al[226]	36	17	—	5.9
+ Vinblastine*		Garewal et al[137]	22	32	5.5	—
+ Vinblastine		Denefrio et al[136]	14	7	—	—
+ Vinblastine		Konits et al[345]	30	40	4.3	—
+ Vinblastine + hexamethyl melamine		Jarowski et al[221]	42	—	—	—
+ Vinblastine + BCNU		Veronesi et al[346]	22	9	—	—
+ Vincristine + Hexamethyl melamine*		Legha et al[179]	27	19	5.0	—
+ Vincristine + BCNU + prednisone		Garewal et al[137]	15	40	8.2	—
+ Vindesine*		Garfield et al[218]	20	10	—	—
Vinblastine (CI)						
+ Methotrexate		Hortobagyi et al[347]	74	23	2.0	6.0
+ Peptichemio		Yap et al[299]	33	33	6.0	—

* One arm of randomized trial
CI, continuous infusion; HD, high dose; Tam, tamoxifen; Halo, fluoxymesterone.

therapy should be precisely defined and the possible use of a new program considered. It can be argued that both the individual and society are best served by the use of experimental programs early in a patient's course, when she is minimally symptomatic, and the use of known effective agents late in the course, at a time when the patient is most in need of palliation.

PRINCIPLES OF THERAPY

Dose Response

It is axiomatic in medical oncology that there is a steep dose-response relationship for most of the cytotoxic agents used in clinical practice.[124] This relationship can be seen most readily in experimental animal tumors, but it is also evident in the treatment of human cancers, especially the leukemias and lymphomas. Even drugs such as doxorubicin, which exhibits a very steep dose response when used to treat AKR leukemia,[130] show some schedule dependency *in vitro*.[358] Doxorubicin is a non–cycle-specific drug, but the cell destruction when the drug is applied to synchronized cells in S-phase is much greater than when the drug is applied to the cells in G_0. Animal tumors and the human tumors in which a dose response has been demonstrated are characterized by a high growth fraction and fairly rapid doubling time. This is in contrast to human breast cancer, which is characterized by a fairly low growth fraction.[359] There is little doubt that breast cancer will demonstrate some dose response to the standard cytotoxic drugs, but the dose-response curve may be much more shallow than in experimental systems. If so, escalation of dose to the maximum tolerated level may be inadequate to have much impact on either the duration of response or survival. New technology, especially the technology of bone marrow transplantation, may permit circumvention of the usual dose-limiting myelosuppression, but it is too early to tell whether the use of this extended dose range will have practical import for the treatment of breast cancer. There is considerable clinical evidence from retrospective surveys and small pilot trials supporting the dose-response effect of chemotherapy for metastatic breast cancer.[360,362,363] Only two randomized trials have been performed, and these have failed to show a clinically important dose effect.[59,364]

One of the first retrospective analyses of dose was performed by the Milan Cancer Institute.[360] Patients with metastatic breast cancer treated with CMF were retrospectively divided into three groups: those given more than 85%, 66% to 84%, or less than 65% of the CMF doses used in the first published report of this regimen. The response rate for those given the highest dose was almost double that of those receiving less than 65% of prescribed protocol doses (study I, Table 13-39). Another group of investigators performing a similar analysis concluded that

Table 13-39
Relationship Between Drug Dose, Patient Performance Status, and Response to Therapy: Retrospective Analysis of Two Studies

	Dose Level as % of Prescribed Full Dose			
	> 85%	*66–84%*	*< 65%*	*All Doses*
Study I[360]				
Dose and Response				
Number of patients	—	—	—	57
Response rate	67%	53%	35%	53%
Study II[361]				
Dose and Response				
Number of patients	14	29	32	75
Response rate	50%	48%	38%	44%
Median duration of response (months)	6	19	14	—
Range	(5–15)	(7–48)	(3–36)	—
Median survival (months)	21	29	26	—
4-year actuarial survival	25%	33%	21%	
Performance Status and Response	*Performance Status (Karnofsky Scale)*			
	>80%		*<80%*	
Response rate	61%		24%	
Complete response rate	24%		6%	
Median duration of response (months)	14		9	
Range	(5–48)		(3–36)	
4-year actuarial survival	41%		14%	

* p value for difference = 0.0001

there was no cause and effect relationship between dose and response.[361] They found that the patient's likelihood of responding and her ability to tolerate a high drug dose were both related to performance status (study II, Table 13-39). Patients given more than 85% of prescribed doses had a somewhat higher response rate than those receiving less than 65% of the dose level, but this difference was not statistically significant, and no correlations between dose and either the duration of response or survival could be made. However, the response rate to CMF was 61% in those patients with a Karnofsky performance status greater than 80% and 24% in those with a performance status less than 80%. A good performance status also correlated with the complete response rate and actuarial survival. These two sets of observations were linked by the fact that 64% of the patients who tolerated high CMF doses had a good Karnofsky performance status, compared with only 57% of patients given the lower dose levels.

In an ECOG trial, patients randomized to CMFP had a significantly longer response and survival than those randomized to receive CMF (see above).[2] Patients treated with CMFP also had less gastrointestinal toxicity and higher nadir white counts, and as a result this group received a significantly higher average dose of each of the cytotoxic drugs in the regimen: cyclophosphamide, methotrexate, and 5-fluorouracil. Although the superior efficacy of the CMFP regimen may be related to an antineoplastic effect of prednisone, it is also possible that the addition of prednisone resulted in less toxicity, higher doses, and a dose-response effect to account for the superiority of the CMFP regimen.

Three groups of investigators have performed small, uncontrolled studies using intense combinations of drugs or drugs and hormones (Table 13-40).[16,362,363] One of these programs used 3 g/m^2 of methotrexate and up to 90 mg/m^2 of doxorubicin combined with more conventional doses of cyclophosphamide and 5-fluorouracil given in a 6-week cycle.[16] Fifty-five patients were treated, and the overall response rate was nearly 80%, the complete response rate 27%. The median time to treatment failure for all patients entered into this study was 21.6 months, almost three times the median time to treatment failure reported with conventional drugs in other trials. A combination of cyclophosphamide, 1200 mg/m^2, on day 1 and 5-fluorouracil, 600 mg/m^2, on days 1 to 5, was given to 30 patients and induced a response in 93%. The complete response rate in this program was also high, 40%, and the median survival time was in excess of 19 months. This represents a 50% increase in median survival time compared with studies using CMF combinations at conventional doses (see Table 13-32). The third of these pilot studies using high-dose regimens employed 11 drugs including doxorubicin, 45 mg/m^2, on day 1 of a 28-day cycle; mitolactol, 135 mg/m^2, on days 2 to 11; methotrexate, 750 mg/m^2, on days 15 and 22; hexamethylmelamine, 2 mg/kg, on days 15 to 26; and bleomycin, 30 units, on days 15 and 22. The high doses of methotrexate were rescued with leucovorin, and the patients were also given vincristine, prednisone, tamoxifen, and fluoxymesterone. Responses in many areas were consolidated with radiotherapy, which was administered after six cycles of this intense chemotherapy program.[363] The overall response rate to this program was 92%, and the complete response rate 73%. The median survival time of patients treated with this program was very similar to that of patients treated with high-dose cyclophosphamide/5-fluorouracil. The complete response rate in each of these trials was higher than is generally reported using conventional doses of chemotherapy, but the increases in complete response rate did not result in a proportionate increase in median survival time.

Other investigators have performed uncontrolled studies using *low* doses of CMF or doxorubicin.[12,64] A

Table 13-40
Three Intensive Programs Used to Treat Metastatic Breast Cancer: Results of Pilot Trials

	"Super-CMF"[16]			*High-Dose CF*[362]			*DAV-MP-HxTHBleo*[363]		
Number of evaluable patients	55			30			23		
Overall response rate (%)	78			93			92		
Complete response rate (%)	27			40			73		
Median time to failure (months)	21.6			12.6			—		
Median survival (months)	—			19.2			17–20		
				Response by Site					
Site	*n*	*RR (%)*	*CR (%)*	*n*	*RR (%)*	*CR (%)*	*n*	*RR (%)*	*CR (%)*
Nodes	15	87	67	9	100	56	15	93	93
Skin	11	54	36	5	100	80	8	100	100
Lung	19	63	37	15	87	53	13	92	85
Liver	13	76	38	12	100	16	3	67	67
Bone	26	89	35	13	85	23	8	88	50

C, cyclophosphamide; M, methotrexate; 5, 5-fluorouracil; D, dibromodulcitol; A, doxorubicin; P, prednisone; Hx, hexamethylmelamine; T, tamoxifen; H, fluoxymesterone; Bleo, bleomycin; RR, total response rate; CR, complete response rate. See text for details regarding dose schedule of regimens.

combination of cyclophosphamide, 50 mg orally on days 1 through 14, and methotrexate, 25 mg, plus 5-fluorouracil, 500 mg, intravenously on days 1 and 8 induced a response rate of 46% and a complete response rate of 13%.[12] Forty-six women were included in this study. Neither this study nor the high-dose studies described above are randomized or large enough to reliably detect even a 50% increase or decrease in response rate, response duration, or survival duration. However, a balanced review of the data from both sets of studies leads to the conclusion that the evidence supporting a dose effect is counterbalanced by data suggesting that at least a moderate reduction in drug dose is not likely to compromise the patient's survival or the palliative potential of the regimen. The scientific validity of the concepts can only be properly evaluated in well-controlled trials.

Two randomized trials with dose as the only or major variable have been performed in patients with metastatic breast cancer.[59,364] The first trial used doxorubicin as a single agent and randomized good-risk patients to receive 75 mg/m^2, 60 mg/m^2, and 45 mg/m^2.[59] Poor-risk patients were randomized to 50 mg/m^2 and 25 mg/m^2. One-hundred and seventy-one patients were included in this study. There was no significant dose effect among patients considered to be a good risk who were randomized to the three highest dose levels. However, the response rate to the 25 mg/m^2 dose among poor-risk patients was only 6%, compared with 24% for those given 50 mg/m^2. These differences were not statistically significant.

High-dose FAC was compared with conventional FAC in a randomized study.[364] In this study, cyclophosphamide doses three times the conventional dose and a doxorubicin dose approximately 50% greater than usual were employed (Table 13-41). Patients treated with the high-dose FAC were also placed in a protected environment and given prophylactic antibiotics (PEPA) to decrease the incidence of infectious complications. At the time of the 3-week evaluation, the response rate to the high-dose FAC was almost twice the response rate to conventional FAC, but at the end of the trial the overall response rates, complete response rates, response durations, and survival of patients treated with high-dose FAC and conventional FAC were not significantly different.

Myelosuppression is the dose-limiting toxicity for almost all of the chemotherapy agents most active in the treatment of metastatic breast cancer. Cyclophosphamide and doxorubicin doses cannot be escalated much higher than described above for FAC-PEPA without some method of protecting the bone marrow. Technically this is possible using bone marrow transplant. The patient's own marrow can be removed prior to the administration of high doses of chemotherapy and reinfused when the cytotoxic drugs have been cleared from the circulation (i.e., autologous bone marrow transplant). This will decrease the duration of myelosuppression, decrease the incidence of serious or life-threatening infections, and permit the administration of higher doses of chemotherapy. A number of the trials using autologous bone marrow transplant have been performed in patients with metastatic breast cancer (Table 13-42). This is difficult research to perform, and the results are difficult to interpret. First, the technology for autologous bone marrow transplant is still complicated, expensive, and limited to a small number of centers. As a result, very few patients can be treated. Second, breast cancer frequently metastasizes to the bone marrow. Reinfusion of marrow from such patients would involve reinfusion of at least some cancer cells. A priori, this is an unattractive prospect even though it is possible that a limited number of cancer cells could be reinfused in this manner without rekindling tumor growth. (Eventually it may be possible to "clean up" the marrow *in vitro* with monoclonal antibodies prior to reinfusion of the marrow into the patient. This technique has been used successfully with some human tumors.) Because of the potential for reinfusion of contaminated bone marrow, most autologous marrow transplant programs exclude patients with known bone

Table 13-41
Prospective Randomized Trial Comparing Two Doses of FAC

		High Dose			*Conventional Dose*	
F		500 mg/m^2 d 1–5			500 mg/m^2 d 1&8	
A		85 mg/m^2 d 1			50 mg/m^2 d 1	
C		1500 mg/m^2 d 1			500 mg/m^2 d 1	
		Response Rate (%)			*Median Duration (Mos)*	
	N	*WK 3*	*PR + CR*	*CR*	*Response*	*Survival*
FAC	28	39	82	32	15	19
FAC-PEPA*	32	70	84	34	11	22
p		0.006	—	—	—	—

* FAC-PEPA, high-dose regimen with PEPA (Protected environment–prophylactic antibiotics)
(Malik R, Blumenschein GR, Legha SS, et al: A randomized trial of high-dose 5-fluorouracil, doxorubicin, and cyclophosphamide versus conventional FAC regimen in metastatic breast cancer. Proc Am Soc Clin Oncol 1:79, 1982)

Table 13-42
Autologous Bone Marrow Transplant Programs Used to Treat Metastatic Breast Cancer

Drug (s)	Dose*	Number of Patients: Total	Number of Patients: With Bone Mets	Number of Patients: Without Prior Chemo.†	Number Responding: Total	Number Responding: CR	Number of Toxic Deaths	Authors
CA	C = 2 g/m^2	1	0	1	1/1	0	0	Tobias et al[365]
CA+VA, ANTM, RT	C = 50–60 mg/kg × 2–4	2	?	?	1/1	1	1	Douer et al[366]
C+RT	C = 60 mg/kg × 2	5	0	0	2/4	2	1	Stewart et al[367]
L-PAM	L-PAM = 40–75 mg/m^2 × 3	3	?	0	2/3	0	0	Lazarus et al[368]
L-PAM	L-PAM = 120–140 mg/m^2	4	1	0	3/4	3	0	Carringham et al[369]
AMSA	AMSA = 200–250 mg/m^2 × 3	16	3	0	2/16	0	0	Tannir et al[370]
MitoC	MitoC = 20–50 mg/m^2	15	1	0	1/15	0	5	Tannir et al[371]
L-PAM	L-PAM = 140–240 mg/m^2	2	0	0	NE	0	2	Maranichi et al[372]
L-PAM	L-PAM = 180 mg/m^2	6	0	0	4/6	1	0	Knight et al[373]
C+P+BCNU	C = 3000–7500 mg/m^2	11	1	2	11/11	4	2	Eder et al[374]
C+P+BCNU or L-PAM	C = 5625 mg/m^2	6	0	?	6/6	6	0	Peters et al[375]

C, cyclophosphamide; A, doxorubicin; VA, vinca alkaloid; ANTM, Antimetabolite, not specified; RT, radiotherapy; L-PAM, L-phenylalanine mustard; AMSA, amsacrine; MitoC, mitomycin C; P, platinum; BCNU, carmustine; NE, not evaluable.
* In studies using drug combinations, the dose of more than one drug may have been escalated, in which case only the dose of the alkylating agent is shown.
† Number of patients without chemotherapy for metastatic disease.
? No data available.

marrow metastases, and this results in the selection of a skewed population of breast cancer patients. Not only must the patient have no evidence of disease to the bone marrow, but these patients are frequently young, have an excellent performance status in order to be able to tolerate the rigors of such intense chemotherapy, and have disease at a limited number of sites. This poses a major problem in interpreting results. With what can these response rates be compared? With what can the survival time of these patients be compared? For this reason, the observations in Table 13-42 must be accepted as a series of anecdotes that are as yet uninterpretable.

Almost all of these regimens have used an alkylating agent, usually as a single agent. One program used amsacrine as a single agent.[370] This is one of the largest studies, and the investigators concluded that even at high doses amsacrine has little potential for the treatment of metastatic breast cancer. In spite of the fact that the duration of myelosuppression is shortened following a bone marrow transplant, the morbidity and mortality associated with this procedure are considerable. In two trials, the toxic deaths exceeded the number of responding patients.[371,372] One of the most successful and largest of these studies used a combination of cyclophosphamide, cisplatin, and carmustine. This regimen was originally designed for a variety of tumors other than breast cancer. However, all of the breast cancer patients treated have responded, and 60% have had a complete response rate. No meaningful response duration or survival data are yet available from these studies.[374,375]

The issue of dose response is one that engenders intense debate. For two reasons, it is difficult to perform controlled trials in which dose is a variable. First, dose response is such a well-established principle in the treatment of other tumors and experimental tumors that many scientists are unwilling to challenge its validity in a tumor such as breast cancer, in which the results of therapy are so difficult to measure. Second, from the available data it seems unlikely that small increments in dose will have a major impact on the survival of patients with metastatic breast cancer. This means that very high doses of drug will be needed, and patients entering these studies will almost certainly experience considerable toxicity. Although reviews and data manipulation from the published literature may support[376] or refute[377] the value of dose response in the treatment of metastatic breast cancer, this issue is not likely to be settled until large, well-designed, and properly controlled randomized trials have been performed.

Schedule Response

The regimen originally described by Cooper was an intensive program involving daily administration of cyclophosphamide throughout the 8-week induction period and daily or weekly injections of the other drugs as well. Subsequent investigators were unable to obtain the high complete response rate originally reported by Cooper, and the question has frequently been raised whether this was due to inappropriate reductions of dose or the use of an intermittent schedule of drug administration. To test this possibility, three of the cooperative research groups in the United States randomized patients to receive either a continuous CMFVP program very similar to that used by Cooper or an intermittent program more akin to the standard CMF regimen.[23,48,307] In each of these studies, use of the continuous regimen resulted in a higher overall response rate and a higher complete response rate but no significant improvement in survival time. In two of these studies, the differences in response rate were statistically significant,[23,48] but in the most recent report the response rate to the two programs was identical.[307] In this study, the median response duration was 9 months after treatment with the continuous program and 7 months following the intermediate program ($p = 0.41$). The median survival time of patients on the continuous program was 16 months, and on the intermediate program 13 months (NS).

Theoretically, an intermittent program should be more effective for any tumor in which dose (or peak dose) is a critical factor. However, it is possible that more frequent administration, or even continuous administration, of drug may be more effective in the treatment of a tumor with a low growth fraction, since the continuously administered drug would more likely be administered at a time when the tumor cell was synthesizing DNA. These theoretical considerations and the higher response rates obtained with the continuous CMFVP regimens provide the rationale for exploring programs that are not only dose intensive but schedule intensive. The DAV-MP-HxTHBleo regimen (Table 13-40) is one example of a high-dose regimen that is also schedule intensive.[363]

The logical extension of schedule intensification is continuous administration of drug. The agent that has been used most frequently as a continuous infusion for metastatic breast cancer is vinblastine. This drug is rapidly cleared from the plasma, and it has an initial half-life of 0.07 hours. It is related to the vinca alkaloid vindesine, and interest in continuous-infusion vinblastine grew out of the observation that vindesine might be more effective as a 48-hour infusion. An early study of vindesine in patients with acute leukemia demonstrated that some patients would respond to a 48-hour infusion after proving refractory to bolus-infusion vindesine.[232] The M.D. Anderson Hospital has now treated more than 100 patients with continuous-infusion vinblastine, and the observed response rate in this group of patients, almost all of whom were refractory to prior chemotherapy programs, is 37%.[378] The observations of the M.D. Anderson researchers have been confirmed by some investigators[379,380] and refuted by others (Table 13-43).[381,382] Continuous-infusion vinblastine has not been compared in a randomized controlled trial with bolus-infusion schedules. However, the response rate to vinblastine given as a bolus 1.7 mg/m^2 for 5 days is 30%, and this is very similar to that obtained with the continuous-infusion regimen.[211] Vindesine has also been administered successfully as a continuous infusion, but the response rate was only marginally higher than the response rate obtained with bolus-infusion vindesine (Table 13-28).[209] The third vinca alkaloid, vincristine, has been used as a continuous infusion and was totally inactive on this schedule.[383]

Other drugs have been used as continuous infusion as well. A 5-day continuous infusion of mitomycin C resulted in only one response among 17 treated patients, and it was concluded that continuous infusion was not likely to improve the therapeutic index for this drug.[384] Doxorubicin has been given as a continuous infusion for periods varying from 24 to 96 hours. In these studies, only the dose schedule and not the dose rate was altered relative to conventional ways of giving this drug. Sixty to 75 mg/m^2 of single-agent doxorubicin was given by continuous infusion and repeated at intervals of 3 weeks. The response rate in previously treated patients was 48%. On the basis of this uncontrolled study, it seems unlikely that continuous-infusion doxorubicin will be less effective than bolus administration. The acute toxicity, especially the gastrointestinal toxicity, of doxorubicin is decreased when it is given as a continuous infusion, and the cardiotoxicity scores obtained from endomyocardial biopsies of patients receiving continuous doxorubicin are significantly less than those of patients treated with doxorubicin on either a weekly or 3-weekly schedule.[385] Although further research needs to be performed to determine whether a continuous infusion of doxorubicin will be more efficacious, these observations regarding the relative toxicity of the continuous-infusion schedule are sufficient to justify the use of this dose schedule on a routine basis.

Table 13-43
Studies of Continuous-Infusion Vinblastine

*Vinblastine Dose**	*Number of Patients*	*Response Rate (%)*	*Authors*
1.4–2.0 mg/m^2/d	106	37	Fraschini et al[378]
1.6 mg/m^2/d	15	0	Ingle et al[381]
1.2–1.8 mg/m^2/d	17	0	Tannock et al[382]
1.6 mg/m^2/d	19	26	Shah et al[380]
2.0–3.0 mg/m^2/d	12	33	Chacon et al[379]

* Administered continuously over 5 days.

Duration of Therapy

The first successful forms of treatment for metastatic breast cancer were endocrine therapies. This modality is thought to affect cancer cells by removing or blocking growth factors, and hormones may be cytostatic rather than cytocidal. (See the section on Endocrine Therapy of Metastatic Disease in Chapter 13.) Continuous administration of hormone may be necessary to suppress tumor growth. Endocrine therapy is also nontoxic, and there are no compelling clinical reasons to discontinue its use. Cytotoxic drugs were introduced in the context of endocrine therapy and were initially used as relatively nontoxic single agents. Therefore, it is not surprising that they were used for an indefinite duration until there was evidence of tumor progression in the same way that endocrine therapy had previously been administered. Until recently, very little thought was given to the idea of discontinuing chemotherapy or changing the chemotherapy regimen after a few cycles of drug.

It is possible—even likely—that the maximum effects of cytotoxic agents are achieved in a very short time following the initiation of drug therapy. A tumor with a long natural history, such as breast cancer, is characterized by multiple tumor clones, each with its own pattern of chemosensitivity and chemoresistance. Additional resistant clones are probably induced following the administration of chemotherapy, and recent work suggests that the induction of chemoresistant clones occurs very rapidly after the first course of therapy.[31] It is possible that the maximum reduction in tumor burden is achieved with two to four cycles of drug. For example, if each cycle of a combination chemotherapy program is 90% cytoreductive, then the initial tumor burden may be reduced from 10^{11} to 10^9 with just two cycles of drug. Subsequent cycles of drug will have little effect if the remaining tumor burden consists predominantly of clones that are resistant to the combination being used. The time when clinical evidence of tumor is again apparent (i.e., the duration of remission) may be completely unaffected by the chemotherapy administered subsequent to the first several cycles.[386] Practically, this means that the patient may have received many months of toxic chemotherapy for no practical gain in either response duration or survival time.

The use of chemotherapy programs of short duration has two potential advantages. First, by definition these would be less toxic since the patient will have a shorter period of time in which to experience the drug toxicities. Second, this would allow for the introduction of new, non–cross-resistant regimens at an early time in the patient's course, and the use of two regimens sequentially (or alternately) may cause greater tumor cell destruction than either regimen alone could achieve.

Several investigators have discontinued chemotherapy in responding patients after a fixed interval and have observed that these responses may be quite durable. In one study, all therapy was discontinued after 15 months regardless of the completeness of the patient's response.[16] Six of 11 complete responders continued in remission off therapy for periods of 12 to 28 months, and several of these patients are now in continuing remission in excess of 6 years, including one patient who originally had liver metastases, had a complete response to chemotherapy, and subsequently developed central nervous system metastases that were successfully treated with radiotherapy. This patient still has no evidence of systemic relapse. Several other investigators have observed that complete responses may be very durable after discontinuing chemotherapy.[24–26] In addition, the response to reinduction chemotherapy may be similar to the response rate to initial chemotherapy. The longest reported follow-up of a patient in complete remission without maintenance chemotherapy is 15 years.[22]

Patients may also continue without progression of disease after a partial response. Twenty-one patients with bone metastases were treated with chemotherapy until a cumulative doxorubicin dose of 450 mg/m² had been administered.[34] Five of these patients relapsed while still on chemotherapy, but 16 completed the course. Six of these 16 relapsed within 4 months; 10 (63% of those who completed the course) continued in remission more than 6 months off therapy. The *median* progression-free survival of this group of patients followed without maintenance therapy is almost 2 years, and the range is 18 to 62 months.

Two randomized trials have addressed the issue of therapy duration.[48,387] In the first of these, patients who were stable after 6 months of CMFVP were randomized to either continue the same therapy or to stop all therapy until evidence of disease progression.[48] There was no significant difference in the survival time of these two groups of patients. In fact, the survival of the group stopping therapy was slightly better (Fig. 13-12). In addition, the patients who progressed after stopping therapy could frequently be re-induced to a secondary response. In the second of these studies, patients with advanced local disease were treated with six cycles of doxorubicin and vincristine prior to radiotherapy of the breast and regional lymph nodes.[387] Patients who were still responding at the end of radiotherapy were subsequently randomized to either another six cycles of doxorubicin/vincristine or no further systemic therapy. Local control was improved among those patients who received the additional chemotherapy, but the incidence of distant metastases and the survival of the two groups was the same. This resulted in a significant difference in the median disease-free survival time, 19 months in the patients receiving further chemotherapy versus 11 months in those patients who stopped therapy ($p = 0.02$). The data from this trial suggest that prolonged chemotherapy may further reduce tumor burden or suppress tumor regrowth but not sufficiently to improve survival time.

FIGURE 13-12. Survival of patients treated with CMFVP who were stable after 6 months of therapy and randomized to continue CMFVP beyond 6 months or to discontinue therapy. (Smalley RV, Murphy S, Huguley CM, et al: Combination versus sequential five-drug chemotherapy in metastatic carcinoma of the breast. Cancer Res 36:3911–3916, 1976.)

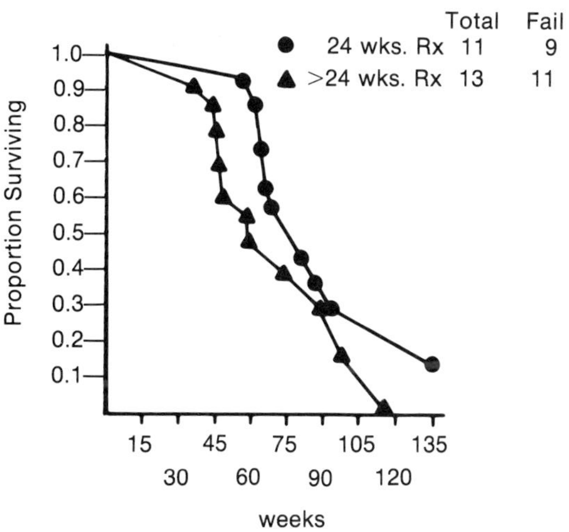

The question of optimal duration of therapy has also been studied in the adjuvant setting, and six independent trials have failed to show a survival advantage for patients treated with a longer duration of chemotherapy. (See the section on Adjuvant Therapy in Chapter 10.) This question deserves further study among patients with metastatic breast cancer. There may be an advantage for prolonged therapy in some patient groups even though this is not readily apparent from the available data, but it is unlikely that prolonged administration of chemotherapy to patients with metastatic breast cancer will result in either clinically important or statistically significant prolongation of survival. Until such data are available, it is both reasonable and prudent to consider short courses of therapy which maximally palliate the patient's symptoms without unduly prolonging the time during which the patient must experience the toxicities of chemotherapy.

Alternating Regimens

If maximum or near maximum cytoreduction from chemotherapy is achieved after several courses of drug therapy, crossover to a non–cross-resistant regimen should further reduce the total tumor burden and either prolong the duration of response or patient survival time. The two most important non–cross-resistant agents for the treatment of breast cancer are cyclophosphamide and doxorubicin. A number of trials have been conducted in which patients were randomized to receive either a cyclophosphamide-containing regimen alone or a cyclophosphamide-containing regimen alternating with a doxorubicin-containing regimen (Table 13-44). In one trial, 100 patients were randomized to receive an initial induction therapy with either the combination CFP or a combination of doxorubicin/L-PAM.[388] After two cycles of treatment with these drugs, all patients were rerandomized to either continue the initial induction regimen or to cross over to the opposite regimen. Patients who crossed over had a marginally higher response rate ($p=0.07$) compared with patients who continued on either CFP or doxorubicin/L-PAM. A slight prolongation of the response duration (16 months versus 12 to 13 months) was not statistically significant, and there was no prolongation of survival time by crossover to the second treatment program. None of the other trials have shown more encouraging results to date, in-

Table 13-44
Randomized Trials Comparing a Single Regimen With Alternating Non–Cross-Resistant Regimens

		Response Rate (%)		*Median Duration (Months) of*		
*Regimen**	*Number of Patients*	*PR + CR*	*CR*	*Response*	*Survival*	*Reference no.*
CFP vs.	23	48	15	12	24	
A/L PAM vs.	27	52	9	13	21	
CFP → A/L-PAM (2) or A/L-PAM → CFP	50	68+	10	16	22	388
CA vs.	26	50	12	10	—	390
CA ⟷ MF (1)	22	55	32	10	—	
CAF vs.	46	63	13	—	—	9
DAV ⟷ CMF (3)	48	71	10	—	—	
CFP vs.	18	18	0	9	14	
CA vs.	42	42	2	12	18	333
CFP ⟷ CA (1)	20	63++	0	11	19	
CMF vs.	47	55	17	8	12	389
CMF ⟷ AV (2)	50	58	22	12++	18+++	
CMFP vs.	135	59	14	11	19	389
CMFP ⟷ AV (2)	176	58	14	10	16	
CAF vs.	66	29	2	8	15	391
CAF ⟷ CAMELEON (3)	91	17+	0	11	16	
CFP vs.	41	46	7	—	18	229
CAP ⟷ CFP (4)	45	49	4	—	11	

C, cyclophosphamide; A, doxorubicin; F, 5-fluorouracil; P, prednisone; L-PAM, L-phenylalanine mustard; M, methotrexate; D, dibromodulcitol (mitolactol); V, vincristine; T, tamoxifen; H, fluoxymesterone; CAMELEON, cytosine arabinoside, methotrexate, leucovorin rescue, vincristine; PR, partial response; CR, complete response; + $p=0.07$–0.08; ++, $p=0.02$–0.03; +++, $p=0.05$; other differences not statistically significant.

* Numbers in parentheses are the cycles before first crossover and/or number of cycles between each subsequent regimen alteration.

cluding a recent study in which patients were randomized to receive either CFP or an alternating program in which patients on one arm received a cisplatin combination followed later by treatment with CFP.[229]

Single Agents Versus Combinations

The theoretical reasons for using a combination of agents rather than a single drug are compelling. It is very unlikely that all or most of the multiple breast cancer clones in the average patient will be sensitive to a single chemotherapeutic agent. It is a well-established principle of medical oncology that a combination of drugs is more effective than a single agent, and this has been an important element of our success in treating leukemias, lymphomas, and testicular cancers. In almost all of the randomized trials comparing the efficacy of a single agent with a drug combination for metastatic breast cancer, the response rate with the drug combination was higher (Table 13-45). There are several exceptions to this rule, and these are best illustrated by the two trials in which cyclophosphamide alone was compared with a combination of either CMF/vinblastine or CMFVP.[49,50] In one of these trials, there was no significant difference in the response rate, the response duration, or the survival of patients on the two treatment arms.[49] In this trial, cyclophosphamide was used at a dose that was equally or even more toxic than the combination CMF/vinblastine. In fact, there was one toxic death on the cyclophosphamide arm and no toxic deaths on the combination chemotherapy arm. In the trial in which the response rate and duration of response to cyclophosphamide alone was significantly lower than to CMFVP, more toxicity was observed with the combination.[50] In three of four randomized trials comparing doxorubicin as a single agent with a combination, either CFP or CMFVP, the response rate to doxorubicin alone was not significantly different from that of the combination. However, the duration of the response to doxorubicin as a single agent was significantly shorter in two of these trials,[23,76] and the complete response rate was lower when doxorubicin was used as a single agent in one of the trials.[23] A survival advantage for the combination over the single agent was seen in only one of the randomized single-agent studies.[98] This may be because secondary treatments given after relapse were able to compensate for the lower response to the initial drug therapy. Alternatively, there may be so little impact of these cytotoxic

Table 13-45
Randomized Trials Comparing the Efficacy of a Single Agent With a Drug Combination

Regimen	*Number of Patients*	*Response Rate (%)*		*Median Duration (Months) of*	
		CR + PR	*CR*	*Response*	*Survival*
5-FU[83]	20	30	—	4.8	—
vs. MFVP	17	29	—	5.5	—
L-PAM[98]	91	20	5	3.3	9
vs. CMF	93	53+	14+	6.3+	12+
Cyclophosphamide[49]	49	55	4	5.5	6
vs. CMF-vinblastine	50	62	2	7.0	6
Cyclophosphamide[50]	24	25	4	7.0	—
vs. CMF-VP	27	63+	19+	13.0+	—
Doxorubicin[75,318]	20	50	—	8.0	—
vs. CFP (±V)	28	46	—	10.5	—
Doxorubicin[76]	32	38	—	7.6	17
vs. CFP	230	43	—	21.3+	21.5
Doxorubicin[23]	79	39	4	4.0	11
vs. CMFVP continuous	106	59+	19+	8.0+	14
vs. CMFVP intermittent	98	40+	8+	10.0	14
F → C → V[51]	30	53	0	—	10.2
vs. CFV	46	43	43	6.0	8.6
F → M → C → V → P[48]	34	18	6	4.0	6
vs. CMF-VP continuous	35	46+	11+	7.0+	12
vs. CMF-VP intermittent	33	27	12	8.5	12
F → C → T_3 P → M[47, 392]	60	33	3	7.7	11.5
vs. CMFP-T_3	61	56+	15+	13.4+	17

T_3, = triiodothyronine; P, prednisone; →, = agent used until response and/or failure, then next agent used; +, difference considered statistically significant. All other differences p>0.05.

agents on the survival of patients with metastatic breast cancer that it is unrealistic to anticipate a survival advantage from any of them, and as a result, it may be unrealistic to anticipate that the survival of patients treated on one arm of a randomized trial will be superior to another (see below).

Time to Response

Measurable lesions in patients with lymphomas, testicular cancer, and small cell carcinoma of the lung often involute within a few days to several weeks following initiation of therapy. This kind of dramatic response may also occur when chemotherapy is given to patients with breast cancer. On occasion, bone pain may dramatically disappear, and incapacitated patients may return to work within a few weeks. More frequently, however, the time to the appearance of a documented response will be much longer. The median time to response in phase II trials varies between 7 and 14 weeks. In some cases, this is the first evidence of any response. The time to response will depend in part on the site of measurable disease (Table 13-46). Disease in the skin, lymph nodes, and lung parenchyma responds most quickly, the median time to evidence of an objective response ranging between 4 and 8 weeks. Lesions in these sites can be measured directly, and shrinkage of tumor does not require "healing." In contrast, the time to evidence of an objective response in lesions of the liver and bone is considerably longer. The median time to response in these organs varied between 15 and 18 weeks in the study outlined in Table 13-46.[19] In some studies it may be even longer.[393] This poses a problem in determining when a patient should be considered "unresponsive" to chemotherapy.

Many oncologists will continue chemotherapy until there is evidence of "progression" of disease. However, even this end point may be difficult to determine precisely. The possibility of a "flare" reaction in patients treated with endocrine therapy is well established. (See the section on Endocrine Therapy of Metastatic Disease in Chapter 13.) This phenomenon has not been as well described in patients receiving chemotherapy. However, patients who respond to chemotherapy have been reported to have a transient increase in both the number and intensity of lesions seen on bone scan during the first months of chemotherapy.[394] A more recently described phenomenon is the transient elevation of the carcinoembryonic antigen (CEA) prior to a response.[395,396] Pretreatment CEA levels greater than 5 ng/ml were found in 42 of 97 (43%) patients entered on an ECOG protocol.[396] Twenty-nine of these patients had a response to chemotherapy. In 15 of the 29 (52%), a response at other sites correlated with a steady fall in the CEA level. In the other 14 patients there was a transient rise in the CEA prior to an eventual fall. The mean peak level seen in these 14 patients was 243% of the pretreatment value, and this peak occurred between 27 and 135 days following initiation of the therapy. The reasons for these transient elevations of CEA are not known, but they are similar to the CEA elevation in patients with a flare from endocrine therapy. It is prudent to continue a chemotherapy program, once initiated, for 3 months, unless there are compelling clinical reasons, such as increased pain, intractable hypercalcemia, or hyperbilirubinemia, that dictate a change in therapy.

SELECTION OF PATIENTS FOR CHEMOTHERAPY

The patients who are most likely to benefit from endocrine therapy are those with relatively indolent disease. Clinical criteria reflecting this disease pattern include a long disease-free interval (i.e., the interval from diagnosis to first evidence of recurrence), a limited number of disease sites, a prior hormone response, and late premenopausal or late postmenopausal status. (See the section on Endocrine Therapy in Chapter 13.) The process of selecting patients for endocrine therapy has been simplified with the discovery of the estrogen and progesterone receptors. Unfortunately, a similar set of criteria and a similar laboratory

Table 13-46
*Time Required to Achieve an Objective Response**

Site	*Number of Patients*	*Response Rate (%)*	*Cumulative Response (%) Week*							
			3	*6*	*9*	*12*	*15*	*18*	*24*	*30*
Skin	22	88	32	73	100					
Nodes	25	86	24	56	88	100				
Lung	21	75		24	71	90	100			
Pleura	10	83	20	40	70	90	100			
Liver	12	75			17	33	58	58	83	100
Bone	24	75		4		29	37	54	75	100

*(Modified from Mattson W, Arwidi A, von Eyben F, et al: Phase II study of combined vincristine, Adriamycin, cyclophosphamide, and methotrexate with citrovorum factor rescue in metastatic breast cancer. Cancer Treat Rep 61:1527–1531, 1977)

test are not available to help in the selection of the patients most likely to benefit from chemotherapy.

A priori, one might expect that the patients most likely to respond to chemotherapy are those with characteristics most *unlike* the endocrine responders. The cells most affected by endocrine therapy are the well-differentiated, end-stage cells. The cells most affected by chemotherapy may be the rapidly dividing, less-differentiated stem cells. *In vitro,* the cell lines most likely to respond to chemotherapy are those with a short doubling time and no estrogen receptors.[397] In a study of five different cell lines, the receptor-positive lines had a doubling time of 32 to 33 hours, and the receptor negative lines 14 to 16 hours. Doxorubicin reduced the cell count and DNA mass in the receptor-positive cells to between 44% and 47% and in the receptor-negative cells to between 9% and 14% of control levels. In the clinic, it has been observed that the average labeling index of patients responding to chemotherapy is almost double that of the nonresponders ($p < 0.01$).[398] This was not observed in an earlier study in which 5-fluorouracil was used as a single agent for patients with breast or colon cancer.[399]

Thymidine kinase has been proposed as a marker of chemoresponsiveness similar to the estrogen receptor for endocrine responsiveness. Tissue thymidine kinase levels have been shown to correlate with the proliferative rate of cancer cells. In a study of 45 patients who had thymidine kinase levels measured and who received chemotherapy, 13 of the 15 tumors (86%) with thymidine kinase levels greater than 80 pmol/mg/minute responded to chemotherapy. Only 4 of 30 (13%) with thymidine kinase levels below 80 pmol/mg/minute responded ($p < 0.001$).[400]

Many attempts have been made to correlate patient characteristics and response to chemotherapy (Table 13-47). Contrary to expectations based on theoretical considerations, the patients most likely to benefit from chemotherapy are quite similar to those likely to benefit from endocrine therapy. In general, these are the patients who have limited disease, who are in an early stage of their illness, and who have relatively few symptoms. Patient performance status is probably the single most important criterion (see Table 13-19).[6,306,324,361,401,402] Patients with a Karnofsky index greater than 70, an ECOG performance level of 0 or 1, and patients who are ambulatory are those most likely to have a durable response and prolonged survival following treatment with chemotherapy. Patients with a long disease-free interval (DFI) are also more likely to respond,[6,15,403,404] and responders with a long DFI are likely to have a more durable remission and prolonged survival.[405] In one literature review, it was observed that the response to chemotherapy in patients with a DFI in excess of 5 years was 68% compared with 55% among those patients with a DFI of less than 2 years.[15] Premenopausal patients may have a slightly higher response rate than postmenopausal women. In one study, the response rates were 68%, 59%, and 61%, respectively, for premenopausal, perimenopausal, and postmenopausal women.[403]

At one time, patients with bone metastases were considered poor candidates for chemotherapy. For example, in some reports bone metastases have been reported to have response rates one-third or less than those at other metastatic sites.[98,406] To some extent this may be an artifact related to the time when a response to therapy is scored. As noted above, the time to evidence of response in some sites, such as bone and liver, is much longer than in others. With intensive chemotherapy programs, the overall response rate in bone metastases has equaled that observed in other sites (see Table 13-40).[16,362,363] However, the complete response rate in bone is approximately half that observed in sites in which a response can be easily and quickly detected, such as lymph nodes and lung parenchyma. There is some evidence that patients with predominantly bone metastases have a more indolent course, and several retrospective analyses have shown that patients with bone metastases who respond to therapy may have a more durable response.[34,402] The Southeastern Group proposed that responses be scored by patterns of metastases, not by the major site of involvement.[407] In their experience, the patients with the lowest response rates were those with pleural involvement on the ipsilateral side, large ulcerative lesions, and bone metastases.

The number of sites involved with metastatic disease is inversely correlated with response.[6,324,402,408,409] It is difficult to separate this factor as a variable independent of the patient's prior exposure to chemotherapy. Patients with

Table 13-47
Factors Associated With Response Rate, Response Duration, and Survival Following Chemotherapy for Metastatic Breast Cancer

Factors Associated With:	
An Increased Probability of Response	*A Decreased Probability of Response*
Good performance status	Bone metastases
Ambulatory status	Liver metastases
Limited number (1–2) of disease sites	Prior chemotherapy
Prior hormone therapy	Prior radiotherapy
Metastases to lymph nodes	Decreased lymphocyte count
An Increased Response Duration or Survival	*A Decreased Response Duration or Survival*
Good performance status	Prior radiotherapy
Disease-free interval	Decreased lymphocyte count
Limited number of disease sites	
Prior hormone therapy	
Prior response to hormone therapy	
Factors Not Associated With Response Rate:	
Age	
Menopausal status	
Dominant disease site	
Carcinoembryonic antigen	

(Henderson IC: Chemotherapy for advanced disease. In Bonadonna G (ed): Breast Cancer: Diagnosis and Management, pp 274–280. New York, John Wiley & Sons, 1984)

multiple metastatic sites are frequently end-stage patients who have a poor performance status as a result of impairment of many organ systems and who have had extensive prior therapy. Patients treated with any form of prior radiotherapy have been found to have a lower response rate to subsequent chemotherapy.[403] This, too, may be related to the stage of the patient's disease. However, one study demonstrated that prior adjuvant radiotherapy postmastectomy significantly reduced the probability of response to chemotherapy ($p = 0.05$), whereas radiation therapy to metastatic sites did not.[408] Decreased lymphocyte count has also been associated with a decreased response rate and decreased survival.[410] This was not specifically correlated with prior radiation therapy, but one might anticipate that patients with extensive prior radiation therapy would have a lower lymphocyte count, and these two variables may be dependent. Prior chemotherapy is the single most important factor for determining response to therapy, and this is consistent through almost all clinical trials (see Tables 13-24, 13-36, 13-38). Potential reasons for this have been discussed above.

A prior response to endocrine therapy does not have predictive value for response to chemotherapy. In most studies, the endocrine responders and nonresponders have an equal response rate.[320,411–413] However, the duration of remission[411,412] and the survival of prior endocrine responders treated with chemotherapy[320] is longer than that of endocrine nonresponders. For example, the overall response rate to chemotherapy was 70% among 53 patients with a prior hormone response and 67% among those patients who had failed previous hormone therapy. The median duration of response among patients who responded to both hormone therapy and chemotherapy was 23 months, compared with only 13 months for the patients who responded to chemotherapy but not to endocrine therapy ($p < 0.01$).[411]

Based on the *preclinical* studies described above, one would anticipate that patients who are estrogen receptor negative would be more likely to respond to chemotherapy than those who are estrogen receptor positive.[414] Based on *clinical* trials, one would expect the estrogen receptor to have no predictive value.[415] In the earliest report correlating estrogen receptor level and response to chemotherapy, the response rate to chemotherapy was 76% among estrogen-receptor-negative patients and 12% among estrogen-receptor-positive patients ($p < 0.0001$).[416] Subsequent studies failed to confirm this early result (Table 13-48).[417–422] Because of this, an extramural analysis was performed with a site visit to all of the institutions involved. The differences in results between studies appeared to be partly related to the scoring of clinical responses, and on extramural review it appeared that in five of the seven institutions the response rate to chemotherapy was actually higher in patients who were estrogen receptor positive.[423] This extramural analysis correlated response with various levels of estrogen receptor but found that regardless of the receptor level chosen, patients who were estrogen receptor positive were more likely to have a response to chemotherapy. It has been suggested that the estrogen receptor is more predictive of a response to nondoxorubicin regimens than to doxorubicin programs.[424] The response rate to nondoxorubicin combinations in estrogen-receptor-positive patients was 67% and in estrogen-receptor-negative patients 31%. The response rate to doxorubicin-containing combinations in estrogen-receptor-positive patients was 52% and in estrogen-receptor-negative patients 61%. The external reviewers were unable to document a relationship between the predictive value of estrogen receptor among patients treated with different chemotherapy combinations.[423] In spite of the elegance of the underlying rationale for using the estrogen receptor as a predictive factor for chemotherapy response, there are insufficient clinical data to justify the use of estrogen receptor values in this way.

The time to appearance of a response may be a predictive factor of the response durability. It was observed in one study that patients who achieved a complete response within 3 months of the initiation of therapy had

Table 13-48
Relationship Between Estrogen Receptor Level and Response to Chemotherapy

	Response Rate in					
	All patients		ER Positive		ER Negative	
Study	Number of Patients	Response Rate (%)	Number of Patients	Response Rate (%)	Number of Patients	Response Rate (%)
NCI[416]	70	53	25	12	45	76*
Minnesota[417]	40	65	19	89	21	43*
Hamburg-Breman[418]	53	45	23	61	30	33
Wayne State[419]	81	69	36	78	45	62
Rochester[420]	44	59	22	50	22	68
Guy's[421]	47	60	33	62	14	57
Tufts[422]	30	60	16	75	14	43*

* Differences between the response rate in estrogen receptor negative and positive patients statistically significant ($p < 0.05$). Other observed differences not statistically significant.

both a more durable remission and longer survival time.[425] In another study, this was found to be true for patients who had disease limited to the soft tissues.[402] However, patients who had a delayed response and who had predominantly bone or visceral disease or both had very durable responses.

The best candidates for chemotherapy are patients who are both symptomatic and are unlikely to benefit from endocrine therapy. It is no longer justified to routinely treat all patients with endocrine therapy before attempting treatment with chemotherapy.[36] Patients with the clinical criteria of endocrine responders or a high level of receptor should be treated with endocrine therapy preferentially, and other patients should be treated with chemotherapy. Endocrine therapy patients should be treated with chemotherapy after they have proved refractory to further endocrine therapy.

COMBINATIONS OF CHEMOTHERAPY AND ENDOCRINE THERAPY

In a tumor characterized by multiple clones, such as breast cancer, it is plausible that some clones will be responsive to endocrine therapy and resistant to chemotherapy and that other clones will be sensitive to chemotherapy and resistant to endocrine therapy. Studies with the estrogen receptor demonstrate that all cells do not have this receptor, and it can be taken as an established principle that even those patients with the most endocrine-sensitive tumors have a mixture of cells that are hormone sensitive and hormone resistant. (See the sections on Endocrine Therapy in Chapter 13 and on Receptors in Chapter 8.) The rationale for developing chemohormonal therapy combinations is that drugs and hormones may be synergistic or additive in their effect on the tumor cell and nonsynergistic in their toxic effects on normal tissues. Whenever possible, myelosuppressive and nonmyelosuppressive drugs are combined, and the use of chemotherapy with hormonal therapy is the most logical extension of this principle. Endocrine therapy is almost nontoxic to normal tissues and should not compromise the dose of chemotherapeutic agents that can be given.

The first trials evaluating combinations of endocrine therapy and chemotherapy were begun almost as soon as chemotherapy was introduced as a new modality for the treatment of metastatic breast cancer (Table 13-49).[426] In almost all of these studies there was an increase in the response rate when a combination of chemotherapy and endocrine therapy was used rather than endocrine therapy alone. If these agents were truly synergistic within each patient, we should see a prolonged duration of response or prolonged duration of survival with the combination, but in most of these studies there is no difference at all in response duration or survival. A recently published report is an exception to all the others.[434] Patients who were estrogen receptor positive were randomized to receive either diethylstilbestrol (DES) or DES plus a combination of cyclophosphamide and 5-fluorouracil. The median survival of patients treated with both hormonal therapy and chemotherapy was more than twice that of the patients treated with DES alone, and the difference was just statistically significant ($p = 0.05$) The authors suggested that one reason they had seen prolongation of survival when it has not been observed by other investigators may have been their limitation of the patient population to those with an estrogen receptor in the tumor cytoplasm. However, a similar study limited to estrogen-receptor-positive patients failed to show any difference in the response rate, response duration, or survival.[435] In this trial, patients were randomized to tamoxifen or tamoxifen plus CMF. Possibly the differences between the results achieved in the two trials reflect greater efficacy for tamoxifen. In two of these studies, patients were randomized after an initial response to endocrine therapy to either continue the endocrine therapy or to have added chemotherapy.[431,432] In both of the studies there was greater evolution to a higher response rate in the patients with added chemotherapy than in those who continued on hormonal therapy alone, but this did not reach levels of statistical significance. The survival time of patients in both groups was identical, even though the duration of first response was significantly longer when chemotherapy was added to oophorectomy in one of the two trials.[432]

In more recent trials evaluating chemohormonal therapy, patients have been randomized to receive chemotherapy alone or chemotherapy plus endocrine therapy (Table 13-50). In more than half of these trials, the response rate to the combination is higher than to chemotherapy alone, and in four trials this difference was statistically significant.[438,440,441,445] One might anticipate that the major difference in response rate would be observed among those patients who were estrogen receptor positive. Estrogen receptor data are available in only three trials. However, the response rate to chemohormonal therapy was greater than to chemotherapy alone among estrogen-receptor-positive patients in only one of those three trials.[441] As in the previous generation of studies, no survival advantage was observed with the combination. In one of the largest of these trials, however, the median survival time of patients treated with CMF was 19 months and with CMF plus tamoxifen 24 months ($p = 0.07$).[445] In this trial, the difference in response rate to the two treatment programs increased with increased patient age. Among women younger than 54 years there was only a 2% difference in response rate. Chemohormonal therapy induced a response in 20% more of the patients in the age-group 50 to 59 years, in 38% more of the patients between the ages of 60 and 64, and in 49% more among women older than 65. Although it might seem likely that the older women received less chemotherapy, a separate analysis of dose reduction failed to find a significant difference in the dose of drugs given to women under and over the age of 60.

A large trial with a three-arm randomization recently reported from Australia must be considered one of the definitive studies on the interactions between chemotherapy and hormonal therapy.[437] Patients in this study were

Table 13-49
Randomized Trials Evaluating Chemotherapy Added to Endocrine Therapy

Study Design	*Authors*	*Number of Patients*	*Response Rate %* 1st†	*Response Rate %* Overall‡	*Median Duration (Months)* Response	*Median Duration (Months)* Survival
Adrenalectomy	Oberfield et al[426]	31	47	—	15.0	20.0
" + TMF			73	—	16.0	19.5
Oophorectomy			18 →	61	5.0	30.0
" + CMFVP*	Falkson et al[427]	145	72‖	72	17.0	26.0
" + C			65	65	16.0	23.0
DES	Kumar et al[428]	44	14 →	43	7.7	15.2
" + CAF			57	57	9.8	20.4
Oophorectomy*	Ahmann et al[429, 430]	76	27 →	42	—	NS
" + CFP			38	38	—	
Tamoxifen§	Glick et al[431]	63	67 →	85	12.0	NS
" + CMF§			55 →	87	19.0	
Oophorectomy*§	Rossof et al[432]	34	50 →	71	6.1	40.4
" + CMF§			55 →	85	17.5‖	41.3
Tamoxifen	Wada et al[433]	82	29 →	38	9.3	24.0
" + tetra-FU			43	43	10.3	36.0
DES†	Kiang et al[434]	40	53		12.0	29.0
" + CF			86		24.0	72.0‖
Tamoxifen†	Bezwada et al[435]	40	63 →	71	12.7	17.7
" + CMF			65		7.4	17.1
Oophorectomy*	Cavalli et al[436]	99	22 →	43	—	21.0
" + LMF (±VPA)			46	46	—	25.3
Tamoxifen	Cavalli et al[436]	297	17 →	33	—	27.5
" + LMF (±VPA)			40	40	—	23.7
Tamoxifen	ANZBCTG[437]	226	22	43	—	21.0
" + AC			51‖	51	—	20.0

T, thiotepa; M, methotrexate; F, 5-Fluorouracil; C, cyclophosphamide; V, vincristine; P, prednisone; A, doxorubicin; L, chlorambucil; tetra-FU, 1-(2-tetrahydrofuryl)-5-fluorouracil; DES, diethylstilbestrol.
* Only premenopausal patients
† Only estrogen receptor positive patients
‡ "1st" is the response rate to the first regimen administered; "overall" is the final response rate based on a response to either the initial regimen or the cross-over regimen.
§ All patients were initially treated with endocrine therapy. Responders were subsequently randomized to either continue on endocrine therapy alone or to have added chemotherapy.
‖ Difference statistically significant, $p \leq 0.05$. Other differences are not statistically significant.

randomized to treatment with either tamoxifen alone, a combination of cyclophosphamide and doxorubicin (CA), or tamoxifen and CA. The initial response rate to tamoxifen alone was significantly less than the response rate to either chemotherapy alone or chemotherapy plus tamoxifen ($p < 0.001$). However, tamoxifen patients were treated with CA on failure, and the overall response rate and survival time of patients on the three study arms were identical.

In all of these studies, the toxicity associated with chemotherapy alone or chemotherapy plus hormonal therapy is greater than with hormonal therapy alone, and this important point is easily overlooked. None has adequately evaluated the quality of life achieved with these two alternative approaches to therapy, in part because quality of life is an extremely difficult parameter to measure objectively. However, the use of chemotherapy and hormonal therapy together may cheat the patient of a very durable response with a nontoxic agent. For example, in the Australian trial the secondary response rate to endocrine therapy after failure to cyclophosphamide/doxorubicin was only 6%.[437] The possibility of combining endocrine therapy and chemotherapy in some meaningful way deserves further exploration. However, until data are available to show that a combination of endocrine therapy and chemotherapy will significantly prolong survival, it is preferable to use endocrine therapy alone in appropriate patients and to use chemotherapy when that patient is clearly refractory to endocrine therapy.

It can be shown *in vitro* that small amounts of estrogen will increase the mitotic rate of MCF-7 cells.[447] There

Table 13-50
Randomized Trials Comparing the Efficacy of Chemotherapy Alone and Chemotherapy Combined With Endocrine Therapy

Design	Author	Number of Patients	Response Rate (%) All Patients	ER+ Patients	ER− Patients	Median Duration (Months) Response	Survival
CMFVP*	Brunner et al[438]	52	43 +	—	—	7.8	13.2
" + oophorectomy			74			9.5	19.9
CMFVP	Brunner et al[438]	96	54	—	—	10.6	19.2
" + DES			63			8.4	26.7
AV/CMF	Rubean et al[439]	69	61	—	—	9.5	15.0
" + Norethisterone			53			9.5	8.0
DA	Tormey et al[440]	122	29 +	—	—	5.3 +	9.0
" + Tamoxifen			50			9.3	11.3
CMF	Cocconi et al[441]	133	51 +	46	71	11.7	27.8
" + Tamoxifen			74	80	76	12.8	19.5
CAF	Kardinal et al[442, 443]	419	55	50	70	14.6	NS
" + Tamoxifen			62	47	54	17.3	
CMF			46	—	—	13.3	22.5
" + Tamoxifen	Viladiu et al[444]	98	71	—	—	16.3	24.7
" + Medroxyprogesterone			68	—	—	12.7	21.7
CMF	Mouridsen et al[445]	220	49 +	—	—	12 ±	19 ±
" + Tamoxifen			75	—	—	18	24
CF*	Kiang et al[434]	31	—	—	29	7.5	16
" + DES			—	—	53	11.0	16
AC	ANZBCTG[437]	226	45	—	—	—	18
" + Tamoxifen			51	—	—	—	20
CFP	Krook et al[446]	125	68	77	—	—	18 ±
" + Tamoxifen			61	50	—	—	13

C, cyclophosphamide; M, methotrexate, F, 5-fluorouracil; V, vincristine; P, prednisone; DES, diethylstilbestrol; D, mitolactol; A, doxorubicin;
+ statistically significant, $p<0.05$; ± marginally significant, $p>0.05$ <0.10;
*All patients premenopausal.
† All patients receptor negative.

is very little evidence that estrogens or other forms of endocrine therapy actually stimulate increased growth of tumors *in vivo*. Labeling indices were determined before and after the administration of physiologic doses of estrogen and progesterone in ten patients with easily accessible skin metastases.[448] This combination of hormones induced a rise in the labeling indices in seven of these ten patients. Interestingly, the increase in labeling index was seen in both estrogen-positive and estrogen-negative tumors. The "flare" phenomenon has often been interpreted as evidence of a stimulatory response to endocrine therapy, but this may occur with the ablation of hormone as well as with the addition. Further, there are very few data to substantiate the widely held notion that flare represents a stimulation of tumor growth. (See the section on Endocrine Therapy in Chapter 13.) Tumors responding to endocrine therapy may actually be less responsive to chemotherapy, since serial biopsies of tumors regressing after treatment with oophorectomy or tamoxifen show a dramatic fall in the labeling index within 1 to 2 weeks following initiation of treatment.[449]

If tumor cells could be synchronized *in vivo* in the same way they are *in vitro,* sequential endocrine therapy and chemotherapy might cause a higher tumor cell kill than either modality alone. This has been attempted in several different ways. The first report used a 10-day course of tamoxifen, 10 mg twice daily, to synchronize cells followed by a 4-day course of estrogen (Premarin 0.625 mg twice daily) to stimulate the cells in a synchronous manner.[450] At the end of the 4-day course of estrogen therapy, the patients were treated with a chemotherapy combination consisting of methotrexate, 200 mg/m^2, followed 1 hour later by 5-fluorouracil, 600 mg/m^2. Methotrexate toxicity was rescued with leucovorin, and this cycle of endocrine and chemotherapy was repeated every 18 days. The initial results were impressive. Seventy-two percent of 25 treated patients responded, and 56% of these patients had a complete response. The median duration

Table 13-51
Trials Evaluating Sequential Endocrine-Chemotherapy Regimens

Regimen	Number of Patients	Response Rate (%) Total	Response Rate (%) Complete	Median Duration (Months)	Author
TAM → Premarin → MF†	25	72	56	>12	Allegra et al[450]
TAM → Premarin → MF†	30	10	3	—	Eisenhauer et al[451]
CA → TAM → Premarin → MF‡	35	65	22	17	Lippman et al[452]
vs. CAMF	32	65	18	14*	
C → DES → EF‡	73	46	18	—	Conte et al[453]
vs. CEF		47	15	—	
AG → EE_2 → FAC†	35	74	36	—	Paridaens et al[454]

TAM, tamoxifen, M, methotrexate; F, 5-fluorouracil; C, cyclophosphamide; A, doxorubicin; DES, diethylstilbestrol; E, 4-epidoxorubicin; AG, aminoglutethimide; EE_2, ethinylestradiol.
* p = 0.009. Other differences in randomized trials not statistically significant.
† Uncontrolled trial
‡ Randomized trial

of response was in excess of 12 months (Table 13-51). This was an uncontrolled trial. Subsequent investigators have been unable to confirm the original results, but this may partially be a result of the fact that patients in subsequent trials were more heavily pretreated with both chemotherapy and endocrine therapy.[451] One theoretical problem with the use of tamoxifen followed by a short course of estrogen is the fact that the half-life of tamoxifen is in excess of 6 weeks,[455] and it is possible that low to moderate doses of estrogens will not overcome the tamoxifen effect quickly.

Two randomized comparisons of sequential chemohormonal therapy with chemotherapy alone have been performed (see Table 13-51). In the first of these, patients were randomized to receive a combination of cyclophosphamide, doxorubicin, methotrexate, and 5-fluorouracil alone (CAMF) or to receive CA on day 1, tamoxifen on days 2 through 6, Premarin on day 7, and methotrexate and 5-fluorouracil on days 8 and 9.[452] The overall response rate was similar on the two treatment arms, but the median duration of response was 3 months longer and the median duration of survival was 5 months longer for patients treated on the sequential arm. These differences were statistically significant. No differences in survival time were observed when patients were randomized to a combination of cyclophosphamide, 4′epidoxorubicin, and 5-fluorouracil versus cyclophosphamide, followed by a course of DES with subsequent 4′epidoxorubicin and 5-fluorouracil.[453] The idea of using aminoglutethimide to synchronize the cells followed by estrogen has considerable appeal because the aminoglutethimide effects can be more rapidly reversed than the tamoxifen effects. In an uncontrolled trial using this sequence followed by FAC, the total response and complete response were impressive but difficult to interpret without an appropriate control arm.[454]

The idea of sequencing hormonal therapy and chemotherapy represents an exciting prospect for the future. At present it has no role in the standard practice of medical oncology.

EFFECT OF THERAPY ON SURVIVAL

The wise clinician will have a well-defined goal for each treatment decision. For patients with metastatic breast cancer, there are two potential goals: palliation of symptoms or the prolongation of survival. Although there are anecdotal reports of survival free of recurrence more than 15 years after treatment for metastatic breast cancer,[22] these are rare exceptions. Almost all patients with a recurrence after primary treatment eventually die with evidence of persistent breast cancer. Endocrine therapy and chemotherapy will palliate the symptoms of metastatic breast cancer very effectively. However, whether either of these therapies prolongs the survival time of patients with overt metastases is a subject of some controversy.

The most scientific method for measuring the effect of treatment on survival is a controlled trial in which half the patients are randomized to receive systemic therapy and the other half to receive no therapy. This would be a reasonable approach in asymptomatic patients, but very few patients continue to be asymptomatic for long. It would be unethical to withhold all endocrine therapy and chemotherapy from patients whose symptoms could best be palliated by these modalities. Therefore, any estimation of the impact of therapy on survival must be made and will continue to be made from indirect observations. Some of these observations have greater validity than others, and all have unique limitations. Three types of data are frequently cited as evidence for or against a survival benefit from therapy:

1. A comparison of the survival time of responders and nonresponders to therapy.

2. Changes in the survival of a defined cohort (usually those seen in one institution) in the years or decades following the introduction of a new therapy.
3. A comparison of the survival time of *all* patients randomized to a regimen with a high response rate to the survival time of patients randomized to a regimen with a low response rate.

Most studies show a statistically significant difference in the survival time of responders and nonresponders to a therapy, and it is assumed that the survivors have lived longer as a result of therapy. An equally likely explanation for this observation is that the responders have responded because of some disease characteristic that is also associated with a better prognosis. Patients who respond to endocrine therapy live longer than patients who fail to respond.[456] Patients with an estrogen receptor are more likely to respond to endocrine therapy than patients without an estrogen receptor. Patients with an estrogen receptor may have a better prognosis than patients without an estrogen receptor *regardless of response* to therapy. (See the section on Receptors in Chapter 8.) In the same vein, patients who respond to chemotherapy live longer than nonresponders.[457] The patients most likely to respond to chemotherapy are those with a good performance status. Patients with a good performance status may have a better prognosis *regardless of response* to chemotherapy (see above and Table 13-39). Because this difference in the survival time of responders and nonresponders has been accepted uncritically by many physicians and is often used as a compelling reason to treat asymptomatic patients, its inclusion in published papers has recently been discouraged and described as more misleading than helpful.[458]

If there were a sound relationship between response and survival time, one might anticipate that patients with a complete response would have a longer survival time than those with a partial response or stable disease. A high complete response rate has been the harbinger of lengthened survival time for other tumor types.[459] However, this has not been true for breast cancer, for which the survival time of patients with a complete response, partial response, and stable disease is almost identical, even though all three of these states are associated with longer survival than that of rapidly progressive disease.[457]

A second method of measuring the impact of therapy on survival time is to look at changes in survival over time. The results from various studies that have attempted to do this are contradictory. When investigators at the Royal Marsden compared the length of survival of patients treated prior to 1974, when chemotherapy was rarely used in that clinic, and the survival time of patients treated after 1974, no significant differences were observed.[460] Similarly, no increase in survival time after first recurrence could be seen in patients treated at Memorial Hospital between 1947–1961 and 1967–1977 (Table 13-52).[461] The 5-year survival in both time periods was less than 10%, and even the 1- and 2-year survivals were almost identical, suggesting that there had not been a transient prolongation in the survival of these patients. It did not seem to make a difference whether the patients had a short or long DFI. Investigators at Yale University looked at the median survival time of patients who presented with evidence of metastases at the time of initial diagnosis between 1920 and 1980 (i.e., patients with a DFI of zero).[462] The median survival of these patients improved from 21 months in 1920 to 41 months in 1970. During this interval, both endocrine therapy and single-agent chemotherapy were introduced. However, between the years 1970 and 1980 there was no further increase in the median survival time or the 5-year survival of patients of this type.

Table 13-52
Survival From First Recurrence: Patients With Metastatic Breast Cancer Treated at Memorial Hospital Between 1947–1961 and 1967–1977

	Number of Patients	Survival After First Recurrence Patients Alive (%) at the end of 1 Year	2 Years	5 Years
All patients				
1947–1961	599	63.3	32.6	6.3
1967–1977	329	69.5	37.5	7.9
Patients With an Initial Disease-Free Interval of < 1 Year				
1947–1961	188	48.9	22.3	3.2
1967–1977	109	51.4	13.8	1.8
Patients With a Disease-Free Interval of > 2 Years				
1947–1961	247	76.9	44.1	9.7
1967–1977	134	85.1	62.7	14.2
Patients With a Disease-Free Interval of > 5 Years				
1947–1961	77	81.8	59.7	14.3
1967–1977	42	88.1	71.4	21.4

(Modified from Kaufman R J: Advanced breast cancer—additive hormonal therapy. Cancer 47:2398–2403, 1981)

Selection factors related to patient referral patterns may have had an important effect on the survival of patients treated in these tertiary centers, such as the Royal Marsden, Yale, and Memorial Hospital. As therapies are shown to be effective, they are administered in community hospitals. Patients who present particularly difficult problems or who are refractory to conventional therapy are more likely to be referred to the major centers. However, a regional study in central and northern Alberta also failed to show much improvement in survival time with the introduction of new therapy.[463] These investigators compared the median survival time of patients who died of breast cancer prior to 1974 with that between the interval of 1974 to 1978. The median survival time of patients in these two time periods was 19 and 18 months, respectively ($p<0.08$).

Other population studies have been somewhat more encouraging. In the city of Stockholm, the median survival time between first evidence of distant metastases and death increased from 9 months in the period 1961–1963 to 13 months in 1971–1973 ($p<0.01$).[464] The survival time of patients registered at the M.D. Andersen between 1956–1966, 1966–1975, and after 1975 were compared, and no differences in overall survival were observed during these three time periods.[465] However, the median survival time of patients in the groups with the highest hazard ratio (i.e., those with evidence of the most aggressive disease and considered the most likely to die early on the basis of their clinical characteristics) was evaluated separately. No differences were seen when patients entering between 1956 and 1966 were compared, but survival almost doubled between 1966 and 1975. These differences were statistically significant ($p=0.05$) for the group with the highest hazard ratio and for the patients with midrange hazard ratios ($p<0.01$).

A third way of assessing the impact of therapy on survival is to compare the survival time of patients treated on a regimen with a high response rate and the survival time of patients treated on a regimen with a low response rate. Throughout this chapter, many such studies have been cited, and a perusal of the tables will indicate that in most cases a doubling of the response rate does not result in a proportionate increase in patient survival (see Tables 13-37, 13-44, 13-45, 13-49, 13-50). The ECOG performed a retrospective analysis of a series of trials in which patients were randomized to receive either a single agent or a combination of drugs.[466] In one of these studies, patients were randomized to receive 5-fluorouracil or 5-fluorouracil plus Premarin. In a second, L-PAM and CMF were compared, and in a third, single-agent doxorubicin was compared with CMF.[10] In these studies, the response rate was lower and the time to treatment failure (TTF) was shorter for patients on the single-agent arm (Table 13-53). The median TTF for patients in single-agent studies was between 1.5 and 3.3, for patients on the combination therapies 5.0 to 7.0 months. However, there was not much difference between the TTF of responders on either program, nor was there a difference in the TTF of nonresponders. If a patient failed to respond to a single agent, she failed as quickly as the patients given a combination. Similarly, the median duration of response was the same whether she received the less effective or the more effective regimen. The difference in response rates resulted in a difference in median survival time of *all* treated patients, but this did not appear to be in excess of 4 months. The survival time of responders and nonresponders to the two different programs was identical. This is consistent with the conclusion reached from the historical comparisons cited above and provides further evidence that the impact of therapy on the survival time of patients with metastatic breast cancer is moderate, at best.

Table 13-53
Relationship Between Response Rate and Survival in Randomized Trials

	Single Agents *5-FU, L-PAM, Adria*	*Combinations* *CMF, CMFP, AV*
Response rate (%)	18–34	45–59
Median time to treatment failure		
All patients	1.5–3.3	5.0–7.0
Responders	5.8–10.3	7.8–10.3
Nonresponders	1.0–4.0	1.0–4.0
Median response duration (months)	3.5–5.8	5.3–7.8
Median survival (months)		
All patients	10.0–14.5	12.5–18.3
Responders	16.8–24.8	18.0–22.5
Nonresponders	7.0–10.8	6.3–8.8

(Tormey DC, Carbone P, Band P. Breast cancer survival in single and combination chemotherapy trials since 1968. Proc Am Assoc Cancer Res 18:64, 1977)

The effect of therapy on survival time may vary from one subset of patients to another. For example, patients with more aggressive forms of the disease and the worst prognosis may benefit more from an aggressive chemotherapy combination than patients with indolent disease. In one series of trials, the difference in the median survival time of responders and nonresponders with visceral metastases was almost three times the difference in the survival time of patients with disease limited predominantly to the bone (Table 13-54).[467] A more valid but less dramatic way of illustrating this point is to compare the impact of more effective therapy with less effective therapy in different patient subsets within a randomized trial. In two trials comparing a combination program and a single agent, only patients with liver metastases had a marked survival advantage as a result of therapy with the combination regimen. The survival of patients with disease of the soft tissues and bone was about the same whether they received the single agent or the combination, even though the response rate to the combination was significantly higher.[47,48] Too often, a poor prognosis is used as a justification for treatment of cancer patients, but it is possible that the benefits of therapy in this group of patients may truly be greater than in other subsets.

A GENERAL APPROACH TO THE TREATMENT OF THE PATIENT WITH METASTATIC BREAST CANCER

The literature of breast cancer is abundant, and the number of promising options for treating these patients is constantly growing. This is confusing for patients and physicians alike. Adherence to a few basic principles may simplify the selection of therapy.

1. Although there may be some survival benefits for treating patients with metastatic breast cancer, the likelihood of such benefits is small and should not serve as the principal determinant of whether a patient should or should not be treated.
2. Almost all of the symptoms of metastatic breast cancer can be effectively palliated, including bone pain, weep-

Table 13-54
Effect of Chemotherapy on the Survival of Patients With Different Dominant Sites of Metatases

Disease Site	Median Survival (Months) From Initiation of Chemotherapy	
	Responders	Nonresponders
Visceral	22	8
Local, nodes, pleura	18	8
Extensive disease:		
bone + viscera	14	7
Bone	19	14

(Fey MF, Brunner KW, Sonntag RW: Prognostic factors in metastatic breast cancer. Cancer Clin Trials 4:237–247, 1981)

ing, malodorous skin lesions, the dyspnea of lymphangitic spread, or even jaundice from liver metastases.

3. Most patients will have three to five major decision points in the years following a diagnosis of metastatic breast cancer. Each therapeutic decision should be considered in light of its effect on future therapeutic options. For example, the use of extensive radiation therapy to palliate symptoms may preclude the future use of chemotherapy. The use of chemotherapy in an asymptomatic patient may induce pleiotropic resistance, thus eliminating the possibility of a response when the patient is symptomatic.
4. When two therapeutic choices are likely to be equally efficacious in a given patient, the least toxic should be chosen (e.g., hormones over chemotherapy). When selecting between regimens that are not equally efficacious, toxicity should not be the primary consideration, since studies on the quality of life suggest that a response is more important than drug toxicity in determining the quality of patient survival.
5. When selecting among combinations of chemotherapeutic agents, it is generally advantageous to consider using a CMF combination and a doxorubicin combination at separate times to ensure that the patient has a possibility of responding to two effective regimens.
6. It is reasonable to consider the use of promising experimental programs early in a patient's course when she is relatively less symptomatic in order to employ the more standard programs to palliate symptoms at a later time.
7. Prolonged courses of chemotherapy are not more effective than short courses. It may be best to use 4- to 8-month courses of chemotherapy repeatedly and only as necessary to palliate symptoms.

REFERENCES

1. Abeloff MD, Ettinger DS: Treatment of metastatic breast cancer with Adriamycin-cyclophosphamide induction followed by alternating combination therapy. Cancer Treat Rep 61:1685–1689, 1977
2. Tormey DC, Gelman R, Band PR, et al: Comparison of induction chemotherapies for metastatic breast cancer. Cancer 50:1235–1244, 1082
3. Brambilla C, DeLena M, Rossi A, et al: Response and survival in advanced breast cancer after two non-cross-resistant combinations. Br Med J 1:801–804, 1976
4. Brambilla C, Valagussa P, Bonadonna G: Sequential combination chemotherapy in advanced breast cancer. Cancer Chemother Pharmacol 1:35–39, 1978
5. Brunner KW, Sonntag RW, Martz G, et al: A controlled study in the use of combined drug therapy for metastatic breast cancer. Cancer 36:1208–1219, 1975
6. Bull J, Tormey D, Li SH, et al: A randomized comparative trial of Adriamycin versus methotrexate in combination drug therapy. Cancer 41:1649–1657, 1978
7. Canellos GP, Devita V, Gold GL, et al: Combination chemotherapy for advanced breast cancer: Response and effect on survival. Ann Intern Med 84:389–392, 1976
8. Muss H, White D, Richards F, et al: Adriamycin versus methotrexate in five-drug combination chemotherapy for advanced breast cancer. Cancer 42:2141–2148, 1978
9. Tormey DC, Falkson G, Simon RM, et al: A randomized comparison of two sequentially administered combination regimens to a single regimen in metastatic breast cancer. Cancer Clin Trials 2:247–256, 1979
10. Carbone PP, Bauer M, Band P, et al: Chemotherapy of disseminated breast cancer. Cancer 39:2916–2922, 1977
11. Creech R, Catalano R, Harris D, et al: Low dose chemotherapy of metastatic breast cancer with cyclophosphamide, Adriamycin, methotrexate, 5-fluorouracil (CAMF) versus sequential cyclophosphamide, methotrexate, 5-fluorouracil (CMF) and Adriamycin. Cancer 43:51–59, 1979
12. Creech RH, Catalano RB, Mastrangelo MJ, et al: An effective low-dose intermittent cyclophosphamide, methotrexate, and 5-fluorouracil treatment regimen for metastatic breast cancer. Cancer 35:1101–1107, 1975
13. Gottlieb JA, Rivkin SF, Spigel SC, et al: Superiority of Adriamycin over oral nitrosoureas in patients with advanced breast carcinoma. Cancer 33:519–526, 1974
14. Gutterman JU, Cardenas JO, Blumenschein GR, et al: Chemoimmunotherapy of advanced breast cancer: Prolongation of remission and survival with BCG. Br Med J 2:1222–1225, 1976
15. Henderson IC, Canellos GP: Cancer of the breast: The past decade. N Engl J Med 302:78–90, 1980
16. Henderson IC, Gelman R, Canellos GP, et al: Prolonged disease-free survival in advanced breast cancer treated with "super-CMF" Adriamycin: An alternating regimen employing high-dose methotrexate with citrovorum factor rescue. Cancer Treat Rep 65:67–75, 1981
17. Hortobagyi GN, Blumenschein GR, Tashima CK, et al: Ftorafur, Adriamycin, cyclophosphamide and BCG in the treatment of metastatic breast cancer. Cancer 44:398–405, 1979
18. Hug V, Hortobagyi GN, Buzdar AU, et al: A phase II study of peptichemio in advanced breast cancer. Cancer 45:2524–2528, 1980
19. Mattson W, Arwidi A, von Eyben F, et al: Phase II study of combined vincristine, Adriamycin, cyclophosphamide, and methotrexate with citrovorum factor rescue in metastatic breast cancer. Cancer Treat Rep 61:1527–1531, 1977
20. Tranum B, Hoogstraten B, Kennedy A, et al: Adriamycin in combination for the treatment of breast cancer. Cancer 41:2078–2083, 1978
21. Tranum B, McDonald B, Thigpen T, et al: Adriamycin combinations in advanced breast cancer. Cancer 49:835–839, 1982

22. Nemoto T: Metastatic breast cancer: Prolonged complete response or possible cure by chemotherapy. Proc Am Soc Clin Oncol 2:110, 1983
23. Hoogstraten B, George SL, Samal B, et al: Combination chemotherapy and Adriamycin in patients with advanced breast cancer. Cancer 38:13–20, 1976
24. Legha SS, Buzdar AU, Smith TL, et al: Complete remissions in metastatic breast cancer treated with combination drug therapy. Ann Intern Med 91:847–852, 1979
25. Decker DA, Ahmann DL, Bisel HF, et al: Complete responders to chemotherapy in metastatic breast cancer. JAMA 242:2075–2079, 1979
26. Abramowitz JW: Long-term complete remissions from chemotherapy +/− hormonal therapy in breast cancer patients. Proc Am Soc Clin Oncol 1:76, 1982
27. DeVita V Jr, Hellman S, Rosenberg SA: Cancer: Principles and Practice of Oncology. Philadelphia: JB Lippincott, 1985
28. Skipper HE, Schabel FM Jr: Tumor stem cell heterogeneity: Implications with respect to classification of cancers by chemotherapeutic effect. Cancer Treat Rep 68:43–61, 1984
29. Skipper HE: Stepwise progress in the treatment of disseminated cancers. Cancer 51:1773–1776, 1983
30. DeVita VT Jr: The relationship between tumor mass and resistance to chemotherapy. Cancer 51:1209–1220, 1983
31. Goldie JH, Coldman AJ, Gudauskas GA: Rationale for the use of alternating non-cross-resistant chemotherapy. Cancer Treat Rep 66:439–449, 1982
32. Curt GA, Clendeninn NJ, Chabner BA: Drug resistance in cancer. Cancer Treat Rep 68:87–99, 1984
33. Emerson WJ, Kennedy BJ, Graham JN, et al: Pathology of primary and recurrent carcinoma of the human breast after administration of steroid hormones. Cancer 6:641–670, 1953
34. Smalley RV, Scogna DM, Malmud LS: Advanced breast cancer with bone-only metastases. Am J Clin Oncol 5:161–166, 1982
35. Priestman T, Baum M, Jones V, et al: Comparative trial of endocrine versus cytotoxic treatment in advanced breast cancer. Br Med J 1:1248–1250, 1977
36. Priestman T, Baum M, Jones V, et al: Treatment and survival in advanced breast cancer. Br Med J 2:1673–1674, 1978
37. Baum M, Priestman T, West RR, et al: A comparison of subjective responses in a trial comparing endocrine with cytotoxic treatment in advanced carcinoma of the breast. In Mouridsen HT, Palshof T (eds): Breast Cancer—Experimental and Clinical Aspects, pp 223–226. Elmsford, New York, Pergamon Press, 1980
38. Hayward JL, Carbone PP, Heuson J, et al: Assessment of response to therapy in advanced breast cancer. Cancer 39:1289–1294, 1977
39. Hoogstraten B, Fabian C: A reappraisal of single drugs in advanced breast cancer. Cancer Clin Trials 2:101–109, 1979
40. Wright JC, Cobb JP, Golomb FM, et al: Chemotherapy of disseminated carcinoma of the breast. Ann Surg 150:221–240, 1959
41. Moore GE, Bross IDJ, Ausman R, et al: Effects of chlorambucil (NSC-3088) in 374 patients with advanced cancer. Cancer Chemother Rep 52:661–666, 1968
42. Nemoto T, Dao TL: 5-Fluorouracil and cyclophosphamide in disseminated breast cancer. NY State J Med 554–558, 1971
43. Kunkler PB, Evans IH, Jones V, et al: Cyclophosphamide in the management of advanced breast cancer. In Forrest APM, Kunkler PB (eds): Prognostic Factors in Breast Cancer, pp 211–217. Edinburgh, E&S Livingston, 1968
44. Coggins P, Eisman SH, Elkins W, et al: Cyclophosphamide therapy in carcinoma of the breast and ovary—a comparative study of intermittent massive versus continuous maintenance dosage regimens. Cancer Chemother Rep 15:3–8, 1961
45. Talley RW, Vaitkevicius VK, Leighton GA: Comparison of cyclophosphamide and 5-fluorouracil in the treatment of patients with metastatic breast cancer. Clin Pharmacol Ther 6:740–748, 1965
46. Piro AJ, Wilson RE, Nevinny HB: Cyclophosphamide therapy in patients with advancing breast cancer following adrenalectomy and 5-fluorouracil. Cancer 27:1342–1345, 1971
47. Chlebowski R, Irwin LE, Pugh RP, et al: Survival of patients with metastatic breast cancer treated with either combination or sequential chemotherapy. Cancer Res 39:4503–4506, 1979
48. Smalley RV, Murphy S, Huguley CM, et al: Combination versus sequential five-drug chemotherapy in metastatic carcinoma of the breast. Cancer Res 36:3911–3916, 1976
49. Rubens RD, Knight R, Hayward JL: Chemotherapy of advanced breast cancer: A controlled randomized trial of cyclophosphamide versus a four-drug combination. Br J Cancer 32:730–736, 1975
50. Mouridsen HT, Palshof T, Brahm M, et al: Evaluation of single-drug versus multiple-drug chemotherapy in the treatment of advanced breast cancer. Cancer Treat Rep 61:47–50, 1977
51. Baker LH, Vaughn CB, Al-Sarraf M, et al: Evaluation of combination versus sequential cytotoxic chemotherapy in the treatment of advanced breast cancer. Cancer 33:513–518, 1974
52. Hurley JD, Trump DS, Flatley TJ, et al: A method of selecting patients for cancer chemotherapy. Arch Surg 83:611–619, 1961
53. Firat D, Olshin S: Treatment of metastatic carcinoma of the female breast with combination of hormones and other chemotherapy. Cancer Chemother Rep 52:743–750, 1968
54. Rundles RW, Laszlo J, Garrison FE Jr, et al: The antitumor spectrum of cyclophosphamide. Cancer Chemother Rep 16:407–411, 1962
55. Wall RL, Conrad FG: Cyclophosphamide therapy. Arch Intern Med 108:456–482, 1961
56. Atkins HL, Gregg HG, Hyman GA: Clinical appraisal of cyclophosphamide in malignant neoplasms. Cancer 15:1076–1080, 1962
57. Edelstyn G, Gleadhill C, Lyons A: Total hypophysectomy for advanced breast cancer. Clin Radiol 19:426–432, 1968
58. Tormey DC: Adriamycin (NSC-123127) in breast cancer: An overview of studies. Cancer Chemother Rep 6:319-327, 1975
59. O'Bryan RM, Baker LH, Gottlieb JE, et al: Dose response evaluation of Adriamycin in human neoplasia. Cancer 39:1940–1948, 1977
60. Ingle J, Ahmann D, O'Fallon J, et al: Randomized phase II trial of rubidazone and Adriamycin in women with advanced breast cancer. Cancer Treat Rep 63:1701–1705, 1979
61. Frederiksen PL, Joergensen ST, Roesdahl K, et al: Activity of Adriamycin in metastatic breast cancer resistant to a combination regimen with cyclophosphamide, methotrexate, 5-fluorouracil, vincristine, and prednisone. Cancer Treat Rep 62:449–450, 1978
62. Bonadonna G, Beretta G, Tancini G, et al: Adriamycin (NSC-123127) studies at the Instituto Nazionale Tumori, Milan. Cancer Chemother Rep 6:231–245, 1975
63. Jones RB, Mass T, Holland JF: Single agent Adriamycin for metastatic breast cancer. Proc Am Soc Clin Oncol 2:107, 1983
64. Creech RH, Catalano RB, Shah MK: An effective low-dose Adriamycin regimen as secondary chemotherapy for metastatic breast cancer patients. Cancer 46:433–437, 1980

65. Creech RH, Catalano RB, Shah MK, et al: A randomized trial of Adriamycin versus mitomycin at low doses in CMF-refractory metastatic breast cancer patients. Proc Am Soc Clin Oncol 1:88, 1982
66. Vaughn CB, O'Bryan R, Reed M, et al: Adriamycin +VP-16 versus Adriamycin alone in advanced adenocarcinoma of the breast, phase II: A Southwest Oncology Group study. Proc Am Assoc Cancer Res 25:184, 1984
67. Dean JC, Griffith KS, Cetas TC, et al: Scalp hypothermia: A comparison of ice packs and the Kold Kap in the prevention of doxorubicin-induced alopecia. J Clin Oncol 1:33–37, 1983
68. Jain KK, Casper ES, Geller NL, et al: A prospective randomized comparison of epirubicin and doxorubicin in patients with advanced breast cancer. J Clin Oncol 3:818–826, 1985
69. Van Oosterom AT, Mouridsen HT, Wildiers J, et al: Doxorubicin (Adm) versus 4′epidoxorubicin (4′epi), a preliminary report: Report of a randomized phase II-III study in pretreated breast cancer patients. In Proceedings, International Symposium on Advances in Anthracycline Chemotherapy: Epirubicin, p 23. Milan, Farmitalia Carlo Erba, 1984
70. Bonfante V, Ferrari L, Brambilla C, et al: New anthracycline analogs in advanced breast cancer. (in press) 1986
71. Osborne CK, Cowan JD, Neidhart JA, et al: The Southwest Oncology Group randomized trial of Novantrone, Adriamycin, and bisantrene in advanced breast cancer. In Coltman CA Jr (ed): The Current Status of Novantrone, pp 55–58. New York, John Wiley & Sons, 1985
72. Henderson IC, Wolff S, Allegra J, et al: A randomized trial comparing mitoxantrone and doxorubicin in patients with metastatic breast cancer. In Coltman CA Jr (ed): The Current Status of Novantrone, pp 45–53. New York, John Wiley & Sons, 1985
73. Neidhart JA, Gochnour D, Roach R, et al: Comparable efficacy of Novantrone and Adriamycin in breast cancer. In Coltman CA Jr (ed): The Current Status of Novantrone, pp 39–43. New York, John Wiley & Sons, 1985
74. Taylor SG IV, Gelber R: Experience of the Eastern Cooperative Oncology Group with doxorubicin as a single agent in patients with previously untreated breast cancer. Cancer Treat Rep 66:1594–1595, 1982
75. Ahmann D, Bisel H, Eagan R, et al: Controlled evaluation of Adriamycin (NSC-123127) in patients with disseminated breast cancer. Cancer Chemother Rep 58:877–882, 1974
76. Nemoto T, Rosner D, Diaz R, et al: Combination chemotherapy for metastatic breast cancer. Cancer 41:2073–2077, 1978
77. Manni A, Trujillo JE, Pearson OH: Sequential use of endocrine therapy and chemotherapy for metastatic breast cancer: Effects on survival. Cancer Treat Rep 64:111–116, 1980
78. Stoll BA: Evaluation of cyclophosphamide dosage schedules in breast cancer. Br J Cancer 24:475–483, 1970
79. Carter SK: Single and combination nonhormonal chemotherapy in breast cancer. Cancer 30:1543–1555, 1972
80. Ravdin RG, Eisman SH: Disseminated breast cancer: Relationship of response to endocrine manipulation, Cytoxan, and fluorouracil. In Segaloff A, Keyer KK, DeBakey S (eds): Current Concepts in Breast Cancer, pp 200–207. Baltimore, Williams & Wilkins, 1967
81. Ansfield FJ, Ramirez G, Mackman S, et al: A ten-year study of 5-fluorouracil in disseminated breast cancer with clinical results and survival times. Cancer Res 29:1062–1066, 1969
82. Chlebowski RT, Pugh RP, Weiner JM, et al: Treatment of advanced breast carcinoma with 5-fluorouracil: A randomized comparison of two routes of delivery. Cancer 48:1711–1714, 1981
83. Lemkin SR, Dollinger MR: Combination vs. single drug therapy in advanced breast cancer. Proc Am Assoc Cancer Res 14:37, 1973
84. Ansfield F, Klotz J, Nealon T, et al: A phase III study comparing the clinical utility of four regimens of 5-fluorouracil. Cancer 39:34–40, 1977
85. Eastern Cooperative Group in Solid Tumor Chemotherapy. Comparison of antimetabolites in the treatment of breast and colon cancer. JAMA 200:110–118, 1967
86. Mackman S, Ramirez G, Ansfield FJ: Results of 5-fluorouracil (NSC-19893) given by the multiple daily dose method in disseminated breast cancer. Cancer Chemother Rep 51:483–489, 1967
87. Moore GE, Bross IDJ, Ausman R, et al: Effects of 5-fluorouracil (NSC-19893) in 389 patients with cancer. Cancer Chemother Rep 52:641–653, 1968
88. Field JB: 5-fluorouracil (NSC-19893) treatment of advanced cancer in ambulatory patients. Cancer Chemother Rep 33:45–49, 1963
89. Kennedy BJ, Theologides A: The role of 5-fluorouracil in malignant disease. Ann Intern Med 55:719–730, 1961
90. Hall BE, Good JW: Treatment of far-advanced cancer with 5-fluorouracil, used alone and in combination with irradiation. Incidence and duration of remission and survival-time data in 223 patients. Cancer Chemother Rep 16:369–386, 1962
91. Eyerly RC: The effects of 5-fluorouracil in patients with incurable cancer. Cancer Chemother Rep 20:89–95, 1962
92. Hall TC, Cavins JA, Khung CL, et al: Time and vehicle studies of a safe and effective method for administration of 5-fluorouracil. Cancer 19:1008–1012, 1966
93. Vaitkevicius VK, Brennan MJ, Beckett VL, et al: Clinical evaluation of cancer chemotherapy with 5-fluorouracil. Cancer 14:131–152, 1961
94. Dao TL, Grinberg R: Fluorinated pyrimidines in treatment of breast cancer patients with liver metastases. Cancer Chemother Rep 27:71–77, 1963
95. Jacobs EM, Luce JK, Wood DA: Treatment of cancer with weekly intravenous 5-fluorouracil. Cancer 22:1233–1238, 1968
96. Silva ARM, Smart CR, Rochlin DB: Chemotherapy of breast cancer. Chemother Breast Cancer 121:494–498, 1965
97. Moore FD, Woodrow SI, Aliapoulios MA, et al: Carcinoma of the breast: A decade of new results with old concepts. N Engl J Med 277:460–468, 1967
98. Canellos GP, Pocock S, Taylor S, et al: Combination chemotherapy for metastatic breast carcinoma. Cancer 38:1882–1886, 1976
99. Buzdar AU, Legha SS, Blumenschein GR, et al: Peptichemio versus melphalan (L-PAM) in advanced breast cancer. Cancer 49:1767–1770, 1982
100. Sears ME, Haut A, Eckles N: Melphalan (NSC-8806) in advanced breast cancer. Cancer Chemother Rep 50:271–279, 1966
101. Yap HY, Blumenschein GR, Yap BS, et al: High-dose methotrexate for advanced breast cancer. Cancer Treat Rep 63:757–761, 1979
102. Sullivan RD, Miller E, Wladyslaw ZZ, et al: Re-evaluation of methotrexate as an anticancer drug. Surg Gynecol Obstet 125:819–824, 1967
103. Vogler WR, Furtado VP, Huguley CM Jr: Methotrexate for advanced cancer of the breast. Cancer 21:26–30, 1968
104. Andrews NC, Wilson WL: Phase II study of methotrexate (NSC-740) in solid tumors. Cancer Chemother Rep 51:471–474, 1967

105. Isacoff WH, Eilber F, Tabbarah H, et al: Phase II clinical trial with high-dose methotrexate therapy and citrovorum factor rescue. Cancer Treat Rep 62:1295–1304, 1978
106. Volger WR, Jacobs J, Moffitt S, et al: Methotrexate therapy with or without citrovorum factor in carcinoma of the head and neck, breast and colon. Cancer Clin Trials 2:227–236, 1979
107. Wilson HE, Louis J: The use of low dosage regimens in the treatments of neoplastic disease. Ann Intern Med 63:918, 1965
108. Schoenbach EB, Colsky J, Greenspan EM: Observations on the effects of the folic acid antagonists, aminopterin and amethopterin, in patients with advanced neoplasms. Cancer 5:1201–1220, 1952
109. Nevinny HB, Hall TC, Haines C, et al: Comparison of methotrexate (NSC-740) and testosterone propionate (NSC-9166) in the treatment of breast cancer. J Clin Pharmacol 8:126–129, 1968
110. Crooke ST, Bradner WT: Mitomycin C: A review. Cancer Treat Rev 3:121–139, 1976
111. Van Oosterom AT, Powles TJ, Hamersma E, et al: A phase II study of mitomycin C in refractory advanced breast cancer. A multi-centre pilot study. In Mouridsen HT, Palshof T (eds): Breast Cancer—Experimental and Clinical Aspects, pp 275–276. Elmsford, New York, Pergamon Press, 1980
112. DeLena M, Jirillo A, Brambilla C, et al: Mitomycin C in metastatic breast cancer resistant to hormone therapy and conventional chemotherapy. Tumori 66:481–487, 1980
113. Pasterz RB, Buzdar AU, Hortobagyi GN, et al: Mitomycin in metastatic breast cancer refractory to hormonal and combination chemotherapy. Cancer 56:2381–2384, 1985
114. Creech RH, Catalano RB, Shah MK, et al: An effective low-dose mitomycin regimen for hormonal- and chemotherapy-refractory patients with metastatic breast cancer. Cancer 51:1034–1040, 1983
115. Zubrod CG, Schneiderman M, Frei E III, et al: Appraisal of methods for the study of chemotherapy of cancer in man: Comparative therapeutic trial of nitrogen mustard and triethylene thiophosphoramide. J Chron Dis 11:7–23, 1960
116. Frei EF III, Carbone PP, Schnider BI, et al: Neoplastic disease. Arch Intern Med 116:846–852, 1965
117. Armstrong JG, Dyke RW, Fouts PJ, et al: Hodgkin's disease, carcinoma of the breast, and other tumors treated with vinblastine sulfate. Cancer Chemother Rep 18:49–71, 1962
118. Goldenberg IS: Vinblastine sulfate (VLB) therapy of women with advanced breast cancer. Cancer Chemother Rep 29:111–113, 1963
119. Wright TL, Hurley J, Korst DR, et al: Vinblastine in neoplastic disease. Cancer Res 23:169–179, 1963
120. Bleehan NM, Jelliffe AM: Vinblastine sulphate in the treatment of malignant disease. Br J Cancer 19:268–273, 1965
121. Grinberg R: Vincristine: Dosage and response in advanced breast cancer. Cancer Chemother Rep 45:57–61, 1965
122. Goldenberg IS: Vincristine (NSC-67574) therapy of women with advanced breast cancer. Cancer Chemother Rep 41:7–9, 1964
123. Gubisch NJ, Norena D, Perlia CP, et al: Experience with vincristine in solid tumors. Cancer Chemother Rep 32:19–22, 1963
124. Frei E III, Canellos GP: Dose: A critical factor in cancer chemotherapy. Am J Med 69:585–594, 1980
125. Schabel FM Jr, Trader MW, Laster WR Jr, et al: Patterns of resistance and therapeutic synergism among alkylating agents. Fundamentals in Cancer Chemotherapy. Antibiot Chemother 23:200–215, 1978
126. Hahn RG, Moertel CG, Schutt AJ, et al: A double-blind comparison of intensive course 5-fluorouracil by oral vs. intravenous route in the treatment of colorectal carcinoma. Cancer 35:1031–1035, 1975
127. Yap HY, Yap BS, Rasmussen S, et al: Treatment for meningeal carcinomatosis in breast cancer. Cancer 49:219–222, 1982
128. Ervin T, Canellos GP: Successful treatment of recurrent primary central nervous system lymphoma with high-dose methotrexate. Cancer 45:1556–1557, 1980
129. Henderson IC: Personal experience.
130. Razek A, Valeriote F, Vietti T: Survival of hematopoietic and leukemia colony-forming cells in vivo following the administration of daunorubicin or Adriamycin. Cancer Res 32:1496–1500, 1972
131. Ritch PS, Occhipinti SJ, Skramstad KS, et al: Increased relative effectiveness of doxorubicin against slowly proliferating sarcoma 180 cells after prolonged drug exposure. Cancer Treat Rep 66:1159–1168, 1982
132. Von Hoff DD, Layard MW, Basa P, et al: Risk factors for doxorubicin-induced congestive heart failure. Ann Intern Med 91:710–717, 1979
133. Torti FM, Bristow MR, Howes AE, et al: Endomyocardial biopsy evidence of reduced cardiotoxicity of doxorubicin delivered on a weekly schedule. Proc Am Assoc Cancer Res 2:26, 1983
134. Jain K, Wittes R, Benedetto P, et al: A randomized comparison of weekly (arm I) vs. monthly (arm II) doxorubicin (DOX) in combination with mitomycin C (MMC) in advanced breast cancer. Proc Am Soc Clin Oncol 2:109, 1983
135. Friedman MA, Marcus FS, Cassidy MJ, et al: 5-Fluorouracil + oncovin + Adriamycin + mitomycin C (FOAM): An effective program for breast cancer, even for disease refractory to previous chemotherapy. Cancer 52:193–197, 1983
136. Denefrio JM, East DR, Troner MB, et al: Phase II study of mitomycin C and vinblastine in women with advanced breast cancer refractory to standard cytotoxic therapy. Cancer Treat Rep 62:2113–2115, 1978
137. Garewal HS, Brooks RJ, Jones SE, et al: Treatment of advanced breast cancer with mitomycin C combined with vinblastine or vindesine. J Clin Oncol 1:772–774, 1983
138. Radford JA, Rubens RD: Mitomycin C (M) and vinblastine (V) in the treatment of advanced breast cancer. Proc Am Soc Clin Oncol 3:114, 1984
139. Luikart SD, Witman GB, Portlock CS: Adriamycin (doxorubicin), vinblastine, and mitomycin C combination chemotherapy in refractory breast carcinoma. Cancer 54:1252–1255, 1984
140. De Lena M, Jirillo A, Villa S, et al: Preliminary results with Adriamycin (A) plus mitomycin (M) combination in metastatic breast cancer. Proc Am Soc Clin Oncol 22:435, 1981
141. Perren TJ, Blackledge G, Mould JJ, et al: Phase II study of vincristine, mitomycin-C and mitoxantrone in advanced breast cancer: A preliminary report of response and toxicity. Invest New Drugs 3:173–177, 1985
142. Glass A, Wieand S, Fisher B, et al: Acute toxicity during adjuvant chemotherapy for breast cancer: The National Surgical Adjuvant Breast and Bowel Project (NSABP) experience from 1717 patients receiving single and multiple agents. Cancer Treat Rep 65:363–376, 1981
143. Mattsson W, Von Eyben F, Hallsten L, et al: A phase II study of combined 5-fluorouracil and mitomycin C in advanced breast cancer. Cancer 49:217–220, 1982
144. Wheeler GP: XIII-4. Alkylating agents. In Holland JF, Frei E III (eds): Cancer Medicine, pp 791–806. Philadelphia, Lea & Febiger, 1974
145. Levine N, Greenwald ES: Mucocutaneous side effects of cancer chemotherapy. Cancer Treat Rev 5:67–84, 1978

146. Buzdar AU, Legha SS, Tahshima CK, et al: Ifosfamide versus cyclophosphamide in combination drug therapy for metastatic breast cancer. Cancer Treat Rep 63:115–120, 1979
147. Forastiere AA, Budman DR, Perry MC: Phase II trials of aclacinomycin-a (A) and bisantrene (B) in advanced breast cancer: CALGB studies. Proc Am Assoc Cancer Res 24:152, 1983
148. Osborne CK, Von Hoff DD, Cowan JD, et al: Bisantrene, an active drug in patients with advanced breast cancer. Cancer Treat Rep 68:357–360, 1984
149. Cavalli F, Gerard B, ten Bokkel Huinink W, et al: Phase II evaluation of bisantrene in metastatic breast cancer. Cancer Treat Rep 69:337–338, 1985
150. Pandya KJ, Muggia FM, Skeel RT, et al: A phase II study of bisantrene in advanced refractory breast cancer. Am J Clin Oncol 8:353–357, 1985
151. Holmes F, Esparza L, Yap H, et al: A comparative study of bisantrene (B) given by single IV dose (s) vs daily for five days (d×5) in patients (pts) with metastatic breast cancer (mbc). Breast Cancer Res Treat 6:170, 1985
152. Yap HY, Yap BS, Blumenschein GR, et al: Bisantrene, an active new drug in the treatment of metastatic breast cancer. Cancer Res 43:1402–1404, 1983
153. Ahmann DL, Bisel HF, Hahn RG: Difficulties designing clinical trials as exemplified by a phase 2 drug evaluation of 5 [3,3-bis(2-chloroethyl)-1-triazenol]-imidazole-4-carboxamide and 1-(2-chloroethyl)-3-cyclohexyl-1-nitrosourea in patients with disseminated breast cancer. Cancer Res 33:1707–1710, 1973
154. Cummings FJ, Gelman R, Skeel RT, et al: Phase II trials of Baker's antifol, bleomycin, CCNU, streptozotocin, tilorone, and 5-fluorodeoxyuridine plus arabinosyl cytosine in metastatic breast cancer. Cancer 48:681–685, 1981
155. Cunningham TJ, Nemoto T, Rosner D, et al: Comparison of 5-azacytidine (NSC-102816) with CCNU (NSC-79037) in the treatment of patients with breast cancer and evaluation of the subsequent use of cyclophosphamide (NSC-26271). Cancer Chemother Rep 58:677–681, 1974
156. Hoogstraten B, Haas CD, Haut A, et al: CCNU and bleomycin in the treatment of cancer: A Southwest Oncology Group study. Med Ped Oncol 1:95–106, 1975
157. Martoni A, Pacciarini MA, Pannuti F: Activity of 4-demethoxydaunorubicin by the oral route in advanced breast cancer. Eur J Cancer Clin Oncol 21:803–9806, 1985
158. Pronzato P, Lionetto R, Gulisano M, et al: A phase-II study with oral 4-demethoxydaunorubicin in metastatic breast cancer. Breast Cancer 6:172, 1985
159. Bastholt L, Ejlertsen B, Dalmark M: A phase II trial of oral 4-demethoxydaunorubicin (DMOR) in patients with measurable advanced carcinoma of the breast. Proc Am Assoc Cancer Res 26:164, 1985
160. Martino S, Samal BA, Vaitkevicius VK, et al: 4′-Deoxydoxorubicin (DxDx) as first line therapy for metastatic breast cancer. Breast Cancer Res Treat 6:171, 1985
161. Leitner SP, Casper ES, Hakes TB, et al: Phase II trial of 4′-deoxydoxorubicin in patients with advanced breast cancer. Cancer Treat Rep 69:1319–1320, 1985
162. Buzdar AU, Goodman A, Chou I, et al: Elliptinium acetate in advanced breast cancer refractory to combination chemotherapy (chemo)—results of phase I-II studies. Breast Cancer Res Treat 4:346, 1984
163. Byrne P, Grady K, Smith F, et al: Phase II clinical trial of 2-n-methyl-9-hydroxy-ellipticium (elliptinium) in patients with advanced breast cancer. Proc Am Soc Clin Oncol 3:127, 1984
164. Einzig AI, Gralla RJ, Leyland-Jones BR: Phase I trial of elliptinium (2-methyl-9-hydroxyellipticinium). Proc Am Assoc Cancer Res 24:166, 1983
165. Juret P, Heron JF, Couette JE, et al: Hydroxy-9-methyl-2-ellipticinium for osseous metastases from breast cancer: A 5-year experience. Cancer Treat Rep 66:1909–1916, 1982
166. Rouesse JG, Le Chevalier T, Caille P, et al: Phase II study of elliptinium in advanced breast cancer. Cancer Treat Rep 69:707–708, 1985
167. Jones WG, Mattsson W: Phase II study of weekly low-dose 4′-epi-doxorubicin in advanced postmenopausal breast cancer. Cancer Treat Rep 68:675–677, 1984
168. Campora E, Nobile MT, Sertoli MR, et al: Phase II study of 4′-epi-doxorubicin in advanced breast cancer. Cancer Treat Rep 68:1285–1286, 1984
169. Hurteloup P, Cappelaere P, Armand JP, et al: Phase II clinical evaluation of 4′-epi-doxorubicin. Cancer Treat Rep 67:337–341, 1983
170. Dawes PJDK: A pilot study of estracyt in advanced breast cancer. Cancer Treat Rep 66:581–582, 1982
171. Sullivan RD, Miller E: The clinical effects of prolonged intravenous infusion of 5-fluoro-2′-deoxyuridine. Cancer Res 25:1025–1033, 1965
172. DeConti RC, Kaplan SR, Papac RJ, et al: Continuous intravenous infusions of 5-fluoro-2′-deoxyuridine in the treatment of solid tumors. Cancer 31:894–898, 1973
173. Wilson WL, Bisel HF, Krementz ET, et al: Further clinical evaluation of 2′-deoxy-5-fluorouridine. Cancer Chemother Rep 51:85–90, 1967
174. Dao TL, Grinberg R: Fluourinated pyrimidines in treatment of breast cancer patients with liver metastases. Cancer Chemother Rep 27:71–77, 1963
175. Ansfield FJ, Curreri AR: Further clinical comparison between 5-fluorouracil (5-FU) and 5-fluoro-2′-deoxyuridine. Cancer Chemother Rep 32:101–105, 1963
176. Wilson WL, Schroeder JM, Bisel HF, et al: Phase II study of hexamethylmelamine (NSC-13875). Cancer 23:132–136, 1969
177. Wilson WL, Bisel HF, Cole D, et al: Prolonged low-dosage administration of hexamethylmelamine (NSC-13875). Cancer 25:568–570, 1970
178. Wampler GL, Mellette SJ, Kuperminc M, et al: Hexamethylmelamine (NSC-13875) in the treatment of advanced cancer. Cancer Chemother Rep 56:505–514, 1972
179. Legha SS, Buzdar AU, Hortobagyi GN, et al: Phase II study of hexamethylmelamine alone and in combination with mitomycin C and vincristine in advanced breast carcinoma. Cancer Treat Rep 63:2053–2056, 1979
180. Denefrio JM, Vogel CL: Phase II study of hexamethylmelamine in women with advanced breast cancer refractory to standard cytotoxic therapy. Cancer Treat Rep 62:173–175, 1978
181. Fabian CJ, Rasmussen S, Stephens R, et al: Phase II evaluation of hexamethylmelamine in advanced breast cancer: A Southwest Oncology Group study. Cancer Treat Rep 63:1359–1361, 1979
182. Ahmann DL, Bisel HF, Hahn RG: Phase II clinical trial of isophosphamide (NSC-109724) in patients with advanced breast cancer. Cancer Chemother Rep 58:861–865, 1974
183. Falkson G, Falkson HC: Further experience with isophosphamide. Cancer Treat Rep 60:955–957, 1976
184. Ingle JN, Brunk SF, Krook JE, et al: Evaluation of mitolactol in women with advanced breast cancer and prior chemotherapy exposure. Cancer Treat Rep 67:955–956, 1983
185. Creech RH, Catalano RB, Dierks KM, et al: Phase II study of mitolactol in chemotherapy-refractory metastatic breast cancer. Cancer 68:1499–1501, 1984

186. Tormey DC, Falkson G, Perlin E, et al: Evaluation of an intermittent schedule of dibromodulcitol in breast cancer. Cancer Treat Rep 60:1593–1596, 1976
187. Tormey DC, Simon R, Falkson G, et al: Evaluation of Adriamycin and dibromodulcitol in metastatic breast carcinoma. Cancer Res 37:529–534, 1977
188. Andrews NC, Weiss AJ, Wilson W, et al: Phase II study of dibromodulcitol (NSC-104800). Cancer Chemother Rep 58:653–660, 1974
189. Smalley R, Gams R: Phase II study of mitoxantrone in patients with metastatic breast carcinoma: A Southeastern Cancer Study Group project. Cancer Treat Rep 67:1039–1040, 1983
190. Levin M, Pandya KJ, Khandekar JD, et al: Phase II study of mitoxantrone in advanced breast cancer: An Eastern Cooperative Oncology Group pilot study. Cancer Treat Rep 68:1511–1512, 1984
191. Mouridsen HT, Cornbleet M, Stuart-Harris R, et al: Mitoxantrone as first-line chemotherapy in advanced breast cancer: Results of a collaborative European study. Invest New Drugs 3:139–148, 1985
192. De Jager R, Cappelaere P, Earl H, et al: Phase II clinical trial of mitoxantrone: 1,4-dihydroxy-5-8-bis (((2-((2-hydroxyethyl)amino)ethyl)amino)9,10 anthracenedione dihydrochloride in solid tumors and lymphomas. Proc Am Soc Clin Oncol 1:89, 1982
193. Knight WA III, Von Hoff D, Tranum B, et al: Phase II trial of dihydroxyanthracenedione (DHAD, mitoxantrone) in breast cancer. A Southwest Oncology Group (SWOG) study. Proc Am Soc Clin Oncol 1:87, 1982
194. Stuart-Harris RC, Bozek T, Pavlidis NA, et al: Mitoxantrone: An active new agent in the treatment of advanced breast cancer. Cancer Chemother Pharmacol 12:1–4, 1984
195. Wilson KS, Paterson AHG: Single-agent mitoxantrone as first line chemotherapy (CT) in advanced breast cancer. Proc Am Soc Clin Oncol 3:117, 1984
196. Yap HY, Blumenschein G, Schell F, et al: Dihydroxyanthracenedione: A promising new drug in the treatment of metastatic breast cancer. Ann Intern Med 95:694–697, 1981
197. Lenzhofer R, Rainer H, Schuster R, et al: Mitoxantrone in the primary treatment of metastasizing breast cancer. Wien Klin Wonchenschr 96:319–326, 1984
198. Bull JM, Anderson T, Lippman ME, et al: A phase II trial of cis-dichlorodiammine platinum II (cis-DDP) in breast and ovarian carcinomas. Proc Am Soc Clin Oncol 19:87, 1978
199. Forastiere AA, Hakes TB, Wittes JT, et al: Cisplatin in the treatment of metastatic breast carcinoma. A prospective randomized trial of two dosage schedules. Am J Clin Oncol 5:243–247, 1982
200. Ostrow S, Egorin M, Aisner J, et al: High-dose cis-diamminedichloro-platinum therapy in patients with advanced breast cancer: Pharmacokinetics, toxicity, and therapeutic efficacy and therapeutic efficacy. 3:23–27, 1980
201. Samal B, Vaitkevicius V, Singhakowinta A, et al: Cis-diamminedichloroplatinum (CDDP) in advanced breast and colorectal carcinomas. Proc Am Soc Clin Oncol 19:347, 1978
202. Yap HY, Salem P, Hortobagyi GN, et al: Phase II study of cis-dichlorodiammineplatinum(II) in advanced breast cancer. Cancer Treat Rep 62:405–408, 1978
203. Mouridsen HT, Kristensen D, Nielsen JH, et al: Phase II trial of prednimustine, 1-1031. (NSC-134087) in advanced breast cancer. Cancer 46:253–255, 1980
204. Lober J, Mouridsen HT, Christiansen IE, et al: A phase III trial comparing prednimustine (LEO 1031) to chlorambucil plus prednisolone in advanced breast cancer. Cancer 52:1570–1576, 1983
205. Currie VE, Camacho F, Wittes R, et al: Phase II evaluation of vindesine in patients with advanced breast cancer. Cancer Treat Rep 64:693–695, 1980
206. Cobleigh MA, Williams SD, Einhorn LH: Phase II study of vindesine in patients with metastatic breast cancer. Cancer Treat Rep 65:659–663, 1981
207. Smith IE, Powles TJ: Vindesine in the treatment of breast cancer. Cancer Chemother Pharmacol 2:261–262, 1979
208. Walker BK, Raich PC, Fontana J, et al: Phase II study of vindesine in patients with advanced breast cancer. Cancer Treat Rep 66:1729–1732, 1982
209. Fleishman GB, Yap HY, Bodey GP, et al: Comparability in therapeutic index with continuous 5-day infusion and 5-day bolus vindesine in the treatment of refractory breast cancer. Proc Am Soc Clin Oncol 1:82, 1982
210. Robins HI, Tormey DC, Skelley MJ, et al: Vindesine: A phase II trial in advanced breast cancer patients. Cancer Clin Trials 4:371–375, 1981
211. Yap HY, Blumenschein GR, Hortobagyi GN, et al: A randomized comparative study of vinblastine (VBL), vindesine (VDS) and vincristine (VCR) in patients (pts) with refractory metastatic breast cancer. Proc Am Soc Clin Oncol 22:441, 1981
212. Dosik M, Winn R, Koven B, et al: Phase II trial of weekly vindesine in early metastatic breast cancer. Proc Am Soc Clin Oncol 22:445, 1981
213. Lokich JJ, Skarin AT, Frei E III: 1,-(2-chloroethyl)-3-cyclohexyl-1-nitrosourea (methyl CCNU) and Adriamycin combination therapy. Cancer 34:1593–1597, 1974
214. Watt RW, Saiki JH, Tranum BL, et al: Adriamycin and CCNU in advanced breast cancer: A Southwest Oncology Group study. Cancer Clin Trials 1:9–11, 1978
215. Waterfield WC, Tashima CK, Hortobagyi GN, et al: Adriamycin and 1-(2-chlorethyl)-3-cyclohexyl-1-nitrosourea (CCNU) in the treatment of metastatic breast cancer. Cancer 41:1235–1239, 1978
216. Presant CA, Van Amburg A III, Klahr C: Adriamycin, 1,3-bis (2-chloroethyl)-1-nitrosourea (BCNU, NSC 409962) and cyclophosphamide therapy of drug-resistant metastatic breast carcinoma. Cancer 40:987–993, 1977
217. Falkson G, Falkson HC: A five-drug combination in the treatment of metastatic breast cancer. Cancer Clin Trials 4:81–85, 1981
218. Garfield D, DiBella N, Fink K, et al: Combination chemotherapy with BCNU, vincristine, mitomycin C and prednisone for patients with adenocarcinoma of the breast refractory to conventional agents. Proc Am Soc Cancer Res 22:437, 1981
219. Salimtschik M, Snel S, Havsteen H, et al: CCNU, melphalan, methotrexate, and prednisone (CAMP) versus cyclophosphamide, methotrexate, and 5-fluorouracil (CMF) in the treatment of advanced breast cancer in postmenopausal women. 64:635–637, 1980
220. Legha SS, Slavik M, Carter SK: Hexamethylmelamine: An evaluation of its role in the therapy of cancer. Cancer 38:27–35, 1976
221. Jarowski CI, Pasmantier M, Coleman M, et al: Hexamethylmelamine, vinblastine and mitomycin in the treatment of refractory adenocarcinoma of the breast. Proc Am Assoc Cancer Res 199, 1978
222. Lawson D, Moore M, Smalley R: An evaluation of hexamethylmelamine, cis-diamminedichloroplatinum, and mitomycin-C in advanced breast cancer: A pilot study of the Southeastern Cancer Study Group. Cancer Clin Trials 3:293–296, 1980
223. Van Amburg AL III, Presant CA, Velez-Garcia E, et al: Phase

I-II study of hexamethylmelamine plus dibromodulcitol in refractory carcinoma of the breast. Cancer Treat Rep 63:141–142, 1979

224. Ingle JN, Green SJ, Brunk SF, et al: Randomized clinical trial of doxorubicin alone or combined with mitolactol in women with advanced breast cancer and prior chemotherapy exposure. Am J Clin Oncol 8:275–282, 1985
225. Cummings FJ, Gelman R, Tormey DC, et al: Adriamycin plus vincristine alone or with dibromodulcitol or ICRF-159 in metastatic breast cancer. Cancer Clin Trials 4:253–260, 1981
226. Falkson G, Gelman RS, Tormey DC, et al: Mitomycin and tamoxifen versus mitolactol, doxorubicin, and tamoxifen in patients with previously treated breast cancer. Cancer Treat Rep 69:755–760, 1985
227. Chang YC, Falkson G, Tormey DC, et al: A pilot study of mitomycin-C and tamoxifen (MT) versus dibromodulcitol, Adriamycin, and tamoxifen (DAT). Am J Clin Oncol 5:521–525, 1982
228. Kolaric K, Roth A, Vukas D, et al: CAP (cyclophosphamide, Adriamycin, platinum) vs. CMFVP (cyclophosphamide, methotrexate, 5-fluorouracil, vincristiine, prednisolone) combination chemotherapy in untreated metastatic breast cancer. A preliminary report of a controlled clinical study. Cancer Chemother Pharmacol 13:142–144, 1984
229. Creagan ET, Green ST, Ahmann DL, et al: A phase III clinical trial comparing the combination cyclophosphamide, Adriamycin, cisplatin with cyclophosphamide, 5-fluorouracil, prednisone in patients with advanced breast cancer. J Clin Oncol 2:1260–1265, 1984
230. Smith IE, Powles TJ, Coombes RC, et al: A controlled randomised trial comparing vindesine and Adriamycin with vincristine and Adriamycin in the treatment of advanced breast carcinoma. In Brade W, Nagel GA, Seeber S (eds): Proceedings International Vinca Alkaloid Symposium—Vindesine, pp 185–194. New York, S Karger, 1980
231. Clarysse A, Heuson JC, Rotmensz N, et al: Cisplatin plus vindesine in multitreated advanced breast cancer—a phase II trial of the EORTC breast cancer cooperative group. Proc Am Soc Clin Oncol 3:114, 1984
232. Mathe G, Misset JL, DeVassal F, et al: Phase II trial with vindesine for remission induction in acute leukemia, blastic crisis of chronic myeloid leukemia, lymphosarcoma, and Hodgkin's disease: Absence of cross-resistance with vincristine. Cancer Treat Rep 62:805–809, 1978
233. Brambilla C, Rossi A, Bonfante V, et al: Phase II study of doxorubicin versus epirubicin in advanced breast cancer. Cancer Treat Rep 70:261–266, 1986
234. Hortobagyi G, Yap H, Aboud A, et al: Doxorubicin (D) vs. 4′-epidoxorubicin (4ed) for metastatic breast cancer (mbc): A prospective randomized study. Proc Am Soc. Clin Oncol 3:121, 1984
235. Rozencweig M, Huinink WB, Cavalli F, et al: Randomized phase II trial of carminomycin versus 4′-epidoxorubicin in advanced breast cancer. J Clin Oncol 2:275–286, 1984
236. Armand JP, Hurteloup P, Hayat M, et al: Phase III chemotherapy comparing FAC vs. FEC in advanced breast cancer. Proc Am Soc Clin Oncol 3:118, 1984
237. Casazza AM: Experimental evaluation of anthracycline analogs. Cancer Treat Rep 63:835–844, 1979
238. Vogel CL, Bennett JM, Byrne P, et al: A randomized multicenter trial of Novantrone versus Adriamycin in combination chemotherapy for metastatic breast cancer. In Coltman CA Jr (ed): The Current Status of Novantrone, pp 59–64. New York, John Wiley & Sons, 1985
239. Stewart DJ, Maroun JA, Hirte W, et al: A randomized comparison of cyclophosphamide-mitoxantrone- 5-fluorouracil vs. cyclophosphamide-doxorubicin-5-fluorouracil in advanced breast cancer: Preliminary observations. Semin Oncol 11:23s–27s, 1984
240. Cowan JD, Osborne CK, Costanzi JJ, et al: Randomized trial of Novantrone (N), bisantrene (b) and Adriamycin (A) in advanced breast cancer. Proc Am Soc Clin Oncol 5:59, 1986
241. Benjamin RS, Chawla SP, Ewer MS, et al: Evaluation of mitoxantrone cardiac toxicity by nuclear angiography and endomyocardial biopsy: An update. Invest New Drugs 3:117–121, 1985
242. Boesen E, Mouridsen HT: Prednimustine in combination with methotrexate and 5-FU (PMF): A pilot study. Cancer Treat Rep 66:2081–2083, 1982
243. Forastier AA, Budman DR, Richards F II, et al: Phase II trial of aclarubicin in advanced breast cancer: A Cancer and Leukemia Group B study. Cancer Treat Rep 67:1137–1138, 1983
244. Gockerman JP, Raney M, Logan T: Phase II evaluation of aclarubicin in advanced breast cancer: A Southeastern Cancer Study Group trial. Cancer Treat Rep 69:1029–1030, 1985
245. Livingston RB, Carter SK: Single agents in cancer chemotherapy. New York, Plenum Publishing, 1970
246. Legha SS, Blumenschein GR, Buzdar AU, et al: Phase II study of 4′-(9-acridinylamino)methanesulfon-m-anisidide (AMSA) in metastatic breast carcinoma. Cancer Treat Rep 63:1961–1964, 1979
247. De Lena M, Rossi A, Bonadonna G: Phase II trial of AMSA in refractory breast cancer. Cancer Treat Rep 66:403–404, 1982
248. Currie VE, Howard J, Wittes R: A phase II evaluation of m-AMSA, 4′-(9-acridinylamino)methanesulfon m-anisidid, in patients with breast cancer. Cancer Clin Trials 4:249–251, 1981
249. Amrein PC, Coleman M, Richards F II, et al: Phase II study of AMSA in patients with metastatic breast cancer: A Cancer and Leukemia Group B study. Cancer Treat Rep 66:1211–1213, 1982
250. Ahmann FR, Meyskens FL, Jones SE, et al: Phase II evaluation of amsacrine (m-AMSA) in solid tumors, myeloma, and lymphoma: A University of Arizona and Southwest Oncology Group study. Cancer Treat Rep 67:697–700, 1983
251. Yap HY, Murphy WK, DiStefano A, et al: Phase II study of anguidine in advanced breast cancer. Cancer Treat Rep 63:789–791, 1979
252. Adler SS, Lowenbraun S, Birch B, et al: A broad phase II study of the Southeastern Cancer Study Group. Cancer Treat Rep 68:423–425, 1984
253. Budman DR, Forastiere A, Perloff M, et al: Aziridinylbenzoquinone (AZQ) in advanced breast cancer: A Cancer and Leukemia Group B phase II trial. Cancer Treat Rep 66:1875–1876, 1982
254. Martino S, Samal B, Singhakowinta A, et al: In-vivo and in-vitro study of AZQ in advanced breast cancer. Proc Am Soc Clin Oncol 3:127, 1984
255. Yap HY, Bedikian AY, Schell FC, et al: Phase II clinical evaluation of AZQ in metastatic breast cancer. Am J Clin Oncol 6:31–33, 1982
256. Bonadonna G, De Lena M, Monfardini S, et al: Clinical trials with bleomycin in lymphomas and in solid tumors. Eur J Cancer 8:205–215, 1972
257. Haas CD, Coltman CA Jr, Gottlieb JA, et al: Phase II evaluation of bleomycin. Cancer 38:8–12, 1976
258. Wiseman CL, Yap HY, Bedikian AY, et al: Phase II trial of bruceantin in metastatic breast carcinoma. Am J Clin Oncol 5:389–391, 1982
259. Booth BW, Weiss RB, Korzun AH, et al: Phase II trial of

carboplatin in advanced breast carcinoma: A Cancer and Leukemia Group B study. Cancer Treat Rep 69:919–920, 1985
260. Baker LH, Kessel DH, Comis RL, et al: American experience with carminomycin. Cancer Treat Rep 63:899–902, 1979
261. Aboud A, Yap HY, Esparza L, et al: Carminomycin: A new anthracycline analog in the treatment of advanced breast cancer. Cancer 53:9–12, 1984
262. Edmonson JH, Rubin J, Kvols LK, et al: Phase II study of chlorozotocin in advanced breast cancer. Cancer Treat Rep 65:537–538, 1981
263. Silver BA, Barlock AL, Lippman ME, et al: Phase II trial of chlorozotocin in malignant melanoma, breast cancer, and other solid tumors. Cancer Treat Rep 66:1229–1230, 1982
264. Samal B, Jones S, Brownlee RW, et al: Chromomycin A_3 for advanced breast cancer: A Southwest Oncology Group study. Cancer Treat Rep 62:19–22, 1978
265. O'Bryan RM, Baker L, Whitecar J, et al: Cyclocytidine in breast cancer. Cancer Treat Rep 62:455–456, 1978
266. Ahmann DL, Bisel HF, Eagan RT, et al: Phase II evaluation of VP-16-213 (NSC-141540) and cytembena (NSC-104801) in patients with advanced breast cancer. Cancer Treat Rep 60:633–635, 1976
267. Thongprasert D, Budman D, Wittes RB, et al: Phase II study of 10-deaza-aminopterin in advanced breast cancer. Proc Am Soc Clin Oncol 2:101, 1983
268. Ahmann DL, O'Connell MJ, Bisel HF, et al: Phase II study of dianhydrogalactitol and ICRF-159 in patients with advanced breast cancer previously exposed to cytotoxic chemotherapy. Cancer Treat Rep 61:81–82, 1977
269. Hoogstraten B, O'Bryan R, Jones S: 1,2:5,6-dianhydrogalactitol in advanced breast cancer. Cancer Treat Rep 62:841–842, 1978
270. Schapira D, Hall TC, Bennett JM, et al: A phase II study of estradiol mustard (NSC-112259) by the Eastern Cooperative Oncology Group. Cancer Clin Trials 1:5–8, 1978
271. Creech RH, Engstrom PF, Harris DT, et al: Phase II study of ICRF-159 in refractory metastatic breast cancer. Cancer Treat Rep 63:111–114, 1979
272. Slavik M: Clinical studies with DTIC (NSC-45388) in various malignancies. Cancer Treat Rep 60:213–214, 1976
273. Blum RH, Wittenberg BK, Canellos GP, et al: A therapeutic trial of maytansine. Cancer Clin Trials 1:113–117, 1978
274. Neidhart JA, Laufman LR, Vaughn C, et al: Minimal single-agent activity of maytansine in refractory breast cancer: A Southwest Oncology Group study. Cancer Treat Rep 64:675–677, 1980
275. Edmonson JH, Rubin J, Kvols LK, et al: Phase II study of maytansine in advanced breast cancer. Cancer Treat Rep 65:536–537, 1981
276. Moore GE, Bross IDJ, Ausman R, et al: Effects of 6-mercaptopurine (NSC-755) in 290 patients with advanced cancer. Cancer Chemother Rep 52:655–660, 1968
277. Ahmann D, Bisel H, Hahn R: A phase II evaluation of 1-(2-chloroethyl)-3-(4-methylcyclohexyl)-1-nitrosourea(NSC 95441) in patients with advanced breast cancer. Cancer Res 34:27–30, 1974
278. Yap HY, Blumenschein GR, Schell F, et al: Phase II evaluation of methyl-GAG in patients with refractory metastatic breast cancer. Cancer Treat Rep 65:465–467, 1981
279. McKelvey EM, Murphy W, Zander A, et al: Neocarzinostatin: Report of a phase II clinical trial. Cancer Treat Rep 65:699–701, 1981
280. Taylor SG, Davis TE, Falkson G, et al: PALA in advanced breast cancer: A phase II pilot study by the ECOG. Am J Clin Oncol 5:627–629, 1982
281. Mann G, Hortobagyi G, Yap H, et al: A comparative study of PALA, PALA/5-FU, and 5-FU in advanced breast carcinoma. Proc Am Soc Clin Oncol 1:76, 1982
282. Kavanagh JJ, Yap HY, Blumenschein GR, et al: Phase II trial of PCNU in refractory advanced breast cancer. Am J Clin Oncol 5:249–251, 1982
283. Martino S, Samal BA, Singhakowinta A: PCNU in advanced breast cancer. Cancer Treat Rep 67:305–306, 1983
284. Palmer RL, Samal BA, Vaughn CB, et al: Phase II evaluation of piperazinedione in metastatic breast carcinoma. Cancer Treat Rep 61:1711–1712, 1977
285. Nichols WC, Kvols LK, Ingle JN, et al: Phase II study of triazinate and pyrazofurin in patients with advanced breast cancer previously exposed to cytotoxic chemotherapy. Cancer Treat Rep 62:837–839, 1978
286. Legha SS, Benjamin RS, Buzdar AU, et al: Rubidazone in metastatic breast cancer. Cancer Treat Rep 63:135–136, 1979
287. Budman DR, Ginsberg S, Perry M, et al: Phase II trial of spirogermanium in breast adenocarcinoma: A Cancer and Leukemia Group B study. Cancer Treat Rep 66:1667–1668, 1982
288. Falkson G, Falkson HC: Phase II trial of spirogermanium for treatment of advanced breast cancer. Cancer Treat Rep 67:189–190, 1983
289. Pinnamaneni K, Yap HY, Legha SS, et al: Phase II study of spirogermanium in the treatment of metastatic breast cancer. Cancer Treat Rep 68:1197–1198, 1984
290. Schein PS, O'Connell MJ, Blom J, et al: Clinical antitumor activity and toxicity of streptozotocin. Cancer 34:993–1000, 1974
291. Pandya KJ, Tormey DC, Davis TE, et al: Phase II trial of 6-thioguanine in metastatic breast cancer. Cancer Treat Rep 64:191–192, 1980
292. Rodriguez V, Richman SP, Benjamin RS, et al: Phase II study with Baker's antifol in solid tumors. Cancer Res 37:980–983, 1977
293. Tirelli U, Franchin G, Crivellari D, et al: Phase II study of VM26 in extensively pretreated breast cancer. Am J Clin Oncol 7:451–452, 1984
294. Falkson G, van Dyk JJ, van Eden EB, et al: A clinical trial of the oral form of 4'-demethyl-epipodophyllotoxin-b-d ethylidene glucoside (NSC 1411540) VP 16-213, Cancer 35:1141–1144, 1975
295. Eagan RT, Ahmann DL, Bisel HF: Evaluation of VP-16 and the combination of Adriamycin and vincristine in advanced breast cancer. Oncology 33:146–148, 1976
296. Nissen NI, Hansen HH, Pedersen H, et al: Clinical trial of the oral form of a new podophyllotoxin derivative, VP-16-213 (NSC-141540), in patients with advanced neoplastic disease. Cancer Chemother Rep 59:1027–1029, 1975
297. Cavalli F, Jungi WF, Brunner KW: Randomisierte phase-II studie mit VP-16-213 (etoposide) in der behandlung vom fortgeschrittenen mammakarzinom. Onkologie 4:80–83, 1981
298. Vaughn CB, Panettiere F, Thigpen T, et al: Phase II evaluation of VP-16-213 in patients with advanced breast cancer: A Southwest Oncology Group study. Cancer Treat Rep 65:443–445, 1981
299. Yap HY, Blumenschein GR, Hortobagyi GN, et al: Combination chemotherapy with continuous infusion vinblastine and peptichemio for patients with advanced metastatic breast cancer. Am J Clin Oncol 5:511–514, 1982
300. Legha SS, Ajani JA, Blumenschein GR, et al: Combination chemotherapy of metastatic breast carcinoma with cyclophosphamide, Adriamycin, and peptichemio. Cancer 53:1836–1840, 1984
301. Buzdar AU, Legha SS, Hortobagyi GN, et al: AMSA and pep-

tichemio in the treatment of advanced metastatic breast cancer: A phase II study. Am J Clin Oncol 5:383–387, 1982
302. Yap HY, Blumenschein GR, Buzdar AU, et al: A randomized comparative study of hormono-chemotherapy with tamoxifen (t) and continuous 48-hour infusion (ci) doxorubicin (A), cyclophosphamide (C) in combination with 5-fluorouracil (F) or VP16-213 (E) in metastatic breast cancer. Proc Am Assoc Cancer Res 24:152, 1983
303. Greenspan EM, Fieber M, Lesnick G, et al: Response of advanced breast carcinoma to the combination of the antimetabolite methotrexate and the alkylating agent thio-TEPA. J Mt Sinai Hosp 30:246–267, 1963
304. Cooper RG: Combination chemotherapy in hormone resistant breast cancer. Proc Am Assoc Cancer Res 10:15, 1969
305. Ramirez G, Klotz J, Strawitz JG, et al: Combination chemotherapy in breast cancer. A randomized study of 4 versus 5 drugs. Oncology 32:101–108, 1975
306. Muss HB, White DR, Cooper R, et al: Combination chemotherapy in advanced breast cancer. A randomized trial comparing a three- vs. a five-drug program. Arch Intern Med 137:1711–1714, 1977
307. Tormey DC, Weinberg VE, Leone LA, et al: A comparison of intermittent vs. continuous and of Adriamycin vs. Methotrexate 5-drug chemotherapy for advanced breast cancer. Am J Clin Oncol 7:231–239, 1984
308. Cummings FJ, Gelman R, Horton J: Comparison of CAF versus CMFP in metastatic breast cancer: Analysis of prognostic factors. J Clin Oncol 3:932–940, 1985
309. Valagussa P, Brambilla C, Bonadonna G: Interim vs. final analysis: Comparability of results in advanced breast cancer trials. Proc Am Soc Clin Oncol 2, 1983
310. Aisner J, Weinberg V, Perloff M, et al: Chemotherapy vs. chemoimmunotherapy (CAF vs. CAFVP vs. CMF each + MER) for metastatic carcinoma of the breast. A CALGB study. (in press) 1986
311. Tormey DC, Weinberg VE, Holland JF, et al: A randomized trial of five and three drug chemotherapy and chemoimmunotherapy in women with operable node positive breast cancer. J Clin Oncol 1:138–145, 1983
312. Canellos GP, DeVita V, Gold GL, et al: Cyclical combination chemotherapy for advanced breast carcinoma. Br Med J 1:218–220, 1974
313. Bonadonna G, Zambetti M, Valagussa P, et al: Adjuvant CMF in node negative breast cancer. Proc Am Soc Clin Oncol 5:74, 1986
314. Jones SE, Durie BGM, Salmon SE: Combination chemotherapy with Adriamycin and cyclophosphamide for advanced breast cancer. Cancer 36:90–97, 1975
315. Smalley R, Carpenter J, Bartolucci A, et al: A comparison of cyclophosphamide, Adriamycin, 5-fluorouracil (CAF) and cyclophosphamide, methotrexate, 5-fluorouracil, vincristine, prednisone (CMFVP) in patients with metastatic breast cancer. Cancer 40:625–632, 1977
316. Segaloff A, Hankey BF, Carter AC, et al: An evaluation of the effect of vincristine added to cyclosphosphamide, 5-fluorouracil, methotrexate, and prednisone in advanced breast cancer. Breast Cancer Res Treat 5:311–319, 1985
317. Tucker WG, Talley RW, Lane M, et al: Treatment of adenocarcinoma with combinations of cyclophosphamide (NSC-26271) and 5-fluorouracil (NSC-19893). Cancer Chemother Rep 59:425–427, 1975
318. Ahmann D, Bisel H, Hahn R, et al: An analysis of a multiple-drug program in the treatment of patients with advanced breast cancer utilizing 5-fluorouracil, cyclophosphamide and prednisone with or without vincristine. Cancer 36:1925–1935, 1975
319. Chlebowski RT, Pugh R, Weiner JM, et al: Doxorubicin and CCNU with or without vincristine in patients with advanced breast cancer. Cancer 52:606–609, 1983
320. Steiner R, Stewart JF, Rubens RD: Results of endocrine therapy do not predict response to chemotherapy in advanced breast cancer. Eur J Cancer Clin Oncol 19:1559–1563, 1983
321. Tattersall MHN, Jackson RC, Connors TA, et al: Combination chemotherapy: The interaction of methotrexate and 5-fluorouracil. Eur J Cancer 9:733–739, 1973
322. Bertino JR, Sawicki WL, Lindquist CA, et al: Schedule-dependent antitumor effects of methotrexate and 5-fluorouracil. Cancer Res 37:327–328, 1977
323. Browman GP: Clinical application of the concept of methotrexate plus 5-FU sequence-dependent "synergy": How good is the evidence? Cancer Treat Rep 68:465–469, 1984
324. Gewirtz A, Cadman E: Preliminary report on the efficacy of sequential methotrexate and 5-fluorouracil in advanced breast cancer. Cancer 47:2552–2555, 1981
325. Tisman G, Wu, SJG: Effectiveness of intermediate-dose methotrexate and high-dose 5-fluorouracil as sequential combination chemotherapy in refractory breast cancer and as primary therapy in metastatic adenocarcinoma of the colon. Cancer Treat Rep 64:829–835, 1980
326. Plotkin D, Waugh WJ: Sequential methotrexate-5 fluorouracil (MF) in advanced breast carcinoma. Proc Am Soc Clin Oncol 1:80, 1982
327. Perrault DJ, Erlichman C, Hasselback R, et al: Sequenced methotrexate (mtx) and 5-fluorouracil (5FU) in refractory metastatic breast cancer: A phase II study. Proc Am Soc Clin Oncol 2:100, 1983
328. Herrmann R, Manegold C, Schroeder M, et al: Sequential methotrexate and 5-FU in breast cancer resistant to the conventional application of these drugs. Cancer Treat Rep 68:1279–1281, 1984
329. Kaye SB, Sangster G, Hutcheon A, et al: Sequential methotrexate plus 5-FU in advanced breast and colorectal cancers: A phase II study. Cancer Treat Rep 68:547–548, 1984
330. Chang JC, Hill G, Ediss G, et al: Sequential chemotherapy of 5-fluorouracil (5-FU) and methotrexate (MTX) in the regimen of cytoxan (CTX), MTX and 5-FU in the treatment of advanced breast cancer. Proc Am Soc Clin Oncol 20:404, 1979
331. Cadman EC, Glick JH, Cross J, et al: Sequential methotrexate and 5-FU in CMFP (cyclophosphamide, methotrexate, 5-FU, and prednisone) therapy for breast cancer. Cancer Treat Rep 68:877–879, 1984
332. Ahmann D, Eagan R, Bisel H, et al: Evaluation of combination therapy with Adriamycin (NSC-123127) and methotrexate (NSC-740) in patients with disseminated breast cancer. Cancer Chemother Rep 6:335–338, 1975
333. Nemoto T, Horton J, Simon R, et al: Comparison of four-combination chemotherapy programs in metastatic breast cancer. Cancer 49:1988–1993, 1982
334. Smalley RV, Lefante J, Bartolucci A, et al: A comparison of cyclophosphamide, Adriamycin, and 5-fluorouracil (CAF) and cyclophosphamide, methotrexate, 5-fluorouracil, vincristine and prednisone (CMFVP) in patients with advanced breast cancer. Breast Cancer Res Treat 3:209–220, 1983
335. Harris MA, Byrne PJ, Smith FP, et al: Treatment of advanced breast cancer with two doxorubicin-containing regimens. Am J Clin Oncol 6:51–58, 1983
336. Tannir N, Yap HY, Hortobagyi GH, et al: Sequential continuous infusion with doxorubicin and vinblastine: An effective chemotherapy combination for patients with advanced breast cancer previously treated with cyclophosphamide,

methotrexate, 5-FU, vincristine, and prednisone. Cancer Treat Rep 68:1039–1041, 1984
337. Yap HY, Blumenschein GR, Barnes B, et al: Sequential combinations of continuous infusion Adriamycin and vinblastine in patients with metastatic breast cancer. Proc Am Soc Clin Oncol 1:78, 1982
338. Perloff M, Hart R, Holland J: Vinblastine, Adriamycin, thiotepa, and halotestin (VATH). Cancer 42:2534–2537, 1978
339. Hart R, Perloff M, Holland J: One-day VATH (vinblastine, Adriamycin, thiotepa, and halotestin) therapy for advanced breast cancer refractory to chemotherapy. Cancer 48:1522–1527, 1981
340. Creech RH, Dayal H, Catalano RB, et al: Combination doxorubicin-mitomycin therapy for hormonal and CMF-refractory metastatic breast cancer. Proc Am Soc Clin Oncol 3:126, 1984
341. Oster MW, Park Y: Vincristine, Adriamycin, and mitomycin (VAm) therapy for previously treated breast cancer. Cancer 51:203–205, 1983
342. Pinnamaneni K, Yap HY, Buzdar AU, et al: Adriamycin, dibromodulcitol, and mitomycin combination chemotherapy for patients with metastatic breast carcinoma previously treated with cyclophosphamide, methotrexate, 5-fluorouracil, vincristine, and prednisone. Cancer 53:1841–1844, 1984
343. Vaughn CB, Maniscalco-Greb E, Lockhard C, et al: VP-16 and Adriamycin in patients with advanced breast cancer. Am J Clin Oncol 5:505–507, 1982
344. Konits PH, Van Echo DA, Aisner J, et al: Doxorubicin plus VP-16-213 for the treatment of refractory breast carcinoma. Am J Clin Oncol 5:515–519, 1982
345. Konits P, Aisner J, VanEcho D, et al: Mitomycin C and vinblastine chemotherapy for advanced breast cancer. Cancer 48:1295–1298, 1981
346. Veronesi A, Tirelli U, Galligioni E, et al: Third-line chemotherapy with mitomycin, vinblastine, and carmustine (BCNU) in refractory breast carcinoma: A pilot study. Cancer Treat Rep 666:559–561, 1982
347. Hortobagyi GN, Yap HY, Blumenschein GR, et al: Phase II evaluation of vinblastine, methotrexate, and calcium leukovorin rescue in patients with refractory metastatic breast cancer. Cancer 51:769–772, 1983
348. Valagussa P, Rossi A, Tancini G, et al: Is there any effective salvage treatment for relapsing operable breast cancer with N+?. Proc Am Soc Clin Oncol 4:56, 1985
349. Rabadi SJ, Haid M, Scanlon EF, et al: Treatment of breast carcinoma recurrent after adjuvant chemoimmunotherapy. J Surg Oncol 26:233–237, 1984
350. Buzdar AU, Legha SS, Hortobagyi GN, et al: Management of breast cancer patients failing adjuvant chemotherapy with Adriamycin-containing regimens. Cancer 47:2798–2802, 1981
351. Bitran JD, Desser RK, Shapiro CM, et al: Response to secondary therapy in patients with adenocarcinoma of the breast previously treated with adjuvant chemotherapy. Cancer 51:381–384, 1983
352. Morris DM, Elias EG, Didolkar MS, et al: The response to further chemotherapy in patients with carcinoma of the breast who progressed while receiving adjuvant therapy. J Surg Oncol 29:154–157, 1985
353. Wendt AG, Jones SE, Salmon SE: Salvage treatments of patients relapsing after breast cancer adjuvant chemotherapy. Cancer Treat Rep 64:269, 1980
354. Schapira D, Velez-Garcia E, Raney M, et al: Salvage therapy for breast cancer patients relapsing after adjuvant therapy. Proc Am Soc Clin Oncol 3:114, 1984
355. Gorton SJ, Zelkowitz L, Agrawal BL, et al: Treatment of breast cancer patients who have failed Cytoxan, methotrexate, and 5-fluorouracil with Cytoxan and 5-fluorouracil. Proc Am Soc Clin Oncol 21:347, 1980
356. Rosner D, Snyderman M, Nemoto T: Potentiating role of previously administered agents in the combination chemotherapy of breast cancer. Oncology 36:160–163, 1979
357. Rosner D: Recycling prior used drugs in sequential combination chemotherapy enhances response and survival in metastatic breast cancer. Proc Am Soc Clin Oncol 1:72, 1982
358. Kim, SH, Kim JH: Lethal effect of Adriamycin on the division cycle of HeLa cells. Cancer Res 32:323–325, 1972
359. Silvestrini R, Daidone MG, Gentili C: Biologic characteristics of breast cancer and their clinical relevance. In Bulbrook RD (ed): Commentaries on Research in Breast Disease, Vol 2, pp 1–40. New York, Alan R Liss, 1981
360. Bonadonna G, Valagussa P: Dose-response effect of CMF in breast cancer. Proc Am Soc Clin Oncol 21:413, 1980
361. Brufman G, Sulkes A, Fuks Z, et al: Cytoxan, methotrexate and 5-fluorouracil (CMF) chemotherapy (chtx) in metastatic breast cancer (mbc): The influence of dose levels (dl) and performance status (ps) upon response rates and survival. Proc Am Soc Clin Oncol 2:103, 1983
362. Israel L, Breau JL, Aguilera J: High-dose cyclosphosphamide and high-dose 5-fluorouracil: A new first-line regimen for advanced breast cancer. Cancer 53:1655–1659, 1984
363. Tormey DC, Kline JC, Palta M, et al: Short-term high-density systemic therapy for metastatic breast cancer. Breast Cancer Res Treat 5:177–188, 1985
364. Malik R, Blumenschein GR, Legha SS, et al: A randomized trial of high-dose 5-fluorouracil, doxorubicin, and cyclophosphamide versus conventional FAC regimen in metastatic breast cancer. Proc Am Soc Clin Oncol 1:79, 1982
365. Tobias JS, Weiner RS, Griffiths CT, et al: Experience with cryopreserved autologous marrow infusion following high-dose chemotherapy. Eur J Cancer 13:269–277, 1977
366. Douer D, Champlin RE, Ho WG, et al: High-dose combined-modality therapy and autologous bone marrow transplantation in resistant cancer. Am J Med 71:973–976, 1981
367. Stewart PS: Autologous bone marrow transplantation in metastatic breast cancer. Breast Cancer Res Treat 2:85–92, 1982
368. Lazarus HM, Herzig RH, Graham-Pole J, et al: Intensive melphalan chemotherapy and cryopreserved autologous bone marrow transplantation for the treatment of refractory cancer. J Clin Oncol 1:359–367, 1983
369. Corringham R, Gilmore M, Prentice HG, et al: High-dose melphalan with autologous bone marrow transplant. Cancer 52:1783–1787, 1983
370. Tannir N, Spitzer G, Schell F, et al: Phase II study of high-dose amsacrine (AMSA) and autologous bone marrow transplantation in patients with refractory metastatic breast cancer. Cancer Treat Rep 67:599–600, 1983
371. Tannir N, Spitzer G, Dicke K, et al: Phase I-II study of high-dose mitomycin with autologous bone marrow transplantation in refractory metastatic breast cancer. Cancer Treat Rep 68:805–806, 1984
372. Maraninchi D, Abecasis M, Gastaut J, et al: High-dose melphalan with autologous bone marrow rescue for the treatment of advanced adult solid tumors. Cancer Treat Rep 68:471–474, 1984
373. Knight WA III, Page CP, Kuhn JG, et al: High-dose L-PAM with autologous bone marrow infusion for advanced, steroid hormone receptor negative, breast cancer. Breast Cancer Res Treat 4:336, 1984
374. Eder JP, Antman KH, Elias A, et al: High-dose combined

alkylating agents (hdca) with autologous bone marrow transplantation (abmt) in metastatic breast cancer. Breast Cancer Res Treat 6:186, 1985
375. Peters WP, Gockerman JP, Olsen GA, et al: High dose combination alkylating agent therapy with autologous bone marrow support as initial therapy for metastatic breast cancer. Breast Cancer Res Treat 6:182, 1985
376. Hryniuk W, Bush H: The importance of dose intensity in chemotherapy of metastatic breast cancer. J Clin Oncol 2:1281–1288, 1984
377. Moore M: Interpretation of results of chemotherapy trials in metastatic breast cancer. J Clin Oncol 4:258, 1986
378. Fraschini G, Yap HY, Hortobagyi GN, et al: Five-day continuous-infusion vinblastine in the treatment of breast cancer. Cancer 56:225–229, 1985
379. Chacon RD, Kotliar ML, Cavarra G, et al: Phase II study with vinblastine continuous infusion. Proc Am Soc Clin Oncol 1:33, 1982
380. Shah MK, Creech RN, Catalano RB, et al: Phase II study of vinblastine infusion in the treatment of refractory advanced breast cancer. Proc Am Soc Clin Oncol 1:73, 1982
381. Ingle JN, Ahmann DL, Gestner JG, et al: Evaluation of vinblastine administered by 5-day continuous infusion in women with advanced breast cancer. Cancer Treat Rep 68:803–804, 1984
382. Tannock I, Erlichman C, Perrault D, et al: Failure of 5-day vinblastine infusion in the treatment of patients with advanced refractory breast cancer. Cancer Treat Rep 66:1783–1784, 1982
383. Hopkins JO, Jackson DV Jr, White DR, et al: Vincristine by continuous infusion in refractory breast cancer: A phase II study. Am J Clin Oncol 6:529–532, 1983
384. Yap HY, Valdivieso M, Blumenschein G, et al: A phase I-II study of continuous 5-day infusion mitomycin-C. Am J Clin Oncol 6:109–112, 1983
385. Legha SS, Benjamin RS, Mackay B, et al: Adriamycin therapy by continuous intravenous infusion in patients with metastatic breast cancer. Cancer 49:1762–1766, 1982
386. Plotkin D, Waugh WJ: Hypothesis: Discontinuous chemotherapy for advanced breast cancer. Am J Clin Oncol 6:375–379, 1983
387. De Lena M, Zucali R, Viganotti G, et al: Combined chemotherapy-radiotherapy approach in locally advanced (T3b-T4) breast cancer. Cancer Chemother Pharmacol 1:53–59, 1978
388. Ahmann D, O'Fallon J, O'Connell MT, et al: Evaluation of a fixed alternating treatment in patients with advanced breast cancer. Cancer Clin Trials 1:219–226, 1978
389. Tormey D, Gelman R, Falkson G: Prospective evaluation of rotating chemotherapy in advanced breast cancer. Am J Clin Oncol 6:1–18, 1983
390. Kennealey GT, Boston B, Mitchell MS, et al: Combination chemotherapy for advanced breast cancer. Cancer 42:27–33, 1978
391. Vogel CL, Smalley RV, Raney M, et al: Randomized trial of cyclophosphamide, doxorubicin, and 5-fluorouracil alone or alternating with a "cycle active" non-cross-resistant combination in women with visceral metastatic breast cancer. A Southeastern Cancer Study Group project. J Clin Oncol 2:643–651, 1984
392. Chlebowski RT, Weiner JM, Ryden V, et al: Factors influencing the interim interpretation of a breast cancer trial. Controlled Clin Trials 2:123–132, 1981
393. Henderson IC, Gelman RS, Canellos GP, et al: Time to first response (IMP), partial response (PR), and complete response (CR) in breast cancer (bc) patients (pts) treated with intensive chemotherapy. Proc Am Soc Clin Oncol 22:445, 1981
394. Gillespie PJ, Alexander JL, Edelstyn GA: Changes in 87m-sr concentrations in skeletal metastases in patients responding to cyclical combination chemotherapy for advanced breast cancer. J Nucl Med 16:191–193, 1975
395. Mughal AW, Hortobagyi GN, Fritsche HA, et al: Serial plasma carcinoembryonic antigen measurements during treatment of metastatic breast cancer. JAMA 249:1881–1886, 1983
396. Loprinzi CL, Tormey DC, Rasmussen P, et al: Prospective evaluation of carcinoembryonic antigen levels and alternating chemotherapeutic regimens in metastatic breast cancer. J Clin Oncol 4:46–56, 1986
397. Franco LA, Shafie SM: Estrogen receptor status, doubling time and sensitivity of breast carcinoma cells to Adriamycin in tissue culture. Proc Am Assoc Cancer Res 22:5, 1981
398. Sulkes, Livingston RB, Murphy WK: Tritiated thymidine labeling index and response in human breast cancer. J Natl Cancer Inst 62:513–515, 1979
399. Wolberg WH, Ansfield FJ: The relation of thymidine labeling index in human tumors in vitro to the effectiveness of 5-fluorouracil chemotherapy. Cancer Res 31:448–450, 1971
400. Zhang HJ, Kennedy BJ, Kiang DT: Thymidine kinase as a predictor of response to chemotherapy in advanced breast cancer. Breast Cancer Res Treat 4:221–225, 1984
401. Rozencweig M, Staquet MJ, Von Hoff DD, et al: Prognostic factors for the response to chemotherapy in advanced breast cancer. Cancer Clin Trials 165–170, 1979
402. Tormey DC, Gelman R, Band PR, et al: A prospective evaluation of chemohormonal therapy remission maintenance in advanced breast cancer. Breast Cancer Res Treat 1:111–119, 1981
403. Swenerton KD, Legha SS, Smith T, et al: Prognostic factors in metastatic breast cancer treated with combination chemotherapy. Cancer Res 39:1552–1562, 1979
404. Valagussa P, Brambilla C, Bonadonna G: Advanced breast cancer: Are the traditional stratification parameters still of value when patients are treated with combination chemotherapy? Eur J Cancer 15:565–571, 1979
405. Hortobagyi GN, Smith TL, Legha SS, et al: Multivariate analysis of prognostic factors in metastatic breast cancer. J Clin Oncol 1:776, 1983
406. Russell J, Baker J, Dady P, et al: Response of metastatic breast cancer to combination chemotherapy according to site. Br Med J 2:1390–1391, 1977
407. Smalley RV, Bartolucci AA: Variations in responsiveness and survival of clinical subsets of patients with metastatic breast cancer to two chemotherapy combinations. In Mouridsen HT, Palshof T (eds): Breast Cancer—Experimental and Clinical Aspects, pp 141–146. Elmsford, NY, Pergamon Press, 1980
408. Aisner J, Weinberg V, Wiernik PH, et al: Frequency and duration of response to combination chemotherapy for metastatic breast cancer: Impact of prior radiotherapy. Proc Am Soc Clin Oncol 20:421, 1979
409. Nash CH III, Jones SE, Moon TE, et al: Prediction of outcome in metastatic breast cancer treated with Adriamycin combination chemotherapy. Cancer 46:2380–2388, 1980
410. Smalley R, Lefante J, Bartolucci A: Multivariate prognostic factor analysis—advanced breast cancer chemotherapy. Proc Am Assoc Cancer Res 22:146, 1981
411. Legha S, Buzdar A, Smith T, et al: Response to hormonal therapy as a prognostic factor for metastatic breast cancer treated with combination chemotherapy. Cancer 46:438–445, 1980

412. Manni A, Trujillo JE, Pearson OH: Sequential use of endocrine therapy and chemotherapy for metastatic breast cancer: Effects on survival. Cancer Treat Rep 64:111–116, 1980
413. Henderson MD, Buroker TR, Samson MK, et al: Response of patients with carcinoma of the breast to hormonal therapy and combination chemotherapy. Surg Gynecol Obstet 141:232–234, 1975
414. Levine RM, Lippman ME: Relationship between estrogen-receptor proteins and response to chemotherapy in breast cancer. Cancer Treat Rep 68:573–576, 1984
415. Kiang DT: Correlation between estrogen-receptor proteins and response to chemotherapy in patients with breast cancer. Cancer Treat Rep 68:577–599, 1984
416. Lippman ME, Allegra JC, Thompson EG, et al: The relation between estrogen receptors and response rate to cytotoxic chemotherapy in metastatic breast cancer. N Engl J Med 298:1223–1228, 1978
417. Kiang DT, Frenning DH, Gay J, et al: Estrogen receptor status and response to chemotherapy in advanced breast cancer. Cancer 46:2814–2817, 1980
418. Jonat W, Maass H, Stolzenbach G, et al: Estrogen receptor status and response to polychemotherapy in advanced breast cancer. Cancer 46:2809–2813, 1980
419. Samal BA, Brooks SC, Cummings G, et al: Estrogen receptors and responsiveness of advanced breast cancer to chemotherapy. Cancer 46:2925–2927, 1980
420. Hilf R, Feldstein ML, Savlov ED, et al: The lack of relationship between estrogen receptor status and response to chemotherapy. Cancer 46:2797–2800, 1980
421. Rubens RD, Hayward JL: Estrogen receptors and response to endocrine therapy and cytotoxic chemotherapy in advanced breast cancer. Cancer 46:2922–2924, 1980
422. Rosenbaum C, Marsland TA, Stolbach L, et al: Estrogen receptor status and response to chemotherapy in advanced breast cancer. Cancer 46:2919–2921, 1980
423. Corle DK, Sears ME, Olson KB: Relationship of quantitative estrogen-receptor level and clinical response to cytotoxic chemotherapy in advanced breast cancer. Cancer 54:1554–1561, 1984
424. Livingston RB: Breast cancer and response to chemotherapy: A possible relationship between hormone receptors and doxorubicin. Cancer Treat Rev 9:229–236, 1982
425. Feldman L, Hortobagyi G, Buzdar A, et al: Duration of chemotherapy to achieve complete remission (CR)—a prognostic factor in metastatic breast cancer (mbc). Proc Am Soc Clin Oncol 3:121, 1984
426. Oberfield RA, Cady B, Pazianos AG, et al: Adrenalectomy-oophorectomy and combined chemotherapy for carcinoma of the breast with metastases. Surg Gynecol Obstet 148:881–886, 1979
427. Falkson G, Falkson HC, Glidewell O, et al: Improved remission rates and remission duration in young women with metastatic breast cancer following combined oophorectomy and chemotherapy: A study by Cancer and Leukemia Group B. Cancer 43:2215–2222, 1979
428. Kumar KS, Ogel CL, Moore MR, et al: Sequential versus concomitant chemo-hormonal therapy in breast cancer. Breast Dis Breast 8:2–7, 1982
429. Ahmann DL, O'Connell MJ, Hahn RG, et al: An evaluation of early or delayed adjuvant chemotherapy in premenopausal patients with advanced breast cancer undergoing oophorectomy. N Engl J Med 297:356–360, 1977
430. Ahmann D, Green S, Bisel H, et al: An evaluation of early or delayed adjuvant chemotherapy in premenopausal patients with advanced breast cancer undergoing oophorectomy. Am J Clin Oncol 5:355–358, 1982
431. Glick JH, Creech RH, Torri S, et al: Tamoxifen plus sequential CMF chemotherapy versus tamoxifen alone in postmenopausal patients with advanced breast cancer. Cancer 45:735–741, 1980
432. Rossof AH, Gelman R, Creech RH: Randomized evaluation of combination chemotherapy vs. observation alone following response or stabilization after oophorectomy for metastatic breast cancer in premenopausal women. Am J Clin Oncol 5:253–259, 1982
433. Wada T, Koyama H, Terasawa T: Tamoxifen versus tamoxifen plus 1-(2-tetrahydrofuryl)-5-fluorouracil in the treatment of advanced breast cancer: A sequential trial. Breast Cancer Res Treat 1:53–58, 1981
434. Kiang DT, Gay J, Goldman A, et al: A randomized trial of chemotherapy and hormonal therapy in advanced breast cancer. N Engl J Med 313:1241–1246, 1985
435. Bezwoda WR, Derman D, DeMoor NG, et al: Treatment of metastatic breast cancer in estrogen receptor positive patients. Cancer 50:2747–2750, 1982
436. Cavalli F, Beer M, Martz G, et al: Concurrent or sequential use of cytotoxic chemotherapy and hormone treatment in advanced breast cancer: Report of the Swiss Group for Clinical Cancer Research. Br Med J 286:5–8, 1983
437. Australian and New Zealand Breast Cancer Trials Group (ANZBCTG): A randomized trial in postmenopausal patients with advanced breast cancer comparing endocrine and cytotoxic therapy given sequentially or in combination. J Clin Oncol 4:186–193, 1986
438. Brunner KW, Sonntag RW, Alberto P, et al: Combined chemo- and hormonal therapy in advanced breast cancer. Cancer 39:2923–2933, 1977
439. Rubens RD, Begent RHJ, Knight RK, et al: Combined cytotoxic and progestogen therapy for advanced breast cancer. Cancer 42:1680–1686, 1978
440. Tormey DC, Falkson G, Crowley J, et al: Dibromodulcitol and Adriamycin plus or minus tamoxifen in advanced breast cancer. Am J Clin Oncol 5:33–39, 1982
441. Cocconi G, DeLisi V, Boni C, et al: Chemotherapy versus combination of chemotherapy and endocrine therapy in advanced breast cancer. Cancer 51:581–588, 1983
442. Kardinal CG, Perry MC, Weinberg V, et al: Chemoendocrine therapy vs. chemotherapy alone for advanced breast cancer in postmenopausal women: Preliminary report of a randomized study. Breast Cancer Res Treat 3:365–372, 1983
443. Kardinal CG, Perry MC, Korzun AH, et al: Response to chemotherapy or chemoendocrine therapy in patients with advanced breast cancer previously treated with adjuvant chemotherapy. Breast Cancer Res Treat 6:185, 1985
444. Viladiu P, Alonso MC, Avella A, et al: Chemotherapy versus chemotherapy plus hormonotherapy in postmenopausal advanced breast cancer patients. Cancer 56:2745–2750, 1985
445. Mouridsen HT, Rose C, Engelsman E, et al: Combined cytotoxic and endocrine therapy in postmenopausal patients with advanced breast cancer. A randomized study of CMF vs. CMF plus tamoxifen. Eur J Clin Oncol 21:219–299, 1985
446. Krook JE, Ingle JN, Green SJ, et al: Randomized clinical trial of cyclophosphamide, 5-FU, and prednisone with or without tamoxifen in postmenopausal women with advanced breast cancer. Cancer Treat Rep 69:355–361, 1985
447. Aitken SC, Lippman ME: Hormonal regulation of net DNA synthesis in MCF-7 human breast cancer cells in tissue culture. Cancer Res 42:1727–1735, 1982
448. Dao TL, Sinha DK, Nemoto T, et al: Effect of estrogen and progesterone on cellular replication of human breast tumors. Cancer Res 42:359–362, 1982
449. Nordenskjold B, Lowhagen T, Westerberg H, et al: 3H-thy-

midine incorporation into mammary carcinoma cells obtained by needle aspiration before and during endocrine therapy. Acta Cytol 20:137–143, 1976

450. Allegra JC, Woodcock TM, Richman SP, et al: A phase II trial of tamoxifen, Premarin, methotrexate and 5-fluorouracil in metastatic breast cancer. Breast Cancer Res Treat 2:93–99, 1982
451. Eisenhauer EA, Bowman DM, Pritchard KI, et al: Tamoxifen and conjugated estrogens (Premarin) followed by sequenced methotrexate and 5-FU in refractory advanced breast cancer. Cancer Treat Rep 68:1421–1422, 1984
452. Lippman ME, Cassidy J, Wesley M, et al: A randomized attempt to increase the efficacy of cytotoxic chemotherapy in metastatic breast cancer by hormonal synchronization. J Clin Oncol 2:28–36, 1984
453. Conte PF, Amadori D, Cortesi C, et al: A randomized study in metastatic breast cancer (mbc) comparing conventional chemotherapy vs chemotherapy with estrogenic recruitment. Breast Cancer Res Treat 6:167, 1985
454. Paridaens R, Blonk van der Wijst J, Julien JP, et al: Medical adrenalectomy and cyclic chemotherapy preceded by estrogenic recruitment in advanced breast cancer. A phase II trial of the EORTC breast cancer cooperative group. Proc Am Soc Clin Oncol 3:130, 1984
455. Fabian C, Sternson L, El-Serafi M, et al: Clinical pharmacology of tamoxifen in patients with breast cancer: Correlation with clinical data. Cancer 48:876–882, 1981
456. Moore FD, VanDevanter SB, Boyden CM, et al: Adrenalectomy and chemotherapy in breast cancer. Surgery 76:376–390, 1974
457. Paterson AHG, Szafran O, Hanson J, et al: Responses to treatment and its influence on survival in metastatic breast cancer. Am J Clin Oncol 8:283–292, 1985
458. Anderson JR, Cain KC, Gelber RD: Analysis of survival by tumor response. J Clin Oncol 1:710–711, 1983
459. Frei E III: Acute leukemia in children: Model for clinical therapeutic research in cancer. Cancer 53:2013–2025, 1984
460. Powles TJ, Smith IE, Ford HT, et al: Failure of chemotherapy to prolong survival in a group of patients with metastatic breast cancer. Lancet 1:580–582, 1980
461. Kaufman RJ: Advanced breast cancer—additive hormonal therapy. Cancer 47:2398–2403, 1981
462. Todd M, Shoag M, Cadman E: Survival of women with metastatic breast cancer at Yale from 1920 to 1980. J Clin Oncol 1:406–408, 1983
463. Paterson AHG, Lees AW, Hanson J, et al: Impact of chemotherapy on survival in metastatic breast cancer. Lancet 2:312, 1980
464. Rutqvist LE: Increasing incidence and constant mortality rates of breast cancer: Time trends in Stockholm County 1961–1973. Breast Cancer Res Treat 4:233–243, 1984
465. Ross M, Buzdar A, Smith T, et al: Improved survival of metastatic breast cancer patients receiving combination chemotherapy—an experience of the past three decades. Proc Am Soc Clin Oncol 2:105, 1983
466. Tormey D, Carbone P, Band P: Breast cancer survival in single and combination chemotherapy trials since 1968. Proc Am Assoc Cancer Res 18:64, 1977
467. Fey MF, Brunner KW, Sonntag RW: Prognostic factors in metastatic breast cancer. Cancer Clin Trials 4:237–247, 1981

Specific Sites of Metastatic Disease and Emergencies

14

Brain Metastases in Patients With Breast Cancer

J. Peter Glass Kathleen M. Foley

The central nervous system (CNS) manifestations of systemic cancer are becoming increasingly evident, particularly as patients live longer. Intracranial metastases represent the most common metastatic complication of systemic cancer. Brain metastases can rarely be cured, but with early diagnosis and aggressive treatment, palliation is likely.

INCIDENCE AND EPIDEMIOLOGY

The overall incidence of brain metastases from breast carcinoma varies from series to series.[1] The range is from 5.9% in a study of 389 cases conducted by Richards and McKissock in 1963 to 39% in a series of 218 cases reported by Chu and Hilaris in 1961. A clinical study conducted at the University of Tokyo in 1981 revealed that 16.2% of 616 patients with breast carcinoma had brain metastases. During the same year, an autopsy study of 1177 cases at Montefiore Hospital and Medical Center in New York demonstrated an incidence of 23.6%..

Brain metastases from breast carcinoma are more likely to occur in women who are premenopausal or those who are less than 5 years postmenopausal and who have advanced disease.[2] A study by Stewart in 1981 showed that estrogen receptor-negative tumors metastasize to the brain more commonly than do those that are estrogen receptor-positive.[3] There has been some evidence to substantiate the premise that the development of brain metastases is delayed in patients who are treated with additive or ablative hormonal therapy for their initial recurrence; however, this has not been found to affect overall survival.[2–4]

PRESENTING SYMPTOMS AND SIGNS

The presenting symptoms and signs of patients with breast carcinoma and brain metastases are similar to those in patients with other solid tumors. The mechanisms by which tumor produces neurologic dysfunction are varied.[5] Localized tumor is, by itself, capable of destroying normal CNS tissue, making possible the identification of the site of metastatic involvement. A brain metastasis may be associated with cerebral edema, which may affect the function of the brain at a site distant from the metastasis. This results in focal symptoms and signs that are more widespread than those caused by the metastasis itself. Likewise, a brain metastasis and its surrounding edema may cause a shift of cerebral structures, thus producing various syndromes of herniation. The two most common types of herniation are cingulate and transtentorial (uncal). When the cingulate gyrus herniates under the falx, it compresses the opposite frontal lobe and both anterior cerebral arteries. Such herniation could produce bilateral frontal lobe infarctions, causing bilateral weakness in the lower extremities, changes in mental status, and urinary incontinence. Herniation of the medial portion of the temporal lobe (uncus) into the tentorial notch compresses the ipsilateral oculomotor nerve, as well as the contralateral cerebral peduncle, causing pupillary dilatation and hemiparesis ipsilateral to the side of the lesion. Uncal herniation may also compress the ipsilateral posterior cerebral artery, resulting in occipital lobe infarction. The brain stem may be displaced downward, causing a decrease in the level of consciousness, and there may be obstruction to the flow of cerebrospinal fluid (CSF), resulting in hydrocephalus.

The onset of symptoms and signs in patients with brain metastases from breast carcinoma is usually insidious, occurring over a period of days to weeks. Breast carcinoma is not hemorrhagic, so a sudden bleed into the tumor that produces a neurologic deficit is highly unlikely, even in the face of thrombocytopenia. Conversely, most metastases occur at the junction of grey and white matter, so that the sudden onset of a focal or generalized seizure disorder is possible. According to Posner, if seizures are excluded, acute or apoplectiform onset of neurologic signs occurs in less than 10% of patients.[6]

The presenting symptoms and signs in 201 patients with brain metastases are summarized in Table 14-1. Of these, perhaps headache should be mentioned in greatest detail.

Headache

Headache is the most common presenting complaint in patients with brain metastases, occurring in approximately 50% of affected patients. It may be either focal or generalized. In only 40% of patients is it the typical "brain tumor headache," which occurs early in the morning—after awakening but before arising—and improves as the day progresses. Left untreated, the headache generally increases in frequency, severity, and duration until it becomes constant, and other signs of increased intracranial pressure, such as drowsiness, nausea, and vomiting, develop.

The most likely explanation for the pathogenesis of headache that occurs with metastatic disease is that it results from increased intracranial pressure with traction on pain-sensitive structures, including the dura, cranial nerves, and large venous sinuses. Occasionally, particularly in patients with cerebellar metastases associated with a marked increase in intracranial pressure, the headache may be paroxysmal, and may be accompanied by neurologic signs, such as visual obscuration, changes in consciousness, nausea, vomiting, and syncope. Paroxysmal headache is thought to be related to sudden, transient increases in intracranial pressure, referred to as plateau waves. Even though the headache caused by metastatic disease is usually accompanied by increased intracranial pressure, the incidence of associated papilledema is not that high, occurring in 25% to 40% of patients.

Table 14-1
Symptoms and Signs in 201 Patients with Brain Metastases

Symptoms	*% of Cases*	*Signs*	*% of Cases*
Headache	45	Impaired cognitive function	42
Behavioral and mental changes	33	Hemiparesis (mild to moderate, 28%, severe, 6%)	34
Focal weakness	21	Aphasia	17
Gait ataxia	22	Unilateral sensory loss	16
Seizures (focal, 7%, generalized, 13%)	20	Papilledema	15
Speech or language disturbances	14	Gait ataxia	14
Limb ataxia	10	Visual field loss	13
Sensory disturbance	10	Limb ataxia	10

(Reproduced with permission from Gamache FW, Jr, et al: Treatment of brain metastases by surgical extirpation. In Weiss L, et al (eds): Brain Metastasis. Copyright © 1980 by Year Book Medical Publishers, Inc., Chicago)

DIAGNOSTIC CONSIDERATIONS

Presently, computed tomography (CT) of the brain remains the radiographic test of choice in establishing the diagnosis of brain metastases. The CT manifestations of brain metastases in 304 patients with breast carcinoma were reviewed by Shi and colleagues in 1982.[7] Metastases were demonstrated in 103 patients. Single lesions were found in 55 patients (53%), and multiple metastases were found in 48 (47%). In 76 of 103 patients (74%), metastases were manifested as areas of decreased density compared with the normal brain on precontrast CT scans. Rounded areas of increased density detected on precontrast scans, were found in 13 patients (12.6%), including 2 patients with calcifications. An isodense area, surrounded by an area of decreased density that presumably was secondary to edema, was seen in seven patients (6.7%). Distortion of the collicular and suprasellar cisterns was the only precontrast finding observed in two patients. Metastasis to the pineal gland in one patient was manifested on a precontrast CT scan by dilatation of the lateral and third ventricles. In three cases (2.6%), precontrast scans were considered normal.

Intravenous iodinated contrast material was administered in 102 patients. All had contrast-enhancing lesions, which were usually smaller than the areas of surrounding edema when edema was present (in 74 patients, or 73%). Metastases exhibiting increased density prior to the infusion of contrast material also demonstrated enhancement following contrast administration.

In Shi's group, cerebral involvement was the first site of metastasis in 16% of patients. Therefore, it might be assumed that 84% of patients with carcinoma of the breast manifest cerebral metastases as part of a more generalized disease process. Cerebral metastases are usually multiple and bilateral. It was surprising to note that CT scanning demonstrated only a single lesion in 53% of the patients included in Shi's series.

To define the maximal extent of metastasis to the brain in a patient with a known primary tumor, rapid, high-dose, delayed CT scanning, using 84.6 g of iodine, should be performed whenever feasible.[8,9] This technique has the potential of demonstrating additional metastases in approximately 11% of cases. This is of particular importance in planning patient management. A single cerebral metastasis that is the only site of involvement might be removed surgically. However, evidence of more than one metastasis alters the approach to treatment. Such patients are more likely to be treated with radiation or che-

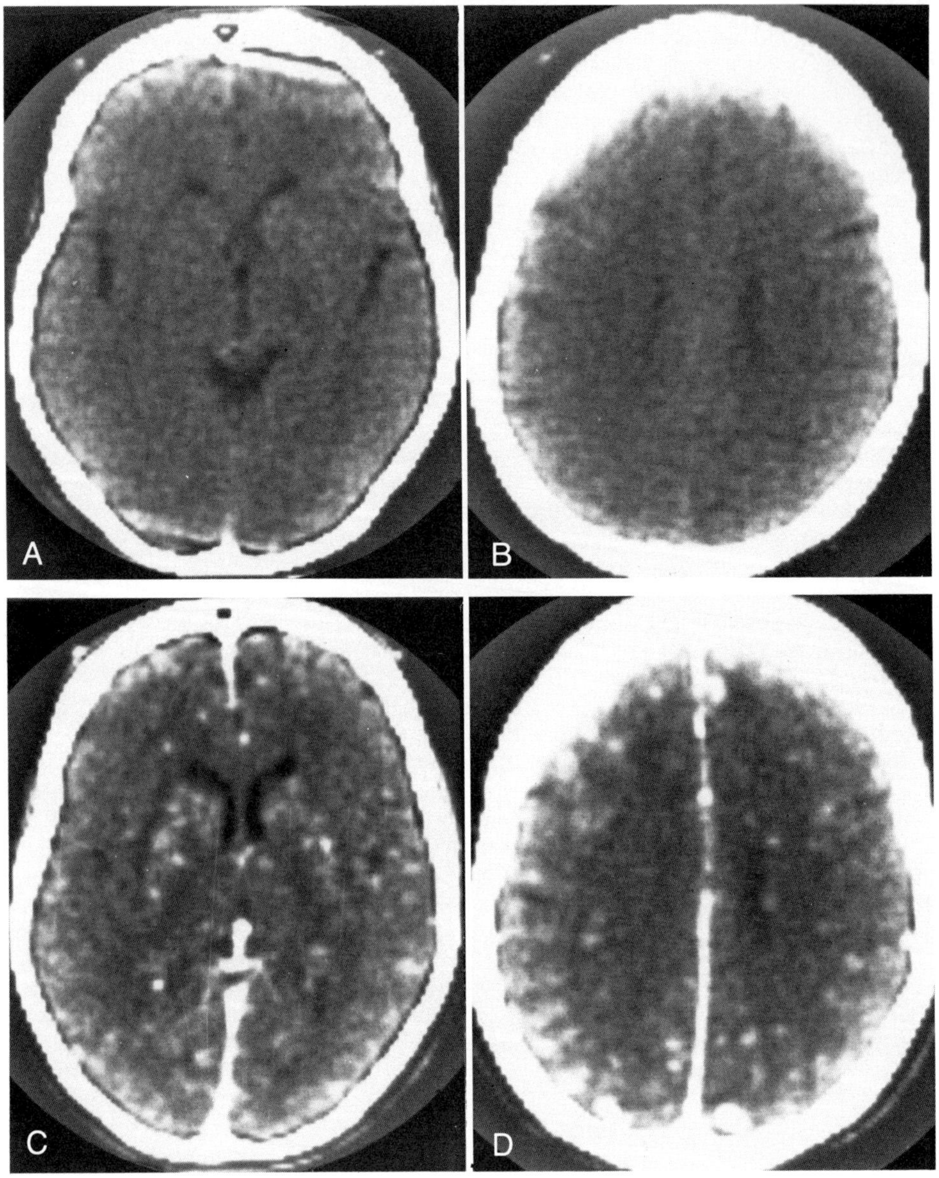

FIGURE 14-1. *(A, B)* A CT scan obtained prior to administration of contrast material in this patient with breast carcinoma appears to be normal. *(C, D)* After the infusion of contrast material, however, multiple metastatic lesions without surrounding edema may be seen. (Reprinted by permission of the publisher from Shield ML et al: Cranial CT of breast carcinoma. J Computed Tomography, 6 [2]: 81, 1982. Copyright © 1982 by Elsevier Science Publishing Co., Inc.)

motherapy, or both. Figures 14-1 and 14-2 demonstrate CT abnormalities in patients with metastatic breast carcinoma.

An association between breast carcinoma and meningioma has been described.[10] Meningioma is a relatively common intracranial tumor, accounting for up to 20% of all malignant disease affecting the CNS. It is twice as common in female patients as in male patients, and symptoms are usually manifested during the fifth and sixth decades of life. Although they are usually solitary, multiple meningiomas may occur in 3% to 5% of all cases.

The importance of differentiating a meningioma from a cerebral metastasis is clear. The clinical presentation of a symptomatic meningioma may be indistinguishable from that of a cerebral metastasis. However, certain radiographic features of meningioma may be helpful in raising the index of suspicion for this complication. Meningiomas occupy certain characteristic sites on radioisotope and CT scans. These include the cerebral convexities, parasagittal areas, tentorium, olfactory groove, perisellar region, and sphenoid ridge. On CT scan studies, a meningioma appears as a homogeneous, high-density area with well-defined borders. It is enhanced by intravenous iodine. Peritumoral edema is usually not very prominent in such cases. In contrast, metastatic breast carcinoma is more likely to be a strictly intraparenchymal lesion, and edema is usually pronounced. Routine x-ray studies of the skull may reveal hyperostosis in the area of a meningioma.

Cerebral arteriography is the most specific test available to help distinguish between meningioma and metastasis. With arteriography, meningioma may be diagnosed

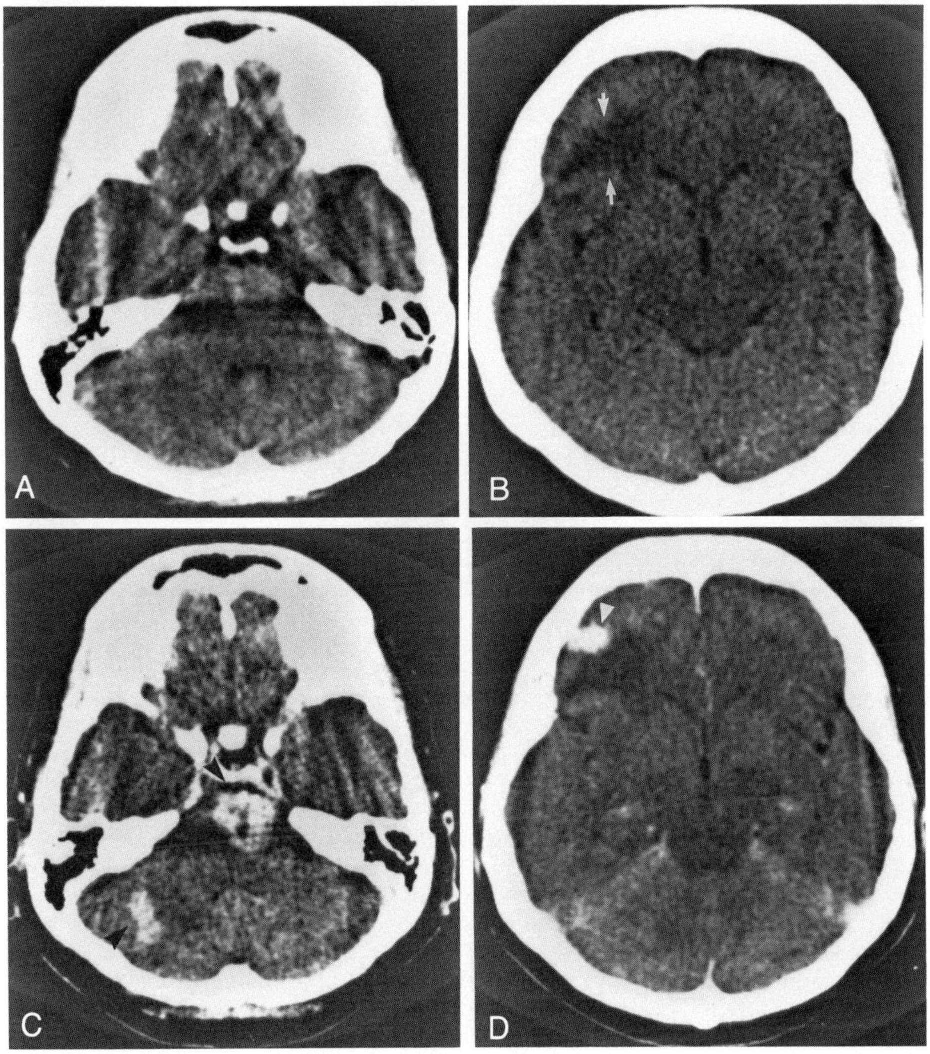

FIGURE 14-2. *(A, B)* A CT scan prior to administration of contrast material reveals an area of edema in the right frontal region *(arrow)*. *(C, D)* After infusion of contrast material, metastatic lesions are seen in the brain stem, right cerebellum, and right frontal lobe *(arrows)*. There is also normal tentorial enhancement.

with a great degree of accuracy if the lesion occupies certain characteristic anatomic territories, is fed by meningeal arteries without early draining veins, and if a typical prolonged vascular stain is produced. In contrast, metastatic lesions occur randomly throughout the brain, are usually fed by cortical arteries, and may show tumor vessels and early draining veins. The tumor stain in metastatic lesions is also likely to be less distinct and of shorter duration.

Magnetic resonance (MR) imaging is the latest technique for visualizing the CNS. However, to date, there are no major studies in which it is compared with CT scanning for accuracy in the diagnosis of metastatic disease (Fig. 14-3).

TREATMENT

A limited number of modalities may be used to treat brain metastases from breast carcinoma or, for that matter, from any other solid tumor. These include radiation therapy, surgery (by itself or in association with radiation), and the use of systemic or intra-arterial chemotherapy. In addition to these modalities, the clinician must also consider the efficacy of steroids (glucocorticoids) and anticonvulsants. It should be mentioned that there has been no prospective, randomized study comparing the results of irradiation alone with those obtained using both surgery and irradiation.

Radiation and Surgical Therapy

The mainstay of the treatment of intracranial metastatic disease is radiation therapy.[11] It is considered to be preferable to surgery when the primary neoplasm is not under control and when there are widespread metastases elsewhere in the body. Of note, however, is the fact that treatment will have little influence upon the ultimate course of the disease or the duration of the patient's survival.

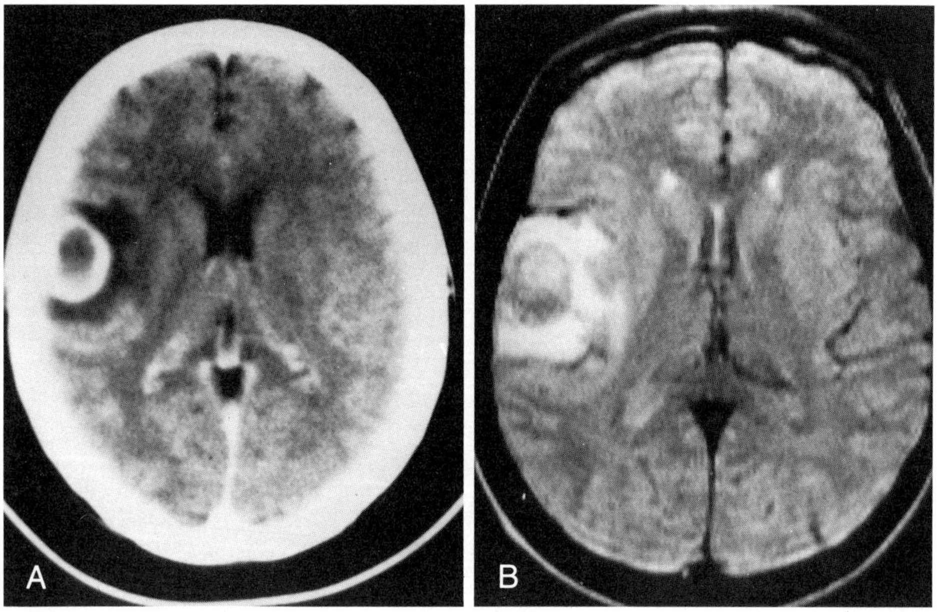

FIGURE 14-3. *(A)* A CT scan with contrast shows a ring-like area of enhancement in the temporal lobe surrounded by a low-density area of edema in this patient with breast cancer. *(B)* MR imaging with a T-2 weighted image in the comparable plane shows an area of hypointensity corresponding to the ring enhancement and increased signal, representing peritumoral edema.

The different time-dose fractionation schemes for delivering whole brain radiation therapy—i.e., 2000 cGy in 5 fractions over a 1-week period, or 4000 cGy delivered in 20 fractions over a period of 4 weeks, or 1500 cGy delivered in 2 fractions within 3 days—have had no influence on overall response rate or duration of response.[12] Median survivals from the time that cerebral metastases are diagnosed until death range from 3 to 6 months. Less than 10% of all patients are alive 1 year after diagnosis.

A pattern has emerged from a review of the overall experience in treating patients with irradiation at Memorial Sloan Kettering Cancer Center in New York.[13–15] Approximately 20% of patients with brain metastases do not complete the prescribed course of radiation therapy because of the rapid deterioration in their general status. Most die of their systemic disease within a short period of time. Approximately 50% of all patients and 75% of those who receive a full course of radiation therapy benefit from it. The use of rapid, high-dose courses of irradiation appears to result in high complication rates.[16] These complications may include headache, nausea, vomiting, fever, and acute cerebral herniation. Most radiation therapists have tended to abandon such regimens.

Re-Treatment

Those patients who redevelop neurologic symptoms and signs after an initial course of irradiation may be re-treated. In a study by Kurup and associates, 56 patients (15 with breast carcinoma) were re-treated.[20] The dosage used ranged from 500 cGy delivered in 1 fraction to 4600 cGy delivered in 20 fractions using 5 fractions per week. Most patients received either 2000 cGy in 5 fractions or 3000 cGy in 10 fractions. The time interval between the first and second courses of radiation therapy ranged from 1 to 46 months, with a median of 5 months.

The second course of irradiation produced a response in 42 of the 56 patients. Improvement in neurologic signs occurred within 1 to 12 months, with a median of 2.5 months. The duration of response was less than 3 months in 26 patients (62%), 3 to 6 months in 12 patients (28.5%), and longer than 6 months in 4 patients (9.5%). The survival data after the second course of radiation treatment were analyzed in 53 patients. Survival ranged from 1 week to 16 months, with a median of 3.5 months. Only 14 patients (25%) survived for more than 6 months after the second course of radiation therapy. Seven patients went on to receive a third course of irradiation, and two patients underwent a fourth treatment course, each time with diminishing responses. No major side effects, such as cerebral radiation necrosis, were reported.

Treatment Results

Cairncross has demonstrated that radiation therapy may be curative and not just palliative in patients with brain metastases.[21] He examined five patients with metastases that had been documented clinically, as well as by radionuclide scan, cerebral arteriography, pneumoencephalography, or CT scan. All were treated with whole-brain irradiation and had no evidence of residual tumor at autopsy. These five patients (1 of whom had breast carcinoma) represented approximately 3% of the patients treated for brain metastases and later examined at autopsy at Memorial Sloan-Kettering Cancer Center between 1968 and 1977. The median survival time of this small group was 9 months, compared with 4 months for those patients in whom tumor was found in the brain at autopsy. Two conclusions were reached: namely, that radiation therapy delivered to brain metastases, particularly in those patients with radiosensitive tumors, may be more than just palliative, and that all nonterminal patients should be offered such treatment. Moreover, it was thought that if some brain metastases could be sterilized with 2400 cGy to 3900 cGy delivered in conventional fractions (palliative radiation), additional lesions would be more likely to be sterilized by higher, "curative" doses. Thus, the standard treatment of brain metastases at Memorial was changed to a course of 3900 cGy delivered in 11 fractions over 17 days (500 cGy in 3 fractions, followed by a 4-day rest, and then 300 cGy in 8 fractions). This regimen delivered the equivalent of approximately 6300 cGy given by conventional means.

Retrospective analyses comparing the results of surgery for brain metastases with those obtained with radiation therapy have generally shown a modest survival advantage for surgery or no difference between the two treatment modalities. The recent literature on the surgical treatment of metastases has been reviewed by Gamache and colleagues.[22] Their series includes 94 patients with single metastases selected for operation from over 1000 patients evaluated for metastatic brain tumors at Memorial Sloan-Kettering Cancer Center, from 1968 to 1977.

Data comparing radiation therapy alone with surgery followed by radiation therapy are not strictly comparable. Patients undergoing surgery are more likely to be in better physical and neurologic condition than are those undergoing irradiation. Also, such patients are more likely to have a single brain metastasis, and are less likely to have extensive systemic disease. Conversely, patients receiving radiation therapy are more likely to have multiple brain metastases and extensive systemic disease. Thus, one might expect the median and long-term survival statistics to be better for patients treated with surgery than for those undergoing irradiation. In Gamache's series, however, approximately 20% of the patients had significant neurologic deficits when surgery was undertaken, and two-thirds of the operated patients were found to have metastatic disease outside the CNS. Despite these facts, the results of this study compare favorably with those from the literature on both radiation and surgical treatment.

The occasional incidence of long-term survival or apparent cure produced by such treatment is frequently used in support of surgical removal of a single brain metastasis. Gamache's series revealed no such prolonged survival. Other series, summarized in Table 14-2, indicate that long-term survival occurs, but that the percentage of patients surviving for a prolonged period is quite small.

Surgical removal of a brain metastasis at least guarantees the accuracy of the pretreatment diagnosis. Since histologic verification of brain metastases treated with irradiation can only be obtained at autopsy, the occasional long-term survivor among patients in the radiation therapy series may be the result of diagnostic error. When Posner reviewed a series of patients who received whole-brain irradiation for presumptive brain metastases and who were examined at autopsy prior to 1971, he discovered a 35% error rate. When strict neurologic criteria, including contrast studies such as cerebral arteriography or computed tomography, were followed in establishing the diagnosis of cerebral metastases, the error rate fell to less than 2%.[23] Thus, if a patient survives for a long period of time after irradiation, it is possible that the diagnosis was incorrect rather than that radiation therapy was effective.

In the absence of a controlled prospective study, it is impossible to determine whether surgery followed by radiation therapy has any advantage over radiation therapy alone in the treatment of brain metastases. The finding that surgically treated patients live somewhat longer may be explained, in part, by the fact that patients considered to be good risks are likely to be treated with surgery and poor-risk patients tend to be treated with irradiation alone.

All patients who undergo surgery should receive postoperative whole-brain irradiation. The purpose of this postoperative treatment is twofold: to treat the bed of the

Table 14-2
Surgical Treatment of Cerebral Metastases

Reference	*No. of Patients*	*30-Day Mortality (%)*	*Survival* Median (mo)	1 Yr	Long-Term	*Neurologic Improvement (%)*
Stortebecker (1954)	125	25 (20 days)	3.6	21	3 (>4 yr)	32*
Richards and McKissock (1963)†	108	32	< 5.0	17	8 (>2 yr)	
Lang and Slater (1964)	208	22	4.0	20	27 (>2 yr)	40‡
Vieth and Odom (1965)	155	15 (14 days)	< 6.0	13.5	12 (>2 yr)	52‡
Raskind et al. (1971)	51	12 (14 days)	< 6.0	30	4 (>3 yr)	79
Haar and Patterson (1972)	167	11	6.0	22	7 (>5 yr)	
Ransohoff (1975)	100	10	6+	38	13 (>2 yr)	
Gamache (1978)	94	8.5	5.5	25	2 (>4 yr)	90

* Patients back to work.
† Total excision only.
‡ Alive and well 6 months following surgery.
(Reproduced with permission from Gamache FW, Jr, et al: Treatment of brain metastases by surgical extirpation. In Weiss L, et al (eds): Brain metastasis. Copyright © 1980 by Year Book Medical Publishers, Inc., Chicago)

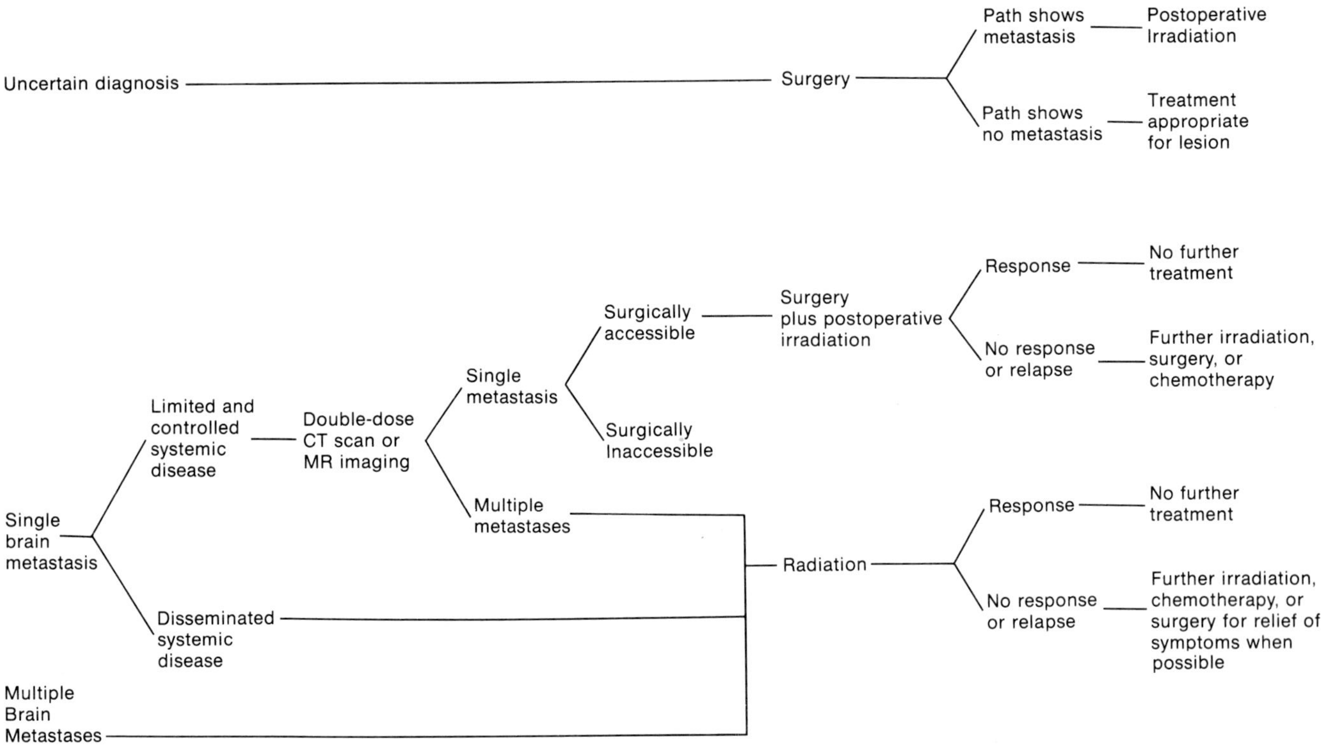

FIGURE 14-4. Treatment approach in patients with brain metastases.

metastasis that was removed, as well as to treat any microscopic disease that might be present elsewhere in the brain. At the time of autopsy in Gamache's series, 68% of the patients were found to have a tumor involving the brain, and about one-third of the patients were found to have local recurrence at the operative site. Nearly 50% of those with brain metastasis documented at autopsy had multiple lesions.

Gamache's study yielded two interesting findings. One was that the longer the interval between the discovery of the primary tumor and the development of brain metastases, the longer the patients survived after surgery. There was no correlation, however, between survival and disease outside the CNS. The median survival of those patients with systemic disease (5 months) was not statistically different from that of patients who had only an isolated brain metastasis (5.75 months).

Our approach to the patient with breast carcinoma and brain metastases is outlined in Figure 14-4. Double-dose, delayed CT scanning or MR imaging is employed in an attempt to establish, as definitively as possible, that a given patient has only a single metastasis. Indications for surgery include an uncertain diagnosis; failure of conservative (radiation) therapy to control symptoms; and surgically accessible, radioresistant tumors that are producing neurologic symptoms and signs. The removal of tumors in patients who are stuporous, comatose, or herniating should be considered only if those patients were in satisfactory medical and neurologic condition prior to their sudden neurologic decompensation.

Chemotherapy

The use of chemotherapeutic agents in the management of brain metastases has been limited for years because it was assumed that the standard antineoplastic drugs, administered systemically, had restricted accessibility to the brain. In recent years, several investigators have produced evidence that the blood–brain barrier is vastly different within brain tumors than it is in normal tissue.[24] This barrier is broken down, in part if not entirely, in the presence of tumor.

A series of recent pharmacokinetic studies with different systemic chemotherapeutic agents has demonstrated that lipid solubility is not a requirement for penetration of the blood–brain barrier.[25] Various drugs, such as 5-fluorouracil, cyclophosphamide, bleomycin, and cisplatin, have been found to enter brain tumors in higher concentrations than in adjacent, normal brain tissue. This factor suggests that tumor growth circumvents the blood–brain barrier, probably through neovascularization.[26]

Rosner reported a series of 66 patients with breast carcinoma and brain metastases treated initially with systemic chemotherapy only.[27] There were three different groups: 36 patients received cyclophosphamide, 5-fluorouracil, and prednisone; 21 patients received cyclophosphamide, 5-fluorouracil, methotrexate, vincristine, and prednisone; and 9 patients received methotrexate, vincristine, and prednisone. An objective response to systemic chemotherapy, as documented by radionuclide brain or CT scans performed both before and after therapy, was seen in 34 of the 66 patients (52%).

The median duration of remission in the 34 responders was 10 months, with a range of 5 to 74+ months. The median survival from the time of initiation of systemic chemotherapy was 13.1 months, again with a range of 5 to 74+ months. The median survival in the 32 nonresponders was 3 months. Eighteen of the 66 patients (27%) survived for longer than 1 year, with a median survival of 18 months.

The prolongation of life was not the only criterion for the success of systemic chemotherapy in Rosner's study. An improvement in quality of life, as well as in functional neurologic status, was noted in 60% of the patients treated. There have also been reports of complete and partial responses in patients treated with intra-arterial carmustine (BCNU),[28] intravenous and intra-arterial cis-platin,[29,30] and oral tamoxifen.[31]

Corticosteroid Therapy

The use of corticosteroids prior to and during whole-brain radiation therapy almost invariably produces immediate and sometimes dramatic improvement in neurologic signs.[17–19] These improvements are short-lived, however, and radiation therapy is necessary to control tumor growth. Steroids are used to stabilize or decrease the edema surrounding cerebral metastases. They have no significant oncolytic effect in most metastatic tumors. Standard doses have not been established, but we recommend administering 10 mg of dexamethasone intravenously as a loading dose in stable patients, followed by administration of 4 mg of the drug intravenously or by mouth every 6 hours with antacid coverage. This treatment regimen should be continued throughout the course of radiation therapy, after which it should be tapered gradually to the lowest dose that will control symptoms. Corticosteroids may successfully be discontinued in more than 50% of patients following radiation therapy for brain metastases.

Anticonvulsant Therapy

In terms of the use of anticonvulsant medication in patients with brain metastases, phenytoin is the drug of choice. The standard dosage is 300 mg to 400 mg per day after an initial loading dose of 15 mg per kg. This regimen should achieve therapeutic blood levels of 10 μg to 20 μg/ml.

Seizures occur in 20% to 30% of patients with brain metastases. It is our belief that anticonvulsants should be administered only to those patients who actually have seizures. This practice eliminates the problems of the obligation to a lifetime of medication, compliance, toxicity, and drug-drug interaction.

SUMMARY

As has been reviewed in this chapter, the diagnosis of brain metastases from breast carcinoma is fairly straightforward, both clinically and radiographically. The treatment of such metastases presently is a much more complex issue. However, with few exceptions, it can be said that prognosis is poor regardless of the treatment modality used. Nevertheless, it is our feeling that patients should be treated aggressively because their quality of life may be excellent, and they may be able to function at home and at work in a meaningful way. New treatment modalities, including the use of surgical lasers, neutron beam therapy, interstitial irradiation, and monoclonal antibodies, must be assessed carefully. These options provide additional hope for the future.

REFERENCES

1. Takakura K, Sano K, Hojo S, et al: Metastatic Tumors of the Central Nervous System, p 113. Tokyo, Igaku-Shoin, 1982
2. Sparrow GEA, Rubens RD: Brain metastases from breast cancer: Clinical course, prognosis, and influence on treatment. Clin Oncol 7:291, 1981
3. Stewart JF, King RJB, Sexton S, et al: Oestrogen receptors, sites of metastatic disease and survival in recurrent breast cancer. Eur J Cancer Clin Oncol 17:449, 1981
4. DiStefano A, Yap HY, Hortobagyi GN, et al: The natural history of breast cancer patients with brain metastases. Cancer 44:1913, 1979
5. Cairncross JG, Posner JB: Neurologic complications of systemic cancer. In Yarbro JW, Bornstein RS (eds): Oncologic Emergencies, pp 73–96. New York, Grune and Stratton, 1981
6. Posner JB: Neurological complications of systemic cancer. Med Clin North Am 63(4):783, 1979
7. Shi M-L, Wallace S, Libshitz HI, et al: Cranial computed tomography of breast carcinoma. J Comput Assist Tomogr 6:77, 1982
8. Hayman LA, Evans RA, Henck VC: Delayed high iodine dose contrast computed tomography. Radiology 136:677, 1980
9. Shalen PR, Hayman LA, Wallace S, et al: Protocol for delayed contrast enhancement in computed tomography of cerebral neoplasia. Radiology 139:397, 1981
10. Smith FP, Slavik M, MacDonald JS: Association of breast cancer with meningioma: Report of two cases and review of the literature. Cancer 42:1992, 1978
11. Cairncross JG, Kim JH, Posner JB: Radiation therapy of brain metastases. Ann Neurol 7:529, 1980
12. Borgelt B, Gelber R, Kramer S, et al: The palliation of brain metastases: Final results of the first of two studies by the radiation therapy oncology group. Int J Radiat Oncol Biol Phys 6:1, 1980
13. Chao JH, Phillips R, Nickson JJ: Roentgen-ray therapy of cerebral metastases. Cancer 7:682, 1954
14. Chu FCH, Hilaris BS: Value of radiation therapy in the management of intracranial metastases. Cancer 14:577, 1961
15. Nisce LZ, Hilaris BS, Chu FCH: A review of experience with irradiation of brain metastases. Am J Roentgenol 111:329, 1971
16. Young DF, Posner JB, Chu FCH, et al: Rapid-course radiation therapy of cerebral metastases: Results and complications. Cancer 34:1069, 1974

17. Galicich JH, French LA: Use of dexamethasone in the treatment of cerebral edema resulting from brain tumors and brain surgery. Am Pract Dig Treat 12:169, 1961
18. Galicich JH, French LA, Melby J: Use of dexamethasone in treatment of cerebral edema associated with brain tumors. Lancet 81:46, 1961
19. Kofman S, Garvin JS, Nagamani D, et al: Treatment of cerebral metastases from breast carcinoma with prednisone. JAMA 163:1473, 1957
20. Kurup P, Reddy S, Hendrickson FR: Results of re-irradiation for cerebral metastases. Cancer 46:2587, 1980
21. Cairncross JG, Chernik NL, Kim J-H, et al: Sterilization of cerebral metastases by radiation therapy. Neurology 29:1195, 1979
22. Gamache FW, Galicich JH, Posner JB: Treatment of brain metastases by surgical extirpation. In Weiss L, Gilbert HA, Posner JB (eds): Brain Metastasis pp 390–414. Boston, GK Hall, 1980
23. Posner JB: Diagnosis and treatment of metastases to the brain. Clin Bull 4:47, 1974
24. Vick NA, Khandekar JD, Bigner DD: Chemotherapy of brain tumors: The "blood-brain barrier" is not a factor. Arch Neurol 34:523, 1977
25. Hasegawa H, Shapiro WR, Posner JB: Chemotherapy of experimental metastatic brain tumors in female wistar rats. Cancer Res 39:2691, 1979
26. Ushio Y, Posner JB, Shapiro WR: Chemotherapy of experimental meningeal carcinomatosis. Cancer Res 37:1232, 1977
27. Rosner D, Nemoto T, Pickren J, et al: Management of brain metastases from breast cancer by combination chemotherapy. J NeuroOncol 1:131, 1983
28. Madajewicz S, West CR, Park MC, et al: Phase II study—Intra-arterial BCNU therapy for metastatic brain tumors. Cancer 47:653, 1981
29. Kolaric K, Roth A, Jelicic I, et al: Phase II clinical trial of cisdichlorodiamine platinum (Cis DDP) in metastatic brain tumors. J Cancer Res Clin Oncol 104:287, 1982
30. Lehane DE, Bryan RN, Horowitz B, et al: Intra-arterial cisplatinum chemotherapy for patients with primary and metastatic brain tumors. Cancer Drug Delivery 1:69, 1983
31. Carey RW, Davis JM, Zervas NT: Tamoxifen-induced regression of cerebral metastases in breast carcinoma. Cancer Treat Rep 65:793, 1981

Breast Cancer and Epidural Spinal Cord Compression: Diagnostic and Therapeutic Strategies

Mark Stillman Kathleen M. Foley

Metastasis to the spinal cord and the cauda equina is a common complication in oncology, occurring in as many as 5% to 10% of all patients with cancer.[1,2] It is particularly common among patients with breast cancer owing to the tendency of breast cancer to metastasize to bone. In several large autopsy and neurosurgical series of cancer patients, adenocarcinoma of the breast is the most common cause of epidural compression of the spinal cord and cauda equina (described here as epidural spinal cord compression, ESCC) (Table 14-3). As in any medical emergency, early diagnosis and appropriate treatment is associated with improved outcome; failure to diagnose or treat this condition invariably leads to paralysis and sphincter dysfunction, and associated morbidity and mortality.[7,8,10,14,15] The clinician caring for patients with cancer must, therefore, recognize the clinical syndrome of ESCC and deal with it effectively and rapidly.

The spinal canal is a closed volume surrounded by the rigid bony structure of the vertebrae. Encroachment on its neural and neurovascular contents by expanding tumor may lead to rapid and irreversible neurologic compromise. There are several routes by which tumor may invade the spinal canal; including hematogenous access (both arterial and venous), cerebrospinal fluid (CSF) pathways, invasion along nerve routes through the intervertebral foramen, and by direct extension from an adjacent vertebral body metastasis. Vertebral body metastases are the most common routes of entry into the epidural space by breast cancer.

Numerous studies have reported the high incidence of bone metastases in breast cancer.[11,16–18] In a combined postmortem, radiographic study of 168 patients with breast cancer, Lenz and Fried reported a 48% incidence of skeletal metastases; 60% of these cases involved the vertebral column.[17] In a more recent study comparing postmortem and antemortem radiographic studies, Fornasier and Horne found a 61% incidence of vertebral metastases among patients with breast cancer,[11] whereas Galasko detected a 73% incidence of osseous metastases in patients with breast cancer using bone scintigraphy.[18]

The distribution of sites of ESCC from breast cancer coincides with the distribution of metastases along the vertebral column. The thoracic spine is the most frequent site in most series, followed by the lumbosacral spine and the cervical spine.[7,9,19] Using x-ray and scintigraphic studies, Harrison and colleagues found a roughly equal distribution of vertebral metastases between the thoracic and lumbosacral spine in 85 patients.[19] Like other researchers, however, they noted the high incidence of multiple sites of vertebral involvement in the individual patient.[6,7,9,15,19]

CLINICAL SYMPTOMS AND SIGNS

Epidural spinal cord compression is heralded by a tetrad of symptoms: pain, weakness, sensory loss, and sphincter disturbance. Numerous studies demonstrate that pain is the presenting complaint in 85% to 97% of cases,[7,8,9,20,21,22] and that it is a presenting symptom in 93% of patients with ESCC secondary to breast cancer.[19] It may be the only symptom evident for months; Gilbert and associates noted a median duration of 7 weeks preceding diagnosis in an oncologic population referred to a large cancer center. Likewise, Cobb and co-workers documented a similar duration of pain of 8 to 10 weeks in a retrospective study of a large referral population with breast cancer. In contrast to these findings, in some patients, the latent interval between the primary diagnosis and the diagnosis of ESCC may be as long as 24 years.[6,7]

The pain associated with ESCC may be of three types: local, radicular, or referred. Nearly all patients report an

Table 14-3
Epidural Metastases

No. of patients	*Chade*[3] *(1976)*	*Brice*[4] *(1965)*	*Constans*[5] *(1983)*	*Stark*[6] *(1982)*	*MSKCC*[7,8] *(1978, 1980)*	*Torma*[9] *(1957)*	*Dunn*[10] *(1980)*	*Fornasier*[11] *(1975)**	*Arseni*[12] *(1959)*	*White*[13] *(1971)*
Total	172	138	600	131	318	226	104	135	231	226
Breast	23(13%)	12(9%)	153(26%)	37(28%)	69(22%)	19(8%)	7(7%)	43(32%)†	27(12%)	37(16%)
Lung	27(16%)	28(20%)	73(12%)	43(33%)	41(13%)	18(8%)	19(18%)	21(16%)	39(17%)	31(14%)
Kidney	25(15%)	3(2%)	20(3%)	4(3%)	20(6%)	21(9%)	8(8%)	1(0.7%)	9(4%)	13(6%)
Thyroid	20(12%)		22(4%)			7(3%)		1(0.7%)	2(0.8%)	8(4%)
Sarcoma		4(3%)	41(7%)		4(1%)	26(12%)				24(11%)
Prostate	19(11%)	8(6%)	11(2%)	5(4%)	33(10%)	10(4%)	21(20%)	4(3%)	16(7%)	23(10%)
Gastrointestinal	8(5%)	3(2%)	28(5%)	5(4%)	15(5%)	11(5%)	6(6%)	7(5%)	15(6%)	11(5%)
Melanoma		1(0.7%)	7(1%)	1(0.8%)	8(3%)			3(2%)	2(0.8%)	8(4%)
Female reproductive	6(3%)		27(5%)		9(3%)			5(4%)	26(11%)	1(0.4%)
Testis		1(0.7%)		3(2%)				1(0.7%)	6(3%)	4(2%)
Bladder		1(0.7%)		4(3%)					3(1%)	1(0.4%)
Head/neck								1(0.7%)	1(0.4%)	8(4%)
Lymphoma		9(7%)			28(9%)	23(10%)	7(7%)	28(21%)	11(5%)	27(12%)
Myeloma		30(22%)			10(3%)	16(7%)	9(9%)	12(9%)		8(4%)
Other (including unknown)	67(39%)	40(29%)	65(11%)	18(14%)	81(25%)	75(33%)	27(26%)	8(6%)	66(29%)	13(6%)

* Autopsy series that studied the thoracic and lumbosacral spine, only.
† The number represents 61% of all patients with breast cancer who underwent autopsy in this series.
MSKCC, Memorial Sloan-Kettering Cancer Center.

aching, continuous pain that is gradual in onset but progressive over time, and that is localized to the vicinity of the block on myelography in nearly 85% of the patients.[7] This pain is caused by periosteal stretching by tumor, or vertebral collapse, and may be followed in time by the intermittent, shooting, radicular pain that accompanies compressed and damaged nerve roots. Both types of pain may increase with coughing, sneezing, or straining, or by assuming a supine position, which causes the vertebral column to lengthen. In the cervical and lumbar spine where there is a wider space to accommodate the cord and nerve roots, the radicular pain is typically unilateral; it is bilateral or bandlike in the less spacious thoracic spine. Referred pain, an infrequently recognized but clinically useful symptom,[23] is a nonradiating pain experienced at a distant site. Midscapular or bilateral shoulder pain may accompany cervicothoracic epidural disease, and bilateral sacroiliac and iliac crest pain may be observed with L-1 vertebral compression.

Weakness is present in as many as 75% of all patients with ESCC at the time of diagnosis, but only rarely is it the presenting symptom.[6,7] It may be segmental, as a result of nerve root damage, or pyramidal in character when the spinal cord itself is damaged. Patients may report heaviness or stiffness in their limbs, unsteadiness, or the dragging of a leg. In the series of Stark and co-workers, which included 37 cases of ESCC from breast cancer, back pain was present at the time of diagnosis in 78%, leg weakness in 84%, sensory symptoms in 49%, and sphincter disturbance in 54%.[6]

Sensory loss is rarely a presenting symptom of ESCC, but a careful history may disclose it in nearly 50% of patients at the time of diagnosis.[6,7] It may be described as numbness, paresthesia, loss of sensation, or a feeling of coldness. Infrequently, it may masquerade as gait unsteadiness secondary to sensory ataxia.

At the time of diagnosis, sphincter disturbances may be apparent in up to 55% of patients with ESCC from cancer.[6,7] Bladder disturbances usually begin with urgency of micturition and nocturia or hesitancy, leading to either urgency incontinence or urinary retention with overflow incontinence, depending on whether the spinal cord or the cauda equina is compressed, respectively. Bowel complaints include constipation or obstipation and, less commonly, fecal incontinence. The characterization of sphincter disturbances is prognostically important as sphincter dysfunction augers a poor prognosis for regaining or preserving ambulatory ability or sphincter control.[4,7,8,15]

A carefully performed physical examination, along with the clinical history of the patient, enables the physician to judge the site(s) and time-course of epidural compression and thereby to direct the work-up expeditiously. Percussion and palpation of the spine may reveal one or multiple sites of tenderness or the presence of a gibbous deformity. Paraspinal muscle spasm may be visible or palpable in an area where there has been root damage. Other mechanical signs, such as straight leg raising, may be present in a patient with radiculopathy from cauda equina disease or nerve root impingement.

Sensory and motor examination help to localize the site of epidural disease to the spinal cord, cauda equina, or the conus medullaris. Lesions that impinge on the spinal cord (corresponding to a *vertebral* lesion above T12-L1) result in classic upper motor neuron signs of variable spastic weakness, hyperactive reflexes, Babinski signs, sensory loss, and sphincter and sexual dysfunction. Spinal cord damage caudal to the T-1 region of the spinal cord results in paraplegia or paraparesis with sparing of the arms, and lesions rostral to the C-5 spinal cord lead to quadriplegia or quadriparesis. As the brachial plexus is derived from C5-T1, partial preservation of function in the arms helps localize the lesion to this vicinity of the spinal cord, and the segmental level is determined by the segmental evaluation of stretch reflexes, motor strength, and sensory dermatomes. Likewise, an examiner may localize a lesion to the area of the spinal cord responsible for the lumbosacral plexus (L1-S5) by performing a segmental examination of the lower extremities. Involvement of the conus medullaris, the distal portion of the spinal cord from which sacral innervation is derived, is a special exception worthy of mention. Lesions in this area are characterized by a rapidly progressive course, with symmetric perineal pain and early loss of autonomic function and saddle (sacral) sensory loss. Finding a sensory level or abdominal reflex loss in the torso is useful in localizing a lesion in the spinal cord territory between the two plexi, since the detection of muscle weakness is difficult in the chest or abdomen. Sensory and motor findings are usually symmetrical in spinal cord lesions, with hemicord disturbances (Brown Séquard syndrome) occurring in less than 5% of the patients in all series.[7,9] Their appearance should suggest bony encroachment on the spinal canal or an alternative diagnosis, such as intradural metastases, intramedullary metastases, or a primary spinal cord tumor.

In contrast, ESCC involving the cauda equina is typically asymmetrical, producing patchy segmental motor and sensory signs in the lower extremities. The findings are typical of lower motor neuron disease: flaccid, not spastic, weakness; diminished or absent reflexes; and no Babinski response. Difficulty might arise in distinguishing a cauda equina lesion from acute spinal cord compression of the lumbar spinal cord because reflexes below the level of compression often are initially absent with acute lesions (spinal shock).

DIAGNOSTIC STUDIES

Abnormalities are found on plain spine x-ray studies in approximately 60% of the general cancer population with ESCC documented by myelography or autopsy.[9,24] Because of breast cancer's proclivity for bone metastasis, the incidence is much higher in patients with this disease.[6,19] Stark and associates studied a large cancer population with ESCC and found that 35 of 37 patients (95%) with breast cancer had abnormal plain spine films. Twenty-three percent had a pedicle abnormality, 92% had a vertebral body abnormality, and 47% had a vertebral body collapse, whereas only 17% had involvement isolated to one vertebral body.[6] In a recent study of 78 symptomatic patients with previously untreated breast cancer, Harrison and colleagues found abnormal spine films in 41 of 42 patients with myelographic evidence of ESCC.[19] Sixty-four percent of these patients had three or more metastatic lesions on x-ray study.

Graus and associates have attempted to categorize plain spine film abnormalities in cancer patients by their ability to predict epidural compression on myelography.[24] Pedicle destruction predicted a positive myelogram in 70% of patients with radicular pain, but only in 34% complaining solely of local pain, whereas ESCC was found in 87% of all patients with vertebral body collapse of greater than 50%, regardless of the nature of their pain. None of 5 patients with negative spine films and positive myelograms had breast cancer.

Radionuclide bone scanning appears to be a less accurate predictor of the presence or absence of ESCC, probably because of its high sensitivity.[24] In the study of Graus and co-workers, bone scans were positive in 16 of 50 patients with negative myelograms. In contrast, Harrison's group found bone scans to be positive along the vertebral column in all 42 previously untreated breast cancer patients with ESCC. Bone scanning, however, may produce false-negative results in areas that have previously been irradiated, which limits its usefulness in this population.[25]

Myelography remains the standard diagnostic test with which all others are compared.[7,8,15,19,24,26,27] It usually successfully distinguishes between intradural and extradural compression, and because it allows visualization of the entire canal, it is able to detect multiple levels of epidural involvement. If a complete block is encountered on lumbar myelography, either a lateral C1-C2 or a cisternal puncture is necessary so that contrast material may be introduced to visualize the upper border of the block. By delimiting the full extent of epidural compression, complete myelography aids in localization in preparation for either surgery or radiotherapy (Fig. 14-5). Finally, an added benefit of myelography is the acquisition of CSF for analysis.

Either iophendylate (Pantopaque), the lipid-based contrast agent, or metrizamide (Amipaque), a water-based contrast agent, may be used. In the cancer population, there is an advantage to using iophendylate in that a small amount (about 5 ml) may be left behind to facilitate refluoroscopic-myelography at a future date (in order to monitor response to therapy or to evaluate a new episode of suspected ESCC). Additionally, iophendylate myelography, unlike metrizamide myelography, may be performed on an outpatient basis as long as an outpatient holding unit is available. The potential, delayed, neurotoxic reactions to intrathecal metrizamide—headache, meningismus, seizures, and encephalopathy—preclude outpatient myelography by this method and necessitate overnight inpatient observation.

The advent of CT scanning and magnetic resonance (MR) imaging has raised the possibility of finding a noninvasive test to replace myelography (Figure 14-6). In contrast to myelography, CT scanning provides transaxial imaging and cannot evaluate the rostral-caudal extent or multiple areas of epidural encroachment unless extensive scanning is performed. The instillation of small amounts

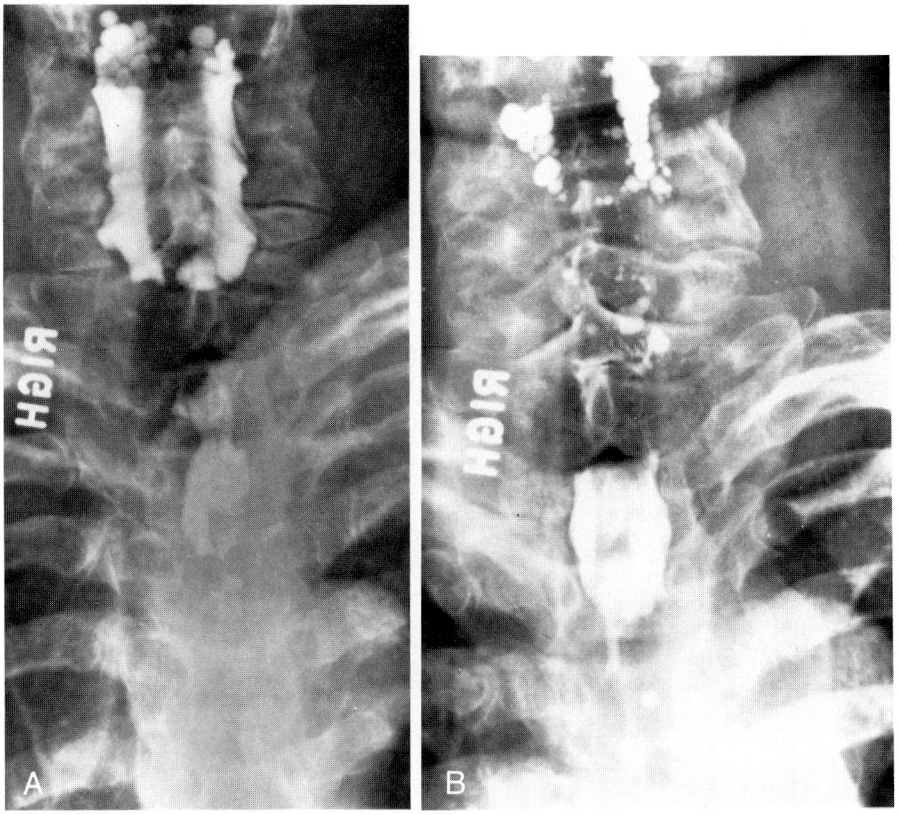

FIGURE 14-5. A 43-year-old woman who had undergone a right radical mastectomy 1 year earlier presented with a 2-month history of interscapular pain radiating to the ulnar aspects of both hands, a right Horner syndrome, weakness and wasting in both hands, and absent triceps and finger jerk reflexes. Epidural spinal cord compression was detected at two levels. *(A)* An iophendylate (Pantopaque) myelogram demonstrates two levels of epidural compromise. The anteroposterior view, feet down, shows right-sided pedicle destruction at T-1 associated with an 80% to 90% block to contrast flow. Another less severe block is seen at T-3. *(B)* A head-down view of the same area demonstrates the lower limit of the high-degree block to be at the lower border of the T-1 vertebral body.

of intrathecal metrizamide enables positive visualization of the subarachnoid space, thereby improving sensitivity, but has the added disadvantages of delayed neurotoxicity, the need for a spinal tap, and overnight in-hospital observation. In two studies, CT scanning underestimated the longitudinal extent of epidural disease in 30% of cases.[21,28] MR imaging, however, may some day replace myelography because of its ability to scan in the sagittal plane. A preliminary study involving 25 cases of ESCC compared MR imaging with myelography and found the overall accuracy of MR imaging to be 76%. MR imaging was unable to quantitate the degree of epidural disease in 4 of 7 cases, particularly in areas of natural kyphosis. Two of these cases involved brachial plexopathies with tumor extension into the spinal canal of the upper thoracic spine.[29] This limitation of MR imaging parallels that seen with CT scanning. In the study by Cascino and colleagues, 6 of 41 patients (15%) with malignant brachial plexopathies had no CT evidence of epidural extension despite positive myelograms.[30] CT scanning and MR imaging, at their present state of technology, therefore, cannot be recommended as procedures that replace myelography; rather, they are adjunct procedures that complement myelography.

DIFFERENTIAL DIAGNOSIS

Back pain with or without neurologic findings in a patient with known carcinoma has a differential diagnosis that includes both neoplastic and nonneoplastic conditions. Given the high incidence of osseous metastases in breast cancer, the most common clinical situation encountered is the patient with a vertebral metastasis but no evidence of ESCC or, alternatively, a patient with multiple painful vertebral metastases, only one of which is causing epidural compromise.

Similar to the general population, cancer patients may develop discogenic disease and spinal stenosis, with symptoms that mimic spinal epidural metastases. Radiographic studies can usually differentiate between these disorders. Much more difficult to distinguish is an epidural abscess; clinically, its presentation parallels that of ESCC, with the additional findings of fever, backache, progression to radicular pain, weakness, and eventual paralysis. Frequently occurring in neurosurgical, immunocompromised, or even immunocompetent patients, it usually extends for several vertebral segments or more, in contrast to the extension in ESCC.[31] A spinal epidural hematoma has an acute onset and identifiable predisposing factors (e.g., coagulopathy, thrombocytopenia, and lumbar puncture), all of which may be present in the patient with (breast) cancer. Also included in the differential diagnosis are transverse myelitis, spinal cord infarction, and spinal arteriovenous malformation (AVM); all are distinguishable clinically and radiographically from ESCC. A more difficult clinical situation presents itself in middle-aged, or elderly women with a history of breast cancer, as well as back pain and osteoporosis with vertebral collapse. The bone

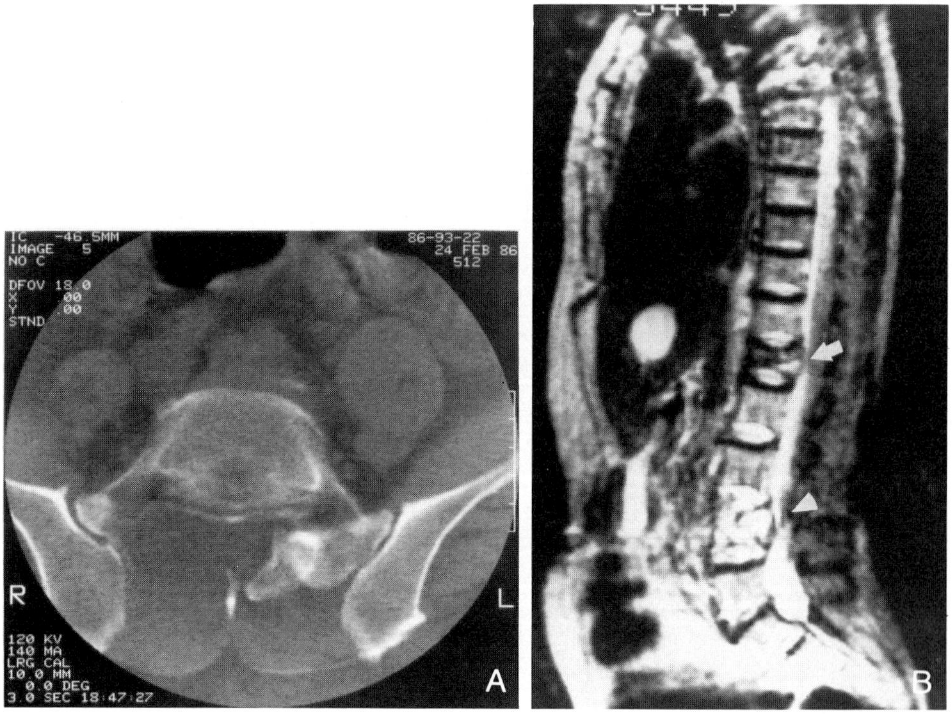

FIGURE 14-6. A CT scan was performed through the sacrum of a 46-year-old woman with low back pain and a history of right-sided S-1 radiation of pain and a left modified radical mastectomy performed 3 years earlier. *(A)* There is destruction of the right side of the sacrum with effacement of the right epidural space. *(B)* Sagittal MR imaging of a 50-year-old woman with metastatic breast cancer and a positive bone scan in the L-1 and L-4 vertebral bodies. Two areas of epidural cord compression are demonstrated. There is approximately a 50% compromise at L-1 *(arrow)* (the thecal sac containing CSF is white in this image), and a smaller area of compromise is seen at L-4 *(arrowhead).*

scan in these patients is usually positive, spine films show preservation of the bony cortex in the setting of diffuse osteopenia, and there is usually no evidence of epidural impingement on myelography.[32] A CT scan through the involved spine should show no paraspinal mass or cortical disruption, but a bone biopsy is sometimes needed to make the diagnosis. Finally, benign intradural extramedullary lesions—meningiomas, neurilemmomas, and neurofibromas—may present diagnostic difficulties. They usually involve a longer clinical course, and myelography and CT scanning readily identify them.

Intramedullary, intradural (leptomeningeal), and paraspinal malignant disease may be more difficult to differentiate. Primary intramedullary spinal tumors—astrocytomas, ependymomas, and lymphomas—have a prolonged, sometimes waxing and waning course, are associated with distinct plain x-ray findings, and present as enlargements of the cord on myelography. Metastatic carcinomas, including breast carcinomas, may reach the cord and cauda hematogenously, or via CSF pathways or nerve roots, with a clinical presentation that is characterized by local or radicular pain (or both), rapidly progressive paraparesis, sensory loss, and sphincter disturbance.[33–36] Though neither the symptoms nor signs distinguish intramedullary from epidural metastases, the rapid tempo of the syndrome, the early loss of sphincter control, the tendency for asymmetric cord signs, and the absence of extradural disease on myelography highlight the disorder. Only two-thirds of affected patients will exhibit cord swelling on myelography.[35] Leptomeningeal carcinomatosis, frequently caused by carcinoma of the breast, may also simulate ESCC, particularly cauda equina compression, but it is not usually associated with an epidural lesion on myelography, and CSF cytology and markers help to confirm the diagnosis.[37] Lastly, patients with metastatic plexopathies and paraspinal masses, which have a high incidence of associated ESCC, may have negative plain films and myelograms, and therefore, may require CT scanning or MR imaging for diagnosis.

MANAGEMENT

Since breast cancer is usually widespread at the time of presentation of ESCC, the therapeutic goal is palliative, aimed at restoring spinal cord function—notably, sphincter control and ambulation—alleviating pain, and restoring the patient to an acceptable quality of life for as long as possible. Many studies spanning the last 40 years address the management of spinal cord compression (Table 14-4), and enormous controversy surrounds the proper use of surgery and radiation therapy. Comparison of all these studies is difficult because of observer variation and bias, inadequate definition of successful responses, inconsistent use of myelography, varying technology and utilization of radiation therapy, and lack of randomization of patients. However, several authors have retrospectively analyzed large groups and have been able to draw useful conclusions regarding management.[7,8,14,15,21] Only one study to date has succeeded at a randomized prospective study comparing neurosurgery and radiation therapy to radiation therapy alone, and although the results agree with the

Table 14-4
Results of Treatment of Epidural Spinal Cord Compression From Metastatic Tumors

Treatment	No. of Patients	Patients Improved No.	%	Mean (%)
I. Surgical Decompression Only*				
Barron et al., 1959	38	11	29	
Wild and Porter, 1963	22	8	36	
Wright, 1963	21	3	14	
Smith, 1965	52	13	25	30
Auld and Buerman, 1966	41	17	41	
Hall and MacKay, 1973	129	39	30	
Brady et al., 1975	24	7	29	
Total	327	98		
II. Radiotherapy Only*				
Mones et al., 1966	41	14	34	
Kahn et al., 1967	82	34	41	
Posner, 1971	75	35	47	
Brady et al., 1975	19	9	47	
Cobb, et al., 1977†	18	9	50	47
Gilbert et al., 1978	170	84	49	
Greenberg et al., 1980	83	47	57	
Young et al., 1980	13	7	54	
Stark et al., 1982	31	11	35	
Total	532	250		
III. Combined Decompression Plus Radiotherapy				
Mullan and Evans, 1957	21	9	43	
Wild and Porter, 1963	23	10	43	
Wright, 1963	17	8	47	51
Brady et al., 1975	90	55	61	
Gilbert et al., 1978	65	29	45	
Young et al., 1980	16	7	43	
Total	232	118		

* I versus II, $p < 0.001$; II versus III, p is not significant.
† Series consists only of patients with breast cancer.
(Adapted from Black P: Spinal metastasis: Current status and recommended guidelines for management. Neurosurgery 5:726, 1979.)

larger retrospective studies, the numbers are too small to be statistically significant.[38]

Corticosteroids, usually dexamethasone, are administered when the diagnosis of ESCC is made or suspected. The theory supporting their use is provided by Ushio and co-workers, who demonstrated steroid-responsive vasogenic edema in the rat spinal cord compression model.[39] In humans, Posner and colleagues reported oncolytic effects of standard doses of dexamethasone in four patients with lymphoproliferative tumors, germinoma, and sarcoma.[40] It is now generally accepted that glucocorticoids, despite their side effects, are necessary to counteract the edema associated with ESCC or its treatment.

Standard therapy consists of intravenous dexamethasone at the time of myelography or before, followed by tapering doses for the duration of treatment, with monitoring of the patient for deterioration. More recently, Greenberg and associates used high doses of dexamethasone, starting with 100 mg intravenously; this regimen was followed by oral treatment at a dosage of 96 mg per day. The dosage was then tapered by halving the dose every 2 to 3 days during treatment. Although the long-term outcome was unchanged from that in studies utilizing conventional doses, Greenberg's group reported dramatic pain relief in a large number of patients, even before radiation therapy was started.[8]

Radiation Therapy

Table 14-4 summarizes the results of several series that demonstrate a success rate for radiation therapy of between 30% and 50%, success being defined as regaining or maintaining ambulation and sphincter function. Using pain as a criterion, radiation therapy was effective in more than 50% of cases,[7,22,38] and Cobb and associates were able to achieve pain relief in 72% of patients with breast carcinoma who were treated with radiation therapy alone.[22]

Factors influencing the prognosis of those patients treated solely with radiation therapy include the radiosensitivity of the tumor and the pretherapy status (in terms of ambulation and sphincter function) of the patient. Patients with radiosensitive tumors fare better than patients harboring radioresistant tumors (response rates of 64% versus 45%) in terms of preserving ambulatory ability and sphincter function.[7,41] Carcinoma of the breast falls into the former category.[7,22]

No controlled studies have determined an optimal radiation dose schedule as it relates to outcome. One study suggests that a protracted, high-dose course (500 cGy every other day for 3 days) is more effective than is protracted low-dose therapy (200 cGy per day for 8 days).[8] A commonly used conventional dose schedule is a total of 4000 cGy delivered in 20 200-cGy-per-day fractions; an alternative schedule calls for a total of 3000 cGy delivered in 10 300-cGy-per-day fractions (which is equivalent to approximately 3800 cGy delivered by conventional doses).

Brachytherapy (internal radiation therapy using surgically implanted radiation seeds) has only recently been applied to the treatment of ESCC.[41] This type of therapy allows large doses of radiation to be directed at tumor, usually paravertebral tumor, without affecting normal structures that are more than 1 mm distant from the tumor. Slatkin and Posner described 14 patients who had previously been irradiated externally and who subsequently relapsed. These patients underwent vertebral body resections followed by brachytherapy; 71% of them improved.[41]

Surgical Therapy

The standard surgical approach for ESCC has been posterior decompressive laminectomy. Earlier surgical series did not include postoperative radiation therapy and produced inferior results when compared to radiation therapy alone.[2,42,43] Wright was the first to demonstrate the synergistic effect of radiation therapy when it followed laminectomy.[42] Comparison of the results in a larger series utilizing laminectomy followed by radiation therapy with the results of radiation therapy alone demonstrates no statistically significant difference in outcome (using ambulation as the criterion), even when the patients are stratified by the severity of neurologic deficit or by the radiosensitivity of the tumor.[7,8,10]

Not surprisingly, factors affecting prognosis after combined laminectomy and radiation therapy are similar to those affecting prognosis when radiation therapy alone is used. These factors include the patient's pretreatment ambulatory status, the nature of the primary tumor (radiosensitive versus radioresistant),[7,15] the rate of onset and progression of signs, and the length of block on myelography.[38] Rapid onset and progression to sphincter incontinence and paraplegia carry a poor prognosis,[4,7,15] and vertebral collapse with angulation has been thought to portend an unfavorable prognosis.[15]

Neurosurgery is associated with complications that are not seen with radiation therapy; operative mortality ranges between 3% and 15%, and operative morbidity, including postoperative neurologic deterioration, vertebral instability, infection and hematoma, may be as high as 30%.[15] The major pitfall of decompressive laminectomy, which accounts for the poor outcome in the surgery-alone series, is the inadequate access it provides to anteriorly situated tumors. A posterior approach does not allow access to the major bulk of compressing tumor and, in fact, further complicates the situation by destabilizing a spine with a destroyed vertebral body.[14,15,44,45]

Barcena and colleagues reviewed 2300 cases of ESCC treated by decompressive laminectomy with or without radiation therapy in order to identify factors favoring radiation therapy over combined surgical and radiation therapy.[14] In this way, they hoped to decrease the surgical morbidity and mortality by improving the selection of surgical candidates. They found two factors to be important in the selection of therapy: the location of the tumor within the spinal canal, which determines which approach (anterior decompression versus posterior laminectomy) is indicated, and the pretreatment condition of the patient.

Their findings underscore the recent interest in anterior decompression that has been evident in the neurosurgical literature.[14,15,44–48] One large and several smaller series describe the technique of vertebral body resection, followed by acrylic and surgical pin fusion stabilization of up to three contiguously involved vertebral bodies. In the series reported by Sundaresan and colleagues, which included 44 patients with ESCC and subacute or chronic decompensation, there was an 84% success rate in pain relief, an improvement in ambulatory status in 15 of 25 patients (60%) who were paraparetic, and only a 4% mortality rate.[44] Similarly, Siegal and associates described the upgrading of 7 of 8 nonambulatory patients (88%) to ambulatory status, which upgrading allowed them to live long enough to die of generalized disease.[47]

Pathologic odontoid fractures and atlantoaxial subluxation from high cervical ESCC deserve special mention. In these instances, metastatic involvement of the odontoid process may lead to cervical spinal instability and acute cervical myelopathy. In one recent study, 12 of 18 such cases were attributable to metastatic breast cancer. Initial treatment consisted of immobilization in a hard (Philadelphia) collar, conventional doses of steroids, and emergency radiation therapy (2000 cGy to 3000 cGy delivered over a 2-week period). Even patients with moderately displaced fractures were treated similarly and showed symptomatic and objective signs of improvement. Patients were considered for surgical fusion if they had severe, symptomatic, atlantoaxial displacement, persistent symptoms following radiation therapy, and a reasonable life expectancy (e.g., those patients with breast cancer).[49]

Guidelines for Management

Management of the patient with ESCC from carcinoma of the breast should begin with early diagnosis to prevent irreversible neurologic damage. Such an approach has also been suggested for the cancer patient with back pain, in general. Rodichok and co-workers[27] and, more recently, Portenoy and colleagues,[50] have attempted to develop algorithms for the management of back pain in cancer patients in order to distinguish between those patients requiring urgent myelography and therapeutic intervention and those patients with pain attributable to some other cause. One such algorithm, adapted for patients with breast cancer, is shown in Figure 14-7. In this diagram, myelography is considered to be the diagnostic test of choice for the evaluation of ESCC. In the future, it may be superseded by MR imaging. This choice is based on several studies that show that CT scanning and MR imaging miss epidural lesions in 26% to 30% of cases,[28,29] In other large series assessing ESCC, 7% to 10% of lesions found on myelography were clinically silent or asymptomatic.[24,27]

The clinical approach to the patient begins with a history that focuses on the site and character of pain, with particular attention being directed toward radicular symptoms, limb weakness, or sphincter dysfunction. A suggestive history for ESCC, as described previously, should be investigated with great urgency, and physical examination should attempt to reveal sites of vertebral tenderness and evidence of segmental and pyramidal weakness, pathologic reflexes, or impaired sensation. An evaluation of sphincter tone and anal sensation should be considered an essential part of the examination.

Patients with evidence of ESCC (myelopathy or myeloradiculopathy), even without progressing signs, should undergo spinal films and be admitted to the hospital for myelography. The patient with signs of impending ESCC should receive dexamethasone, 100 mg intravenously, before myelography.

For the patient with back pain and a normal neurologic examination, or back pain and radiculopathy without myelopathy or sphincter disturbance, the first step should be plain films of the spine. Both the bone scan and the

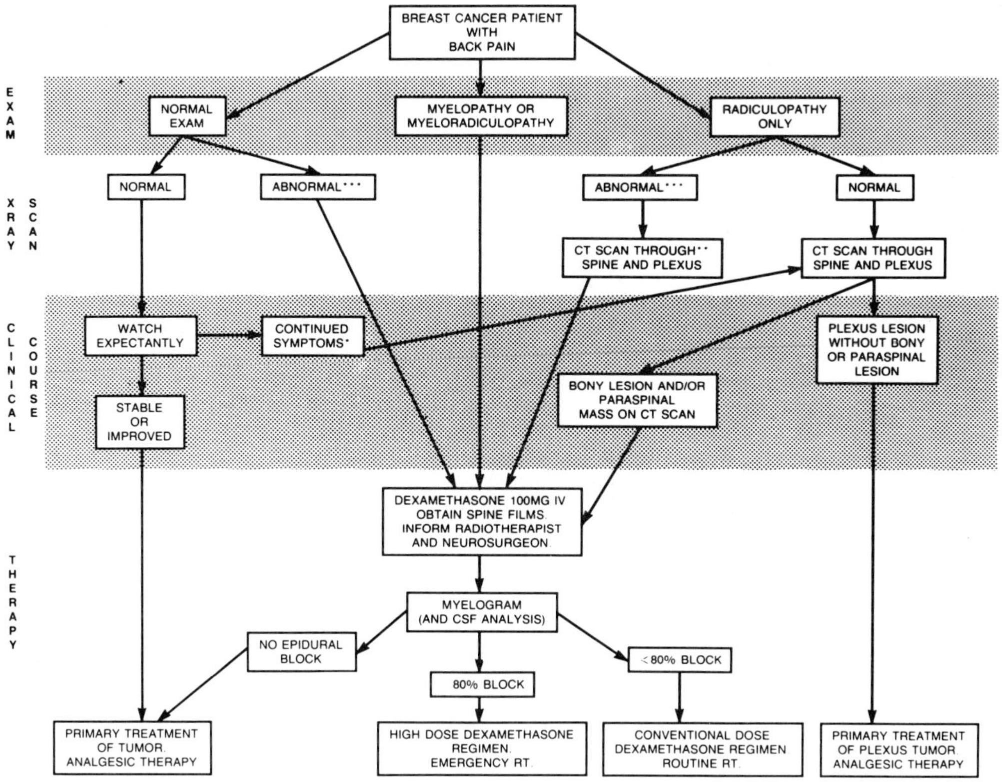

* If plain films and CT are negative, then myelogram is done to pursue intramedullary or meningeal (intradural) disease.
** If plexus is lesion found in addition to epidural disease, RT port is extended to include plexus as well as spine.
*** Abnormal X-ray is defined as vertebral metastasis, with or without pedicle erosion or vertebral body collapse greater than 50%.

FIGURE 14-7. Algorithm for the management of a breast cancer patient with back pain. The captions to the left of the diagram (exam, x-ray/scan, clinical course, and treatment) describe the steps taken in the work-up of a patient. The management of any particular patient progresses vertically in the diagram.

spine series may be used as screening tests in the patient with a normal neurologic examination; if the results are negative, the patient may be followed expectantly.[27] If the patient's symptoms worsen or fail to improve, CT scanning through the symptomatic area might successfully reveal retroperitoneal, paraspinal, or, less commonly, epidural disease as the cause. Progressive symptoms, however, will eventually warrant myelography if the results of radiographic studies prove to be negative. This approach allows investigation of the possibility of epidural or leptomeningeal disease. The exception to this guideline is the patient who has received previous radiation therapy; bone scans may be falsely negative in previously irradiated sites, despite progressive disease, so CT scanning should be utilized in these patients. The CT scan has proved to be the most sensitive test for the detection of metastatic bone disease.[32]

Patients with radiculopathy should routinely undergo a CT scan if the results of plain film or bone scan studies prove to be negative. Brachial and lumbosacral plexopathy, particularly when associated with paraspinal masses, may invade the epidural space without evidence of bony involvement.[51–53] Graus and colleagues describe a 29% incidence of epidural metastases secondary to paraspinal disease and a 5% incidence of epidural extension from lumbosacral plexus disease in patients having negative results on spinal film study.[24] Myelography should, therefore, be performed in patients with back pain and radiculopathy who have a paraspinal mass or early bony involvement detected on CT scan, even if the results of spinal films and bone scans are negative. In situations in which the patient is either unable or unwilling to undergo contrast myelography, CT scanning or MR imaging may be substituted, with the knowledge that 24% to 30% of epidural lesions may be overlooked.

The likelihood of ESCC in patients with back pain and normal examination but abnormal spinal films may be predicted from the recent studies of Graus and co-workers.[24] A vertebral body collapse of greater than 50% is associated with a likelihood of greater than 85% that ESCC will be found on myelography. Pedicle destruction or vertebral metastasis without collapse in the patient whose only symptom is back pain is associated with an incidence of 31% and 7%, respectively. However, in the patient with local back and radicular pain, the incidence is much higher (75% and 42,%, respectively). Hence, patients with abnormal spinal films but nonprogressive signs and no evidence of myelopathy should be treated with steroids and scheduled for myelography as soon as possible.

The decision regarding therapy is simpler for breast cancer than for other carcinomas since breast cancer responds well to radiation therapy.[14,22] Patients with breast cancer should be treated with appropriate supportive measures, and dexamethasone therapy should be tapered gradually, with close monitoring for neurologic deterioration. The indications for surgical intervention in these patients are the same as those in patients with ESCC caused by other carcinomas:

Further clinical deterioration during radiation therapy
Recurrence in a previously irradiated area
Bony encroachment on the spinal canal and spinal instability (usually requiring anterior decompression and spinal stabilization)
A questionable diagnosis

The specific surgical approach is determined by the site of the tumor (anterior versus posterior), with anterior decompression and stabilization being the currently favored approach in patients who have failed with radiation therapy.

In summary, ESCC is an important complication of breast cancer. Early diagnosis and treatment are facilitated by the appropriate diagnostic studies, and prevention of irreversible neurologic injury is possible.

REFERENCES

1. Patchell RA, Posner JB: Neurological complications of systemic cancer. Neurol Clin North Am 3:729, 1985
2. Barron KD, Hirano A, Araki A, et al: Experiences with metastatic neoplasms involving the spinal cord. Neurology 9:91, 1959
3. Chade HO: Metastatic tumours of the spine and the spinal cord. In Vinken PJ, Bruyn GW (eds): Handbook of Clinical Neurology, vol 20, pp 415–433. Amsterdam, North-Holland Publishing Co, 1976
4. Brice J, McKissock W: Surgical treatment of malignant extradural spinal tumors. Br Med J 1:1341, 1965
5. Constans JP, DeDivitis E, Donzelli R, et al: Spinal metastases with neurological manifestations. J Neurosurg 59:111, 1983
6. Stark RJ, Henson RA, Evans SJW: Spinal metastases, a retrospective survey from a general hospital. Brain 105:189, 1982
7. Gilbert RW, Kim J-H, Posner JB: Epidural spinal cord compression from metastatic tumor: Diagnosis and treatment. Ann Neurol 3:40, 1978
8. Greenberg HS, Kim J-H, Posner JB: Epidural spinal cord compression from metastatic tumor: Results with a new treatment protocol. Ann Neurol 8:361, 1980
9. Torma T: Malignant tumors of the spine and spinal extradural space. Acta Chir Scand (Suppl)225:1, 1957
10. Dunn RC, Kelly WA, Wohns RNW, et al: Spinal epidural neoplasia. J Neurosurg 52:47, 1980
11. Fornasier VL, Horne JG: Metastases to the vertebral column. Cancer 36:590, 1975
12. Arseni CN, Simionescu MD, Horwath L: Tumors of the spine. Acta Psychiatr Neurol Scand 34:398, 1959
13. White WA, Patterson RH, Bergland RM: Role of surgery in the treatment of spinal cord compression by metastatic neoplasm. Cancer 27:558, 1971
14. Barcena A, Lobato RD, Rivas JJ, et al: Spinal metastatic disease: Analysis of factors determining functional prognosis and the choice of treatment. Neurosurgery 15:820, 1984
15. Black P: Spinal metastasis: Current status and recommended guidelines for management. Neurosurgery 5:726, 1979
16. Hendrickson FR, Sheinkop MB: Management of osseous metastases. Semin Oncol 2:399, 1975
17. Lenz M, Fried J: Metastases to the skeleton, brain and spinal cord from cancer of the breast and the effect of radiotherapy. Ann Surg 93:278, 1931
18. Galasko CSB: Bone metastases. In Weiss L, Gilbert HA (eds): The Anatomy and Pathway of Skeletal Metastases, pp 49–63. Boston, GK Hall, 1981
19. Harrison KM, Muss HB, Ball MR, et al: Spinal cord compression in breast cancer. Cancer 55:2839, 1985
20. Khan FR, Glicksman AS, Chu FCH, et al: Treatment by radiotherapy of spinal cord compression due to extradural metastases. Radiology 89:495, 1967
21. Bernat JL, Greenberg ER, Barrett J: Suspected epidural compression of the spinal cord and cauda equina by metastatic carcinoma. Cancer 51:1953, 1983
22. Cobb C, Leavens ME, Eckles N: Indications for nonoperative treatment of spinal cord compression due to breast cancer. J Neurosurg 47:653, 1977
23. Foley KM: Pain syndromes in patients with cancer. In Bonica JJ, Ventafridda V (eds): Advances in Pain Research and Therapy, vol 2, pp 59–75. New York, Raven Press, 1979
24. Graus F, Krol G, Foley KM: Early diagnosis of spinal epidural metastasis: correlation with clinical and radiological findings. J Clin Oncol (in press)
25. Kanner RM, Martini N, Foley KM: Incidence of pain and other clinical manifestations of superior pulmonary sulcus (Pancoast) tumors. In Bonica JJ, Ventafridda V (eds): Advances in Pain Research and Therapy. New York, Raven Press, 1982
26. Rodriguez M, Dinapoli R: Spinal cord compression with special reference to metastatic epidural tumors. Mayo Clin Proc 55:442, 1980
27. Rodichok LD, Harper GR, Ruckdeschel JC, et al: Early diagnosis of spinal epidural metastases. Am J Med 70:1181, 1981
28. Wang AM, Lewis ML, Rumbaugh CL, et al: Spinal cord or nerve root compression in patients with malignant disease: CT evaluation. J Comput Assist Tomogr 8:420, 1984
29. Krol G, Heier L, Becker R, et al: MRI and myelography in the evaluation of epidural extension of primary and metastatic tumors. International Excerpta Medica (in press)
30. Cascino TL, Kori S, Krol G, et al: CT of the brachial plexus in patients with cancer. Neurology 33:1553, 1983
31. Baker AS, Ojemann RG, Swartz MN, et al: Spinal epidural abscess. N Engl J Med 293:463, 1975
32. Kori SH, Krol G, Foley KM: Computed tomographic evaluation of bone and soft tissue metastases. In Weiss L, Gilbert HA (eds): Bone Metastases, Metastases Monograph Series, Vol 3, pp 245–257. Boston, GK Hall, 1981
33. Edelson RN, Deck MDF, Posner JB: Intramedullary spinal cord metastases: Clinical and radiographic findings in nine cases. Neurology 22:1222, 1972
34. Costigan DA, Winkelman MD: Intramedullary spinal cord metastasis. J Neurosurg 62:227, 1985

35. Jellinger K, Kothbauer P, Sunder-Plassmann E, et al: Intramedullary spinal cord metastases. J Neurol 220:31, 1979
36. Henson RA, Urich H: Involvement of the vertebral column and spinal cord. In Henson RA, Urich H (eds): Cancer and the Nervous System. Oxford, Blackwell Scientific Publications, 1983
37. Wasserstrom WR, Glass PJ, Posner JB: Diagnosis and treatment of leptomeningeal metastases from solid tumors: Experience with 90 patients. Cancer 49:759, 1982
38. Young RF, Post EM, King GA: Treatment of spinal epidural metastases: Randomized prospective comparison of laminectomy and radiotherapy. J Neurosurg 53:741, 1980
39. Ushio Y, Posner R, Kim J-H, et al: Treatment of experimental spinal cord compression caused by extradural neoplasms. J Neurosurg 47:380, 1977
40. Posner JB, Howieson J, Cvitkovic E: "Disappearing" spinal cord compression: Oncolytic effect of glucocorticoids (and other chemotherapeutic agents) on epidural metastases. Ann Neurol 2:409, 1977
41. Slatkin NE, Posner JB: Management of spinal epidural metastases. Clin Neurosurg 30:698, 1983
42. Wright RL: Malignant tumors in the extradural space—Results of surgical treatment. Ann Surg 157:227, 1963
43. Brady LW, Antoniades J, et al: The treatment of metastatic disease of the nervous system by radiation therapy. In Seydel HG (ed): Tumors of the Nervous System. New York, John Wiley & Sons, 1975
44. Sundaresan N, Galicich JH: Treatment of spinal metastases by vertebral body resection. Cancer Invest 2:383, 1984
45. Sundaresan N, Galicich JH, Bains MS, et al: Vertebral body resection in the treatment of cancer involving the spine. Cancer 53:1393, 1984
46. Harrington KD: The use of methylmethacrylate for vertebral body replacement and anterior stabilization of pathological fracture-dislocations of the spine due to metastatic malignant disease. J Bone Joint Surg 63:36, 1981
47. Siegal T, Siegal T, Robin G, et al: Anterior decompression of spine for metastatic epidural cord compression: Is it a promising avenue of therapy? Ann Neurol 11:28, 1982
48. Overby MC, Rothman AS: Anterolateral decompression for metastatic epidural spinal cord tumors. J Neurosurg 62:344, 1985
49. Sundaresan N, Galicich JH, Lane JM, et al: Treatment of odontoid fractures in cancer patients. Neurosurgery 54:187, 1981
50. Portenoy RK, Lipton RB, Foley KM: Back pain in the cancer patient: An algorithm for evaluation and management. Neurology (in press)
51. Kori SH, Foley KM, Posner JP: Brachial plexus lesions in patients with cancer: 100 cases. Neurology 31:45, 1981
52. Jaeckle KA, Young DF, Foley KM: The natural history of lumbosacral plexopathy in cancer. Neurology 35:8, 1985
53. Thomas JE, Cascino TL, Earle JD: Differential diagnosis between radiation and tumor plexopathy of the pelvis. Neurology 35:1, 1985

Carcinomatous Meningitis

J. Peter Glass Kathleen M. Foley

Carcinomatous meningitis, meningeal carcinomatosis, or more properly, leptomeningeal metastasis is defined as diffuse or widespread multifocal involvement of the subarachnoid space by metastatic tumor. Carcinomatous involvement of the leptomeninges had been described by Eberth in the German literature as early as 1870,[1] but its metastatic nature had not been appreciated.

Beerman first used the term meningeal carcinomatosis in the English literature in an article published in 1912.[2] He described the course of a 62-year-old woman without known malignant disease who developed generalized headaches approximately 6 weeks prior to being hospitalized. In the hospital, she was noted to be confused, had visual hallucinations, and became progressively less responsive. She died 3 months after the onset of her illness. At autopsy, there were no gross abnormalities of the CNS, but microscopic examination of the brain revealed diffuse involvement of the pia-arachnoid with neoplastic cells.

There is limited information available today with respect to the incidence of leptomeningeal tumor. Gonzales-Vitale reviewed a series of 13,500 consecutive autopsies in a search for cases of leptomeningeal involvement exclusive of leukemia or lymphoma.[3] Eighteen cases were found in which there were metastases to the subarachnoid space alone. These represented 6% of the 306 cases with metastatic involvement of the CNS. The incidence of leptomeningeal tumor at autopsy at Memorial Sloan-Kettering Cancer Center in New York is between 8% and 10%.[4]

EPIDEMIOLOGY AND DISEASE CHARACTERISTICS

Although there are no epidemiologic studies on its clinical incidence, there is evidence to support the conclusion that leptomeningeal metastasis is increasing in frequency, particularly as a complication of certain solid tumors—namely, adenocarcinoma of the breast and lung and malignant melanoma. The reason for this increase may be twofold. First, treatment of systemic cancer has improved, with resultant longer survival, particularly in patients with breast carcinoma, probably without the ability of the systemic chemotherapeutic agents used to affect the CNS. Second, clinicians are becoming more aware of leptomeningeal metastasis, and a lumbar puncture is often done as a screening procedure to determine the extent of disease in a given patient.

The natural history of leptomeningeal metastasis is one of progressive neurologic dysfunction involving multiple CNS sites and leading to death in a matter of 4 to 6 weeks.[5,6] Patients lapse into stupor and coma because of widespread but strategically placed microscopic tumor infiltrates that involve the lower cranial nerves and brain stem. They may also develop cardiac arrythmias, pulmonary emboli, aspiration pneumonia, and septicemia.

There is no sexual predisposition for leptomeningeal metastasis except for that of the underlying malignant process. Forty-six of 90 patients with solid tumors studied by Wasserstrom had breast carcinoma, and ranged in age from 30 to 74.[7] The interval from diagnosis of the primary tumor to diagnosis of leptomeningeal involvement in these patients was usually between 6 months and 3 years, but in two patients with breast carcinoma, leptomeningeal metastasis was the presenting condition, and the primary tumor was only found later. Also in two patients with breast carcinoma, leptomeningeal metastasis appeared more than 10 years after the primary tumor had been diagnosed and treated, and it was the only evidence of disease.

Several mechanisms for the involvement of the leptomeninges by tumor cells have been postulated.[8] Direct, hematogenous spread via the capillary structure of the choroid plexus is possible.[9] Tumor deposits along the perivascular (Virchow-Robin) spaces of penetrating vessels may extend outward to infiltrate the subarachnoid space.[10] Alternatively, rupture of cerebral metastases into the ventricular system may occur, subsequently involving the subarachnoid space.[11] In addition, deposits of cerebral subdural tumor may extend directly into the underlying meninges, or spinal epidural deposits of tumor may infiltrate along nerve roots through the intervertebral foramina and into the subarachnoid space.[12]

SYMPTOMS AND SIGNS

Patients with breast carcinoma and leptomeningeal metastasis may present in any number of ways. There are two important aspects of the patient's history and examination that suggest the diagnosis: symptoms and signs of structural disease involving the neuraxis at more than one anatomic site, and neurologic signs indicating more prominent and widespread dysfunction than the symptoms alone.

The symptoms and signs of leptomeningeal tumor are best divided according to three major sites: cerebral, cranial nerve, and spinal cord, including nerve roots. The pathophysiology of these symptoms and signs may be related to any number of factors, including the development of hydrocephalus secondary to obstruction of CSF pathways, interference with the blood supply to the parenchyma, metabolic competition between tumor cells and CNS cells, and direct invasion of the nerves, nerve roots, and the parenchyma itself.

Forty-five of 90 patients in Wasserstrom's series initially presented with cerebral symptoms. Headache was the most frequent symptom, affecting 30 patients (73%). It was usually severe and intractable, unrelieved by common analgesics, and often associated with nausea, vomiting, and a stiff neck. The second most common symptom reported was a change in mental status. This occurred in 15 patients, and consisted of lethargy, confusion, or memory loss. Cognitive abnormalities were found in 28 patients on initial examination. Five patients had seizures at presentation, and 13 eventually developed seizures (which were focal in 5 and generalized in 8 patients). Five patients had papilledema on initial examination, and one had a hemiparesis. Twelve patients reported difficulty in walking and had wide-based, ataxic gaits (Table 14-5).

Fischer-Williams stated that cranial nerve paralysis was the single most consistent feature of leptomeningeal metastasis.[13] Cranial nerve symptoms were the initial complaint in 35 of 90 patients (38%) in Wasserstrom's series. The most common symptoms were double vision, hearing loss, facial numbness, and a decrease in visual acuity. In three patients, blindness was the presenting symptom. On initial examination, cranial nerve abnormalities were found in 50 patients. Ocular muscle pareses were the most common of these abnormalities, followed by facial weakness, hearing loss, and visual loss (Table 14-6).

Spinal cord and nerve root symptoms were also common. The most common of these symptoms was weakness, usually in the lower extremities, followed by paresthesias, back pain, radicular pain, and bowel or bladder dysfunction. Approximately 70% of the patients had signs of nerve root involvement detected on initial examination, primarily characterized by deep tendon reflex asymmetry. Thirty patients had signs of a cauda equina syndrome characterized by a lower motor neuron lesion that caused flaccid weakness of the lower extremities, a decrease or loss of deep tendon reflexes, mute or flexor plantar responses, sensory deficits from L-1 down, and bowel or bladder incontinence, or both. The syndrome took from 2 to 36 weeks to develop in the 12 patients who manifested it after

Table 14-5
Cerebral Symptoms and Signs in 90 Patients With Leptomeningeal Metastases from Solid Tumors

Symptoms	*No. Patients*	*Signs*	*No. Patients*
Headache	30	Mental change	28
Mental change	15	Seizures	5
Difficulty in walking	12	Generalized	3
Nausea/vomiting	10	Focal	2
Unconsciousness	2	Papilledema	5
Dysphasia	2	Diabetes insipidus	2
Dizziness	2	Hemiparesis	1
	Total: 45 Patients		

(Glass PJ, et al: Diagnosis and treatment of leptomeningeal metastases from solid tumors: Experience with 90 patients. Cancer 49:759, 1982)

Table 14-6
Cranial Nerve Symptoms and Signs in 90 Patients With Leptomeningeal Metastases from Solid Tumors

Symptoms	*No. Patients*	*Signs*	*No. Patients*
Diplopia	18	Ocular muscle paresis (III, IV, VI)	18
Hearing loss	7	Facial weakness (VII)	15
Visual loss	5	Diminished hearing (VIII)	9
Facial numbness	5	Optic neuropathy (II)	5
Decreased taste	3	Trigeminal neuropathy (V)	5
Tinnitus	2	Hypoglossal neuropathy (XII)	5
Hoarseness	2	Blindness	3
Dysphagia	1	Diminished gag (IX, X)	3
Vertigo	1		
	Total: 50 Patients		

(Glass PJ, et al: Diagnosis and treatment of leptomeningeal metastases from solid tumors: Experience with 90 patients. Cancer 49:759, 1982)

Table 14-7
Spinal Symptoms and Signs in 90 Patients With Leptomeningeal Metastases from Solid Tumors

Symptoms	*No. Patients*	*Signs*	*No. Patients*
Lower motor neuron weakness	34	Reflex asymmetry	64
Paresthesias	31	Weakness	54
Radicular pain	19	Sensory loss	24
Back/neck pain	23	Straight leg raising	11
Bowel/bladder dysfunction	12	Decreased rectal tone	10
		Nuchal rigidity	7
	Total: 74 Patients		

(Glass PJ, et al: Diagnosis and treatment of leptomeningeal metastases from solid tumors: Experience with 90 patients. Cancer 49:759, 1982)

Table 14-8
CSF Findings in 90 Patients With Leptomeningeal Metastases from Solid Tumors

Finding	*Initial Finding (No. of Patients)*	*Subsequent Finding (No. of Patients)*
Pressure > 160 mm CSF	45	64
Cells > 5 mm^3	51	65
Protein > 50 mg/dl	73	80
Glucose < 40 mg/dl	28	37
Positive cytology	49	82
Normal	3	1

(Glass PJ, et al: Diagnosis and treatment of leptomeningeal metastases from solid tumors: Experience with 90 patients. Cancer 49:759, 1982)

the diagnosis of leptomeningeal involvement (Table 14-7).

DIAGNOSTIC CONSIDERATIONS

Lumbar puncture is the single most useful test in the diagnosis of leptomeningeal metastasis. The CSF profile includes elevated pressure, increased protein, substantially decreased glucose levels (hypoglycorrhachia), a cellular response that is predominantly lymphocytic, positive cytology, and persistently negative cultures. All 90 of the patients in Wasserstrom's series underwent a lumbar puncture, some as many as 7 times before a diagnosis could be made. Abnormalities were found in the CSF in 89 patients (Table 14-8); one patient's CSF remained persistently within normal limits. Cerebrospinal fluid findings included a pressure that ranged from 60 mm to 450 mm of CSF, protein levels of 24 mg to 2485 mg/dl, glucose levels of 2 mg to 244 mg/dl, and a white blood cell count of 0 to 1800 cells/mm^3. Eighty-two patients (90%) had a positive CSF cytology (Fig. 14-8). In 8 patients (10%), CSF cytology remained negative throughout the course of the disease.

Biochemical tumor markers may be measured in the CSF of patients with leptomeningeal metastasis.[14–17] Levels considered to be abnormal are β-glucuronidase levels of

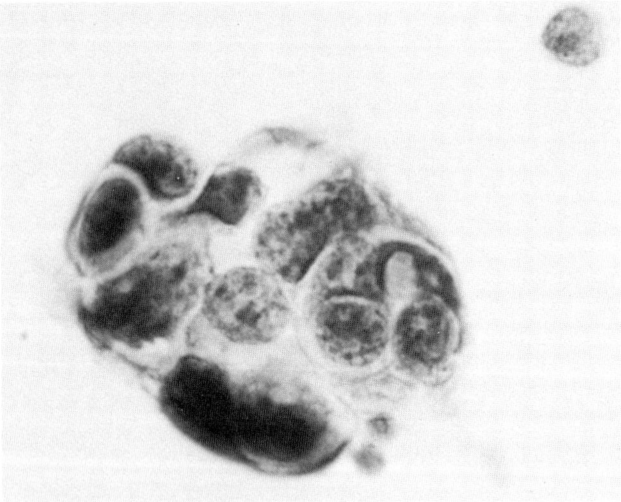

FIGURE 14-8. Bizarre, multinucleated, clumped cells of a patient with breast carcinoma are seen in this CSF specimen stained with toluidene blue.

greater than 80 mμ/liter, carcinoembryonic antigen (CEA) levels of greater than 1.5 ng/ml with a serum level of less than 100 ng/ml, and lactic dehydrogenase (LDH) isoenzyme LDH-5/LDH-1 levels of greater than 15% (Table 14-9). At the present time, these markers should not be used alone to establish the diagnosis. Cerebrospinal fluid samples should be collected for analysis prior to performing myelography or instilling any chemotherapeutic agent into the subarachnoid space because some of these markers are made by white blood cells and may become falsely elevated in the face of chemical meningitis or arachnoiditis.

Neuroradiographic studies that may be helpful in the diagnosis of leptomeningeal metastasis are myelography[18] and CT scanning.[19–21] Myelographic results are positive in 25% to 30% of patients, revealing irregular filling defects in the subarachnoid space owing to thickening and nodularity of nerve roots, particularly in the cauda equina (Fig. 14-9). This finding may occasionally yield unequivocal evidence of leptomeningeal disease when CSF analysis is unrewarding. Lee and colleagues identified four basic CT abnormalities that occurred in approximately 35% of patients with leptomeningeal disease: sulcal-cisternal enhancement; ependymal-subependymal enhancement; widened, irregular tentorial enhancement; and communicating hydrocephalus (Figs. 14-10 and 14-11).[20]

There are few positive findings in the gross examination of the brain and spinal cord in patients with leptomeningeal metastasis. The most common one is thickening and opacification of the leptomeninges, which usually occurs at the base of the brain, but also may occur over the convexities. There may be enlargement of the ventricular system secondary to obstruction of the flow of CSF. Tumor nodules, along with swelling and matting together of new roots, may be seen most prominently in the cauda equina (Fig. 14-12).

On microscopic examination, the leptomeninges show either diffuse or multifocal infiltration by tumor cells, with occasional reactive fibrosis and a lymphocytic infiltrate. There is usually a concentration of tumor in the subarachnoid cisterns along the ventral surface of the brain stem as well as deep within the sulci. The choroid plexus is involved in a substantial number of cases. Tumor cells may extend along the perivascular spaces of penetrating vessels down to capillary levels (Fig. 14-13). Invasion of the subpial parenchyma has occurred, both in the brain and spinal cord. In certain cases, tumor cells have invaded nerves and nerve roots, but more commonly, they tend to encase the perineurium, causing ischemia and subsequent degeneration of nerve fibers.

TREATMENT

Radiation Therapy

The treatment of leptomeningeal metastasis in patients with breast carcinoma (solid tumors)[22–24] is basically a carry-over from the treatment of malignant cells in the CSF of children with acute lymphoblastic leukemia (ALL).[25–30] Patients are irradiated to the area of symptomatic involvement—that is, the whole brain is irradiated if there is cerebral or cranial nerve dysfunction, or the particular spinal cord segment that is most involved clinically (cervical, thoracic, or lumbosacral) may be treated. We do not separate whole-brain from base-of-skull irradiation for two reasons. Despite cranial nerve involvement at the base of the skull, when patients with leptomeningeal disease are examined at autopsy, the entire subarachnoid space over the convexities, brain stem, and spinal cord is filled with malignant cells.[31] For that reason and to prevent cerebral symptoms from developing later, the entire brain is irradiated. In addition, it is difficult for the radiation therapist to patch radiation portals for the cerebral hemispheres onto the portals of a previously irradiated base of skull because of overlap and the potential for later development of cerebral radiation necrosis. Irradiating the entire spinal cord would not be feasible in adults with systemic disease because this could destroy as much as 40% of the patient's bone marrow, making it more difficult to administer systemic chemotherapy. The total radiation dose is 2400 cGy to 3000 cGy delivered in 8 to 10 fractions over a period of 10 to 14 days. Steroids (dexamethasone) are administered during irradiation, usually at a dosage of 16 mg per day (in divided doses) with antacid coverage. The dose is then tapered slowly, usually without problems, by 2 mg every other day until it is discontinued.

Intraventricular/Intrathecal Chemotherapy

The second modality for the treatment of leptomeningeal metastasis is intraventricular/intrathecal chemotherapy. As a result of the development of the Ommaya reservoir in 1963,[32] a much more uniform distribution of chemotherapeutic agents can be injected into the ventricular system,

Table 14-9
Biochemical Tumor Markers in the CSF of 90 Patients With Leptomeningeal Metastases from Solid Tumors

Primary Tumor	*β-Glucuronidase (No. of patients with levels > 80 mμ/1)*	*Carcinoembryonic Antigen (CEA) (No. of patients with levels > 1 ng/ m1)**	*Lactic Dehydrogenase Isoenzymes (No. of patients with LDH-5/LDH-1 levels > 15%)*	*One Abnormal Marker*
Breast	13/17	10/17	9/12	15/17
Lung	6/9	8/9	3/5	8/9
Melanoma	2/4	1/4	3/3	3/4

* Serum CEA < 100.

(Glass PJ, et al: Diagnosis and treatment of leptomeningeal metastases from solid tumors: Experience with 90 patients. Cancer 49:759, 1982)

with tumoricidal concentrations lasting for 48 to 72 hours.[33] Also as a result of this development, samples of CSF can easily be obtained, chemotherapeutic agents may be injected, and the patient is spared the trauma of multiple lumbar punctures.

The reservoir is usually placed through a burr hole in the right frontal region so that the intraventricular catheter sits in the frontal horn of the right lateral ventricle, close to the foramen of Monro (Fig. 14-14). It may be inserted before, during, or after whole-brain irradiation. There are few complications,[34] although a CT scan should always be performed prior to placement.

A limited number of chemotherapeutic agents may be injected into the subarachnoid space without causing permanent damage to the CNS. These include methotrexate, cytosine arabinoside, steroids, thiotepa, and derivatives of 5-fluorouracil. Methotrexate alone or in combination with cytosine arabinoside or thiotepa is the drug regimen that is most commonly used to treat leptomeningeal metastasis from breast carcinoma. The dosage of methotrexate varies from 7 mg to 12 mg/m^2. The dosages for cytosine arabinoside and for thiotepa are 100 mg/treatment and 10 mg/m^2, respectively. When methotrexate is administered, it enters the systemic circulation, and may have an effect upon the rapidly dividing cells of the oropharynx, gastrointestinal tract, and bone marrow. Therefore, citrovorum factor is administered orally, 9 mg every 12 hours, for 4 days after therapy. This drug blocks the action of methotrexate on the enzyme dihydrofolate reductase and allows for continued pyrimidine synthesis systemically. Treatment is initiated twice per week for 4 to 6 weeks until the patients stabilize or improve neurologically and their CSF parameters begin to return to normal. If patients do not respond in the first 4 weeks, chemotherapeutic agents may be changed; in all likelihood, however, these patients will not respond to any agent. After 4 to 6 weeks, the chemotherapeutic regimen is changed to a once weekly course; this time interval is doubled for every three consecutively negative CSF cytologic studies. The patient, however, is obligated to a lifetime of treatment, with the longest acceptable time interval between treatments being 2 months.

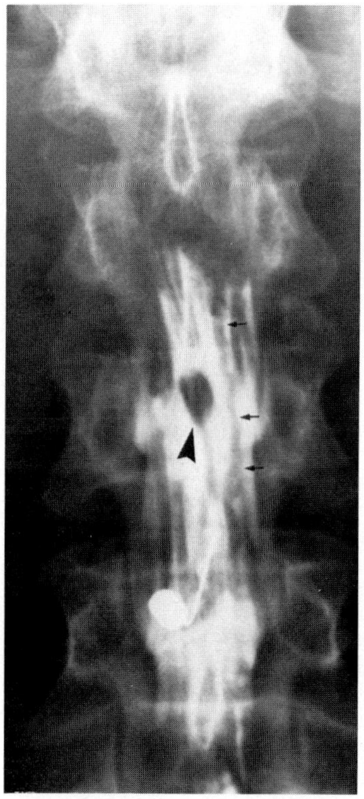

FIGURE 14-9. A myelogram reveals an intradural filling defect *(arrowhead)* and a swollen nerve root *(arrows)* in a patient who developed a cauda equina syndrome.

Treatment Complications

There are acute and chronic toxicities associated with the medications injected intraventricularly, particularly meth-

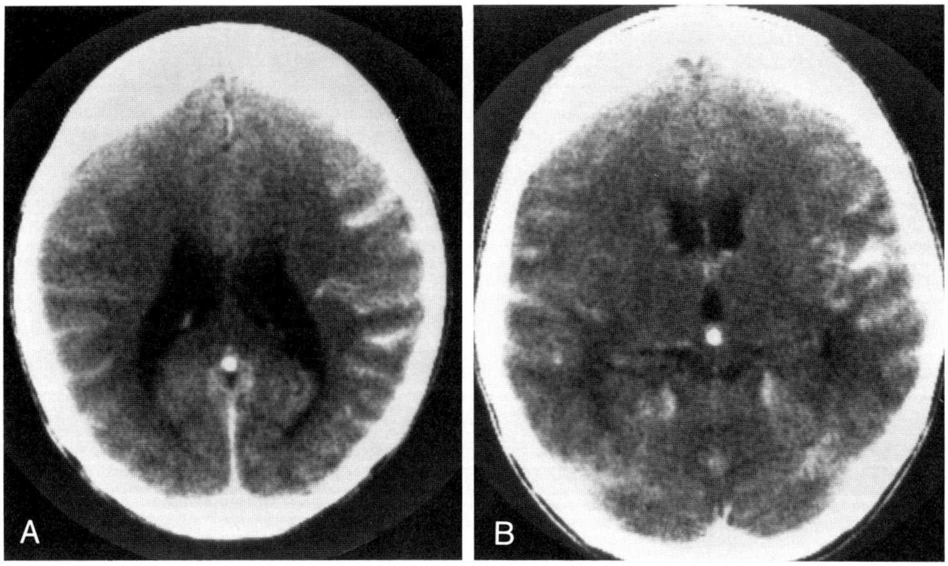

FIGURE 14-10. *(A, B)* Diffuse sulcal enhancement in breast carcinoma. Obliteration of the cortical sulci by leptomeningeal enhancement associated with communicating hydrocephalus. (Taveras JM: Cranial computed tomographic abnormalities in leptomeningeal metastasis. AJNR 5:559, 1984)

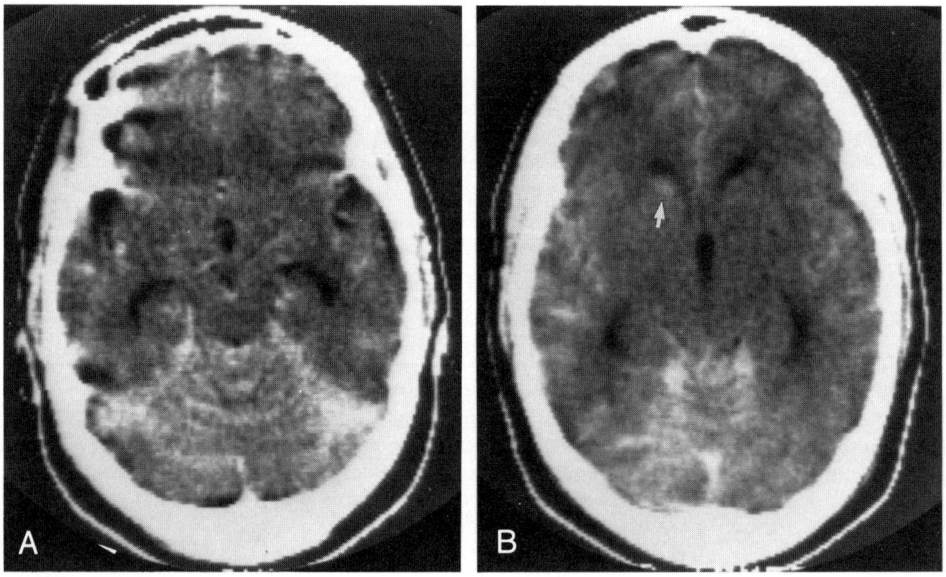

FIGURE 14-11. *(A, B)* Diffuse tentorial enhancement in breast carcinoma. Associated sulcal enhancementandanependymal-subependymal lesion in the head of the right caudate nucleus *(arrow)*. (Taveras JM: Cranial computed tomographic abnormalities in leptomeningeal metastasis. AJNR 5:559, 1984)

otrexate. On an acute basis, this drug may produce a chemical meningitis, with headache, fever, stiff neck, confusion, disorientation, and hallucinations being reported. This occurs in approximately 10% of patients and resolves within 24 to 72 hours. The CSF may reveal an elevated protein and an increased white cell count. Such a reaction does not preclude further therapy and, as a matter of fact, in the 9 patients in Wasserstrom's series who developed acute toxicity, it was a one-time phenomenon.

Chronic, methotrexate-induced leukoencephalopathy is a more difficult problem. It may occur when methotrexate is administered alone intraventricularly, or when it is combined with either whole-brain irradiation or whole-brain irradiation and systemic chemotherapy. The approximate incidence of this condition has been delineated in a Venn diagram by Bleyer (Fig. 14-15).[35] The total dose of intraventricular methotrexate usually exceeds 140 mg. White matter changes seen on CT scan, which are usually diffuse and associated with ventricular enlargement, may be the only manifestation of leukoencephalopathy. Or, more commonly, there may also be changes in mental status in addition to the CT findings. Chronic, methotrexate-induced leukoencephalopathy is reversible, but the drug must first be discontinued. Normalization occurs slowly, and the possibility of recurrent leptomeningeal disease must be considered.

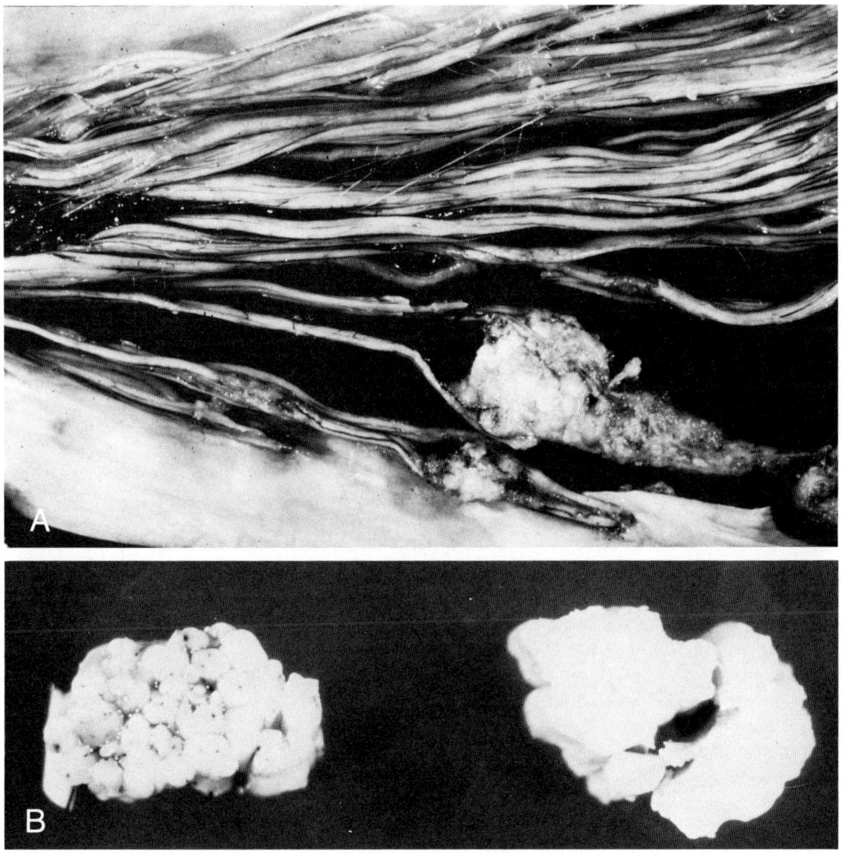

FIGURE 14-12. *(A)* Gross autopsy specimen of the cauda equina of a patient with breast carcinoma and leptomeningeal metastasis. Multiple tumor nodules are present. *(B)* A cross section of a normal cauda equina is shown on the left and one of a patient with leptomeningeal metastasis is depicted on the right. The nerve roots of the latter are matted together, swollen, and infiltrated by tumor.

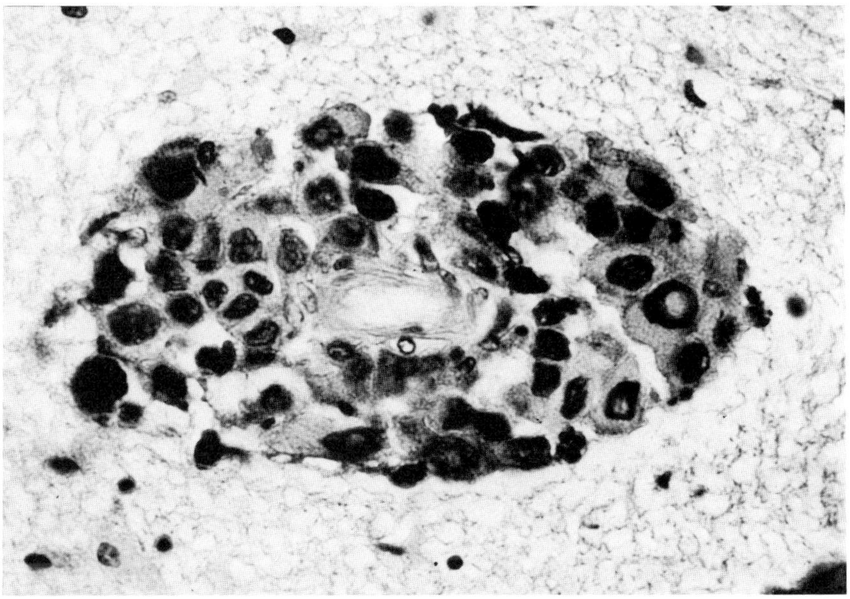

FIGURE 14-13. Microscopic section of tumor cells occupying the perivascular space of Virchow-Robin.

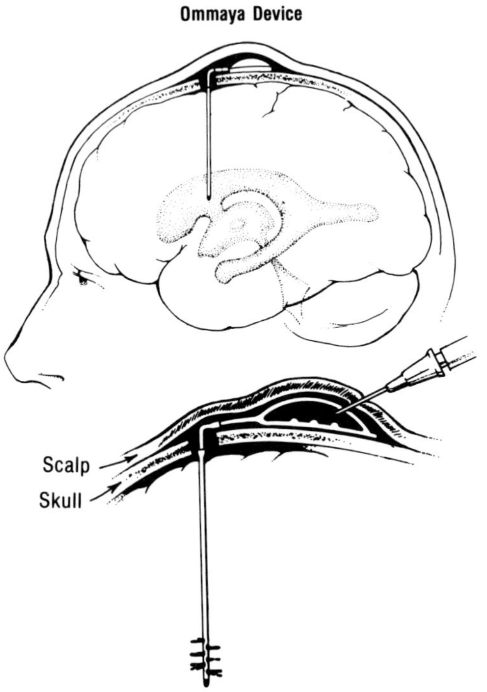

FIGURE 14-14. Diagram of an Ommaya reservoir attached to an intraventricular catheter. The device sits just below the scalp with the catheter in the frontal horn of the right lateral ventricle.

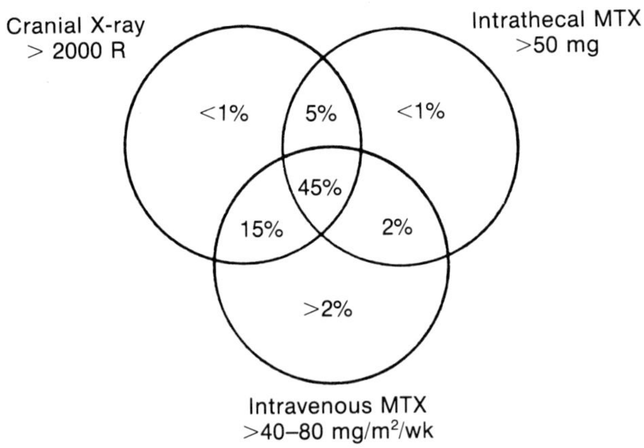

FIGURE 14-15. Venn diagram giving the approximate incidence of leukoencephalopathy for three major treatment modalities. (MTX, methotrexate)

Treatment Results

Given the above treatment regimen of the combination of radiation and intraventricular/intrathecal chemotherapy, the majority of patients with breast carcinoma stabilize or improve both clinically and with respect to their CSF. Median survival with aggressive therapy is approximately 7 months from the time of diagnosis. This is quality survival

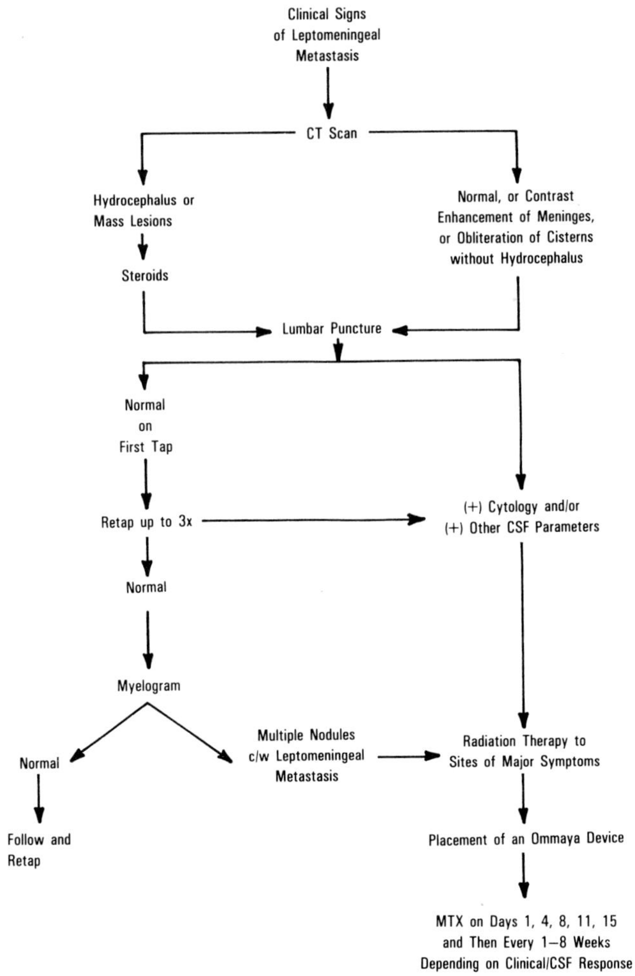

FIGURE 14-16. Treatment approach to the patient with leptomeningeal metastasis. (MTX, methotrexate)

and represents an improvement over previous studies, and certainly over the survival associated with untreated disease. In patients without evidence of systemic disease, median survival increases to up to 10 months. Ten percent of patients are alive 1 year or longer after diagnosis.

Other Considerations

In patients with clinical and CT evidence of obstructive hydrocephalus, whole-brain irradiation without intraventricular chemotherapy should be considered in an attempt to provide return of flow of CSF through the arachnoid villi, as well as through the foramina of Luschka and Magendie. The other major consideration is placement of a ventriculoperitoneal shunt with an on-off valve.

Whole-brain radiation therapy is usually administered via a portal that resembles a German helmet. Such a portal does not include the orbits or the optic nerves. If patients with leptomeningeal metastasis begin to develop decreased visual acuity, the most likely cause is infiltration of the optic nerves by tumor cells. The portal must then be changed to include the optic nerves.

Since one-third of patients with leptomeningeal metastasis present with or develop signs of a cauda equina syndrome, myelography must be considered for all patients in an attempt to document asymptomatic disease or to empirically irradiate the lumbar spine from L-1 through L-5.

Using the combination of radiation and intraventricular/intrathecal chemotherapy, the majority of patients with leptomeningeal metastasis either stabilize or undergo neurologic remission. Some of them relapse again, but over 40% may be stabilized until recurrence of systemic disease causes their death, often without the reappearance of disabling neurologic symptoms. However, even by the most optimistic standards, the treatment of the disease is, for most patients, poor and ineffective. More effective chemotherapeutic agents are needed that can either cross the blood–brain barrier in sufficient concentrations to kill the tumor in the CNS or that can be injected directly into the subarachnoid space in tumoricidal doses.[36,37] What is also needed is a method of diagnosis to discover whether early or even prophylactic treatment of the nervous system might prevent the development of neurologic symptoms and signs. Figure 14-16 outlines our approach to the patient with signs and symptoms of leptomeningeal involvement.

REFERENCES

1. Eberth CJ: Zur entwicklung des epitheliomas (cholesteatoms) der pia und der lung. Virchow Arch 49:51, 1870
2. Beerman WF: Meningeal carcinomatosis. JAMA 58:1437, 1912
3. Gonzales-Vitale JC, Garcia-Bunuel R: Meningeal carcinomatosis. Cancer 37:2906, 1976
4. Posner JB, Chernik NL: Intracranial metastases from systemic cancer. Adv Neurol 19:579, 1978
5. Little JR, Dale AJD, Okazaki H: Meningeal carcinomatosis: Clinical manifestations. Arch Neurol 30:138, 1974
6. Olson M, Chernik NL, Posner JB: Infiltration of the leptomeninges by systemic cancer: A clinical and pathologic study. Arch Neurol 30:122, 1974
7. Wasserstrom WR, Glass JP, Posner JB: Diagnosis and treatment of leptomeningeal metastasis from solid tumors: Experience with 90 patients. Cancer 49:759, 1982
8. Kokkoris CP: Leptomeningeal carcinomatosis. How does cancer reach the pia arachnoid? Cancer 51:154, 1983
9. Grain GO, Karr JP: Diffuse leptomeningeal carcinomatosis: Clinical and pathologic characteristics. Neurology 5:706, 1955
10. Globus JH, Meltzer T: Metastatic tumors of the brain. Arch Neurol Psychiatry 48:163, 1942
11. Dinsdale HB, Taghavy A: Carcinomatosis of the meninges. J Can Med Assoc 90:505, 1964
12. Griffin JW, Thompson RW, Mitchinson MJ, et al: Lymphomatous leptomeningitis. Am J Med 51:200, 1971
13. Fischer-Williams M, Bosanquet FD, Daniel PM: Carcinomatosis of the meninges. Brain 78:42, 1955
14. Shuttleworth E, Allen N: CSF B-glucuronidase assay in the diagnosis of neoplastic meningitis. Arch Neurol 37:684, 1980
15. Schold SC, Wasserstrom WR, Fleisher M, et al: Cerebrospinal fluid biochemical markers of central nervous system metastases. Ann Neurol 8:597, 1980
16. Wasserstrom WR, Schwartz M, Fleisher M, et al: Cerebrospinal fluid biochemical markers in central nervous system tumors: A review. Ann Clin Lab Sci 11:239, 1981
17. Fleisher M, Wasserstrom WR, Schold SC, et al: Lactic dehydrogenase isoenzymes in the cerebrospinal fluid of patients with systemic cancer. Cancer 47:2654, 1981
18. Guyer PB, Westbury H, Cook PL: The myelographic appearance of spinal cord metastases. Br J Radiol 41:615, 1968
19. Ascheri GF, Hilal SK, Brisman R: Computed tomography of disseminated meningeal and ependymal malignant neoplasms. Neurology 31:567, 1981
20. Lee YY, Glass JP, Geoffray A, et al: Cranial computed tomographic abnormalities in leptomeningeal metastasis. AJNR 5:559, 1984
21. Jaeckle KA, Krol G, Posner JB: Evolution of computed tomographic abnormalities in leptomeningeal metastases. Ann Neurol 17:85, 1985
22. McKelvey EM: Meningeal involvement with metastatic carcinoma of the breast treated with intrathecal methotrexate. Cancer 22:576, 1968
23. Yap HY, Yap BS, Tashima CK, et al: Meningeal carcinomatosis in breast cancer. Cancer 42:293, 1978
24. Ongerboer de Visser BW, Somers R, Nooyen WH, et al: Intraventricular methotrexate therapy of leptomeningeal metastasis from breast carcinoma. Neurology 33:1565, 1983
25. Wang JJ, Pratt CB: Intrathecal arabinosyl cytosine in meningeal leukemia. Cancer 25:531, 1970
26. Aur RJ, Husto HO, Verzosa M, et al: A comparative study of "prophylactic" craniospinal irradiation in 94 children with acute lymphocytic leukemia (ALL). Proc AACR/ASCO 12:5, 1971
27. Simone J, Aur RJ, Husto HO, et al: "Total therapy"—Studies of acute lymphocytic leukemia in children. Cancer 30:1488, 1972
28. Price RA, Johnson WW: The central nervous system in childhood leukemia. I. The arachnoid. Cancer 31:520, 1973
29. Bank PR, Holland JF, Bernard J, et al: Treatment of central nervous system leukemia with intrathecal cytosine arabinoside. Cancer 32:744, 1973
30. Bleyer WA, Poplack DG: Intraventricular versus intralumbar methotrexate for central-nervous-system leukemia: Prolonged remission with Ommaya reservoir. Med Pediatr Oncol 6:207, 1979
31. Glass JP, Melamed M, Chernik N, et al: Malignant cells in cerebrospinal fluid (CSF): The meaning of a positive CSF cytology. Neurology 29:1369, 1979
32. Ommaya AK: Subcutaneous reservoir and pump for sterile access to ventricular cerebrospinal fluid. Lancet 2:983, 1963
33. Shapiro WR, Young DF, Mehta BM: Methotrexate: Distribution in cerebrospinal fluid after intravenous, ventricular, and lumbar injection. N Engl J Med 293:161, 1975
34. Obbens EAMT, Leavens ME, Beal JW, et al: Ommaya reservoirs in 387 cancer patients: A 15-year experience. Neurology 35:1274, 1985
35. Bleyer WA: Current status of intrathecal chemotherapy for human meningeal neoplasms. Natl Cancer Inst Monogr 46:171, 1977
36. Ushio Y, Posner JB, Shapiro WR: Chemotherapy of experimental meningeal carcinomatosis. Cancer Research 37:1232, 1977
37. Seeldrayers P, Hildebrand J: Treatment of neoplastic meningitis. Eur J Cancer Clin Oncol 20:449, 1984

Choroidal Metastases from Breast Cancer

Mary Ann Rose Edward L. Feldman

Metastatic disease to the choroid of the eye was first reported in 1872 by Perls, who described bilateral deposits at the time of autopsy in a 43-year-old man.[1] Since that time, clinicians have recognized that the symptom of decreased visual acuity in cancer patients mandates rapid diagnosis and treatment, for few complications of metastatic cancer are as debilitating as blindness. Choroidal metastases in women occur most commonly in patients with primary tumors of the breast and thus are of special interest to the physician caring for these patients. This chapter will briefly outline the incidence, diagnostic procedures, and therapeutic options for treating choroidal metastases from breast cancer.

INCIDENCE

In a 15-year review of the literature, Albert and co-workers found that breast cancer was the primary site for 64% of patients with metastasis to the choroid.[2] Ferry and Font reported that breast cancer accounted for 77% of the cases observed in women.[3]

The actual clinical incidence of this entity is somewhat difficult to determine. An autopsy series reported by Nelson and associates at Duke University revealed a 6.6% incidence of ocular metastasis in patients dying of breast cancer.[4] Albert and colleagues studied the frequency with which choroidal metastases became evident in the clinical setting of metastatic breast cancer over a two-year period. Four cases of choroidal metastases were seen in 52 women with breast cancer (7.7%). In an earlier report, Cade found 11 cases of choroidal metastases in 135 women who had undergone adrenalectomy for metastatic breast cancer (8.1%).[5] These reports included patients who were not necessarily symptomatic from their disease. Two clinical series which attempted to define the incidence of symptomatic choroidal metastasis occurring in all women with breast cancer seen in these institutions yielded an incidence of 0.4% and 2%, respectively.[6,7]

The occurrence of synchronous or metachronous bilateral choroidal metastasis is also well described. Brady and colleagues reported a 19% incidence of bilateral disease in their review and commented on the predilection of breast cancer metastases to occur bilaterally.[8] Series that report specifically on breast cancer state that 40%[9] to 50%[7] of cases exhibit bilateral disease. In patients with breast cancer, choroidal metastases were often the first signs of disseminated disease.[10,11]

Metastatic disease of the choroid is presumed to be caused by hematogenous spread. Tumor emboli may enter the choroid through the short posterior ciliary arteries, the ophthalmic arteries, and the internal carotid arteries. The incidence of concomitant or subsequent brain metastasis is of therapeutic significance.

Thatcher and Thomas reported that only 5 of 42 patients in their series developed brain metastasis during their life.[6] Similarly, Maor reported that cerebral deposits developed in only 3 of 42 patients.[11] In a more recent series, however, Mewis reported that 30 of 67 patients had concomitant or subsequent CNS spread.[9] These figures probably reflect the increasingly routine use of CT scans in recent years. Certainly, evidence of concomitant brain metastasis warrants brain treatment, as well as specific therapy to treat the intraocular disease.

DIAGNOSIS

The principal symptoms leading to the diagnosis of choroidal metastases are decreased visual acuity and visual field changes.[10,11] Other, less common symptoms include metamorphopsia, pain, and photophobia. Lesions in the posterior portion of the globe on the temporal side of the macula are usually symptomatic.[11] These lesions appear as discrete, pale yellow areas in the choroid which are slightly elevated, with mottled retinal pigment epithelium on the surface (See Color Plate 4, Chapter 3).[8,11] There is often serous detachment of the retina (See Color Plate 5, Chapter 3),[8] with shifting of the subretinal fluid relative to the patient's head position. The latter is an important diagnostic sign that helps to distinguish retinal detachment due to choroidal metastases from a typical rhegmatogenous detachment.

Individuals in whom the diagnosis is suspected should undergo careful, indirect ophthalmoscopy, slit-lamp examination, and visual fields testing. Although the lesions are usually characteristic, occasionally, further diagnostic studies are indicated. A-scan and B-scan ultrasonography usually confirms the degree of retinal detachment and the underlying choroidal mass seen clinically.[12] Recently, high-resolution CT scanning has been shown to be a better method for further delineating choroidal lesions and any extrascleral extension.[13] On CT scans, the lesions appear as focal areas of enhancement, and the orbit is well visualized. Recently, Sternberg and co-workers reported on controlled aspiration of subretinal fluid using scleral depression for the diagnosis of choroidal metastasis, a technique that warrants further investigation.[14] Serial dilated fundus examinations remain the most effective diagnostic tool.

TREATMENT

The modalities used to treat choroidal metastasis from breast cancer include radiation therapy, hormonal therapy, chemotherapy, and, less commonly, cryosurgery and enucleation. Because of reports in the literature of worsening vision following cryotherapy,[15] this approach is not frequently utilized. There is little, if any, role for enucleation or orbital exenteration except in patients with painful eyes who are not responsive to other therapeutic maneuvers.

Radiation Therapy

Radiation therapy using external beam irradiation is generally regarded as the most effective means of treating choroidal metastases. A palliative dose of 3000 cGy, administered over a period of 3 weeks, is adequate to control tumor in most cases, although doses and fractionation vary from institution to institution.

The radiation technique most commonly employed is a direct lateral field on the involved side. The field usually measures 4 × 4 cm, with the anterior border at the bony canthus of the lateral orbital wall, thus sparing the lens. The field is angled 5 degrees posteriorly to avoid irradiating the lens of the opposite eye. In patients with bilateral disease, opposing lateral fields may be used. Other techniques may be indicated in specific clinical situations. For example, an anterior field may be added if there is any question about anterior structure involvement. Chu and colleagues, at Memorial Sloan-Kettering Cancer Center, used high-energy electrons to treat small choroidal metastases in an effort to further reduce the dose delivered to normal tissues.[10]

The results of recent radiation therapy series are illustrated in Table 14-10. Most series report response rates in the range of 80% to 94%. Responses were usually defined as improvement in visual acuity. In patients who responded with improved vision, similar improvements were seen funduscopically, with a decrease in the size of the masses or in the volume of subretinal fluid. Conversely, however, funduscopic improvement did not always result in visual improvement.[6] The median survival in all series was short, ranging from 7[6] to 12 months,[10] although in all series, there were several long-term survivors. Dose-response relationships remain unclear, although Maor found that doses of less than 3000 cGy resulted in tumor regrowth.[11] Similarly, Thatcher reported that all patients who had a complete response received more than 3250 cGy.[6] Chu recommended the administration of a somewhat higher dose (4000 cGy delivered over 3 weeks).[10] Some patients in these series received concomitant chemotherapy or hormonal therapy, or both; the effective contribution of these modalities cannot be assessed. Complications secondary to radiation therapy occurred infrequently; cataract formation or radiation retinitis were rarely a problem. No enucleations were required as a result of therapy or therapeutic failure.

Chemotherapy

Chemotherapy has been less frequently used than other modalities in the treatment of choroidal metastases from breast cancer. In 1972, Orenstein reviewed several case reports of responses to single-agent chemotherapy.[15] More recently, Brinkley reported complete regression of a choroidal metastasis in a 32-year-old woman undergoing five-drug combined chemotherapy (with cyclophosphamide, methotrexate, 5-fluorouracil, vincristine, and prednisone) for widespread metastases.[16] She died of systemic metastases 6 1/2 months after initiation of chemotherapy; no evidence of disease in the eye was found. Letson and coworkers reported on six patients (representing eight involved eyes) with choroidal metastases from breast cancer who were treated with various drug combinations.[17] Tumor regressed in all eight eyes, and visual improvement was reported in five cases. The three eyes with good initial acuity maintained their acuity level. In their opinion, chemotherapy seems to be as effective as irradiation in the treatment of this entity, and it has the advantage of avoiding the complication of cataract formation. However, further investigation is certainly needed.

Hormonal Therapy

The response of patients with choroidal metastases from breast cancer to hormonal manipulation has been addressed specifically in a few reported cases. Cade, in 1957, described regression of intraocular tumors in 11 cases following adrenalectomy for metastatic disease, although the nature of the lesions was not described.[5] Many patients who received radiation therapy or chemotherapy, or both,

Table 14-10
Radiation Therapy for Treatment of Choroidal Metastases

Author	*No. Patients*	*Recommended Dose (cGy)*	*% Bilateral Disease*	*Response Rate (%)*	*Median Survival (Mo)*
Thatcher[6]	42	≥ 3250	41	80	7
Rottinger[7]	26	3000	50	80	9.5
Maor[11]	42	≥ 3000	36	89	10
Chu[10]	46	4000	24	63	12
Mewis[9]	67	2500–3000	40	94.2	9

for choroidal metastasis have also undergone hormonal manipulation. The relative contribution of this modality of treatment, therefore, remains unknown. Retinal detachment with decreased visual acuity represents an urgent clinical situation, and treatment delays resulting from relatively slow responses to hormonal therapy may have catastrophic consequences for the patient.

SUMMARY

In conclusion, choroidal metastasis in women with breast cancer may result in blindness and pain if a diagnosis is not actively sought at the time the first symptoms of decreased visual acuity appear. The exact clinical incidence of this complication of metastatic breast cancer is unknown, but it may occur in as many as 6% to 8% of women during the course of their disease. Bilateral choroidal metastases, either synchronous or metachronous, may be seen in approximately one-third of patients. The mainstay of diagnosis is the funduscopic exam with serial retinal photographs, although CT scan, ultrasonography, and even subretinal aspiration may be helpful in some cases.

Radiation therapy is the treatment of choice for choroidal metastases, resulting in improvement in visual acuity in 80% to 90% of patients in most series. Recent reports of complete responses to combination chemotherapy are encouraging, but further investigation of this treatment modality is required. It may be that small, asymptomatic lesions in patients who are about to commence systemic treatment for widespread metastasis may simply be observed for response. The importance of vision preservation in these patients cannot be underestimated and, for most patients, prompt initiation of radiation therapy affords a high chance of success, with minimal risk to the patient.

REFERENCES

1. Perls M: Beitrage zur pathologie der Geshwolste. Arch Pathol Anat 56:437, 1872
2. Albert DM, Robinstein RA, Scheie HC: Tumor metastasis to the eye, Part I. Am J Ophthalmol 63:723, 1967
3. Ferry AP, Font RL: Carcinoma metastatic to the eye and orbit. I. A clinicopathologic study of 227 cases. Arch Ophthalmol 92:276, 1974
4. Nelson CC, Spector B, Klintworth GK: Incidence of ocular metastases in patients dying with cancer: An autopsy study (meeting abstr). Lab Invest 46(1):61A, 1982
5. Cade S: Presented at the annual scientific session of the American Cancer Society, Inc., New York, October, 1956
6. Thatcher N, Thomas PRM: Choroidal metastases from breast carcinoma: A survey of 42 patients and the use of radiation therapy. Clin Radiol 26:549, 1975
7. Rottinger EM, Heckemann R, Scherer E, et al: Radiation therapy of choroidal metastases from breast cancer. Albrecht V. Graefes Arch Klin Exp Ophthalmol 200:243, 1976
8. Brady LW, Shields JA, Augsburger JJ, et al: Malignant intraocular tumors. Cancer 49:578, 1982
9. Mewis L, Young SE: Breast carcinoma metastatic to the choroid: Analysis of 67 Patients. Ophthalmology 89(2):147, 1982
10. Chu FCH, Huh SH, Nisce LZ, et al: Radiation therapy of choroid metastasis from breast cancer. Int J Radiat Oncol Biol Phys XX(2):273, 1977
11. Maor M, Chan R, Young SE: Radiotherapy of choroidal metastases. Breast cancer as primary site. Cancer 40:2081, 1977
12. Dallow RL, Coleman DJ: Ultrasonic evaluation of orbital disorders. In Jakobiec FA (ed): Ocular and Adnexal Tumors, pp 311–340. Birmingham, Aesculapius, 1978
13. Hessselink JR, Davis KR, Weber AL, et al: Radiological evaluation of orbital metastases, with emphasis on computed tomography. Radiology 137:363, 1980
14. Sternberg P, Tiedeman J, Hickingbotham D, et al: Controlled aspiration of subretinal fluid in the diagnosis of carcinoma metastatic to the choroid. Arch Ophthalmol 102:1622, 1984
15. Orenstein MM, Andersonn DP, Stein JJ: Choroid metastases. Cancer 29:1101, 1972
16. Brinkley JE: Response of a choroidal metastasis to multiple-drug chemotherapy. Cancer 45:1538, 1980
17. Letson AD, Davidorf FH, Bruce RA: Chemotherapy for treatment of choroidal metastases from breast carcinoma. Am J Ophthalmology 93:102, 1982

Local Recurrence

Abram Recht Daniel F. Hayes

DEFINITION OF LOCAL RECURRENCE

The terms "local recurrence" and "local-regional recurrence" refer to the reappearance of breast cancer adjacent to or in areas previously treated by either mastectomy or local irradiation (with or without conservative surgical resection of the primary tumor). Authors differ on the exact sites they consider to constitute local recurrence. We will define local recurrence as being any reappearance of cancer in the ipsilateral breast, the chest wall, the skin overlying the chest wall, the ipsilateral axillary lymph nodes, the supraclavicular lymph nodes, the infraclavicular lymph nodes, or the internal mammary lymph nodes. An "isolated" (or "solitary") local recurrence refers to the reappearance of breast cancer in these areas in the absence of other disease on routine evaluation for metastases. Recurrence in the breast after primary radiation therapy carries with it a substantially different prognosis and treatment than local recurrence after mastectomy; hence, we will discuss local recurrence in these two patient groups separately.

LOCAL RECURRENCE FOLLOWING MASTECTOMY

Incidence of Local Recurrence

The incidence of local recurrence after definitive surgery depends on many factors, the most important of which appears to be the pathologic status of the axillary lymph nodes. The chance of a local relapse following radical mastectomy with pathologically negative axillary nodes is from 3% to 8%. Approximately two-thirds of these are isolated local recurrences, and the remainder are simultaneous with or follow the development of distant metastases. When the axillary lymph nodes are positive, however, the incidence of local relapse increases to 19% to 27%.[1–3] The chance of local recurrence also increases with the number of positive nodes. In two series, when eight or more nodes were involved the incidence of recurrence in the chest wall increased to 35% to 40% for Columbia Stage A and B patients.[1,3]

Other factors also influence the incidence of local recurrence. These include the size of the primary tumor, the histologic grade of the tumor, the presence of skin fixation or invasion clinically, invasion of the deep fascia, ulceration of the skin, and breast edema.[3–5] Pathologically positive internal mammary nodes are associated with an increase in the incidence of local recurrence, but the effect is minor when corrected for the presence of positive axillary lymph nodes.[6] Patients whose primary tumors are negative for estrogen receptors appear in one series to have a greater risk of axillary or supraclavicular nodal recurrence than patients with positive receptors. However, there is no difference between these groups in the incidence of chest wall recurrences.[7]

Whether the extent of the initial surgical procedure determines the rate of local recurrence has been highly controversial. Two randomized series comparing radical mastectomy with modified radical mastectomy have shown a trend toward an increased rate after modified radical mastectomy, although the differences did not reach statistical significance.[8,9] Various technical aspects of radical mastectomy, such as the size of the skin flaps, the thickness of the skin flaps, whether a skin graft is used or not, and the size of the resected skin margin, do not cause any substantial differences in the rate of chest wall or other forms of local recurrence.[3,4,10–16]

The use of postoperative radiation therapy after mastectomy substantially reduces the incidence of local recurrence in high-risk patients but (at least in the absence of effective adjuvant systemic therapy) does not appear to increase overall cure rates.[17] Although adjuvant chemotherapy alone does appear to improve survival, it decreases the incidence of local recurrence only minimally, if at all.[18]

Mechanisms of Local Recurrence

Numerous mechanisms have been proposed to explain local recurrence after mastectomy.[3,5,10–12] The recurrence of cancer in internal mammary, supraclavicular, infraclavicular, and axillary lymph nodes has been thought by most authors to represent residual cancer cells in unremoved nodes. Most local recurrences, however, are in the chest wall or the skin overlying it. There has been no widespread consensus concerning the many theories advanced for this. These theories have led to changes in treatment technique and philosophy, and hence the controversy surrounding them is of some importance.

Theories about chest wall recurrence fall into three categories: (1) Tumor cells are left on the surface of the chest wall or in the skin flaps at the time of mastectomy, including possible tumor implantation at the time of surgery due to the use of contaminated instruments or showers of tumor emboli ("inadequate surgery"); (2) Tumor cells continue to reside in intercostal lymphatics or the muscles of the chest wall after surgery and are beyond the reach of standard radical operations ("retrograde dissemination"); (3) Recurrence in the chest wall is simply another form of systemic spread from the primary tumor rather than a result of direct extension or lymphatic involvement ("hematogeneous spread").

Evidence in favor of the "inadequate surgery" hypothesis includes the difference in local recurrence rates between radical mastectomy and modified radical mastectomy.[8,9] However, as noted before, the recurrence rate does not appear to be influenced by the type of surgical closure or skin flap utilized. Even meticulous separation of the epidermis from dermal and subdermal tissues (the so-called "dermal dissection" technique) does not eliminate chest wall recurrences.[12] Moreover, the incidence of microscopic involvement of the skin or subcutaneous tissues in patients with operable breast cancer is low. In one study there were no malignant cells in 146 skin biopsies overlying the tumor,[19]; in another, 42 of 946 patients had microscopic involvement of the dermis or dermal lymphatics.[20] In neither study, however, was local recurrence found to correlate with the presence or absence of skin involvement. Similarly, the skin margins of mastectomy appear to make no difference to the likelihood of recurrence in the chest wall.[3,13,14]

The intercostal lymphatics are a known site of drainage of the breast. One study showed that 17 of 23 patients who died with breast cancer had disease in the chest wall.[21] Disease was situated in all levels of the deep fascial tissues, in the intercostal tissues, and in some of the endolymphatic spaces. However, as in all autopsy studies, this probably does not reflect the initial distribution of disease, because these 17 patients had widespread distant metastases as well. Only one patient initially relapsed with a local recurrence, and only one other patient had a clinical local recurrence at the time of death. Only one of the six patients studied who died without widespread metastases was found to have disease of the chest wall. Therefore, much of this chest wall involvement may represent late hematogeneous spread.

Almost all patients with local recurrence will also develop distant bloodborne metastases either before, simultaneously with, or after the development of a local recurrence (see below). Further, the time course to development of either distant metastases or local recurrence appears to be almost identical.[22] However, this would seem at least as likely to reflect a similarity in the growth rates of subclinical distant metastases and local recurrences as it would a common mechanism of spread from the primary tumor.

Presenting Symptoms and Signs of Local Recurrence

The first manifestation of local recurrence is usually an asymptomatic nodule in the axilla, in the supraclavicular fossa, or in or under the skin of the chest wall. A parasternal mass or occasionally an erythematous skin rash may also be the first sign. Approximately one-half of all local recurrences involve only the chest wall or the overlying skin. The axilla alone is involved in approximately 10% of patients. Isolated supraclavicular recurrences are rare in most series but account for 5% to 13% in some series.[23,24] Isolated parasternal recurrences will occur in 0% to 36% in most series. Infraclavicular recurrences are very unusual. Simultaneous recurrence in chest wall and lymph node sites will occur in approximately 30% of patients.[4–6,25,26] The distribution of recurrence sites appears similar whether radical mastectomy or modified radical mastectomy is performed.[27] Postoperative radiation therapy possibly decreases the ratio between the number of internal mammary and supraclavicular node recurrences (when these areas are treated) and the number of chest wall recurrences.[28,29] However, the total incidence of local recurrences after radiotherapy is small.

The number of separate nodules initially found on the chest wall is usually small. In one analysis of 60 patients, 62% had only a single nodule, 15% had two skin nodules, 13% had three or four nodules, and 10% had five or more nodules.[26] These nodules will usually be located in or near the scar of the mastectomy or skin graft, with most others in the skin flaps.[25,26] Some nodules appear to originate in the thoracic wall without direct involvement of the skin itself, probably as a result of intercostal lymphatic deposits.[12,25] A few patients will present with diffuse chest wall involvement with multiple nodules; this however seems most common in patients who had locally advanced tumors originally.[12]

Carcinoma en cuirasse is a distinct form of diffuse infiltration of the skin or subcutaneous tissues of the chest wall, with woody induration and spread of tumor well beyond the limits of standard surgical or radiation therapy boundaries (See Color Plate 6, Chapter 3). Nodules and ulcerations are often present. It was first described (and named) by Velpeau in 1838[1] and was again discussed at length by Billroth.[29a] They both observed that the natural history of carcinoma en cuirasse differs from that of other breast cancers: "... deposits in internal organs are late and restricted...; the total duration may vary from 3 to 6 or 8 years, or even longer."[29a] There are scant modern data available on this phenomenon, which now appears almost always to be a late development in the course of uncontrolled local recurrence or, rarely, untreated primary breast tumors. It is resistant to both local and systemic therapy.[30]

As is the case with distant metastases, approximately 80% to 90% of local recurrences will manifest themselves by 5 years after mastectomy, with almost all remaining recurrences occurring before the end of 10 years after surgery.[3,4,10,11,16,22,25,31–33] However, local recurrences 15 years and more after initial surgery are well known and have been previously summarized.[34] It is often difficult or impossible to show that these patients did not have a new primary tumor, but well-documented cases with intervals of 28 years,[11] 32 years,[34,35] and 37 years (personal communication, CD Haagensen) between mastectomy and local recurrence have been described. The longest reported interval is 50 years.[34] The time to local recurrence after mastectomy is affected by several factors: the type of surgery, with the interval being shorter after modified radical mastectomy as compared with radical mastectomy[27]; whether the axillary nodes were pathologically positive initially[1,2]; and the initial stage of the primary tumor.[1,26,36,37] The time to development of local recurrence after initial postoperative radiation therapy appears to be similar.[38]

Approximately one-quarter to one-third of patients with local recurrence will have had preceding distant metastases.[39–42] Another one-quarter of patients will develop distant metastases within a few months of the discovery of local recurrence.[26,39] Thus, only about one-half of these patients will have an "isolated" local recurrence. This appears true as well for patients whose first recurrence occurs more than 5 years after initial surgery.[43]

Subsequent Course and Prognosis After Development of Local Recurrence

At initial presentation, the majority of patients with local recurrences are asymptomatic. It is unclear how often patients would develop significant symptoms due to their local recurrence in the absence of any specific treatment. Most patients who do receive treatment will not suffer significant morbidity due to their local recurrence. In a group of 57 patients variously treated for local recurrence at the Lahey Clinic from 1965 to 1972, 42 of 57 patients (74%) had either no problems or only minor problems requiring minor outpatient care.[39] Despite treatment, local recurrence caused major problems requiring hospitalization or a change in treatment in 15 of 57 patients (26%). Local recurrence was, however, the direct cause of death in only one patient. Tumor penetrated the chest wall, resulting in an effusion and pneumothorax.[39] In a group of 100 patients with *uncontrolled* disease, 62 had one or more significant symptoms before death: 47 patients had bleeding or ulceration that required a daily dressing change; 17 patients had pain requiring narcotics; 7 patients had arm edema; and 3 patients had brachial plexus paralysis.[40] Thus, although local recurrence is rarely a cause of death in itself[44,45] and many patients will likely die before they have significant symptoms due to the local recurrence itself, a substantial group may suffer extremely distressing local complications that can be very difficult to manage.

The development of a local recurrence at one site often will be followed by recurrences in other chest wall or lymph node sites. From 1964 to 1977, 157 patients with isolated local recurrence were seen at the Mallinckrodt Institute, Washington University, St. Louis.[40] Because of changing treatment policies and different patient presentations, some patients received radiation only to small

Table 14-11
Sites of Further Local Recurrence

Site	No Radiotherapy	Elective Radiotherapy
Chest wall*	43% (17/40)	8% (1/13)
Supraclavicular nodes†	28% (17/60)	7% (2/28)
Axillary nodes	6% (5/78)	6% (2/31)
Internal mammary nodes	4% (3/82)	0% (0/36)

* $p < 0.02$ (chi-squared test)
† $p < 0.025$
(Adapted from Bedwinek JM, Fineberg B, Lee J, et al: Analysis of failures following local treatment of isolated local-regional recurrence of breast cancer. Int J Radiat Oncol Biol Phys 7:581–585, 1981)

fields encompassing the observable recurrence but others (usually patients with more extensive disease) were electively treated with radiation to larger fields including the entire chest wall and draining lymph nodes. A substantial proportion of patients treated with small fields developed a clinical recurrence in another local site. Large-field irradiation, however, prevented most of these subsequent recurrences (Table 14-11). Other series usually support[4,37,46,47] but occasionally refute[27] these findings. Thus, even patients with only small amounts of clinically evident disease may have fairly widespread subclinical deposits in the chest wall and regional lymph nodes.

Despite aggressive local treatment, almost all patients with an isolated local recurrence will eventually develop distant metastases. The 5-year overall survival rate is 0% to 50%, with 10-year survival from 0% to 26% (Table 14-12). The more recent series have higher survival rates, possibly because of better staging (excluding patients with occult distant metastases), as well as better systemic treatment (see below). The median survival time for patients with isolated local recurrence is 2 to 3 years. However, only a fraction of these survivors will be free from further disease altogether. In a series of patients treated from 1968 to 1978 at the Joint Center for Radiation Therapy (JCRT), 5- and 10-year actuarial survival rates were 50% and 26%, but freedom from distant metastases after local recurrence was 30% at 5 years and only 7% at 10 years.[48,49] It is yet unclear whether the use of systemic chemotherapy will improve the overall or disease-free survival times in these patients (see below). Occasional patients have enjoyed extraordinarily long disease-free intervals after treatment of local recurrence. Patients surviving without disease 15 years and 21 years[24] after treatment with radiation therapy have been described, and two patients are reported alive and without disease at 13 years[50] and 24 years[32] after radical surgical procedures following recurrence. Even these patients may ultimately succumb to breast cancer. Morton[35] describes a patient who had a local recurrence 16 years after treatment (and apparent cure) of a chest wall recurrence.

Several factors have been proposed as influencing the disease-free interval and length of survival time after the discovery and treatment of an isolated local recurrence. Among these are the interval between mastectomy and local recurrence, the initial stage of the tumor, the grade of the primary tumor, the initial extent of axillary nodal involvement,[31] the number and location of local sites involved at recurrence, whether the patient had treatment for a previous local recurrence, the effectiveness and type of local therapy, and the use of adjuvant systemic therapy. Many of these factors appear related and may reflect the biology of breast carcinomas more than treatment modalities (e.g., time to local recurrence, initial stage, and grade).[42] Multivariate statistical tests have rarely been used in the analysis of these factors. In the JCRT series, only a few of these could be examined because of the limitations of patient numbers and available information. The disease-free interval after mastectomy clearly influenced subsequent survival ($p = 0.002$, Cox regression analysis), but age, prior local recurrence, the type of mastectomy, and whether the recurrence could be completely excised did not (JCRT, unpublished data). The biologic and clinical heterogeneity of breast cancer, coupled with shifting treatment policies and techniques in the available studies, prevents drawing firm conclusions regarding the true impact of treatment on the history of patients with locally recurrent disease.

The grade of the primary tumor has been examined as an influence on prognosis in only one series. A group of 73 patients with isolated local recurrence seen at Guy's Hospital, London, from 1948 to 1975 were observed for a minimum of 8 years or until death.[42] Histologic slides could be reviewed in 65 cases. The average disease-free interval from mastectomy decreased with increasing grade, but the extent of recurrence (single or multiple nodules) was not changed by tumor grade. Actuarial survival at 5 years after local recurrence was 44% in grade 1, 36% in grade 2, and 0% in grade 3. These differences were statistically significant only between grades 1 and 3.

The interval between mastectomy and local recurrence is probably the most reliable indicator of the length of subsequent survival time, regardless of whether effective local or systemic therapy is used. This again may simply reflect the intrinsic growth rate of the tumor cells. Patients treated at the University of California at San Francisco from 1918 to 1947 who had a recurrence less than 2 years after mastectomy had a median survival of 13 months, compared with 31 months for those patients who had a recurrence from 2 to 5 years after surgery and 57.5 months (average, 64 months) for 12 patients who had a recurrence more than 5 years after surgery.[32] However, in another older series, the average survival of 45 patients whose initial isolated recurrence occurred 5 years or more after surgery was only 24 months (range, 3 to 72 months). Unfortunately, information was available for only 24 of the 45 patients.[25] The same trend is found in patients treated with aggressive radiation therapy. At the JCRT, the relapse-free survival at 3 years was 20% for 32 patients who had isolated local recurrence less than 24 months after initial surgery, compared with 36% in 58 patients who had isolated local recurrence at 24 months or longer after surgery.

Table 14-12
Survival Following Isolated Local Recurrence After Mastectomy

Institution	*Dates*	*Number of Patients*	*Median Survival (Months)*	*5-Year Survival*	*10-Year Survival*	*Authors*
Roswell Park	1958–61	13		0%		Dao and Nemoto[13]
UCSF	1918–47	98	23	10%		Shimkin et al[32]
Christie Hosp.	1949–55	81*	19	10%		Jackson [23]
MDAH	1944–77	60		18%	5%	Gilliland et al[26]
MSKCC	1950s–60s	215	30	21%	5%	Chu et al[24]
Athens Univ.	1968–76	150	24	26%		Karabali-Dalomaga et al[22]
Milan NCI	1955–65	120	24	28%		DiPietro et al[31]
Guy's Hosp.	1948–75	73	32	30%	13%	Fentiman et al[42]
Pittsburgh	1970–79	107		35%		Deutsch et al[53]
Mountain States Tumor Institute	1970–79	121		35% (20%)	23% (12%)	Beck et al[51]
Washington Univ.	1964–77	157	32	36%		Bedwinek et al[40]
Miami	1966–78	121	41	38% (26%)	26% (15%)	Toonkel et al[37]
JCRT	1968–78	90	60	50% (30%)	30% (7%)	Aberizk et al[48]

* All patients had recurrences only in the supraclavicular nodes.
Numbers in parentheses represent disease-free survival.

The respective 5-year survival rates were 33% versus 58%, and 10-year survival 7% versus 36%.[48,49] Similar results have been found in most[24,27,31,37,51–53] but not all[47] other radiotherapy series.

The initial surgical stage of the patient also influences the time of subsequent survival and development of distant metastases.[26,37,51] For example, one series shows 5-year survival rates of approximately 60%, 35%, and 15% for Stages I, II, and III patients, respectively.[51] Other series do not show this trend, however.[42,47] In addition, there appears to be a correlation between more advanced stage and the other factors that may influence survival after local recurrence, such as the overall time to isolated local recurrence, the grade of the tumor, and the number of local recurrences found at presentation.[42]

The presence of single or multiple sites of recurrence on the chest wall and draining lymph nodes may be prognostically significant, with superior 5- and 10-year survivals in patients who have only a single site of recurrence.[24,27,42] It is unclear whether the particular site of local recurrence (i.e., in lymph nodes alone, in the chest wall alone, in a combination of these, or in specific lymph nodes) rather than the total volume of disease plays a substantial role in prognosis. Although in some series patients with only chest wall disease have better survival rates than patients with isolated or concurrent involvement of the regional lymph nodes,[48,52,53] other series suggest the opposite[24,27] or no substantial difference.[47] Although the presence of recurrence in the supraclavicular lymph nodes is, in general, a grave sign, median and long-term survival after this event appears no different than in other patients with local recurrence,[47] and in fact a few long-term survivors have been reported.[23] In one series, 19 patients with isolated internal mammary node recurrences had a better prognosis than other patients (median disease-free interval, 60 months).[47]

There is little information about whether those patients who develop a local recurrence despite postmastectomy radiotherapy have a different prognosis after local recurrence than patients never irradiated. In one series, there was a trend toward decreased survival at 10 years (but not 5 years) in 36 patients who had previous radiation therapy (20%) as compared with 85 patients who had no radiation therapy before treatment of their isolated local recurrence (35%). However, the difference did not reach statistical significance.[37]

Other factors, such as the patient's age[48,49,52] and menopausal status,[31,42] have also not consistently been shown to affect prognosis after local recurrence. Prior adjuvant chemotherapy also does not worsen prognosis or response to local treatment.[52,54]

In view of the many variables that may influence outcome, evaluating the effectiveness of either local or systemic therapies from the available retrospective studies is very difficult. No prospective randomized studies have been conducted to show whether such interventions will change ultimate survival rates or the time course of distant recurrence. These problems will be examined in greater detail below.

PRETREATMENT EVALUATION

Occasionally, other benign or malignant conditions may mimic a local recurrence. The most common of these is a foreign body cyst around suture material. Sometimes a bony nodule develops on a rib or costal cartilage as a result of surgical trauma.[1] Radiation-induced sarcomas of the bones or soft tissues of the chest wall usually appear 8 or more years after postoperative treatment.[55] Although quite rare, this diagnosis must be considered in irradiated patients.[56]

We believe that a biopsy should be obtained in all cases of suspected local recurrence, both in order to establish the diagnosis and also to obtain tissue for estrogen and progesterone receptor assays. Several authors suggest that the estrogen receptor status of the primary tumor and that of subsequent metastases will be the same in only 75% to 85% of patients.[57,58] Intervening hormonal therapy may account for these phenotypic changes by selecting for cells that are estrogen receptor negative.[57] However, such disconcordance can occur without intervening therapy.

CT scanning of the chest wall may show areas of previously unexpected tumor, which may alter planned radiation fields or the overall goals and means of treatment. Twenty-one of 42 patients (50%) with chest wall or nodal recurrences examined at the Massachusetts General Hospital had additional sites of involvement discovered only on CT scan.[59] The most common site of unsuspected disease was in the internal mammary nodes (12 of 33 patients with only clinical chest wall involvement). None of these was definitely observable on chest x-ray film. Other sites of disease detected *only* on CT scan included sternal erosion (three patients, all with internal mammary node disease), mediastinal adenopathy (three patients), axillary adenopathy (two patients), rib metastasis (one patient), and brachial plexus root and chest wall involvement (one patient). Fishman and associates[60] found unsuspected axillary node involvement in 7 of 25 patients studied with CT scan. Four of these 25 patients had contralateral axillary involvement. The incidence of such findings in *unselected* patients with isolated local recurrence, and hence the overall value of CT scans in treatment planning, is at present uncertain. Clearly, however, even preliminary reports of this sort imply strongly that the CT scan should be routinely used in pretreatment evaluation.

The patient should also have a complete restaging to find occult distant metastases, which may be present in a substantial number of patients.

The use of circulating tumor markers for the diagnosis and evaluation of patients with breast cancer has been of great interest. Circulating levels of carcinoembryonic antigen (CEA) are elevated in 35% to 70% of patients with metastatic or recurrent breast cancer.[61–63] The CEA value tends to reflect the total disease burden and, perhaps, sites of metastases.[64] Elevated levels of CEA are observed less frequently in patients with isolated local recurrences than in patients with metastatic disease.[61–64] Thus, an elevated CEA value suggests the possibility of occult distant metastases and is an indication for thorough restaging. Serial changes in initially elevated CEA values can be useful in monitoring the course of disease.[64–66] Other circulating tumor-related molecules have also been proposed as markers for breast cancer (see Chapter 5). None of these has yet gained widespread clinical utility. Recently, investigators have reported the presence of components of the human milk fat globule in the sera of breast cancer patients. These antigens are easily detectable with monoclonal antibodies. One such antigen, detected with the monoclonal antibody DF3, is elevated in 75% of all patients with metastatic breast cancer.[67] Changes in levels correspond to the clinical course of the patient. Like CEA, DF3 levels are not frequently elevated in patients with evidence of only local recurrence. Investigations are currently under way to increase the sensitivity, and hence the clinical utility, of such assays.

TREATMENT OF LOCAL RECURRENCE

Radiation Therapy

As noted above, effective local treatment may have an enormous impact on the overall quality of a patient's life after the appearance of an isolated local recurrence. Numerous series of patients treated for local recurrence with radiation therapy have been published (Table 14-13). In general, most patients have complete regression of disease initially. However, a disappointingly large number have suffered a further appearance of disease within the treated area or, if not treated prophylactically, in adjacent untreated sites. For example, the actuarial 5-year sustained local control rate was only 43% in the JCRT series.[48,49] Differences in patient populations and analysis make comparisons of these published series difficult. However, they do appear to indicate which radiotherapy techniques, fields, and doses are likely to be most effective.

Patients with a recurrence in one portion of the chest wall or draining lymph node areas are likely to develop a further local recurrence if treatment is not given to the entire chest wall and all draining nodes, as discussed above (see also Table 14-11). When large fields are used, the majority of subsequent local failures will be in the radiation fields, or "re-recurrences" (29 of 39 in the JCRT series), with most of these in-field failures being at the original site of disease (25 of 29).[49] In general, the higher the dose of radiation delivered, the less likely the patient is to have an in-field recurrence.[24,27,40,68] The volume of disease being treated is also important. As shown in Table 14-13, patients in whom disease can be completely excised have a higher rate of in-field control than those with residual disease on the chest wall. Nonetheless, doses of at least 4500 centiGray (cGy) are required even in the setting of complete excision of disease in order to achieve reasonably low rates of in-field recurrence. When gross residual disease is present, boost treatment to the local area to more than 6000 cGy is needed. Hence for most patients, dose to the entire chest wall and draining lymph nodes of 4500 to 5000 cGy in 4 1/2 to 5 weeks appears reasonable, followed by a boost to areas of previous gross residual disease to a total dose of 6000 to 6500 cGy, depending on the exact circumstances of the individual patient.

Even when large fields are used, failures in the adjacent chest wall or other areas at the edges of the fields

Table 14-13
Effectiveness of Radiation Therapy in Treatment of Local Recurrence After Mastectomy

Institution	Dates	Number of Patients	Initial CR	Further Local Recurrence: Total	Proportion In-Field	Authors
Ellis Fischel	1940–58	24	79%			Donegan et al[3]
MDAH	1956–81	194		36%	75%	Chen et al[47]
MSKCC	1950s–60s	215	67%			Chu et al[24]
Maryland	1963–77	102		44%		Patanaphan et al[27]
Washington Univ.	1964–77	132		61%	70%	Bedwinek et al[40]
Miami	1966–78	124		31%*	66%	Chen et al[47]
JCRT	1968–1978	90	97%	45%†	73%	Aberizk et al[49]
Pittsburgh	1970–79	107	79%	44%		Deutsch et al[53]
Mountain States Tumor Institute	1970–79	43	63%			Beck et al[51]
Thomas Jefferson	1972–80	72	71%	54%‡	74%	Danoff et al[52]

CR: complete response.
All proportions are crude. Further local recurrence is based on patients with CR.
* Actuarial 10-year total recurrence rate (of CRs): 54%.
† Actuarial 5-year and 10-year: 61% and 68%.
‡ Actuarial 3-year: 65%.

Table 14-14
Radiation Dose, Extent of Surgery, and Chance of In-Field Recurrence

Dose (cGy)	Complete Excision	Gross Residual Tumor
≤4000	50% (10/20)	73% (32/44)
4001–4500	12% (1/8)	50% (8/16)
4501–5000	0% (0/16)	39% (14/36)
>5000	0% (0/2)	17% (3/18)

(Adapted from Bedwinek JM, Fineberg R, Lee J, et al: Analysis of failures following local treatment of isolated local-regional recurrence of breast cancer. Int. J Radiat Oncol Biol Phys 7:581–585, 1981)

can occur. These "marginal misses" appear to be more likely in patients with the larger or more numerous recurrences. In the JCRT series, nine of ten marginal misses were located on the adjacent chest wall (one was nodal). In patients with complete excisional biopsy of their recurrences (i.e., who had small amounts of disease), the incidence of marginal misses was 1 of 29; for the remaining patients, the incidence was 9 of 58.[49]

Thus, the volume of disease probably influences relapse both inside and outside the fields. The actuarial 5-year total local failure rate (both in-field and out-of-field) in the JCRT series (in patients who received doses of 4000 cGy or higher) was 43% for patients who could have complete excision versus 76% for those who could not ($p = 0.03$).[49]

The ability to achieve local control with radiotherapy also appears to be related to the specific sites involved. Most series show higher local control rates when only the chest wall or lymph nodes are involved, rather than both.[47,49] Survival rates are also lower when multiple sites are involved.[53] Some series show that local control is also easier to achieve for supraclavicular or internal mammary node disease than chest wall or axillary disease,[47] but this finding is not universal.[49] Recurrences in the mastectomy scar itself may be harder to eradicate than other chest wall recurrences.[37] Control of inflammatory-type skin recurrences may also be difficult (personal communication, ED Montague).

Orthovoltage techniques are clearly outmoded because of the enormous dose given to the skin relative to the deeper tissues. There are no clear differences in local control between the different megavoltage photon or electron treatment techniques, and the selection of these is probably dictated by individual preference and facilities.

At the JCRT, we employ 4- or 6-MV photons (or, for patients with large chest walls, 8-MV photons occasionally) using the same corner-block technique used for primary radiation therapy of the intact breast (for appropriate references, see Chapter 10). Radionuclide lymphoscintigraphy or CT scan is employed to localize the internal mammary nodes; if these are not available, the fields are extended 3 cm across the midline. The lateral border of the tangential fields is usually at the midaxillary line. However, if tumor is located close to this edge, then it may be wise to move the border posteriorly. The placement of the matchline between the tangential and supraclavicular/axillary fields must also be done carefully, as it is preferable to avoid putting this in an area of gross disease. Although we prefer to use bolus over the chest wall every day so that the skin receives a full dose of radiation, this may be impossible because of skin reaction. At a minimum, gross lesions should be covered with bolus. Boosts are usually done with electrons, making sure to cover the entire depth of the lesion. Occasionally orthovoltage, molds, or implants may be technically advantageous. Many patients at the JCRT were treated in past years with 225-cGy fractions given four times weekly. Although this technique is effective, these patients often developed significant telangiectasia and skin fibrosis. Therefore, we now recommend 180-cGy to 200-cGy fractions given five times weekly.

Treatment can also be given with electron beams alone. At the M.D. Anderson Hospital, several large fields are matched to one another and irradiated with 7-MeV or 9-MeV electrons.[69] The use of lower-energy electrons has sometimes resulted in avoidable parasternal recurrences.[47] Because the thickness of the chest wall varies considerably, CT scanning is very helpful in avoiding misses of this sort while also minimizing the amount of lung irradiated.[70] In the past, doses of 5000 cGy to 5500 cGy in 4 weeks were given, followed by 1000-cGy to 1500-cGy boosts.[69] At present, such patients are treated with twice-daily fractions of 150 cGy to a dose of 4500 cGy in 3 weeks, with a boost of 1500 cGy, also given with twice-daily fractionation. (Bolus is applied to the chest wall during every treatment when photons are used.) Because of the potential complications, the previously dissected axilla is *not* irradiated unless clinically involved or at high risk of recurrence (Personal communication, ED Montague). Techniques using electron arcs or rotational motions have also been described.[68,71,72]

The incidence of complications after radiation therapy for local recurrence is difficult to estimate because of the often limited life expectancy of patients and the confounding effects of persistent or recurrent local disease. Such information has only rarely been reported. In a group of 82 patients who had recurrences in lymph nodes and received 6000 cGy to 7000 cGy to small areas, one patient suffered radionecrosis leading to a surgical resection, two patients had soft tissue necrosis, and one patient had a symptomatic rib fracture (total incidence of moderate to severe complications, 5%).[46] In another series, 4 of 63 patients (6%) developed chest wall ulcers, but two patients had undergone previous radiation therapy, and two of these four patients died less than 2 months after treatment.[68]

There is little information on re-treating patients after postoperative chest wall radiation or previous radiation therapy for recurrences. In one series, 36 patients who had previous radiation therapy had lower rates of local control (36% versus 68%) and survival at 10 years (20% versus 35%) than 88 patients with no previous radiation therapy. These differences were not statistically significant, however.[37] Chen and colleagues[47] report similar findings. Patients in these two series did not, however, undergo re-irradiation of previously treated areas because of fear of complications. (Interestingly though, no nodal failures were seen in 28 patients who had postmastectomy elective irradiation of only lymph nodes.[47]) No evidence of soft tissue necrosis was seen in 13 patients re-treated with an additional 4000 cGy to 6000 cGy in 4 to 6 weeks using electrons, after previously receiving 4000 cGy to 5000 cGy to the entire chest wall.[73] The electron field sizes were not reported, though. Although 9 of 13 patients were described as having local control for their remaining lifetime or follow-up, one of these patients died 6 months after treatment and three of the remaining eight had further chest wall recurrences outside the re-treated volume. Another group of seven patients who had previous postoperative radiation therapy were re-treated with 4-MeV to 6-MeV electrons to small fields, giving a dose of 4000 cGy to 5000 cGy, sometimes with a 1000-cGy to 1500-cGy boost.[74] They were also treated with an aggressive regimen of skin grafting, silver nitrate, and dressings to control local disease. Some patients received hormonal therapy or chemotherapy. Two of seven patients were alive without evidence of disease 2.5 to 15 years after treatment, and all patients had control of pain. At death or last follow-up, five of nine patients had a complete response to treatment with full healing of the chest wall, and eight of nine patients had stable or controlled disease. One patient suffered osteomyelitis. Most patients had only mild complications, which were slow to resolve, however. Thus, the role of re-treatment of patients who received prophylactic postmastectomy radiation therapy is not well established. However, for selected patients with significant local symptoms, re-treatment with moderate to high doses with small fields may be warranted.

Local control of isolated local recurrences is more difficult to achieve when previous local excision or low-dose radiotherapy only has been tried and has failed.[49] The ability to attain local control is not affected by whether a patient has received postmastectomy adjuvant chemotherapy.[52] (The role of systemic therapy given at the time of recurrence in improving local control will be discussed below.)

Finally, does aggressive radiotherapy change the natural history or outcome in these patients? Some series suggest that patients who achieve a complete response or maintain local control after aggressive radiotherapy for an isolated local recurrence have longer survival times than patients who do not.[24,47,51,52] However, neither survival nor freedom from distant metastases was so affected for patients treated at the JCRT.[49] Many factors that affect whether local control can be achieved, such as tumor bulk and number of sites involved, probably also reflect the likely length of survival. Hence, although effective local treatment alone may increase survival time, this is by no means certain, and even those patients who achieve local control will almost certainly die of distant metastases eventually.

Surgery

The role of either local or radical forms of surgery in patients with isolated local recurrences is difficult to evaluate. Obviously, only individuals with relatively circumscribed lesions can be considered for definitive surgical procedures. Even wide local excision (in conjunction with radiotherapy) can be used in only about one-third of patients.[49]

Local Excision

Local control with radiotherapy appears to be improved in patients who can undergo complete local excisions.[40,49] However, local excision *alone* has been used in only a few patients, and the details are not usually well described (Table 14-15). In selected patients, local excision alone sometimes yields long-term local control and, rarely, long survival time free of further recurrences. As discussed above, since local control with radiotherapy may be harder to achieve in the setting of re-recurrence after limited surgery, the use of complete local excision alone appears warranted only rarely.

Radical Surgery

Radical resection for chest wall recurrences has been practiced since the late 19th century but did not come into wide use until the late 1940s.[50,75] The full thickness of the chest wall is removed en bloc, including the parietal pleura and sometimes a portion of or (occasionally) the entire sternum. The resulting defect may sometimes be closed primarily, but more often some form of covering or graft is needed. This has been done with ox fascia, Marlex mesh, a full-thickness skin flap, a pedicle or rotated flap from the other breast, a latissimus dorsi myocutaneous flap, a rectus abdominus myocutaneous flap, a pectoralis flap, omentum covered with a skin graft, or the diaphragm.[76–81] For selected patients, local control is usually obtained, with a number of patients surviving 5 years or more (Table 14-16). Survival time appears longer in patients in whom chest wall resection is used as the initial treatment of a local recurrence than in patients who are treated because of persistent disease after irradiation.[76] Since the group initially chosen to receive radiotherapy is likely to contain the larger or more aggressive tumors, the significance of this observation for treatment selection is not clear.

Complication rates are described as low in experienced hands but are only rarely reported in detail. In a recent series of 43 patients who underwent chest wall resection for breast cancer (33 patients) and/or the complications of prior treatment (28 patients), 4 patients (9%) required operative revisions, 12 patients (28%) had minor wound problems, and 2 deaths occurred within 1 month of surgery (1 from pulmonary embolus and 1 from respiratory failure). No flail chests were seen.[77] Five of 26 patients (who received postoperative chest wall irradiation) in another series developed small areas of necrosis at the edges of their flaps, and these healed with conservative treatment.[81]

Clearly, patients who undergo radical chest wall resections must be carefully selected from the entire group of patients with local recurrence. Few patients will probably be best served with such treatment. Nonetheless, such surgery appears to be a useful form of treatment and palliation for patients in whom more conservative measures have failed. Most authors recommend that only patients with a life expectancy of 1 year or more be submitted

Table 14-15
Results of Complete Excision Alone for Local Recurrence After Mastectomy

Institution	*Dates*	*Number of Patients*	*Local Control*	*Survival*	*Authors*
MDAH	1944–77	15	43%	2-yr: 53%	Tough[36]
Ellis Fischel	1948–58	15	27%	1/15, 17 mo	Donegan et al[3]
Washington Univ.	1964–77	25	24%	?	Bedwinek et al[40]
Mountain States Tumor Institute	1970–79	11	27%	1/11, 118 mo	Beck et al[51]

Table 14-16
Results of Chest Wall Resection for Local Recurrence After Mastectomy

Institution	*Dates*	*Number of Patients*	*Local Control*	*Survival Rate*	*Authors*
Mayo Clinic	1945–61	76	75%	5-yr: 18%	Snyder et al[50]
MSKCC	1950–72	47	?	5-yr: 31%	Shah and Urban[76]
MDAH	1977–82	32	88%	40-mo: 9%	McKenna et al[77]

for operation. However, the presence of distant metastases, in itself, is not an absolute contraindication to surgery.

Systemic Therapy

Systemic Therapy and Survival

Although several mechanisms of local recurrence have been proposed, most studies suggest that, for nearly all patients, local relapse follows or is soon followed by the appearance of disseminated disease. The recent success of adjuvant chemotherapy in improving both disease-free survival time and overall survival time in premenopausal women with nodal metastases at the time of primary breast cancer therapy has been encouraging.[18] Thus, the use of chemotherapy or hormonal therapy has been proposed for women rendered locally disease free after local recurrence.[27,82–84] However, no controlled clinical trials have been conducted to investigate this question in patients with an isolated local recurrence. Investigators at M.D. Anderson Hospital have suggested that local control, distant disease-free survival, and overall survival time all are significantly improved in patients treated with Adriamycin-containing regimens plus radiotherapy or surgery, compared with historical controls treated with chemotherapy or radiotherapy alone.[85] The addition of chemotherapy to irradiation increased the 5-year survival rate to 56%, from 42% for irradiation alone. The respective disease-free survival rates were 37% and 26%. Although the differences are statistically significant, fewer patients in the combined-modality treatment group (15%) than in the radiotherapy-only group (36%) had four or more positive lymph nodes. Interestingly, the survival rate was similar in a group of patients with isolated visceral metastases, also treated with aggressive chemotherapy and surgery or radiotherapy at M.D. Anderson Hospital, but not in a group of patients with bone metastases.[84] In another series, patients with local relapse who received radiotherapy only were compared with a second group who were treated with either chemotherapy (12 patients) or hormonal therapy (30 patients).[51] The group treated with radiotherapy had clearly superior local control. However, the group receiving systemic therapy enjoyed an improved overall 5-year survival rate (35% versus 13%) and disease-free survival rate (23% versus 5%) compared with 43 patients treated with radiotherapy alone. Patients were selected for treatment in a nonrandom manner, however.

Several considerations argue against the routine use of adjuvant systemic treatment in this setting. These include the absence of efficacy in several subgroups in the primary breast cancer adjuvant trials,[18] the potential acute and chronic toxicity of systemic therapy (especially chemotherapy), and the often prolonged survival time after only local treatment of breast cancer relapse (see Table 14-12). Some authors suggest that patients who have metastatic breast cancer and who are treated with intensive chemotherapy enjoy a prolonged survival time and that a certain number of them are cured,[86] but most investigators disagree.[87] Whether adjuvant systemic therapy following eradication of local breast cancer relapses can prolong disease-free or overall survival time is an intriguing question. Because so many variables can influence survival in these patients, this would be best answered by a large, multi-institutional, randomized, stratified trial with control arms offering no systemic treatment.

Systemic Therapy and Local Control

So far, no data clearly show that the use of adjuvant chemotherapy or hormonal therapy in addition to radiotherapy at the time of local recurrence markedly increases or lengthens local control. However, small improvements in local control so produced have been described. In one recent report, radiotherapy alone resulted in local control in 52% of 73 patients, whereas combined radiotherapy and Adriamycin-containing chemotherapy yielded 66% local control in 49 patients.[85] Eleven patients in another series were treated with large-field radiation therapy to doses of greater than 4500 cGy, and also with hormonal therapy or chemotherapy.[41] The lifetime local control in this small group was 73%. Both series are retrospective, and differences in patient population and selection make these findings hard to interpret. One small randomized study has shown improved local control from the concurrent use of actinomycin D and irradiation.[88] Local control was reported as 80% (12 of 15) when chemotherapy was given, as opposed to 59% (10 of 17) when it was not. Similar results were seen in a nonrandomized group of 124 patients. However, the median follow-up in this series was only 15 to 18 months, and radiotherapy field sizes were not described. Thus, although systemic chemotherapy may improve local control when given in combination with radiotherapy, at present such effects, if real, appear to be modest.

Very little information is available on the ability of systemic chemotherapy or hormonal therapy to control local disease without the use of radiotherapy or surgery. Bedwinek and colleagues[40] reported lifetime local control in 2 of 7 patients who received various chemotherapeutic agents; however, 23 other patients who received only chemotherapy were not evaluable.. The Southwest Oncology Group treated 53 patients with local recurrence with Adriamycin or cyclosphosphamide-Adriamycin-fluorouracil combinations, without irradiation.[89] Complete response was obtained in 34%, and partial response in 28% of patients. The duration of these responses is not given. Response rates (complete plus partial) of local disease to various hormonal manipulations have been reported in 30% to 40% of patients in older series, in which hormone-receptor levels were not known.[3,16,26] The median duration of response ranges from 8 to 19 months[3,16,51]; Bedwinek and colleagues[40] found that 4 of 11 patients had lifetime local control. One study showed a surprisingly high complete response rate of 64% and partial response rate of 21% in 42 patients treated with either chemotherapy (12 patients) or hormone therapy (30 patients), with 6 patients still in complete response at 3 years.[51] In general, however, systemic treatment alone is unlikely to cause local disease to regress permanently.

Hyperthermia

Hyperthermia has been used deliberately in the treatment of human malignancies for as long as radiotherapy has.[90] However, the success of ionizing radiation and the primitive technology available for hyperthermia hampered the progress of the latter until the past two decades. Quantitative investigations of the biologic responses to hyperthermia, coupled with progress in the technical delivery of therapeutic thermal radiation, have recently stimulated a number of studies that suggest that this modality may hold great promise for the treatment of human malignancies.[91–92] Not only is hyperthermia cytotoxic when applied alone, but its lethal effects are synergistic with ionizing radiation and certain drugs.[91,92]

Manning and colleagues[93] observed that 11 of 14 patients (79%) with metastatic adenocarcinoma of the chest wall, of whom 7 had breast cancer, achieved either complete or partial response with external heat alone, external heat in combination with radiotherapy, or hyperthermia given as interstitial thermoradiotherapy. The complication rate was 5% to 10%. Jabboury and colleagues[94] used ultrasonic energy delivery in 30 patients, all of whom had locally recurrent or advanced breast carcinoma. They observed complete responses in 15%, partial responses in 33%, and minor regressions in 33% in a population of heavily pretreated patients. Interestingly, several patients received concurrent chemotherapy, but tumor regression was observed only in the area of hyperthermia. The Radiation Therapy Oncology Group has studied the combination of hyperthermia and 6000 cGy to 6600 cGy of radiation.[95] Recently this has been reported to cause complete regression in 88% of 33 patients with locally recurrent adenocarcinoma of the breast.[96] Five of seven evaluable patients remain free of disease at 30 months. Again, severe thermal blisters and poorly healing skin ulcers were observed in 5% to 10% of patients in these two studies.

In summary, hyperthermia is a promising modality for the treatment of locally recurrent breast cancer. The optimal means of delivery is not yet determined. The best results may be achieved when hyperthermia is combined with either radiotherapy or chemotherapy. The incidence of severe complications, including thermal burns and tumor necrosis with ulceration, is currently 5% to 10%. Whether hyperthermia will improve local control rates over what can be achieved by high-dose, large-field radiotherapy alone is unclear. Much longer observation of these patients is needed. Studies to answer these questions are in progress.[91] The use of hyperthermia for the treatment of locally recurrent breast cancer should be considered investigational pending the results of these trials.

Topical and Miscellaneous Treatments

Meticulous topical treatments may provide adequate control of local infections and pain. The use of 0.5% silver nitrate-soaked dressing with local debridement and skin grafts has been described elsewhere.[74] Such aggressive local management, similar to the management of burn patients, may palliate symptoms in many patients for their remaining life. Local infections can also be vigorously treated with frequent changes of povidine or saline-wetted gauze bandages. Broad-spectrum oral antibiotics may be helpful. Metronidazole has been effective in treating foul-smelling ulcerated lesions, suggesting the involvement of anaerobic organisms.[97]

The use of superficial laser therapy has been reported for 31 patients with 87 sites of recurrent breast cancer.[98] Treatment was given with a pulsed laser of wavelength 1016 nm, with a fluence of 300 to 450 joules/cm^2, depending on the depth of recurrence. All sites of treatment were free of further relapse from 6 months to 3 years after exposure. None of these patients had involvement of the muscles or deeper structures of the chest wall, however.

"Photoradiation therapy," using hematoporphyrin derivatives as a photosensitizing agent for high-intensity xenon arc lamps or lasers (wavelengths 600 to 700 nm), has also been employed in patients with local recurrences.[99–101] The initial response rates are excellent (34 of 35 patients in one series); however, with longer observation a large number of these patients may have in-field recurrences (10 of 16 evaluable patients).[99] Some patients can be successfully re-treated in this event. Photoradiation therapy can, however, cause considerable pain, which may prevent the completion of treatment.[99] The advantages of photoradiation therapy over laser treatment alone, if any, are unclear from the available data.

RECOMMENDATIONS FOR TREATMENT OF LOCAL RECURRENCES FOLLOWING MASTECTOMY

There are no controlled, well-conducted, prospective clinical trials involving treatment of isolated local recurrences that are comparable to those that have been so valuable in determining the management of primary tumors. Hence, these guidelines represent only one of many possible approaches to the treatment of these patients.

For the overwhelming majority of patients, local recurrence following mastectomy unfortunately will be accompanied by either preexisting, simultaneous, or later development of distant metastases. Currently, only a handful of patients who develop isolated local recurrence may be eventually cured of their breast cancer through aggressive local treatment alone. Many patients, however, may live for years after local recurrence, especially if they had small primary tumors, a long interval between primary therapy and local recurrence, and minimal local disease at recurrence. The side effects of uncontrolled local recurrence may be unbearable, although only rarely will they lead directly to the death of the patient. Hence, we believe that aggressive treatment of local recurrences after mastectomy is reasonable in those patients in whom there is no evidence of distant metastases. Patients who instead are first treated with systemic chemotherapy or hormonal therapy (or with observation alone) should be carefully observed for progression of local disease, since local control with radiotherapy is probably easier when the local tumor burden is minimal. Radiation therapy should encompass the entire chest wall and the internal mammary and supraclavicular lymph nodes. Treatment of the dissected axilla may cause an increase in the likelihood of arm edema, and this risk must be weighed against the potential benefits for each patient. When an axillary recurrence is present or the chances of it are substantial, such therapy is undoubtedly warranted. Other cases are less clear-cut. A chest CT scan is useful in planning treatment because of the chance of unsuspected bilateral internal mammary node or sternal involvement. It is also useful in examining other sites of occult disease. Initial doses of 4500 cGy to 5000 cGy in conventional fractionation are appropriate, with a boost of 1000 cGy to 1500 cGy to areas of gross disease and biopsy scars. Complete local excision of the recurrences, if feasible, appears to increase the likelihood of long-term local control with lower radiation doses, but only a minority of patients will qualify for such resection. Previously irradiated patients can be retreated only with small fields. Local control is less likely, and complication rates higher, than for patients not previously irradiated. However, re-treatment may be of benefit to selected patients.

Whether systemic chemotherapy or hormonal therapy will ultimately increase the length of disease-free or overall survival time in patients with isolated local recurrences is not yet sufficiently established. However, preliminary results of such use of combination chemotherapy are encouraging. The use of systemic treatment with radiotherapy appears warranted in patients with isolated local recurrence in an investigational setting. These candidates must be willing to tolerate the potential side effects of these modalities and must understand the limitations of current knowledge of the final results of such treatment.

In patients who develop distant metastases before or concurrently with local recurrence, whose life expectancy is limited, it is less clear that the benefits of palliative radiation therapy outweigh its costs. We prefer to treat these patients with chemotherapy or hormonal therapy as indicated for their systemic metastases, reserving radiation therapy for patients with progressive local symptoms or perhaps for the occasional patient with a complete response to systemic treatment and long disease-free interval after mastectomy. Hormonal therapy and chemotherapy alone will not usually lead to permanent control of local disease, however.

Complete local excision of lesions without radiation therapy may occasionally result in long-term control and may enhance the quality of life but in general will not prevent further local recurrences. Radical chest wall resection is sometimes warranted for palliation and also, perhaps, in an attempt to cure selected patients. It is unclear what role, if any, chest wall resection should play in the *initial* management of the patient with an isolated local recurrence because the same results are probably achieved with fewer risks by aggressive radiation therapy. For patients who have had previous high-dose irradiation, however, the use of chest wall resection as the initial management of localized disease seems reasonable. Such surgery should be performed only by a surgical team familiar with the approach.

Finally, meticulous nursing care of the chest wall and judicious use of antibiotics may substantially relieve pain and decrease the rate of infection in these patients when no specific therapy for their breast cancer remains. New treatment techniques such as hyperthermia, laser excision, and photoradiation therapy are promising potential adjuncts to conventional treatment, but their true usefulness is still largely unknown.

LOCAL RECURRENCE FOLLOWING PRIMARY RADIATION THERAPY

Incidence of Local Recurrence

The incidence of local recurrence after primary radiation therapy for breast cancer depends on many factors. These include whether a complete gross excision of the primary tumor is performed, the extent of surgery in the breast, the histologic features of the primary tumor, the radiation dose to the entire breast and the region of the primary tumor, and the radiotherapy technique used. (For details, see Chapter 10.) For patients with clinical Stage I–II breast cancer in whom a "lumpectomy" or larger excision is performed, the local recurrence rate at 5 years in most series is 5% to 10%, [102–110] with a range of 2%[111] to 20%.[112,113]

The incidence of recurrence in the breast in patients treated without excisional biopsy is substantially higher, ranging from about 30% at 5 years[102,103] to 40% or 50% at 10 years[105,112] for patients with clinical Stage II cancers. Recurrence rates may be higher yet for patients with Stage III breast cancers.[105,112] Recurrence of the primary tumor or, possibly, the appearance of a new primary tumor has been seen up to at least 15 years after treatment.[114,115] The risk of breast recurrence in these series with a minimum 15-year follow-up appears fairly constant through this interval. However, these patients were treated with techniques somewhat different from those used at present, and the time course to local recurrence may be different for patients treated more recently with more effective methods, such as iridium implants.[107]

In the great majority of patients with a local relapse after primary radiation therapy, tumor will reappear only in the breast, rather than in lymph nodes or on or in the chest wall. Approximately 5% of patients will simultaneously have clinically evident axillary nodes. Pathologic involvement of the axilla is observed in a few additional patients on mastectomy.[102,107] Isolated axillary recurrences will be seen in at most 1% to 2% of patients in series in which most or all patients undergo axillary dissection.[102,105,110,116] The role of axillary irradiation in preventing this, in addition to the axillary dissection, is not clear. Supraclavicular recurrences have been reported but are rare.[105,113] Recurrences in the skin overlying the breast without an underlying mass have been found in two JCRT patients[102] and also in other series.[113] Isolated or concomitant parasternal recurrences are exceedingly uncommon at the JCRT (1 of 525 patients).[102] Unlike the situation following mastectomy, local recurrence after the development of distant metastases in patients treated initially with primary radiation therapy is rare, with only three such patients in the experience of the JCRT.[103] (The true incidence may be higher than we have observed, as careful examination of the breast and follow-up mammograms are often not performed after patients develop distant metastases.)

As discussed extensively in the chapter on primary radiation therapy for breast cancer, we believe that most relapses in the breast are due to a failure to control the primary tumor. However, failures in other quadrants of the breast are seen, especially with continued observation.[103,116,117] We believe these may represent new primary tumors.

Presenting Symptoms and Signs of Local Recurrence

Primary radiation therapy may cause changes in physical examination, such as thickening and masslike regions of fibrosis, which may be difficult to distinguish from a local recurrence.[118] The radiologic changes taking place in the treated breast are highly variable but often include skin edema, thickening of the fibroglandular and suspensory apparatus of the breast, the appearance of coarse calcifications, and occasionally, the appearance of a mass-like effect. Changes on mammogram usually stabilize within 4 months to a year after treatment.[119–121] Malignant-appearing changes, such as a mass or microcalcifications, may also occasionally be seen.[122] It may therefore be necessary to biopsy patients in whom there is a question of recurrence. We have found that open biopsies of greater than 1 ml in volume have a false-negative rate of 3% (1 of 31 cases), as opposed to 14% (2 of 14) for smaller biopsies (mostly needle biopsies). A modest-sized open biopsy (1 to 10 ml appears reasonable) does not appear to create complications or worsen cosmetic results.[122]

There have been 40 recurrences in the treated breast, as the first site of failure, in a series of 536 breast cancers treated from 1968 to 1980 at the JCRT, with median follow-up of 51 months.[102] Most of these (30 of 38 evaluable patients, or 79%) were detectable by physical examination. In 22 cases, a mass was clearly palpable. In eight patients, however, there was only a thickening or fullness and no mass. Two of five mammograms from these patients were suspicious for malignancy. Only 25 patients had mammograms at the time of recurrence, of which 17 (68%) were considered positive. In seven patients, only a mass could be seen, in seven patients there were microcalcifications but no mass, and in three patients there were both a mass and microcalcifications. Only 9 of 25 patients (36%) were detected to have a recurrence by both physical examination and mammography, with 8 recurrences (32%) being detectable only by physical examination and 8 being detectable only on mammograms.

The majority of recurrences will be located at or near the site of the primary tumor. With time, recurrence will be seen in other quadrants or in regions at least several centimeters from the area of the boost field. In the JCRT series, 5 of the 40 patients failing in the breast developed such a recurrence ("elsewhere in the breast") from 26 to 100 months after treatment.[102] In a group of 16 patients who had a recurrence after conservative treatment at the M.D. Anderson Hospital, 12 tumors were in the same quadrant as the first cancer and 4 were in other quadrants. These latter four tumors recurred after at least 6 years.[110] The Marseilles Cancer Institute has found a similar pattern.[116] These recurrences elsewhere in the breast may be histologically either similar to or different from the patient's original primary tumor.[117]

A small proportion of patients will have concurrent distant metastases when the tumor recurrence is discovered in the treated breast. This occurred in 3 of 40 and 2 of 43 patients in the JCRT[102] and Marseilles[116] series, respectively. Occasionally, locally extensive recurrences occur that preclude surgery (2 of 40 and 5 of 43 patients in these two series); these patients will usually develop metastases soon after. Two of 40 JCRT patients developed recurrences in the skin overlying the breast without a tumor being found in the breast itself.[102] The pretreatment evaluation of the patient with a local recurrence after mastectomy is therefore also applicable to those with local recurrence after primary radiation therapy.

As with patients treated with irradiation following mastectomy, sarcomas must be considered in the differential diagnosis of a breast mass appearing long after primary radiation therapy. These are likely to be very rare, however, as only one such case was seen in a group of 289 patients surviving at least 10 years after irradiation.[115] Other cases following primary radiation therapy have also been reported.[123]

Subsequent Course and Prognosis After Development of Local Recurrence

Local recurrence after primary radiation therapy has a much better prognosis than local recurrence after mastectomy. As noted above, a small proportion of patients will have either distant metastases or locally extensive disease at the time of discovery of local recurrence. Most patients can be cured with mastectomy or other surgery, however. Forty-five percent to 70% of all patients with breast recurrences in recent series were alive after 5 years.[102,105,109,110,114,116] Approximately 50% of all patients were free of distant metastases. No distant recurrences were found later than 6 years after initial local recurrence in a group of patients with long follow-up.[114] This is substantially better than the prognosis of patients after local recurrence following mastectomy as primary treatment. Salvage may be as high as 75% of those patients who can undergo mastectomy.[102,116] Patients who originally had pathologically positive lymph nodes and then a recurrence in the breast appear to have a very poor prognosis in one series.[109] This is not true of the JCRT experience, however (JCRT, unpublished data).

There is little difference in prognosis whether or not the axillary lymph nodes are involved clinically or pathologically at the time of breast recurrence (JCRT, unpublished data).[114] However, the number of patients in this group is small. Salvage of patients with isolated axillary recurrences seems comparable to salvage of breast recurrence. The time between primary treatment and recurrence also seems to make little difference in subsequent prognosis (JCRT, unpublished data).[114]

The prognosis after recurrence appears influenced by whether invasive cancer is present or not at breast relapse and whether the recurrence is palpable or not. Recurrence consisted of intraductal carcinoma without invasion in 6 of 25 patients who were treated at the JCRT and for whom mastectomy specimens were available for review. All six patients are alive without disease following salvage mastectomy. Four of these patients had their recurrence detected only by mammography. In addition, 2 more of these 25 patients also had their recurrence detected only on mammography. Their tumors at recurrence consisted primarily of ductal carcinoma in situ with only focal invasion. These two patients also remain free of further disease after salvage mastectomy. Follow-up on these patients is still short, however.[117]

Two patients in the JCRT series have had recurrences in the skin of the breast without an underlying mass being found clinically or on mastectomy. Both patients have died of distant metastases despite vigorous systemic treatment.[102] Recurrence in the chest wall following salvage mastectomy has occurred in 2 of 24 patients at the JCRT.[102]

Treatment of Local Recurrence

The majority of patients with breast cancer relapse can be salvaged by mastectomy. Whether mastectomy is superior to lesser procedures in this setting is unclear. Patients have occasionally refused mastectomy or have been medically inoperable. At least some of these patients appear to be cured by conservative excision. Four of eight patients treated only with excisional biopsy after failing primary radiation therapy at the JCRT continue to be alive and without disease, as does one patient treated only with an iridium implant. Follow-up on these patients is short, however.[102] Fifty-five patients with breast cancer recurrence have been treated with wedge excisions at the Marseilles Cancer Institute. These patients had mobile lesions less than 2 cm in size and had no skin involvement. However, these constituted only 35% of all patients undergoing salvage procedures between 1961 and 1979. With median follow-up of 4 years (range, 1 to 13 years), actuarial 5-year survival was 82%, with an actuarial disease-free survival of 79% at 5 years and 66% at 8 years. Eight patients (14.5%) had further breast or regional recurrences noted 9 to 50 months following the first recurrence. Further surgery was able to control disease locally in five of eight patients. Two patients were inoperable at that time.[124] Such second breast cancer recurrences may be due to widespread or multicentric involvement of the breast by tumor at the initial recurrence. Four of 18 (22%) evaluable mastectomy specimens at the JCRT showed unsuspected gross or microscopic foci of carcinoma in quadrants other than those in which the recurring tumor was initially identified.[117] It is therefore possible that selected patients (after careful clinical and radiologic evaluation to rule out multifocal disease) might be treated as well with wide local excision as with mastectomy. At present, however, we strongly believe that mastectomy is the treatment of choice for all operable patients with breast cancer recurrence following primary radiation therapy.

Eleven patients in the JCRT series underwent ipsilateral axillary sampling or dissection at the time of their breast recurrence. In four cases, metastatic carcinoma was found. There were no complications related to the redissection of the axilla in the four patients who had undergone a prior axillary dissection.[117] Postoperative complications following mastectomy are rare in these patients. One patient who suffered trauma to the chest wall after mastectomy developed a nonhealing ulcer 4 months postoperatively, and this required a transpositional pedicle flap to cover the area.[117] Morbidity from wide local excision as a salvage procedure has been reported as negligible.[124] Many of our patients currently undergo simultaneous mastectomy and breast reconstruction using a rectus abdominis flap.[125] The flap appears to promote healing, and so far we have not seen recurrences underneath such a flap.

The role of chemotherapy or hormonal manipulation after local recurrence following primary radiation therapy is unclear. In our experience at the JCRT there appears to be little difference in outcome whether or not such treatment is given, but the number of patients treated is small (JCRT, unpublished data). However, it would appear reasonable to give adjuvant systemic therapy to patients if the axillary nodes are positive at the time of recurrence, the surgical margins are positive, muscle invasion is found, extensive blood vessel or lymphatic vessel invasion is found in the specimen, or the skin of the breast is involved. The role, if any, of re-treatment of patients who have received prior hormonal or chemotherapy is unknown.

There is very little experience with giving further radiation therapy after local recurrence, either as a primary means of treatment or as adjuvant treatment after mastectomy. However, in patients with an intact breast previously treated with a high dose, such treatment will almost certainly lead to severe cosmetic deformities, and chest wall and skin necrosis would be likely.

REFERENCES

1. Haagensen CD: Diseases of the breast, 2nd rev ed. Philadelphia, WB Saunders, 1971
2. Valagussa P, Bonadonna G, Veronesi U: Patterns of relapse

and survival following radical mastectomy: Analysis of 716 consecutive patients. Cancer 41:1170–1178, 1978
3. Donegan WL, Perez-Mesa CM, Watson FR: A biostatistical study of locally recurrent breast carcinoma. Surg Gynecol Obstet 122:529–540, 1966
4. Zimmerman KW, Montague ED, Fletcher GH: Frequency, anatomical distribution and management of local recurrences after definitive therapy for breast cancer. Cancer 19:67–74, 1966
5. Carter RL: Significance of local recurrence. In Stoll BA (ed): Secondary spread in breast cancer, pp 31–44. London, William Heinemann, 1977
6. Donegan WL: The influence of untreated internal mammary metastases upon the course of mammary cancer. Cancer 39:533–538, 1977
7. Campbell FC, Blamey RW, Elston CW, et al: Oestrogen-receptor status and sites of metastasis in breast cancer. Br J Cancer 44:456–459, 1981
8. Maddox WA, Carpenter JT, Laws HL, et al: A randomized prospective trial of radical (Halsted) mastectomy versus modified radical mastectomy in 311 breast cancer patients. Ann Surg 198:207–212, 1983
9. Turner L, Swindell R, Bell WG, et al: Radical versus modified radical mastectomy for breast cancer. Ann R Coll Surg Engl 63:239–243, 1981
10. Oliver DR, Sugarbaker ED: The significance of skin recurrences following radical mastectomy. Surg Gynecol Obstet 85:360–367, 1947
11. Demaree EW: Local recurrence following surgery for cancer of the breast. Ann Surg 134:863–867, 1951
12. Auchincloss H: The nature of local recurrence following radical mastectomy. Cancer 11:611–619, 1958
13. Dao TL, Nemoto T: The clinical significance of skin recurrence after radical mastectomy in women with cancer of the breast. Surg Gynecol Obstet 117:447–453, 1963
14. Deck KB, Kern WH: Local recurrence of breast cancer. Arch Surg 111:323–325, 1976
15. White WC: The problem of local recurrence after radical mastectomy for carcinoma. Surg 19:149–153, 1946
16. Helman P: Breast cancer: Aspects of local recurrence. South Afr Med J 35:197–202, 1961
17. Bedwinek J: Adjuvant irradiation for early breast cancer: An on-going controversy. Cancer 53:729–739, 1984
18. Bonadonna G, Valagussa P, Rossi A, et al: Ten year experience with CMF-based adjuvant chemotherapy in resectable breast cancer. Breast Cancer Res Treat 5:95–115, 1985
19. Roberts MM, Blumgart LH, Davies M, et al: Simple versus radical mastectomy: Preliminary report of the Cardiff breast trial. Lancet 1:1073–1076, 1973
20. Fisher ER, Gregorio RM, Fisher B, et al: The pathology of invasive breast cancer. A syllabus derived from the findings of the National Surgical Adjuvant Breast Project (protocol no. 4). Cancer 36:1–85, 1975
21. Roth D, Bayat H: The role of residual tumor in the chest wall in the late dissemination of mammary cancer. Ann Surg 168:887–890, 1968
22. Karabali-Dalamaga S, Souhami RL, O'Higgins NJ, et al: Natural history and prognosis of recurrent breast cancer. Br Med J 2:730–733, 1978
23. Jackson SM: Carcinoma of the breast—the significance of supraclavicular lymph node metastases. Clin Radiol 17:107–114, 1966
24. Chu FCH, Lin FJ, Kim JH, et al: Locally recurrent carcinoma of the breast: Results of radiation therapy. Cancer 37:2677–2681, 1976
25. Pawlias KT, Dockerty MB, Ellis FH: Late local recurrent carcinoma of the breast. Ann Surg 148:192–198, 1958
26. Gilliland MD, Barton RM, Copeland EM: The implications of local recurrence of breast cancer as the first site of therapeutic failure. Ann Surg 197:284–287, 1983
27. Patanaphan V, Salazar OM, Poussin-Rosillo H: Prognosticators in recurrent breast cancer: A 15-year experience with irradiation. Cancer 54:228–234, 1984
28. Weichselbaum RR, Marck A, Hellman S: The role of postoperative irradiation in carcinoma of the breast. Cancer 37:2682–2690, 1976
29. Fisher B, Redmond C, Fisher ER, et al: Ten-year results of a randomized clinical trial comparing radical mastectomy and total mastectomy with or without radiation. N Engl J Med 312:674–681, 1985
29a. DeMoulin D: A Short History of Breast Cancer, p 76. Boston, Martinus Nijhoff, 1983
30. Neumann-Redlin E, Horstschafer W: A rare case of cancer en cuirasse in an untreated breast carcinoma of 24 years duration (in German). Zentralbl Bakteriol (Orig B) 91:568–572, 1975
31. Di Pietro S, Bertario L, Piva L: Prognosis and treatment of loco-regional breast cancer recurrences: Critical considerations on 120 cases. Tumori 66:331–338, 1980
32. Shimkin MB, Lucia EL, Low-Beer VA, et al: Recurrent cancer of the breast: analysis of frequency, distribution, and mortality at the University of California Hospital, 1918 to 1947, inclusive. Cancer 7:29–46, 1954
33. Spratt JS: Locally recurrent cancer after radical mastectomy. Cancer 20:1051–1053, 1967
34. Danckers UF, Hamann A, Savage JL: Postoperative recurrence of breast cancer after thirty-two years: A case report and review of the literature. Surgery 47:656–662, 1960
35. Morton JJ, Morton JH: Cancer as a chronic disease. Ann Surg 137:683–703, 1953
36. Tough ICK: The significance of recurrence in breast cancer. Br J Surg 53:897–900, 1966
37. Toonkel LM, Fix I, Jacobson LH, et al: The significance of local recurrence of carcinoma of the breast. Int J Radiat Oncol Biol Phys 9:33–39, 1983
38. Bruce J, Carter DC, Fraser J: Patterns of recurrent disease in breast cancer. Lancet 1:433–435, 1970
39. Marshall KA, Redfern A, Cady B: Local recurrences of carcinoma of the breast. Surg Gynecol Obstet 139:406–408, 1974
40. Bedwinek JM, Fineberg B, Lee J, et al: Analysis of failures following local treatment of isolated local-regional recurrence of breast cancer. Int J Radiat Oncol Biol Phys 7:581–585, 1981
41. Bedwinek JM, Munro D, Fineberg B: Local-regional treatment of patients with simultaneous local-regional recurrence and distant metastases following mastectomy. Am J Clin Oncol (CCT) 6:295–300, 1983
42. Fentiman IS, Matthews PN, Davison OW, et al: Survival following local skin recurrence after mastectomy. Br J Surg 72:14–16, 1985
43. Papaioannou AN, Tanz FJ, Volk H: Fate of patients with recurrent carcinoma of the breast: Recurrence five years or more after initial treatment. Cancer 20:371–376, 1967
44. Hagemeister FB, Buzdar AU, Luna MA, et al: Causes of death in breast cancer: A clinicopathologic study. Cancer 46:162–167, 1980
45. Cho SY, Choi HY: Causes of death and metastatic patterns in patients with mammary cancer: Ten-year autopsy study. Am J Clin Pathol 73:232–234, 1980
46. Madoc-Jones H, Nelson AJ, Montague ED: Evaluation of the

effectiveness of radiotherapy in the management of early nodal recurrences from adenocarcinoma of the breast. Breast 2:31–34, 1976
47. Chen KKY, Montague ED, Oswald MJ: Results of irradiation in the treatment of locoregional breast cancer recurrence. Cancer 56:1269–1273, 1985
48. Aberizk WJ, Silver B, Hellman S, et al: The results of radiation therapy for locally recurrent breast carcinoma after mastectomy (abstr). Int J Radiat Oncol Biol Phys (suppl 2)10:78–79, 1984
49. Aberizk WJ, Silver B, Henderson IC, et al: The results of radiotherapy in patients with isolated local-regional recurrence of breast carcinoma after mastectomy. Cancer 58:1214–1218, 1986
50. Snyder AF, Farrow GM, Masson JK, et al: Chest-wall resection for locally recurrent breast cancer. Arch Surg 97:246–253, 1968
51. Beck TM, Hart NE, Woodard DA, et al: Local or regionally recurrent carcinoma of the breast: Results of therapy in 121 patients. J Clin Oncol 1:400–405, 1983
52. Danoff BF, Coia LR, Cantor RI, et al: Locally recurrent breast carcinoma: The effect of adjuvant chemotherapy on prognosis. Radiology 147:849–852, 1983
53. Deutsch M, Parsons J, Mittal B: Local-regional recurrent breast cancer—treatment with radiotherapy (abstr). Int J Radiat Oncol Biol Phys (suppl 1)11:101–102, 1985
54. Valagussa P, Rossi A, Tancini G, et al: Is there any effective salvage treatment for relapsing operable breast cancer with N+? (abstr). Proc Am Soc Clin Oncol 4:56, 1985
55. Kim K, Tidrick RT, Skeel RT, et al: Fibrosarcoma of the chest wall following mastectomy and radiation therapy for mammary carcinoma. Breast 6:26–30, 1980
56. Friedman IH, Mori K, Kabakow B: Radiation-induced extraskeletal fibrosarcomas simulating locally recurrent carcinoma of the breast. NY State J Med 77:1932–1935, 1977
57. Allegra JC, Barlock A, Huff KK, et al: Changes in multiple or sequential estrogen receptor determinations in breast cancer. Cancer 45:792–794, 1980
58. Campbell FC, Elston CW, Blamey RW, et al: Quantiative oestradiol receptor values in primary breast cancer and response of metastases to endocrine therapy. Lancet 2:1317–1319, 1981
59. Lindfors KK, Meyer JE, Busse PM, et al: CT evaluation of local and regional breast cancer recurrence. AJR 145:833–837, 1985
60. Fishman EK, Zinreich ES, Jacobs C, et al: CT of the axilla—normal anatomy and pathology—impact on radiation therapy planning (abstr). Int J Radiat Oncol Biol Phys (suppl 1)11:94, 1985
61. Chu TM, Nemoto T: Evaluation of carcinoembryonic antigen in human mammary carcinoma. J Natl Cancer Inst 51:1119–1122, 1973
62. Steward A, Nixon D, Zamcheck N, et al: Carcinoembryonic antigen in breast cancer patients: Serum levels and disease progress. Cancer 33:1246–1252, 1974
63. Varnavides L, O'Higgins N, Clark C: CEA in mammary disease: a clinical evaluation. Clin Oncol 4:329–337, 1978
64. Lamerz R, Leonhardt A, Erhart H, et al: Serial CEA determinations in the management of metastatic breast cancer. Oncodev Biol Med 1:123–135, 1980
65. Tormey D, Waalkes T, Snyder JJ, et al: Biological markers in breast carcinoma: III. Clinical correlations with CEA. Cancer 39:2397–2404, 1977
66. Lokich J, Zamcheck N, Lowenstein M: Sequential CEA levels in the therapy of metastatic breast cancer. Ann Intern Med 6:902–906, 1978
67. Hayes DF, Sekine H, Ohno T, et al: Use of a murine monoclonal antibody for detection of circulating plasma DF3 antigen levels in breast cancer patients. J Clin Invest 75:1671–1678, 1985
68. Lo TCM, Salzman FA, Wright KA, et al: Megavolt electron irradiation in the treatment of recurrent carcinoma of the breast on the chest wall. Acta Radiol Oncol 22:97–99, 1983
69. Tapley NV, Fletcher GF, Montague ED: Breast. In Tapley NV (ed): Clinical Applications of the Electron Beam, pp 199–232. New York, John Wiley & Sons, 1976
70. Badcock PC: CT scanning: Its value in the planning of radiotherapy of the chest wall. Strahlentherapie 158:558–562, 1982
71. Peacock LM, Leavitt DD, Gibbs FA, et al: Electron arc therapy: Clinical experience with chest wall irradiation. Int J Radiat Oncol Biol Phys 10:2149–2153, 1984
72. Leavitt DD, Peacock LM, Gibbs FA, et al: Electron arc therapy: Physical measurement and treatment planning techniques. Int J Radiat Oncol Biol Phys 11:987–999, 1985
73. Laramore GE, Griffin TW, Parker RG, et al: The use of electron beams in treating local recurrence of breast cancer in previously irradiated fields. Cancer 41:991–995, 1978
74. Elkort RJ, Kelly W, Mozden PJ, et al: A combined treatment program for the management of locally recurrent breast cancer following chest wall irradiation. Cancer 46:647–653, 1980
75. Beardsley JM, Cavanaugh CR: Radical excision of malignant chest wall tumors. J Thorac Surg 29:582–596, 1955
76. Shah JP, Urban JA: Full thickness chest wall resection for recurrent breast carcinoma involving the bony chest wall. Cancer 35:567–573, 1975
77. McKenna RJ, McMurtrey MJ, Larson DL, et al: A perspective on chest wall resection in patients with breast cancer. Ann Thorac Surg 38:482–487, 1984
78. Larson DL, McMurtrey MJ, Howe J, et al: Major chest wall reconstruction after chest wall irradiation. Cancer 49:1286–1293, 1982
79. Larson DL, McMurtrey MJ: Musculocutaneous flap reconstruction of chest-wall defects: An experience with 50 patients. Plastic Reconstr Surg 73:734–740, 1984
80. Tsur H, Lieberman Y, Heim M: Diaphragm mobilization for closure of chest wall defects. Ann Plast Surg 13:234–238, 1984
81. Nieminen S, Hietanen T, Nordman E: Surgical treatment of local recurrences of breast carcinoma in the skin and subcutaneous tissues. Acta Chir Scand 145:463–465, 1979
82. Stefanik D, Goldberg R, Byrne P, et al: Local-regional failure in patients treated with adjuvant chemotherapy for breast cancer. J Clin Oncol 3:660–665, 1985
83. Buzdar AU, Blumenschein GR, Smith TL, et al: Adjuvant chemoimmunotherapy following regional therapy for isolated recurrences of breast cancer (stage IV NED). J Surg Oncol 12:27–40, 1979
84. Blumenschein GR, Pinnamaneni K, Buzdar AU, et al: Combined regional and systemic therapy in breast cancer patients with an isolated metastases with or without chemotherapy. In Jones SE, Salmon SE (eds): Adjuvant Therapy of Cancer, IV, pp 311–318. New York, Grune & Stratton, 1984
85. Janjan NA, McNeese MD, Buzdar AU, et al: Loco-regional recurrent breast cancer treated with radiation or a combination of radiation and chemotherapy (abstr). Int J Radiat Oncol Biol Phys (suppl 1)11:152–153, 1985
86. Ross M, Buzdar A, Smith T, et al: Improved survival of patients with metastatic breast cancer receiving combination chemotherapy. Cancer 55:341–346, 1985
87. Henderson IC, Canellos G: Cancer of the breast: The past decade. N Engl J Med 302:17–30, 78–90, 1980
88. Olson CE, Ansfield F. Richards M, et al: Review of soft tissue

recurrence of breast cancer irradiated with and without actinomycin D. Cancer 39:1981–1984, 1977

89. Hoogstraten B, Gad-el-Mawla N, Malone TR, et al: Combined modality therapy for first recurrence of breast cancer: a Southwest Oncology Group study. Cancer 54:2248–2256, 1984
90. Warren S: Preliminary study of the effect of artificial fever upon hopeless tumor cases. Am J Roentgen 33:75–87, 1935
91. Stewart JR, Gibbs FA: Hyperthermia in the treatment of cancer: Perspectives on its promise and its problems. Cancer 54:2823–2830, 1984
92. Hahn GM: Hyperthermia and Cancer. New York, Plenum Press, 1982
93. Manning M, Cetas T, Miller R, et al: Clinical hyperthermia: Results of a phase I trial employing hyperthermia alone or in combination with external beam or interstitial radiotherapy. Cancer 49:205–216, 1982
94. Jabboury K, Corry P, Armour E, et al: Local hyperthermia in the management of superficial lesions in breast cancer (abstr). Proc Am Soc Clin Oncol 3:123, 1984
95. Perez C, Nussbaum G, Emami B, et al: Clinical results of irradiation combined with local hyperthermis. Cancer 52:1597–1603, 1983
96. Scott RS, Perez CA, Johnson R, et al: Hyperthermia and radiotherapy in the treatment of recurrent adenocarcinoma of the breast (abstr). Int J Radiat Oncol Biol Phys (suppl 1)11:120, 1985
97. Ashford R, Plant G, Maher J, et al: Letter: Double blind trial of metronidazole in malodorous ulcerating tumours. Lancet 1:1232–1233, 1984
98. Moskalik KG, Dymarsky LYU, Kozlov AP, et al: Treatment of breast cancer recurrence by pulsed laser radiation (in Russian). Vopr Onkol 29:25–28, 1983
99. Dougherty TJ: Photoradiation therapy for cutaneous and subcutaneous malignancies. J Invest Dermatol 77:122–124, 1981
100. Wile AG, Coffey J, Nahabedian MY, et al: Laser photoradiation therapy of cancer: An update of the experience at the University of California, Irvine. Lasers Surg Med 4:5–12, 1984
101. Berns MW, Coffey J, Wile AG: Laser photoradiation therapy of cancer: Possible role of hyperthermia. Lasers Surg Med 4:87–92, 1984
102. Recht A, Silver B, Harris JR: The patterns of failure within the treated breast following primary radiation therapy (abstr). Int J Radiat Oncol Biol Phys (suppl 2)10:79, 1984
103. Recht A, Silver B, Schnitt S, et al: Breast relapse following primary radiation therapy for early breast cancer. I: Classification, frequency, and salvage. Int J Radiat Oncol Biol Phys 11:1271–1276, 1985
104. Clark RM: Alternatives to mastectomy—the Princess Margaret Hospital experience. In Harris JR, Hellman S, Silen W (eds): Conservative Management of Breast Cancer, pp 35–46. Philadelphia, JB Lippincott, 1983
105. Calle R, Pilleron JP, Vilcoq JR, et al: Breast carcinoma: Experience of the Curie Institute. In Ames FC, Blumenschein GR, Montague ED (eds): Current Controversies in Breast Carcinoma, pp 121–128. Austin, University of Texas Press, 1984
106. Sarrazin D, Le M, Rouesse J, et al: Conservative treatment versus mastectomy in breast cancer tumors with macroscopic diameter of 20 millimeters or less: The experience of the Institut Gustave-Roussy. Cancer 53:1209–1213, 1984
107. Pierquin B, Otmezguine Y, Lobo PA: Conservative management of breast carcinoma: The Creteil experience. Acta Radiol Oncol 22:101–107, 1983
108. Fisher B, Bauer M, Margolese R, et al: Five-year results of a randomized clinical trial comparing total mastectomy and segmental mastectomy with or without radiation in the treatment of early breast cancer. N Engl J Med 312:665–673, 1985
109. Danoff BF, Pajak TF, Solin LJ, et al: Excisional biopsy, axillary node dissection and definitive radiotherapy for stages I and II breast cancer. Int J Radiat Oncol Biol Phys 11:479–483, 1985
110. Montague ED: Conservation surgery and radiation therapy in the treatment of operable breast cancer. Cancer 53:700–704, 1984
111. Veronesi U, Del Vecchio M, Greco M, et al: Results of quadrantectomy, axillary dissection, and radiotherapy (QUART) in T1N0 patients. In Harris JR, Hellman S, Silen W (eds): Conservative Management of Breast Cancer, pp 91–100. Philadelphia, JB Lippincott, 1983
112. Amalric R, Santamaria F, Robert F, et al: Radiation therapy with or without primary limited surgery for operable breast cancer: A 20-year expreience at the Marseilles Cancer Institute. Cancer 49:30–34, 1982
113. Osborne MP, Ormiston N, Harmer CL, et al: Breast conservation in the treatment of early breast cancer: A 20-year follow-up. Cancer 53:349–355, 1984
114. Harris JR, Recht A, Amalric R, et al: Time course and prognosis of local recurrence following primary radiation therapy for early breast cancer. J Clin Oncol 2:37–41, 1984
115. Kurtz JM, Amalric R, Delouche G, et al: The second ten years: Long-term risks of breast conservation (abstr). Int J Radiat Oncol Biol Phys (suppl 1):11, 184–185, 1985
116. Kurtz JM, Spitalier JM, Amalric R: Late breast recurrence after lumpectomy and irradiation. Int J Radiat Oncol Biol Phys 9:1191–1194, 1983
117. Schnitt S, Connolly J, Recht A, et al: Breast relapse following primary radiation therapy for early breast cancer. II: Detection, pathologic features, and prognostic significance. Int J Radiat Oncol Biol Phys 11:1277–1284, 1985
118. Silen W, Botnick LE: Physical examination of the treated breast. In Harris JR, Hellman S, Silen W (eds): Conservative Management of Breast Cancer, pp 261–264. Philadelphia, JB Lippincott, 1983
119. Berenberg AL, Levene MB, Tonnesen GL: Mammographic examination of the postirradiated breast. In Harris JR, Hellman S, Silen W (eds): Conservative Management of Breast Cancer, pp 91–100. Philadelphia, JB Lippincott, 1983
120. Paulus DD, Libshitz HI: Breast. In Libshitz HI (ed): Diagnostic roentgenology of radiotherapy change, pp 55–68. Baltimore, Williams & Wilkins, 1979
121. Paulus DD, Libshitz HI, Montague ED: Malignant masses in the therapeutically irradiated breast. AJR 135:789–795, 1980
122. Recht A, Harris JR: Negative breast biopsies after primary radiation therapy: Safety and accuracy (abstr). Int J Radiat Oncol Biol Phys (suppl 1)11:131, 1985
123. Kuten A, Sapir D, Cohen Y, et al: Postirradiation soft tissue sarcoma occurring in breast cancer patients: Report of seven cases and results of combination chemotherapy. J Surg Oncol 28:168–171, 1985
124. Kurtz JM, Amalric R, Brandone H, et al: A second chance to preserve the breast: Results of wide excision after lumpectomy and irradiation (abstr). Int J Radiat Oncol Biol Phys (suppl 1)11:103, 1985
125. Dinner MI, Dowden RV: The operative technique of the transverse abdominal island flap for breast reconstruction. Clin Plast Surg 11:317–331, 1984

Management of Pathologic Fractures

Charles N. Cornell Joseph M. Lane

Life expectancy in patients with carcinoma of the breast and skeletal metastases is generally longer than that seen with other primary tumors. Roentgenographic evidence of bone metastases is seen in 20% to 60% of patients with metastatic breast cancer and in 80% of autopsy specimens.[1,2] In a review of 63 patients with a single pathologic fracture resulting from breast cancer, Marcove found that 40% of patients survived 6 months, and 34% lived longer than 1 year.[3] Of those with multiple pathologic fractures, 39% lived up to 6 months, and 26% survived for longer than 1 year. These survival statistics are from a group of surgically treated patients, but are quite similar to those from other series in which both operative and nonoperative treatment of pathologic fractures was used.[1–4] Recent reviews of survival in patients with skeletal metastases from carcinoma of the breast at Memorial Sloan-Kettering Cancer Center revealed a median survival time of 5.6 months; 20% of these patients survived for 1 year after diagnosis of metastases.

This prolonged survival underscores the need for skilled, effective fracture management in these patients. Many women with metastatic breast cancer have led close to normal lives up until the time of fracture. Immobilization of the affected area, rather than definitive surgical treatment, may lead to narcotic dependency, hypercalcemia, increased risk of thromboembolic disease, and decubitis formation. Moreover, in many cases, pathologic fractures will fail to unite if treated nonoperatively.[7,8] Therefore, these patients require rapid treatment that will restore their mobility, relieve any pain, and maintain their quality of life in the face of a terminal illness.[5,6,9,10]

FRACTURE MANAGEMENT

In recent years, the treatment of pathologic fractures has improved considerably as a result of advancements in internal fixation and prosthetic devices. Basic to these advances has been the introduction of methyl methacrylate bone cement, which enables the surgeon to achieve instantaneous, rigid bonding of the fractured parts and the internal fixation device. This is the key to achieving stability in cases in which severe bone destruction has occurred, making fixation by other means impossible, especially in fractures involving the weight-bearing skeleton.

As a result of the experience at Memorial Hospital over the last decade, a philosophy of pathologic fracture management has been formulated and implemented. The magnitude of the surgery involved in fixation of pathologic fractures is significantly greater than that for nonpathologic fractures. Blood loss is greater, partially because of the large dissections needed for exposure and the enhanced vasculature of certain metastatic lesions (such as thyroid or renal lesions). Preoperative embolization may be indicated in selected cases. Adequate supplies of packed cells, fresh frozen plasma, and occasionally, platelets should be available. In cases in which methyl methacrylate is used, patients should be well hydrated and well oxygenated, with any lost blood fully replaced with blood products prior to cement insertion. In the postoperative period, the risk of deep venous thrombosis and pulmonary embolism is present, as it is in all orthopedic procedures involving the lower extremities, but anticoagulation is often contraindicated in patients receiving postoperative radiation or chemotherapy. Moreover, these patients are often debilitated and nutritionally depleted by their disease process and treatment programs. During the postoperative period, early mobilization and aggressive pulmonary toilet are essential. Prophylactic antibiotics should be administered, and use of suction drains to prevent hematoma formation should be routine. Ideally, the surgeon who performs this type of surgery plans the operative procedure well in advance, organizing a multidisciplinary approach that includes nursing, physical therapy, and medical consultation to assist the patient in the postoperative period.

In addition, we have found that multiple metastases often appear in a single bone at different times, giving rise to a predictable risk of secondary fracture through newly apparent lesions which may develop proximal or distal to fixation devices (Fig. 14-17). Revision of the devices to stabilize these subsequent fractures may be extremely difficult, and in many cases, impossible if methyl methacrylate has been used.

The Bone Tumor Service at Memorial Hospital advocates the following principles:

1. Operative fixation of pathologic fractures involves extensive, major surgery. Patients should be medically able to withstand prolonged, stressful procedures. Patients with a life expectancy of less than 1 month should probably be treated nonoperatively.
2. The bone involved by a pathologic fracture is prone to refracture. The entire bone should be stabilized by an appropriate internal fixation device, and methyl methacrylate should be used to achieve initial stability.
3. Pathologic fractures will usually not heal. The fixation devices implanted must outlive the patient.

The most common sites of metastatic spread of breast cancer are the spine, pelvis, femur, and humerus, in that order. Techniques for fixation of each of these fractures, as applied by the Bone Tumor Service staff at Memorial Hospital, will be discussed in the remainder of this chapter section.

Prophylactic Fixation

Prophylactic fixation of impending fractures is an unsettled issue in the literature. To date, no randomized, prospective trials have been performed that conclusively indicate

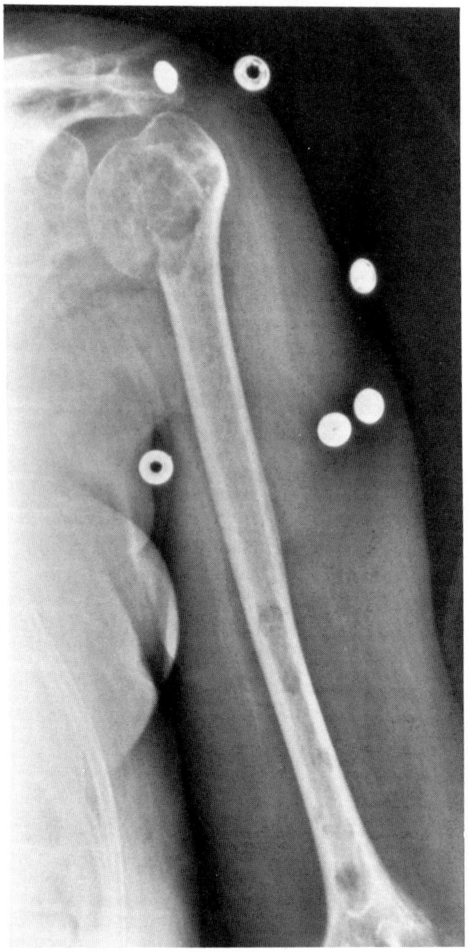

FIGURE 14-17. An example of a pathologic fracture of the proximal humerus with multiple additional distal metastases that may lead to further pathologic fractures in the future.

which patients might benefit from surgery and which would benefit from conservative management using hormonal therapy and chemotherapy or radiation. Many surgical reviews advocate prophylactic fixation for lesions which measure greater than 2.5 cm or 50% of the bone diameter, or for those that involve the cortex or are painful, regardless of location.[8,9] Osteoblastic metastases from breast carcinoma appear to be associated with a reduced risk of fracture; because of this, the need for prophylactic fixation of bone lesions may not be warranted. Furthermore, breast metastases to bone are often quite radiosensitive, and several reports of palliative radiotherapy definitely demonstrate, over short-term follow-up, that many of these lesions may be rendered adequately asymptomatic using this modality.[2,11]

In our experience, the choice of prophylactic internal fixation versus conservative management (which may include radiotherapy) is based on definite selection criteria. Small lesions that are intramedullary and osteoblastic are initially treated by conservative means. Painful, large, lytic lesions involving the cortex and causing significant destruction, as well as those lesions that involve regions of the cortex in which fracture fixation would be technically difficult (e.g., a lesion involving the subtrochanteric femur) are approached with early prophylactic fixation.

Although the series reported by the Radiation Therapy Oncology Group supports initial nonoperative treatment,[11] only 60% of the patients who eventually present with fractures and undergo surgery at Memorial Hospital have received prior radiotherapy to the fracture site. However, data regarding the use of radiation therapy in the prevention of fractures is not complete. As yet, we are unaware of a prospective study that conclusively demonstrates the relative value of radiotherapy in the prevention of pathologic fractures once a symptomatic lesion has appeared. In any case, if nonoperative management is chosen initially, careful follow-up with orthopedic consultation should be instituted to optimize future treatment if a fracture occurs. Persistent pain 6 to 8 weeks following radiotherapy may indicate the presence of a complete, nondisplaced fracture.

Fractures of the Hip

Hip fractures occur in 10% of patients with metastatic breast cancer to bone. In addition, approximately 1.4% of all patients with breast cancer will ultimately sustain a pathologic hip fracture. Pathologic fractures of the hip are particularly disabling, and are known to shorten life expectancy significantly if treated conservatively. Operative treatment of fractures in this region are difficult for several reasons. Severe bone destruction as a result of tumor makes stable reduction an arduous task, and the various muscle attachments about the hip often lead to wide displacement of fractured fragments.[12]

Several methods of stabilizing pathologic fractures of the hip have been advocated. Hip screws and other devices, supplemented with cement, have been successful.[5,13] Zickel has advocated the use of his device for subtrochanteric fractures.[14] In a series of 45 patients treated in this manner, he achieved early mobilization in all patients, and approximately 60% became ambulatory.[14] Healing of fractures was observed in most long-term survivors of breast cancer, and Zickel concluded that this device was particularly suitable for patients with breast cancer. In this series, the tumor was not curetted and bone was not grafted, nor was cement used to supplement fixation. At Memorial Hospital, we recently reviewed 17 patients with 20 subtrochanteric fractures that were treated using the Zickel device.[15] Fifty percent of the Zickel devices used were cemented (Fig. 14-18). Seventy-one percent of these patients had complete pain relief following treatment, and 65% regained community ambulatory status. Seven of 10 impending fractures were converted to complete fractures by the process of device insertion, but no adverse effect was observed. None of these patients experienced loss of fixation. In Zickel's series, 4 of 45 patients with unce-

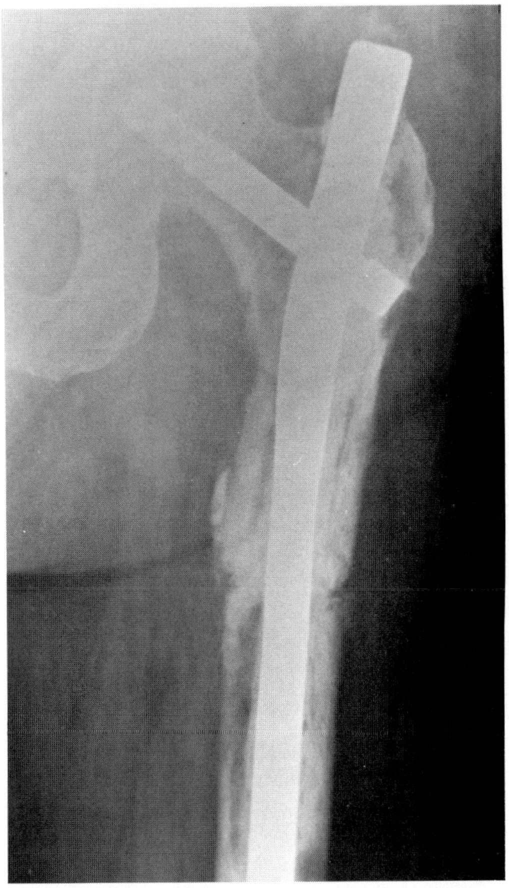

FIGURE 14-18. Subtrochanteric pathologic fracture of the femur treated by open reduction and internal fixation using the Zickel nail and methyl methacrylate.

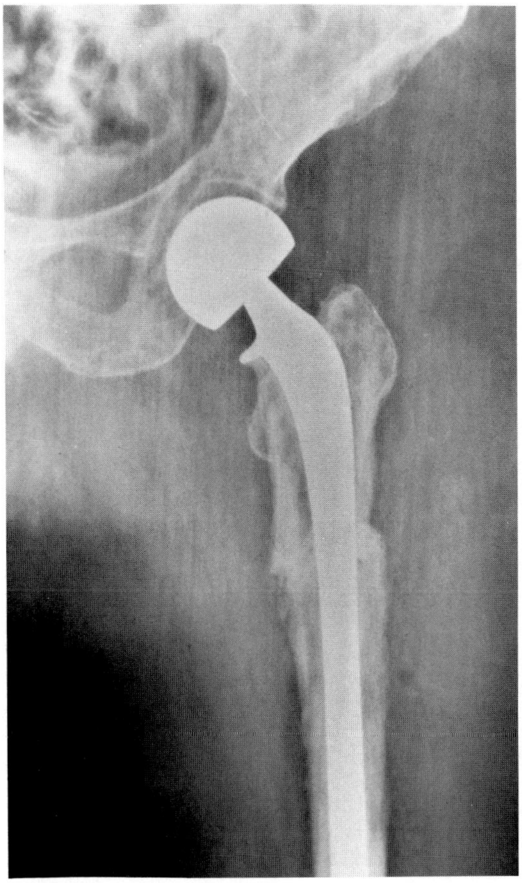

FIGURE 14-19. Subtrochanteric pathologic fracture of the femur treated by a long-stem, cemented, bicentric prosthesis. This treatment approach accomplishes fracture fixation as well as stabilization of the entire femoral shaft, providing durable fixation even in the presence of progressive local disease.

mented devices experienced loss of fixation as a result of proximal migration or spread of tumor, leading to cut-out of the flanged nail in the femoral head and neck. We believe that cementing may prevent migration and augment stability when the Zickel device is used.

At Memorial Hospital, cemented, long-stem hemiarthroplasty is the method of fixation that is most commonly used for pathologic fractures of the proximal femur (Fig. 14-19). In our experience, the femur is usually diffusely involved, and in patients with breast cancer in whom life expectancy may be prolonged, additional metastases may occur, compromising fixation at the proximal and distal ends of more limited devices. In addition, significant stress concentrations may occur at the tips of devices at the site of junction with the remaining bone, and spontaneous fractures may appear, especially in those debilitated patients in whom bone quality is poor. Long-stem, cemented hemiarthroplasty avoids these possible complications by splinting the entire bone and by achieving instant and durable fixation that will persist throughout the patient's life, even when local bony involvement progresses.

An initial series using the Austin-Moore type of hemiarthroplasty has been reported from Memorial Hospital,[1] but since 1980, these unipolar devices have been replaced by bipolar devices. Since 1980, 101 long-stem, bipolar hemiarthroplasties have been performed for fractures of the hip and proximal femur.[16] Fifty percent of these fractures resulted from metastatic breast cancer. The Bateman or Gilberty devices were used exclusively. The average postoperative survival for this group was 8.6 months. Thirty-four percent and 17% of these patients were alive after 1 and 2 years, respectively. Postoperatively, 87% of these patients were ambulatory with excellent pain relief; only 62% required mild analgesics. These results represented a significant improvement over those achieved prior to 1980 when unipolar Austin-Moore devices were used. Bipolar devices appear to provide better pain relief and an improved overall rate of return of ambulatory function.

The postoperative complications encountered in this series included a 3% incidence of deep venous thrombosis, with one case of nonfatal pulmonary embolism. A 3% incidence of wound infection was also noted. The high incidence of pseudofat embolic complications may represent a major limitation of cemented, long-stem devices. Since 1980, we have experienced four instances (4%) of sudden, intraoperative hypotension and death during or immediately after insertion of the prosthesis and cement, the exact etiology of which is unclear. The use of long-stem devices with large quantities of cement may lead to extremely high intramedullary pressures, with an increased risk of embolization of fat and marrow into the central circulation.[17–20] This problem seems to be exacerbated with the use of long-stem devices, since this complication is seen very rarely in short-stem total hip replacements. A review of these intraoperative deaths suggests that patients with severe cardiopulmonary disease related to coronary artery disease, valvular heart disease, or chronic obstructive pulmonary disease, patients with pulmonary metastases, and those who have received extensive radiotherapy to the chest are at increased risk. The likelihood of this complication may be decreased by ensuring adequate fluid and blood resuscitation during the procedure,[18] and by the use of 100% inspired oxygen just before cement insertion.[21,22] In patients who are at increased risk, venting the femur by drill holes (4 cm proximal to the distal tip of the prosthesis) may be advisable to relieve pressure buildup during component insertion and cement polymerization.

Despite these complications, long-stem bipolar devices do provide immediate fracture fixation and an intramedullary splint in the face of extensive and potentially progressive disease. In our opinion, the benefits of pain relief and secure ambulation outweigh the potential complications of this procedure.

Acetabular Fractures

When the acetabulum is the predominant site of involvement, with bone destruction and medial or superior migration of the femoral head, total hip arthroplasty is required. This condition occurs relatively uncommonly, and it should be recognized that the subchondral plate of the acetabulum may be the strongest remaining bone of the acetabulum. In many cases, we have found bipolar hemiarthroplasty to be effective, despite acetabular involvement. However, when extensive periacetabular destruction has occurred, total hip arthroplasty may be necessary. In these cases, sufficient bone stock for conventional seating of the acetabular component may not be present. In terms of fixation durability, previous reports document the inadequacy of both methyl methacrylate (used alone) to reconstruct bone loss and seating of the acetabular cup in a migrated position.[23,24] Harrington has advocated use of acetabular rings with wires and pins that reinforce the cement and transmit loads onto the remaining bone, which is functionally capable of withstanding weight-bearing forces (Fig. 14-20).[25] He has reported good to excellent results 6 months after surgery in 67% of 58 patients treated by these methods.[25] After 2 years of follow-up, 45% of the

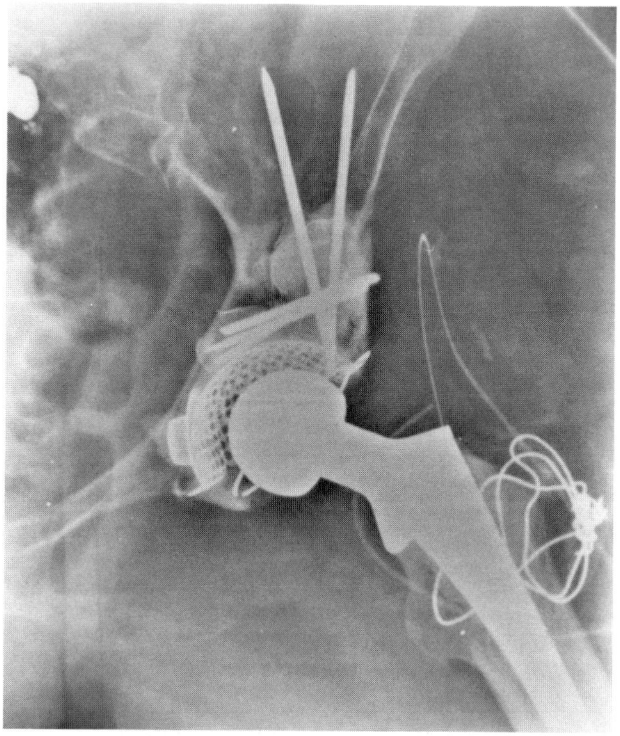

FIGURE 14-20. An example of acetabular reconstruction made necessary by extensive pelvic and acetabular metastases. Mesh, supplementary Kirsčhner-wires, and methyl methacrylate are used to accomplish fixation to the uninvolved bone.

patients in his series were still ambulatory and were considered to have excellent results.

Fractures of the Femoral Shaft

Femoral shaft fractures may easily be treated using intramedullary rod devices augmented with cement.[13] Again, in keeping with our approach, if proximal lesions are noted to be bicentric, long-stem hemiarthroplasty, which bridges the diaphyseal fracture, is advocated. If the fracture has occurred through an isolated lesion in the diaphysis, a fluted, intramedullary rod without cement is a suitable device that provides support even when severe bone destruction has occurred. In addition, these devices may easily be removed if conversion to an endoprosthesis is necessary.

Metastatic Disease of the Spine

The most common site of deposit of metastatic breast cancer to the skeleton is the thoracic spine. Several factors contribute to this predilection. Batson described the valveless network of vertebral veins that communicate with the lumbar and intercostal veins, providing a direct route of spread between the breast and the thoracic spine.[26] The vertebral bodies contain red marrow throughout life, and this may provide an environment that is conducive to tumor growth.

Spinal cord compression is a consequence of metastatic spread in the spine that necessitates urgent treatment. Spinal cord compression may occur secondary to enlarging extradural deposits, pressure resulting from fracture-dislocation, or severe kyphosis resulting from vertebral collapse. Pressure resulting from intradural metastases is very rare.[27]

In planning treatment, it is important to determine the exact location and extent of the tumor. Myelography and CT scanning may readily provide this information. The experience at Memorial Hospital, as well as elsewhere, clearly documents the fact that most lesions resulting in spinal cord compression are located in the vertebral body and exert anterior extradural pressure.[28,29] Our extensive experience also demonstrates that posterior decompression and stabilization has a high complication rate, incompletely decompresses the cord, and also fails to improve neurologic function.[28–30]

The anterior approach to the spine was developed for the treatment of Pott's disease. In 1960, Hodgson and Stock reported on their experience in a series of 100 patients.[31] They concluded that the anterior approach allowed better visualization of the lesion and complete excision of all diseased tissues, provided excellent dural decompression, and permitted immediate stabilization by bone grafts. In 1967, Scoville described the use of vertebral body resection for metastatic cancer.[32] In 1981, Harrington reported a series of 14 patients who were treated with resection of the vertebral body and stabilized, using methyl methacrylate reinforced with Steinmann pins.[29] Pain relief was achieved in 13 of these patients, and neurologic improvement was noted in 10.

Over a 5-year period, more than 100 vertebral body resections have been performed for metastatic disease at Memorial Hospital. Following this procedure, 78% of these patients became ambulatory, 80% reported significant postoperative pain relief, and 60% of the patients who were nonambulatory preoperatively regained the ability to walk postoperatively. The mortality rate was 9% overall and was 10% in those patients who experienced postoperative complications. This figure reflects the progression of cancer in a debilitated population. We believe that the postoperative complications were, in most cases, related to preoperative treatment with steroids, intensive chemotherapy, and radiation. In *de novo* cases, the morbidity and mortality were nil.

In view of these results, we believe that surgical decompression by the anterior approach is the preferred treatment for single or adjacent vertebral body metastases with resulting pain, mechanical instability, or neurologic compromise in patients in whom high-dose steroids and radiation therapy have failed (Fig. 14-21). The procedure is probably more beneficial if performed early after the

FIGURE 14-21. Anteroposterior and lateral radiographs demonstrate an example of the use of methyl methacrylate and Steinmann pins in the reconstruction of a thoracic vertebral body after anterior decompression and resection of a metastatic lesion.

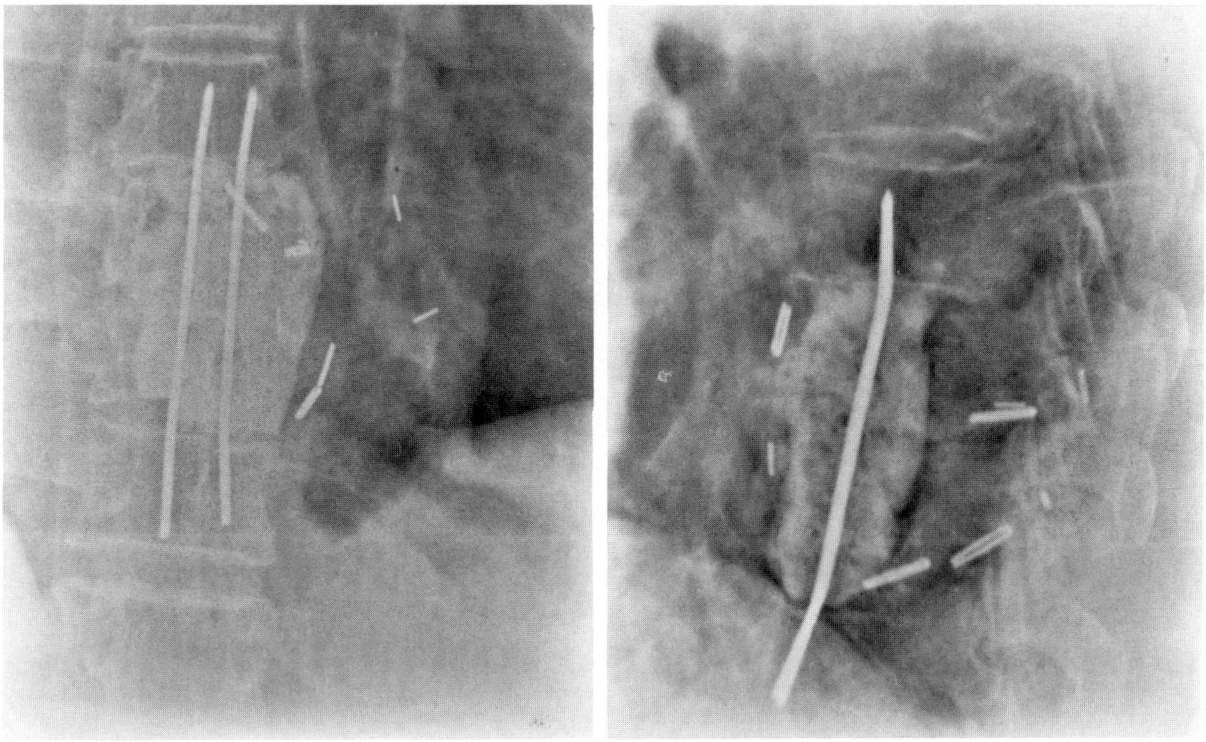

onset of symptoms. In light of our experience at Memorial Hospital, we believe that this procedure warrants reappraisal as the initial mode of treatment for spinal metastases. At this time, no prospective randomized study has been conducted that would clearly indicate the preferred order of treatment (i.e., surgical decompression or radiotherapy).

Humeral Fractures

Metastatic deposits to the upper extremities most commonly involve the proximal humerus and humeral diaphysis. Pathologic fractures of the upper extremities have traditionally been managed by conservative, nonoperative means.[9,13] Conservative treatment implies immobilization, usually with a plaster-reinforced sling and swathe dressing. Sarmiento has recently reported excellent results using functional bracing for nonpathologic fractures of the humeral shaft.[33] At Memorial Hospital, the functional brace has been used to treat pathologic fractures as well. Between 1982 and 1984, 26 patients with pathologic fractures of the humeral shaft were treated by application of a humeral fracture brace, followed by early and aggressive occupational therapy (Fig. 14-22). All patients experienced significant pain relief immediately upon application of the brace, and most were able to begin using the extremity. Eighty-nine percent of those patients surviving longer than 1 month were able to perform light activities of daily living. In 36% of the fractures, union was achieved, and in all of those patients, the fracture healed with satisfactory alignment. In only 4 of the original 26 patients who were treated using the brace was the outcome considered to be poor; these patients were considered to be early failures of treatment by this method. One late complication of cast bracing in this series was a high refracture rate. Of the 12 patients who lived longer than 3 months after treatment, 5 developed refractures of the same humerus within 5 to 15 months.

Despite the good early results of closed treatment obtained in this series, there are many patients for whom only operative treatment is suitable. Operative management of humeral fractures is most appropriate in patients with involvement of the lower extremities who require use of the upper extremities for weight-bearing. In many obese patients, closed methods are not effective in stabilizing such fractures, and patients with very proximal or distal fractures are not suitable for cast bracing. In addition, as pointed out earlier, patients with reasonable life expectancies may be expected to have refractures or additional fractures develop with time; these patients are best

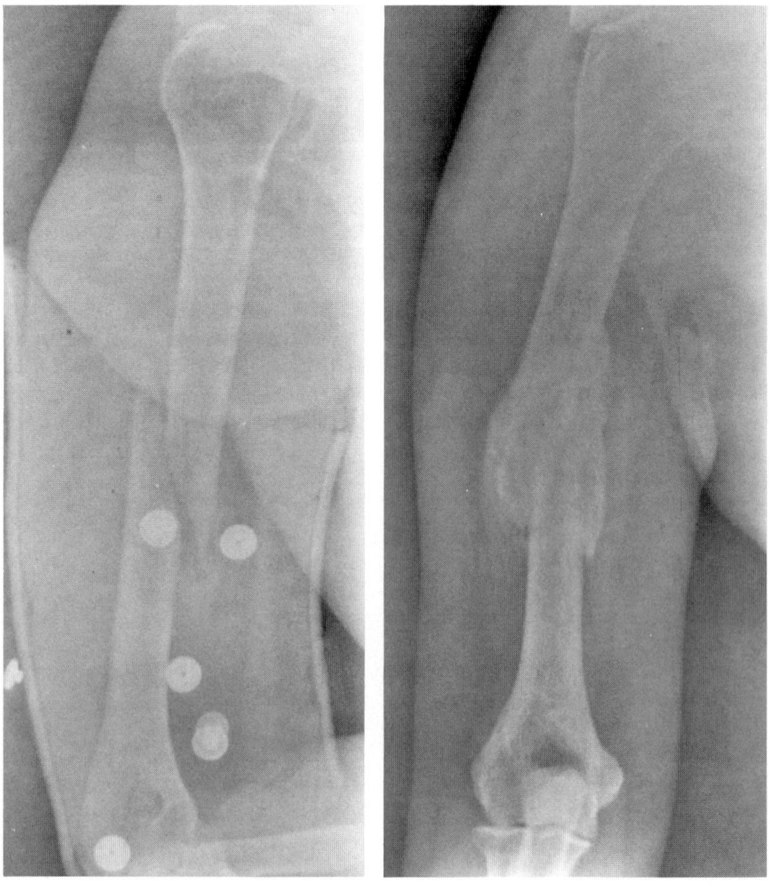

FIGURE 14-22. A pathologic fracture of the humeral shaft that is well controlled by a humeral fracture brace. Healing with satisfactory alignment was achieved in this patient.

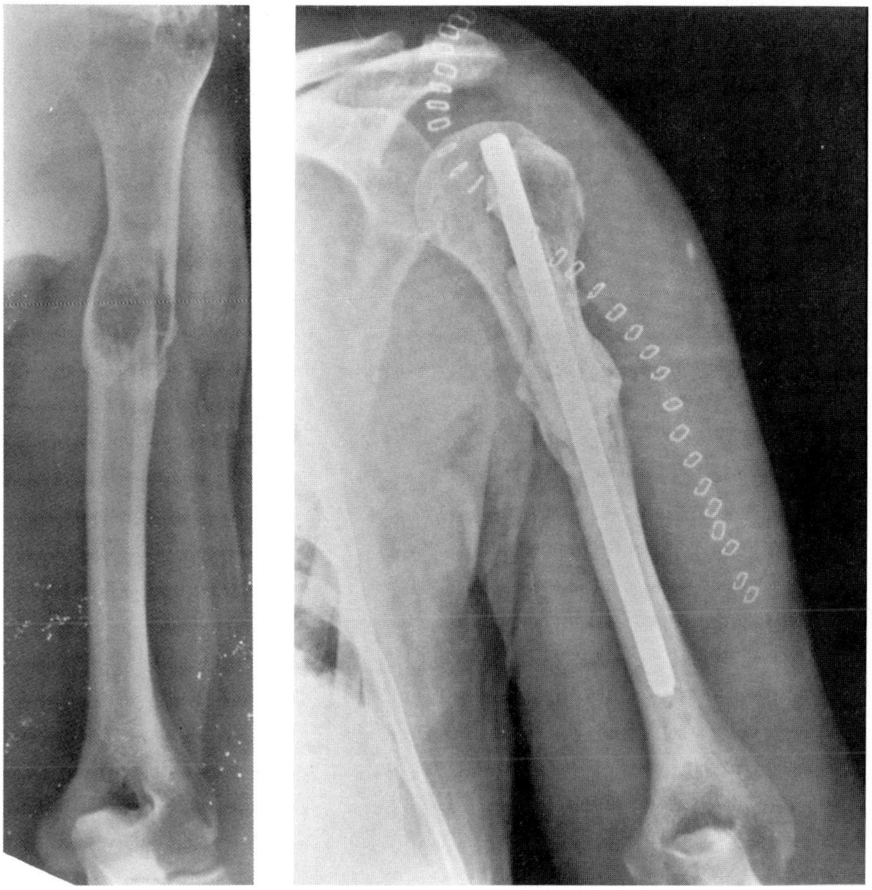

FIGURE 14-23. Solitary metastatic lesion of the humeral shaft treated by insertion of a Küntschner rod with adjunctive use of methyl methacrylate.

treated with complete stabilization of the bone, as is the case with patients with fractures of the lower extremities.

Our current protocol for treatment of pathologic fractures of the humerus involves an assessment of the location of the fracture, as well as an assessment of the patient's prognosis for survival. Patients with a life expectancy of less than 3 months are generally treated nonoperatively. Fractures of the metaphysis and diaphysis in this group of patients are treated by functional bracing. Metaphyseal fractures require a deltoid extension of the brace over the shoulder for additional support. Patients who are expected to survive longer than 3 months, those who require the upper extremities for weight-bearing, and those in whom closed treatment fails are treated operatively, employing the principle of complete stabilization of the entire bone using an intramedullary device and cement (Fig. 14-23). Patients with diffuse humeral involvement and those with fractures of the humeral head and neck are treated with cemented, long-stem hemiarthroplasties of the Neer type. Isolated diaphyseal lesions may be treated with intramedullary rods and cement in the region of the fracture. We prefer using Sampson and Küntschner rods for diaphyseal lesions. For fractures secondary to distal metaphyseal lesions, we employ rush rods that are inserted in retrograde fashion akin to the modified Hackethal procedure.[34,35] In the Memorial Hospital experience, of 137 patients in whom pathologic fractures of the humerus were treated surgically, 86% reported excellent pain relief and 51% achieved satisfactory postoperative function. There were four postoperative complications in this group, including three transient nerve palsies and one secondary fracture below a Sampson rod.

SUMMARY

Pathologic fractures are devastating complications of disseminated breast cancer. The resultant pain and suffering and loss of function may significantly shorten a patient's remaining life, increasing the morbidity of the disease. We believe that aggressive surgical treatment provides prompt return of function and pain relief in most cases, and we generally only withhold surgery from patients who are terminally ill with life expectancies of less than 1 month.

We abide by the principle that the patient is best served by splinting the entire bone and by using cement for instantaneous and durable fixation that will endure, even in the presence of progressive, adjacent disease. We have found that application of these principles, coupled with vigorous rehabilitation in the postoperative period, restores function, relieves pain, and allows patients to return to their homes and families.

REFERENCES

1. Lane JM, Sculco TP: Treatment of pathologic fractures of the hip by endoprosthetic replacement. J Bone Joint Surg 62A:954, 1980
2. Cheng DS, Seitz CB, Eyre HJ: Nonoperative treatment of femoral, humeral, and acetabular metastases in patients with breast carcinoma. Cancer 45:1533, 1980
3. Marcove RC, Yang DJ: Survival times after treatment of pathologic fractures. Cancer 20:2154, 1967
4. Perez CA, Bradfield JS, Morgan HC: Management of pathologic fractures. Cancer 29:684, 1972
5. Coran AG, Banks HH, Aliapoulios MA, et al: The management of pathologic fractures in patients with metastatic carcinoma of the breast. Surg Gynecol Obstet 127:1225. Dec, 1968
6. Schurman DS, Amstutz HC: Orthopaedic management of patients with metastatic carcinoma of the breast. Surg Gynecol Obstet 137:831, 1973
7. Lane JM, McCormack RR, Sundareson N, et al: Treatment of pathologic fractures. In Current Concepts of Diagnosis and Treatment of Bone and Soft Tissue Tumors, pp 203–212. Berlin, Springer-Verlag, 1984
8. Ryan JR, Rowe DE, Salcicuolio GG: Prophylactic internal fixation of the femur for neoplastic lesions. J Bone Joint Surg 58A:1071, 1976
9. Parrish FF, Murray JA: Surgical treatment for secondary neoplastic fractures. J Bone Joint Surg 52A:665, 1970
10. Takita R, Watne AL: Operative treatment of pathologic fractures. Surg Gynecol Obstet 116:683, June, 1963
11. Tong D, Gillick L, Hendrickson FR: The palliation of symptomatic osseous metastases—Final results of the study by the Radiation Therapy Oncology Group. Cancer 50:893, 1982
12. Springfield DS, Brower TD: Pathologic fractures. In Rockwood CA, Green DF (eds): Fractures, pp 295–312. Philadelphia, JB Lippincott, 1984
13. Harrington KD, Sim FH, Enis JE, et al: Methylmethacrylate as an adjunct in internal fixation of pathological fractures. J Bone Joint Surg 58A:1047, 1976
14. Zickel RE, Nouradian WH; Intermedullary fixation of pathological fractures and lesions of the subtrochanteric region of the femur. J Bone Joint Surg 58A:1061, 1976
15. Gebhart M, Lane JM, Glasser DB: The Zickel device and bicentric hemiarthroplasty in pathologic fractures of the proximal femur. In Orthoped Trans (in press)
16. Bockner R, Lane JM, Glasser DB, et al: Endoprosthetic replacement for pathologic fractures of the hip. In Orthoped Trans (in press)
17. Herndon JH, Bechtel CO, Crickenberger DP: Fat embolism during total hip replacement. J Bone Joint Surg 56A:1350, 1974
18. Peltier LF: Fat embolism. An appraisal of the problem. Clin Orthoped 187:3, 1984
19. Johansen I, Benumof JL: Methylmethacrylate: A myocardial depressant and peripheral dilator. Anesthesiology 51S:77, 1979
20. Kallos T, Enis JE, Gollan F, et al: Intramedullary pressure and pulmonary embolism of femoral medullary contents in dogs during insertion of bone cement and a prosthesis. J Bone Joint Surg 56A:1363, 1974
21. Kallos T: Impaired arterial oxygenation associated with the use of bone cement in the femoral shaft. Anesthesiology 42:210, 1975
22. Wong KC, Martin WE, Kennedy WF, et al: Cardiovascular effects of total hip placement in man. With observations on the effects of methylmethecrylate on the isolated rabbit heart. Clin Pharmacol Ther 21:709, 1977
23. Johnson JTH: Reconstruction of the pelvic ring following tumor resection. J Bone Joint Surg 60A:747, 1978
24. Scales JT: Massive bone and joint replacement involving the upper femur, acetabulum and iliac bone in the hip. Proc Third Open Scientific Meeting of the Hip Society, pp 245–275. St. Louis, CV Mosby, 1975
25. Harrington KP: The management of acetabular insufficiency secondary to metastatic malignant disease. J Bone Joint Surg 63A:653, 1981
26. Batson DV: The function of vertebral veins and their role in the spread of metastases. Ann Surg 112:138, 1940
27. Edelson RN, Deck MD, Posner JB: Intramedullary spinal cord metastases: Clinical and radiographic findings in nine cases. Neurology 22:1222, 1972
28. Boland PJ, Lane JM, Sundareson N: Metabolic disease of the spine. Clin Orthoped 169:95, 1985
29. Harrington KD: The use of methylmethacrylate for vertebral body replacement and anterior stabilization of pathological fracture—Dislocations of the spine due to metabolic disease. J Bone Joint Surg 63A:36, 1981
30. Hall AJ, Mackay NN: The results of laminectomy for compression of the cord or cauda equina by extradural malignant tumor. J Bone Joint Surg 55B:497, 1973
31. Hodgson AR, Stock FE: Anterior spine fusion for the treatment of tuberculosis of the spine. The operative findings and results of treatment in the first one hundred cases. J Bone Joint Surg 42A:295, 1960
32. Scoville WB, Palmer AH, Samra K, et al: The use of acrylic plastic for vertebral replacement or fixation in metastatic disease of the spine. A technical note. J Neurosurg 27:274, 1967
33. Sarmiento A, Kinman PB, Galvin EG, et al: Functional bracing of fractures of the shaft of the humerus. J Bone Joint Surg 59A:596, 1977
34. Hackethal KH: Die Bundel-Nageling. Berlin, Springer-Verlag, 1961
35. Foster RJ, Dixon GL, Bach AW, et al: Internal fixation of fractures and non-unions of the humeral shaft. Indications and results in a multicenter study. J Bone Joint Surg 67A:857, 1985

Brachial Plexopathy in Patients with Breast Cancer

Kathleen M. Foley

In patients with cancer, brachial plexus signs may be attributable to unrelated acute brachial neuritis,[1] trauma to the plexus during surgery or anesthesia,[2] metastatic spread of tumor,[3] a second primary tumor,[4] transient or permanent radiation injury,[5,6] or radiation-induced plexus tumors.[7] In patients with breast cancer, metastatic spread of tumor and radiation injury to the plexus are the most common causes of such signs. Tumor infiltration of the brachial plexus from breast cancer is common because of the contiguous relationship of the plexus to the draining mammary lymph nodes, yet this diagnosis represented only 3% of the neurologic consultations evaluated by one neuro-oncology consultation service,[8] and only 2.8% of the metastatic complications of breast cancer in one series.[9] Early and accurate diagnosis is critical in preventing irreversible nerve damage and chronic pain and in determining both prognosis and treatment of tumor. There is a group of clinical symptoms and signs, electrodiagnostic studies, and radiographic procedures that may be helpful in diagnosing the etiology of a brachial plexopathy.

TUMOR INFILTRATION OF THE BRACHIAL PLEXUS (METASTATIC BRACHIAL PLEXOPATHY)

Clinical Symptoms

Pain is the most common symptom, often preceding neurologic signs or symptoms for up to 9 months,[8] and its distribution depends upon the site of plexus involvement. Eighty-five percent of patients with tumor infiltration present with pain, which is moderate to severe, beginning in the shoulder girdle and radiating to the elbow, medial side of the forearm, and the fourth and fifth fingers. In some patients, pain is localized to the posterior aspect of the arm or to the elbow. Some patients complain of a burning or freezing sensation and hypersensitivity of the skin along the ulnar aspect of the arm. This distribution of pain is consistent with involvement of the lower plexus (C7, C8, T1). In certain patients, the pain is restricted to either the shoulder girdle or the tips of the fingers (either the index finger or thumb). In these patients, infiltration of the upper plexus (C5-6), often in the supraclavicular fossa, is the site of nerve compression. By the time of diagnosis of a brachial plexus lesion, 98% of patients have pain which is most often reported as severe. In Kori's series,[8] 2 of 78 patients with tumor infiltration of the brachial plexus had pain as the only symptom or sign of tumor recurrence; exploration and biopsy of the plexus established the diagnosis of tumor recurrence when there were no other signs of metastatic disease or objective signs of plexus disorder.

Paresthesias occur as a presenting symptom in 15% of patients in this group, most commonly affecting the ulnar distribution from infiltration of the lower plexus, with median distribution being more common in lesions of the upper plexus. Lymphedema is rarely a presenting symptom of tumor infiltration of the brachial plexus, but it does occur in about 10% of patients, most commonly in patients who have had previous radiation therapy to the plexus and who subsequently develop recurrent tumor.

Clinical Signs

Focal weakness, atrophy, and sensory changes in the distribution of the C7, C8, and T1 roots occur in more than 75% of patients. Twenty-five percent of patients in one series presented with whole-plexus motor weakness (panplexopathy).[8] Of note is the fact that these patients had epidural deposits at C5-6 that mimicked the involvement of the plexus at that level. Horner syndrome, which occurs in over 50% of patients with tumor infiltration of the plexus, is an ominous sign because it suggests paraspinal and epidural extension. In 12 of 78 patients with tumor infiltration of the brachial plexus included in the Kori series, the plexus lesion was the only evidence of tumor, and other metastases appeared only after several months.[8] In two patients, the plexus lesion was the only sign of recurrence for 4 years. In one patient, surgical exploration after 2 years of plexus signs proved to be normal, but because of progressive worsening of neurologic signs, a second exploration was carried out, confirming tumor recurrence.

Electrodiagnostic Studies

Electromyography reveals fibrillation potentials and positive waves characteristic of denervation in the distribution of the brachial plexus, and results are usually consistent with plexus signs and symptoms.[9,10,11] Cervical paraspinal muscles are normal, excluding the presence of root disease. Myokymia has not been reported in patients with tumor infiltration of the brachial plexus.[12] Median somatosensory-evoked potentials have been used in the evaluation of patients with brachial plexopathy, and may be reliable in confirming the presence of an abnormality in the brachial plexus, the C5-T1 roots, or the epidural space rostral to the second vertebral body. In a study of 23 patients with tumor infiltration of the brachial plexus, vertebral body disease, and radiation fibrosis,[13] median somatosensory-evoked potentials detected myelopathy in nine patients with epidural disease, but reported myelopathic changes in four patients with negative myelograms. In this study, the median somatosensory-evoked potentials did not distinguish tumor infiltration of the brachial plexus from radiation injury. This test is of clinical usefulness in patients with pain but without evidence of objective neurologic findings who are at risk for tumor infiltration of the brachial plexus. Abnormal median somatosensory-evoked potentials are an indication for exploration of the plexus in patients without evidence of diffuse metastatic disease.

Radiographic Findings

Computed Tomography

Radiographic studies other than CT scans are of little help in determining the etiology of brachial plexopathy in patients with breast cancer.[11] The CT scan provides both soft tissue and bony definition in a two-dimensional anatomic plane, and in each CT study, the symptomatic plexus may be compared with the asymptomatic one, rendering it a valuable diagnostic technique. In studies of patients with tumor involving the brachial plexus, the CT scan was abnormal in 89% of patients; all but one had a circumscribed mass in the region of the brachial plexus.[11] Paravertebral extension and tumor erosion of bone were frequently demonstrated despite normal plain radiographs and bone scans. In fact, plain radiographs of the spine were abnormal in only 4 of 39 patients, whereas CT scanning detected spine abnormalities in 13 of 41 patients. Similarly, bone scans were not helpful and were falsely negative, especially in patients who had received prior radiation therapy. In fact, in patients who had been irradiated previously, the radionuclide bone scan was usually negative, even in areas of proven metastases. Plain radiographs, such as chest radiographs, are sometimes helpful if there is an associated apical mass or radiation fibrosis of the lung, but again, CT scanning provides better definition of these abnormalities. In Cascino's study, CT studies were reviewed for four abnormalities: soft tissue density changes in the region of the brachial plexus, paravertebral extension of soft tissue masses, bony erosion, and epidural extension.[11] Forty-one of 46 patients with metastatic plexopathy had abnormalities in the region of the symptomatic brachial plexus. Five patients had a completely normal CT scan despite proven metastatic plexopathy. All other diagnostic studies (bone scans, myelograms, or cervical spine radiographs) in four of these patients were negative, as well. One patient had an epidural tumor at C7, detected on myelography, which was found, during surgery, to extend out and invade the plexus. Two patients had negative surgical explorations of the brachial plexus through an anterior approach. Postoperative CT scans demonstrated a mass deep in the brachial plexus. Repeat exploration of the abnormality revealed by CT scanning demonstrated a tumor at biopsy. Figures 14-24 and 14-25 represent typical findings on CT scans in patients with breast cancer.

Myelography

A myelogram is the only diagnostic radiographic test that defines a specific abnormality better than the CT scan. In Cascino's series, which explored the role of CT studies in the evaluation of patients with brachial plexopathies, CT scanning did not detect epidural extension of tumor

FIGURE 14-24. A CT scan shows diffuse infiltration of soft tissues with loss of normal tissue planes in a patient without a history of previous radiation therapy. Exploration revealed diffusely infiltrating tumor.

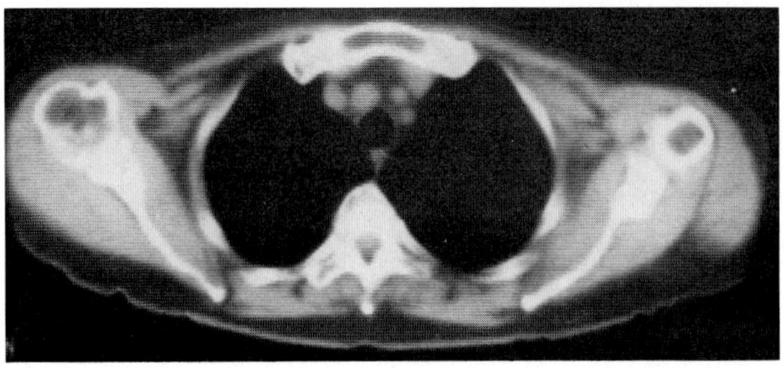

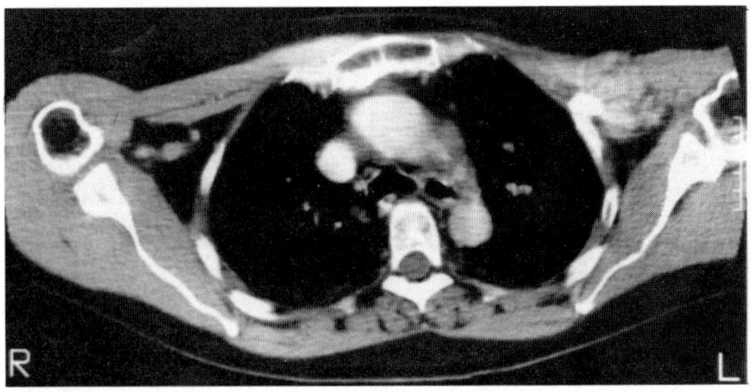

FIGURE 14-25. A CT scan shows a circumscribed mass in a patient with breast cancer and recent onset of symptoms of a C7-T1 plexopathy.

in six patients with proven epidural metastases. Myelography is indicated if epidural spinal cord compression is suspected clinically. Patients with brachial plexus lesions are at high risk for developing epidural cord compression from direct tumor infiltration along the plexus into the epidural space, or from hematogenous spread of tumor to the vertebral body.[8,11,14] Certain clinical findings are commonly associated with this complication, including panplexopathy, Horner syndrome, vertebral body erosion or collapse at the C7-T1 levels, or a paraspinal mass detected on CT scanning . Such patients may have no signs of myelopathy despite escalating pain. Myelography should be performed to define the appropriate radiation ports. Improved resolution of CT scans and the concomitant use of contrast agents, such as metrizamide, may change this approach.

Treatment

The treatment of tumor infiltration of the brachial plexus depends upon the status of the patient's disease, the extent of neurologic involvement, and any prior history of radiation therapy to the brachial plexus. In patients with tumor infiltration of the brachial plexus with evidence of metastatic disease in other sites, systemic chemotherapy is a reasonable approach. In those who have undergone previous radiation therapy to the region, chemotherapy may offer the only reasonable antitumor treatment. However, if the neurologic signs are rapidly progressive, or if there is evidence of epidural spinal cord compression, radiation therapy is the procedure of choice. As stated, CT scans and myelograms should be used to define the exact radiation ports. The dose of radiation therapy employed varies. In the reported series, a dose of 3000 cGy, delivered over a 3-week period, or 5000 cGy delivered over a period of 5 weeks represents the most commonly used dose ranges.[6,8,9,15] There is anecdotal evidence to suggest that steroids provide pain relief in patients with tumor infiltration of the brachial plexus, and they are often used to provide analgesia during therapy. If the diagnosis of brachial plexus tumor infiltration is made early and effective therapy is instituted, the patient's neurologic symptoms should resolve, and a marked reduction in pain should be noted. Ampil reviewed the literature, summarizing the results of external irradiation and his own experience, and reported that the total amount of delivered dose, rather than the width of the therapy port, was the most important factor in determining successful outcome.[15] In the series by Nisce and Chu, 12 of 47 patients (25.5%) with metastatic brachial plexopathy and breast cancer had complete pain relief for a mean duration of 15 months, and 23 (49%) had partial pain relief for a mean duration of 6 months.[16] These researchers suggested that higher doses of irradiation (5000 cGy) were more effective than lower doses. However, if neurologic signs have progressed and the pain has a burning, dysesthetic component, effective tumor therapy may not be associated with a marked improvement in pain. This results, in part, from the fact that nerve injury is not reversible and that a causalgia or deafferentation pain has developed.[17] This type of pain results from injured nerve, and analgesic treatment modalities in these cases are significantly limited. In Kori's review, the treatment of metastatic plexopathy was disappointing.[8] Radiation therapy, in doses of 2000 cGy to 5000 cGy delivered to the plexus, relieved pain in only 46% of cases. Neurologic improvement was minimal, and persistent, chronic pain was the most significant problem.

RADIATION INJURY TO THE BRACHIAL PLEXUS

Transient Radiation Injury

Two distinct clinical syndromes—reversible brachial plexopathy and radiation fibrosis or radiation injury to the brachial plexus—have been reported in patients with breast cancer. Both are rare clinical entities, each with a characteristic clinical presentation and course. Reversible or transient brachial plexopathy was reported to occur in 8 of 565 patients (1.4%) who were treated with moderate doses (5000 cGy in 5 weeks) of super voltage radiation therapy. The clinical symptoms included paresthesias in the arm and hand and, less commonly, weakness and pain, with the onset of symptoms occurring 3 to 14 months following irradiation (a median of 4.5 months). Seven of 8 patients received adjuvant chemotherapy; in 6 patients, symptoms began following drug treatment. There was a temporal clustering of these cases, suggesting a neurotropic viral component. The symptoms and signs of paresthesias and weakness did not conform to any anatomical pattern, but most commonly affected the distributions of the lower plexus. Weakness occurred in 5 of 8 patients, and was profound in 2 of them. All patients regained full strength. In 3 patients, residual paresthesias persisted.

Radiation Fibrosis

In contrast, radiation fibrosis of the brachial plexus results in progressive and irreversible neurologic dysfunction of the brachial plexus. This entity has been well described in the literature. Its salient clinical features are summarized in the following sections.

Clinical Symptoms

Pain is a presenting symptom in less than 20% of patients with radiation injury to the brachial plexus. It is commonly described as mild discomfort associated with aching pain in the shoulder or hand. Other symptoms include paresthesias in the entire hand in over 50% of affected patients, swelling and heaviness of the arm in 50% of patients, and proximal weakness of the arm in the deltoid distribution in all patients. The paresthesias are commonly reported to occur in the thumb and forefinger, but often involve the entire hand. These symptoms are often confused with carpal tunnel syndrome, but may be differentiated clinically and by electromyography. At the time of diagnosis, 65% of patients will report discomfort or pain in the arm; in 35%, it is severe.[8] Several series of patients with radiation injury to the brachial plexus have been reported.[5,8,10,18–20]

Clinical Signs

Typically, a C5-6 distribution of motor weakness occurs in patients with radiation injury. In Kori's series, 5 of 22 patients with radiation injury and breast cancer had involvement of the whole plexus, which had occurred over a period of several years. Lymphedema and swelling of the ipsilateral arm, observed in 16 of 22 of these patients with radiation fibrosis, were significant and important signs of this disorder. Radiation skin changes were noted in approximately one-third of the patients with radiation injury, but these changes were not predictive of an underlying plexopathy.[8]

Radiation Factors

In the Kori series, the interval from the last dose of radiation to the first symptoms of plexus disorder in patients with radiation fibrosis ranged from 3 months to 26 years, with a median of 4 years and an average of 5.5 years.[8] In 7 of 22 patients, symptoms appeared within 1 year after the completion of radiation therapy. Kori attempted to correlate the latency in the development of radiation injury and the reason for initial radiation therapy. Five of 7 patients in his series who received radiation therapy because of local disease developed radiation damage within 1 year, whereas 13 of 15 patients who received radiation therapy to the plexus as prophylaxis developed symptoms after 1 year. There is no good explanation for this finding. The radiation doses that are associated with radiation injury have usually been reported to be greater than 6000 cGy[5,18,19] but there are numerous factors that appear to play a role.

Pathophysiology of Radiation Injury

The peripheral nervous system has been thought to be relatively radioresistant, but a series of experimental studies have demonstrated that, under certain conditions, the peripheral nerves are sensitive to radiation therapy. Sensitivity to a given dose of radiation is dependent upon several factors, including age, the radiation dose, the size of the port, and especially, the premorbid state of the irradiated nerve.[21,22] In cases of radiation injury to the brachial plexus, the predominant findings are in the upper plexus.

When the anatomic relationship of the brachial plexus to the surrounding lymph nodes is considered, these findings are not surprising. In 73 of 78 patients with metastatic plexopathy in the Kori series, the initial tumor was located in an area that drains into the lateral group of axillary lymph nodes, which are in close contact with the division of the lower trunk of the plexus, whereas the upper trunk and its divisions are remarkably free of lymph nodes. Thus, when metastatic plexopathy is a result of the spread of tumor through lymphatics, the roots affected are C8 and T1. On the other hand, the divisions of the lower trunk run a shorter course through the radiation port, are partially protected by the clavicle, and are less likely to be damaged by irradiation than are the divisions of the upper trunk.

There are three possible types of peripheral nerve damage after radiation therapy.[22] First, a very high dose of radiation may cause direct damage to a segment of a nerve trunk or may injure the nerve trunk by causing severe vascular damage. This type of peripheral nerve damage occurs within months to 2½ years after irradiation. Second, a peripheral nerve trunk situated within intact tissue that is treated by a high dose of irradiation may be damaged, but only if extensive fibrosis of the adjacent and overlying connective tissues has been present for many years. Finally, a peripheral nerve trunk situated in tissue previously subjected to surgical dissection may also be damaged by a course of irradiation after extensive fibrosis of the adjacent connective tissues has been present for a period of a few months to a few years. The trauma of surgically removing subcutaneous and connective tissues, irradiation, and the subsequent decreased vascularity are all contributing factors in facilitating the development of early and extensive fibrosis of the adjacent connective tissues around the nerve trunk. This fibrosis and decreased vascularity over a period of months to years may destroy peripheral nerves and prevent the regeneration of their proximal normal portions. The degree of connective tissue injury at the time of or preceding radiation therapy may be important in influencing the subsequent development of connective tissue fibrosis.

Electrodiagnostic Procedures

Electrodiagnostic procedures in patients with radiation fibrosis have been demonstrated to show signs of fibrillation and positive waves associated with denervation, and myokymia has also been reported to occur in this group of patients.[12] Median somatosensory-evoked potentials cannot distinguish between patients with brachial plexus dysfunction from tumor infiltration and those with radiation fibrosis, but they can detect abnormal nerve function.[13]

Radiographic Findings

The typical appearance of radiation fibrosis of the plexus on CT studies is a diffuse infiltration and loss of tissue planes without a mass lesion (Fig. 14-26). There is often associated lymphedema in the arm, evident on CT, and occasionally, radiation necrosis of the clavicle or rib occurs at the adjacent level. Tumor infiltration of the plexus cannot be differentiated from radiation fibrosis by CT studies when diffuse infiltration is noted. Plain x-ray films of the chest and spine may be useful in demonstrating both radiation fibrosis of the apex of the lung or clavicle, or both, and rib erosion from radiation necrosis. Myelography is not indicated in these patients.

Treatment

The management of patients with radiation fibrosis begins with the establishment of an accurate diagnosis to rule out metastatic disease. There are no proven methods to reverse neurologic damage. Splinting the arm at the chest wall, preventing subluxation of the shoulder joint, and using a Jobst machine to manage lymphedema are all common approaches to managing the musculoskeletal pain syndromes associated with this disorder. Pain treatment with amitriptyline has anecdotally been reported to be of some benefit in patients with significant dysesthesias.[23] Rarely, patients have been treated with a forequarter amputation of the limb for relief of the discomfort of a lymphedematous, functionless arm, but this approach is not successful in providing significant pain relief.

Differential Diagnosis

The differential diagnosis of tumor infiltration of the brachial plexus, especially as distinguished from radiation injury to the plexus, may be made in the majority of cases using the clinical criteria summarized in Table 14-17. However, if these diagnostic approaches fail to detail the nature of the neurologic disorder, exploration of the plexus

FIGURE 14-26. A CT scan shows diffuse soft tissue changes with loss of normal tissue planes and fibrosis of the apex of the lung. Exploration revealed diffuse fibrosis, and the history was consistent with radiation injury.

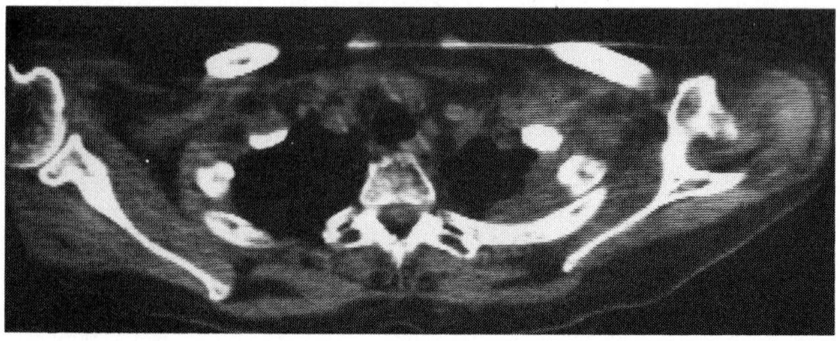

Table 14-17
Clinical Features of Brachial Plexus Syndromes in Patients with Breast Cancer

	Tumor Infiltration	*Radiation Fibrosis*	*Reversible Radiation Injury*
Incidence of pain	89%	18%	40%
Location of pain	Shoulder, upper arm, elbow, radiating to 4th and 5th fingers	Shoulder, wrist, hand	Hand, forearm
Nature of pain	Dull aching in shoulder; lancinating pain in elbow and ulnar aspect of hand; occasional dysesthesias, burning, or freezing sensations	Aching pain in shoulder; paresthesias in C5, C6 distribution in hand	Aching pain in shoulder. Paresthesias in hand and forearm
Severity of pain	Moderate to severe (severe in 98% of patients)	Mild to moderate; severe in 35% of patients	Mild
Course	Progressive neurologic dysfunction; atrophy and weakness with C7–T1 distribution; persistent pain; Horner syndrome	Progressive weakness with C5, C6 distribution; stabilizing pain with appearance of weakness	Transient weakness and atrophy affecting C6–C7, T1; complete resolution of motor findings
CT scan findings	Circumscribed mass with diffuse infiltration of tissue planes	Diffuse infiltration of tissue planes	Normal
EMG findings	Segmental slowing; no myokymia	Myokymia	Segmental slowing; no myokymia.

should be considered. Such exploration should be undertaken only under the following circumstances:

1. The CT scan is normal or shows no evidence of change from before the onset of symptoms.
2. The site of neurologic involvement is certain (for example, a lesion that can be localized to either the upper or lower plexus). This factor is important in determining the appropriate surgical approach. Upper plexus dysfunction may best be assessed through a supraclavicular approach, whereas involvement of the lower plexus is best assessed through a posterior scapular approach or a high posterior thoracotomy, commonly used to explore apical tumors of the lung.[24]
3. A work-up establishing the full extent of disease has been completed and shows no evidence of diffuse metastatic disease.
4. The onset of symptoms and signs occurs several years after completion of successful antitumor therapy or treatment for the presumed primary tumor does not appear to be effective. Both second primary tumors (of the lung)[4] and radiation-induced peripheral nerve tumors[7] have been reported in patients with breast cancer presenting with brachial plexopathy. In the Kori study, there were no adverse effects of surgical exploration of the plexus, but the procedure requires an expert surgeon who can carefully distinguish fibrous tissue from nerve tissue using intraoperative neurophysiological approaches.

REFERENCES

1. Tsairis P, Dyck P, Mulder D: Natural history of brachial plexus neuropathy. Arch Neurol 27:109, 1972
2. Jackson L, Kebts AS: Mechanisms of brachial plexus palsy following anesthesia. Anesthesiology 26:190, 1965
3. Moersch HJ, Henshaw HG, Wilson IH: Apical lung tumors or so-called superior pulmonary sulcus tumor. Minn Med 23:221, 1940
4. Payne R, Foley KM: Exploration of the brachial plexus in patients with cancer (abstr). Neurology 36 (suppl 1): 329, 1986
5. Stoll BA, Andrews JT: Radiation-induced peripheral neuropathy. Br Med J 1:834, 1966
6. Salner AL, Botnick LE, Herzog AG, et al: Reversible brachial plexopathy following primary radiation therapy for breast cancer. Cancer Treat Rep 65:797, 1981
7. Foley KM, Woodruff JM, Ellis FT, et al: Radiation-induced malignant and atypical peripheral nerve sheath tumors. Ann Neurol 7:288, 1980
8. Kori SH, Foley KM, Posner JB: Brachial plexus lesions in patients with cancer: 100 cases. Neurology 31:45, 1981
9. Son Y: Effectiveness of irradiation therapy in peripheral neuropathy caused by malignant disease. Cancer 20:1447, 1967
10. Bagley FH, Walsh JW, Cady B, et al: Carcinomatous versus

radiation-induced brachial plexus neuropathy in breast cancer. Cancer 41:2154, 1978
11. Cascino TL, Kori SH, Krol G, et al: CT scans of the brachial plexus in cancer patients. Am Soc Clin Oncol 1:5, 1982
12. Albers JW, Allen AH, Bashow JA, et al: Limb myokimia. Muscle Nerve 4:494, 1981
13. Rapoport S, Stacy C, Foley KM: Median nerve somatosensory-evoked potentials are useful in the diagnosis of metastases to the brachial plexus and adjacent spinal roots and epidural space. Ann Neurol 14:143, 1983
14. Gilbert RW, Kim TH, Posner JB: Epidural spinal cord compression from metastatic tumor diagnosis and treatment. Ann Neurol 3:40, 1978
15. Ampil FL: Radiotherapy for carcinomatous brachial plexopathy: A clinical study of 23 cases. Cancer 56:2185, 1985
16. Nisce LZ, Chu FC: Radiation therapy of brachial plexus syndrome from breast cancer. Radiology 91:1022, 1968
17. Tasker RJ: Deafferentation. In Wall PD, Melzack R (eds): Textbook of Pain, pp 305–331. New York, Churchill Livingston, 1984
18. Thomas JE, Colby MY: Radiation-induced or metastatic brachial plexopathy? JAMA 222:1392, 1972
19. Basso-Rici S, della Costa C, Viganotti G, et al: Report on 42 cases of post-irradiation lesions of the brachial plexus and their treatment. Tumori 66:117, 1980
20. Maruyama Y, Mylrea MM, Logothetis J: Neuropathy following irradiation. Am J Roentgenol 101:216, 1967
21. Cavanagh, JB: Effects of x-irradiation on the proliferation of cells in peripheral nerve during wallerian degeneration in the rat. Br J Radiol 41:275, 1968
22. Glass JP, Foley KM: Harmful effects of radiation. In Asbury AK, McKhann GM, McDonald WI (eds): Diseases of the Nervous System, pp 1108–1202. Philadelphia, WB Saunders, 1985
23. Walsh TD: Antidepressants in chronic pain. Clin Neuropharmacol, 6:271, 1983
24. Kline DG, Kott J, Barnes G, et al: Exploration of selected brachial plexus lesions by the posterior subscapular approach. J Neurosurg 49:872, 1978

Lymphangitic Spread of Carcinoma of the Breast

William David Henner

Lymphangitic carcinoma is defined as metastatic carcinoma that predominantly or exclusively involves the lymphatic system of the lungs. This mode of lung involvement by metastasis was described in the 19th century by Virchow[1] and Wagner.[2] Histologic findings include diffuse permeation of the lung lymphatics by tumor cells and a surrounding fibrous reaction.[3] The surface of the lung may show a network of fine, whitish lines caused by the enlarged superficial lymphatics. In advanced cases of disease, the lung may be reduced in volume and resistant to distention. Enlargement of the lymphatics tends to be more pronounced in the lower lobes.[3]

EPIDEMIOLOGY AND PATHOPHYSIOLOGY

Breast carcinoma is the most frequent diagnosis associated with lymphangitic carcinomatosis, accounting for 35% of such cases.[4] In autopsy series of patients with breast cancer, pulmonary lymphangitic carcinoma is found in 24% to 34% of cases.[5,6] This frequency is roughly equivalent to that of pulmonary nodules in the same series. However, the clinical diagnosis of lymphangitic carcinoma is made much less frequently, as only about 20% of cases are diagnosed ante mortem.[6]

The pathway by which breast carcinoma cells enter the pulmonary lymphatics is not well established. The autopsies of 26 patients who died of disseminated breast carcinoma indicate that the frequency of mediastinal node involvement was greater ipsilateral to the primary breast cancer, suggesting a role for local-regional spread in the development of this entity.[7] The greater incidence of involvement of the parenchymal pleural lymphatics in comparison to that of the parietal pleural lymphatics also suggests that lymphatic involvement usually occurs first in the mediastinum, spreading centrifugally through the visceral lymphatics to the pleura.[7,8] No identifiable group of patients with breast cancer appears to be particularly prone to the development of lymphangitic metastases, and this entity occurs with equal frequency in patients of all age groups. Infiltrating ductal carcinoma is the most common histologic type reported.[6]

SIGNS AND SYMPTOMS

The presenting symptoms of lymphangitic breast cancer are progressive dyspnea, nonproductive cough, general physical deterioration, and, in advanced cases, cyanosis. Often, there is a paucity of physical findings to explain the severe dyspnea.[9] The most common radiographic finding is diffuse reticular-nodular pulmonary infiltrates (Fig. 14-27). About 50% of affected patients will have a characteristic radiographic appearance of Kerley A or B lines (or both), with small, nodular densities in several lung zones and enlargement of the hilar nodes. Often, a tumor mass or pleural effusion will also be present.[3] Pleural effusions are more common in patients with breast cancer dying with lymphangitic metastases (63%) than in those without (41%), and these effusions occur somewhat more frequently on the side ipsilateral to the primary carcinoma. Lymphangitic spread of breast cancer is usually associated with bilateral enlargement of the hilar nodes;[10] invariably, chest x-ray films are abnormal bilaterally.[5]

DIAGNOSIS

The diagnosis of lymphangitic metastases may be difficult. In a series of patients with histologic evidence of lymphangitic metastases at autopsy, the diagnosis was established prior to death in only 20%.[6] Because neither the symptoms nor the radiographic appearance of lymphangitic metastases are specific, many patients will require further studies to establish the diagnosis.[5] Pulmonary function studies in patients with lymphangitic carcinoma demonstrate decreased tidal volume, increased respiratory rate, diminished inspiratory capacity, diminished vital ca-

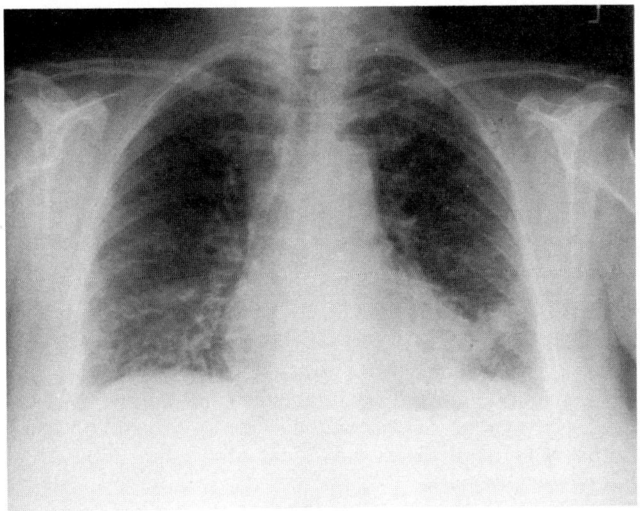

FIGURE 14-27. Lymphangitic metastases from breast carcinoma developed in a 65-year-old woman 18 months following excision and primary radiation therapy to the left breast.

pacity, diminished maximal breathing capacity, and diminished expiratory reserve volume. Goldsmith and co-workers suggested that these findings differentiate lymphangitic metastases from all similar conditions except radiation fibrosis.[6]

Because the radiographic findings associated with lymphangitic carcinoma may be mimicked by those of treatable conditions, such as congestive heart failure, opportunistic infections, and pulmonary reactions to antineoplastic drugs,[5] histologic confirmation of the diagnosis may be warranted, provided the patient's overall medical condition permits. For example, the rapid onset of lymphangitic-like infiltrates, the absence of other evidence of recurrent breast cancer, and the presence of fever would all be relative indications for early biopsy.

Bronchoscopy is the procedure of choice in the biopsy of suspected lymphangitic breast cancer. In one reported series, transbronchial biopsy was diagnostic in all of 6 cases of lymphangitic breast carcinoma.[11] In those patients whose infiltrates cannot be diagnosed by less invasive methods and whose clinical condition permits, a wedge biopsy of the lung during thoracotomy may be performed to rule out an infectious etiology for the pulmonary infiltrates. Patients with breast cancer whose symptoms and radiographic studies are interpreted as congestive heart failure may benefit from Swan-Ganz catheterization. Measurement of a normal capillary wedge pressure would eliminate heart failure from the differential diagnosis and would suggest the diagnosis of lymphangitic carcinomatosis.[12]

PROGNOSIS

The prognosis for patients with breast cancer who develop lymphangitic spread was reported by Kreisman and coworkers for a group of patients treated between 1975 and 1979.[5] Survival was dependent on whether lymphangitic tumor was the initial or subsequent site for the development of metastases. In patients with lymphangitic disease as the initial metastatic site, survival was 80% at 1 year and 30% at 2 years from diagnosis. However, when the development of lymphangitic disease occurred subsequent to the development of either thoracic or extrathoracic metastases, the one-year survival was only 31%, and the two-year survival rate was only 5%. In both groups, survival was moderately less than that in patients with other forms of intrathoracic metastases.[5] There has been relatively little recent improvement in the prognosis of patients with lymphangitic spread of breast cancer. The duration of survival from the time of diagnosis of lymphangitic metastases for a group of 20 patients treated during the 1960s was similar to that reported in a recent series, with 30% and 20% surviving one and two years, respectively.[6]

TREATMENT

No specific local therapy has proved to be useful in the treatment of lymphangitic carcinoma of the breast. Treatment should be directed toward palliation of the patient's symptoms of dyspnea, usually accomplished through the use of systemic therapy. Unfortunately, there is a dearth of information available concerning the response of lymphangitic breast carcinoma to systemic hormonal or cytotoxic chemotherapy. Therefore, a reasonable approach to the treatment of such patients would be to use the same systemic treatment that would be chosen for metastases to other visceral sites.

REFERENCES

1. Virchow R: Trois observations de tumeurs epitheliales generalisees. Gazette medical Paris 3 ser 10:208, 1855
2. Wagner E: Der Krebs der Lymphgefasse der Pleura und der Lungen. Arch Heilk 4:538, 1863
3. Trapnell DH: Radiological appearances of lymphangitis carcinomatosa of the lung. Thorax 19:251, 1964
4. Lange VS, Minck C: Lymphangiosis carcinomatosa der Lungen beim metasierenden Mammakarzinom. ROFO 140:408, 1984
5. Kreisman H, Woklove N, Finkelstein HS, et al: Breast cancer and thoracic metastases: Review of 119 patients. Thorax 38:175, 1983
6. Goldsmith HS, Bailey HD, Callahan EL, et al: Pulmonary lymphangitic metastases from breast carcinoma. Arch Surg 94:483, 1967
7. Thomas JM, Redding WH, Sloane JP: The spread of breast cancer: Importance of the intrathoracic lymphatic route and its relevance to treatment. Br J Cancer 40:540, 1979
8. Schattenberg HJ, Ryan JR: Lymphangitic carcinomatosis of the lungs. Case report with autopsy findings. Ann Intern Med 14:1710, 1941
9. Hauser TE, Steer A: Lymphangitic carcinomatosis of the lungs: Six case reports and a review of the literature. Ann Intern Med 34:881, 1951
10. Yang S-P, Lin C-C: Lymphangitic carcinomatosis of the lungs:

The clinical significance of its roentgenologic classification. Chest 62:179, 1972

11. Aranda C, Sidhu G, Sasso LA, et al: Transbronchial lung biopsy in the diagnosis of lymphangitic carcinomatosis. Cancer 42:1995, 1978
12. Koenigs KP, Campbell DR, Magrina J, et al: Pulmonary lymphangitic carcinomatosis from vaginal carcinoma presenting as congestive heart failure. Obstet Gynecol 61:760, 1983

Malignant Effusions in Breast Cancer

William David Henner

Effusions are a frequent problem encountered in the treatment of patients with metastatic breast carcinoma. Approximately 50% of patients with metastatic breast cancer will develop a pleural effusion during the course of their disease.[1,2] Breast carcinoma is second only to carcinoma of the lung as a cause of both malignant pleural effusions[3,4] and pericardial effusions.[5,6] Peritoneal effusions in patients with breast cancer are approximately fourfold less frequent than pleural effusions, but may also be the cause of significant chronic morbidity and become difficult management problems for the oncologist.[7]

PATHOGENESIS OF MALIGNANT PLEURAL EFFUSIONS IN PATIENTS WITH BREAST CANCER

Metastatic spread to the pleura in patients with breast cancer might be expected to occur either hematogenously or in a local-regional manner through the chest wall via the lymphatic pathways described earlier (see chapters 1 and 7). Both the external and the internal intercostal muscles have lymphatic connections to the parietal pleura.[8] The external intercostal lymphatics connect to the lymphatics from the posterior portion of the parietal pleura at the posterior intercostal lymph nodes; the internal intercostal lymphatics drain the lymphatics from the parietal pleura and, in turn, drain anteriorly into the internal mammary nodes.

Several authors have noted the predominance of ipsilateral over contralateral malignant pleural effusions in patients with breast cancer.[9,10] A compilation of seven published series[3,9–14] yields 566 cases of malignant pleural effusion secondary to breast cancer, 344 of which are effusions that are ipsilateral to the primary cancer, 145 of which are contralateral, and 77 of which are bilateral. The preponderance of ipsilateral cases is highly significant ($p < 0.001$) and sufficient to conclude that at least one-fifth of pleural effusions attributable to breast cancer arise by local-regional spread. Factors that may predispose a patient to development of pleural effusion through local spread include a medial location of the primary tumor[12] and the development of a chest wall recurrence.[9]

The accumulation of fluid in either the pleural, pericardial, or peritoneal space is governed by the principles of hydrostatic forces first described by Starling in 1898.[15] The pathogenesis of pleural effusions secondary to breast carcinoma appears to involve a combination of increased capillary permeability as a result of inflammation and disruption of the capillary endothelium at tumor sites on the pleura, as well as decreased lymph flow due to tumor obstruction.[4] The amount of fluid accumulation required to produce symptoms is dependent on the site. Rapid accumulation of as little as 250 ml of pericardial effusion may produce cardiac tamponade, whereas up to 1000 ml may accumulate gradually before symptoms occur. Usually, more than 1 liter of fluid must accumulate in the pleural or peritoneal cavity before severe symptoms develop. However, the severity of dyspnea may not be proportional to the volume of effusion when there is substantial involvement of the pleura by tumor. Other symptoms and physical findings all result from effusion compressing either the lung, heart, or gut.

PRESENTATION AND DIAGNOSIS OF MALIGNANT PLEURAL EFFUSIONS

Symptoms are usually present in patients with malignant pleural effusions and may include dyspnea, nonproductive cough, and chest pain. The physical examination will often reveal dullness in response to percussion, decreased breath sounds on the involved side, and occasionally, deviation of the trachea. When the history or physical examination suggests the presence of pleural effusion, the diagnosis should be ascertained by chest x-ray films. If the anteroposterior view suggests the presence of pleural effusion, lateral decubitus views should be obtained. As little as 100 ml of fluid may be detected in this position.[16] In some cases, especially in those patients in whom the pleural effusion is loculated, x-ray findings may be equivocal. In these cases, ultrasonography should be used to confirm the presence, location, and volume of pleural effusions.[17,18]

Effusion is only rarely the initial presentation of the patient's breast cancer.[19] However, effusions frequently provide the initial evidence of metastic breast carcinoma, and may be present without other evidence of recurrent disease. In most patients with breast cancer who develop pleural effusion, and especially in those who were not previously known to have metastatic disease, the etiology of the effusion should be determined.

Several factors may make the diagnosis of effusions in patients with known breast cancer difficult; for this reason, cytologic confirmation of malignant disease is usually necessary. The first of these factors is the long interval between the initial diagnosis and the development of effusion. In two series of patients who developed malignant pleural effusions secondary to breast cancer, the average interval from initial diagnosis to the development of effusion was 48 and 54 months.[5,20] The second factor complicating diagnosis of effusions in patients with breast cancer is the development of effusions as a complication of therapy. Patients who have received radiation doses in excess of 4000 cGy to a significant volume of heart are at risk for development of pericarditis[21] and pericardial effusion. Such effusions almost always occur (in 92% of the cases) within the first 12 months following therapy.[22] Following excisional biopsy and definitive radiation therapy for primary breast carcinoma, the incidence of both pericarditis and pleural effusion is 1%.[23] Pleural effusions have also been reported as a complication of systemic hyperthermia.[24] Effusion may also occur as a result of congestive heart failure secondary to the administration of doxorubicin. Empyema must also be considered in a patient with neutropenia secondary to chemotherapy.

Thus, depending on the clinical setting, the differential diagnosis of effusion must include congestive heart failure, infection, radiation pericarditis and pleuritis, and other malignant processes in addition to metastatic breast carcinoma.

The first steps in the diagnostic evaluation of pleural effusions in patients with breast cancer should be a careful history, review of symptoms, physical examination, and staging for breast cancer. This sequence should identify those patients whose effusions are likely to stem from either radiation pneumonitis, congestive heart failure, or other treatment-related disease. For some patients in whom a nonmalignant etiology for effusion is strongly suspected, observation or symptomatic treatment may be worth a trial. When a nonmalignant etiology is unlikely, or if the patient fails to improve, thoracentesis usually is required. The initial thoracentesis may be both diagnostic and therapeutic because a small percentage of patients (10%) whose effusions are drained will not have a recurrence.

The fluid obtained during the initial thoracentesis should be analyzed for protein and glucose levels and cell count, submitted for cytologic analysis, and cultured for both bacteria and mycobacteria. In effusions secondary to breast cancer, the fluid is almost always an exudate and is usually bloody.[25] No single laboratory test can reliably distinguish between exudates and transudates. Exudates will generally have a specific gravity of > 1.015 g/ml and a protein content of > 3.0 g/dl. Light and co-workers have shown that when the ratio of pleural fluid to serum, protein, or LDH concentrations is > 0.5, or when the LDH level of the pleural fluid is > 200 u/ml, the effusion is reliably classed as an exudate.[26]

Cytologic examination of the effusion is the most specific test available for the diagnosis of malignant effusion. False-positive results are very rare. Although there are no absolute criteria by which neoplastic cells in effusions may be identified as arising from breast carcinoma, breast cancer cells are often characterized by "Indian filing" or balls of cells.[5] If possible, at least 250 ml of fresh pleural effusion should be submitted to the cytology laboratory. Smaller volumes or stored specimens are less likely to allow an adequate study.[27] In malignant pleural effusions attributable to carcinoma of the breast, 71% of the initial cytologic analyses will be positive for carcinomatous cells.[28] This percentage may be increased somewhat (to 85%) by analysis of the fluid from multiple thoracenteses and needle biopsy of the pleura.[29] However, because false-negative cytologic results are common, it is important to emphasize that a negative cytology report does not rule out the diagnosis of malignant effusion.

In those patients with known or suspected breast cancer whose effusion remains undiagnosed following one or more fluid examinations, the physician should consider submitting the fluid for measurement of CEA levels and estrogen receptor protein (ERP) levels. Titers of CEA may be determined from samples of effusion fluid, and are generally higher in malignant effusions than they are in benign effusions.[30–33] Although most effusions secondary to carcinoma will have a CEA titer of > 10 ng/ml, false-positive titers do occur in benign effusions.[30,31,33] A further limitation to the usefulness of the CEA titer is the strong positive correlation between positive cytology reports and elevations of CEA.[30] Estrogen receptor protein levels may be determined from pleural fluid cells.[34,35] However, as noted above for CEA levels, ERP levels are usually only positive when substantial numbers of malignant cells are present on cytologic examination. In those patients whose primary tumor is of unknown ERP status and in whom knowledge of the ERP status would be important in the selection of therapy, Levine and co-workers have described a thoracoscopic technique that has been successful in obtaining tissue for histologic analysis in 5 of 6 patients and for determination of ERP levels in 4 of 6 cases.[36]

New technologic methods may eventually prove useful in patients in whom the diagnosis is not established by repeated cytologic evaluation of pleural fluid. Submission of fluid for cytogenetic evaluation or electron microscopy[37] occasionally will yield a diagnosis of malignant disease. In addition, some monoclonal antibodies are capable of distinguishing adenocarcinoma from mesothelial cells.[38] However, none of these techniques can yet be recommended on a routine basis. Some effusions may resist diagnosis and remain idiopathic even at autopsy.[39]

PRESENTATION AND DIAGNOSIS OF MALIGNANT PERICARDIAL EFFUSIONS

The symptoms and physical findings associated with malignant pericardial effusion are similar, regardless of tumor type. The initial symptoms of pericardial effusion, including fatigue and weakness, may be difficult to distinguish from the systemic effects of malignant disease. Substernal pain, dyspnea, and orthopnea may be present. Tachycardia is almost invariably present. Other findings may include a pericardial friction rub, neck vein engorgement that is more prominent with inspiration, and hepatic enlargement. With the accumulation of 250 ml to 1000 ml of pericardial effusion, tamponade may occur, accompanied by hypotension. Pulsus paradoxus often occurs at the onset of tamponade.

The presence of pericardial effusion may be suggested by an enlarged cardiac silhouette or by decreased voltage on the QRS complex of the electrocardiogram. Ultrasonography is the optimal procedure for detection and measurement of pericardial effusions, and may be used to localize the effusion for diagnostic or therapeutic pericardiocentesis. When the pericardium is involved by malignant tumor, the ultrasonographer may be unable to determine whether effusion, constriction, or both are the cause of tamponade. In some cases, right heart catheterization and pressure tracings following pericardiocentesis may be needed to rule out constriction.[40]

The various methods used to obtain pericardial fluid will be discussed below under the section on therapy. When fluid is available, the same analyses as described for pleural effusions should be performed. The cytologic analysis of malignant pericardial effusions from breast cancer will demonstrate malignant cells in only 30% to 58% of cases.[5,41,42] Again, it is important to emphasize that a negative cytology report by no means rules out the diagnosis of a malignant pericardial effusion.

PROGNOSIS OF PATIENTS WITH MALIGNANT EFFUSIONS SECONDARY TO BREAST CANCER

When planning treatment for patients with malignant effusions secondary to breast cancer, the physician must have an accurate picture of the prognosis of such patients. Patients with breast cancer effusions have a significantly better prognosis than do patients with malignant effusions attributable to any other solid tumor.[3,7] In various series, the median survival of patients with malignant pleural effusions secondary to breast cancer was 7.3 months,[3] 14 months,[43] and 20 months.[44] In a series reported in 1983 by Poe and co-workers, patients with breast cancer who presented with malignant pleural effusion as the only evidence of metastasis had a median survival of 48 months, whereas patients with additional sites of metastases had a median survival of only 12 months.[45] One case report described a 5-year survival in a patient with malignant effusion secondary to breast cancer who was treated only with a single pericardiocentesis.[46] Clearly, pleural effusion secondary to breast cancer is not necessarily a terminal event.

There is less information about the natural history of breast cancer in patients who develop pericardial effusions or ascites. The available information suggests that the prognosis of patients with effusion at these sites is somewhat worse than the prognosis for patients with pleural effusions.[7] Median survival with pericardial effusion or ascites and breast cancer was 10 months[5] or 6 months,[47] respectively. Again, the presence of disease at other sites was an unfavorable prognostic sign. When ascites was accompanied by hepatomegaly or jaundice, there were no survivors beyond 3 months. When tamponade accompanied pericardial effusion, median survival was 1 week, compared to a median survival of 1 year in the absence of tamponade.[48,49] In patients with pericardial involvement by breast carcinoma, this involvement is a primary or contributory cause of death in all but 15% of cases.[50]

TREATMENT OF PLEURAL EFFUSIONS SECONDARY TO BREAST CANCER

When choosing therapy for a patient with effusion due to breast cancer, the physician should consider several factors: the prognosis and medical condition of the patient, the availability of effective systemic therapy, and the severity of symptoms. For example, patients who are terminal, very elderly, or who have comorbid disease are not candidates for aggressive approaches, such as pleurectomy, despite the effectiveness of this procedure, because of its high morbidity and mortality. If systemic hormonal or cytotoxic chemotherapy is expected to be effective and immediate relief of symptoms is not necessary, a trial of systemic therapy should be undertaken prior to local treatment.

Thoracentesis and Thoracostomy

For most patients, thoracentesis will be both the initial diagnostic and therapeutic maneuver for pleural effusion. However, only 10% of patients will have their effusion controlled by the first thoracentesis. Complications of thoracentesis include pneumothorax, empyema, and bleeding. Each patient should have a chest x-ray study performed following thoracentesis to determine the extent of drainage and whether pneumothorax has occurred. In those patients with loculated effusions, thoracentesis, performed with ultrasonographic guidance, may reduce the risk of pneumothorax.[17,18] Following thoracentesis, some patients will develop re-expansion pulmonary edema.[51] If $\leq$ 1000 ml are drained during one procedure, this complication is less likely to occur. Repeated thoracenteses of large fluid volumes may result in hyponatremia and hypoalbuminemia.

Although repeated thoracenteses may provide palliation in some patients, most patients will require other local therapy. The mainstay of local therapy for pleural effusions is the use of thoracostomy drainage of the effusion with installation of medication into the chest tube. The mechanism by which chest tube drainage prevents reaccumulation of the pleural effusion is unknown. Several authors have speculated that the same inflammation and disruption of the pleural surfaces that causes the effusion may result in sclerosis when the two pleura are apposed by drainage of the fluid. Indeed, 22% to 53% of effusions will be controlled by chest tube drainage alone without instillation of drug into the pleural cavity.[4,19]

Instillation Therapy

A variety of pharmacologic agents have been instilled into the pleural space to cause sclerosis and to improve the results of chest tube thoracostomy. These include the radioisotopes gold-198 and chromic phosphate-32;[52] the anticancer drugs nitrogen mustard,[4,53] thiotepa,[53] 5-fluorouracil,[44] bleomycin,[54] and doxorubicin;[55] and other agents, including quinacrine,[56] talc,[57,58] tetracycline,[56,59] and Coparvax (a preparation of formalin-killed *Corynebacterium parvum*).[60]

The comparative benefits of various forms of instillation therapy for malignant pleural effusions has recently been reviewed by Hausheer and Yarbro.[4] These authors reviewed 85 published studies that included more than 3500 patients whose responses could be assessed according to the following criteria. An objective response was scored when the patient survived and underwent follow-up for at least 1 month, during which time the fluid did not reaccumulate and no thoracentesis was required. A failure was scored when more than 50% of the original effusion volume reaccumulated or when thoracentesis was required within 1 month. When these criteria were applied, the response rate to chest tube drainage was found to be 22%. Only a moderate increase in the response rate occurred with intrapleural instillation of the alkylating agents nitrogen mustard (48%) or thiotepa (52%). Intrapleural instillation of the radioisotopes gold-198 or chromic phosphate-32 was used extensively for treatment of malignant effusions in the 1950s,[61] and a response rate of 59% was observed in patients with pleural effusions.[4] The expense and inconvenience of such therapy and the possibility of radiation exposure to family and staff have severely restricted the use of this therapy.[4,62] Other anticancer agents for which the objective response rates to intrapleural instillation therapy are known include bleomycin (90%), 5-fluorouracil (66%), and doxorubicin (80%).[4,55,62]

The mechanisms by which instillation therapy of anticancer agents promotes sclerosis may not be related to the antitumor action of these drugs, but rather to their role in producing inflammation of the pleural surfaces. This hypothesis has led a number of investigators to use agents that produce inflammation and sclerosis without necessarily producing an antitumor response. These agents and their accompanying objective response rates include talc suspension (96%), quinacrine (86%), tetracycline (69%–87%), and Coparvax (100%).[4,56,57,59,60,63–65] What factors determine whether an agent will achieve effective palliation of pleural effusion by instillation therapy? It has been suggested that tetracycline sclerosis might be effective simply because of the acidic *p*H of the solution. However, a randomized controlled trial has shown tetracycline therapy to be more effective than a solution of the same *p*H and buffering capacity.[59]

The specific frequency of response in patients with breast cancer treated for pleural effusions may be assessed in some series.[64] The objective response rate for breast cancer effusions appears to be similar to the overall average frequency of response for effusions due to a variety of tumor types.[55]

Although the type of tumor has relatively little influence on the effectiveness of instillation therapy, the condition of the patient, stage of disease, and history of prior treatment are all important factors in determining response. Although nitrogen mustard is a sclerosing agent of only moderate effectiveness, it has been reported to be 90% effective in patients who have received no prior therapy. Similarly, there is a marked positive correlation between the patients' responses to local sclerosing therapy and their subsequent response to systemic therapy.[19,28]

A number of agents used in instillation therapy have been compared in randomized controlled trials. Some trials have shown significant differences in the outcome achieved with these agents. For example, talc,[57] Coparvax,[60,64] and doxorubicin[55] have all been shown to be superior to nitrogen mustard, whereas tetracycline and quinacrine were found to be approximately equally effective.[56] On what criteria then, should a physician base the selection of an agent for instillation when choosing among several agents with a response rate ranging from 75% to 100% (including tetracycline, quinacrine, Coparvax, talc, and doxorubicin)? As the response rates are equivalent, the agent with the least side effects and most convenience should be chosen. Although quinacrine and tetracycline are equally effective, quinacrine is associated with a greater incidence of postinstillation pain and fever.[56] Talc or Coparvax are not generally available in the U.S. in preparations suitable for instillation. In view of all these factors, tetracycline (1 g in 50 ml of normal saline) would be optimal instillation therapy for malignant pleural effusions.

If local therapy for malignant pleural effusions in breast cancer is to be improved, it will likely be through reduction in the morbidity and expense of treatment for this problem. Only a very large, randomized, and carefully stratified study could be expected to demonstrate the superiority of any sclerosing agent over tetracycline. Only 13% to 17% of patients fail to respond to tetracycline.[4,64] Because the major morbidity of this procedure is related to the thoracostomy, future studies should seek to develop methods to eliminate the discomfort and expense of this procedure.

Poudrage or Pleurectomy

In a few patients, thoracostomy drainage and instillation therapy may fail to control the malignant pleural effusion. In these patients, thoracotomy with either talc poudrage or pleurectomy should be considered. This is a highly effective mode of treatment, as evidenced by the low recurrence rate of effusion (0% to 4%).[43,66] It is also a morbid procedure, with an operative mortality in the range of 6%.[66] Still, some patients with breast cancer and resistant effusions who are in otherwise good medical condition have been afforded long-term (greater than 2 years) palliation with this procedure.

TREATMENT OF MALIGNANT PERICARDIAL EFFUSIONS

Local treatment of malignant pericardial effusions is usually necessary only when cardiac tamponade seems imminent as a result of a progressive increase in effusion volume. Despite the reduction in morbidity afforded by the use of echocardiographic and electrocardiographic guidance, pericardiocentesis is still associated with a high morbidity rate and is optimally performed only by a physician well-trained in this procedure.[67] Accordingly, in patients with breast cancer, pericardiocentesis should be limited to the prevention of tamponade, to those cases in which the diagnosis of recurrent carcinoma cannot be made by other methods, and to those patients in whom pericardial effusion secondary to bacterial or fungal infection is strongly suspected. When pericardiocentesis is required, a flexible, indwelling catheter may be placed, which may be left in place for several days with little increase in morbidity.[68] This catheter facilitates the collection of additional fluid if the initial cultures and cytologic studies are negative; it also allows instillation therapy to be initiated if malignant disease is diagnosed as the etiology.

The results of instillation therapy for malignant pericardial effusions are difficult to assess. Many series combine the results of instillation therapy for pericardial effusions with the results of the much larger series of pleural effusions so treated. However, there are series of 6 and 7 patients who were treated with instillation of either tetracycline or nitrogen mustard. None of these 13 patients had a recurrence of their effusion.[48,68–70] With the instillation of tetracycline, complications included transient chest pain and fever. Nitrogen mustard produced minimal side effects with the exception of one patient who developed an arrhythmia and died soon after instillation.[70] Instillation of methotrexate, cisplatin, gold-198, chromic phosphate-32, or talc into malignant pericardial effusions has also been reported.[61,71–73] However, the number of reported patients treated with these agents is too few to evaluate effectiveness.

In those patients in whom pericardial effusions recur following instillation therapy or whose effusions cannot be drained safely by pericardiocentesis, a surgical procedure to provide permanent drainage should be considered. Such surgical procedures involve the creation of a pericardial "window" (either pericardiocutaneous or pleuropericardial) or pericardial "stripping."[67,74,75] A subxiphoid technique for placement of a pericardiocutaneous window was described by Berman.[76] This procedure may be performed using local anesthesia and without entering the pleural cavity.[67,74,77] Recurrence rates are low (0 of 17 patients). However, this procedure is complicated by high rates of infection. Pleuropericardial window placement avoids direct communication of the pericardium with the skin, but requires general anesthesia and has a high frequency of closure with recurrence of effusion.[75,78] Pericardial "stripping" has also been used for control of malignant pericardial effusions.[75] This procedure, involving thoracotomy, is associated with a high morbidity rate in patients with malignant disease, and for this reason, cannot be recommended.[74]

It should be noted that radiotherapy is sometimes effective in controlling malignant pericardial effusions. In the series reported by Cham and co-workers, 11 of 16 pericardial effusions secondary to breast cancer were controlled by a 2500-cGy to 4000-cGy dose of external beam radiotherapy.[20] Radiotherapy should be considered in those patients for whom pericardiocentesis with instillation therapy has not proved to be effective and for whom a surgical "window" or "stripping" is contraindicated. Because the development of congestive heart failure is a complication of radiotherapy to the mediastinum, previous or planned doxorubicin therapy must be considered to be a relative contraindication to this therapy.

TREATMENT OF MALIGNANT ASCITES

Malignant ascites is a less common problem in patients with breast cancer than is malignant pleural effusion, and consequently, there is less information available concerning treatment. If the same principles that govern other types of malignant ascites, particularly those resulting from ovarian carcinoma, may be applied, then several recommendations concerning management may be made. If a patient with breast cancer is suspected of having ascites on the basis of physical findings, such as abdominal distention, shifting dullness, symptoms of bloating, early satiety, or dyspnea, an abdominal x-ray study should be obtained. If ascites is present, the x-ray film may show the typical "ground glass" appearance. If any question remains concerning the diagnosis of ascites, an abdominal ultrasonogram should be obtained. In most cases of breast cancer associated with the development of ascites, the diagnosis should be established by peritoneocentesis. The fluid should be analyzed as described above for pleural effusions. False-negative cytologic exams are common and so the presence of malignant ascites cannot be ruled out by this method.

Treatment of malignant ascites secondary to breast cancer may be either systemic or local. Systemic therapy is preferred when ascites is only one of several sites of progressive metastatic disease, or if hepatic metastases are contributing to the ascites. Local therapy should be considered for those patients in whom the peritoneum is the primary site of metastatic disease or in whom massive ascites produces respiratory embarrassment. Temporary relief of symptoms may be achieved through peritoneocentesis and removal of up to 1000 ml of fluid. Removal of larger volumes of fluid may cause hypotension as the intravascular volume becomes depleted with reaccumulation of the fluid. Unfortunately, the effectiveness of this procedure is limited by the rapid recurrence of fluid build-up. Tube drainage of ascites cannot be recommended[79] as it rarely induces sclerosis sufficient to prevent recurrence, and it is frequently complicated by bacterial peritonitis, hypoalbuminemia, and hyponatremia.

Several forms of intraperitoneal therapy have been used for the treatment of malignant ascites, including colloidal gold-198 and chromic phosphate-32 radiotherapy. However, these agents are not as effective in preventing recurrence of malignant ascites as they are in preventing recurrence of malignant pleural effusions.[80,81] Additional limitations associated with the use of intraperitoneal radioisotopes are the requirement for skilled personnel to administer the agents and the risk of contamination of staff or family. These limitations have led to a decline in the use of this modality. Several types of chemotherapeutic agents may be administered by intraperitoneal injection, including 5-fluorouracil,[82] methotrexate,[83] bleomycin,[54] doxorubicin,[84] and cisplatin,[85] yielding response rates ranging from 30% to 50%. For some drugs, intraperitoneal instillation may provide a higher therapeutic index for achieving local response. If care is taken to obtain an even distribution of the drug throughout the peritoneal cavity, instillation of cisplatin into the peritoneal cavity achieves a 30-fold greater exposure of peritoneum to drug than does the systemic route.[85] However, no information is available as to whether any drug is more effective in treating ascites due to breast cancer when administered intraperitoneally rather than systemically.

Selected patients with chronic malignant ascites that is unresponsive to either systemic or intraperitoneal therapy may benefit from placement of a peritoneovenous shunt of either the LeVeen or Denver types.[86,87] Both of these types of shunts afford a direct connection between the abdominal cavity and the superior vena cava. A one-way valve prevents venous blood from entering the abdominal cavity. Complications of shunt placement include fever and fluid overload immediately following placement. Essentially all patients with functioning peritoneovenous shunts will develop laboratory evidence of disseminated intravascular coagulation.[88] The risk of bleeding complications is higher in those patients with severe hepatic dysfunction.[89,90] Another frequent problem with the use of peritoneovenous shunts in the treatment of malignant ascites is shunt failure. Clotting occurs most often in patients with bloody ascites and high concentrations of malignant cells and protein in ascitic fluid.[81,88,91,92] If patients are carefully selected, some patients with breast cancer will achieve effective palliation for 4 or more months from this procedure.[93]

Another surgical procedure that has been used for palliation in patients with ascites secondary to ovarian cancer is ileoentectropy. A loop of small bowel is separated from the gastrointestinal tract and everted to provide a mucosal surface for absorption of ascitic fluid.[94,95] To date, however, reports on this procedure are still insufficient to determine its effectiveness.

PHARMACOKINETIC CONSIDERATIONS IN PATIENTS WITH EFFUSIONS

Many patients with effusions will require systemic chemotherapy. The comparative pharmacokinetic parameters for plasma and pleural fluids have been determined for several anticancer agents. For most agents, there is a delay in entry of drug from plasma into effusion, so that peak levels occur later. Often, efflux from the effusion is also slow, which may result in a prolonged terminal half-time for the drug in both effusion and plasma. For some drugs, such as 5-fluorouracil, the alteration in pharmacokinetics has little or no clinical significance. The prolonged terminal half-time does not substantially alter the area under the plasma concentration $\times$ time curve.[96] Although peak concentrations of 5-fluorouracil in effusion are substantially lower than those in plasma, the area under the concentration $\times$ time curve for effusion is approximately 50% of the area for plasma. In contrast, the same alteration in the pharmacokinetics of methotrexate by an effusion may markedly increase the toxicity of high-dose methotrexate. Toxicity of high-dose methotrexate is associated with concentrations of greater than $9 \times 10^{-7} M$ 48 hours after infusion. The prolongation of terminal half-life by an effusion may result in frequent and severe toxicity.[97,98] If the clinical situation warrants the use of methotrexate in the presence of an effusion, several steps may be taken to prevent toxicity: the fluid should be drained prior to treatment, the patient should be kept well hydrated, and methotrexate levels should be monitored. If elevated levels are present at 48 hours, then leucovorin may be administered at high doses for a prolonged period.

REFERENCES

1. Friedman MA, Slater E: Malignant pleural effusions. Cancer Treat Rev 5:49, 1978
2. Leff A, Hopewell PC, Costello J: Pleural effusion from malignancy. Ann Intern Med 88:532, 1978
3. Chernow B, Sahn SA: Carcinomatous involvement of the pleura. Am J Med 63:695, 1977
4. Hausheer FH, Yarbro JW: Diagnosis and treatment of malignant pleural effusion. Semin Oncol 12:54, 1985
5. Yazdi HM, Hajdu SI, Melamed MR: Cytopathology of pericardial effusions. Acta Cytol 24:401, 1980
6. Bisel HF, Wroblewski F, LaDue JS: Incidence and clinical manifestations of cardiac metastases. JAMA 153:712, 1953
7. Yamada S, Takeda T, Matsumoto K: Prognostic analysis of malignant pleural and peritoneal effusions. Cancer 51:136, 1983
8. Haagensen CD, Feind CR, Herter FP, et al: The lymphatics in cancer, pp 331–332. Philadelphia, WB Saunders, 1972
9. Weichselbaum R, Marck A, Hellman S: Pathogenesis of pleural effusion in carcinoma of the breast. Int J Radiat Oncol Biol Phys 2:963, 1977
10. Porter EH: Pleural effusion and breast cancer. Br Med J 1:251, 1965
11. Goldsmith HS, Bailey HD, Callahan EL, et al: Pulmonary lymphangitic metastases from breast carcinoma. Arch Surg 94:483, 1967
12. Fentiman S, Mellis R, Sexton S, et al: Pleural effusion in breast cancer. A review of 105 cases. Cancer 47:2087, 1981
13. Stoll BA, Ellis F: Treatment by oestrogens of pulmonary metastases from breast cancer. Br Med J 2:796, 1953
14. Kreisman H, Woklove N, Finkelstein HS, et al: Breast cancer and thoracic metastases: Review of 119 patients. Thorax 38:175, 1983
15. Starling EH: On the absorption of fluids from the connective tissue spaces. J Physiol (Lond) 19:312, 1898
16. Peterson JA: Recognition of infrapulmonary pleural effusion. Radiology 74:34, 1960
17. Gryminski J, Krakowka P, Lypaceqicz G: The diagnosis of

pleural effusion by ultrasonic guidance and radiologic technique. Chest 70:33, 1976
18. Ravin CE: Thoracentesis of loculated pleural effusions using grey scale ultrasonic guidance. Chest 71:666, 1977
19. Izbicki R, Weyhing BT, Baker L, et al: Pleural effusion in cancer patients: A prospective randomized study of pleural drainage with the addition of radioactive phosphorus versus pleural drainage alone. Cancer 36:1511, 1975
20. Cham WC, Freiman AH, Carstens PH, et al: Radiation therapy of cardiac and pericardial metastases. Radiology 114:701, 1975
21. Stewart JR, Cohn KE, Fajardo LF, et al: Radiation-induced heart disease: A study of twenty-five patients. Radiology 89:302, 1967
22. Martin RG, Ruchdeschel JC, Chang P, et al: Radiation-related pericarditis. Am J Cardiol 35:216, 1975
23. Danoff BF, Pajak TF, Solin LJ, et al: Excisional biopsy, axillary node dissection and definitive radiotherapy for Stages I and II breast cancer. Int J Radiat Oncol Biol Phys 11:479, 1985
24. Stark P, Guthrie AM, Bull J: Thoracic radiographic changes after systemic hyperthermia for advanced cancer. Radiology 154:55, 1985
25. Hirsch A, Ruffie P, Nebut M, et al: Pleural effusion: Laboratory tests in 300 cases. Thorax 34:106, 1979
26. Light RN, MacGregor MI, Luchsinger PC, et al: Pleural effusions: The diagnostic separations of transudates and exudates. Ann Intern Med 77:507, 1972
27. Leff A, Hopewell PC, Costello J: Pleural effusion from malignancy. Ann Intern Med 88:532, 1978
28. Anderson CB, Philpott GW, Ferguson TB: The treatment of malignant pleural effusions. Cancer 33:916, 1974
29. Salyer WR, Eggleston JC, Erozan YS: Efficacy of pleural needle biopsy and pleural fluid cytopathology in the diagnosis of malignant neoplasm involving the pleura. Chest 67:536, 1975
30. Rittgers RA, Loewenstein MS, Feinerman AE, et al: Carcinoembryonic antigen levels in benign and malignant pleural effusions. Ann Intern Med 88:631, 1978
31. Booth SN, Lakin G, Dykes PN, et al: Cancer-associated proteins in effusion fluids. J Clin Pathol 30:537, 1977
32. Faravelli B, D'Amore E, Nosenzo M, et al: Carcinoembryonic antigen in pleural effusion: Diagnostic value in malignant mesothelioma. Cancer 53:1194, 1984
33. Nystrom JS, Dyce B, Wada J, et al: Carcinoembryonic antigen titers on effusion fluid: A diagnostic tool? Arch Intern Med 137:875, 1977
34. Murakami T, Kitamura S, Ohsawa N: A rapid, sensitive method for estrogen receptor analysis of cells from malignant pleural effusions in recurrent breast cancer. Chest 83:936, 1983
35. McCarty KS Jr, Wortman J, Moore JO, et al: Malignant effusions in recurrent breast cancer: Steroid hormone receptor analysis of effusion-derived cells. Cancer 45:1609, 1980
36. Levine MN, Young JEM, Ryan ED, et al: Pleural effusion in breast: Cancer thoracoscopy for hormone receptor determination. Cancer 57:324, 1986
37. Mukherjee TM: The role of electron microscopy in the diagnosis of neoplastic cells in effusion fluids. J Submicrosc Cytol 14:717, 1982
38. Szpak CA, Johnston WW, Lottich SC, et al: Patterns of reactivity of four novel monoclonal antibodies (B72.3, DF3, B1.1, and B6.2) with cells in human and benign effusions. Acta Cytol 28:356, 1984
39. Wade JL, Little AG, Vogelzang NJ, et al: Idiopathic pericardial effusions in patients with malignancy. Proc Annu Meeting Am Soc Clin Oncol 3:15, 1984
40. Mann T, Brodie BR, Grossman W, et al: Effusive-constrictive hemodynamic pattern due to neoplastic involvement of the pericardium. Am J Cardiol 41:781, 1978
41. Zipf RE, Johnston WW: The role of cytology in the evaluation of pericardial effusions. Chest 62:593, 1972
42. King, DT, Nieberg, RK: The use of cytology to evaluate pericardial effusions. Ann Clin Lab Sci 9:18, 1979
43. Martini N, Bains MS, Beattie EJ: Indications for pleurectomy in malignant effusion. Cancer 35:734, 1975
44. Suhrland LG, Weisberger AS: Intracavitary 5-fluorouracil in malignant effusions. Arch Intern Med 116:431, 1965
45. Poe RH, Qazi R, Israel RH, et al: Survival of patients with pleural involvement by breast carcinoma. Am J Clin Oncol (CCT) 6:523, 1983
46. Hirsch DM, Nydick I, Farrow JH: Malignant pericardial effusion secondary to metastatic breast carcinoma: A case of long-term remission. Cancer 9:1269, 1966
47. Fentiman IS, Rubens RD, Hayward JL: Ascites in breast cancer. Br Med J 287:1023, 1983
48. Theologides A: Neoplastic cardiac tamponade. Semin Oncol 5:181, 1978
49. Smith FE, Lane M, Hudgins PT: Conservative management of malignant pericardial effusion. Cancer 33:47, 1974
50. Thurber DL, Edioards JE, Achor RWP: Secondary malignant tumors of the pericardium. Circulation 26:228, 1962
51. Sprung CL, Elser B: Reexpansion pulmonary edema. Chest 84:788, 1983
52. Rose RG: Intracavitary radioactive colloidal gold: Results in 257 cancer patients. J Nucl Med 3:323, 1962
53. Fracchia AA, Knapper WH, Carey JT, et al: Intrapleural chemotherapy for effusion from metastatic breast carcinoma. Cancer 26:626, 1970
54. Paladine W, Cunningham JJ, Sponzo R, et al: Intracavitary bleomycin in the management of malignant effusions. Cancer 38:1903, 1976
55. Kefford RF, Woods RL, Fox RM, et al: Intracavitary Adriamycin, nitrogen mustard and tetracycline in the control of malignant effusions: A randomized study. Med J Aust 2:447, 1980
56. Bayly TC, Kisner DL, Sybert A, et al: Tetracycline and quinacrine in the control of malignant pleural effusions, a randomized trial. Cancer 41:1188, 1978
57. Fentiman IS, Rubens RD, Hayward JL: Control of pleural effusions in patients with breast cancer. Cancer 52:737, 1983
58. Rinaldo JE, Owens GR, Rogers RM: Adult respiratory distress syndrome following intrapleural instillation of talc. J Thorac Cardiovasc Surg 85:523, 1983
59. Zaloznik AJ, Oswald SG, Langin M: Intrapleural tetracycline in malignant pleural effusions: A randomized study. Cancer 51:752, 1983
60. Editor: Coparvax for malignant effusion? Drug Ther Bull 21:79, 1983
61. O'Bryan RM, Talley RW, Brennan MJ, et al: Critical analysis of the control of malignant effusions with radioisotopes. Henry Ford Hosp Med J 16:3, 1968
62. Austin EH, Flye MW: The treatment of recurrent malignant pleural effusion. Ann Thorac Surg 28:190, 1979
63. Srinwasan Y, Beroff RL, Goldberg E, et al: Intrapericardial instillation of sodium hydroxide: Failure to produce pericardial symphysis. Angiology 35:22, 1984
64. Millar JW, Hunter AM, Horne NW: Intrapleural immunotherapy with *Corynebacterium parvum* in recurrent malignant pleural effusions. Thorax 35:856, 1979
65. Webb HE, Oaten SW, Pike DP: Treatment of malignant ascitic and pleural effusions with *Corynebacterium parvum.* Br Med J 1:338, 1978
66. Jensik R, Cagle JE, Milloy F, et al: Pleurectomy in the treatment of pleural effusion due to metastatic malignancy. J Thoracic Cardiovasc Surg 46:322, 1963
67. Fredriksen RT, Cohen LS, Mullins CB: Pericardial windows or

pericardiocentesis for pericardial effusions. Am Heart J 82:158, 1971
68. Rubinson RM, Bolooki H: Intrapleural tetracycline for control of malignant pericardial effusion. South Med J 65:847, 1972
69. Davis S, Sharma SM, Blumberg ED, et al: Intrapericardial tetracycline for the management of cardiac tamponade secondary to malignant pericardial effusion. N Engl J Med 299:1113, 1978
70. Terpenning M, Orringer M, Wheeler R, et al: Intrapericardial nitrogen mustard with catheter drainage for the treatment of malignant effusions. Proc Annu Meeting Am Assoc Cancer Res 20:286, 1979
71. Kilpatrick ZM, Chapman CB: On pericardiocentesis. Am J Cardiol 16:722, 1965
72. Markman M, Howell SB: Intrapericardial instillation of cisplatin in a patient with a large malignant effusion. Cancer Drug Delivery 2:49, 1985
73. Golman BS, Pearson FG: Malignant pericardial effusion; Review of hospital experience and report of a case successfully treated by talc poudrage. Can J Surg 8:157, 1965
74. Harkins JR, Satterfield JR, Aisner J, et al: Pericardial window for malignant pericardial effusion. Arch Thorac Surg 30:465, 1980
75. Williams G, Soulter L: Pericardial tamponade. Arch Intern Med 94:571, 1954
76. Berman K, Fielding LP, Richi AA: Diagnosis and treatment of malignant pericardial effusion: The subxiphoid approach. Conn Med 48:701, 1984
77. Lajos TZ, Black HE, Cooper RG, et al: Pericardial decompression. Ann Thoracic Surg 19:47, 1975
78. Hill GJ, Cohen BI: Pleural pericardial window for palliation of cardiac tamponade due to cancer. Cancer 26:81, 1970
79. Memon A, Zawadzki ZA: Malignant effusions: Diagnostic evaluation and therapeutic strategy. Curr Probl Cancer 5:3, 1981
80. Dybecki J, Balchum OJ, Meneely GR: Treatment of pleural and peritoneal effusion with intracavitary colloidal radiogold (Au^{198}). Arch Intern Med 104:802, 1959
81. Jacobs ML: Radioactive colloidal chronic phosphate to control pleural effusion and ascites. JAMA 166:597, 1958
82. Speyer JL, Collins JM, Dedrick RL, et al: Phase I and pharmacologic studies of 5-fluorouracil administered intraperitoneally. Cancer Res 40:565, 1980
83. Jones RB, Collins JM, Myers CE, et al: High volume intraperitoneal chemotherapy with methotrexate in patients with cancer. Cancer Res 41:55, 1981
84. Ozols RF, Young RC, Speyer JL, et al: Intraperitoneal (IP) Adriamycin (ADR) in ovarian carcinoma (OC). Proc Annu Meeting Am Assoc Cancer Res 40:565, 1980
85. Casper ES, Kelsen DP, Alcock NW, et al: IP cisplatin in patients with malignant ascites: Pharmacokinetic evaluation and comparison with the IV route. Cancer Treat Rep 67:235, 1983
86. Le Veen NH, Wapnik S, Grosberg S, et al: Further experience with peritoneovenous shunt for ascites. Ann Surg 184:574, 1976
87. Lund RH, Newkirk JB: Peritoneo-venous shunting system for surgical management of ascites. Contemp Surg 14:31, 1979
88. Harmon DC, Demirjian Z, Ellman L, et al: Disseminated intravascular coagulation with the peritoneovenous shunt. Ann Intern Med 90:774, 1979
89. Ragni MV, Lewis JH, Spero JA: Ascites-induced LeVeen shunt coagulopathy. Ann Surg 198:91, 1983
90. Lokich J, Reinhold R, Silverman M, et al: Complications of peritoneovenous shunt for malignant ascites. Cancer Treat Rep 64:305, 1980
91. Qazi R, Savlov ED: Peritoneovenous shunt for malignant ascites. Cancer 49:600, 1982
92. Souter RG, Tarin D, Kettlewell MG: Peritoneovenous shunts in the management of malignant ascites. Br J Surg 70:478, 1983
93. Reinhold RB, Lokich JJ, Tomashefski J, et al: Management of malignant ascites with peritoneovenous shunting. Am J Surg 145:455, 1983
94. McCann WJ, Cagalletti RR, Neuman CG: Ileoentectropy for ascites associated with ovarian tumors. Obstet Gynecol 32:482, 1968
95. Neuman CG, Brunwald NS, Hinton JW: The absorption of ascitic fluid by a pedicled flap of intestinal mucosa exposed within the peritoneal cavity. Ann Surg 184:574, 1976
96. Wagner T: Die Pharmakokinetik von 5-Fluorouracil und seine Permeation in Pleuraergusse bei der Therapie des metastassierenden Mamma-Karzinoms. Onkologie 7:22, 1984
97. Wan SH, Huffman DH, Azarnoff DL, et al: Effect of route of administration and effusion on methotrexate pharmacokinetics. Cancer Res 34:3487, 1974
98. Chabner BA, Stoller RG, Hande KR, et al: Methotrexate disposition in humans: Case studies in ovarian cancer and following high-dose infusion. Drug Metabol Rev 8:107, 1978

Gastrointestinal and Hepatic Metastases

Stacey M. Gore Steven E. Come

GASTROINTESTINAL METASTASES

Metastases from breast carcinoma have been found along the entire alimentary canal from the tip of the tongue to the rectum.[1] Autopsy series report a 14% to 35% incidence of gastrointestinal metastases in patients with breast cancer, and approximately one-third of these have multiple sites of involvement (Table 14-18).[2–8] Certain histologic types of breast cancer may have a predisposition to gastrointestinal metastases. Merino found that patients with signet ring cell carcinoma of the breast have a propensity for metastasis to the serosal surfaces, with an associated, marked, desmoplastic reaction. Multiple metastatic lesions of the stomach, small and large intestine, and pancreas were noted in several patients.[9] Cormier reported a relationship between lobular carcinoma of the breast and the subsequent development of a linitis plastica pattern of gastric metastases.[10]

Although postmortem diagnosis is not uncommon, gastrointestinal metastases are often unsuspected clinically. In Hagemeister's study, gastrointestinal involvement was noted in 35% of patients with breast cancer, but the diagnosis was established ante mortem in only 8%.[3] The diagnosis of metastases to the gastrointestinal tract is difficult for several reasons. Gastrointestinal metastases usually occur in patients with advanced disease whose clinical picture may be dominated by other sites of involvement. Furthermore, symptoms, when present, are often not specific and may mimic those of radiation or chemotherapeutic toxicity, hypercalcemia, or comorbid conditions, such as gastritis, peptic ulcer disease, or primary neoplasms of the gastrointestinal tract.[11] In a review of 35 patients with

Table 14-18
Autopsy Incidence of Gastrointestinal Metastases From Carcinoma of the Breast *

Organ	*Incidence (%)*
Esophagus	4–6
Stomach	6–18
Small and large intestine	5–14
Rectum	1–2
Liver	54–71
Biliary tract	4
Mesentery	18–25
Pancreas	13–17
Spleen	15–17

* Compiled data, modified from Lee YY-TN: Breast carcinoma: Pattern of metastasis at autopsy. J Surg Oncol 23:175, 1983.

breast cancer who had gastrointestinal metastases, the prominent symptoms were abdominal pain (31%), vomiting (31%), nausea (25%), hematemesis (19%), dysphagia (18%), melena (15%), weight loss (12%), and anorexia (6%).[12]

Radiographic procedures may fail to clarify the nature of the gastrointestinal symptoms, as the appearance of metastatic breast cancer may be difficult to distinguish from that of several primary gastrointestinal disorders. Frequently, the diagnosis of gastrointestinal metastases can only be made with certainty by examining tissue obtained either endoscopically or surgically. Pathologic confirmation is most important in patients in whom apparent gastrointestinal involvement is the first sign of disseminated breast cancer. This may occur many years after the initial diagnosis of breast cancer; intervals of more than 10 years between the primary diagnosis and gastrointestinal recurrence have been reported.[11]

Esophageal Metastases

Esophageal involvement by metastatic breast carcinoma is found in 4% to 6% of autopsy cases,[5,6] and ante mortem diagnosis has been reported by several authors.[6,11,13–16] The peak incidence of symptomatic esophageal metastases occurs 4 to 5 years after the primary diagnosis of breast cancer.[14] Dysphagia is the most common symptom, followed by vomiting, epigastric pain, and weight loss.[6,11,14,15,17] Hoarseness, reflecting mediastinal extension and recurrent laryngeal nerve involvement, may also occur.[11,15] Barium swallow studies typically reveal a short, symmetrical stricture with smooth borders located in the middle one-third of the esophagus.[11,14] This region appears to be particularly prone to metastases from the breast because of connecting lymphatic channels.[16]

The differential diagnosis suggested by these clinical and radiographic findings include radiation or reflux esophagitis with stricture formation, primary carcinoma of the esophagus, and esophageal diverticulum.[11,15] Rarely, a clinical picture that is indistinguishable from idiopathic achalasia is produced by metastatic breast cancer.[11] The results of endoscopic biopsy may be negative owing to the serosal and submucosal location of tumor. Deeper biopsies are associated with a risk of perforation,[16] and open biopsy may be required in patients without other evidence of metastases. Although esophageal involvement frequently occurs late in the course of breast cancer, significant palliation has been achieved with radiation, chemotherapy, or surgical intervention.[6,11,13]

Gastric Metastases

Metastases to the stomach are found in up to 18% of patients with breast cancer at autopsy.[2,5,6,16,18] In a series of 31 patients with linitis plastica caused by metastatic lobular carcinoma of the breast, 74% developed gastric metastases within 5 years of their initial diagnosis of breast cancer; however, several women had disease-free intervals of more than 10 years.[10] In 45%, gastric involvement, alone or in association with other metastases, provided the first sign of disseminated disease. Two-thirds of these patients presented with weight loss, nausea, and vomiting. Other symptoms included epigastric pain (50%), early satiety (30%), and gastrointestinal hemorrhage (10%). A minority of patients were asymptomatic.[10]

Upper gastrointestinal x-ray studies most often disclose a linitis plastica pattern which is characterized by gastric rigidity, decreased or absent peristalsis, thickening of the gastric wall and narrowing of the lumen.[18] Histologic examination in these cases reveals diffuse intramural tumor infiltration, primarily involving the submucosa and muscularis propria. Although the mucosa is generally spared, superficial ulcerations may occasionally occur. Less commonly, the gastric roentgenogram may demonstrate single or multiple filling defects that represent well-circumscribed, nodular, metastatic lesions.[10,12,18] Rarely, the radiographic study may be entirely normal.[10,19]

Several patients have been treated effectively with systemic cytotoxic therapy with or without the addition of hormonal agents.[11,12] In one series, survival of up to 4 years from the time of diagnosis of gastric involvement was noted, with one-third of patients surviving in excess of 2 years, despite extensive metastatic disease.[10]

Intestinal Metastases

Involvement of the small intestine by breast cancer occurs with an incidence of approximately 10% in autopsy series.[2,5,6] Usually, small bowel involvement is secondary to metastatic seeding of the peritoneum. Symptoms related to intestinal obstruction occur in almost 50% of patients as a result of the marked desmoplastic reaction associated with submucosal metastases. Gastrointestinal bleeding and weight loss are present in approximately one-third of cases.[6,11,16,20] Rarely, intussusception from an intraluminal mass may occur.[11,21] Localized involvement of the terminal ileum by metastatic breast cancer may cause clinical signs similar to regional enteritis.[11]

The radiographic features of small bowel metastases include thickening of the intestinal wall and extrinsic compression, fixation and angulation of the bowel loops, and displacement by neoplastic masses. Multiple lesions are frequently observed.[11,22–25]

Mammary carcinoma metastasizes to the colon as frequently as it does to the stomach.[6,8] In both locations, a linitis plastica pattern predominates, and the metastases are often histologically derived from lobular or signet ring cell carcinomas of the breast.[26,27]

Colorectal metastases are usually symptomatic, mimicking either primary colorectal cancer or an inflammatory colitis.[27–30] A palpable abdominal mass is present in 15% of patients.[16] Barium studies characteristically demonstrate mucosal thickening and nodularity, multiple strictures, and loss of a haustral pattern. Long segments of bowel may be involved. Mucosal ulcerations and intraluminal defects, which are common in primary colorectal cancer, are rare.[11,26,29,31–33]

Breast cancer metastases may involve the veriform appendix. Five of the 12 cases described by Burney presented with acute appendicitis within an average of 35 months after the initial breast carcinoma was diagnosed (a range of 6 to 72 months).[34] Two of these patients had no prior evidence of metastatic disease. An additional five patients were incidentally found to have appendiceal metastases at the time of oophorectomy. Patients with breast cancer who are otherwise subjected to laparotomy should undergo prophylactic appendectomy.

BILIARY TRACT METASTASES

Extrahepatic biliary obstruction from metastatic breast carcinoma has been reported by several groups.[11,35,36] Popp described seven such patients who presented with jaundice and pruritus, but without significant hepatomegaly, within an average of 40 months after the initial diagnosis of breast cancer (a range of 9 months to 8 years).[35] Liver scans were normal in six of the patients. In all of these cases, nodal metastases produced the extrahepatic biliary obstruction, and the liver was free of metastases in 5 of the 7 patients. Local treatment with surgery, transhepatic catheter drainage, or radiation therapy relieved the jaundice in 6 of 7 patients, and prolonged survival occurred in 3. Extrahepatic biliary obstruction may also result from direct infiltration of the common bile duct by metastatic carcinoma.[11,36]

LIVER METASTASES

The liver is the second most frequent site of metastatic disease in patients with breast cancer, occurring with an incidence of 54% to 71% in autopsy series.[2–5,37–39] Hepatic metastases generally occur in the setting of widely disseminated disease. Isolated liver metastases are found in only 2% to 12% of patients with breast cancer.[40,41]

Hepatic involvement in patients with advanced breast cancer carries a poor prognosis, with a reported median survival of 6 months.[42] A median 30-day survival has been observed in patients with jaundice or ascites.[43] Hepatic failure is a major cause of death in 20% of patients with breast cancer.[3]

Clinical Findings

Early liver metastases are generally asymptomatic.[44,45] However, with progressive disease, symptoms directly related to hepatic involvement may evolve. In addition, constitution symptoms are often present. Of a large series of patients with hepatic metastases reported by Fenster and Klatskin, 67% had symptoms referable to the liver, with more than 50% seeking medical attention because of abdominal pain.[46] Increased abdominal girth was noted in 30% of patients. The majority of patients also reported nonspecific symptoms, such as weight loss (80%) and anorexia (69%).[46,47] Fever was present in 25% of patients with liver metastases.[46] Although generally low-grade, fevers as high as 102° F to 106° F with associated night sweats may occur.[46,48] Infectious etiologies must be excluded before fever may be ascribed to hepatic metastases.[49]

Sixty-five percent of patients with hepatic metastases have palpable livers, and the majority have significant hepatomegaly.[46] However, 10% of patients with extensive metastases have no hepatic enlargement. A friction rub is audible in 10% of cases, and is considered pathognomonic of hepatic metastases. Jaundice is generally accompanied by other signs of advanced hepatic involvement, and its isolated occurrence suggests extrahepatic biliary obstruction. Patients with breast cancer who have liver metastases will occasionally present a clinical picture that mimics cirrhosis, with portal hypertension, ascites, spider angiomata, and esophageal varices. Histologic examination in these cases reveals diffuse fibrosis of the hepatic parenchyma and perivascular tumor infiltration.[44]

Diagnosis

A variety of biochemical, immunologic, and imaging techniques are useful in the detection and assessment of hepatic metastases. Serum alkaline phosphatase levels remain the single best screening test, as elevated levels are present in approximately 80% of patients with breast cancer who have liver involvement.[46,50–52] Since an elevation of the alkaline phosphatase level may also reflect osseous metastases or benign conditions, correlation with other tests enhances the positive diagnostic accuracy. Liver metastases have been documented in more than 90% of patients with abnormalities in alkaline phosphatase, glutamic oxalacetic transaminase, and serum albumin levels.[53] Elevation of the enzyme 5′-nucleotide phosphodiesterase isozyme-V is present in 95% of patients with breast cancer who have other clinical signs of hepatic metastases, but the specificity of this test is only 67%.[45,54]

Carcinoembryonic antigen (CEA) levels are elevated in 70% of patients with metastatic breast cancer, and abnormalities are most common in, but not limited to, those with hepatic involvement.[55–58] The combination of an increased CEA level and an abnormal hepatic radionuclide scan is essentially diagnostic of liver metastases.[59,60]

Radionuclide imaging of the liver utilizing technetium-99m sulfur colloid has an overall accuracy rate of 67% to 89%, with false-positive rates of 5% to 42% and false-negative rates of 10% to 25% in patients with breast cancer who have hepatic metastases.[45,60–64] The scintigraphic pattern of breast cancer that is metastatic to liver may be a heterogeneous distribution of radiocolloid, with or without focal defects.[65] The appearance of abnormalities on liver scanning tends to follow the emergence of clinical and laboratory evidence of hepatic involvement; for this reason, several researchers argue against routine liver scanning in patients with breast cancer.[66–69] Hepatic scintigraphy is most useful as a confirmatory test in the subset of patients with clinical evidence of hepatic metastases and as a means of serially assessing the response of liver metastases to therapy.

Ultrasonography and CT scanning may also assist in the diagnosis and follow-up of hepatic metastases. Ultrasonography is particularly useful in clarifying defects seen on ^{99m}Tc sulfur colloid scan, such as the differentiation of a solid from a cystic mass, and in assessing the biliary tract.[64,70] Computerized tomography with the administration of intravenous contrast material facilitates the detection of small metastatic foci, and may help to differentiate benign vascular lesions from metastases.[70] In a recent prospective collaborative study by Alderson, CT scanning was more accurate than scintigraphy or ultrasonography in diagnosing hepatic metastases.[71]

Histologic diagnosis remains the "gold standard" for confirming the presence of hepatic metastases. Blind percutaneous liver biopsies have a significant false-negative rate owing to sampling error.[46] The yield is greatly improved when biopsy is performed under ultrasonographic or CT guidance.

Treatment

Treatment of patients with breast cancer who have liver metastases is palliative and of limited efficacy. Endocrine therapy is generally not attempted in these patients, as observed response rates are low, averaging 13%.[72,73] Determination of estrogen receptor (ER) status may identify a subset of patients who benefit from hormonal maneuvers. Johnson found that 27% of the liver metastases assayed were ER-positive. In this subset of patients, the response rate to endocrine ablation was 75%.[74] However, others have reported a poor response of liver metastases to endocrine ablation therapy in ER-positive patients.[75]

Systemic chemotherapy is the cornerstone of treatment for patients with hepatic metastases. Multiple therapeutic trials in patients with metastatic breast cancer have suggested that hepatic involvement exerts an independent negative prognostic effect on treatment response.[76–78] Kemeny recently reviewed the response of hepatic metastases from breast cancer to chemotherapy and noted a cumulative response rate of 46% for patients with liver metastases, compared to 53% for those without hepatic involvement ($P = 0.04$).[79]

Combination chemotherapy appears to produce response rates, response durations, and survival rates that are superior to those achieved with single-agent therapy in patients with breast cancer who have hepatic metastases.[72,77,80] In addition, the highest response rates reported have been with the use of doxorubicin-containing programs.[81–83]

Since most patients with breast cancer develop hepatic metastases in the setting of widely disseminated disease, regional therapy alone does not result in substantial benefit. Intrahepatic arterial chemotherapy has not been found to improve upon results achieved with systemically delivered treatment.[84] Similarly, surgical resection of apparently isolated hepatic metastases secondary to breast cancer has not been rewarding.[85]

Radiation therapy may provide useful palliation of hepatic metastases. Although the liver is a relatively radiosensitive organ, patients may receive 1800 cGy to 2500 cGy with a resulting decrease in hepatic distention and pain. In a study by Turek-Maischeider of patients with symptomatic metastatic liver disease, 73% had complete relief of symptoms and an additional 18% achieved moderate palliation without any evidence of radiation hepatitis at autopsy.[86]

REFERENCES

1. Fink J, Garb J: Carcinoma of the tip of the tongue: A case of metastasis from a malignant tumor of the breast. Am J Surg 62:138, 1943
2. Cho SY, Choi HY: Causes of death and metastatic patterns in patients with mammary cancer: Ten-year autopsy study. Am J Clin Pathol 73:232, 1980
3. Hagemeister FB Jr, Buzdar AU, Luna MA, et al: Causes of death in breast cancer. A clinicopathologic study. Cancer 46:162, 1980
4. Amer MH: Chemotherapy and patterns of metastases in breast cancer patients. J Surg Oncol 19:101, 1982
5. Cifuentes N, Pickren JW: Metastases from carcinoma of the mammary gland. An autopsy study. J Surg Oncol 11:193, 1979
6. Asch MJ, Wiedel PD, Habif DV: Metastases from carcinoma of the breast. Autopsy study and 18 cases requiring operative intervention. Arch Surg 96:840, 1968
7. Abrams HL, Spiro R, Goldstein N: Metastases in carcinoma. Analysis of 1000 autopsied cases. Cancer 3:74, 1950
8. Graham WP, Goldman L: Gastro-intestinal metastases from carcinoma of the breast. Ann Surg 159:477, 1964
9. Merino JJ, Livolsi VA: Signet ring carcinoma of the female breast: A clinicopathologic analysis of 24 cases. Cancer 48:1830, 1981

10. Cormier WJ, Gaffey TA, Welch JM, et al: Linitis plastica caused by metastatic lobular carcinoma of the breast. Mayo Clinic Proc 55:747, 1980
11. Chang SF, Burrell MI, Brand MH, et al: The protean gastrointestinal manifestations of metastatic breast carcinoma. Radiology 126:611, 1978
12. Marshall ME: Gastrointestinal metastases from carcinoma of the breast. J Ky Med Assoc 81:154, 1983
13. Anderson MF, Harell GS: Secondary esophageal tumors. AJR 135:1243, 1980
14. Holyoke ED, Nemoto T, Dao TL: Esophageal metastases and dysphagia in patients with carcinoma of the breast. J Surg Oncol 1:97, 1969
15. Conklin EF: Some unusual complications of metastatic carcinoma of the breast. Ann Surg 159:489, 1964
16. Caramella E, Bruneton JN, Roux P, et al: Metastases of the digestive tract. Report of 77 cases and review of the literature. Eur J Radiol 3:331, 1983
17. Polk HC Jr, Camp FA, Walker AW: Dysphagia and esophageal stenosis: Manifestation of metastatic mammary carcinoma. Cancer 20:2002, 1967
18. Joffe N: Metastatic involvement of the stomach secondary to breast carcinoma. AJR 123:512, 1975
19. Menuck LS, Amberg JR: Metastatic disease involving the stomach. Am J Dig Dis 20:903, 1975
20. Meyers MA, McSweeney J: Secondary neoplasms of the bowel. Radiology 105:1, 1972
21. Fawaz F, Hill GJ III: Adult intussusception due to metastatic tumors. South Med J 76:522, 1983
22. Meyers MA: Metastatic seeding along the small bowel mesentery. Roentgen features. AJR 123:67, 1975
23. Smith SJ, Carlson HC, Gisvold JJ: Secondary neoplasms of the small bowel. Radiology 125:29, 1977
24. Zornoza J, Goldstein HM: Cavitating metastases of the small intestine. AJR 129:613, 1977
25. Libshitz HJ, Lindell MM, Dodd GD: Metastases to the hollow viscera. Radiol Clin North Am 20:487, 1982
26. Fayemi AO, Ali M, Braun EV: Metastatic carcinoma simulating linitis plastica. Am J Gastroenterol 71:311, 1979
27. Koos L, Field RE: Metastatic carcinoma of the breast simulating Crohn's disease. Int Surg 65:359, 1980
28. Melnick GS, Rosenholtz MJ: Metastatic breast carcinoma simulating ulcerative colitis. Report of a case. AJR 86:702, 1961
29. Meyers MA, Oliphant M, Teixidor H, et al: Metastatic carcinoma simulating inflammatory colitis. AJR 123:74, 1975
30. Weisberg A: Metastatic adenocarcinoma of the breast masquerading as Crohn's disease of the colon. Am J Proctol Gastroenterol Colon Rectal Surg 33:10–15, 22, 1982
31. Ginaldi S, Lindell MM, Zornoza J: The striped colon: A new radiographic observation in metastatic serosal implants. AJR 134:453, 1980
32. Balthazar EJ, Rosenberg HD, Davidian MM: Primary and metastatic scirrhous carcinoma of the rectum. AJR 132:711, 1979
33. Vigh R, Tapley NV: Metastatic lesions to the large intestine. Radiology 70:222, 1958
34. Burney RE, Koos N, Goldenberg IS: Acute appendicitis secondary to metastatic carcinoma of the breast. A report and review of two cases. Arch Surg 108:872, 1974
35. Popp JW, Schapiro RH, Warshaw AL: Extrahepatic biliary obstruction caused by metastatic breast carcinoma. Ann Intern Med 91:568, 1979
36. Engel JJ, Trujillo YY, Spellberg M: Metastatic carcinoma of the breast. A case of obstructive jaundice. Gastroenterology 78:132, 1980
37. Haagensen CD: Diseases of the Breast, p 426. Philadelphia, WB Saunders, 1971
38. Viadana E, Cotter R, Pickren JW, et al: An autopsy study of metastatic sites of breast cancer. Cancer Res 33:179, 1973
39. Lee Y-TN: Breast carcinoma: Pattern of metastasis at autopsy. J Surg Oncol 23:175, 1983
40. Viadana E, Bross IDJ, Pickren JW: An autopsy study of some routes of dissemination of cancer of the breast. Br J Cancer 27:336, 1973
41. Viadana E, Aui KL: Patterns of metastases in adenocarcinomas of man: An autopsy study of 4728 cases. J Med 6:1, 1975
42. Cutler SJ, Asire AJ, Taylor SG: Classification of patients with disseminated cancer of the breast. Cancer 24:861, 1969
43. Jaffe BM, Donegan WL, Watson F, et al: Factors influencing survival in patients with untreated hepatic metastases. Surg Gynecol Obstet 127:1, 1968
44. Borja ER, Hori JM, Pugh RP: Metastatic carcinomatosis of the liver mimicking cirrhosis. Case report and review of the literature. Cancer 35:445, 1975
45. Tsou KC, Lo KW, Rosato EF, et al: Evaluation of 5′-nucleotide phosphodiesterase isozyme-V as a predictor for liver metastasis in breast cancer patients. Cancer 50:191, 1982
46. Fenster LF, Klatskin G: Manifestations of metastatic tumors of the liver. A study of eighty-one patients subjected to needle biopsy. Am J Med 31:238, 1961
47. Cady B: Natural history of primary and secondary tumors of the liver. Semin Oncol 10:127, 1983
48. Chawla SP, Buzdar AU, Hortobagyi GN, et al: Tumor-associated fever in breast cancer. Cancer 53:1596, 1984
49. Aderka D, Kidron D, Weinberger A, et al: Absence of correlation between liver metastases and unexplained fever episodes. Cancer 55:2830, 1985
50. Donegan WC, Lewis JD: Clinical diagnosis and staging of breast cancer. Semin Oncol 5:373, 1978
51. Baker RR: Preoperative assessment of the patient with breast cancer. Surg Clin North Am 64:1039, 1984
52. White DR, Maloney JJ III, Mass HB, et al: Serum alkaline phosphatase determination: Value in staging of advanced breast cancer. JAMA 242:1147, 1979
53. Castagna J, Benfield JR, Yamada H, et al: The reliability of liver scans and function tests in detecting metastasis. Surg Gynecol Obstet 134:463, 1972
54. Tsou KC, Creech RH, Inouye WY, et al: 5′-Nucleotide phosphodiesterase isozyme-V as a marker for liver metastases in breast cancer patients. Cancer 54:1788, 1984
55. Tormey DC, Waalkes TP, Ahmann D, et al: Biological markers in breast carcinoma. I. Incidence of abnormalities of CEA, HCG, three polyamines and three minor nucleosides. Cancer 35:1095, 1975
56. Tormey DC, Waalkes TP, Snyder JJ, et al: Biological markers in breast carcinoma. III. Clinical correlations with carcinoembryonic antigen. Cancer 39:2397, 1977
57. Waalkes TP, Tormey DC: Biologic markers and breast cancer. Semin Oncol 5:434, 1978
58. Coombes RC, Powles TJ, Gaze JC, et al: Screening for metastases in breast cancer: An assessment of biochemical and physical methods. Cancer 48:310, 1981
59. Sugarbaker PH, Beard JO, Drum DE: Detection of hepatic metastasis from cancer of the breast. Am J Surg 133:531, 1977
60. McCartney WH, Hoffer PB: Carcinoembryonic antigen assay: An adjunct to liver scanning in hepatic metastasis detection. Cancer 42:1457, 1978
61. Lee YY-TN: Liver scanning in patients with malignancy: Rationale, results and limitations. Cancer Treat Rep 62:1183, 1978

62. Nomura Y, Kondo H, Yamagata J, et al: Evaluation of liver and bone scanning in patients with early breast cancer, based on results obtained from more advanced cancer patients. Eur J Cancer 14:1129, 1978
63. Ostfeld DA, Meyer JE: Liver scanning in cancer patients with short interval autopsy correlation. Radiology 138:671, 1981
64. Smalley RV, Malmud LS, Ritchie WGM: Preoperative screening: Evaluation for metastatic disease in carcinoma of the breast, lung, colon, bladder, and prostate. Semin Oncol 7: 358, 1980
65. Drum DE, Beard JM: Scintigraphic criteria for hepatic metastases from cancer of the colon and breast. J Nucl Med 17:677, 1976
66. Rosenthal S, Kaufman S: The liver scan in metastatic disease. Arch Surg 106:656, 1973
67. Sears HR, Gerber FH, Sturtz DL, et al: Liver scan and carcinoma of the breast. Surg Gynecol Obstet 140:409, 1975
68. Wiener SN, Sachs SH: An assessment of routine liver scanning in patients with breast cancer. Arch Surg 113:126, 1978
69. Arnstein NB, Harbert JC, Byrne PJ: Efficacy of bone and liver scanning in breast cancer patients treated with adjuvant chemotherapy. Cancer 54:2243, 1984
70. Clouse ME: Roentgenographic techniques for the diagnosis and management of liver tumors. Semin Oncol 10:159, 1983
71. Alderson PO, Adams DF, McNeil BT, et al: Computerized tomography, ultrasound and scintigraphy of the liver in patients with colon or breast carcinoma. A prospective comparison. Radiology 149:225, 1983
72. Henderson JC, Canellos GP: Cancer of the breast: The past decade. N Engl J Med 302:17–30, 78–90, 1980
73. Kennedy BJ: Hormonal therapies in breast cancer. Semin Oncol 5:119, 1974
74. Johnson FE, Rosen PP, Menedez-Botet C, et al: Estrogen receptor protein in visceral metastases from breast cancer. Am J Surg 142:252, 1981
75. Moseley HS, Fletcher WS, Leung BS, et al: Predictive criteria for the selection of breast cancer patients for adrenalectomy. Am J Surg 128:143, 1974
76. George SL, Hoogstraten B: Prognostic factors in the initial response to therapy by patients with advanced breast cancer. J Natl Cancer Inst 60:731, 1978
77. Canellos GP, Pocock SJ, Taylor SJ III, et al: Combination chemotherapy for metastatic breast carcinoma. Cancer 38:1882, 1976
78. Nash CH III, Jones SE, Moon TE, et al: Prediction of outcome in metastatic breast cancer treated with Adriamycin combination chemotherapy. Cancer 46:2380, 1980
79. Kemeny N: The systemic chemotherapy of hepatic metastases. Semin Oncol 10:148, 1983
80. Chlebowski RT, Irwin LE, Pugh RP, et al: Survival of patients with metastatic breast cancer treated with either combination or sequential chemotherapy. Cancer Res 39:4503, 1979
81. Smalley RV, Carpenter T, Bartolucci A, et al: A comparison of cyclophosphamide, Adriamycin, 5-fluorouracil (CAF) and cyclophosphamide, methotrexate, 5-fluorouracil, vincristine, prednisone (CMFVP) in patients with metastatic breast carcinoma. Cancer 40:625, 1977
82. Creech RH, Catalano RB, Harris DT, et al: Low-dose chemotherapy of metastatic breast cancer with cyclophosphamide, Adriamycin, methotrexate, 5-fluorouracil (CAMF) versus sequential cyclophosphamide, methotrexate, 5-fluorouracil and Adriamycin. Cancer 43:51, 1979
83. Bull JM, Tormey DC, Li S-H, et al: A randomized comparative trial of Adriamycin versus methotrexate in combination drug therapy. Cancer 41:1649, 1978
84. Peetz M, Swanson J, Moseley HS, et al: Endocrine ablation and hepatic artery infusion in the treatment of metastasis to the liver from carcinoma of the breast. Surg Gynecol Obstet 155:395, 1982
85. Foster JH: Survival after liver resection for secondary tumors. Am J Surg 135:389, 1978
86. Turek-Maischeider M, Kazem I: Palliative irradiation for liver metastasis. JAMA, 232:625, 1975

Hypercalcemia in Breast Cancer

Lowell E. Schnipper Steven E. Come

Malignant disease accounts for 35% of all cases of hypercalcemia.[1] In patients with neoplasia, hypercalcemia may be subdivided into three categories. One of these, the humoral hypercalcemia of malignant disease, occurs in the setting of solid tumors without discernible bone metastases,[2] and is most commonly observed with squamous cell carcinomas of the lung, head, or neck, and with carcinoma of the kidney. A second group, consisting of hematologic malignant processes, such as plasma cell dyscrasias (predominantly, multiple myeloma), T-cell lymphomas, and Burkitt's lymphoma, constitutes 20% of the cases of hypercalcemia associated with malignant disease.[3] Approximately 70% of the cases of malignant hypercalcemia occur in patients with solid tumors that are metastatic to bone, and breast cancer accounts for 40% of this group.

PATHOGENESIS

Bone metastases develop in 80% of women with advanced breast cancer, and hypercalcemia develops in as many as 40%. Two components of bone resorption by metastatic disease have been proposed. One results from osteoclast stimulation by tumor cells in a process mediated by prostaglandins.[4] A second postulated mechanism is direct resorption of bone by tumor cells.[5] *In vitro,* cultured, human breast cancer cells have the capacity to resorb bone directly, independent of osteoclast stimulation, and this process is closely associated with the release of hydrolytic enzymes.[5,6] Breast cancer cells have receptors for 1,25-dihydroxy-vitamin-D, and this may be related to their mineral-transporting ability.[7,8] Another factor that may be important in the hypercalcemia of breast cancer is the cellular immune response that is sometimes present at the site of a bone metastasis.[9,10] In this setting, the accumulation of activated lymphocytes and monocytes, which can release the lymphokine osteoclast activating factor (OAF), may stimulate osteoclasts. This mechanism has best been documented in cases of hypercalcemia associated with multiple myeloma.

Although the major pathophysiologic component of malignant hypercalcemia is bone resorption, renal function may also be an important factor in the precipitation of hypercalcemia.[11] Many patients with extensive lytic bone metastases are normocalcemic, presumably as a result of their ability to maintain normal calcium concentrations through homeostatic mechanisms, including diminished absorption of calcium from the gastrointestinal tract[12] and hypercalciuria.[13] Compromised renal function may result in a decrease in the filtered calcium load or an increase in proximal tubular reabsorption of calcium, owing to a decline in the glomerular filtration rate (GFR), since sodium and calcium reabsorption in the renal tubules are closely linked.[14] Such a decrease in GFR often occurs in patients with cancer because of fever, dehydration, vomiting, or infections, thereby precipitating hypercalcemia.

Only rarely is the humoral hypercalcemia of malignant disease associated with breast cancer.[15] Consequently, no renal phosphate wasting is observed, urinary levels of cyclic adenosine monophosphate (cAMP) are normal, and immunoreactive parathyroid hormone (PTH) levels are depressed.[2]

Selective hormonal therapy for the treatment of breast cancer may precipitate hypercalcemia in patients with metastatic bone disease as part of a flare response that may also include worsening of bone pain (see Chapter 13). Serum calcium (Ca^{++}) levels should be monitored closely during the initial 2 to 4 weeks of endocrine therapy. Approximately 15% of ER-positive women will develop acute and severe hypercalcemia when treated with pharmacologic doses of estrogens.[16,17] Two percent of women with ER-positive breast cancer treated with an antiestrogen, such as tamoxifen or nafoxidine, will develop hypercalcemia.[18] Consistent with this fact is the observation that estrogens and antiestrogens stimulate bone resorption *in vitro*. Prostaglandin E_2 (PGE_2) may be an important mediator of this effect since bone resorption activity, stimulated by 17-beta-estradiol, is inhibited by indomethacin.[16] The importance of PGE_2 as a mediator in the *in vivo* setting is unclear.

The development of hypercalcemia as part of a flare reaction poses the difficult question of whether hormonal therapy should be discontinued (see Chapter 13). Since the flare response is generally self-limited and followed by tumor regression, it is important to decide whether hypercalcemia may be managed effectively without cessation of hormonal treatment. No firm guidelines exist, but if the Ca^{++} level is under 15 mg/dl and there are no cardiac or dire neurologic signs (confusion, stupor, or coma), it is appropriate to institute hypocalcemic measures, while maintaining systemic therapy. In the event of failure to control the serum Ca^{++} level, or in patients with an initial level in excess of 15 mg/dl, it is prudent to withhold hormones until the metabolic problem is under control. At that point, endocrine therapy may be resumed cautiously.

CLINICAL FEATURES AND DIAGNOSIS

The common clinical features of hypercalcemia are nausea, constipation, weakness, confusion, and lethargy. These symptoms are nonspecific and may easily be confused with those of the underlying disease, but their recognition is important since hypercalcemia is usually reversible.

Gastrointestinal symptoms, generally manifested when the calcium level is greater than 13 mg/dl, may include constipation secondary to bowel hypomotility, nausea, and vomiting. Pancreatitis more frequently occurs as a complication of hypercalcemia secondary to primary hyperparathyroidism rather than to breast cancer.[19] Diminished muscle tone may be observed, along with the neuropsychiatric findings of confusion, personality change, drowsiness, and, at times, stupor or coma associated with a rapidly rising serum calcium level.

Polyuria and polydipsia result from the ability of calcium to impair the effect of antidiuretic hormone on the collecting tubules of the kidneys.[20,21] Calcium ions also have an important role in determining the contractility of cardiac muscle. In acute hypercalcemia, the heart rate is slowed and ventricular systole is shortened. The QT interval is shortened with moderate calcium elevations,[22] but is prolonged with calcium elevations exceeding 16 mg/dl.[23] Special caution must be exercised when using digitalis in patients with hypercalcemia because its toxic effects may be potentiated by the drug.

Certain features of chronic hypercalcemia—band keratopathy, hypertension, and pruritis—that are common in primary hyperparathyroidism are infrequently associated with malignant hypercalcemia. Since the clinical manifestations of hypercalcemia relate to the rapidity with which the calcium level rises, patients with malignant disease often exhibit symptoms with even modest elevations in serum calcium, whereas those with primary hyperparathyroidism in whom hypercalcemia develops gradually may tolerate high calcium levels with a minimum of clinical sequelae.[12]

The differential diagnosis of hypercalcemia in the setting of breast cancer is quite limited. Since most patients will have destructive skeletal metastases, the absence of bone lesions should suggest other etiologies, such as primary hyperparathyroidism. More unusual causes of hypercalcemia to be considered when the prior two possibilities have been excluded are thyrotoxicosis, vitamin D intoxication, sarcoidosis, and the milk-alkali syndrome.

The diagnostic studies that are important in evaluating hypercalcemia in patients with breast cancer are corrected serum calcium, serum phosphorus, chloride, and bicarbonate levels; bone scans, and skeletal x-ray films of areas demonstrating increased radionuclide uptake. The ionized serum calcium level is the closest physiological correlate with the clinical manifestations of hypercalcemia. This level may be measured directly, although it may also be calculated by correcting for the binding of calcium to serum proteins.[24,25] The corrected serum calcium level is the sum of the measured total serum calcium, plus 4, minus the concentration (conc.) of serum albumin, times 0.8 (e.g., Ca^{++} = serum Ca + [4-(conc. serum albumin) (0.8)]). Albumin is used in this correction because 75% of protein-bound serum calcium is bound to albumin and only 25% is bound to globulins. Acid-base balance also affects the ionized calcium level, which is increased in the presence of acidosis and decreased at *p*H levels of greater than 7.4. The serum phosphorus level may be elevated, normal, or depressed, and the serum chloride level is generally less than 103 mEq/liter in patients with malignant hypercalcemia. Radioimmunoassay for PTH is primarily

Table 14-19
Management of Hypercalcemia in Breast Cancer

Serum Calcium Level	*Symptoms*	*Treatment**	*Comments*
> 13 mg/dl	Present or absent	Acute management	
		1. Fluids, IV normal saline, 150–200 ml/hr	1–2 mg/dl decrement within 24 hours
		2. Furosemide, 80–100 mg q 1–2 hrs	Watch for electrolyte imbalance; this may be the sole therapy if the condition is not life-threatening.
		3. Calcitonin, 100–400 MRC units q 12 hr, plus hydrocortisone, 100 mg IV q 6 hr, then taper	Use with fluids if Ca^{++} levels are > 15 mg/dl, or if life-threatening signs are present. This regimen will lower the Ca^{++} level in 4–6 hr
		4. Phosphate, 1.5 g (IV) infused over 6–8 hr	Extremely dangerous; justified only if death appears imminent and conventional measures have failed
		Chronic management	
		5. Mithramycin, 15 μg/kg IV	For semi-acute or chronic management of patients with Ca^{++} levels > 13 mg/dl; onset of hypercalcemic effect within 36–48 hr; treatment with mithramycin usually not more than twice weekly
		6. Oral phosphate, 1–3 g/day in divided doses	Serum PO_4 levels should be < 4 mg/dl; regimen is useful for chronic treatment once acute hypercalcemia has been controlled.
> 10.5 < 13 mg/dl	Present	As above	
	Absent	1. Try oral phosphates	Patient should be treated nonurgently; avoid IV hydration unless the Ca^{++} level rises or symptoms develop.
		2. Calcitonin/glucocorticoids	

* The suggested treatment approach is presented in order of preference. (IV, intravenous; Ca^{++} serum calcium; PO_4, phosphate)

reserved for situations in which primary hyperparathyroidism is being considered as a diagnosis. A low or normal value for urinary AMP makes the diagnosis of primary hyperparathyroidism very unlikely.

TREATMENT

The severity of hypercalcemia may be judged by the level of the ionized calcium (or the corrected serum calcium) and the rate at which hypercalcemia has developed. The relationship between symptoms and calcium elevation is important in deciding when to institute therapy, as well as in determining the specific therapy to be employed (Table 14-19). In general, patients with a corrected serum calcium level of greater than 13 mg/dl, whether symptomatic or not, should be regarded as having an urgent medical problem that requires prompt therapy. At lower serum calcium levels, the presence of symptoms should be the stimulus for prompt initiation of therapy. In asymptomatic patients with Ca^{++} levels of less than 13 mg/dl, it is prudent to institute nonurgent hypocalcemic measures, since rapid rises in the level of Ca^{++} may occur without warning.

Reduction of tumor burden is the ultimate goal of therapy since it is the only long-term measure for reversing hypercalcemia.

Fluids and Diuretics

Fluids are a mainstay in the initial treatment of hypercalcemia for several important reasons (see Table 14-18). Many patients are dehydrated at the time of clinical presentation. In addition to repleting intravascular volume, the administration of intravenous normal saline promotes calciuresis because sodium and calcium excretion are linked.[26,27] The resulting natriuresis promotes a calcium diuresis.[27] Although its effects are temporary, infusions of intravenous saline (150 ml to 200 ml/hr, after fluid repletion) will reliably reduce the serum calcium level within 12 to 24 hours. Concurrently, these patients should be studied carefully for other electrolyte problems—notably, hypokalemia and hypophosphatemia. This approach must be modified for patients with marginal myocardial and renal function, and other measures should be instituted earlier.

Mundy and co-workers have identified a risk for developing hypernatremia during vigorous rehydration of patients with hypercalcemia.[11] This condition has occurred in individuals who are semi-conscious or who have an impaired thirst mechanism. Owing to their relative resistance to antidiuretic hormone, these patients continue to excrete a dilute urine even after being given intravenous normal saline. If not recognized, this problem may result in hyperosmolality and neurologic sequelae that may compound those of hypercalcemia.

Loop diuretics, used in conjunction with intravenous normal saline, have gained wide acceptance in the treatment of hypercalcemia although their efficacy has not been established in a rigorously performed randomized study. Suki and co-workers have administered 80 mg to 100 mg of furosemide every 1 to 2 hours, combined with careful fluid and electrolyte replacement.[28] This regimen has resulted in excretion of 1000 mg of calcium per day. Meticulous attention to potassium and magnesium losses are essential with this form of therapy, and it is not established whether this approach is justifiable considering the risks involved, except in the most dire circumstances. If adequate rehydration is not maintained, the diuretic effect of the drug will exceed the hypercalciuric effect; failure to correct extracellular volume depletion may then result in increased calcium resorption.

Calcitonin

Calcitonin is a naturally occurring polypeptide, secreted by the C cells of the thyroid gland, which has potent inhibitory effects on bone resorption.[29,30] When used to treat hypercalcemia, its effect is observed within a few hours and persists for 1 to 3 days.[31] After serial administration of calcitonin, an "escape phenomenon" develops in some patients, making them refractory to its hypocalcemic effect.[31] This may be related to down-regulation of calcitonin receptors on bone cells, and may be prevented through the use of glucocorticoids.[32] As a result, many clinicians employ calcitonin and glucocorticoids jointly, which together produce a hypocalcemic effect within 4 to 6 hours in about 80% of the patients.[33] Salmon calcitonin is the most potent of the available preparations; the other types are of porcine and human origin. The usual dose is 4 MRC units/kg, administered subcutaneously or intramuscularly every 12 hours. When used in conjunction with glucocorticoids, the usual treatment regimen is hydrocortisone hemisuccinate, 100 mg, administered intravenously every 6 hours, with the dose being tapered subsequently. Calcitonin is virtually free of toxicity, and this factor, combined with its relatively rapid onset of action, makes it an attractive treatment modality, particularly in patients with life-threatening calcium elevations (see Table 14-19).

Mithramycin

Mithramycin is a cytotoxic antibiotic that is useful in managing hypercalcemia by virtue of its direct inhibitory effect on osteoclasts, and possibly, its cytotoxic effect on bone cells.[34,35] The hypocalcemic effect of mithramycin becomes apparent within 36 to 48 hours, and may persist for 1 week or longer.[36] The dose may be repeated after 48 hours if no discernible hypocalcemic effect is observed. Thereafter, mithramycin should not be used repeatedly, but should be withheld until hypercalcemia recurs. The primary concern with its use relates to its potential toxicity, the risk for which appears to increase as a function of the number of doses employed. The drug may cause nausea and vomiting, but the major toxic effects are thrombocytopenia, a bleeding diathesis, hepatocellular cytotoxicity, and nephrotoxicity.[37–39] Moreover, its use may increase the risks associated with cytotoxic chemotherapeutic agents being utilized to treat the underlying disease; therefore, careful consideration of the alternatives for treating hypercalcemia is appropriate prior to selecting mithramycin.

Phosphate

Intravenous inorganic phosphate should be reserved for hypercalcemia that is life-threatening and unresponsive to more conventional measures. Intravenous phosphate will reduce urinary calcium excretion, but the decline in serum calcium reflects sequestration of calcium throughout the body.[40–45] Calcification in the heart, kidneys, and lens has been observed, sometimes in association with hypocalcemia, hypotension, and renal failure.[45,46] In addition to precipitation of calcium in extraskeletal tissues, *in vitro* studies have demonstrated that inorganic phosphate may function as an inhibitor of bone resorption.[47] When used, the dose should not exceed 50 mmol (1.5 g of phosphorus) infused over a 6- to 8-hour period.[48] In general, only one dose per 24 hours is required; the serum calcium level may decline promptly, but this reduced level may persist for days following the infusion.

Oral phosphate is an extremely useful modality in the management of chronic hypercalcemia (see Table 14-19). It interferes with absorption of calcium from the gastrointestinal tract and may promote soft tissue calcifications.[48] It should not be administered to patients whose serum phosphorus levels are greater than 4 mg/dl. The usual daily dose is 1 g to 3 g, by mouth, with the maximum effect being observed after several days. The salutory effects of oral phosphate treatment must be balanced by its associated morbidity (i.e., diarrhea, nausea, and vomiting).

Glucocorticoids

Glucocorticoids are capable of inhibiting bone resorption and, therefore, have a hypocalcemic effect.[49–51] In specific tumors, such as in lymphoproliferative disorders, these agents may decrease serum calcium levels by exerting a cytolytic effect on tumor cells. Steroids interfere with the absorption of calcium through the gastrointestinal tract, but this is not likely to be important in treating the hypercalcemia of breast cancer since calcium absorption is already decreased. It is uncertain whether their unpredictable hypocalcemic effect in breast cancer (an approximate response rate of 30%) is related to suppression of adrenal estrogen synthesis, a direct effect on neoplastic cells, or osteoclasts. The large doses of steroids that are usually required may have significant medical consequences; therefore, long-term use of steroids in the treatment of hypercalcemia in patients with breast cancer should be undertaken only after careful consideration of the alternatives.

Inhibitors of Prostaglandin Synthesis

Despite the fact that specific prostaglandins, such as PGE_2, have been implicated as mediators of malignant hypercalcemia associated with metastatic bone disease, pharmacologic agents, such as indomethacin or aspirin, rarely provide clinical benefit.[52] Lack of utility precludes this category of agents from being used in the early treatment of hypercalcemia, and their use should only be considered when all other measures deemed more likely to be effective have failed.

Diphosphonates

Diphosphonates are inhibitors of osteoclastic bone resorption and function as synthetic analogues of inorganic phosphate, a naturally occurring inhibitor of hydroxyapatite crystal growth.[53–55] The three diphosphonates under clinical study at this time are ethane-1-hydroxy-1,1-diphosphonate (EHDP); dichloromethylene diphosphonate (CL_2MDP); and amino-hydroxypropylidine diphosphonate (ADP). All are active inhibitors of osteoclast activity and, when used intravenously, EHDP has been effective in producing a hypocalcemic effect in patients with the hypercalcemia of malignant disease.[56] In an interesting preliminary study, Van Breukelen treated seven patients who had refractory malignant hypercalcemia with ADP.[57] In all cases, the serum calcium level was normalized in conjunction with diminished calcium excretion in the urine. In addition, seven other patients in the study who had bone lesions but no hypercalcemia had reduced bone resorption as assessed by urine calcium and hydroxyproline excretion. These findings raise the possibility that ADP may be useful in treating normocalcemic patients with metastatic bone disease.

The major risk associated with diphosphonate therapy is osteomalacia resulting from defective mineralization of normal bone. Further treatment trials are necessary in order to provide a more detailed assessment of the clinical utility and risks associated with this promising class of compounds before they may be recommended for routine use in treating the hypercalcemia of breast cancer or any other malignant disease.

REFERENCES

1. Mundy GR, Cove DH, Fisken R: Primary hyperparathyroidism—Changes in the pattern of clinical presentation. Lancet 1:1317, 1980
2. Stewart AF, Horst R, Deftos LJ, et al: Biochemical evaluation of patients with cancer-associated hypercalcemia. Evidence for humoral and non-humoral groups. N Engl J Med 303:1377, 1980
3. Myers WPL: Hypercalcemia in neoplastic disease. Arch Surg 80:308, 1960
4. Galasko CSB, Bennett A: Relationship of bone destruction in skeletal metastases to osteoclast activation and prostaglandins. Nature 263:508, 1976
5. Eilon G, Mundy GR: Direct resorption of bone by human breast cancer cells *in vitro*. Nature 276:726, 1978
6. Eilon G, Mundy GR: Effects of inhibition of micro-tubule assembly on bone mineral release and enzyme release by human breast cancer cells. J Clin Invest 67:69, 1981
7. Eisman JA, Martin TJ, MacIntyre I, et al: 1,25-dihydroxy-vitamin D_3 receptor in breast cancer cells. Lancet 2:1335, 1979
8. Eisman KA, Martin TJ, MacIntyre I, et al: 1,25-dihydroxy-vitamion D_3 receptor in a cultured human breast cancer cell line (MCF 7 cells). Biochem Biophys Res Commun 93:9, 1980
9. Salmon SE, Hamburger AW: Immunoproliferation in cancer: A common macrophage derived promoter substance. Lancet 1:1289, 1978
10. Underwood JCE: Lymphoreticular infiltration in human tumors: Prognostic and biological implications: A review. Br J Cancer 30:538, 1974
11. Mundy GR, Martin TJ: The hypercalcemia of malignancy: Pathogenesis and treatment. Metabolism 31:1247, 1982
12. Coombes RC, Ward MK, Greenberg PB, et al: Calcium metabolism in cancer: Studies using calcium isotopes and immunoassay for parathyroid hormone and calcitonin. Cancer 38:2111, 1976a
13. Marx SJ, Spiegel AM, Brown EM, et al: Divalent cation metabolism: Familial hypocalciuric hypercalcemia versus typical primary hyperparathyroidism. Am J Med 65:235, 1978
14. Walser M: Calcium clearance is a function of saline clearance in the dog. Am J Physiol 200:1099, 1961
15. Galasko CSB, Burn JI: Hypercalcemia in patients with advanced mammary cancer. Br Med J 3:573, 1971
16. Valentin-Opran A, Eilon G, Saez S, et al: Estrogens and antiestrogens stimulate release of bone resorbing activity by cultured human breast cancer cells. J Clin Invest 75:726, 1985
17. Kennedy BJ, Tibbetts DM, Nathanson IT, et al: Hypercalcemia, a complication of hormone therapy of advanced breast cancer. Cancer Res 13:445, 1953
18. Patterson JS, Baum M: Safety of tamoxifen. Lancet 1:105, 1978
19. Mixter CG Jr, Klynes WM, Chir M, et al: Further experience with pancreatitis as a diagnostic clue to hyperparathyroidism. N Engl J Med 266:265, 1962
20. Zeffen JL, Heinemann HO: Reversible defect in renal concentrating mechanism in patients with hypercalcemia. Am J Med 33:54, 1962
21. Epstein FM: Calcium and the kidney. Am J Med 45:700, 1968
22. Shiner PT, Harris WS, Weissler AM: Effects of acute changes in serum calcium levels on the systolic time intervals in man. Am J Cardiol 24:42, 1969
23. Bronsky D, Dubin A, Waldstein SS, et al: Calcium and the electrocardiogram: II. The electrocardiographic manifestations of hyperparathyroidism and of marked hypercalcemia from various etiologies. Am J Cardiol 7:833, 1961
24. Berry EM, Gupta MM, Turner SJ, et al: Variation in plasma calcium with induced changes in plasma specific gravity, total protein and albumin. Br Med J 4:640, 1973
25. Payne RB, Little AJ, William RB, et al: Interpretation of serum calcium in patients with abnormal serum proteins. Br Med J 4:643, 1973
26. Massry SG, Friedler RM, Coburn JW: Excretion of phosphate

and calcium: Physiology of their renal handling and relation to clinical medicine. Arch Intern Med 131:828, 1973
27. Massry SG, Kleeman CR: Calcium and magnesium excretion during acute rise in glomerular filtrate rate. J Lab Clin Med 80:654, 1972
28. Suki WN, Yium JJ, Von Minden M, et al: Acute treatment of hypercalcemia with furosemide. N Engl J Med 283:836, 1970
29. Friedman JL, Au WYW, Raisz LG: Responses of fetal rat bone to thyrocalcitonin in tissue culture. Endocrinology 82:149, 1968
30. Hirsch PF, Munson PL: Thyrocalcitonin. Physiol Rev 49:548, 1969
31. Wener JA, Gorton SJ, Raisz LG: Escape from inhibition of resorption in cultures of fetal bone treated with calcitonin and parathyroid hormone. Endocrinology 90:752, 1972
32. Tashjian AH Jr, Wright DR, Ivey JL, et al: Calcitonin binding sites in bone. Relationships to biological response and escape. Recent Prog Horm Res 34:285, 1978
33. Binstock ML, Mundy GR: Effect of calcitonin and glucocorticoids in combination in malignant hypercalcemia. Ann Intern Med 93:269, 1980
34. Raisz LG, Trummel CL, Simmons H: Induction of bone resorption in tissue culture: Prolonged response after brief exposure to parathyroid hormone or 25-hydroxycholecalciferol. Endocrinology 90:744, 1972a
35. Minkin C: Inhibition of parathyroid hormone stimulated bone resorption in vitro by the antibiotic mithramycin. Calcif Tiss Res 13:249, 1973
36. Parsons V, Baum M, Self M: Effect of mithramycin on calcium and hydroxyproline metabolism in patients with malignant disease. Br Med J 1:474, 1967
37. Kofman S, Medrek TJ, Alexander RW: Mithramycin in the treatment of embryonal cancer. Cancer 17:938, 1964
38. Brown JH, Kennedy BJ: Mithramycin in the treatment of disseminated testicular neoplasms. N Engl J Med 272:111, 1965
39. Ryan WG, Schwartz TB, Northrop G: Mithramycin in Paget's disease of bone. JAMA 213:1153, 1970
40. Fulmer DH, Dimich AB, Rothschild EO, et al: Treatment of hypercalcemia: Comparison of intravenously administered phosphate, sulphate, and hydrocortisone. Arch Intern Med 129:923, 1972
41. Goldsmith RS, Ingbar SH: Inorganic phosphate treatment of hypercalcemia of diverse etiologies. N Engl J Med 274:1, 1966
42. Dent CE: Some problems of hyperparathyroidism. Br Med J 2:1495, 1962
43. Shackney S, Hasson J: Precipitous fall in serum calcium, hypotension, and acute renal failure after intravenous phosphate therapy for hypercalcemia: Report of two cases. Ann Intern Med 66:906, 1967
44. Breuer RI, LeBauer J: Caution in the use of phosphates in the treatment of severe hypercalcemia. J Clin Endocrinol Metab 27:695, 1967
45. Carey RW, Schmitt GW, Kopald HH, et al: Massive extraskeletal calcification during phosphate treatment of hypercalcemia. Arch Intern Med 122:150, 1968
46. Dudley FJ, Blackburn CRB: Extraskeletal calcification complicating oral neutral-phosphate therapy. Lancet 2:628, 1970
47. Raisz LG, Niemann I: Effect of phosphate, calcium and magnesium on bone resorption and hormonal responses in tissue culture. Endocrinology 85:446, 1969
48. Goldsmith RS, Ingbar SH: Phosphate, sulphate, and hypercalcemia. Ann Intern Med 67:463, 1967
49. Lazor MZ, Rosenberg LE: Mechanisms of adrenal steroid reversal of hypercalcemia in multiple myeloma. N Engl J Med 270:749, 1964
50. Myers WPL: Cortisone in the treatment of hypercalcemia in neoplastic disease. Cancer 11:83, 1958
51. Walser M: Treatment of hypercalcemias. Mod Treat 7:662, 1970
52. Williams GH, Dluhy RG, Thorn GW: Diseases of the adrenal cortex. In Petersdorf RG, Adams RD, Braunwald E, et al (eds): Harrison's Principles of Internal Medicine, pp 634–657. New York, McGraw-Hill, 1983
53. Fleisch H, Russell RGG, Francis MD: Diphosphonates inhibit hydroxyapatite dissolution in vitro and bone resorption in tissue culture and in vivo. Science 165:1262, 1969
54. Russell RGG, Muhlbauer RC, Bisaz S, et al: The influence of pyophosphate, condensed phosphates, phosphonates, and other phosphate compounds on the dissolution of hydroxyapatite in vitro and on bone resorption induced by parathyroid hormone in tissue culture and in thyroparathyroidectomized rats. Calcif Tiss Res 6:183, 1970
55. Francis MD, Russell RGG, Fleisch H: Diphosphonates inhibit formation of calcium phosphate crystals in vitro and pathological calcification in vivo. Science 165:1264, 1969
56. Jung A: Comparison of two parenteral diphosphonates in hypercalcemia of malignancy. Am J Med 72:221, 1982
57. Van Breukelen FJM, Bijvoet OLM, Van Oosterom AT: Inhibition of osteolytic bone lesions by (3-amino-1-hydroxypropylidene)-1,1-biphosphonate (A.P.D.). Lancet 1:803, 1979

Myelophthisic Anemia

Steven E. Come   Lowell E. Schnipper

Myelophthisic anemia is a state of diminished bone marrow function associated with encroachment of the marrow cavity by proliferating cells and the appearance of red blood cell and granulocytic precursors in the peripheral blood. Often, this condition is alternatively described as leukoerythroblastic anemia. In 215 cases of leukoerythroblastic anemia at the Mayo Clinic, approximately 50% occurred in patients with hematologic malignant disease and myeloproliferative syndromes. Metastatic carcinoma was the most frequent nonhematologic etiology in that series and accounted for 8 of the 13 cases in Vaughn's original report.[1,2] Carcinomas of the breast, prostate, stomach, and lung are the most common primary sites.[3]

The pathogenesis of myelophthisic anemia in malignant disease is incompletely understood. Displacement of normal marrow elements by tumor cells probably contributes to the condition; however, myelophthisic anemia is seen in only 12% to 45% of patients with marrow metastases, and the degree of anemia does not correlate with the extent of tumor in the marrow.[4–6] A desmoplastic response to the intramedullary metastases appears to be an important factor in the myelophthisic process. Myelofibrosis is found in 80% of patients with myelophthisic anemia secondary to marrow metastases.[5,6] Tumor or fibrosis, or both, not only replace the marrow space but also may interfere with hematopoiesis by disrupting the marrow microvasculature. Distortion of the endothelial sinuses permits nondeformable early red cells and granulocytes, normally confined to the marrow, to escape into the circulation.[3,7] A corresponding increase in the level of colony-forming unit–cultures (CFU-Cs) in the peripheral blood has also been reported in patients with myelophthisic anemia.[8] These circulating immature marrow cells give rise to or reflect the presence of extramedullary hepatosplenic hematopoiesis, which is a frequent, probably secondary, pathologic finding in patients with myelophthisic anemia and malignant disease.[5,9]

BONE MARROW METASTASES IN PATIENTS WITH BREAST CANCER

Bone marrow metastases in breast cancer are associated with a spectrum of clinical and hematologic manifestations. At one end of this spectrum are patients with clinically localized breast cancer and occult micrometastases to the marrow. Using an immunocytochemical stain for epithelial membrane antigen, tumor cells were detected in marrow aspirates taken from 28% of women with primary breast cancer in one recent report.[10] In this series, 22% of patients with T1 or T2 tumors and 39% with T3 or T4 tumors had carcinoma cells present in marrow smears. Further, 5 of 6 women with positive axillary nodes, intratumoral vascular invasion, and a negative estrogen receptor had marrow metastases.

Thirty to 60 percent of patients with metastatic breast cancer have marrow involvement.[11–14] Two-thirds of these patients with marrow metastases have an abnormal complete blood count (CBC). Anemia is the most frequent abnormality, with 40% to 60% of patients with Stage IV disease and bone marrow involvement having a hemoglobin of less than 12 g/dl, compared to 14% of Stage IV patients with no marrow involvement.[4,11] However, the presence of anemia is not diagnostic of marrow metastases since the "anemia of chronic disease" is a common additional cause of decreased red cell production in this setting. Leukopenia or thrombocytopenia, or both, are seen in only 12% to 25% of Stage IV patients with a positive bone marrow.[4,11,15] One-third of patients with metastatic breast cancer and marrow metastases have normal CBCs.[4,11,15] Thus, routine hematologic parameters are of limited usefulness in predicting bone marrow involvement. However, in patients with advanced breast cancer, metastatic involvement of the marrow correlates well with the presence of cortical bone involvement. Ingle found marrow metastases in 55% of patients with positive bone films or scans.[11] Moreover, multiple series have demonstrated that only 6% to 8% of patients with Stage IV breast cancer and marrow metastases have no evidence of skeletal involvement on combined radiographic and radionuclide studies.[4,11,12,16,17]

A proportion of patients with advanced breast cancer and marrow involvement have more prominent hematologic abnormalities. Myelophthisic anemia has been reported in 12% to 50% of patients with marrow metastases.[4,5,6,18] A very small number of patients with breast cancer who have myelophthisic anemia will develop an associated microangiopathic hemolytic anemia. This syndrome of mechanical intravascular hemolysis occurs when there is a large tumor burden with extensive marrow infiltration and tumor microemboli in the pulmonary and other vascular beds.[19] Another rare occurrence in patients with breast cancer that is metastatic to the bone marrow is the appearance of tumor cells in the peripheral blood. This carcinoma cell leukemia (carcinocythemia) has been observed in patients with underlying myelophthisic anemia and accompanying microangiopathic hemolysis. In some of these patients, prior incidental splenectomy or splenic atrophy has been postulated to diminish the clearance of circulating tumor cells, permitting their accumulation to levels that may reach 25,000 per mm^3.[20,21] In peripheral smears, these cells are larger (25 μ to 30 μ) than leukemic blasts, often appear in clusters, and have vacuolated basophilic cytoplasm. Intracellular mucin is present, and the periodic acid-Schiff (PAS) stain is positive.

CLINICAL FINDINGS AND DIAGNOSTIC EVALUATION OF MYELOPHTHISIC ANEMIA

Myelophthisic anemia may occur at any point in the course of breast cancer. Webster has estimated that the incidence of leukoerythroblastosis in the total breast cancer population is 0.5% per year.[22] In that series, three patients presented with myelophthisic anemia; evaluation revealed the primary breast tumor. Conversely, two patients developed myelophthisic anemia 7 and 12 years after the primary diagnosis. Kiely reported myelophthisic anemia occurring as early as 3 months and as late as 21 years after the initial diagnosis of breast cancer.[9] Patients with myelophthisic anemia may be slightly younger than the overall population of patients with breast cancer.[22]

Symptoms

The most common symptoms of myelophthisic anemia in patients with breast cancer are those of anemia, including congestive heart failure in the elderly, and bone pain. The latter may reflect the associated cortical bone metastasis or marrow necrosis that is secondary to the myelophthisic process itself.[3,9] The accompanying physical findings may include tachycardia, signs of increased cardiac output, pulmonary congestion, edema, and focal or diffuse bony tenderness. Although extramedullary hematopoiesis is usually present on pathologic examination, marked splenomegaly is less common, occurring in only 12% to 25% of patients.[2,9] Additional symptoms and signs related to other sites of metastases may be present.

Laboratory Findings

The most common hematologic abnormality is a normocytic normochromic anemia. Although some patients will have a leukoerythroblastic peripheral smear without anemia, the mean hemoglobin level reported in three series was 7.8 g/dl to 8.9 g/dl, with ranges from 6.2 g/dl to 11.6 g/dl.[9,22,23] The reticulocyte count is usually slightly increased, but the reticulocyte index is low.[3,9,23] Thrombocytopenia occurs in 70% to 90% of patients; platelet counts are less than 100,000 per mm^3 in more than 50% of patients.[9,22,23] Thrombocytosis is seen in less than 10% of cases. The white blood count may be elevated or slightly decreased, but is usually normal.

Examination of the peripheral smear in patients with myelophthisic anemia reveals nucleated red blood cells numbering from 1 to 135 per 100 white blood cells.[9,23] Immature granulocytes, constituting 1% to 30% of the total white blood cell count, are also seen.[9,23] Other morphologic abnormalities may include tear drop poikilocytosis, anisocytosis, red cell stippling, polychromatophilia, giant platelets, and megakaryocytic fragments.[3] Schistocytes, helmut cells, and burr cells may be present if there is associated microangiopathic hemolysis.[19]

Other frequent laboratory abnormalities appearing in patients with breast cancer who have myelophthisic anemia include elevation of LDH and alkaline phosphatase levels. Hypercalcemia is occasionally present. Hyperbilirubinemia and evidence of disseminated intravascular coagulation are common in patients with superimposed microangiopathic hemolysis.

Bone Marrow Examination

In patients with breast cancer, the bone marrow biopsy is more useful than is an aspirate smear or clot section in establishing marrow involvement. In Ingle's series from the National Cancer Institute, biopsy results were positive in 89% of patients with marrow metastases, and biopsy was the only procedure yielding positive results in 33% of patients.[11] Results of clot sections and aspirate smears were positive in 30% to 85% of patients, but rarely revealed tumor when the biopsy results were negative.[4,11]

The presence of the characteristic peripheral blood findings of myelophthisic anemia in a patient with known metastatic breast carcinoma is essentially diagnostic of marrow involvement.[1] Bone marrow aspiration and biopsy are confirmatory procedures. The bone marrow aspiration in patients with myelophthisic anemia may be a dry tap. The biopsy reveals fibrosis and nests of tumor cells, in addition to normal hematopoietic tissue. The relative proportions of tumor and fibrosis are variable.

DIFFERENTIAL DIAGNOSIS OF MYELOPHTHISIC ANEMIA IN PATIENTS WITH BREAST CANCER

The detection of carcinomatous cells by bone marrow examination establishes the etiology of myelophthisic anemia and eliminates other diagnoses that may be associated with a leukoerythroblastic peripheral smear, including primary hematologic or lymphoreticular malignant disease, tuberculosis, sarcoidosis, histoplasmosis, and lipid storage diseases. However, when the biopsy reveals extensive fibrosis without abundant carcinomatous cells, differentiation of marrow metastases from agnogenic myeloid metaplasia may be difficult.[9] This differential diagnosis is most important in patients who have previously been treated for primary breast cancer and who were without evidence of metastases prior to the development of myelophthisic anemia. Since intramedullary metastases are highly correlated with cortical bone involvement, the presence of skeletal pain or evidence of bone metastases on radiographic studies often helps to establish this distinction.[9] In addition, Kiely found that patients with marrow metastases and myelophthisic anemia had less marked splenomegaly than did patients with agnogenic myeloid metaplasia. Leukocytosis, basophilia, tear drop poikilocytosis, giant platelets, and platelet fragments were more pronounced in agnogenic myeloid metaplasia, whereas normoblastosis was more prominent in patients with marrow metastases.[9] Marked leukocytosis or thrombocytosis is rare in myelophthisic anemia associated with malignant disease.[3,9,22,23]

Determination of the level of urinary hydroxyproline excretion may also be useful in establishing the diagnosis. Elevated levels have been found in patients with breast cancer who have myelophthisic anemia, whereas normal values were reported in patients with breast cancer but without marrow metastases, as well as in those with agnogenic myeloid metaplasia.[24]

Myeloproliferative syndromes, which may arise as a consequence of the treatment of breast cancer with alkylating agents or radiation therapy, must also be considered in the differential diagnosis of myelophthisic anemia secondary to marrow metastases. A cumulative risk of approximately 1.5% has recently been reported for acute leukemia and myeloproliferative syndromes following adjuvant chemotherapy for breast cancer.[25] Pancytopenia and increased reticulin fibrosis in the marrow are common features of these treatment-induced hematologic neoplasms.[26–28] Dysplastic and cytogenetic changes in hematopoietic cells, and an absence of carcinomatous cells on marrow examination, allow a distinction to be made between this entity and myelofibrosis associated with marrow metastases.

PROGNOSIS OF PATIENTS WITH BREAST CANCER AND BONE MARROW METASTASES

The prognosis reported for patients with breast cancer who have marrow metastases is variable. In a large series from Sweden, Landys observed a highly significant increased "death risk" in patients with marrow metastases, compared to those without marrow metastases.[12] In contrast, other studies have found that positive results on bone marrow biopsy have no correlation to the response rate, duration of response, or survival in patients with advanced breast cancer.[13–15] In part, this discrepancy likely results from differences in characteristics among patients, as several factors influence the prognosis of patients with marrow metastases. The extent of marrow involvement is important as an indicator of the overall tumor burden and hence, the patient's potential resistance to treatment. Further, the degree of marrow compromise may govern the intensity of therapy. In a multivariate analysis of prognostic factors in patients with metastatic breast cancer, a pretreatment hemoglobin of less than 11 g/dl and a platelet count of less than 200,000 per mm^3 were found to have a statistically significant negative effect on both response to chemotherapy and survival.[29] A decrease in response rate and survival in patients with marrow metastases who require reductions in chemotherapeutic dose has also been reported.[13] The extent of concurrent metastases to other sites is another prognostic factor in patients with marrow metastases, with the combination of visceral, osseous, and soft tissue involvement having a particularly adverse impact.[30] The disease-free interval from the time of the initial diagnosis of breast cancer to the onset of metastases, the timing of the metastases with respect to menopause, the hormone receptor status of the tumor, and the history of prior treatment are additional prognostic variables in patients with marrow metastases.[4]

Differences in these factors undoubtedly contribute to the wide range of response and survival rates recorded in the subset of patients with breast cancer who have marrow metastases and myelophthisic anemia. West reported a median survival of 72 days in 18 patients with breast cancer and myelophthisic anemia at Memorial Hospital. The seven responding patients had a mean survival of 4.8 months, compared to a mean survival of 1.1 months for those who did not respond.[23] In contrast, Kiely's observations were more optimistic, with 5 of 6 patients surviving for at least 1 year after the onset of myelophthisic anemia; 3 of these patients survived 2 to 4 years.[9] Similarly, Webster reported a two-year survival in 40% of patients with breast cancer and leukoerythroblastosis.[22] In that series, all patients with disease-free intervals of 0 or greater than 1 year responded to treatment, whereas no responses were observed in patients with disease-free intervals of 1 year or less from the time of the primary diagnosis and the onset off myelophthisic anemia.

TREATMENT OF PATIENTS WITH BONE MARROW METASTASES AND MYELOPHTHISIC ANEMIA

The therapeutic approach to patients with breast cancer who have marrow metastases consists of both supportive measures and treatment of the underlying neoplasm. In patients with anemia or thrombocytopenia, transfusions may be necessary before and during therapy. Antibiotics are indicated in patients with fever and neutropenia that occurs as a consequence of either marrow involvement or its treatment. Both hormonal manipulation and chemotherapy may be efficacious in patients with marrow metastases. The choice between these modalities is based on the considerations that apply in general to the management of patients with advanced breast cancer (see Chapter 13).

Endocrine Therapy

Budd found that 54% of patients with breast cancer who had marrow involvement had estrogen receptor-positive tumors, and that an additional 11% had tumors with borderline levels of receptor.[17] Thus, the majority of patients with marrow metastases are potential candidates for endocrine therapy, which may have a particularly high therapeutic ratio when marrow involvement is extensive, such as in those with myelophthisic anemia. Patients with metastases limited to the marrow or with associated osseous or soft tissue involvement who have hormone receptor-positive tumors and disease-free intervals of 0 or in excess of 2 years should receive endocrine therapy. Indeed, endocrine manipulation may be more effective in patients with myelophthisic anemia than in the overall population with advanced breast cancer. Although approximately 40% of patients with advanced breast cancer will respond to endocrine therapy, patients with myelophthisic anemia have reported response rates of 50% to 85%.[22]

In premenopausal patients with breast cancer and myelophthisic anemia, oophorectomy has produced response rates ranging from 25% to 100%, with response durations frequently exceeding 2 years.[22,23] Tamoxifen is a potential alternative to oophorectomy in premenopausal women and is the initial treatment of choice in postmenopausal patients. Other endocrine maneuvers, including adrenalectomy and hypophysectomy, have also produced response rates in excess of 50% in patients with marrow metastases.[31–33] Androgenic steroids may have a dual role in patients with myelophthisic anemia, providing both an antineoplastic effect and potential stimulation of the residual normal marrow.[3,22]

Chemotherapy

Chemotherapy is indicated in patients with breast cancer and marrow metastases who have hormone receptor-negative tumors, who have become refractory to hormone maneuvers, or who have clinical features, such as a short disease-free interval, rapid progression of disease, or involvement of multiple visceral sites, that are unfavorable for the use of endocrine therapy. In particular, patients with pulmonary lymphangitic metastases or microangiopathic hemolytic anemia require prompt initiation of chemotherapy.

Studies from the National Cancer Institute and from the M.D. Anderson Hospital have assessed the impact of chemotherapy on patients with marrow metastases.[13,15] Using a combination of cyclophosphamide, 5-fluorouracil, and either methotrexate or doxorubicin, Ingle achieved response rates of 67% in patients with advanced breast cancer and marrow metastases, compared to a response rate of 71% in those without bone marrow involvement.[15] The median duration of response was also comparable for patients with and without marrow involvement. However, patients with bone marrow involvement had a greater requirement for hematologic support and a higher incidence of infection. Forty-six percent of patients with marrow metastases required transfusion, compared to only 21% of those without bone marrow involvement. Twenty percent of the group with marrow involvement developed sepsis, which occurred in only 7% of the group without marrow metastases. In this study, chemotherapeutic doses were decreased for patients with leukopenia and thrombocytopenia; 50% of the full dose or less was given when the white blood cell count was below 3000 per mm^3 or the platelet count was below 75,000 per mm^3. Patients with bone marrow involvement had lower white blood cell counts for the first two cycles of therapy and lower platelet counts for the first three cycles of therapy than did those without marrow metastases. Thereafter, for the duration of the 10-cycle treatment plan, the white blood cell and platelet counts were comparable in the two groups.

Rodriguez-Kraul treated 48 patients with metastatic breast cancer and marrow metastases with a combination of doxorubicin, cyclophosphamide, methotrexate, 5-fluorouracil, and bacille Calmette Guérin (BCG) vaccine or levamisole.[13] In this series, dose reduction was permitted only for infection or hemorrhage, rather than in cases of myelosuppression. Sixteen of 21 patients (76%) receiving full doses of chemotherapy achieved a response, including 8 (38%) who experienced complete marrow remissions. In contrast, 14 of 27 patients (52%) receiving less than full doses responded, and only 3 (11%) had complete resolution of marrow metastases. Compared to similarly treated patients without marrow metastases, the patients with marrow involvement had more frequent and more severe myelosuppression. Hematologic support was required in 60% of patients with bone marrow involvement, compared to 26% of those without bone marrow metastases. Eleven of 48 patients with marrow metastases were hospitalized at least once for fever and neutropenia. Five episodes of sepsis and three infectious deaths occurred in these patients. The patients with bone marrow involvement had a median duration of response of 16 months, which was equivalent to that in patients without marrow metastases.

Both of these reports demonstrate that chemotherapy with vigorous supportive care may achieve good results in patients with marrow metastases. However, it is likely that the extent of marrow involvement in these patients was relatively minimal, as marrow metastases were detected by biopsies performed as routine staging procedures rather than as procedures to evaluate cytopenias or abnormal peripheral smears. Only 40% of the patients in Ingle's series were anemic, 27% were leukopenic, and 13% were thrombocytopenic when positive results were obtained from marrow biopsy.[15] Only 15 of 48 patients with marrow metastases in Rodriguez-Kraul's study had hematologic abnormalities. However, other researchers have demonstrated the feasibility and effectiveness of chemotherapy in patients with more advanced marrow involvement.[34–36] Using a combination of vincristine, doxorubicin, and prednisone, Dady obtained four responses, three of which were complete, in patients with both marrow metastases and profound, pretreatment thrombocytopenia.[34] Kiang reported a complete response in a patient with leukoerythroblastic anemia, thrombocytopenia, myelofibrosis, and splenomegaly.[35] During treatment with cyclophosphamide, methotraxate, 5-fluorouracil, vincristine, prednisone, and halotestin, all abnormalities, including dense reticulin and collagen fibrosis in the marrow, resolved.

In patients with severely compromised marrow function, initial doses of chemotherapy must be reduced, and the necessity of intensive hematologic support can be anticipated. Early in treatment, infection, including sepsis, is common, and neutropenic febrile patients require hospitalization and antibiotics. However, with response to therapy, the hematologic parameters and the safety of ongoing treatment improve.

REFERENCES

1. Weick JK, Hagedorn AB, Linman JW: Leukoerythroblastosis: diagnostic and prognostic significance. Mayo Clin Proc 49:110, 1974
2. Vaughn MJ: Leukoerythroblastic anemia. J Pathol Bacteriol 42:541, 1938
3. Zucker S: Anemia associated with foreign cells in the marrow (myelophthisis). In Lichtman MA (ed): Hematology and Oncology: The Science and Practice of Clinical Medicine, pp 42–44. New York, Grune and Stratton, 1980
4. Westberg M, Armitage JD, Corder MP: Bone marrow involvement in breast cancer—Unexpected clinical findings. Proc Am Soc Clin Oncol 1:85, 1982
5. Delsol G, Guiu-Godfrin B, Guiu M, et al: Leukoerythroblastosis and cancer: Frequency, prognosis and physiopathologic significance. Cancer 44:1009, 1979
6. Rubins JM: The role of myelofibrosis in malignant leukoerythroblastosis. Cancer 51:308, 1983
7. Lazlo J: Anemia associated with marrow infiltration. In Williams W, Beutler E, Erslev R, et al (eds): Hematology, pp 528–532. New York, McGraw-Hill, 1983
8. Delforge A, DeCaluwe JP, Ronge-Collard E, et al: Increased levels of myeloid progenitor cells in the blood of patients with metastatic invasion of the marrow. Scand J Haematol 31(3):275, 1983
9. Kiely JM, Silverstein MN: Metastatic carcinoma simulating agnogenic myeloid metaplasia and myelofibrosis. Cancer 24:1041, 1969
10. Redding WH, Coombes RC, Monaghan P, et al: Detection of micrometastases in patients with primary breast cancer. Lancet 2:1271, 1983
11. Ingle JN, Tormey DC, Tan HK: The bone marrow examination in breast cancer: Diagnostic considerations and clinical usefulness. Cancer 41:670, 1978
12. Landys K: Prognostic value of bone marrow biopsy in breast cancer. Cancer 49:513, 1982
13. Rodriguez-Kraul R, Hortobagyi GN, Buzdar AU, et al: Combination chemotherapy for breast cancer metastatic to bone marrow. Cancer 48:227, 1981
14. Mendoza CB, Moore GE, Crosswhite LH, et al: Prognostic significance of tumor cells in the bone marrow. Surg Gynecol Obstet 129:483, 1969
15. Ingle JN, Tormey DC, Bull JM, et al: Bone marrow involvement in breast cancer: Effect on response and tolerance to combination chemotherapy. Cancer 39:104, 1977
16. DiStefano A, Tashima CK, Yap Y, et al: Bone marrow metastases without cortical bone involvement in breast cancer patients. Cancer 44:196, 1979
17. Budd GT: Estrogen receptor profile in patients with breast

cancer metastatic to the bone marrow. J Surg Oncol 24:167, 1983
18. Contreras E, Ellis LD, Lee RE: Value of bone marrow biopsy in the diagnosis of metastatic carcinoma. Cancer 29:778, 1972
19. Antman KH, Skarin AT, Mayer RJ, et al: Microangiopathic hemolytic anemia and cancer: A review. Medicine 58:377, 1979
20. Carey RW, Taft PD, Bennett JM, et al: Carcinocythemia (carcinoma cell leukemia): An acute leukemia-like picture due to metastatic carcinoma cells. Am J Med 60:273, 1976
21. Myerowitz RL, Edwards PA, Sartiano GP: Carcinocythemia (carcinoma cell leukemia) due to metastatic cancer of the breast. Cancer 40:3107, 1977
22. Webster DJT, Preece PR, Bolton PM, et al: Leucoerythroblastosis in breast cancer. Clin Oncol 1:315, 1975
23. West LD, Ley NB, Pearson DH: Myelophthisic anemia in cancer of the breast. Am J Med 18:923, 1955
24. Wang JC, Aung MK, Tobin MS: Urinary hydroxyproline excretion in myelofibrosis. Blood 55:383, 1980
25. Fisher B, Rockette H, Fisher ER, et al: Leukemia in breast cancer patients following adjuvant chemotherapy or postoperative radiation: The NSABP experience. J Clin Oncol 3:1640, 1985
26. Sultan C, Sigaux F, Imbert M, et al: Acute myelodysplasia and myelofibrosis: A report of eight cases. Br J Haematol 49:11, 1981
27. Feuilhade F, Brun B, Tuhran A, et al: Acute leukemia and breast cancer: Apropos of 12 cases observed in the department of oncology at the Henri Mondor Hospital. Bull Cancer (Paris) 70:389, 1983
28. Soffer T, Chan WC, Arynes RK, et al: Myeloproliferative disorder with profound hypereosinophilia associated with chemotherapy for breast cancer. Cancer 54:2356, 1984
29. Hortobagyi GN, Smith TL, Legha SS, et al: Multivariate analysis of prognostic factors in metastatic breast cancer. J Clin Oncol 1:776, 1983
30. Valagussa P, Brambilla C, Bonadonna G: Advanced breast cancer: Are the traditional stratification parameters still of value when patients are treated with chemotherapy? Eur J Cancer 15:565, 1979
31. Frazer ID, Talbot CH: The response to adrenalectomy of a leucoerythroblastic process due to metastatic carcinoma of the breast. Lancet 1:690, 1961
32. Akinsete FI, Kernohaw IR, Dawson AA: Pituitary ablation for leucoerythroblastosis in carcinoma of the breast. Lancet 2:1050, 1973
33. Hortling H, Malmio K, Bjor Keston GA, et al: Leuko-erythroblastic anaemia in breast cancer treated by hypophysectomy. Acta Med Scand 162:387, 1958
34. Dady PJ, Sugarbaker PH, Robertson NH: Combination chemotherapy for thrombocytopenia and bone marrow metastases from breast cancer. Br Med J 1:554, 1977
35. Kiang DT, McKenna RW, Kennedy BJ: Reversal of myelofibrosis in advanced breast cancer. Am J Med 64:173, 1978
36. Kiang DT, Greenberg LJ: CEA in designing chemotherapy for advanced breast cancers. Proc Am Soc Clin Oncol 2:104, 1983

Special Therapeutic Problems

15

Management of Locally Advanced Breast Cancer

Thomas A. Sheldon
Leroy M. Parker Blake Cady

Locally advanced, noninflammatory carcinoma of the breast is a heterogeneous disease with a poor prognosis. Although this group includes only about 5% of patients with breast cancer, it presents some of the most difficult treatment problems. As defined by the combined International Union Against Cancer–American Joint Committee on Cancer Staging (UICC–AJC) in 1977, Stage III patients have T3 or T4 primary tumors or N2 or N3 axillary nodes, or both, without evidence of metastatic involvement to distant sites.

Based on the work of Halsted, radical mastectomy was established as the standard treatment for breast cancer at the turn of this century. Halsted's report on the use of radical mastectomy primarily included patients who had locally advanced breast cancer.[1] Although this report showed that radical mastectomy could be performed without immediate local recurrence, there was little understanding at that time as to which patients ultimately benefited from its use. In an attempt to determine this, the records from a series of 1135 patients treated with radical mastectomy at the Presbyterian Hospital in New York between 1915 and 1942 were analyzed by Haagensen and Stout.[2] They identified clinical features associated with an extremely poor outcome. Table 15-1 lists clinical features, each of which was associated with a greater than 50% risk of local recurrence and the absence of clinical cure 5 years after diagnosis. These features became the basis of the Columbia Clinical Class D or inoperable group. A second group of features, shown in Table 15-2, were designated "grave signs of breast cancer." These signs by themselves did not indicate inoperability, but were associated with an increased rate of local recurrence, as well as a poor survival rate. A single grave sign placed a patient in Columbia Clinical Class C, whereas patients with two or more grave signs were considered to be inoperable and were assigned to Class D. In the presence of any two grave signs, 42% of patients in the Presbyterian series developed local recurrence, and only one (2%) was free of disease at 5 years. This study was the first to delineate the limits of operability for radical mastectomy and to define a group of patients with locally advanced, but apparently localized, breast cancer.

RADIATION THERAPY

The high incidence of local-regional recurrence following the surgical treatment of patients with locally advanced breast cancer resulted in radiation therapy assuming a major role in the treatment of these patients. In patients with locally advanced breast cancer, radiation therapy may be used either as definitive treatment after minimal biopsy or, in some cases, in conjunction with mastectomy. Definitive treatment of locally advanced tumors following minimal biopsy requires radiation doses that are greater than those used for early-stage tumors. There are many reports in the literature in which low doses of irradiation have been delivered to patients with locally advanced breast cancer, resulting in local control rates of only 11% to 38%.[3–8] Although a dose of 5000 cGy has been shown to be effective in controlling microscopic amounts of tumor, doses well in excess of 6000 cGy are required for gross tumor control. Baclesse was one of the first to show that tumor control was achievable when sufficiently high radiation doses were used.[9] This is true even in the case of unresected primary tumors larger than 6 cm in diameter. A similar approach was described by Fletcher and Mon-

Table 15-1
Clinical Features of Breast Cancer Associated With Poor Results Following Radical Mastectomy

Clinical Feature	*No. of Patients*	*Local Recurrence (%)*	*5-Year Clinical Cure (%)*
Extensive edema of skin over breast	51	61	0
Satellite nodules	7	57	0
"Inflammatory" carcinoma of the breast	25	60	0
Distant metastases	10	20	0
Parasternal or supraclavicular node metastases	16	56	0
Edema of the arm	4	50	0

(Haagensen CD: Diseases of the Breast, 2nd rev ed, p 623. Philadelphia, WB Saunders, 1971.)

Table 15-2
Grave Signs of Breast Cancer

Clinical Feature	*No. of Patients*	*Local Recurrence (%)*	*5-Year Clinical Cure (%)*
Edema of the skin of the breast (less than one-third)	75	32	23
Skin ulceration	14	14	36
Solid fixation of the tumor to the chest wall	20	40	5
Axillary lymph node greater than 2.5 cm in diameter	24	13	38
Fixed axillary nodes	8	13	13

(Haagensen CD: Diseases of the Breast, 2nd rev ed, pp 625–628. Philadelphia, WB Saunders, 1971.)

tague, who obtained a 72% local control rate in patients with inoperable breast cancer who were given 6000 cGy in 8 weeks.[10]

In cases in which high doses of radiation therapy are required, interstitial implantation appears to play an important role. In a recent update of the experience at the Joint Center for Radiation Therapy (JCRT),* 192 patients with Stage III breast cancer were treated with primary radiation therapy, 65% of whom underwent interstitial implantation. The actuarial local-regional failure rate (uncensored for distant failure) was 27% at 5 years (Fig. 15-1). The rate of failure in the breast was related to the radiation dose delivered to the primary site. The use of 6000 cGy or greater was associated with an improvement in the local-regional control rate at 5 years (76% vs 57%, $p = 0.03$). This improvement in local-regional control with an increased radiation dose was particularly significant for patients who had undergone less-than-excisional biopsy (74% vs 40%, $p = 0.006$). These results suggest that the use of interstitial implantation is a useful means of delivering the high dose of radiation required in these situations.

* Sheldon TA, Silver B, Harris JR, unpublished data, 1985.

Both radiation dose to the primary site and primary tumor size are important factors in achieving local control with radiation therapy. Baclesse achieved complete disappearance of tumor (proven by biopsy in more than 50% of cases) in 27 of 33 patients (82%) with tumors 4 to 6 cm in diameter, and in 25 of 42 patients (60%) with tumors larger than 6 cm in diameter. Similarly, 20 of 33 patients (61%) receiving a dose of less than 7000 cGy had complete disappearance of tumor, as compared to 34 of 42 patients (81%) who received 7000 cGy or more. When a dose of 9000 cGy or more was used, 16 of 17 patients (94%) had complete resolution of their tumors. Similar results were obtained in a study from the Princess Margaret Hospital and the Institut Gustave-Roussy.[11] This retrospective study included 242 patients who had tumors that were too advanced locally to be excised or who were unfit for general anesthesia. Only 20% of the patients in this series had Stage I or II disease. Patients who did not have at least a partial tumor response (12% to 15%) were excluded. Both

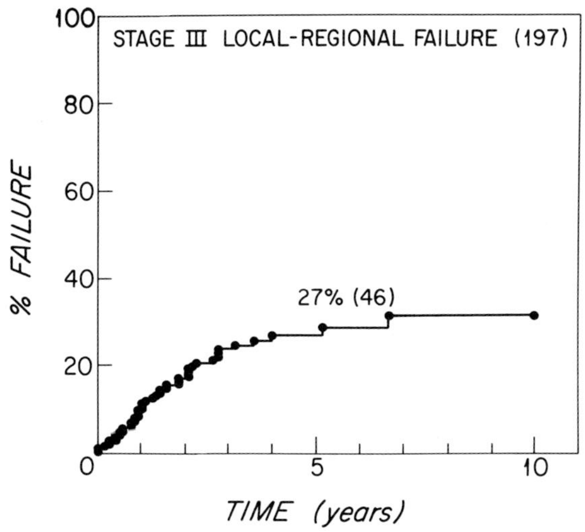

FIGURE 15-1. Uncensored local-regional failure rates for 192 patients (five with bilateral disease) with Stage III breast cancer treated by primary radiation therapy (JCRT).

radiation dose to the primary site and primary tumor size changed the relative risk of local recurrence. However, whereas changes in tumor size were associated with a twofold change in the relative risk, radiation dose was associated with a 10-fold change. Moreover, the intrinsic value of tumor size as a factor influencing local control decreased when other factors, such as tumor and nodal fixation, were taken into account. This study also indicated that a dose level of greater than 7000 cGy was required to achieve a high rate of local control. The series from Washington University also emphasized the importance of radiation dose.[12] The vast majority of patients in this series were treated with a dose of 7000 cGy or less to the primary site. Under these circumstances, primary tumor size was a very important predictor of local failure. In contrast, in recent results from the JCRT,* a dose of 7000 cGy or more to the primary site yielded a 5-year actuarial breast failure rate of 18% in patients with tumors smaller than 7 cm in diameter, and 16% in those with tumors 7 cm in diameter or larger. These results indicate that primary tumor size may be an important variable at lower radiation dose levels; however, when adequate radiation doses are delivered, a high rate of local control may be achieved, even in those patients with large tumors.

The use of high doses of radiation may be associated with significant complications. Moderate to severe complications were observed in 15 patients (8%) at the JCRT. Six patients had arm edema, four had brachial plexopathy (which was transitory in three of them) and four had restricted shoulder motion. Of interest was the lack of breast ulceration or necrosis in patients who did not have ulceration at presentation. Significant fibrosis occurred in several patients, but was not functionally important, and therefore, was considered to reflect a poor cosmetic result rather than a true complication. This is in contrast to the M.D. Anderson experience in which Spanos and co-workers found a high rate of fibrosis and necrosis in the breast.[13] Among patients treated with doses of 8100 rad or more, these problems continued to appear at an undiminished rate, even after 10 years. Of note, only 20 of 158 patients underwent interstitial implantation as a boost technique, and 13 of their 17 cases of necrosis had occurred by 6 years. Longer follow-up periods in the JCRT series may reveal some late breast necrosis as well, although the median follow-up in the current JCRT series is over 5 years.

* Sheldon TA, Silver B, Harris JR, unpublished data, 1985.

SYSTEMIC THERAPY

Although the results obtained by radiation therapy represented an improvement over those obtained by radical mastectomy in regard to local tumor control, the long-term survival rate was still poor. Among patients treated at the JCRT with only primary radiation therapy, for example, the 5-year survival rate was only 38%. This poor survival is attributable to the high probability of systemic disease in these patients. As a result, systemic therapy, usually combination chemotherapy, is now routinely used to treat patients with locally advanced breast cancer. These treatments are given either prior to local therapy as "neoadjuvant" therapy, or immediately following surgery or irradiation, in the same manner as adjuvant chemotherapy is given in patients with Stage I or II breast cancer. The use of adjuvant chemotherapy in patients with Stage III disease has been based on the good results seen in patients with Stage I and II disease. The ideal clinical trial for testing the value of initial systemic therapy has not yet been performed, however. In such a trial, precisely the same combination of hormones or chemotherapy would either be given initially or be withheld until used to treat the symptoms of systemic disease.

Since there is, as yet, no proof that the cure rate for locally advanced breast cancer has been improved by initial combined modality treatment, three potential benefits may be evaluated based on retrospective analysis: prolongation of median survival, prolongation of disease-free survival, and improvement in local control. A variety of regimens, originally developed and tested for their effect on metastatic disease, have now been tested as components of initial therapy for locally advanced breast cancer. Hormonal therapy has been added to some of these regimens or used alone as the sole systemic therapy in other trials. Chemotherapeutic regimens that have been evaluated in both retrospective and prospective studies include Adriamycin-vincristine (AV); cyclophosphamide, methotrexate, and 5-fluorouracil with or without prednisone (CMF or CMFP); cyclophosphamide, Adriamycin, and 5-fluorouracil (CAF or FAC); as well as more intensive regimens, such as cyclophosphamide, Adriamycin, methotrexate, and 5-fluorouracil (CAMF) in conjunction with calcium leucovorin, added as "rescue." Alternating, "non–cross-resistant" combinations have also been employed in the treatment of locally advanced breast cancer.

CHEMOTHERAPY

Use in Local Disease

Patients with intact primary tumors allow for the direct measurement of response to chemotherapy in locally advanced breast cancer. In their initial study of 74 patients, DeLena and co-workers reported a complete or partial response of 86% to four cycles of AV given prior to local irradiation.[14] Their follow-up study indicated a total response rate of only 54%.[15] Thalmo and colleagues reported 3 complete and 4 partial responses in 16 patients who had been treated with two cycles of CAF.[16] Mastectomy was performed in 14 cases, revealing residual microscopic tumor in 2 of 3 complete responders. Hortobagyi and associates reported an 83% overall response rate to a similar combination of drugs in 52 patients with locally advanced breast cancer who were able to be evaluated.[17] In a larger study of 69 patients from the same institution, Feldman and co-workers described 11 patients with grossly negative mastectomy specimens; of these, only 3 patients had no microscopic evidence of tumor.[18] From these data, one might estimate a clinical complete response rate of 10% to 15% to the best available chemotherapy, and a cell-kill approximating one log of tumor cells. A more impressive response rate was reported from the National Cancer Institute by Sorace and colleagues.[19] In a study which included equal numbers of patients with inflammatory carcinoma and other locally advanced forms of breast cancer, there was a 33% complete response rate, documented pathologically, following treatment with CAMF-leucovorin rescue plus premarin and tamoxifen. This response rate was determined by needle biopsy of the area that had previously been involved by tumor.

With this relatively modest degree of cytotoxic activity, it is not surprising that the evidence for improvement in local control by chemotherapy is equivocal. In a prospective study conducted at the M.D. Anderson Hospital,[17] patients were treated initially with FAC chemotherapy, subsequently undergoing primary radiation therapy after either a complete response or no response, or undergoing mastectomy plus radiation therapy after a partial response. Following local therapy, further FAC or CMF chemotherapy was administered. Local recurrence rates were similar for the two arms of the study (22% for radiation therapy and 19% for surgery plus radiation therapy). The 52 patients in this series were matched with 52 historical controls treated without chemotherapy, and no improvement in local control was seen. Balawajder and co-workers reviewed the sequence of combined modality therapy in a retrospective study of the experience at Mt. Sinai Hospital in New York.[20] They found that when a radiation dose of 5000 to 6000 rad was employed, local control rates could be improved from 38% to 55% by the addition of either mastectomy or chemotherapy to the treatment regimen. Their best local control rate was achieved when all three modalities were combined. Bruckman and colleagues conducted a retrospective comparison of matched patients who received or did not receive chemotherapy (or ablative endocrine therapy) and reported an improvement in local control from 65% to 85% at 4 years in patients receiving adjuvant systemic therapy.[21] Although a subsequent study using multivariate analysis suggested similar results,[22] an update of this series* indicated that the local control rate was not improved by chemotherapy.

Impact on Survival

A summary of seven large series using radiation therapy alone as initial therapy reveals a range of survival rates of 13% to 30% at 5 years.[5,9,23–27] This variation in 5-year survival rates may be the result of patient selection, improvements in the treatment of metastatic disease, or differences in the effectiveness of local treatment. The median survival time reported for three of these series was identical at 24 to 25 months. The 5-year survival rate for patients treated at the JCRT with either radiation only or radiation with single-agent chemotherapy was 38% (Fig. 15-2).* Although there was a trend toward improved survival in patients receiving CMF or an Adriamycin-containing regimen, the difference at 5 years was not statistically significant (51% versus 38%, $p = 0.16$). Moreover, the linear downward trend of both curves reflects a constant force of mortality. This implies that neither treatment is curative. Improvements in median survival time have been reported for patients who receive chemotherapy as part of their initial therapy. Sponzo and associates added CFP to radiation therapy in 13 patients. They reported a 92% complete response rate and a median duration of complete response of more than 38 months.[28] Median survival time in DeLena's study, in which AV therapy preceded radiation therapy, was 36 months.[14] Using the same chemotherapeutic program, Rubens randomly assigned women with locally advanced breast cancer to regimens of initial or delayed breast irradiation.[25] Median survival time for these patients was also 36 months. Hortobagyi and associates treated 52 women with FAC, BCG vaccine, and irradiation.[17] They, too, achieved an 83% response rate, a median duration of remission of 24 months, and a median survival time of 65 months. Long-term survival after relapse in this group of patients may well be attributable to endocrine-responsive tumors, as 75% were initially determined to be estrogen receptor-positive. The most aggressive chemotherapeutic and radiotherapeutic regimen reported to date (by LoPrinzi and co-workers[29])

* Sheldon TA, Silver B, Harris JR, unpublished data, 1985.

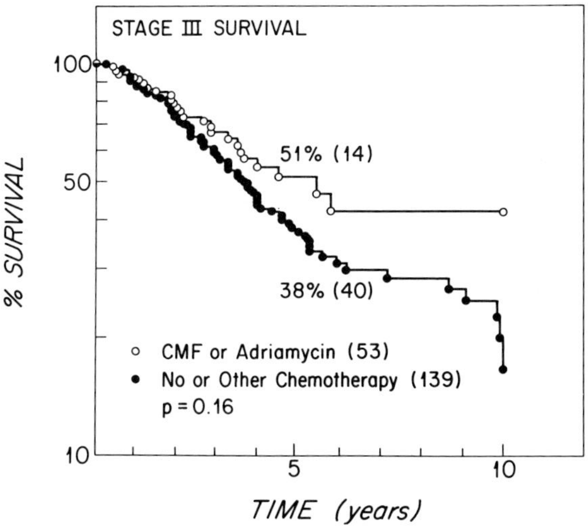

FIGURE 15-2. Actuarial survival rates for patients with Stage III breast cancer treated with primary radiation therapy with or without chemotherapy (JCRT). (CMF, cyclophosphamide, methotrexate, and 5-fluorouracil)

employed surgery, irradiation, and a chemotherapeutic regimen of cyclophosphamide, methotrexate, 5-fluorouracil, prednisone, and tamoxifen (CMFPT) alternating with AVT. This regimen succeeded in producing a median disease-free survival of only 30 months, which was, in part, related to the toxicity and morbidity associated with the regimen.

As noted earlier, it is only by reference to historical controls that we can gauge the benefits in disease-free or overall survival attributable to the use of adjuvant systemic therapy. The results indicate that there is a modest improvement in disease-free survival with the addition of adjuvant systemic therapy. Unless substantially better chemotherapeutic regimens are developed, the next task for those involved in clinical research on the treatment of locally advanced breast cancer will be to determine which subgroups benefit from such systemic therapy.

HORMONAL THERAPY IN LOCALLY ADVANCED BREAST CANCER

The use of hormonal therapy as the sole treatment for locally advanced breast cancer was reported by Veronesi and associates.[30] In this study, 46 postmenopausal women with locally advanced breast cancer received tamoxifen as initial therapy. Response occurred in only 14 patients (30%); median survival was 17.5 months in those who responded and 9 months in the nonresponders. These results appear to be worse than those seen in patients undergoing local treatment. As a result, it seems reasonable to restrict this approach to older women with tumors rich in estrogen receptors. In younger populations, it becomes more important to integrate local treatment, either surgery or irradiation, with hormonal or systemic therapy.

SURGERY

Inoperability, as defined by Haagensen and Stout, may be further classified as clinical or technical inoperability. Tumors that are not resectable with clear margins are considered to be technically inoperable. These include primary tumors that are fixed to the chest wall or associated with satellite skin nodules outside the operative field. Nodal lesions that are technically inoperable include any N3 lesions (involving the supraclavicular or infraclavicular nodes), or advanced N2 lesions with fixation within the axilla. Lesions with clinical features associated with a high rate of local recurrence may be operable with clear margins; therefore, they are technically operable but clinically inoperable. Such lesions include primary tumors associated with skin edema (including inflammatory carcinoma), ulceration, or cutaneous metastases within the operative field. "Early N2" lesions that have lymph nodes matted together but not fixed within the axilla are also technically operable, but clinically inoperable. Of note is the fact that patients with T3N0–1 tumors are generally considered to be operable, and have been categorized as having Stage III disease because of the poor prognosis associated with large primary lesions. In the most recent version of the UICC-AJC staging system (1986), these tumors have been reclassified as Stage II lesions.

The options for surgical treatment of locally advanced breast cancer range from incisional biopsy as a diagnostic procedure prior to radiation therapy to an extended radical mastectomy. In some patients with T3N0 or N1 breast cancer, the primary tumor may be resected in such a way that the breast remains cosmetically attractive; these patients may thus be treated with primary radiation therapy in a manner similar to those with Stage I or II lesions. The majority of these T3N0 or N1 cases have a sufficiently large primary cancer that the ultimate cosmetic result mitigates against the use of lumpectomy and radiation therapy. In the absence of the Columbia Clinical Classification's "grave signs," the results following mastectomy are quite satisfactory, with 5-year survival rates approaching 50% and 10-year survival rates being slightly lower.[31] Indeed, if the pathologic evaluation in such patients reveals that axillary lymph nodes are uninvolved, the prognosis is somewhat improved. Radical mastectomy may be performed, but a total mastectomy and partial axillary dissection with preservation of the pectoral muscle is more appropriate if the tumor is anterior to the pectoral fascia.[32]

Most patients with Stage III breast cancer are considered to be either clinically inoperable, based on a high rate of local recurrence following mastectomy, or technically inoperable because the tumor cannot be resected with clear margins. In these patients, mastectomy may be combined with other therapy (chemotherapy or radiation therapy). If the tumor involves a large portion of the pectoral muscle, a radical mastectomy in the traditional Halstedian fashion should be performed, including sacrifice of the entire pectoralis major and pectoralis minor muscles with radical axillary dissection. In most cases, however, preservation of all or most of the pectoral muscle may be achieved. The relative merits of mastectomy and primary radiation therapy will be discussed below.

MASTECTOMY VERSUS RADIOTHERAPY FOR LOCAL CONTROL

The role of primary radiation therapy as compared to mastectomy was addressed in a prospective trial from the National Cancer Institute in Milan, Italy.[15] This trial randomized patients to groups undergoing either radical mastectomy or definitive radiation therapy following four initial cycles of AV therapy. The patients then received six or seven additional courses of AV. Patients treated in a similar manner in a previous study were included for analysis of the irradiation arm. Therefore, more patients undergoing radiation therapy (126) were evaluated than were patients treated with surgery (79), and the group receiving radiation therapy had a longer median follow-up time. Patients were treated with 6000 cGy delivered to the entire breast over a 6-week period, and 70% received a boost of 1000 cGy to the primary site by external beam radiotherapy. Interstitial implantation was not used. The rates of local tumor control at 5 years were 75% for the group receiving radiation therapy and 82% for the group undergoing surgery. No statistically significant differences in 5-year distant disease or overall survival rates were observed between the groups. Progression of disease was continual in both groups. This result emphasizes the comparable, but poor, results seen with both forms of local therapy, even with vigorous systemic therapy.

The use of initial chemotherapy in conjunction with mastectomy is now favored at many institutions. This approach has been recommended because it avoids the high doses of radiation therapy required to treat such tumors primarily, and because it can avoid interruption in the use of systemic therapy. In many institutions, radiation therapy is used after mastectomy to help ensure local tumor control. This approach is described in greater detail in the following section.

SURGERY PLUS RADIATION THERAPY

Radiation therapy has also been used both preoperatively and postoperatively with mastectomy to treat patients with locally advanced breast cancer. Local control rates, when reported, have ranged from 55% to 97%.[3–5,12,23,24,33–38] Retrospective studies comparing mastectomy combined with postoperative radiation therapy to primary radiation therapy have generally shown that better local control rates have been achieved with the combined approach.[3,20,24,35,39] However, the local control rates achieved with the combined approach are similar to those obtained in the high-dose radiation therapy series discussed earlier. Furthermore, the selection of cases may be biased in favor of a surgical approach. This bias is suggested by the results of two nonrandomized studies comparing surgery alone and surgery plus radiation therapy.[39,40] In both studies, better local tumor control and 5-year survival rates were achieved in the group treated with surgery alone compared to the group that underwent surgery and radiotherapy. Results from the M.D. Anderson Hospital for their "group III" patients also demonstrate the importance of such case selection.[41] In this series, treatment consisted of a total or extended total mastectomy followed by 5000 cGy of external beam radiotherapy delivered over 5 weeks, with an additional 1000 cGy to 1500 cGy delivered to areas of increased risk. Of the patients included in this series, 195 were considered to have tumors that were clinically inoperable but technically resectable. The crude incidence of local recurrence in these patients was 11%, compared to 22% in 117 patients whose tumors were considered resectable but without clear margins. Even with aggressive combined surgery and radiation therapy, the extent of local disease is important in predicting the rate of local control.

Prospective clinical trials comparing primary radiation therapy alone and mastectomy plus radiation therapy are not available. The patients included in the nonrandomized prospective study from the M.D. Anderson Hospital[17] received initial FAC chemotherapy and were subsequently stratified, based on response, between radiation therapy for complete responders and nonresponders, and surgery plus radiation therapy for partial responders. Local recurrence rates were comparable for the two treatment groups. Given the selection biases in such a treatment approach, no definitive statement may be made regarding the relative efficacy of these two approaches.

THE TREATMENT APPROACH AT THE JCRT

Patients with locally advanced and inoperable disease who have been referred to the JCRT are treated after undergoing minimal biopsy to establish their hormone receptor status and histologic diagnosis. Currently, patients typically receive initial systemic therapy for approximately 4 months. Radiation therapy is then begun, using opposed tangential fields to the entire breast. Beam-modifying wedges are used as tissue compensators, and the dose is specified 1.5 cm inside the deepest edge of the fields. Bolus is used in patients with skin involvement, but it is limited as much as possible in order to maximize the cosmetic result. A dose to the whole breast of 4500 cGy to 5000 cGy is delivered at a rate of 900 cGy to 1000 cGy per week in five fractions. This is typically followed by an interstitial implant to the primary site for an additional 2500 cGy to 3000 cGy, bringing the total dose to the primary site to 7000 cGy to 8000 cGy. Since the peripheral radiation from interstitial implantation will also raise the dose to the whole breast, the whole breast dose by external beam is now typically restricted to 4500 cGy. Ipsilateral axillary and supraclavicular areas are treated with an anterior field to a total dose of 4600 cGy in 5 weeks. In patients with gross palpable axillary adenopathy, an en face or posterior axillary boost is added, bringing the total axillary dose to 5600 cGy. With this approach, axillary failure is uncommon (8% at 5 years), even in patients with initial gross lymphadenopathy in the absence of axillary dissection.*

SURGERY FOR LOCAL RECURRENCE

When a mastectomy is performed for recurrence following radical radiation therapy, the irradiated skin is frequently inelastic, stiff, and unsuitable for creating proper flaps to obtain primary closure. In these cases, plastic surgical techniques that bring new tissue from a latissimus dorsi or rectus abdominus myocutaneous flap may then be used. These flaps provide adequate skin replacement and a modest breast reconstruction for cosmetic appearance. The preoperative evaluation should include a critical appraisal of the amount of skin to be sacrificed. The skin margins, as well as other margins, should be checked by frozen section in the operating room before final determinations about closure are made. For this reason, and because of uncertainty regarding the degree of skin flexibility, it is frequently difficult to predict the ability to achieve primary closure preoperatively. It is, therefore, wise to consult a plastic surgeon preoperatively and to prepare for a pedicle flap unless the recurrence is localized and requires minimal skin sacrifice.

Local tumor recurrence sometimes involves the chest wall, and chest wall resection might be indicated to provide the best chance of local control. In these situations, resection of a total block of the chest wall, including several ribs or portions of the sternum, may be required to achieve pathologically disease-free margins. Such full-thickness chest wall resections, although not to be undertaken lightly, should be considered in any patient in whom there seems to be fixation by recurrent tumor. Major postoperative morbidity is not usually observed provided the chest wall defect is stabilized with heavy, flexible, surgical wires that are placed through the cut ends of the ribs and sternum to provide a scaffolding for the placement of the pedicle flap from the rectus abdominus or latissimus dorsi donor site.

SUMMARY

The results presented in this chapter section indicate that locally advanced breast cancer is a heterogeneous disease that is associated with a high rate of local recurrence and poor median and long-term survival rates. When compared to historical controls, the results obtained with multi-agent chemotherapy and local therapy suggest an improvement in the median disease-free interval and overall survival rate compared to those obtained with local therapy alone. On this basis, multi-agent chemotherapy is recommended in conjunction with local treatment for most patients with locally advanced breast cancer. In some older patients with estrogen receptor-rich tumors, hormonal therapy, either alone or in conjunction with local treatment, may have a similar role. Systemic therapy has not been shown to improve the cure rate, nor has a consistent improvement in local control been seen when this mode of therapy has been used in conjunction with local treatment.

Appropriate local treatment of locally advanced breast cancer is still controversial. A minority of patients with early Stage III breast cancer may be treated in a manner similar to that used in treating Stage I and II breast cancer—that is, mastectomy or conservative surgery and radiotherapy. For patients with technically operable breast cancer who respond favorably to initial systemic therapy, reasonable approaches include mastectomy with or without radiation therapy or high-dose radiation therapy alone. In the absence of improved cure rates for patients with technically operable breast cancer, we continue to view primary radiation therapy as the standard local treatment. In patients with technically inoperable breast cancer or in patients who do not respond favorably to initial systemic therapy, primary radiotherapy is generally preferred. Ongoing randomized trials may provide some insight into the indications for these various approaches to local management. The major emphasis in research, however, is on the development of better systemic therapy, which will require a reassessment of all local treatment options.

* Sheldon TA, Silver B, Harris JR, unpublished data, 1985.

REFERENCES

1. Halsted WS: The results of radical operations for the cure of cancer of the breast. Ann Surg 46:1, 1907
2. Haagensen CD, Stout AP: Carcinoma of the breast: Criteria of operability. Ann Surg 118:859–870, 1032–1051, 1943
3. Atkins HL, Horrigan WD: Treatment of locally advanced carcinoma of the breast with roentgen therapy and simple mastectomy. AJR 85:860, 1961
4. DelaRue NC, Ash CL, Peters V, et al: Preoperative irradiation in management of locally advanced breast cancer. Arch Surg 91:136, 1965
5. Langlands AO, Kerr GR, Shaw S: The management of locally advanced breast cancer by x-ray therapy. Clin Oncol 2:365, 1976
6. Golding P: The treatment of inoperable carcinoma of the breast in Portsmouth 1960–1969. Proc R Soc Med 69:701, 1976
7. Rubens RD, Armitage P, Winter PJ, et al: Prognosis in inoperable stage III carcinoma of the breast. Eur J Cancer 13:805, 1977
8. Treurniet-Donker AD, Hop WCJ, den Hoed-Sijtsema S: Radiation treatment of stage III mammary carcinoma: A review of 129 patients. Int J Radiat Oncol Biol Phys 6:1477, 1980
9. Baclesse F: Roentgen therapy as the sole method of treatment of cancer of the breast. AJR 62:311, 1949
10. Fletcher GH, Montague ED: Radical irradiation of advanced breast cancer. Am J Roentgenol Radium Ther Nucl Med 93:573, 1965

11. Arriagada R, Mouviesse H, Sarrazin D, et al: Radiotherapy alone in breast cancer. I. Analysis of tumor parameters, tumor dose, and local control. The experience of the Gustave-Roussy Institute and the Princess Margaret Hospital. 1986 Int J Radiat Oncol Biol Phys 11:1751, 1985
12. Bedwinek J, Rao DV, Perez C, et al: Stage III and localized stage IV breast cancer: Irradiation alone vs irradiation plus surgery. Int J Radiat Oncol Biol Phys 8:31, 1982
13. Spanos WJ, Montague ED, Fletcher GH: Late complications of radiation only for advanced breast cancer. Int J Radiat Biol Phys 6:1473, 1980
14. DeLena M, Zucali R, Viganotti G, et al: Combined chemotherapy-radiotherapy approach in locally advanced (T3b-T4) breast cancer. Cancer Chemother Pharmacol 1:53, 1978
15. DeLena M, Varini M, Zucali R, et al: Multimodal treatment for locally advanced breast cancer. Results of chemotherapy-radiotherapy versus chemotherapy-surgery. Cancer Clin Trials 4:229, 1981
16. Thalmo W, Sand J, Marti J, et al: Clinical and pathological (Path) findings in locally advanced breast cancer (LABC) treated with cyclophosphamide-Adriamycin-5-FU (CAF). (Abstr) Proc Am Soc Clin Oncol 3:127, 1984
17. Hortobagyi GN, Blumenschein GR, Spanos W, et al: Multimodal treatment of locally advanced breast cancer. Cancer 51:763, 1983
18. Feldman L, Hortobagyi G, Buzdar A, et al: Pathologic complete remission in patients with inflammatory breast cancer and locally advanced breast cancer. Proc Am Assoc Cancer Res 3:121, 1984
19. Sorace RA, Bagley CS, Lichter AS, et al: Management of nonmetastatic locally advanced breast cancer using primary induction chemotherapy with hormonal synchronization followed by radiation therapy with or without debulking surgery. World J Surg 9:775, 1985
20. Balawajder I, Antich PP, Boland J: An analysis of the role of radiotherapy alone and in combination with chemotherapy and surgery in the management of advanced breast carcinoma. Cancer 51:574, 1983
21. Bruckman JE, Harris JR, Levene MB, et al: The results of treating stage III carcinoma of the breast by primary radiation therapy. Cancer 43:985, 1979
22. Harris JR, Sawicka J, Gelman R, et al: Management of locally advanced carcinoma of the breast by primary radiation therapy. Int J Radiat Oncol Biol Phys 9:345, 1983
23. Fletcher GH: Local results of irradiation in the primary management of localized breast cancer. Cancer 29:545, 1972
24. Zucali R, Uslenghi C, Kenda R, et al: Natural history and survival of inoperable breast cancer treated with radiotherapy and radiotherapy followed by radical mastectomy. Cancer 37:1422, 1976
25. Rubens RD, Sexton S, Tong D, et al: Combined chemotherapy and radiotherapy for locally advanced breast cancer. Eur J Cancer 16:351, 1980
26. Treurniet-Donker AD, Hop WCJ, den Hoed-Sijtsema, S: Radiation treatment of stage III mammary carcinoma: A review of 129 patients. Int J Radiat Oncol Biol Phys 6:1477, 1980
27. Golding P: The treatment of inoperable carcinoma of the breast in Portsmouth 1960–1969. Proc R Soc Med 69:701, 1976
28. Sponzo RW, Gray R, Damsker JI, et al: The management of nonresectable (stage III) breast cancer. Proc Am Soc Clin Oncol 2:110, 1983 (C-430)
29. LoPrinzi CL, Carbone PP, Tormey DC, et al: Aggressive combined modality therapy for advanced local-regional breast carcinoma. J Clin Oncol 2:157, 1984
30. Veronesi A, Frustaci S, Tirelli U, et al: Tamoxifen therapy in postmenopausal advanced breast cancer: Efficacy of the primary tumor site in 46 evaluable patients. Tumori 67:235, 1981
31. Valagussa P, Bonadonna G, Veronesi U: Patterns of relapse and survival following radical mastectomy. Analysis of 716 consecutive patients. Cancer 41:1170, 1978
32. Cady B: Total mastectomy and partial axillary dissection. Surg Clin North Am 53:313, 1973
33. McWirther R: Simple mastectomy and radiotherapy in the treatment of breast cancer. Br J Radiol 28:128, 1955
34. Bouchard J: Advanced cancer of the breast treated primarily with irradiation. Radiology 84:823, 1965
35. Yaram J, Assa J, Robinson E: The survival of inoperable breast cancer treated with radiotherapy and radiotherapy followed by mastectomy. J Surg Oncol 9:203, 1977
36. Tarz JJ, Romero CA, Kay S, et al: Preoperative radiotherapy for stage III carcinoma of the breast. Surg Gynecol Obstet 147:497, 1978
37. Arnold DJ, Lesnick GJ: Survival following mastectomy for stage III breast cancer. Am J Surg 137:362, 1979
38. Cody HS, Bretsky SS, Urban JA: The continuing importance of adequate surgery for operable breast cancer. Significant salvage of node-positive patients without adjuvant chemotherapy. Cancer 32:242, 1982
39. Valagussa P, Zambetti M, Piguami P, et al: T3b–T4 Breast cancers: Factors affecting results in combined modality treatments. Clin Exp Metastasis 1:191, 1983
40. Fracchia AA, Evans JF, Eisenberg BL: Stage III carcinoma of the breast: A detailed analysis. Ann Surg 192:705, 1980
41. Montague ED: Radiation management of advanced breast cancer. Int J Radiat Oncol Biol Phys 4:305, 1978

Inflammatory Breast Cancer

Leroy M. Parker
Thomas A. Sheldon Blake Cady

Inflammatory carcinoma of the breast is the most lethal of the variants of locally advanced breast cancer. A description of the clinical findings that appeared in Bell's surgical textbook in 1816 is often quoted and remains true today: "When a purple color is on the skin over the tumor accompanied by shooting pains, it is a very unpropitious beginning."[1] A pathologic correlate, the presence of tumor cell "emboli" in subdermal lymphatics, was described in 1889.[2] The term inflammatory carcinoma was coined by Lee and Tannenbaum in 1924.[3] Prior to that, a number of other terms had been used, including acute carcinoma, carcinoma mastoides, and mastitis carcinomatosa gravidarum et lactantum. The unique clinical syndrome and poor prognosis associated with inflammatory carcinoma justify its separate consideration in this and other treatises on breast cancer.

DEFINITION

Inflammatory carcinoma of the breast has been defined by taking into account the clinical, pathologic, and biological features of the disease. Haagensen has provided the following description of this entity: "... in its fully evolved state [there is] enlargement and generalized induration of the breast and redness and edema of the skin over it."[4] These clinical findings should be accompanied by infiltrating mammary carcinoma that diffusely permeates the dermal lymphatics. Finally, the disease has been viewed as rapidly evolving—that is, as biologically aggressive—with a short duration of symptoms and a short, almost uniformly fatal outcome.

The 1986 UICC-AJC system for the staging of cancer specifies both clinical and pathologic criteria for all presentations of breast cancer.[5] The current clinical definition for inflammatory carcinoma is diffuse, brawny induration of the skin of the breast with an erysipeloid edge, usually without a palpable mass. (See Color Fig. 1 in Chapter 3.) Between 1983 and the 1986 revision, the AJC staging manual had no clinical description of inflammatory carcinoma, making it a purely pathologic diagnosis based upon a skin biopsy demonstrating plugging of subdermal lymphatics by breast cancer cells.[6] The rationale for the 1983 classification scheme rested upon the work of Ellis and Teitelbaum[7] and Saltzstein.[8] The former reviewed the pathologic findings of seven patients reported to have survived 5 years following initial treatment; these survivors accounted for only 4% of 173 patients included in the three series from which they were derived.[9–11] Only 1 of the 7 patients had evidence of subdermal lymphatic involvement, which led to the conclusion that clinical examples of inflammatory breast cancer lacking subdermal lymphatic involvement also lacked the essential feature of biologic aggressiveness. Saltzstein described four rapidly fatal cases of breast cancer with subdermal lymphatic involvement of the skin of the breast but without clinical evidence of "inflammation;" he termed this "occult" inflammatory carcinoma. Others have disputed the primacy of a pathologic definition of inflammatory carcinoma, and a return to a clinicopathologic definition is justified by the findings of Lucas and Perez-Mesa,[12] Droulias and co-workers,[13] Nussbaum and associates[14] and Fastenberg and colleagues.[15] The latter developed criteria by which they hoped they might accurately select examples of so-called "classic" inflammatory cancer and distinguish them from the "common" variety, which lacked some or all of the classic features (Table 15-3). Although there was a trend toward improved survival in patients with a common presentation or those who had no dermal involvement, the difference was not statistically significant. From the data from four studies in which the prognostic importance of dermal involvement was analyzed, it appears (Table 15-4) that there is no justification for separating cases that exhibit dermal involvement from those that lack it; the prognosis is very poor in either case.

In our opinion, it is probable that dermal lymphatic involvement by breast cancer cells is an important, perhaps essential, feature in the pathophysiology of inflammatory breast cancer. Accordingly, in its earliest stage, one would expect to find dermal lymphatic involvement prior to the appearance of inflammatory features.[8,12,13] Likewise, in its more advanced stage, one would expect to see not only subdermal lymphatic involvement, but dermal involvement with ulceration, in addition to inflammation. These findings have been reported and do not substantially worsen the prognosis.[12,13]

Inflammatory carcinoma is classified as Stage IIIB disease along with other locally advanced breast cancers having a poor prognosis, including other T4 lesions or those with N3 nodal involvement.

Table 15-3
Clinical, Radiographic, and Pathologic Features of Inflammatory Breast Cancer

Feature	*Classic Form*	*Common Form*
Erythema, *peau d'orange,* ridging	Present	Present
Duration of symptoms	< 3 Months	> 3 Months*
Mass detected on mammography	Absent	Present*
Dermal lymphatic involvement	Present	Absent*

* Patients with the common form of this disease have one or more of these features.

Table 15-4
Survival for Patients With the Clinical Features of Inflammatory Carcinoma With and Without Dermal Lymphatic Involvement

Invasion Present		*Invasion Absent*		
No. Patients	*Survival (mo)*	*No. Patients*	*Survival (mo)*	*Reference*
39	18	19	14.5	(12)
27	18	18	14.5	(14)
31	21	32	29.0	(15)

CLINICAL CHARACTERISTICS

Age and Menopausal Status

In the United States, inflammatory carcinoma occurs with an incidence of 1% to 4% among all presenting stages of breast cancer (Table 15-5). The average age of onset is 52 years, and approximately one-third of affected patients are premenopausal. Despite the term mastitis carcinomatosa gravidarum et lactantum, only 6 of 335 patients included in seven series were pregnant or lactating, constituting an incidence of only 2%. These findings are in sharp contrast to those in patients with "rapidly progressing breast cancer," encountered in Tunisia.[19] These latter patients, who have many of the features of inflammatory breast cancer and account for 55% of the patients with breast cancer

Table 15-5
Incidence, Age, and Peripartum Incidence of Inflammatory Breast Cancer

Study	*Dates*	*No. Patients*	*Patients with Inflammatory Breast Cancer (no./%)*	*Age Range (yr)*	*Mean Age (yr)*	*No. Patients Pregnant*	*Reference*
Pondville	1927–37	885	38/4.0	33–84	53	2	(16)
Pennsylvania	1926–52	1,774	46/2.6	26–80	50	1	(10)
Mayo Clinic	1933–45	7,000	74/1.0	32–72	53	1	(9)
Mayo Clinic	1946–56	3,200	53/1.7	25–78	52	1	(11)
Johns Hopkins	1946–55	697	19/2.7	36–65	43	1	(17)
Emory University	1937–75	3,039	75/2.4	27–83	53	NS	(18)
Duke University	1951–71	1,458	30/2.0	30–67	48	0	(13)
Total		17,168	335/2.0	25–84	52	6	

seen at the Institute Salah Azaiz in Tunis, also exhibit a strong correlation with pregnancy and lactation.[20]

Symptoms

Haagensen noted that the typical symptoms of inflammatory breast cancer were reported by patients with the following frequency: a mass (51%); breast or nipple pain (26%); breast enlargement (43%); and redness of the skin (51%). Less frequently, women reported increased skin warmth, edema, nipple retraction, itching or discharge, axillary pain, arm swelling, or bone pain. The median duration of these symptoms prior to diagnosis was 2½ months. In an Italian series, the median duration was 45 days.[21] This rapidity of onset has previously been noted as a characteristic of the classic presentation of inflammatory breast cancer. It is one of the features that distinguishes this entity from so-called "neglected" primary breast cancer.

Physical Findings

The most striking physical findings in patients with inflammatory breast carcinoma relate to the skin. Skin color varies from a light pink blush to a purplish hue, which is almost ecchymotic in nature. Comparison with erysipelas is easily made, as the skin is often warmer than the opposite breast in cases of inflammatory breast cancer, a finding which can be documented thermographically.[22] Furthermore, as with erysipelas, a superficial, palpable ridge is evident between "normal" skin and the most distal border of the inflammatory change in the skin of the breast. The term normal is placed in quotations because it is unwise to assume that any skin in the vicinity of a breast involved by inflammatory cancer is totally uninvolved. The presence of edema is evident from the increased size of the affected breast and the possible *peau d'orange* appearance. On deep palpation, one has the impression that the entire breast is involved. This, however, describes the "classic" presentation. As we have previously stated, the findings may vary from a state in which the inflammatory changes are almost imperceptible[8] to one in which dermal involvement with ulceration is present. If a mass is present, the clinical history protracted, and the patient exhibits a pathological element of denial, then one may be dealing with an advanced T4B or T4C lesion, the progression of which may be slower.

Axillary lymph node involvement is almost universal in inflammatory breast cancer. In Haagensen's series, it was present in 81 of 89 patients (91%).[4] Despite this fact, the disease was considered to be "technically operable" in 70% of patients whose nodal involvement did not exceed the N2 level. In this series, evidence of N3 nodal involvement (arm edema, involvement of the supraclavicular nodes) was found in 13%. The opposite breast was involved synchronously in 2% and metachronously in 28%. In the early series of Taylor and Meltzer, cancer developed in the opposite breast in 21 of 38 patients (55%).[16] Involvement of the opposite breast does not worsen the prognosis of inflammatory carcinoma.[16]

Radiographic and Laboratory Findings

The hallmark of mammographic findings in inflammatory carcinoma is an increase in skin thickness.[22,23] A second finding is asymmetric widening of the subcutaneous lymphatic vessels. Equal in importance is the detection of increased tissue density in the affected breast. All of these findings may be overlooked if the radiologist is not aware of the symptoms and clinical findings. These radiologic images form the now-classic mammographic pattern of inflammatory breast cancer. Other patients may present with a breast mass and radiologic findings typical of a scirrhous cancer with or without malignant microcalcifications.

Breast thermography in patients with inflammatory breast cancer produces an asymmetric thermal image with a generalized increase in heat reflected from the affected breast. Although this procedure would be considered superfluous in the contemporary evaluation of a patient with inflammatory carcinoma, it has been used with some success in evaluating response to therapy.[24]

Differential Diagnosis

Infection and abscess rarely occur in other than the lactating breast. Despite this, patients referred to our center with inflammatory carcinoma have often been treated initially and inappropriately with antibiotics. Although mammary duct ectasia may mimic a localized inflammatory process in the nonlactating breast, the greatest difficulty for the clinician is the accurate distinction between inflammatory carcinoma and other locally advanced breast cancers that involve the skin.

Histopathology

The usual histologic types of breast cancer are found in inflammatory carcinoma. The majority are poorly differentiated. In addition to subdermal lymphatic involvement, the small vessels of the breast are also frequently involved by tumor cell emboli.

Hormone Receptor Status

The relative rarity of inflammatory carcinoma and the possible reluctance of clinicians to perform incisional surgical biopsy have made it difficult to accumulate information on the frequency and prognostic importance of estrogen receptors (ER) and progesterone receptors (PR). DeLarue and co-workers have reported on a series of 59 patients, comparing their results with those obtained in 496 patients with "operable tumors;" for unexplained reasons, they have excluded patients who reported rapidly growing tumors. Using a cut-off of 100 fmol/g of tissue, they found the following frequency of receptor combinations: ER+PR+, 28%; ER−PR+, 5%; ER+PR−, 19%; ER−PR−, 48%. The frequency of ER−PR− tumors was significantly higher among patients with inflammatory carcinoma than among patients with operable tumors ($P < 0.02$). Patients with inflammatory breast cancer without metastases at diagnosis who had ER+ tumors had median disease-free survivals that were significantly longer than those for similar patients with ER− tumors (>36 months versus 15 months, respectively, $P > 0.001$). Harvey and associates presented data from 16 patients seen at four different U.S. medical centers.[26] Defining a positive assay as greater than 10 fmol/mg of cytosol protein, they found 5 patients with ER+ tumors, with levels ranging from 21 to 83 (with a median of 43). It is not yet possible to determine whether patients with the "common" presentation of inflammatory breast cancer are more likely to have ER+ tumors. It seems clear, however, despite the paucity of data, that receptor values will be important both in providing prognostic information as well as in improving the care for appropriately selected patients. Every effort, therefore, should be made to obtain adequate tissue for determination of receptor levels.

TREATMENT

Role of Mastectomy

Although radiation therapy should be viewed as the standard therapy for achieving local control in inflammatory breast cancer, mastectomy has an important historical role and a potential—and experimental—role in the management of these patients. There are only a small number of nonrandomized, retrospectively reviewed, mastectomy series, each of which contains only a few patients (Table 15-6). The largest series is that of Haagensen.[4] The 29 patients he reviewed were among those upon which he and Stout based their conclusion that inflammatory breast cancer should be considered categorically inoperable. This conclusion was based on the fact that surgical treatment was not curative, and that at least 50% of patients suffered local recurrence. Despite this, some authors continue to recommend mastectomy as the principle modality for achieving local control. Hagelberg and colleagues reported a retrospective review of 33 patients with inflammatory carcinoma, 28 of whom fulfilled both the clinical and pathologic criteria for the diagnosis.[34] It is probable that patient selection would best explain why the 5-year survival (25%) and local recurrence rate (25%) for these patients is in such sharp contrast to Haagensen's results; patients undergoing mastectomy were more likely to have clinically negative axillae and a well-defined mass than were their nonsurgically treated counterparts.

Today, mastectomy is more commonly used as adjunctive treatment to achieve local control. This treatment approach has been tested by those who recognize the systemic nature of inflammatory breast cancer and wish to avoid protracted courses of irradiation which may both postpone chemotherapy and limit the total dose of myelosuppressive therapy that can be delivered. A pilot study of 13 consecutive patients by Wiseman and co-workers utilized an extended simple mastectomy (removal of the breast and axillary contents lateral to the pectoralis minor muscle) or simple mastectomy following hematologic recovery from the second or third cycle of CAF chemotherapy.[35] Chemotherapy was resumed 1 to 2 weeks after mastectomy. The theoretical advantage of this approach was the removal of bulk disease and thus, its potential to generate resistant tumor cells, which could improve both local and systemic control. Chest wall irradiation was subsequently administered after approximately 8 months of chemotherapy. The follow-up study by Fastenberg and colleagues included a nonrandomized comparison of results in 21 patients undergoing irradiation and mastectomy with those obtained in 41 patients receiving irradiation alone.[15] This study did not demonstrate an advantage to adding

Table 15-6
Survival of Patients With Inflammatory Breast Cancer Treated By Radical Mastectomy or Radiation Therapy

	No. Patients	Average Survival (mo)	No. 5-Year Survivors (%)	Reference
Radical Mastectomy Alone				
	4	15	0	(3)
	6	21	0	(16)
	29	19	1	(4)
	2	8	0	(17)
	8	12	–	(21)
Total	49	17	1(2%)	
Radiation Therapy Alone				
	13	11	0	(3)
	19	9	0	(15)
	9	16	0	(27)
	24	16	1	(10)
	3	4	0	(28)
	29	15	0	(4)
	23	21	2	(29)
	17	20	0	(30)
	53	23	3	(13)
	86	—	3	(31)
	10	18	0	(18)
	70	15	–	(32)
	19	20	0	(12)
	62	18	2	(33)
	20	17	–	(21)
Total	457	18	11(3%)	

mastectomy in terms of either local control or survival. At present, the role of mastectomy in the management of inflammatory breast cancer remains unproven and requires further testing (in a randomized setting) before it can be recommended.

Role of Radiation Therapy

Between 1924 and 1981, more than 450 patients with inflammatory carcinoma treated by radiation therapy alone were reported (see Table 15-6). Survival of patients treated with irradiation averaged 18 months, and less than 5% survived 5 years. Today, we recognize both the importance and the limitations of local therapy. Aggressive radiation therapy using high doses or vigorous fractionation schedules appears to be the most important factor in gaining local control of inflammatory carcinoma. Many of the studies referred to in Table 15-6 have concentrated on survival without regard to local-regional control rates.[3,10,12,13,16,18,32] The series reported by Wang and Griscom in 1964 noted that only one-third of patients achieved complete disappearance of their primary tumor or permanent local control during their lifetime;[29] the dose employed averaged 2600 roentgens, delivered mostly by orthovoltage technique. A more recent group of 62 patients from the same institution was treated with low-dose megavoltage technique, with most receiving only 4500 roentgens to the breast fields.[33] A similar local control rate of 31% was achieved.

Bruckman and associates reported a 65% actuarial probability of local control in 18 patients with inflammatory carcinoma.[36] These same patients had an actuarial relapse-free survival of only 13%, with most relapses occurring outside the treated area. Local control was achieved in 11 of 13 patients (85%) who received greater than 6000 cGy to the primary site, compared to only 1 of 5 patients (20%) who received less than 6000 cGy. Recent data from the JCRT, which extended the series to 42 patients, show an 88% five-year actuarial local-regional control rate. This rate is similar to that for noninflammatory, locally advanced breast cancer.*

Results from the M.D. Anderson Hospital also suggest the benefit of more aggressive radiation therapy.[31,37,38] Barker and colleagues reported on the results in 86 patients treated with a standard, once-per-day regimen prior to 1972.[31,,37] A 54% local-regional control rate was achieved using either kilovoltage (in 45 patients) or megavoltage (in 24 patients) techniques. After 1972, a more aggressive, twice-per-day regimen was used; this resulted in a 73% local-regional control rate in 11 patients treated with radiation alone and a 75% rate in 32 patients treated with the same radiation therapy program plus FAC chemotherapy. A comparable, improved rate of local control was seen in 6 patients treated twice daily at the Massachusetts General Hospital, as reported by Chu and associates.[33] Neither the nonrandomized studies described above nor the more recent experience of the JCRT indicate that the addition of chemotherapy improves the chances for local control.

A recent, randomized, concurrently controlled trial of radiation therapy alone versus irradiation plus chemotherapy in patients with locally advanced and inflammatory carcinoma has provided a careful description of its local control rates.[39] The complete response rate in 45 patients receiving radiation therapy alone was 75%; in a second group of 34 patients who received 12 months of CMF after radiation therapy, the response rate was 71%. In a third group of 39 patients receiving alternating cycles of AV and CMF therapy, the response rate was 26% after two cycles, 64% after the radiation therapy that followed, and 71% after further chemotherapy. Local recurrence was observed in 28% of patients who had complete remission; the rate of local recurrence was not different in any of the three groups. If the local recurrences (in 24 of 86 patients who responded completely) and the 19 "regrowths" that occurred in the 32 partial responders or nonresponders are combined, a 36% rate of local progression or recurrence

*JCRT, unpublished data

results. However, only 14 of 118 patients (12%) in the study were said to experience local discomfort.

Technique of Radiation Therapy for the Treatment of Inflammatory Breast Carcinoma at the JCRT

At the JCRT, the breast involved with inflammatory carcinoma is treated with opposed tangential fields adjusted so that the posterior field edges are parallel. The essential difference between the treatment of locally advanced inflammatory carcinoma and that of T1 or T2 lesions is the need to increase markedly the dose that the skin receives in the former. To accomplish this, bolus material is placed on the breast and chest wall over one-half to one-third of the treatment course. Using beam-modifying wedges that act as tissue compensators, the dose is specified 1.5 cm inside the deepest edge of the field. A radiation dose of 4500 cGy to 5000 cGy is delivered at a rate of 900 cGy to 1000 cGy per week in five fractions (1 cGy = 1 rad). External beam treatment is followed by an interstitial implant to the primary site for an additional 2500 cGy to 3000 cGy, bringing the total dose delivered to the primary tumor to 7000 cGy to 8000 cGy. The peripheral radiation from interstitial implantation also contributes to the whole-breast dose. The ipsilateral axillary and supraclavicular areas are treated with an anterior field or with an additional posterior or (rarely) en face field for gross axillary disease.

Role of Endocrine Therapy

Systemic endocrine therapy, either surgical ablation or additive hormonal therapy, has been tested in small numbers of patients with inflammatory breast cancer. Dao and McCarthy were the first to report two responses in three patients treated by combined adrenalectomy-oophorectomy.[28] Fracchia and co-workers observed responses in 7 of 22 patients with inflammatory breast cancer after the same treatment.[40] Yonemoto and colleagues noted that 5 of 6 premenopausal patients and only 2 of 8 postmenopausal patients responded, but the median survival of 22 months for this series was little different from that reported for patients treated with radiation therapy.[41]

In the era of hormone receptor determination, there have been few attempts to use either the antiestrogen tamoxifen, megestrol, aminoglutethemide-hydrocortisone, or oophorectomy in appropriate patients. In their retrospective review, Harvey and associates noted one partial response to oophorectomy among five ER+ patients; only 3 of these patients received endocrine therapy.[26] Levine and co-workers found that premenopausal Tunisian women with "rapidly progressive" breast cancer (with inflammatory features) had low ER levels, and suggested that the standard management in that country—oophorectomy—be changed.[42] However, in properly selected patients, these nontoxic approaches may have a favorable impact on median survival, even if they do not eradicate the disease.

Table 15-7
Response Rate of Patients With Inflammatory Carcinoma to Chemotherapy

Agents	No. Patients	CR	PR	<PR	PROG	Total (CR+PR) (%)	Reference
		No. Responders					
CAF	62	9	34	17	2	68	(15)
AVMF	15	3	11	1	–	93	(24)
AV	36	7	17	10	2	67	(43)
AV + CMF	39	10					(39)

CR, complete response; PR, partial response; <PR, less than partial response; PROG, progression; CAF, cyclophosphamide, Adriamycin, and 5-fluorouracil; AVMF; Adriamycin, vincristine, methotrexate, and 5-Fluorouracil; AV, Adriamycin and vincristine; AV + CMF, Adriamycin and vincristine plus cyclophosphamide, methotrexate, and 5-fluorouracil.

Role of Chemotherapy

Chemotherapy has been used both before, concurrently, and following radiation therapy in patients with inflammatory carcinoma. When used as initial therapy, one can judge the overall effectiveness of treatment; as expected, it is similar to that observed in metastatic disease. Most standard drug regimens have been explored (Table 15-7). The first large series of patients treated with combined modes of therapy was reported by DeLena and associates.[43] They administered four cycles of AV chemotherapy before and after radiation therapy. The complete response rate to chemotherapy alone was 19%; only 2 patients (6%) progressed while receiving chemotherapy. Zylberberg and colleagues reported a 93% overall response rate, but only 20% of the patients in their series were complete responders.[24] The addition of CMF to AV in alternating cycles prior to radiation therapy resulted in a complete response rate of 26%.[39] At the M.D. Anderson Hospital, the use of CAF therapy resulted in a 14% complete response rate. Thus, there is no evidence for the superiority of one regimen over another, although all regimens that have been tested adequately have contained Adriamycin as one of the components.

Nonrandomized and retrospective trials of chemotherapy suggest an improvement in median relapse-free survival, median survival, and 5-year survival when compared with the survival rates reported for historical or literature controls (Table 15-8). Most of the reports have involved no more than 5 years of follow-up. Median relapse-free survival has ranged from 15 to 30 months when reported. Median survivals in these studies exceed 36 months, with 5-year survival rates of 31% to 60% being reported.

Despite these optimistic trends, a more sobering view

Table 15-8
Nonrandomized and Pilot Studies Employing Chemotherapy, Radiation Therapy, and Mastectomy for Inflammatory Carcinoma

	Relapse-Free and Overall Survival					
	No. Patients		Median Survival (mo)		5-Year Survival	
Series and Date	LABC	IC	RFS	S	(%)	Reference
Milan, 1978	74	36	15	36		(43)
Hospital Bichat, 1982		15		>56		(24)
Wisconsin, 1984	23	9	30	>24		(44)
M.D. Anderson, 1985		63	24	43	31	(15)
Vanderbilt, 1985		11			60	(45)

LABC, locally advanced breast cancer. IC, inflammatory cancer; RFS. relapse-free survival; S, survival.

emerges from the single randomized and controlled trial performed in Holland between 1977 and 1980.[39] In this three-arm study (Table 15-9), it was possible to compare the effect of chemotherapy given before or after radiation therapy as an "adjuvant," with the same chemotherapy administered in a delayed fashion at the time of relapse. Tamoxifen, 30 mg/day, was administered in both chemotherapy arms of the study. The 5-year survival rate was 37% in all three study arms. There was a trend in median relapse-free survival that favored the addition of chemotherapy, but the difference was not statistically significant ($p = 0.11$). The authors concluded that their findings did not support the routine use of adjuvant chemotherapy and endocrine therapy for inoperable breast cancer.

Table 15-9
A Randomized Trial Comparing Irradiation With and Without Chemotherapy in Locally Advanced and Inflammatory Breast Cancer

			Survival	
Group	Treatment	No. Patients	Median RFS (mo)	5-Year Survival (%)
I	Irradiation alone	45	14	37
II	Irradiation and a 12-month course of CMF + tamoxifen	34	26*	37
III	AV-CMF prior to and after irradiation + tamoxifen	39	20*	37

*Arm I versus II + III (p = 0.11).
RFS, relapse-free survival; CMF, cyclophosphamide, methotrexate and 5-fluorouracil; AV, Adriamycin and vincristine.
(Schaake-Koning C, van der Linden EH, Hart G, et al: Adjuvant chemotherapy and hormonal therapy in locally advanced breast cancer: A randomized clinical study. Int. J Radiat Oncol Biol Phys 11:1759, 1985.)

SUMMARY

Inflammatory carcinoma remains a major challenge to oncologists treating breast cancer. Although its presentation may vary, patients with either the clinical findings of inflammation, the pathologic findings of tumor emboli in subdermal lymphatics, or both of these criteria, have a rapidly progressive illness that should be considered systemic at the outset. Radiation therapy should be considered to be the standard therapy for local control. When proper attention is paid to radiation dose, most patients should be able to achieve symptomatic local control without resorting to mastectomy. Although chemotherapy, with or without the addition of endocrine therapy, is routinely administered in an adjuvant fashion to patients with inflammatory carcinoma, there is little evidence to support its use as initial treatment (as opposed to its delayed use in the treatment of metastatic disease). Improved methods of patient selection using hormone receptor assays may lead to less toxic initial therapy for certain subsets of patients. More effective systemic therapy is required for inflammatory breast cancer, as well as for other forms of locally advanced and metastatic breast cancer.

REFERENCES

1. Bell C: A System of Operative Surgery, Vol 2, p 136. Hartford, Hale and Hosmer, 1816
2. Bryant T: Diseases of the Breast, vol 4, pp 35–322. New York, Wood's Medical and Surgical Monographs, 1889
3. Lee BJ, Tannenbaum NE: Inflammatory carcinoma of the breast: A report of twenty-eight cases from the breast clinic of the Memorial Hospital. Surg Gynecol Obstet 39:580, 1924
4. Haagensen CD: Diseases of the Breast, 2nd ed, pp 576–584. Philadelphia, WB Saunders, 1971
5. TNM Classification of Malignant Tumours (in press)
6. Harmer MH (ed): TNM Classification of Malignant Tumours, 3rd ed rev. Geneva, 1982
7. Ellis DL, Teitelbaum SL: Inflammatory carcinoma of the breast: A pathologic definition. Cancer 33:1045, 1974
8. Saltzstein SL: Clinically occult inflammatory carcinoma of the breast. Cancer 34:382, 1974

9. Meyer AC, Dockerty MB, Harrington SW: Inflammatory carcinoma of the breast. Surg Gynecol Obstet 87:417, 1961
10. Rogers CS, Fitts WT: Inflammatory carcinoma of the breast: A critique of therapy. Surgery 39:367, 1956
11. Barber KW, Dockerty MB, Clagett OT: Inflammatory carcinoma of the breast. Surg Gynecol Obstet 112:406, 1961
12. Lucas FV, Perez-Mesa C: Inflammatory carcinoma of the breast. Cancer 41:1595, 1978
13. Droulias CA, Sewell CW, McSweeney MB, et al: Inflammatory carcinoma of the breast: A correlation of clinical, radiologic and pathologic findings. Ann Surg 184:217, 1976
14. Nussbaum H, Kagan AR, Gilbert H, et al: Management of inflammatory breast carcinoma. Breast 3:25, 1977
15. Fastenberg NA, Buzdar AU, Montague ED, et al: Management of inflammatory carcinoma of the breast: A combined modality approach. Am J Clin Oncol 8:134, 1985
16. Taylor GW, Meltzer A: "Inflammatory carcinoma" of the breast. Am J Cancer 33:33, 1938
17. Richards GJ, Lewison EF: Inflammatory carcinoma of the breast. Surg Gynecol Obstet 113:729, 1961
18. Stocks LH, Patterson FMS: Inflammatory carcinoma of the breast. Surg Gynecol Obstet 143:885, 1976
19. Tabbane F, Muenz LR, Jaziri M, et al: Clinical and prognostic features of a rapidly progressing breast cancer in Tunisia. Cancer 40:376, 1977
20. Mourali N, Muenz LR, Tabbane F, et al: Epidemiologic features of rapidly progressing breast cancer in Tunisia. Cancer 46:2741, 1980
21. Bozzetti F, Saccozzi R, De Lena M, et al: Inflammatory cancer of the breast: Analysis of 114 cases. J Surg Oncol 18:355, 1981
22. Buchanan JB, Bland KI, Kuhns JG: Inflammatory mammary carcinoma. Breast 5:22, 1979
23. Berger SM: Inflammatory carcinoma of the breast. AJR 88:1109, 1962
24. Zylberberg B, Salat-Baroux J, Ravina JH, et al: Initial chemoimmunotherapy in inflammatory carcinoma of the breast. Cancer 49:1537, 1982
25. DeLarue JC, May-Levin F, Mouriesse H, et al: Oestrogen and progesterone cytosolic receptors in clinically inflammatory tumours of the human breast. Br J Cancer 44:911, 1981
26. Harvey HA, Lipton A, Lawrence BA, et al: Estrogen receptor status in inflammatory breast carcinoma. J Surg Oncol 21:42, 1982
27. Chris SM: Inflammatory carcinoma of the breast: Report of 20 cases and review of the literature. Br J Surg 38:163, 1950
28. Dao TL, McCarthy JD: Treatment of inflammatory carcinoma of the breast. Surg Gynecol Obstet 105:289, 1957
29. Wang CC, Griscom NT: Inflammatory carcinoma of the breast. Clin Radiol 15:168, 1964
30. Spratt JS, Donegan WL: Cancer of the Breast, p 167. Philadelphia, WB Saunders, 1967
31. Barker JL, Nelson AJ, Montague ED: Inflammatory carcinoma of the breast. Radiology 121:173, 1976
32. Zucali R, Uslenghi C, Kenda R, et al: Natural history and survival of inoperable breast cancer treated with radiotherapy and radiotherapy followed by radical mastectomy. Cancer 37:1422, 1976
33. Chu AM, Wood WC, Doucette JA: Inflammatory breast carcinoma treated by radical radiotherapy. Cancer 45:2730, 1980
34. Hagelberg RS, Jolly PC, Anderson RP: Role of surgery in the treatment of inflammatory breast carcinoma. Am J Surg 148:125, 1984
35. Wiseman C, Jessup JM, Smith TL, et al: Inflammatory breast cancer treated with surgery, chemotherapy and allogeneic tumor cell/BCG immunotherapy. Cancer 49:1266, 1982
36. Bruckmann JE, Harris JR, Levene MB, et al: Results of treating Stage III carcinoma of the breast by primary radiation therapy. Cancer 43:985, 1979
37. Barker JL, Montague ED, Peters LJ: Clinical experience with irradiation of inflammatory carcinoma of the breast with and without elective chemotherapy. Cancer 45:625, 1980
38. Buzdar AU, Montague EP, Barker JL, et al: Management of inflammatory carcinoma of breast with combined modality approach—An update. Cancer 47:2537, 1981
39. Schaake-Koning C, van der Linden EH, Hart G, et al: Adjuvant chemotherapy and hormonal therapy in locally advanced breast cancer: A randomized clinical study. Int J Radiat Oncol Biol Phys 11:1759, 1985
40. Fracchia AA, Randall HT, Farrow JH: The results of adrenalectomy in advanced breast cancer in 500 consecutive patients. Surg Gynecol Obstet 125:747, 1967
41. Yonemoto RH, Keating JL, Byron RL, et al: Inflammatory carcinoma of the breast treated by bilateral adrenalectomy. Surgery 68:461, 1970
42. Levine PH, Tabbane F, Muenz LR, et al: Hormone receptors in rapidly progressing breast cancer. Cancer 54:3012, 1984
43. DeLena M, Zucali R, Viganotti G, et al: Combined chemotherapy-radiotherapy approach in locally advanced (T3b-T4) breast cancer. Cancer Chemother Pharmacol 1:53, 1978
44. LoPrinzi CL, Carbone PP, Tormey DC, et al: Aggressive combined modality therapy for advanced local-regional breast carcinoma. J Clin Oncol 2:157, 1984
45. Sherry MM, Johnson DH, Page DL, et al: Inflammatory carcinoma of the breast: Clinical review and summary of the Vanderbilt experience with multimodality therapy. Am J Med 79:355, 1985

Male Breast Cancer

David W. Kinne

Breast cancer in males is an uncommon disease, occurring less than 1% as often as in females.[1] According to the American Cancer Society, an estimated 900 male breast cancers are diagnosed each year in the United States and 300 men die of the disease.[2] Breast cancer represents less than 1% of all malignancies developing in males.

EPIDEMIOLOGY

Family histories in male breast cancer patients have been poorly documented. In a collective series, Crichlow found 10 cases of carcinoma of the breast in female blood relatives of 79 males with breast cancer, but doubted the significance of such low numbers.[3] However, rare families have been reported in which several males have developed breast cancer.[4–9] Although most of these cases occurred in brothers, two of the reports involve father and son, with one study describing bilateral breast cancer in both.[9]

Hyperestrogenism has been implicated as a risk factor. Patients with Klinefelter syndrome (sex chromosomes XXY) have a 6% incidence of breast cancer, approaching the risk for females.[10] This syndrome consists of hypogonadism, with seminiferous tubule dysgenesis, aspermatogenesis, increased urinary gonodotropin, and usually normal urinary 17-ketosteroid excretion. The breasts of these patients are hypertrophic, showing not only gynecomastia but also occasionally the development of acini and lobules as seen in female breasts.[11] This may be further increased if a family history of female breast cancer exists. Breast cancer has also been reported in an XX male.[12,13]

In Egypt, schistosomiasis is associated with male breast cancer, which accounts for 6% of all breast cancers.[14] This disease causes liver damage and hyperestrogenism. Breast cancer is more common than prostate cancer in Egypt, unlike most western countries, leading to the hypothesis that hyperestrogenism may be an etiologic factor in developing breast cancer and protecting against the development of prostate cancer. However, prostate cancer is a disease with a late age incidence, and developing countries such as Egypt have a smaller proportion of elderly persons compared with developed countries. In most of 77 populations in whom the age-standardized incidence of prostate and male breast cancers were compared, Sobin and Sherif noted a direct, not an inverse, relationship between these two malignancies, extending from a very low incidence of both in Japanese to the highest rates for U.S. blacks.[15]

Exogenous administration of estrogen leads to breast enlargement and the development of acini and true lobules.[11,16,18] In males undergoing this therapy for metastatic prostate cancer, breast malignancies originally thought to be primary cancers were shown to be metastatic.[19,20] Crichlow[3] reviewed four separate cases in which primary breast cancer developed in males receiving exogenous estrogen,[21,23] indicating that this is a relatively rare occurrence.

Studies of estrogen metabolism have been carried out in males with breast cancer. Zumoff and colleagues[24] tested 6 males with breast cancer and 16 normal controls. Following administration of radioactive-labeled estradiol, 72-hour urine collections showed elevated estriol production and lower levels of estrone, 2-hydroxyestrone, and 2-methoxyestrone in patients with carcinoma. Scheike and colleagues, however, noted no differences in the excretion patterns of urinary estrogen metabolites in control patients compared with 19 men with breast cancer.[25] However, Dao and colleagues[26] reported the same patterns of excretion as Zumoff. They suggested a testicular origin of these endogenous estrogens, explaining the beneficial effect of orchiectomy frequently observed in males with advanced breast cancer.

Gynecomastia, although frequently not mentioned in reports, does not seem to be a clinical entity preceding or associated with the development of breast cancer. In a collective review, Crichlow[3] reported 625 breast cancer patients in whom the presence or absence of gynecomastia was noted, and there were only 17 cases of gynecomastia. However, the microscopic appearance of gynecomastia (fibroepithelial hyperplasia and stromal hypertrophy) may be more common. In a recent Memorial Hospital series of male breast cancer reported by Heller and colleagues,[27] histologic material was reviewed by Rosen, who noted that 40% of 70 patients who had sufficient tissue for review showed microscopic evidence of gynecomastia.

Radiation exposure has been reported in 11 patients with male breast cancer. Greene and colleagues[28] summarize nine cases and report another. Although radiation therapy doses were unknown in most instances, the risk in males seemed similar to that accepted in females. Exposure above doses as low as 50 to 100 cGy increases the risk of breast cancer in females incrementally, and the risk is greater if exposure occurs at a young age.[29–31] These males developed breast cancer 12 to 36 years after radiation exposure for a variety of conditions (four for thymic enlargement). Of interest is that 5 of 10 had clinical gynecomastia. The patient reported by Greene and colleagues had a family history of four generations of various pathologically confirmed cancers (including one female breast cancer) and did not have Klinefelter syndrome. Skin biopsies from the patient and family members indicated that colony-forming ability of cultured skin fibroblasts had increased sensitivity to irradiation and to bleomycin, a radiomimetic drug. Abnormalities were noted in his mother and sister also, suggesting that a genetic susceptibility affected the risk of radiation-induced cancer in this patient. The final report is of a male who had undergone repeated fluoroscopy for tuberculosis at age 25 and who developed breast cancer on that side at age 63.[32]

A history of trauma has been elicited in some patients with breast cancer, but as noted by Crichlow,[3] the association is unclear. Most clinicians believe that trauma called attention to or was coincident with the development of a breast tumor. An antecedent history of trauma was present in 30 of 532 patients, or just 6%.

NATURAL HISTORY

The median age at which male breast cancer develops is several years later than in females. In the Crichlow series, it was 59.6 years.[3] The earlier Memorial Hospital series reported by Holleb and colleagues[33,34] gave a median age of 56, but in the more recent series it was 65 years.[27] It has been stated to occur in patients as young as 5 and as old as 93.[3] The reported incidence of bilateral breast cancer, 1.4% in 1158 patients, is lower than in females. This may be due to a poorer prognosis from the primary cancer and the later age of development, with patients dying of other causes.

Male breast cancer patients usually present in a more advanced stage of disease than females.[35,36] This may be due in part to a longer duration of symptoms demonstrated in males. In older series (prior to 1951), an average delay of 18 months between onset of symptoms and treatment was described.[3] In the later collected series of 587 cases, an average delay of 10 months occurred.

The left breast is more commonly involved with cancer in males than the right, with a ratio of 1.07:1.[3] This approximates the ratio seen in females.

PATHOLOGY

Stewart[37] noted that the only type of breast cancer seen in females but not documented in males, in the Memorial Hospital material, was lobular carcinoma. In a series of male breast cancers reviewed pathologically by Rosen[27] and compared with his review of female breast cancers (Table 15-10), some interesting differences were seen. Although the majority of both sexes had infiltrating ductal carcinoma (87% in males), with about the same percentage having *in situ* disease (5% versus 3.8%), a significantly higher percentage of women had intraductal carcinoma within the infiltrating lesions than did men (64% versus 47%). Conversely, more men had pure infiltrating duct carcinoma than did females (40% versus 15%). These differences relate to the pathologic stage of disease; males having an intraductal component had significantly earlier stages of disease than those with infiltrating duct disease alone (Table 15-11). Intracystic papillary carcinoma was associated with a 5-year survival rate of 100%.

The 15% of other carcinomas in the female series (see Table 15-10) includes lobular lesions, which were not observed in this series of male breast cancer. However, lobular carcinoma (invasive) has been noted in males,[38] although it has not been seen in the *in situ* form. All other types of breast cancer, including medullary, papillary, colloid, lobular, and Paget's disease, have been reported in males.[39]

More than 50 cases of Paget's disease in males have been reported,[40] but only 25 have had histologic confirmation.[41] In the later collective review by Gupta and colleagues,[41] the disease seemed more aggressive than in females. Most patients were treated by radical mastectomy, and only four patients were alive and free of disease 5 years after treatment.

Inflammatory breast carcinoma in males was stated by Treves[42] to be present in 2% of men with breast cancer. This is a slightly higher incidence than that found in females, but the same poor prognosis was noted.

HORMONE RECEPTORS

There are data to suggest that estrogen receptor (ER) protein is present in male breast cancer in a higher percentage of patients than in females with breast carcinoma. Rosen and colleagues[43] reported ER-positive tumors in six of eight male breast cancer patients. One of eight patients with gynecomastia had ER-positive breast disease. Other series, confirming this, have found positive progesterone receptors (PgR) in about 75% of cases and no correlation between positive ER and age of the patients, size and histologic grading of the tumors, or stage and nodal involvement.[44,45,46] In a collected series of 47 patients, 80% had ER-positive cancers,[47] and more than 80% with metastatic disease responded to hormonal manipulation, usually orchiectomy. Each institution represented in this series had somewhat different definitions of receptor positivity.

Everson and colleagues[48] indicated that 29 of 34 males with breast cancer had ER-positive tumors. Although several institutions were represented, comparable assay techniques were employed and all contributors had had considerable experience in performing such assays on samples from females. The quantity of ER protein showed some correlation with PgR levels, disease-free interval, and duration of response among responders, but without statistical significance. PgR-positive tumors were present in 9 of 14 patients, and several patients had androgen receptor or glucocortical receptor activity.

Although these authors observed a tendency for patients with low ER-positive cancers to have unfavorable responses to orchiectomy and for patients with high ER-positive tumors to respond more favorably, the available data do not justify basing therapeutic intervention in male breast cancer on ER levels alone.

Table 15-10
Comparison of Pathologic Types of Breast Carcinoma in Groups of Men and Women at Memorial Hospital

Type of Carcinoma	*Men*	*Women*
Intraductal (ID)	(4) 5%	3.8%
Intraductal and infiltrating duct (ID + IFDC)	(37) 47%	64.0%
Infiltrating duct (IFDC)	(31) 40%	15.0%
Intracystic papillary	(4) 5%	
Colloid	(1) 1%	1.4%
Tubular	(1) 1%	
Not reviewed	(19)	15.0% (other)*

* Includes lobular carcinoma, medullary carcinoma, and others.
(Heller KS, Rosen PP, Schottenfeld D, et al: Male breast cancer: A clinicopathologic study of 97 cases. Ann Surg 188:60–65, 1978)

Table 15-11
Relationship of Extent of Disease to Pathologic Type in Men With Breast Cancer

	Pathologic Stage			*Lymph Node Status**	
	I	*II*	*III*	*Neg.*	*Pos.*
ID + IFDC	13	17	3	19	16
IFDC	3	14	4	8	18

* Patients with ID component had higher percentage with negative nodes than those with pure IFDC, $p<.001$.
(Heller KS, Rosen PP, Schottenfeld D, et al: Male breast cancer: A clinicopathologic study of 97 cases. Ann Surg 188:60–65, 1978)

DIAGNOSIS

The majority of males with breast cancer present with a unilateral mass, usually firm and painless. In contrast to female breast cancer patients, male patients rarely present with an occult primary tumor and axillary lymph node metastases.[3]

Sanguineous or serosanguineous nipple discharge is an ominous sign in males, as reported by Treves and colleagues.[49] It was associated with early symptoms of breast cancer in 80% of cases. Nipple discharge occurred in 13.7% of all cases of male breast cancer in this series. Nipple or areolar ulceration was observed in 28% of older collected series,[3] but is not commonly seen today.

The principal differential diagnosis is with gynecomastia. A history of appropriate drug or hormone ingestion, excessive alcohol intake, bilaterality, and a discoid or sharply-marginated or tender mass all favor gynecomastia. However, unilateral gynecomastia is not uncommon. Mammographic criteria can distinguish these lesions, as reported by Kalisher and Peyster.[50] A pattern of increased ducts only, ductal hyperplasia similar to adenosis, small ducts with stromal proliferation, and fatty replacement favor gynecomastia. The radiographic appearance of carcinoma is more dense, with irregular spiculated margins. An example of this pattern is shown in Figure 15-3, a palpable mass that proved to be carcinoma in a male. However, as is true in females, patients with clinically dominant masses should undergo biopsies, even if the mammographic pattern suggests benign disease.

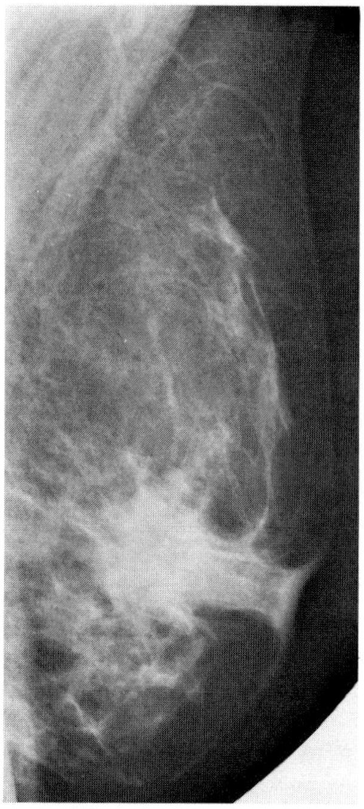

FIGURE 15-3. Central carcinoma seen on lateral oblique mammographic view (left breast) in a male.

Dershaw has reported a case of occult nonpalpable male breast cancer detected by mammography in a patient who had undergone mastectomy on the other side.[51] With improved techniques facilitating mammography in males, this diagnostic test should be used in males at high risk for breast cancer.

Clinical assessment of axillary lymph node status is incorrect as in males commonly as in females. In the Memorial Hospital experience,[27] pathologic evaluation of nodes agreed with the clinical impression in 74% of patients. They were false-negative in 18% and false-positive in 8% of cases.

TREATMENT OF THE PRIMARY TUMOR

The standard approach in most reported series has been radical mastectomy. This is due to the proximity of these tumors to the pectoralis major muscle (perhaps involving muscle) and, especially in earlier experience, to the more advanced stage of disease with which these patients present. In the past 7 years at our institution, modified radical mastectomy has been performed in 27 of 36 cases. Earlier stage of disease at presentation and excision of portion of the pectoralis major muscle beneath the tumor have led to this change.

Adjuvant therapy in most cases has been radiotherapy, either preoperative or (more often) postoperative. The impact of this is difficult to assess, although most authors[3] suggest that improved local control with no effect on survival has been achieved with this therapy. Recently, adjuvant systemic therapy has been advised for patients with pathologically involved nodes. At our institution, this involves combination chemotherapy (similar to that given in female breast cancer) with antiestrogen therapy in patients who are ER positive.

Analysis of the result of treatment in male breast cancer patients is difficult because of the need to review collective series. Because males develop this disease at an older age than females, many die of other causes, and 5-year results are given in many reports.

In Crichlow's collective series,[3] most results indicated that males with breast cancer had a poorer prognosis than females. The 5-year survival rate was 49% overall, ranging from 79% in the node-negative group to 28% if nodes were involved. In the few series in which 10-year results were given, overall survival was 35% (62% if nodes were negative and only 4.3% in the node-positive subgroup). Pathologically involved axillary lymph nodes were observed in 55% of specimens. Since then, several reports have suggested that breast cancer in males carries a poorer prognosis than in females,[52–60] whereas others indicated similar outcomes in each group.[61–66] The Memorial Hospital series reported by Heller and colleagues[27] noted 5- and 10-year results by clinical and pathologic stage and compared these results in males with an earlier experience in females reported by Schottenfeld.[67] The overall survival rate at 10 years was 40% for males compared with 62% for females. No difference at 5 years was noted. This difference in 10-year survival rates was limited to Stage II patients with positive nodes; the 10-year survival rate of males with Stage I (T1N0M0) disease was 89%, the same as in females. Based on this result, we do not advise adjuvant therapy in this subgroup of patients. Patients with pathologic Stage II disease did poorly whether male or female, with 10-year survival rates of 25% versus 35% noted. However, the survival rate at 10 years for males with Stage II disease was only 12%, compared with 68% in the female series. There were similar percentages of patients with pathologically negative nodes in these series of male and female patients (46% versus 48%), similar involvement of level I nodes only (17% versus 19%) and level II–III nodal involvement (28% versus 32%). The total number of nodes involved could not be analyzed in this retrospective review, but Rosen and colleagues have shown a close correlation between the highest level of axillary node involvement and the total number of metastatic nodes.[68] Therefore, this difference in survival rate of Stage II male and female patients is probably not due to an increased number of involved nodes in males. We agree with Crichlow,[69] who suggested that the central location of all male breast cancers in the presence of pathologically involved axillary nodes increases the likelihood of internal mammary lymph node involvement. To our knowledge, these nodes have not been evaluated or treated in any systematic manner. Our present policy is to advise all male breast cancer patients with positive axillary nodes to undergo adjuvant systemic therapy. It would not seem unreasonable to add radiation therapy to the internal mammary lymph node chain in these patients.

No significant experience has been reported with primary radiation therapy for male breast cancer. Also, the experience with systemic adjuvant therapy in males with positive nodes has not been reported. In our experience, with small numbers of patients and short duration of follow-up, these patients seem to be doing better than would be expected in females with similar node involvement. This is a preliminary and anecdotal assessment, but the experience with adjuvant therapy will be of interest.

TREATMENT OF METASTATIC DISEASE

Treves reported objective remission of advanced male breast cancer in 28 of 42 patients treated by orchiectomy,[70] following an earlier report on a single patient by Farrow and Adair.[71] More recent experience with 23 patients showed an objective response rate of 48%.[72] Median survival time in responders was 58 months. Few of these patients underwent subsequent hormone ablation, but Patel and colleagues[73] reported a 50% response rate to orchiectomy and, after subsequent relapse, an 80% remission rate to adrenalectomy in ten patients.

Patterson and colleagues reported 31 males treated with tamoxifen at 16 centers.[74] Complete or partial response was observed in 48% of patients. ER data in eight patients showed that four out of five ER-positive patients responded and none of three ER-negative patients responded. This compared favorably with the 38% response rate to diethylstilbestrol reported earlier by Ribeiro[75] and without the undesirable side effects of estrogen therapy in males. Similar response rates reported subsequently[76–81] document regression in patients who have not undergone orchiectomy. Isolated reports suggest an improved duration of response if orchiectomy is carried out in tamoxifen responders after they relapse.[82] Additional reports of response to progestational agents[83,84] and antiandrogen therapy[85] indicate the increasing role of additive hormonal therapy. Orchiectomy would still seem to have a role, either as initial therapy or as a second hormonal approach in tamoxifen responders, but major hormonal ablation by adrenalectomy or hypophysectomy will be carried out less than in earlier years. However, orchiectomy may have a valid alternative in sequential additive hormonal therapies. In a recent report of 35 endocrine trials in 14 males with disseminated breast cancer, Lopez and colleagues[86] reported an overall response rate of 43%. Remissions were noted with the use of tamoxifen, estrogens, cyproterone acetate, progesterone, and androgens, and also with medical adrenalectomy with aminoglutethimide. Patients responding to one form of hormonal treatment had a greater likelihood of responding to a second hormonal manipulation. Further experience needs to be accumulated with additive hormonal therapies.

The results with single agent or combination chemotherapy in males with metastatic breast cancer has not been reported frequently.[87,88] A collected series of 62 trials in 48 patients[88] demonstrated an overall response rate of 32%, which is considered lower than in female breast cancer. However, patients with far advanced disease and visceral predominant sites are entered in these trials, probably because of promising results with several additive hormonal agents as noted above. When patients with less advanced metastatic disease were analyzed, a 50% regression rate to chemotherapy was noted.

REFERENCES

1. Treves N, Holleb AI: Cancer of the male breast: A report of 146 cases. Cancer 8:1239–1250, 1955
2. Silverberg E, Lubera J: Cancer statistics 1986. CA 36:9–25, 1986
3. Crichlow RW: Carcinoma of the male breast. Surg Gynecol Obstet 134:1011–1019, 1972
4. Anderson DE: Genetic considerations in breast cancer. In Breast Cancer: Early and Late, pp 27–36. Chicago, Year Book Medical Publishers, 1970
5. Everson RB, Li FP, Fraumeni JF, et al: Familial male breast cancer. Lancet 1:9–12, 1976
6. Marger D, Urdaneta N, Fisher JJ: Breast cancer in brothers. Cancer 36:458–461, 1975
7. Schottenfeld D, Lilienfeld AM, Diamond H: Some observations on the epidemiology of breast cancer among males. Am J Public Health 53:890–897, 1963
8. Teasdale C, Forbes JF, Baum M: Familial male breast cancer. Lancet i:360–361, 1976
9. Schwartz RM, Newell RB, Hauch JF, et al: A study of familial male breast carcinoma and a second report. Cancer 46:2697–2701, 1980

10. Jackson AW, et al: Carcinoma of the male breast in association with the Klinefelter syndrome. Br Med J 1:223–225, 1965
11. Lynch HT, Kaplan AR, Lynch JF: Klinefelter syndrome and cancer. A family study. JAMA 229:809–811, 1974
12. Giammarini A, Rocchi M, Zennaro W, et al: XX male with breast cancer. Clin Genet 18:103–108, 1980
13. Decker JP, Lerner HJ, Schwartz I: Breast carcinoma in a 46, XX true hermaphrodite. Cancer 49:1481–1484, 1982
14. El-Gazayerli MM, Abdel-Aziz AS: On bilharziasis and male breast cancer in Egypt: A preliminary report and review of the literature. Br J Cancer 17:566, 1963
15. Sobin LH, Sherif M: Relation between male breast cancer and prostate cancer. Br J Cancer 42:787–790, 1980
16. Sandison AT: An Autopsy Study of the Adult Human Breast. Natl Cancer Inst Monograph No 8. Washington, DC, US Government Printing Office, 1962
17. Scarff RW, Smith CP: Proliferative and other lesions of the male breast with notes on two cases of proliferative mastitis in stilboestrol workers. Br J Surg 29:393, 1942
18. Schwartz S, Wilens SL: The formation of acinar tissue in gynecomastia. Am J Pathol 43:797, 1963
19. Benson WR: Carcinoma of the prostate with metastases to breasts and testis; critical review of the literature and report of a case. Cancer 10:1235, 1957
20. Campbell JH, Cummins SD: Metastases simulating mammary cancer, in prostatic carcinoma under estrogenic therapy. Cancer 4:303, 1951
21. O'Grady WP, McDivitt RW: Breast cancer in a man treated with diethylstilbestrol. Arch Pathol 88:162, 1969
22. Baierl W: Zur Frage der Mammacarcinom-Manifestierung nach Cyren-B-Behandlung beim. Mann Med Klin 35:1284, 1953
23. Symmers W St C: Carcinoma of the breast in transsexual individuals after surgical and hormonal interference with the primary and secondary sex characteristics. Br Med J 2:83, 1968
24. Zumoff B, Fishman J, Cassouto J, et al: Estradiol transformation in men with breast cancer. J Clin Endocrinol Metab 26: 960, 1966
25. Scheike O, Svenstrup B, Frandsen VA: Metabolism of Oestradiol-17^B in men with breast cancer. J Steroid Biochem 4:489–501, 1973
26. Dao TL, Morreal CE, Nemoto T: Urinary estrogen excretion in men with breast cancer. N Engl J Med 289:138–140, 1973
27. Heller KS, Rosen PP, Schottenfeld D, et al: Male breast cancer: A clinicopathologic study of 97 cases. Ann Surg 188:60–65, 1978
28. Greene MH, Goedert JJ, Bech-Hansen NT, et al: Radiogenic male breast cancer with in vitro sensitivity to ionizing radiation and bleomycin. Cancer Invest 1:379–386, 1983
29. Tokunga M, Norman JE, Asano M, et al: Malignant breast tumors among atomic bomb survivors. J Natl Cancer Inst 62:1342–1359, 1979
30. McGregor DH, Land LE, Choi K, et al: Breast cancer incidence among atomic bomb survivors. J Natl Cancer Inst, 59:799–811, 1977
31. Boice JD, Monson RR: Breast cancer in women after repeated fluoroscopic examinations of the chest. J Natl Cancer Inst 59:823–832, 1977
32. Cohen R, Schauer PK: Male breast cancer following repeated fluoroscopy. Am J Med 76:929–930, 1984
33. Holleb AI, Freeman HP, Farrow JH: Cancer of male breast. Part I. NY State J Med 68:544–553, 1963
34. Holleb AI, Freeman HP, Farrow JH: Cancer of male breast, Part II. NY State J Med 68:656–661, 1968
35. Donegan WL, Perez-Mesa CM: Carcinoma of the male breast. Arch Surg 10:273–279, 1973
36. Langlands AO, Maclean N, Kerr GR. Carcinoma of the male breast: Report of a series of 88 cases. Clin Radiol 27:21–25, 1976
37. Stewart FW: Tumors of the breast: In Atlas of Tumor Pathology, Section IX, Fascicle 34, p 7. Washington, DC, Armed Forces Institute of Pathology, 1950
38. Giffler RF, Kay S: Small-cell carcinoma of the male mammary gland: A tumor resembling infiltrating lobular carcinoma. Am J Clin Pathol 66:715, 1976
39. Visfeldt J, Scheike O: Male breast cancer. I. Histologic typing and grading of 187 Danish cases. Cancer 22:985–990, 1973
40. Lancer HA, Moschella SL: Paget's disease of the male breast. Am Acad Dermatol 7:393–396, 1982
41. Gupta S, Khanna NN, Khanna S, et al: Paget's disease of the male breast: A clinicopathologic study and a collective review. J Surg Oncol 22:151–156, 1983
42. Treves N: Inflammatory carcinoma of the breast in the male patient. Surgery 34:810, 1953
43. Rosen PP, Menendez-Botet CJ, Nisselbaum JS, et al: Estrogen receptor protein in lesions of the male breast. Cancer 37:1866–1868, 1976
44. Ruff SJ, Bauer JE, Keenan EJ, et al: Hormone receptors in male breast cancer. J Surg Oncol 21:55–59, 1981
45. Gupta N, Cohen JL, Rosenbaum C, et al: Estrogen receptors in male breast cancer. Cancer 46:1781–1784, 1980
46. Pegoraro RJ, Nirmul D, Joubert SM: Cytoplasmic and nuclear estrogen and progesterone receptors in male breast cancer. Cancer Res 42:4812–4814, 1982
47. Friedman MA, Hoffman PG Jr, Dandolos EM, et al: Estrogen receptors in male breast cancer: Clinical and pathologic correlations. Cancer 47:134–137, 1981
48. Everson RB, Lippman ME, Thompson EB: Clinical correlations of steroid receptors and male breast cancer. Cancer Res 40:991–997, 1980
49. Treves N, Robbins GF, Amoroso WL: Serous and serosanguinous discharge from the male nipple. Arch Surg 73:319–329, 1956
50. Kalisher L, Peyster RG: Xerographic manifestations of male breast disease. Am J Roentgenol 125:656–661, 1975
51. Dershaw DD: Male mammography. Am J Radiol 146:127, 1986
52. Hudson MJR, Smart CJ: Carcinoma of the male breast. Br J Surg 61:440–444, 1974
53. Ramantanis G, Besbeas S, Garas JG: Breast cancer in the male: A report of 138 cases. World J Surg 4:621–624, 1980
54. Gupta S, Paut GC, Gupta S: Male breast cancer. J Surg Oncol 16:149–157, 1981
55. Ajaxi DVS, Osegbe DN, Ademiluyi SA: Carcinoma of the male breast in West Africans and a review of world literature. Cancer 50:1664–1667, 1982
56. Appelqvist P, Salmo M: Prognosis in carcinoma of the male breast. Acta Chir Scand 148:499–502, 1982
57. Axelsson J, Andersson A: Cancer of the male breast. World J Surg 7:281–287, 1983
58. Erlichman C, Murphy KC, Elhakim T: Male breast cancer: A 13 year review of 89 patients. J Clin Oncol 2:903–909, 1984
59. Hodson GR, Urdaneta LF, Al-Jurf AS, et al: Male breast carcinoma. Am Surg 51:47–49, 1985
60. Spence RA, Mackenzie G, Anderson JR, et al: Long-term survival following cancer of the male breast in Northern Ireland. Cancer 55:648–652, 1985
61. Scheike O: Male breast cancer—six factors influencing prognosis. Br J Cancer 30:261–271, 1974

62. Morgan GW: Carcinoma of the male breast in East Anglia 1960–1976. Clin Oncol 5:331–339, 1979
63. Carlsson G, Hafstrom L, Jonsson P: Male breast cancer. Clin Oncol 7:149–155, 1981
64. Vercoutere AL, O'Connell TX: Carcinoma of the male breast—an update. Arch Surg 119:1301–1304, 1984
65. Ouriel K, Lotze MT, Hinshaw JR: Prognostic factors of carcinoma of the male breast. Surg Gynecol Obstet 159:373–376, 1984
66. Van Geel AN, van Slooten EA, Mavrunac M, et al: A retrospective study of male breast cancer in Holland. Br J Surg 72:724–727, 1985
67. Schottenfeld D, Nash AG, Robbins GJ, et al: Ten-year results of the treatment of primary operable breast carcinoma. A summary of 304 patients evaluated by the TNM system. Cancer 38:1001–1007, 1976
68. Rosen PP, Lesser ML, Kinne DW, et al: Discontinuous or "skip" metastases in breast carcinoma. Analysis of 1228 axillary dissections. Ann Surg 197:276–283, 1983
69. Crichlow RW, Kaplan EL, Kearney WH: Male mammary cancer: An analysis of 32 cases. Ann Surg 175:489–494, 1972
70. Treves N: The treatment of cancer, especially inoperable cancer of the male breast by ablative surgery (orchiectomy, adrenalectomy, and hypophysectomy) and hormone therapy (estrogens and corticosteroids): An analysis of 42 patients. Cancer 12:820–832, 1959
71. Farrow JH, Adair FE: Effect of orchiectomy on skeletal metastases from cancer of the male breast. Science 95:664, 1942
72. Kraybill WG, Kaufman R, Kinne D: Treatment of advanced male breast cancer. Cancer 47:2185–2189, 1981
73. Patel JK, Nemoto T, Dao TL: Metastatic breast Cancer in males. Assessment of endocrine therapy. Cancer 53:1344–1346, 1984
74. Patterson JS, Battersby LA, Bach BK: Use of tamoxifen in advanced male breast cancer. Cancer Treat Rep 64:801–804, 1980
75. Ribeiro GC: The result of diethylstilbestrol therapy for recurrent and metastatic carcinoma of the male breast. Br J Cancer 33:465–467, 1976
76. Becher R, Hoffken K, Pape H, et al: Tamoxifen treatment before orchiectomy in advanced breast cancer in men. N Engl J Med 305:169–170, 1981
77. Abele R, Alberto P: Letter: Tamoxifen before orchiectomy for breast cancer in men. N Engl J Med 305:1091–1092, 1981
78. Tirelli E, Tumolo S, Talamini R, et al: Tamoxifen before and after orchiectomy in advanced male breast cancer. Cancer Treat Rep 66:1882–1883, 1982
79. Ribeiro GG: Tamoxifen in the treatment of male breast carcinoma. Clin Radiol 34:625–628, 1983
80. Hilliard DA, Wilbur DW, Camacho ES: Tamoxifen response following no response to orchiectomy in metastatic male breast cancer: A case report. J Surg Oncol 25:42–43, 1984
81. Kantarjian H, Yap H-Y, Hortobagyi G, et al: Hormonal therapy for metastatic male breast cancer. Arch Intern Med 143:237–240, 1983
82. Tirelli U, Tumulo S, et al: Tamoxifen before and after orchiectomy in advanced male breast cancer. Cancer Treat Rep 66:1882–1883, 1982
83. Pannuti F, Martoni A, Busutti L, et al: High-dose medroxyprogesterone acetate in advanced male breast cancer. Cancer Treat Rep 66:1763–1765, 1982
84. Mitsuyasu R, Bonomi P, Anderson K, et al: Response to megestrol in male breast carcinoma. Arch Intern Med 141:809–810, 1981
85. Lopez M, Barduagni A: Cyproterone acetate in advanced male breast cancer. Cancer 49:9–11, 1982
86. Lopez M, DiLauro L, Lazzaro B, et al: Hormonal treatment of disseminated male breast cancer. Oncology 42:345–349, 1985
87. Yap H-Y, Tashima CK, Blumenschein GR, et al: Chemotherapy for advanced male breast cancer. JAMA 243:1739–1741, 1980
88. Lopez M, DiLauro L, Papaldo P, et al: Chemotherapy in metastatic male breast cancer. Oncology 42:205–209, 1985

Cystosarcoma Phyllodes

Jeanne A. Petrek

Cystosarcoma phyllodes (or phylloides) is a rare distinctive fibroepithelial tumor of the breast without counterpart in any other organ. The entity produces a spectrum of diseases ranging from benign, with a significant risk of local recurrence, to malignant, with rapidly growing metastases. During the past 150 years, since given its classical description by Johannes Müller (1838),[1] cystosarcoma phyllodes has had at least 62 synonymous designations.[2] Even though the tumor had been described several times in the preceding decades, his description was so definitive that subsequent generations often ignored his chosen term "cystosarcoma phyllodes" and simply called it "Müller tumor." He believed the tumor was entirely benign and stressed its difference from routine breast cancer and apparently chose the term "sarcoma" not to indicate malignancy but merely to describe the fleshy appearance.

It was only in 1931 that Lee and Pack[3] at Memorial Hospital described the first case of metastatic cystosarcoma phyllodes. Nevertheless, the name overstates the malignant potential of the vast majority of such tumors and is thus unduly alarming to patients and physicians alike. Of course, the term "cystosarcoma" is not objectionable when it refers to malignant and borderline malignant varieties, both of which are infrequent. "Cysto" implies either that the lesion is related to cystic disease or that it contains macroscopic cysts, although this is not always the case.

As concerns other terms, "fibroadenoma phyllodes" would be appropriate, especially if applied only to those tumors that are deemed, after careful pathologic study, almost certainly to be benign. It has the merits of alerting surgeons that they are dealing with an unusual tumor that shares some characteristics with fibroadenoma but not with sarcoma. If this term is used for tumors that have a local recurrence rate of nearly 20%[4] but that rarely undergo malignant alteration, the term seems acceptable. The malignant category could still be called "malignant cystosarcoma phyllodes." The borderline category of this tumor, however, is still a problem, since this term does not imply the possibility. The alternative name "giant fibroadenoma" used as a synonym, especially in the recent past, reflects this problem. Giant fibroadenoma implies that the tumor is identical to ordinary fibroadenoma except for its size and underrates both the metastatic potential of cystosarcoma phyllodes as well as the potential for local recurrence.

Perhaps this entity should merely be called "phyllodes tumor" and qualified according to the pathologist's assessment of its microscopic appearance and likely behavior. The tumor would thus remain under a single heading, a situation that would be appreciated insofar as the separation of benign from malignant tumors is concerned. Moreover, this term conforms with the emerging nomenclature in parts of western Europe. Third, the term is not entirely new and merely reminds one of the original term (cystosarcoma phyllodes). Nevertheless, the term "cystosarcoma phyllodes" is firmly embedded in the literature and, for the sake of uniformity and clarity, may have to remain.

MACROSCOPIC APPEARANCE

The size of the tumor is variable, ranging from 1 cm[5] to greater than 40 cm[6].

Most cystosarcoma phyllodes tumors, benign or malignant, are well circumscribed in the gross, although they lack a true capsule. This may occur because, being so hypercellular, they present a hard barrier compressing and pushing the softer surrounding breast tissue. Müller[1] described the lesion as grayish-white and resembling a head of cauliflower. The barely visible surface projections make complete surgical excision difficult, since inadvertent amputation predisposes to tumor recurrence. The cut surface is slimy or mucoid and tends to bulge outward. Firm fibrous areas alternate with soft fleshy areas and occasionally with cysts filled with clear or semisolid bloody fluid. Yellow fatty areas as well as areas of hemorrhage and necrosis can occur. Leaflike (phyllodes) papillary protrusions of stromal connective tissue lined with epithelium often extend into the cystic areas.

MICROSCOPIC APPEARANCE

Histologically, cystosarcoma phyllodes, like fibroadenoma, is composed of epithelial elements and a connective tissue stroma. Cuboidal epithelium, resembling ductal epithelium of the surrounding breast tissue, lines the canaliculi, which appear as ductal spaces. These epithelial areas can become irregularly flattened in rapidly growing lesions, presumably by the pressure of the enlarging stroma. The epithelium may be hyperplastic, with varying degrees of atypia in benign or malignant cystosarcoma phyllodes.[5,6] Apocrine and squamous metaplasia of the epithelial elements, although rare, have also occurred.[5] There have been at least two cases in which epithelium was atypical enough to be designated as carcinoma.[6]

Characteristics of the stroma alone, however, determine whether a cystosarcoma phyllodes should be classified as benign or malignant, just as the appearance of the connective tissue distinguishes cystosarcoma phyllodes from fibroadenoma (Fig. 15-4). In general, stroma from malignant cystosarcoma phyllodes contains marked cellularity, severe nuclear atypia, and increased mitotic activity (Fig. 15-5).[7] Often the malignant areas are focal and can be overlooked if multiple samples are not reviewed.[8,9]

McDivitt and colleagues[5] reported that there are two common stromal patterns. In the first type, cells are spindle shaped, resembling a fibrosarcoma. In the second, the cells are looser and myxoid in appearance, resembling a myxoliposarcoma. Both patterns are usually found intermixed in the same tumor. The stroma can also show differentiation into other mesenchymal elements, which are, in order of frequency, fibrosarcoma, liposarcoma, chondrosarcoma, osteosarcoma, and muscle sarcoma.[5]

FIGURE 15-4. Benign cystosarcoma phyllodes. *(A)* Low-power view showing characteristic epithelium-lined clefts, which outline islands of stroma composed of spindle cells and collagen. *(B)* High magnification showing thin layers of benign epithelial cells and benign stroma. Mitoses and nuclear pleomorphism are absent from the stroma.

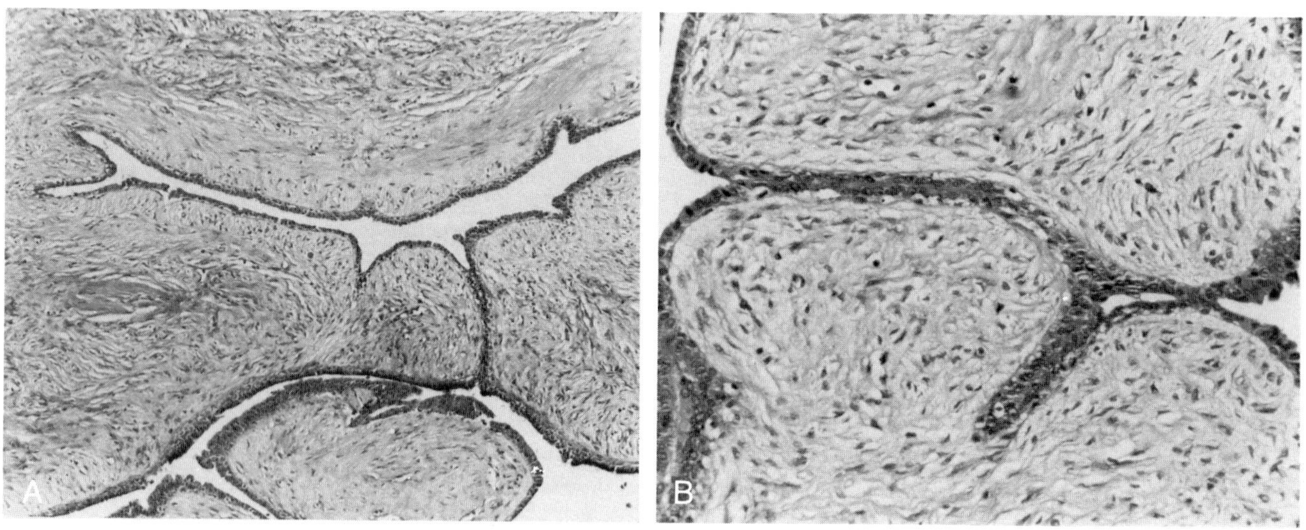

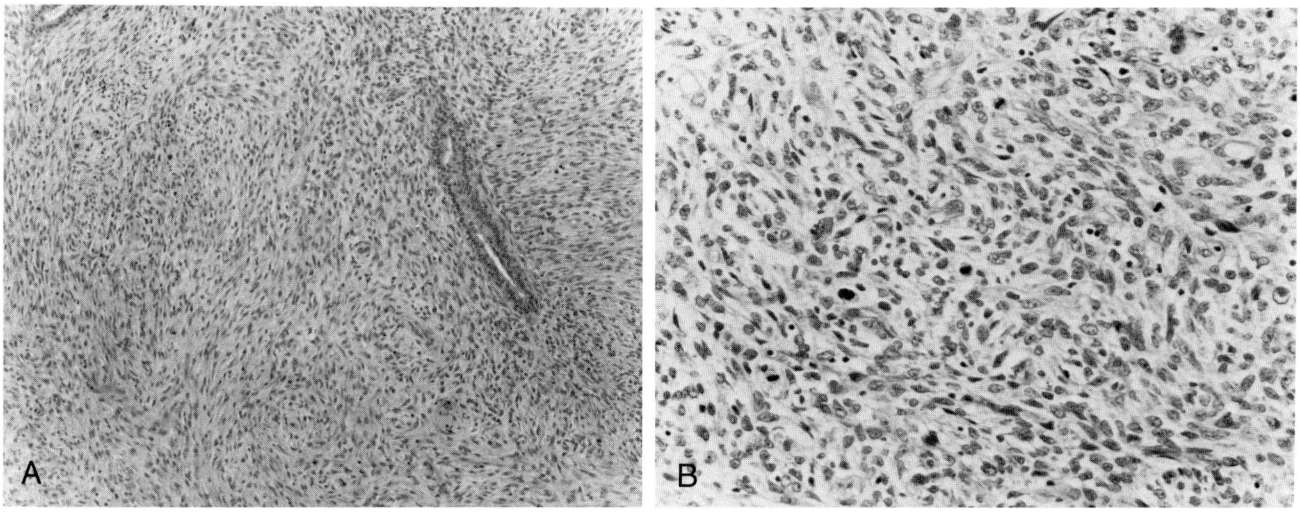

FIGURE 15-5. Malignant cystosarcoma phyllodes. *(A)* Low-magnification view exhibiting very cellular stroma and relatively inconspicuous epithelium. *(B)* At higher magnification, the very cellular stroma features considerable nuclear pleomorphism and several mitotic figures.

HISTOLOGIC DISTINCTION OF BENIGN FROM MALIGNANT

The association of histologic appearance with the clinical course has been studied in several retrospective surveys. In the 1950s, the large series of Lester and Stout[9] (58 patients) and that of Treves and Sunderland[10] (77 patients) tried to relate the clinical behavior of cystosarcoma phyllodes to two characteristics of the stroma—cellular atypia and increased mitotic activity. Both groups found this classification unreliable, since many patients with characteristics of malignancy had a benign course, and worse, some patients with metastases had tumors with only benign or borderline characteristics.

In 1967, Norris and Taylor[11] employed the same two characteristics—cellular atypia and mitotic activity—and added a third, tumor margin (pushing versus infiltrating), as determinants of malignant potential. These three criteria, when considered together, are somewhat more reliable than the first two alone. Increasing mitotic activity (number of figures in 10 high-power fields [HPF]) resulted in increased rates of recurrence and death.

Pietruszka and Barnes,[12] refining the criteria of Norris and Taylor, attempted to correlate clinical behavior with classification as benign (0 to 4 mitoses in 10 HPF), borderline (5 to 9 mitoses in 10 HPF, pushing or infiltrating margins, minimal stromal cellular atypia), or malignant (10 or more mitoses in 10 HPF, infiltrating margins, moderate to marked stromal cellular atypia). Even though mitotic rate was still the most important determinant, they found a close relationship with the three criteria. Metastases occurred only in the malignant category, with 23.5% of patients demonstrating systemic disease.

More recently, Grigoni and colleagues[13] added the ratio of mesenchymal over epithelial tissue to cell atypia, mitotic activity, and tumor margin. He also correlated the longer history of a palpable abnormality with the greater likelihood of its being benign. Ultrastructural observations have not contributed to the differentiation of benign from malignant.[14] A detailed evaluation of criteria used to classify malignant cystosarcoma phyllodes is beyond the scope of this chapter, and the reader is referred to a recent comprehensive review by Azzopardi.[15]

Probably because of the diverse criteria used to determine malignancy, the percentage of all cystosarcoma phyllodes so classified ranges between 23%[10] and 50%.[15] One review article concluded that the accepted incidence of histologically malignant tumors is about 25%.[16] Metastases occur in between 6.2%[17] and 22%[18] of all cases. The wide range in the literature results from pathologists' distinguishing hypercellular fibroadenoma from cystosarcoma phyllodes and malignant cystosarcoma phyllodes with sarcomatous differentiation from stromal sarcoma. Classification by individual pathologists into benign, borderline, and malignant further widen the range. Referral patterns may weigh in favor of malignancy in series from specialized institutions, such as Memorial Sloan-Kettering Cancer Center[5,10] or the Armed Forces Institute of Pathology.[11] Haagensen[17] believes that the most realistic figure is that from his series (6.2%), originating in a general surgical center.

HISTOGENESIS

The site of origin of cystosarcoma phyllodes has been difficult to investigate, presumably because of its relative rarity and because small tumors and microscopic disease are rarely encountered. Many authors believe that most cystosarcoma phyllodes arises in preexisting fibroadenoma.[3,7,19,20,21] Patients have noted small lumps in their breasts for as long as 45 years before growth of the nodule, biopsy, and diagnosis of cystosarcoma phyllodes.[22] In some tumors, the more dense fibrous parts appear localized into a distinctly ovoid outline, an appearance that has been interpreted as the residual benign fibroadenoma that gave rise to cystosarcoma phyllodes.[17] Accordingly, cystosarcoma phyllodes may be the only breast tumor that can become malignant from a previously benign entity,[8] although causative factors are unknown. Some authors feel that the lesion can also arise *de novo* from breast parenchyma.[7,8,23]

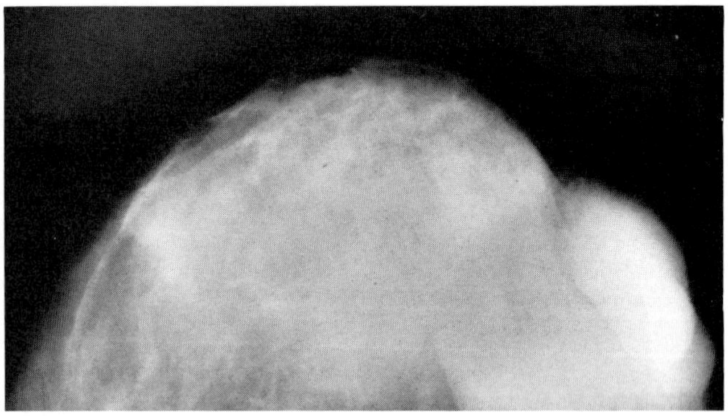

FIGURE 15-6. Craniocaudad mammographic view demonstrating the smooth, multinodular contours of cystosarcoma phyllodes, which compresses the surrounding breast tissue.

STEROID RECEPTORS

Estrogen and progesterone receptor analysis has recently been performed on tumor tissue from patients with cystosarcoma phyllodes. Initial reports suggested the presence of these receptors.[24] In a subsequent detailed study of six tumors, no specific receptors were found.[14] The variability has been enlarged by three recent studies[26,27,28]; 9 of 17 tumors were estrogen receptor positive, and 7 of 7 were progesterone receptor positive. These variable observations may reflect in part the relative amounts of epithelium and stroma in individual cystosarcoma phyllodes.

CLINICAL AND RADIOLOGIC FEATURES

In almost all cases, cystosarcoma phyllodes is discovered as a painless breast mass that is smooth, multinodular, bulky, and rounded. Some patients have a long duration of continuous growth, although many patients have had rapid growth in a previously stable, long-standing nodule. The tumor is often large, although this is not an essential criterion. When it grows to a large size, it often does so rapidly, but this does not necessarily imply malignancy. The shiny, stretched, and attenuated skin with varicose veins over a massive-sized tumor is well known. In these circumstances, skin ulceration is due to stretching and extreme pressure, and unlike adenocarcinoma of the breast, ulceration occurs only with sufficient size of the cystosarcoma phyllodes. Dimpling and *peau d'orange* do not occur. A large tumor may produce erythema as a result of necrosis as it outgrows its blood supply. Prominent veins on the surface, distended and occasionally clotted, are also part of the clinical picture. The nipple may be effaced but is not invaded or retracted. A notable feature of cystosarcoma is the usual absence of suspicious axillary lymph glands, despite a large-sized mass, a situation that is infrequent with adenocarcinoma of the breast. On the other hand, axillary lymph node enlargement can occur (20% of patients studied by Norris and Taylor[11]), although it is important to recognize that this is virtually never due to metastatic disease. Necrotic tumor or infected, ulcerated tumor causes enlarged lymph nodes as a result of hyperplasia much more frequently than does metastatic disease. (Unless one appreciates that regional lymphadenopathy is rarely caused by metastases, one could consider axillary dissection a necessary part of treatment.)

On mammography, the appearance of cystosarcoma phyllodes is very much like that of fibroadenoma, with smooth, polylobulated margins, although some margins may be irregular, suggesting local invasion (Fig. 15-6).[29] Likewise, on ultrasonography these tumors cannot be differentiated from fibroadenomas and well-circumscribed malignancies. However, fluid-filled elongated spaces or clefts may be found within an otherwise solid mass, thereby suggesting the diagnosis. Cystosarcoma phyllodes, therefore, should be one of the considerations if cysts are demonstrated within a solid, circumscribed lesion.[30]

PATIENT CHARACTERISTICS

Cystosarcoma phyllodes is rare, ranging from 2% to 2.9%[8,9,17] to 4.4%[7] of all fibroadenomas (diagnosed at the same institution).

The mean age of patients in large series is in the fourth decade,[5,10,12,31] which is 10 to 20 years older than the mean age for diagnosis of fibroadenoma. A wide age range is recorded in most series, and cystosarcoma phyllodes has been recorded in prepubertal[32,33,34] and adolescent[35,36,37] females. The mean age of patients with benign lesions shows a slight trend toward younger patients when compared with malignant tumors. McDivitt and colleagues (1967)[38] found the mean age of patients with malignant tumors at Memorial Hospital to be 3 years older than those with benign tumors, agreeing with the earlier study (1951).[5] Metastatic malignant cystosarcoma phyllodes before the age of 20 is very rare, and only one case has been reported.[36]

Bilaterality is rare with either benign[11,17] or malignant tumors.[19,39,40] The rate of 30% bilaterality found by McDonald and Harrington[41] is a notable exception.

McDivitt and colleagues[38] reported that 60% of patients with benign cystosarcoma were parous, compared with 30% of those with malignant tumors, with no differences between the mean age at diagnosis. In another series, 33% of the patients with benign or malignant cystosarcoma were nulliparous.[42] The importance of these observations is unknown.

Cystosarcoma phyllodes is rarely, if ever, found in males. It would appear that the only two adequately documented cases in males had preceding gynecomastia.[43,44] It has been noted that the normal male breast does not contain lobular-alveolar units and therefore should be incapable of developing cystosarcoma.[44]

Intraductal cancer,[11,17,45,46] infiltrating duct cancer,[46,47] lobular carcinoma *in situ* (lobular neoplasia) either within the tumor or in adjacent breast tissue[8,17,45] and squamous carcinoma[48] all have been described. The Memorial Sloan-Kettering Cancer Center experience of carcinoma associated with cystosarcoma phyllodes was fully reviewed in 1975.[45] The study concludes that cystosarcoma phyllodes patients should be carefully observed, not only for local recurrence of the original tumor but also for potential development of cancer in either breast. Nevertheless, an associated carcinoma is quite rare, and principles of management for cystosarcoma phyllodes should generally not take this possibility into account.

NATURAL HISTORY

Benign cystosarcoma phyllodes recurs locally 20% of the time,[4,38] probably because the tumor was unrecognized as cystosarcoma phyllodes at the time of the initial surgical therapy and was therefore not completely excised. The recurrence may either be as readily excised as the original lesion or, rarely, may be quite aggressive, invading the chest wall and thoracic cavity.[10,49] One-half of patients with metastatic disease also have an aggressive local recurrence.[16] However, when considering malignant cystosarcoma phyllodes (not necessarily metastatic), Hajdu and colleagues at Memorial Hospital found an 8% local recurrence rate. This probably results from more extensive surgical procedures performed because of less favorable histologic findings. Most locally recurrent tumors arising from cystosarcoma phyllodes are histologically similar to the original. Hajdu and colleagues,[4] however, reported that 2 of the 28 benign lesions had histologic "malignant transformation." Other authors either do not comment or simply note its rarity.[17,42,50] Hajdu and colleagues[4] also reported earlier recurrences when the original lesion was classified as malignant (6 to 24 months) rather than as benign (18 to 24 months).

Regional lymph node metastases very rarely occur from cystosarcoma phyllodes. Clinical enlargement of the lymph nodes is present in 16%.[11] Pathologic nodal metastases have been reported in approximately 15% of cases of metastatic cystosarcoma.[16,51,52] It appears that only one patient with axillary lymph node metastases has been reported as cured.[52]

To date, all metastatic lesions except one[34] have resembled sarcomas, being devoid of all the epithelial elements. Approximately 5% of cystosarcoma phyllodes (benign and malignant) metastasize. Almost one-fourth of those histologically classified as malignant metastasize.

Metastatic lesions have been reported as early as the initial diagnosis of the primary tumor and as late as 12 years after diagnosis.[16] In a review of all reported cases of metastatic cystosarcoma phyllodes in the English literature until 1972 (67 cases), Kessinger and colleagues[16] found that the average survival time was 30 months. The longest survival time with metastatic disease was 14.5 years. The most common site of distant metastases is the lungs, in 66% of cases. Osseous metastases occur in 28%, and rarely are liver, heart, distant lymph nodes and other sites involved, as reviewed by Kessinger and colleagues.[16]

MANAGEMENT CONSIDERATIONS

Because of the rarity of cystosarcoma phyllodes and its similarity to fibroadenoma on physical examination and mammography, the former are often excised with no margin—a standard treatment for fibroadenoma. In general, a visible margin of only 1 to 2 mm for cystosarcoma phyllodes will lead to a local recurrence rate variously recorded as 20%,[4] 28%,[17] and 33%.[11] Resection with 2 cm of visibly normal tissue is recommended by Haagensen.[17]

Frozen section for identification of possible cystosarcoma phyllodes has been recommended in order to perform a wide rather than a close excision as the initial surgical procedure. Apart from the expense and time of frozen sections on all apparent fibroadenomas, the sarcomatous element in cystosarcoma phyllodes can be mistakenly diagnosed as an undifferentiated carcinoma, thereby leading to an unnecessary radical procedure. Frozen sections are difficult to interpret, and the pathologist often lacks the whole gross lesion for examination of its distinctive characteristics.

Frozen sections might be used selectively. For example, bisection of every removed specimen permits the surgeon to become adequately familiar with the bland gross characteristics of the fibroadenoma so as to recognize the typical characteristics of the rarer cystosarcoma phyllodes. Of course, with a small enough tumor and large enough breast, all benign tumors including fibroadenomas could ideally be excised with 2 cm of normal tissue, making frozen section unnecessary.

For the local recurrence of a benign cystosarcoma phyllodes, re-excision with at least a 2- or 3-cm margin is advised. As noted, almost all recurrences retain the histologic pattern of the primary tumor, and more aggressive treatment for the small possibility of malignant transformation is not advised. Often, especially with a large tumor relative to breast size, the recommended margin will necessitate a mastectomy whether the primary tumor or a local recurrence is being treated. Sometimes the mastectomy (or even wide excision) may include the pectoralis fascia or some muscle directly behind the lesion, if these structures are within the recommended margin.

Most authors agree on initial wide excision for benign cystosarcoma phyllodes. However, for histologically malignant cystosarcoma phyllodes, most authors[7,11,16,22,23,34,38,50] recommend total mastectomy (with some pectoralis major muscle if necessary for margins) and either a low or no axillary dissection. Certainly, low axillary dissection (or more) is advisable if suspicious nodes exist.

Haagensen,[17] although acknowledging that no patient treated by simple mastectomy had a recurrence, points out that when local recurrence followed local excision, mastectomy was successful at that time. Haagensen believes that in patients with malignant cystosarcoma, aggressive initial treatment would not have saved the patients, as bloodborne metastases to the lungs appeared within a few months.

Thus far, therapy of metastatic disease has proved discouraging, with no sustained remissions from radiation,[9,10,34,54] additive hormones,[10] castration,[38,53] or chemotherapy.[16,34] At the opposite end of the spectrum are the rare tumors that prove fatal by direct extension without distant metastases.[12,54] As with sarcomas in general, distant pulmonary metastases may be resectable.[52,55]

REFERENCES

1. Müller J: Uber den feineran Bau and die Forman der krankhaften Geschwilste. Berlin, G. Reimer, 1838
2. Fiks A: Cystosarcoma phyllodes of the mammary gland—Müller's tumor. Virchows Arch [A] 392:1–6, 1981
3. Lee B, Pack G: Giant intracanalicular fibroadenomyxoma of the breast. Am J Cancer 15:2583–2595, 1931
4. Hajdu S, Espinosa MH, Robbins GF: Recurrent cystosarcoma phyllodes—a clinicopathologic study of 32 cases. Cancer 38:1402–1406, 1976
5. McDivitt RW, Urban JA, Farrow JH: Cystosarcoma phyllodes. Johns Hopkins Med J 120:33–45, 1966
6. Lee B, Pack G: Giant intracanalicular myxoma: The so-called cystosarcoma phyllodes mammae of Johannes Muller. Ann Surg 93:250–268, 1931
7. Dyer NH, Bridger JE, Taylor RS: Cystosarcoma phyllodes. Br J Surg 53:450–455, 1966
8. Treves N: A study of cystosarcoma phyllodes. Ann NY Acad Sci 114:922–935, 1964
9. Lester J, Stout A: Cystosarcoma phyllodes. Cancer 7:335–353, 1954
10. Treves N, Sunderland D: Cystosarcoma phyllodes of the breast: A malignant and a benign tumor. Cancer 4:1286–1332, 1951
11. Norris HJ, Taylor HB: Relationship of histologic features to behavior of cystosarcoma phyllodes. Analysis of ninety-four cases. Cancer 20:2090–2099, 1967
12. Pietruszka M, Barnes L: Cystosarcoma phyllodes. A clinicopathologic analysis of 42 cases. Cancer 41:1974–1983, 1978
13. Grigoni WF, Santini D, Grassigli A, et al: A clinico-pathologic study of cystosarcoma phyllodes. Twenty case reports. Arch Anat Cytol Pathol 30:303–306, 1982
14. Kesterson GHD, Georgiade N, Seigler HF, et al: Cystosarcoma phyllodes. A steroid receptor and ultrastructure analysis. Ann Surg 190:640–647, 1979
15. Azzopardi JG: Sarcomas of the breast. In Bennington JL (ed): Problems in Breast Pathology. Vol. II, Major Problems in Pathology. Philadelphia, WB Saunders, 1979
16. Kessinger A, Foley JF Lemon HM, et al: Metastatic cystosarcoma phyllodes: A case report and review of the literature. J Surg Oncol 4:131–145, 1972
17. Haagensen CD: Diseases of the Breast. 2nd ed, pp 227–249. Philadelphia, WB Saunders, 1975
18. Oberman HA: Cystosarcoma phyllodes. A clinicopathologic study of hypercellular periductal stromal neoplasms of the breast. Cancer 18:697–710, 1965
19. Notley RG, Griffiths HJL: Bilateral malignant cystosarcoma phyllodes. Br J Surg 52:360–362, 1965
20. Cooper WG, Ackerman LV: Cystosarcoma phyllodes with a consideration of its more malignant variant. Surg Gynecol Obstet 77:279–283, 1943
21. Hill RP, Stout AP: Sarcoma of the breast. Arch Surg 44:723–759, 1942
22. Maier WP, Rosemond GP, Wittenberg R, et al: Cystosarcoma phyllodes mammae. Oncology 22:145–158, 1968
23. Hafner D, Mezger E, Wylie JH Jr: Cystosarcoma phyllodes of the breast. Surg Gynecol Obstet 115:29–34, 1962
24. Rao BR, Meyer JS, Fry CG: Most cystosarcoma phyllodes and fibroadenomas have progesterone receptor but lack estrogen receptor: Stroma-localization of progesterone receptor. Cancer 47:2016–2021, 1981
25. Raynaud JP: Estrogen and progestin receptors in human breast cancer. In McGuire WL,Raynaud J-P, Baulieu E-E et al (eds): Progress in Cancer Research and Therapy, Vol. 4. New York, Raven Press, 1977
26. Pashof T: Estradiol binding protein in cystosarcoma phyllodes of the breast. Eur J Cancer Clin Oncol 16:591–593, 1980
27. Porton WM, Poortman J: Estrogen receptors in cystosarcoma phyllodes of the breast. Eur J Cancer Clin Oncol 17:1147–1148, 1981
28. Brentani MM, Nagai MA, Oshima CTF, et al: Steroid receptors in cystosarcoma phyllodes. Cancer Detect Prev 5:211–219, 1982
29. Dorsi CJ, Feldhaus L, Sonnenfeld M: Unusual lesions of the breast. Radiol Clin North Am 21:67–80, 1983
30. Cole-Beuglet C, Soriano R, Kurtz AB, et al: Ultrasound, x-ray mammography, and histopathology of cystosarcoma phyllodes. Radiology 146:481–486, 1983
31. Contarini O, Urdaneta LF, Hagan W, et al: Cystosarcoma phyllodes of the breast: A new therapeutic proposal. Am Surg 48:157–166, 1982
32. Amerson JR: Cystosarcoma phyllodes in adolescent females. A report of seven patients. Ann Surg 171:849–858, 1971
33. Gibbs BF Jr, Roe RD, Thomas DF: Malignant cystosarcoma phyllodes in a pre-pubertal female. Ann Surg 167:229–231, 1968
34. West L, Weiland LH, Clagett OT: Cystosarcoma phylloides. Ann Surg 173:520–528, 1971
35. Simpson TE, Van Dervoort RL, Lynn HB: Giant fibroadenoma (benign cystosarcoma phylloides): Report of a 13-year-old girl. Surgery 65:341–342, 1969
36. Hoover HG, Trestioreanu A, Ketcham AS: Metastatic cystosarcoma phylloides in an adolescent girl, an unusually malignant tumor. Ann Surg 181:279–282, 1975
37. Stromberg GV, Golladay ES: Cystosarcoma phyllodes in the adolescent female. J Pediatr Surg 13:423–426, 1978
38. McDivitt RW, Stewart FW, Berg JW: Tumors of the breast. In Atlas of Tumor Pathology, 2nd Series, Fascicle 2. Washington, DC, Armed Forces Institute of Pathology, 1968
39. Bader E, Isaacson C: Bilateral malignant cystosarcoma phyllodes. Br J Surg 58:519–521, 1961
40. Reich T, Solomon C: Bilateral cystosarcoma phyllodes, malignant variant with 14 year follow-up case report. Ann Surg 147:39–43, 1958

41. McDonald JR, Harrington SW: Giant fibro-adenoma of the breast—cystosarcomas phylloides. Ann Surg 131:243–251, 1950
42. Al-Jurf A, Hawk WA, Crile G Jr: Cystosarcoma phyllodes. Surg Gynecol Obstet 146:358–364, 1978
43. Reingold IM, Ascher GS: Cystosarcoma phyllodes in a man with gynecomastia. Am J Clin Pathol 53:852–856, 1970
44. Pantoja E, Llobet RE, Lopez E: Gigantic cystosarcoma phyllodes in a man with gynecomastia. Arch Surg 111:611, 1976
45. Rosen PP, Urban JA: Coexistent mammary carcinoma and cystosarcoma phyllodes. Breast 1:9–15, 1975
46. Klausner JM, Lelcuk S, Ilia B, et al: Breast carcinoma originating in cystosarcoma phyllodes. Clin Oncol 9:71–74, 1983
47. Philip PJ: Carcinosarcoma of the breast. J R Coll Surg Edinb 21:229–232, 1976
48. Cornog JL, Mobini SE, Enterline HT: Squamous carcinoma of the breast. Am J Clin Pathol 55:410–417, 1971
49. Ross DE: Malignancy occurring in cystosarcoma phyllodes. Am J Surg 88:243–245, 1954
50. Rix DB, Tredwell SJ, Forward AD: Cystosarcoma phyllodes (cellular intracanalicular fibroadenoma). Clinicopathologic relationships. Can J Surg 14:31–37, 1971
51. Rhodes RY, Kenneth AF, Davis LD, et al: Metastatic cystosarcoma phyllodes. A report of two cases presenting with neurological symptoms. Cancer 41:1179–1187, 1978
52. Fernandez BB, Hernandez FJ, Spindler W: Metastatic cystosarcoma phyllodes: A light and electron microscopic study. Cancer 37:1737–1746, 1976
53. Geist D: Cystosarcoma phyllodes of the female breast. Am Surg 30:105–108, 1964
54. Aronson W: Malignant cystosarcoma phyllodes with liposarcoma. Wis Med J 65:184–187, 1966
55. Hart WR, Bauer RC, Oberman HA: A clinicopathologic study of twenty-six hypercellular periductal stromal tumors of the breast. Am J Clin Pathol 70:211–216, 1978

Paget's Disease of the Nipple

Robert T. Osteen

In 1874 Sir James Paget[1] described a "disease of the mammary areola preceding cancer in the mammary gland." (See Color Plate 2 in Chapter 3.) The condition of the areola and nipple was a "very acute, diffuse eczema, or like that of an acute balanitis." Copious, yellow, clear, viscid exudate was associated with tingling, itching, and burning. This condition differed only from persistent eczema or psoriasis in that cancer of the mammary gland followed within at most 2 years and usually within 1 year. The cancer never occurred in the skin and always was seen in the substance of the breast beneath or not far from the nipple. Paget believed that the superficial skin change was benign and that it somehow induced the cancer below it. Unna[2] in 1896 agreed with Paget's interpretation that the changes in the nipple somehow prepared the ground for cancer to develop but felt that the skin lesion was neither eczema nor cancer. Darier[3] described the typical Paget cells in 1889 but believed that they were parasitic and not malignant. Jacobeus[4] was the first person to conjecture that the nipple change was carcinoma arising from the glandular epithelium of the terminal ducts.

THEORIES OF HISTOGENESIS

The classical Paget cell (Fig. 15-7) is "large, ovoid, possessive of an abundant clear to opaque pale-staining cytoplasm, with a large round or ovoid nucleus." It tends to shrink during fixation and is most frequently located in the malpighian layer of the epidermis.[5] Toker[6] described histologically benign clear cell infiltrates in 31 of 340 nipples from cancerous breasts and 23 of 190 normal controls. The clear cell aggregates occasionally form tubular structures resembling mammary ductules within the nipple epidermis. Toker[6] cautioned against confusing these benign cells with Paget cells (Fig. 15-8).

By the end of the 1930s, the possible relationships between malignant cells in the nipple and malignant cells in the breast had been investigated, and each theory had its adherents. Inglis[7] believed that the cancer began at the junction of the lactiferous duct with the epidermis and spread downward in the epithelial lining of the duct wall. Muir[8] showed that there could be upward spread from the duct to the surface. In some cases, Muir demonstrated normal ductal tissue between the invasive breast cancer and the surface lesion, and he thus postulated that the growths were ordinarily due to extension from independent foci of intraductal carcinoma.

The comparative benignity of the Paget cells in the nipple was deduced from the lack of invasive spread from the areola into the substance below and from the absence of Paget cells in metastases to axillary lymph nodes.

FIGURE 15-7. Paget's disease of the nipple in a 57-year-old woman who presented with an ulcerated nipple. Mastectomy revealed intraductal carcinoma of lactiferous ducts in nipple and intraductal carcinoma in the lower outer quadrant. This photograph shows the junction of normal epidermis on the left and the zone of Paget's disease on the right. Epidermal hyperplasia and lymphocytic infiltration of dermis are commonly seen in Paget's disease. Adenocarcinoma cells appear to lie in spaces within the squamous epithelium and have clear cytoplasm. Note that nuclei of Paget cells have cytological features of tumor cells *(inset)*.

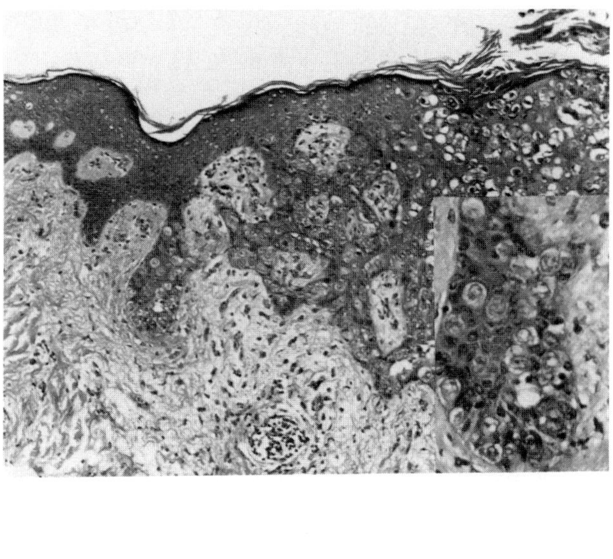

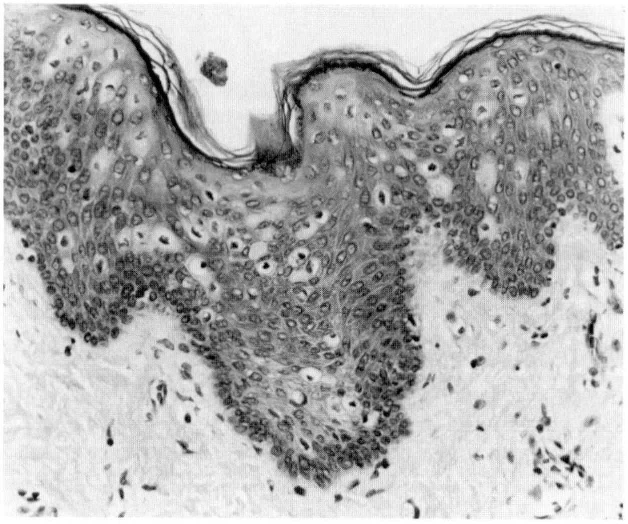

FIGURE 15-8. Clear cells in epidermis of nipple of a 50-year-old woman which may be mistaken for Paget cells. Note small, punctate nuclei which lack cytological appearance of carcinoma cells. The specimen was obtained from a mastectomy performed for lobular carcinoma *in situ*.

Orr and Parish[9] argued that Paget cells are reactive, not neoplastic cells and that they may represent altered melanocytes. Five arguments were offered for their position: (1) Paget cells do not invade the deeper tissues. (2) Paget cells do not show a proportionate increase in their contribution to the epidermal cell population in advanced as compared with early cases. (3) There is an inflammatory infiltration of the superficial part of the underlying dermis. (4) The damaged muscle and connective tissue of the nipple appear to be related to a damaging agent rather than neoplastic invasion. (5) Dendritic cells that are argyrophilic and DOPA positive appear to be closely related to Paget cells and sometimes appear to be identical with them, suggesting that the Paget cells may be altered melanocytes.

The resemblance of Paget cells to some of the subjacent, invasive, cancer cells favors a theory of malignant origin. Greenwood and Minkowitz[10] reported a case in which typical Paget cells spread within the skin of the arm, which was directly invaded by a metastastic infiltrating ductal carcinoma.

Three possible sources of malignant cells in the epidermis have been described: (1) The Paget cells may be a malignant infiltrate of the dermis from the ducts and stroma below. (2) The malignant cells may originate in the skin and descend along the ducts, causing invasive cancer within the breast. (3) Paget's disease may be an *in situ* carcinoma arising from keratinocytes, melanocytes, or clear cells in the skin of the nipple. Each theory for the origin of Paget cells emphasizes some clinical characteristic of the disease.

Although intraductal carcinoma is usually present in the nipple, nipple changes with minimal intraductal tumor or even without any demonstrable subjacent change have been recorded.[6,11,12] Analysis of the time course of the disease does not fit with the hypothesis of a premalignant change in the nipple progressing to intraductal carcinoma and finally to invasive cancer.

Occasional cases of minimal invasion of the nipple by a well-developed, invasive mass have been reported by a number of investigators[11,12,14,15,16] since Muir[8] and provide direct evidence for the hypothesis that at least one mechanism for the development of Paget's disease is direct upward spread of malignant cells. Paget-type cells are seen in other apocrine, epidermal malignancies[17] and in metastatic breast cancer to the skin.[10]

Evidence for epidermotropic migration of Paget cells was presented by Toker,[18] who examined more than 1000 serial sections of the ductal system from a breast containing a tumor located 3 cm from the surface of the nipple. Paget cells could be traced from the tumor within the epithelium of a single duct to the nipple. The intraepithelial permeation preserved the integrity of the superficial layer of the duct lining and the basement membrane. This pattern of spread was distinctly different from the progressing core of tumor seen filling the ducts with intraductal carcinoma. Descent of Paget cells down a branch off of the main route of progression was also noted, showing that the Paget cells could infiltrate in either direction along a duct.

Finally, an invasive breast cancer may be at some distance from the nipple, and a direct line of communicating cells may be difficult or impossible to demonstrate. This observation tends to argue in favor of two separate disease foci of intraductal carcinoma, perhaps stimulated by the same etiologic agent but with infiltrative carcinoma arising from the parenchymal focus. No one theory seems to fit all cases of Paget's disease.

Histochemical studies have given some indication of the nature of Paget cells. Culberson and Horn[19] observed pigment granules in 10 of 25 cases including four black patients. No pigment was seen in tumor cells within the breast or in metastases to axillary lymph nodes. Although the four cases of extramammary Paget's disease reported by Dockerty and Pratt[17] were all mucicarmine positive, none of the Paget cells from the patients in the study of Culberson and Horn[19] stained positively with mucicarmine.

Toker[18] reported that some but not a majority of Paget cells stained with periodic acid-Schiff (PAS) and occasional cells were strikingly positive. Ashikari and colleagues[12] noted strongly PAS-positive, diastase-resistant Paget cells, indicating a high content of neutral mucopolysaccharides. PAS positivity favors a theory of glandular rather than epidermal origin for the Paget cells.

Further evidence for glandular origin of Paget cells was supplied by Nadji and colleagues,[20] who used an immunoperoxidase technique to demonstrate the presence of carcinoembryonic antigen within the cytoplasm or on the cell surface membrane of the tumor but not keratinocytes or melanocytes from seven cases of Paget's disease. An immunoperoxidase technique with two monoclonal antibodies was used by Kirkham and colleagues[21] to demonstrate milk fat globular membrane antigens in 12 cases of mammary Paget's disease. The Paget cells showed a cytoplasmic staining pattern similar to that of intraductal and invasive carcinoma, supporting the contention that the Paget cells are related to malignant ductal cells. Lagios and colleagues[13] combined information from electron microscopy with the immunoperoxidase staining pattern from an antiestradiol antibody to conclude that Paget cells arise *in situ*. Those authors identified intermediate cells, possibly abnormal keratinocytes, with a staining pattern for the antiestradiol antibody similar to that of the Paget cells.

Desmosomes between Paget cells and between adjacent epidermal cells were reported by Sagebiel[22] and by Lagios and colleagues.[13] Sagebiel[22] noted that alteration of epidermal cells adjacent to Paget cells suggested *in situ* transformation of epidermal cells to Paget cells.

In summary, the origin of Paget cells is still controversial. There is evidence that Paget cells can ascend within the epithelium of a duct, descend within the epithelium of a duct, and originate *de novo* within the epithelium of the nipple. Some histochemical evidence points toward origin from glandular epithelium, whereas ultrastructural studies suggest *in situ* transformation of skin cells. Toker[6] has suggested that the clear cells of the nipple epidermis may provide an anatomical basis for the development of Paget's disease as a primary intraepidermal malignancy. It is possible that several of these explanations are correct and that the clinical and microscopic appearance of Paget's disease can arise from multiple circumstances.

AGE AND INCIDENCE

The incidence of overt Paget's disease in patients with breast cancer is low, ranging from 0.7% reported by Dockerty and Harrington[14] to 2.3% reported by Ashikari and colleagues.[12] Among the 9000 patients in the Philadelphia County Breast Cancer Study, the incidence was 1.5%.[23] Among 138 breast cancers reported by Ramantanis and colleagues,[25] there were only two cases of Paget's disease. Although the disease occurs in males, it is very rare.[24] The age range for patients with Paget's disease corresponds to that of other forms of breast cancer. No racial predisposition has been described, and no predisposing factors are known. Subclinical involvement of the nipple with Paget's disease, described by Muir[8] and by Dockerty and Harrington,[14] may be common. Lagios and colleagues[15] noticed pagetoid changes in the nipples of 12 of 149 mastectomy specimens. Only 1 of the 12 was clinically evident.

SIGNS AND SYMPTOMS

A majority of patients complain of an eczematoid change in the nipple or a mass in the breast with an unnoticed nipple change or a change that the patient feels is too insignificant to warrant attention. Maier and colleagues[23] recorded crusting, scaling, erosion, or discharge of the nipple in 62% of the patients in their series. A bloody discharge was the first sign of abnormality in approximately 15%. Weeping, eczematoid lesions are accessible for cytologic examination. Positive cytologic findings indicate the need for mammography and a definitive diagnosis. Negative cytologic findings should not be considered a definitive diagnosis of suspicious nipple lesions, and a biopsy is still indicated.

Long delays in diagnosis are common, with an average duration of symptoms greater than 1 year in most series. Nance and colleagues[26] were unable to correlate duration of symptoms with survival. In Maier and associates'[23] series, patients who waited longer than 6 months before treatment had a better 5-year survival rate than those who were treated earlier. A significant age difference between patients who presented with a mass and those who presented without a mass was shown by Kister and Haagensen.[11] Patients with a mass presented at an average age of 49 years, and those without a mass at an average age of 58 years. The "earlier" presentation in older patients suggests that progression from nipple involvement to an invasive breast cancer is not a common model for the disease.

PAGET'S DISEASE OF THE NIPPLE AND INVASIVE BREAST CANCER

The prognosis in Paget's disease is related to the presence or absence of invasive cancer and the tendency of the cancer to metastasize, as demonstrated by spread to axillary lymph nodes. Paget changes in the nipple are frequently associated with invasive breast cancer and are almost invariably associated with noninvasive breast cancer. The invasive component may be occult but more often presents as a mass. Prognosis depends on the presence or absence of invasive cancer. A mass associated with Paget changes of the nipple must be considered suspicious.

In 15 series from the literature reporting a total of 890 patients, 54% of patients had a mass and 46% presented without a mass (Table 15-12). The 5-year survival rate was 88% among patients who had nipple changes only and 38% in those patients with a mass. Of patients who presented with nipple changes only, 42% (129 of 308) had infiltrating carcinomas. The survival rate of patients with intraductal carcinoma only is close to 100%, and the mortality of patients without a palpable mass is entirely due to spread from clinically occult, histologically demonstrable, invasive cancer.

Positive axillary lymph nodes adversely affect survival (Table 15-13). The survival rate of 160 patients reported in the literature with a mass and positive lymph nodes was 22% compared with the 5-year survival rate of 68% for patients who presented with a mass but were not found to have metastasis to the axillary lymph nodes. The incidence of positive lymph nodes in patients who did not have a mass was low (8%) among 330 patients reported. The highest incidence of lymph node metastases in patients without a mass was reported by Maier and colleagues[23] to be 20% in 40 patients. Several series had no example of positive axillary lymph nodes in a patient who presented without a mass. It should be noted that most reported series of patients with Paget's disease an-

Table 15-12
Relationship of Survival to the Presence of a Palpable Mass

	No Palpable Mass			Mass	
Author	Number of Cases	Infiltration*	Survival†	Number of Cases	Survival†
Culberson and Horn[19]	13	2/13	4/4	12	3/8
Helman and Kliman[34]	15	2/15	5/7	12	10/15
Salvadori et al[30]	41	33/41	38/41	50	19/50
McGregor and McGregor[36]	14	1/14	7/9	7	1/5
Ashikari et al[12]	96	33/96	88/96	113	48/113
Solheim[38]	46	36/46	30/46	25	5/25
Freund et al[29]	19		18/19	10	4/10
Kister and Haagensen[11]	26		21/26	59	28/47
Rissanen and Holsti[37]	13		10/12	13	0/9
Paone and Baker[27]	19		19/19	31	15/31
Nance et al[26]	21	2/21	16/16	32	9/29
Kay[33]	7	1/7	5/5	16	3/16
Colcock and Sommers[32]	15	5/15	8/8	8	1/8
Maier et al[23]	56	14/40	28/40	81	18/48
West and Nickel[28]	5		3/3	15	1/8
Totals	406	129/308 (42%)	300/351 (85%)	484	165/435 (38%)

* Number of cases in which infiltrating carcinoma was found and number examined.
† Number of patients surviving 5 years and number of patients observed for 5 years.

tedate the era of high-quality mammography. In a recent series, Paone and Baker[27] reported finding five occult tumors in six patients who underwent mammography after presenting with nipple changes only.

TREATMENT

Different authors have chosen to emphasize different aspects of the pathobiology of Paget's disease in their recommendations for therapy. Although the incidence of positive axillary lymph nodes in the absence of a mass is low, it is high enough to persuade several authors to recommend mastectomy and axillary node dissection to all patients with or without a mass. In much of the literature preceding the popularity of pectoral muscle preservation, standard radical mastectomy was the recommendation.[11,20,23,28] Other authors have concluded that in the absence of a palpable mass or palpable axillary lymph nodes, a modified radical mastectomy could be performed with immediate examination of the specimen and removal of the pectoral muscles if invasion of the breast parenchyma or lymph node metastasis is found.[12,30,31] The very low incidence of positive lymph nodes in patients without a mass in their individual series have led some authors[26,32,33] to recommend radical mastectomies for patients with a mass and simple mastectomies for patients with only nipple changes. Paone and Baker,[27] citing their comparable results for modified radical and standard radical mastectomy in the treatment of breast cancer without Paget changes of the nipple, recommended modified radical mastectomy in patients with a mass and simple mastectomy for patients with a nipple lesion without a mass. Helman and Kliman[34] reported such dismal results for the treatment by radical mastectomy of patients with a mass that they believed that all such patients should be treated "palliatively" with simple mastectomy and radiation therapy. The results with simple mastectomy and radiation in patients without a mass were so good that they did not recommend a more radical procedure. The obvious disadvantage of that treatment plan is the loss of information regarding prognosis that is obtained from examination of the axillary lymph nodes.

A few patients have been treated for cure with breast-conserving surgery with or without radiation therapy. Table 15-14 describes 46 such cases collected from the literature. These patients were treated with excisions less than mastectomy, either because of patient's demands or the surgeon's preferences. Among the 46 patients, three local recurrences were noted (one after 6 years). All patients who were followed for 5 years or longer were still alive and, except for the one local recurrence, were free

Table 15-13
Relationship of Survival to Nodal Status

Author	*Number With Mass*	*Number With Mass (+) Nodes*	*5-Year Survival Mass (+) Nodes*	*Number With Mass (−) Nodes*	*5-year Survival Mass (−) Nodes*	*Number With Nipple Only*	*Number With Nipple Only (+) Nodes*	*5-Year Survival Nipple Only (+) Nodes*
Culberson and Horn[19]	8	6	1/5	2	2/2	5	1	0/1
Helman and Kliman[34]	12	7	0/3	5	0/4	15	0	
Salvadori et al[30]	48	42		6		32	0	
Ashikari et al[12]	113	74	19/74	39	28/39	96	13	8/13
Freund et al[29]	10	5		5		19	2	
Kister and Haagensen[11]	59	33	9/33	26	19/26	56	3	1/2
Rissanen and Holsti[37]	13	10		3		13	0	
Paone and Baker[27]	31	20	4/20	11	8/11	14	0	
Nance et al[26]	18	9		9		21	0	
Kay[33]	16	11	1/11	5	2/5	5	0	
Colcock and Sommers[32]	8	7	1/7	1		15	0	
Maier et al[23]						40	8	2/8
West and Nickel[28]	15	8	0/7	7	2/3	2	0	
Totals	351	232 (66%)	35/160 (22%)	119 (34%)	61/90 (68%)	333	27 27/333 = (8%)	11/24 (46%)

Table 15-14
Limited Local Therapy for Paget's Disease

Author	*Number of Cases*	*Procedure*	*Radiation*	*Result*
Colcock and Sommers[32]	2	Excision of nipple-areola	0	NED 10 mo, 14 yr
Malak and Tapolcsanyi[31]	18	Excision of nipple-areola	16 cases	15 NED 5 yr
	2	Excision of nipple-areola and tumor		2 NED 10 yr
Paone and Baker[27]	5	Excision of nipple-areola and wedge of breast	0	5 NED 10 yr
Lagios et al[13]	4	Excision of nipple-areola	0	4 NED 16–55 mo
	1	Nipple biopsy, axillary dissection	0	Nipple recurrence. NED 31 mo after nipple resection
Helman and Kliman[34]	2	Biopsy	Yes	NED 1 yr, 10 yr
McGregor and McGregor[36]	2	Excision of nipple-areola	1	NED 2 yr, 8 yr
Rissanen and Holsti[37]	6	Local excision	2400–3100 cGy	5 NED, 1 local recurrence
	1	Local excision	0	Local recurrence 4 yr

of disease. The criteria for patient selection, other than having no palpable mass, were not described. Lagios and colleagues[13] reported a series of patients selected for breast conservation because of nipple changes without a mass and negative mammograms. Patients underwent excision of the nipple-areolar complex and a wedge of underlying breast tissue. Histologically, the disease was found to be limited to the nipple in all cases. With an average follow-up of 50 months, all five of these highly selected patients were free of disease.

In theory, Paget's disease that is limited to the skin of the nipple or to the skin and ducts of the nipple should be curable by local excision. The risk of subsequent development of other foci of intraductal or invasive carcinoma within such breasts is unknown. Very limited involvement of only the skin of the nipple is rare, accounting for only a small percentage of all patients with Paget's disease and approximately 6% of all patients with disease without a palpable mass. Nance and colleagues[26] detected only 1 of 53 cases without underlying intraductal or invasive cancer. The incidence of Paget's disease of the nipple with limited involvement of the terminal lactiferous ducts is more difficult to assess but may represent a significant population of patients who, if they could be identified, could be adequately treated by limited surgery. The five patients reported by Lagios and colleagues[13] fall into this category. Maier and colleagues[23] were able to find only two patients with disease limited to the major ducts from the 60 pathology specimens examined. There were 3 instances of pre-invasive ductal cancer in 17 patients reported by Cheatle and Cutler[35] and 5 of 39 reported by Muir. Diffuse intraductal carcinoma throughout the breast is probably a more common phenomenon and is probably best treated by prophylactic mastectomy prior to the development of invasive cancer. Ashikari and colleagues[12] reported 6 of 214 patients with Paget's disease of the nipple without underlying intraductal carcinoma, or 6.25% of those without a palpable mass.

Too few authors have mapped the location of parenchymal masses with respect to the nipple to estimate the possibility of breast conservation therapy, which would involve resection of the nipple-areolar complex and an underlying mass with or without leaving residual multifocal invasive or noninvasive carcinoma. Unfortunately, the only selection criteria for such patients would be preoperative mammography and examination of the specimen for evidence of multifocality. Little statistical basis for prediction of diffuse disease is available in the literature. Presumably, even with postexcision radiation therapy, residual intraductal or invasive disease after excision would pose a hazard to the patient. Of the seven palpable masses reported by McGregor and McGregor,[36] four were subareolar and three were elsewhere in the breast. Six of the 31 palpable breast masses reported by Paone and Baker[27] were 2 cm or more away from the areola.

Reports of radiation therapy for definitive treatment of Paget's disease are few. Radiation therapy to control local diseases in the face of metastatic cancer may be helpful but can hardly contribute to long-term survival. Helman and Kliman[34] used radiation therapy in association with simple mastectomy, but it is difficult to evaluate their results since most of their patients probably did not have axillary metastasis or residual chest wall disease. Although Rissanen and Holsti[37] recommended local excision and radiation therapy, the doses that they used (2400 to 3100 cGy) were so low as to be of questionable value.

The efficacy of radiation therapy against residual intraductal carcinoma is unknown, and one of the main problems with breast-conserving surgery for Paget's disease is the risk of leaving residual intraductal carcinoma after resection of the known disease. Unless radiation therapy can be proved to be an effective treatment for intraductal carcinoma, nipple-areolar excisions should be limited to highly selected patients without evidence of diffuse intraductal disease. Patients with diffuse and multifocal intraductal carcinoma throughout the breast are probably best treated by total mastectomy with or without axillary node dissection. A carefully monitored trial of treating selected patients with Paget's disease of the nipple and limited infiltrating carcinoma by conservative surgery and radiation therapy would be interesting. Large centrally located lesions, masses at a distance from the nipple, and infiltrating carcinomas associated with diffuse intraductal carcinoma are best treated with modified radical mastectomy.

REFERENCES

1. Paget J: Disease of the mammary areola preceding cancer of the mammary gland. St Bart Hosp Rep 10:89, 1874
2. Unna PG: The Histopathology of the Diseases of the Skin. Edinburgh, WF Clax, 1896
3. Darier J: La maldie de Paget du mamelon. CR Soc Biol Paris. 1:224, 1889
4. Jacobeus HC: Paget's Disease und sein Verhältnis zum Milchdrünsenkarzinom. Virchows Arch Pathol Anat 178:124, 1904
5. McDivitt RW, Stewart FW, Berg JW: Tumors of the Breast. Atlas of Tumor Pathology. AFIP Fascicle #2. 1967
6. Toker C: Clear cells of the nipple epidermis. Cancer 25:601–610, 1970
7. Inglis K: Paget's Disease of the Nipple. New York, Oxford University Press, 1936
8. Muir R: Further observations on Paget's disease of the nipple. J Pathol Bacteriol 49:299–312, 1939
9. Orr JW, Parish DJ. The nature of the nipple changes in Paget's disease. J Pathol Bacteriol 84:201–208, 1962
10. Greenwood SM, Minkowitz S: Paget's disease in metastatic breast carcinoma. Arch Dermatol 104:312–315, 1971
11. Kister SJ, Haagensen CD: Paget's disease of the breast. Am J Surg 119:606–609, 1970
12. Ashikari R, Park K, Huvos AG, et al: Paget's disease of the breast. Cancer 26:680–685, 1970
13. Lagios MD, Westdahl PR, Rose MR, et al: Paget's disease of the nipple. Cancer 54:545–551, 1984
14. Dockerty MB, Harrington SW: Preclinical Paget's disease of the nipple. Surg Gynecol Obstet 93:317–320, 1951
15. Lagios MD, Gates EA, Westdahl PR, et al: A guide to the frequency of nipple involvement in breast cancer. Am J Surg 138:135–141, 1979
16. Morimoto T, Komaki K, Inui K, et al: Involvement of nipple and areola in early breast cancer. Cancer 55:2459–2463, 1985

17. Dockerty MB, Pratt JH: Extramammary Paget's disease. Cancer 5:1161–1169, 1952
18. Toker C: Some observations on Paget's disease of the nipple. Cancer 14:653–672, 1961
19. Culberson JD, Horn RC: Paget's disease of the nipple. Arch Surg 72:224–231, 1956
20. Nadji M, Morales AR, Girtanner RE, et al: Paget's disease of the skin. Cancer 50:2203–2206, 1982
21. Kirkham N, Berry N, Jones DB, et al: Paget's disease of the nipple: Immunohistochemical localization of milk fat globule membrane antigens. Cancer 55:1510–1512, 1985
22. Sagebiel RW: Ultrastructural observations on epidermal cells in Paget's disease of the breast. Am J Pathol 57:49–64, 1969
23. Maier WP, Rosemond P, Harasym EI, et al: Paget's disease in the female breast. Surg Gynecol Obstet 128:1253–1263, 1969
24. Lancer HA, Moschell SL: Paget's disease of the male breast. J Am Acad Dermatol 7:393–396, 1982
25. Ramantanis G, Besbeas S, Garas JG: Breast cancer in the male: A report of 138 cases. World J Surg 4:621–624, 1980
26. Nance FC, DeLoach DH, Welsh RA, et al: Paget's disease of the breast. Ann Surg 171:864–874, 1970
27. Paone JF, Baker R: Pathogenesis and treatment of Paget's disease of the breast. Cancer 48:825–829, 1981
28. West JP, Nickel WF: Paget's disease of the nipple. Ann Surg 116:19–25, 1942
29. Freund H, Maydovnik M, Laufer N, et al: Paget' disease of the breast. J Surg Oncol 9:93–98, 1977
30. Salvadori B, Fariselli G, Saccozzi R: Analysis of 100 cases of Paget's disease of the breast. Tumori 62:529–536, 1976
31. Malak G, Tapolcsanyi L: Characteristics of Paget's carcinoma of the nipple and problems of its negligence. Oncology 30:278–293, 1974
32. Colcock BP, Sommers SC: Prognosis in Paget's disease of the breast. Surg Clin North Am 35:773–783, 1954
33. Kay S: Paget's disease of the nipple. Surg Gynecol Obstet 123:1010–1014, 1966
34. Helman P, Kliman M: Paget's disease of the nipple: A clinical review of 27 cases. Br J Surg 43:481–486, 1956
35. Cheatle GL, Cutler M: Tumors of the breast. Philadelphia, JB Lippincott, 1931
36. McGregor JK, McGregor DD: Paget's disease of the breast: A twenty-year survey of cases presenting at a large general hospital. Surgery 45:562–568, 1959
37. Rissanen PM, Holsti P: Paget's disease of the breast: The influence of the presence or absence of an underlying palpable tumor on the prognosis and on the choice of treatment. Oncology 23:209–216, 1969
38. Solheim O: Paget's sykdom; papilla mammae. Nord Med 64:1442–1446, 1960

Other Cancers in the Breast

Jeanne A. Petrek

STROMAL SARCOMAS

The term "stromal sarcoma" was coined by Berg and colleagues in 1962 to describe the rather homogeneous group of primary mesenchymal malignant tumors with "fibrous, myxoid, and fatty patterns," excluding malignant cystosarcoma phyllodes, lymphomas, and angiosarcomas.[1] Since then, the term "stromal sarcoma" has been used as if it adequately classified all breast sarcomas. However, primary mesenchymal breast malignancies should be reported, as far as possible, in standard histogenetic terms (i.e., liposarcoma, fibrosarcomas, and so on) and a histologic grade should be assessed. Breast sarcomas would then be categorized uniformly with sarcomas arising from other organs, and the term "stromal sarcoma" would be reserved for very rare malignancies arising from the specialized hormone-responsive stroma of the breast.[2] Since the restricted use of the term "stromal sarcoma" is not frequent, this chapter will apply as Berg and colleagues[1] defined it and as it is commonly understood.

Incidence and Pathology

Stromal sarcoma constitutes 0.5%[3] to 1%[4] of primary breast cancers. The relative incidence of cystosarcoma phyllodes (both benign and malignant) to stromal sarcoma is about 3 to 1.[4,5]

When listed in histogenetic terms, the most commonly described tumors are fibrosarcoma (including malignant fibrous histiocytomas), liposarcoma, and undifferentiated high-grade sarcoma.[1,6,7] In diagnosing fibrosarcomas in particular, there is always the possibility that the benign epithelial elements, identifying the lesion as a malignant cystosarcoma phyllodes, will be overlooked. Leiomyosarcoma[8,9] and sarcomas with bone and cartilage[10,11] seem to be about equally infrequent. Leiomyosarcoma of the breast may originate from the blood vessels, the myoepithelium, or the nipple musculature. With only eight reported cases of this neoplasm by 1978,[8] men and women appear equally affected by this neoplasm.[12,13] Liposarcoma, in a pure form not associated with cystosarcoma, is extremely rare, with only 11 cases reported by 1982.[6,14,15] Although it is accepted that rare breast sarcomas may show cartilaginous, osseous, and muscular metaplasia, the admonition of Stewart in 1950[16] that many apparent cases of "sarcoma" probably represent carcinoma with osseous and cartilaginous metaplasia remains valid today.

Clinical and Radiographic Features

The physical findings in stromal sarcoma probably vary greatly from one subgroup to another. Mesenchymal tumors are usually firm, painless, mobile masses that grow slowly, seldom invade the overlying skin, and in general develop over a period of years. As a consequence, a misdiagnosis of benign tumor, such as fibroadenoma, frequently occurs. Although nipple discharge and dermal lymphatic involvement may be present, they are noted much less often than with similar-sized carcinomas. Spontaneous hemorrhage occurs infrequently. In two typical series, the median age was 51 years[6] and 54 years,[2] and the median tumor size was 5.0 cm (range 3 cm to 15 cm)[6] and 4.0 cm (range 1 cm to 20 cm).[2]

The diagnosis of malignant mesenchymal tumor was never made in any of the patients subjected to mammography.[7] Breast sarcomas usually appear to have well-defined margins (not typically spiculated like those of carcinomas), and fibroadenoma may be mistakenly diagnosed. As opposed to carcinoma, the palpated size of a sarcoma is very close to its radiographic size. Sarcomas are usually quite dense and, even in breasts with severe fibrocystic disease, are easily discernible.[17]

Prognosis and Treatment

The prognosis of mammary sarcoma is uncertain because of its infrequent occurrence and imprecise terminology, among other factors. Excluding well-differentiated fibrosarcomas, a recent study,[3] by combining 11 previous reports, observed a 59% 5-year survival rate. In the recent report from Memorial Sloan-Kettering Cancer Center,[2] 8 of 32 (25%) patients died of disease, a figure comparable to 29% of the patients in another recent series.[6]

For the 25 patients treated initially at Memorial Sloan-Kettering Cancer Center, the 5-year actuarial survival rate was 91%. None received adjuvant chemotherapy, and only one received postoperative radiation therapy. Twenty-two patients had a total mastectomy; three patients underwent a partial mastectomy. There was one local recurrence in each group.

Norris and Taylor[5] suggested various histologic parameters that might identify tumor aggressiveness, including tumor size, microscopic contour, degree of cellular atypia, and frequency of mitotic activity. Barnes and Pietruszka[6] confirmed the last three characteristics, but they and others[7] found no correlation between tumor size and outcome.

The relatively favorable prognosis of mammary sarcomas (as compared with sarcomas arising at other sites) may relate to the smaller size of these easily detected, superficial lesions and the fact that wide local excision—usually in the form of mastectomy—can be easily accomplished.

The recent Memorial Hospital series[2] included a review of four series[1,4,6,7] in order to evaluate local recurrence of breast sarcoma according to extent of primary resection. When at least a total mastectomy was the initial treatment, only 8% of 71 patients had local recurrence, as contrasted to 53% of 32 patients who underwent partial mastectomy. Radiation therapy was used in only 11 patients, and chemotherapy in no patients. In the partial mastectomy group, and even in the total mastectomy group, however, it is not known whether the surgical margins were involved. Since excellent local control (with its probable influence on survival) is readily available by mastectomy alone, partial mastectomy with radiation or other adjuvant therapy should be applied judiciously, if at all.

Regional lymph node metastases are virtually unheard-of.[1,2,7,18] Axillary lymphadenectomy is indicated only when it is technically necessary to achieve local clearance of the primary tumor or in the rare patient whose lymph nodes are clinically positive.

For most breast sarcomas, simple mastectomy is adequate therapy. Adjuvant radiation may be necessary for close margins or in the investigational setting when combined with partial mastectomy. Although adjuvant chemotherapy regimens appear promising for extremity sarcoma,[19] their role has yet to be defined for breast sarcomas.

ANGIOSARCOMA—A SPECIAL CASE

Angiosarcoma, a rare malignant mesenchymal tumor, seems to occur disproportionately more often in the breast than in other body sites. Memorial Sloan-Kettering Cancer Center treated more breast angiosarcomas[20] than all stromal sarcomas[2] combined. Nevertheless, it is a rare disease, with Stewart[16] reporting (1950) one angiosarcoma for every 2000 to 3500 breast cancers.

Pathology

The tumor appears to be composed of interanastomosing vascular channels with an endothelial layer that may have bland single cells or papillary projections, with hemorrhage, necrosis, and solid spindle-cell sarcomatous elements. Often a variable papillary pattern is seen beyond the microscopic limits of the tumor.[22] The deceptively benign appearance has caused a mistaken diagnosis of hematoma, hemangioma, or lymphangioma in more than a third of cases,[23] with correct diagnosis determined only after one or more local recurrences.[23] Every vascular tumor of the breast should be seriously evaluated, since angiosarcoma appears to be more common than benign hemangioma of the breast.[20,24]

Stewart[16] named the rare perilobular capillary angioma that is incidentally identified in the 1.2% of breast biopsies or mastectomy specimens[23] as the site of origin, although other authors[2] do not agree.

Clinical Features

About 100 cases have been reported in the medical literature of this century. The median age of patients is in the late 30s or early 40s.[2,20,21,22,25] Bilateral synchronous[20,25] and metachronous primary tumors[2,20] have been described, including several cases diagnosed during pregnancy.[2,20,21,26,27,28] Two probable cases have been described in males.[29,30]

Angiosarcoma usually presents as a rather soft, painless, rapidly enlarging, ill-defined mass. Local tumor fixation and axillary adenopathy are unusual.[31] Occasionally, ecchymosis around and within the tumor can cause local discomfort.[32]

Prognosis and Treatment

Before the 1980s, only one series[21] (consisting of ten patients) attempted to correlate histologic features with clinical behavior. The authors concluded that tumor size and duration of symptoms were more important factors. More recently, the largest reported series[20] (36 patients) from Memorial Hospital found that three general histologic pat-

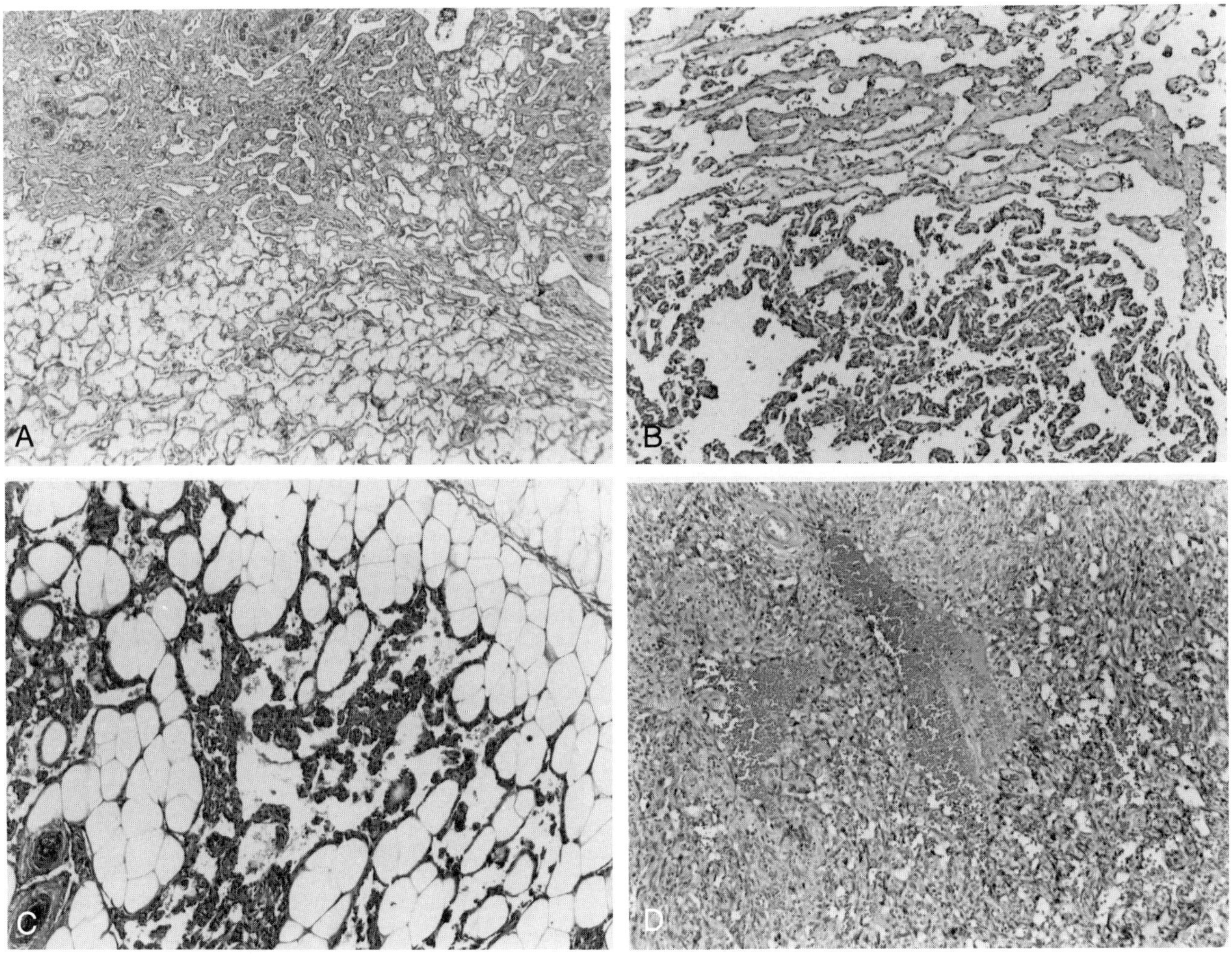

FIGURE 15-9. Angiosarcoma has diverse growth patterns ranging from very orderly vascular proliferation to high-grade sarcoma. *(A)* Type I, or low-grade, angiosarcoma composed of anastomosing vascular channels lined by a single layer of endothelial cells. *(B)* Type II angiosarcoma is composed largely of type I channels, seen in the upper part of the picture, and focal areas of papillary endothelial proliferation, seen in the lower portion of the picture. *(C)* High-power view of type II area, exhibiting papillary growth of endothelium. *(D)* Type III, or high-grade, angiosarcoma composed of solid sheets of anaplastic cells with focal areas of hemorrhagic necrosis. Small vascular channels are evident in the tumor on the right side of the picture.

terns of growth were closely correlated with prognosis (Fig. 15-9). Whereas 10 of 13 patients with type I were alive and free of disease, with an average follow-up of nearly 6 years, only 2 of 16 with type III were free of disease, and two have died. The six patients with type II had a survival rate similar to those with type I. The Memorial Sloan-Kettering Cancer Center series of 40 cases showed a 41% 3-year disease-free survival rate. A review of 87 cases from the world literature until 1980[22] revealed a 14% 3-year and 6% 5-year disease-free survival rate. Until this series, there were only eight reported cases with a greater than 5-year survival time.[21,32,33,34,35,36,37] More than half of these resulted in a late recurrence.[32,33,35,37] An even more recent small series (15 patients) confirmed that histologic patterns (characterized as well to poorly differentiated) correlated closely with prognosis.[38]

Because of the exceptional difficulty of microscopically determining a clear margin, a total mastectomy is almost always necessary, and occasional muscle or extensive skin excision is required for adequate margins. Axillary dissection is necessary only to achieve adequate margins in the axilla, since only one case of lymph node metastases has been reported.[32] Seven patients (of 36 patients) developed local recurrence after simple (2 patients), modified radical (2 patients), or radical (3 patients) mastectomy in the Memorial Hospital series.[20]

The earliest recurrence after primary therapy was at 5 months and the latest at 2 years. Four of these patients died with metastatic disease within 2 to 17 months after local recurrence.

The effectiveness of radiation in primary treatment is unknown, although it can be beneficial for palliation.[37] Endocrine influences on angiosarcoma are unknown, although estrogen receptor status was negative in the one patient who was analyzed.[38] Because of poor results from standard therapy, newer protocols have been evaluating multimodal therapy, which has already proved useful in sarcomas.[38]

LYMPHOMA

The diagnosis of primary breast lymphoma requires the recognition, in close association, of normal breast tissue and lymphomatous infiltrate in patients with neither previous lymphoma nor concurrent lymphoma in another site.[40]

Pathology

Since a uniform lymphoma classification system has not been used in the rare primary breast lymphomas, the frequency of various types is indeterminable. Microscopically, lymphoma cells infiltrate among the quite normal breast lobules and ducts. In histiocytic lymphoma, the cells are of moderate size and are uniform, although pleomorphism, giant cells, and atypia are also found. The well-differentiated lymphocytic lymphomas are composed of small, mature, monotonous lymphocytes. The poorly differentiated lymphocytic lymphomas demonstrate marked nuclear pleomorphism and cellular immaturity, sometimes with sheets of pure lymphoblasts.[40] Occasionally, the primary breast lymphoma may be difficult to differentiate from pseudolymphoma,[41,42] granulocytic sarcoma,[43,44] and, less often, from medullary or poorly differentiated carcinomas.[18] Electron microscopy is particularly helpful in the last case.[45]

Clinical and Radiographic Features

Median age at diagnosis is late 30s.[40] Even though only small numbers are involved, occurrence during pregnancy and the postpartum period seems frequent. Lymphoma has tended to involve the right breast more often than the left in some series.[40,46,47]

Several case reports and review articles indicate that the incidence of primary breast lymphoma is 0.05% to 0.53% of the total breast malignancies, and bilateral breast involvement occurs in about 15% of cases.[40,46,48,49]

Mammographically,[17] the nodular lymphomas tend to present as a distinct mass, whereas the diffuse group tends to appear as increased parenchymal density and skin thickening. The discrete form can closely mimic benign tumors such as fibroadenoma.

Prognosis and Treatment

For 33 cases of breast lymphoma, the 5-year survival rate, based on data from the End Results Group of Cancer Registries, was 35%.[50] Many series, however, report worse survival rates. The excellent 5-year survival rate (64%) reported from Memorial Sloan-Kettering Cancer Center in 1962[46] may be due to the inclusion of several follicular lymphomas, with their good prognosis. A recent, comprehensive article[48] from M.D. Anderson Hospital reports a 5-year survival rate of 49%. In Mambo and colleagues' M.D. Anderson report, all patients eventually received chemotherapy, either following radiotherapy or immediately after biopsy/excision of the mass. Only four patients had mastectomies.

A search for lymphoma elsewhere may include chest x-ray, bipedal lymphangiography, computerized tomography, bone marrow aspiration/biopsy, chest tomography, isotope scanning of bone or liver, and biopsy of equivocal adenopathy. Treatment of primary breast lymphoma should be performed by an experienced hematologist according to the treatment of the same lymphoma occurring elsewhere. Such treatment will probably include adequate open biopsy with material for touch prep, cell surface markers, and possibly for electron microscopy. Further treatment of breast lymphoma, depending on the cell of origin, will usually involve radiation or chemotherapy or both.

PSEUDOLYMPHOMA

More than 8000 consecutive mastectomies and quadrantectomies revealed only five patients with pseudolymphoma.[51] The median age was 36 years. Grossly, the tumor was a solid, firm nodule with accompanying fat necrosis in some cases. Microscopically, the lymphoid infiltrate had a nodular pattern with no atypical cells and often displayed germinal centers. No tumors recurred following local excision alone. It is postulated that, similar to lung pseudolymphoma, this lesion may represent an overwhelming local response to injury, especially since breast injury had occurred in half of the breast pseudolymphoma patients. This entity should be differentiated from malignant lymphoma by expert consultations, so that patients are not subjected to unnecessary mastectomy, radiation, or chemotherapy.

METASTASES TO THE BREAST

Incidence and Origin

Metastases to the breast range from 0.8% to 6.6% of all breast malignancies,[52,53,54] with the variation presumed to be due to inclusion of leukemia/lymphoma in some series and the increased incidence found in autopsy versus clinical material.[52]

Metastases can occur through cross-lymphatic channels (metastatic from the contralateral breast) or can be bloodborne. Diffuse hematologic malignancies—such as lymphoma and leukemia—are considered a subgroup of bloodborne. Opposite-breast primary tumors, followed by hematopoietic primary tumors (lymphomas and leukemias), are the lesions most commonly metastatic to the breast.[52,53,54] Excluding those malignancies, melanoma was the next most common source, 28% in one of the largest single series.[52] Metastases from the lung (particularly oat cell) and stomach are also frequent. Less common, but included in any large series, have been metastases from the ovary, kidney, prostate, and carcinoid lesions.

To distinguish metastatic disease of the breast from primary breast cancer, the former should have a periductal or perilobular distribution of malignant cells in the absence of intraductal carcinoma or lobular carcinoma *in situ*. In some cases (e.g., suspected melanoma metastases) electron microscopy can be helpful.

Clinical and Radiographic Features

Cancers metastatic to the breast are often superficial, sharply limited, solitary masses with a predilection for the upper, outer quadrant.[52,53,55,56] Multiple lesions, bilateral involvement, and diffuse disease are less common. Although one large report found pain or discomfort in more than half of the patients,[52] other series found it absent.[53,54,55] One series found these usually superficial tumors adherent to the skin in about one-half of the cases.[52]

Nodular lesions were the most common finding on mammography in most series,[52,53,54,55,57] although diffuse skin thickening was most common in one.[58] Spiculation is distinctly absent, since there is little desmoplasia associated with these lesions. None of the metastases had microcalcifications, except three cases of metastatic ovarian cancer,[57,59,60] which contained psammoma bodies. Therefore, the presence of calcifications in the nodule virtually rules out the diagnosis of metastatic disease.

Prognosis and Treatment

The breast abnormality was the first sign of malignancy in about one-third of these patients.[58] Nonetheless, the discovery of breast involvement from a distant primary neoplasm likely indicates widespread dissemination. In 1962, Hajdu and Urban[52] found that 41 of 51 patients died within 1 year. A recent series (1983) had similar results, with 13 of 16 dead in one year.[58] Treatment of metastatic cancer to the breast is obviously directed at the primary tumor. It may, however, be rarely necessary to obtain local control by excision, radiotherapy, or both.

REFERENCES

1. Berg JW, DeCosse JJ, Fracchia AA, et al: Stromal sarcomas of the breast. A unified approach to connective tissue sarcomas other than cystosarcoma phyllodes. Cancer 15:418–424, 1962
2. Callery CD, Rosen PP, Kinne DW: Sarcoma of the breast. A study of 32 patients with reappraisal of classification and therapy. Ann Surg 201:527–532, 1985
3. Tang PM, Petrelli M, Robechek PJ: Stromal sarcoma of the breast. A light and electron microscopic study. Cancer 43:209–217, 1979
4. Oberman HJ: Sarcomas of the breast. Cancer 18:1233–1243, 1965
5. Norris HJ, Taylor HB: Sarcomas and related mesenchymal tumors of the breast. Cancer 22:22–28, 1968
6. Barnes L, Pietruszka M: Sarcomas of the breast. Cancer 40:1577–1585, 1977
7. Salvadori B, Greco M, Galluzzo D, et al: Surgery for malignant mesenchymal tumors of the breast: A series of 31 cases. Tumori 68:325–329, 1982
8. Hernandez FJ: Leiomyosarcoma of the male breast originating in the nipple. Am J Surg Pathol 2:299–304, 1978
9. Chen KT, Kuo T-T, Hoffman KD: Leiomyosarcoma of the breast: A case of long survival and late hepatic metastasis. Cancer 47:1883–1886, 1981
10. Benediktsdottir K, Lagerberg F, Lundell L, et al: Osteogenic sarcoma of the breast. Acta Pathol Microbiol Scand 88:161–168, 1980
11. Jernstrom P, Lindberg AL, Meland, ON: Osteogenic sarcoma of the mammary gland. Am J Clin Pathol 40:521–526, 1963
12. Visfeldt J, Sheike O: Male breast cancer. I. Histologic typing and grading of 187 Danish cases. Cancer 32:985–990, 1973
13. Pardo-Mindan J, Garcia-Julian G, Altuna MD: Leiomyosarcoma of the breast; report of a case. Am J Clin Pathol 62:477–480, 1974
14. Menon M, Van Venthoven PCM: Liposarcoma of the breast. A case report. Arch Pathol 98:370–375, 1974
15. Arbabi L, Narhol MJ: Pleomorphic liposarcoma following radiotherapy for breast carcinoma. Cancer 49:878–880, 1982
16. Stewart FW: Tumors of the Breast, Atlas of Tumor Pathology, Section 9, Fascicle 34, pp 75–87. Washington, DC, Armed Forces Institute of Pathology, 1951
17. D'Orsi CJ, Feldhaus L, Sonnenfeld M: Unusual lesions of the breast. Radiol Clin North Am 21:67–80, 1983
18. Lattes R: Sarcomas of the breast. JAMA 201:531–532, 1967
19. Rosenberg SA, Tepper J, Gladstein E, et al: Prospective randomized evaluation of adjuvant chemotherapy in adults with soft tissue sarcoma of the extremities. Cancer 52:424–434, 1983
20. Donnell RM, Rosen PP, Lieberman PH, et al: Angiosarcoma and other vascular tumors of the breast. J Surg Pathol 5:629–642, 1981
21. Steingaszner LC, Enzingert M, Taylor HP: Hemangiosarcoma of the breast. Cancer 18:352–361, 1965
22. Chen KTK, Kirkegaard DD, Bocian JJ: Angiosarcoma of the breast. Cancer 46:368–371, 1980
23. Rosen PP, Ridolfi RL: The perilobular hemangioma. Am J Clin Pathol 68:21–23, 1977
24. Alvarez-Fernandez E, Salinero-Paniagua E: Vascular tumors of the mammary gland. Virchows Arch (Pathol Anat) 394:31–47, 1981
25. Barber KW, Harrison EJ, Clagett OT, et al: Angiosarcoma of the breast. Surgery 48:869–878, 1960
26. Batchelor GB: Hemangioblastoma of the breast associated with pregnancy. Br J Surg 46:647–649, 1959
27. Tibbs D: Metastasizing hemanomata. A case of malignant endothelioma. Br J Surg 40:465–470, 1953
28. Enticknap JB: Angioblastoma of the breast complicating pregnancy. Br Med J 2:51, 1946

29. Procter DSC: Angioma of the male breast with malignant characteristics. S Afr Med J 32:407–409, 1958
30. Yadav RVS, Saharian S, Mittal MS, et al: Angiosarcoma of the male breast. Int Surg 61:453–464, 1976
31. Haagensen CD: Diseases of the Breast, 2nd ed, pp 227–249. Philadelphia, WB Saunders, 1971
32. Gulesserian HP, Lawton HPO: Angiosarcoma of the breast. Cancer 24:1021–1026, 1969
33. Horne WI, Percival WL: Hemangiosarcoma of the breast. Can J Surg 18:81–84, 1975
34. Masse SR, Mongeau CH, Rioux A: Angiosarcoma of the breast. Can J Surg 20:341–343, 1977
35. Gross GF: Angiosarcoma of the breast. Am Surg 43:734–736, 1977
36. Myerowitz RL, Pietruszka M, Barnes EL: Primary angiosarcoma of the breast. JAMA 239:403, 1978
37. Savage R: The treatment of angiosarcoma of the breast. J Surg Oncol 18:129–134, 1981
38. Merino MJ, Berman M, Carter D: Angiosarcoma of the breast. Am J Surg Pathol 7:53–60, 1983
39. Antman KH, Corson J, Greenberger J, et al: Multimodality therapy in the management of angiosarcoma of the breast. Cancer 50:2000–2003, 1982
40. Wiseman C, Liao KT: Primary lymphoma of the breast. Cancer 29:1705–1712, 1972
41. Fisher ER, Palekar AS, Paulson JD: Pseudolymphoma of breast. Cancer 44:258–263, 1979
42. Nakano A, Hamada Y, Hirono M: Differentiation between pseudo- and malignant lymphoma of the breast. Jpn J Surg 12:76–78, 1982
43. Banerjee D, Silva E: Mediastinal mass with acute leukemia. Myeloblastoma masquerading as lymphoblastic lymphoma. Arch Pathol Lab Med 105:126–129, 1981
44. Sears HF, Reid J: Granulocytic sarcoma. Local presentation of a systemic disease. Cancer 37:1808–1813, 1976
45. Navas JJ, Battifora H: Primary lymphoma of the breast. Ultrastructural study of two cases. Cancer 39:2025–2032, 1977
46. DeCosse JJ, Berg JW, Fracchia AA, et al: Primary lymphosarcoma of the breast. A review of 14 cases. Cancer 15:1264–1268, 1962
47. Lawler MR, Richie RE: Reticulum cell sarcoma of the breast. Cancer 20:1438–1446, 1967
48. Mambo NC, Burke JS, Butler JJ: Primary malignant lymphomas of the breast. Cancer 39:2033–2040, 1977
49. Jernstrom P, Sether JM: Primary lymphosarcoma of the mammary gland. JAMA 201:503–506, 1967
50. Freeman C, Berg JW, Cutter SJ: Occurrence and prognosis of extranodal lymphomas. Cancer 29:252–260, 1972
51. Lin JJ, Farha GJ, Taylor RJ: Pseudolymphoma of the breast in a study of 8654 consecutive tylectomies and mastectomies. Cancer 45:973–978, 1980
52. Hajdu SI, Urban JA: Cancers metastatic to the breast. Cancer 29:1691–1696, 1972
53. Toombs BD, Kalisher L: Metastatic disease to the breast. Clinical, pathologic, and radiographic features. Am J Roentgenol 129:673–676, 1977
54. Sandiston AT: Metastatic tumors in the breast. Br J Surg 47:54–58, 1959
55. Charache H: Metastatic tumors in the breast. Surgery 33:385–390, 1953
56. Harriet T, Kalisher L: Breast metastasis: An unusual manifestation of a malignant carcinoid tumor. Cancer 40:3102–3111, 1977
57. Paulus DD, Libshitz HI: Metastasis to the breast. Radiol Clin North Am 20:561–568, 1982
58. McCrea ES, Johnston C, Haney DJ: Metastases to the breast. AJR 141:685–690, 1983
59. Moncada R, Cooper RA, Garces M: Calcified metastases from malignant ovarian neoplasm. Radiology 113:31–35, 1974
60. Royen PM, Ziter FMH: Ovarian carcinoma metastatic to the breast. Br J Radiol 47:356–357, 1974

Breast Cancer and Pregnancy

Jeanne A. Petrek

INCIDENCE

The relationship of breast cancer to pregnancy is problematic. Although reports note that pregnancy and lactation may be concurrent with as much as 1% to 2% of all breast cancer,[1] the percentage associated with breast cancer is actually much higher, given that the occult preclinical phase of tumor growth can require several years.[2,3] That is, a large percentage of breast cancers in younger women may have been present during previous pregnancy. However, this report is typical in considering breast cancer as associated with pregnancy only if the diagnosis was made during the pregnant period or within 1 year afterward.

Diagnosed breast cancers occur in between 10 and 39 cases per 100,000 deliveries,[4,5] making the malignancy approximately as common as that of the uterine cervix.[6] Although only 1% to 2% of all breast cancer patients are pregnant or postpartum, the incidence among breast cancer patients less than 40 years old is at least 15%.[1,7]

One investigator,[8] noting an even higher coincidence among young women, has reported that 10% of 67 patients less than 35 years old were pregnant at the time of diagnosis and that an additional 15% had been pregnant within the previous year. With more women bearing children later in life, this incidence will probably rise.

DIAGNOSIS

A thorough breast examination is especially important at the first obstetric visit, since with the progression of pregnancy there is increasing firmness, nodularity, and hypertrophy, which may obscure a subtle mass lesion. Masses may feel similar to and are readily attributed to the thickness produced by normal hypertrophy during pregnancy. This process may disguise and cover the masses, creating the illusion that they have resolved.

The hyperemia and increased water content of the breasts during pregnancy contribute to a generalized radiographic density, with loss of the contrasting fatty tissue that usually helps to define tumor masses.[9] Even though there is virtually no risk of ionizing radiation to a developing infant—particularly if the abdomen is shielded—mammograms are not routinely performed to visualize a palpable mass. On the other hand, because of natural variation due to the individual breasts and stage of pregnancy, mammograms may be helpful in a particular patient. Breast ultrasonography, although not posing any radiation risks, has not been routinely performed and there are no standards for its interpretation in the breast of a pregnant woman. Nevertheless, it should be accurate—as it is in nonpregnant women—in differentiating cyst from solid.

Aspiration of masses with a fine needle readily serves to differentiate cysts or galactoceles from solid tumors. Benign lesions during pregnancy, in decreasing order of frequency, include fibroadenomas, lipomas, papillomas, fibrocystic disease, galactoceles, and inflammatory lesions.[10] In Byrd's[11] series of 105 benign biopsies, 71% of patients had conditions also found in nonpregnant women and 29% had changes peculiar to gestation, such as lobular hyperplasia, galactocele, lactational mastitis, and so on. Moreover, localized breast infarcts can cause mass lesions during pregnancy, either from overgrowth of a preexisting fibroadenoma[12] or spontaneously.[13]

Inflammatory cancer probably arises no more frequently in pregnant patients than in others,[1,14] despite earlier opinions to the contrary.[4,15] Notwithstanding referral patterns that might attract more severe cases, only 3% of pregnant patients with breast cancer at Memorial Hospital had inflammatory breast cancer.[16] Nevertheless, the surgeon must not make the dire error of mistaking inflammatory cancer for the quite common lactational mastitis or abscess.[17] White made the simple suggestion more than 30 years ago to perform a biopsy on all lactational abscesses at the time of incision and drainage.[15]

Many authors have attributed to delay of diagnosis the advanced disease and poor prognosis often characteristic of gestational breast cancer. One of the first reports[18] noted that pregnant or lactating patients delayed 6 months before seeking a physician and that the physician waited an average of 3 months before biopsy. More recent reports[7,19,20] similarly note delays of several months. One such report[21] compared delay in pregnant or lactating patients with that in other women in the same institution and found that the former delayed an average of 7 months longer than the latter. Only one author[11] states that delays are not different from those in nongestational patients. However, considering that pregnant women are in routine contact with their obstetricians, it is not surprising to note that the majority of the delay before biopsy has been attributed to physician procrastination.[11]

A study of 63 breast cancer patients referred to Memorial Hospital between 1960 to 1980 and diagnosed while pregnant or one year postpartum seems to reveal particular reluctance toward performing a biopsy during pregnancy.[16] Less than 20% of such patients were diagnosed and treated during pregnancy. Almost half were diagnosed and treated within 12 weeks after delivery for a mass often documented during pregnancy. Even in those with previously undocumented masses, the large size of the cancers at the time of postpartum diagnosis (median of 3 cm) makes it likely that a smaller mass was palpable during pregnancy.

SPECIAL PROBLEMS OF BREAST BIOPSY DURING PREGNANCY AND LACTATION

Even more so than on the nongestational breast, biopsy of the breast of a pregnant or lactating woman calls for careful hemostasis because of increased vascularity. Biopsy of the lactating breast further requires meticulous attention to sterility, given the good culture medium provided by milk. Local anesthesia is theoretically safer, although general anesthesia is acceptable, especially in the later phases of pregnancy (see the section on teratogenesis, below).

In the earlier literature, Byrd[11] reported only one fetal demise in 134 biopsies on pregnant patients under general anesthesia. (Follow-up on the delivery and physical condition of the infants was not made.) Nevertheless, the administration of drugs pre-, intra-, and postoperatively requires special knowledge and caution. Obstetric consultation is probably advisable in every case. All patients in Byrd's series were prepared for immediate mastectomy in the event of malignancy, as was more common then.

Since doctors and patients realize the value of a routine two-stage procedure (in the event that breast cancer is found), local anesthesia for breast biopsy during pregnancy seems even more attractive. The preparatory work necessary before definitive treatment usually militates against proceeding under the biopsy anesthetic. A brief delay between biopsy and mastectomy or other definitive treatment affords the surgeon time to plan with oncologic and obstetric members of the team and allows the patient and her family to consider the pregnancy in light of the proposed cancer treatment.

Although excisional biopsies under local anesthesia during pregnancy may occasionally be difficult, depending on the individual breast, an incisional biopsy can be an excellent choice. Liberal use of electrocautery and other hemostatic techniques will be useful. Since extraneous drugs are always avoided in pregnancy, prophylactic antibiotics probably should not be given, despite a presumed higher infection rate without them. In the absence of literature on the subject, there appears to be no contraindication to core needle biopsy nor to needle aspiration on the breast of the pregnant woman. As is the case in nonpregnant patients, the needle technique runs the risk of missing the mass unbeknownst to the surgeon.

Because of the risk of infection and milk fistula, the breast should cease milk production before scalpel or core needle biopsy is performed. Some kinds of hormonal manipulation for "drying up" breast milk, such as lowering the level of prolactin by the use of bromocriptine, have not been associated with breast cancer.[22] Nevertheless, it may be wisest to stop milk production "naturally" by instructing the patient to cease breastfeeding. Binding the breasts and using ice packs may be folkloric but cannot do any harm. If a woman will not stop nursing but will accept the risk of fistula or infection (best recorded in writing), the surgeon can proceed with biopsy, depending on individual factors such as location of the lump and so on. Although there appear to be no data on the subject, it is surmisable that the risk of milk fistula rises from almost nonexistent in peripheral biopsies to significant in central biopsies.

As concerns infection, if the woman stops nursing for 2 days, a dose of preoperative prophylactic antibiotics can be given. The milk, containing the mother's antibiotics, can be expressed by breast pump during this period and discarded. After a brief period of bottle feeding, the infant may then resume breastfeeding, assuming a benign diagnosis.

CONSIDERATIONS OF THE DEVELOPING FETUS IN DIAGNOSTIC TESTS AND TREATMENT

In cancer diagnosis and treatment, dangers to the developing fetus include those influencing development, such as teratogenicity caused by radiation, chemotherapy, and general anesthesia. In addition to possible congenital abnormalities, various other risks such as intrauterine growth retardation resulting in low birth weight and possible postnatal neoplasia must also be considered.

Radiation Risks

Most knowledge regarding the effects of ionizing radiation on the embryo and fetus comes from experiments with mice and rats. Although one must always exercise caution in extrapolating these animal data to humans, existing human information correlates with observations in rodents.

In both rodents and humans, the principal effect of radiation during the preimplantation period (from conception to days 10 to 14) is embryo death. The second period, that of organogenesis (lasting from days 10 to 14 through the eighth week), is undoubtedly the most sensitive to ionizing radiation. There is a 20% incidence of severe malformations (often involving the central nervous system) in mice with exposures as low as 18 cGy and a 100% incidence with 200 cGy.[23] In the pregnant women of Hiroshima and Nagasaki, an air dose of 1 to 9 cGy during weeks 6 through 11 of pregnancy resulted in an 11% incidence of microcephaly and mental retardation in children, compared with 4% in a Japanese nonirradiated control population.[24] However, two factors related to the atomic bomb probably accounted for a greater proportion of malformations than would occur with a similar amount of medical irradiation: (1) A certain unknown proportion of the radiation was neutron, which has a greater biologic effect than the same amount of gamma irradiation. (2) The single-dose exposure would have a greater biologic effect than the same dose received over a protracted period.

Radiation exposure during the fetal period of gestation (from 8 weeks to term) is much less likely to produce congenital abnormalities than during the organogenesis period. The only observed developmental effect in mice is stunted growth.[23] In humans, microcephaly has been observed after radiation exposures during the early fetal period, but, dose-for-dose, the incidence is four to five times less than after exposure during the earlier organogenesis period.[24] After about 30 weeks of gestation, radiation-induced congenital defects are extremely rare.[25]

Accordingly, the atomic bomb experience and animal experimentation urge the conclusion that 5 cGy is the dose level at which radiation-induced anomalies become meaningful. The American Academy of Pediatrics (1978) and other organizations support the recommendation of the American College of Radiology that interruption of pregnancy on the basis of radiation risk is not justified if the fetus or embryo was exposed to less than 5 cGy.[1]

Another theoretical risk of radiation is carcinogenesis in the offspring. Although some retrospective studies indicate an association between pre-natal x-ray exposure (usually via maternal pelvimetry) and future childhood cancers, it is not clear that the x-ray exposure was the cause of the increased incidence. Even so, the risk of leukemia at 10 years following a 2-cGy exposure is only 1:2000 versus 1:3000 in unexposed controls.[26] Therefore, the risk of future carcinogenesis should be kept in perspective.

STAGING PROCEDURES DURING PREGNANCY

Accurate staging and appropriate treatment depend on comprehensive evaluation for metastatic disease. Since ultrasonography is not applicable in most organs and magnetic resonance (MR) imaging is preliminary, most techniques for diagnosing distant metastases use roentgen rays and radionuclides.

Although the calculation of the possible embryonic or fetal dose should be individualized, published estimates of the approximate fetal and maternal exposures are available.[27] The radiation dose to the embryo, fetus, or even a particular fetal organ can be calculated by a medical physicist trained in nuclear medicine when the relevant parameters are known (amount, chemical form and radiation characteristics of the radionuclide, maternal health and size, stage of gestation, and so on[28]).

Some guidelines can be made for recommended staging tests. There is no contraindication to a chest x-ray. Appropriate abdominal and pelvic shielding may be valuable, especially during the organogenesis and early fetal periods. Late in pregnancy, with the gravid uterus directly under the diaphragm, fetal shielding will obscure the lower lung parenchyma. Nevertheless, exposing the fetus to less than 1 cGy with a chest x-ray should be no problem, since in late pregnancy the fetus is resistant to developmental malformation. As regards evaluation for bone metastases, serum alkaline phosphatase can be elevated due to pregnancy itself. Conventional radiography, excluding the pelvis and lumbosacral spine, can evaluate some areas (e.g., ribs, long bones) and should always be performed if there are symptoms. For example, an extremity film of the pregnant patient results in 1 mRad estimated average fetal dose, compared with 275 mRad estimated fetal dose for lumbar-spine films. Examination of the patient's skull produces 4 mRad fetal dosage compared with 300 mRad for the patient's hip films.[25]

There is no adequate substitute for a bone scan, one of the tests used most for staging breast cancer. However, the bone scan may be deleted from preoperative staging in many individuals, since data gathered from 12 studies have shown only a 3% true-positive yield in Stage I, 7% in Stage II, and 25% in Stage III.[29] Therefore, if a patient with Stage I or II disease has no special indications such as bone pain, bone scan is usually avoided. For Stage III pregnant patients, the increased possibility of early detection of bone metastases may provide a rational approach to treatment plans if it yields proof of incurability. Calculations by the nuclear medical physicist can estimate the absorbed fetal dosage. Therefore, the benefit of the test must be weighed against the small risk of teratogenesis.

If neurologic symptoms or evaluating late-stage disease renders evaluation of the brain necessary, a head CT scan with abdominal shielding provides negligible x-ray exposure to the fetus. The circulating radionuclide of a brain scan would provide greater radiation exposure to the fetus. If liver scan is indicated, ultrasonography can be performed instead, although the radionuclide scan or liver CT scan may still be indicated if ultrasonography is equivocal. If the pregnancy is in its very early stage, it may be possible to perform a liver CT scan in the upper abdomen with appropriate pelvic shielding.

RADIOTHERAPY AS AN ALTERNATIVE TO MASTECTOMY

It is important to discuss the topic of breast preservation as an alternative to mastectomy, irrespective of pregnancy, while bearing in mind the unacceptability of dosages greater than 5 cGy to a developing human fetus. The fetal dose can be estimated by thermoluminescent dosimeters placed in an anatomical phantom constructed similar to the individual or by measurement on the individual woman with external abdominal shielding. However, as explained below, a standard external radiotherapy course of 5000 cGy will expose the fetus to at least 10 to 15 cGy, and primary radiotherapy should be discarded as a treatment option in currently pregnant women.

The developing fetus receives from several tenths of a percent to several percent of the breast dose, depending on the distance from the center of the radiation field, the field size, the individual radiotherapy unit, and the radiation energy used. Leakage from the radiotherapy unit and internal scatter from within the body account for most of the fetal irradiation. The radiation leakage should not exceed 0.1% of the direct beam exposure rate, as measured at a distance of 1 m from the radiation source.[30] Therefore, as the fetus nears the radiation field center, the radiation received will increase. The amount of fetal exposure due to radiation leakage can be reduced by external abdominal shielding.

The radiation reaching the fetus from internal scatter by the mother's tissues cannot be reduced by external shielding. The quantity of such radiation depends on (1) the distance of the fetus from the field center, (2) the field size, and (3) the energy of the radiation. The first two factors are self-evident. Higher energies produce less fetal dosage because less radiation is scattered toward the fetus—that is, a 6-meV linear accelerator produces less fetal dose by scatter than a 1.25-meV cobalt-60 unit.

For example, when the fetus is less than 12 weeks (i.e., is still in the true pelvis and perhaps 40 cm from field center), the dose from a field that is 10 cm × 10 cm and is produced by a 4-meV unit would be in the range of 0.2% to 0.3% of the tumor dose. This results in 10 to 15 cGy for a treatment course of 5000 cGy. Toward the end of pregnancy, if a fetal part is 10 cm distant from the center, it will receive 200 cGy for the same treatment course.[1]

Likewise, adjuvant radiation after mastectomy poses the same hazard to the fetus. Since routine postmastectomy irradiation is of arguable benefit in Stages I and II in the nonpregnant woman, it should be avoided in similar-staged pregnant women. Although some physicians may feel strongly about internal mammary lymph node irradiation in a medially located lesion, it is wisest to postpone the treatment course until after the pregnancy. Irradiation in Stage III and Stage IV is often indicated because of the high risk of local recurrence. Nevertheless, it is probably wisest to delay the radiotherapy until the patient is no longer pregnant. If local recurrence occurs prior to delivery, it should be excised to the extent possible to enable further postponement of irradiation at least until late in pregnancy. In the last trimester, the risk of teratogenesis is greatly lessened. However, a tumor dose of 5000 cGy to the breast or chest wall will result in at least 10 to 20 cGy of fetal exposure, depending on the beam energy, field size, radiotherapy unit, and size of the patient and fetus.

CHEMOTHERAPY

Chemotherapeutic agents are minimally selective and usually affect rapidly proliferating cells, which makes the developing fetal cells a prime target for teratogenesis.[25] However, the human incidence of congenital anomaly after *in utero* chemotherapy exposure appears small. Whether it is truly small or whether the collection of case reports (on which incidence is estimated) is biased is unknown.

The fetal effect is related to drug dosage, to gestational age, to synergism when combined with other drugs or radiation, and to the individual drugs—working, as they do, through different mechanisms and at different molecular sites. The placenta may create a biologic barrier to some antineoplastic agents,[31] although most apparently readily traverse the placenta.[32]

In general, antimetabolites, and particularly folic acid antagonists such as methotrexate, carry a significant risk of producing congenital anomalies.[33] Therefore, no particular agent, much less a combination, can be considered safe. Recent reports of several successful pregnancies[34–40] almost all involve leukemia and lymphoma.

There are several excellent reviews of fetal effects.[41–44] Nicholson reviewed 185 pregnancies reported prior to 1967 and suggested that fewer than 8% of infants had an obvious congenital malformation when the drugs were administered in the first trimester and later exposure was not associated with increased congenital malformation.[43] A decade later, Sweet suggested in his review[41] that if aminopterin, a known abortifacient, were excluded from the analysis, the risk of congenital anomalies was about 5%, similar to that of nonexposed infants. Nevertheless, in this series (and one other[43] as large), 40% of infants exposed to chemotherapy *in utero* were of low birth weight. The concern is thus one of subtle anomalies undetected at birth and of future slow development. In summary, the decision to treat with chemotherapy—whether adjuvant or palliative—must be made by the patient after due deliberation over risks and benefits.

METASTATIC DISEASE IN THE FETUS AND PLACENTA

Only melanoma and choriocarcinoma have been reported to cause actual fetal metastases.[45] Placental metastases have been reported in only 30 patients with solid tumor.[46] Microscopic examination of the placenta—especially of the intervillous space—is important as only half the patients had visible metastases.[47]

ANESTHETIC CONSIDERATIONS

General anesthesia is necessary for a mastectomy or axillary dissection, and sometimes even for an adequate tumorectomy. There is a plethora of conditions that make general anesthesia of pregnant women difficult. These include increased blood volume, increased heart rate and cardiac output, increased platelet count and fibrinogen level, supine positional hypotension, decreased pulmonary functional residual capacity, elevated diaphragms, prolonged gastric emptying, hypervascularity of the respiratory tract mucosa, and so on. As compared with the risks of teratogenesis from radiation and chemotherapy, those associated with the general anesthetic drugs are small. As is well known, the most critical time is that of the organogenesis period, from day 14 to day 56 of gestation. Despite the fact that nitrous oxide and halothane interfere *in vitro* with nucleic acid synthesis,[48,49] no deleterious effects can be detected in humans.[48] These potent inhalational agents have the theoretical advantage of relaxing uterine musculature and forestalling premature labor. In fact, premature labor seems to depend more on the surgical site—being more common with lower abdominal or pelvic operations—than on anesthetic technique and is not likely with breast operations. In any event, obstetricians have several drugs for reversal of premature labor. Barbiturates, including common drugs such as Pentothal, are known to protect the monkey and rat fetus against hypoxic brain damage. With respect to narcotics, studies of offspring of narcotics addicts indicate no fetal effects other than low birth weight.

In summary, balanced narcotic or inhalation anesthesia may be chosen with careful attention to dosage (often reduced in pregnancy) and adequate oxygenation. Fetal monitoring should be used whenever possible, so that patterns of fetal distress may be followed immediately by fine adjustments of anesthetic technique.

THE QUESTION OF THERAPEUTIC ABORTION

The traditional older view of concurrent breast cancer and pregnancy as an especially dreaded situation may have contributed to zealous enthusiasm for abortion, usually combined with oophorectomy. For example, Haagensen and Stout (1943)[50] recommended refusing operation to any breast cancer patient diagnosed during pregnancy or lactation as categorically incurable (although they later changed their opinion).[51] In 1953, Adair[52] at Memorial Hospital noted longer crude survival rates associated with therapeutic abortion, especially for patients with axillary lymph node involvement (these differences were not statistically significant).

Gradually thereafter, both the opinion on the uniformly lethal nature of concurrent breast cancer and pregnancy and the unquestioned value of therapeutic abortion began to change. Holleb and Farrow,[53] also at Memorial Hospital, reported in 1962 on 24 patients treated with radical mastectomy; half underwent abortion and half did not. In this instance, the 5-year clinical cure rate of the patients who underwent abortion was inferior to that of patients who were allowed to deliver normally. The difference was 17% versus 33%, but again it was not significant. The most recent reports from the mid-1980s[54,55] also do not show any advantage in survival rate with therapeutic abortion. In all these data, reported numbers are small, cases are not precisely staged, and selection is an important biasing factor (with advanced cases more likely to undergo therapeutic abortion). Nevertheless, when combined with standard therapy, the benefit of routine therapeutic abortion cannot be demonstrated. There is a growing tendency to minimize pregnancy and treat the patient similarly to her nonpregnant counterpart. Byrd[11] summed up this attitude after a review of material at Vanderbilt University: "In the face of general enthusiasm for terminating the pregnancy, we believe the evidence is that the cancer should be terminated."

On the other hand, therapeutic abortion may be strongly recommended because of the danger to the fetus from the proposed chemotherapy or radiation treatments. If a hormone receptor assay by a laboratory experienced in gestational breast cancer suggests hormone responsivity of an individual tumor, therapeutic abortion might also be advised. Moreover, rapid advancement of the disease during pregnancy might also constitute clinical evidence for the value of therapeutic abortion in the individual case. In the end, it is the parents' responsibility to make an informed decision about their family.

TREATMENT DELAY

In view of the above, it is generally agreed that modified radical mastectomy (and sometimes radical mastectomy for pectoralis invasion, bulky nodes, and so on) without delay is indicated for potentially curable stages of breast cancer, regardless of the trimester of pregnancy or decision for therapeutic abortion. However, one author[56] believed that patients whose cancer was discovered in the third trimester should have been allowed to deliver before mastectomy, if the tumor was not aggressive and if a prolonged delay was not involved. Even though patients thus treated had a good survival rate in the retrospective study, this is likely to be the result of selection, in that only the more favorable patients were delayed. Certainly, a policy of significant delay entails risk for the patient and places an exceptional burden of responsibility on the physician. With the safety afforded by advances in obstetrics, anesthesia, and surgery, significant delay before mastectomy in the routine pregnancy cannot be condoned. Comments and speculation on the advisability and timing of therapeutic abortion, castration, chemotherapy, and radiotherapy are found above.

PROGNOSIS

Since the earliest reports more than a century ago, the prognosis for patients with breast cancer during pregnancy has gradually improved. Kilgore and Bloodgood[57] in 1929 reported a 17% 5-year survival rate. Haagensen and Stout[50] reported no survivors, and White's collective series (1953)[4] showed only an 8.6% overall 5-year survival rate.

At about the same time, Harrington[58] is credited with starting to revive optimism about treatment. He reported on 92 patients operated on at the Mayo Clinic; there was a 61% 5-year survival rate among those without axillary metastases. Unfortunately, presentation with lymph node metastases is common. Three-fourths (74%) of Montgomery's[59] 70 patients had axillary metastases. Seventy-two percent of Holleb and Farrow's (1964)[53] group had axillary metastases, as did 75% of Applewhite's (1973)[21] group.

Eight papers published during the 1960s,[11,53,56,60,61,62,63,64,65] reporting numbers of patients ranging from 29 to 117, found a rate of positive lymph nodes ranging from 53% to 74% (median of 65%). Four similar papers[5,21,66,67] published during the 1970s found a rate of positive lymph nodes from 56% to 81%. Only several studies have attempted to put these percentages into the context of the patient's age, time period, and institution by designating a nonpregnant comparison group.

The pregnant and 1-year postpartum patients with technically operable tumors (AJC Stages I/II/III) diagnosed at Memorial Hospital between 1960 and 1980 were compared with a nonpregnant group of the same age, diagnosed during the same time period.[16] Sixty-one percent of the pregnancy-associated patients had positive lymph nodes versus 38% of their nonpregnant counterparts ($p > 0.05$). Only 31% of the pregnant patients had pathologic T1 tumors versus 50% of their counterparts ($p>0.05$). (The further studies on these Memorial Hospital patients are similar to other studies[7,8,55,61,68,69] which also include a "control" group.) Only four Memorial Hospital patients were lost before 5-year follow-up (and one patient before a 10-year follow-up). These five were known to have recurrent disease.

The 23 Memorial Hospital pregnancy-associated patients with negative lymph nodes had a 79% 5-year survival rate compared with 82% in their nonpregnant counterparts. The 29 patients with positive lymph nodes had a 46% 5-year survival rate compared with 58% in their counterpart. Eleven of the 63 patients presented with technically inoperable primary tumors or distant metastases and had a median survival of 1 year. Among pregnancy-associated patients who were eligible, there was a 76% 10-year survival rate for those with negative lymph nodes and a 25% rate for those with positive lymph nodes. In comparison, the 10-year survival rate was 75% for the nonpregnant patients with negative nodes and 42% for the nonpregnant patients with positive nodes. The differences in survival times are not statistically significant.

The series of Haagensen,[19] of Peters,[61] and of Bunker and Peters[56] are valuable because of the personally supervised treatment of gestational breast cancer and excellent follow-up. Stage for stage, the survival times are either equivalent between the pregnancy-associated patients and the "control" group, or the pregnancy-associated group has a somewhat inferior survival time, although the difference is not statistically significant.

Several authors[8,19,69] suggest that gestational breast cancer patients have an increased incidence of synchronous and metachronous contralateral tumors. Incidence in the Memorial Hospital series was 7 patients out of 63, which is only slightly higher than in nonpregnant patients of the control group.[16]

STEROID HORMONE RECEPTORS

Little is known about the accuracy and ultimate value of steroid hormone receptor status during pregnancy. The results of a small collected series of ten pregnant patients showed eight to be estrogen receptor negative, and 2 to be low positive.[1] Pregnancy may depress levels of estrogen/progesterone receptor detectable in breast cancer cytosol fractions and result in false negatives. Circulating levels of estrogens in pregnancy exceed those of the normal menstrual cycle by a factor of ten or more, and levels of progesterone late in pregnancy by a factor of three or more. Such high levels should cause receptor translocation into the nucleus and should occupy all the cytoplasmic receptor. In the nonpregnant state, only up to 36% of cytosol receptor was occupied by endogenous steroid, so that most was available for assay.[70] When the receptor assay is performed during pregnancy, unbound estrogen should first be removed by treatment of cytosol with dextran-charcoal.[71] Exchange assays should then be performed to detect occupied estrogen receptor within cytosol[72] and nuclei.[73] Since most laboratories are not experienced in these techniques, the frozen tissue should be shipped to a laboratory where the procedures are routinely performed. No retrospective data on pregnant patients with accurate hormone receptor status now exist for formulating recommendations on therapeutic abortions, hormonal manipulation, or subsequent pregnancies.

EFFECT OF SUBSEQUENT PREGNANCY ON BREAST CANCER PROGNOSIS

Many more breast cancer patients will be seeking medical advice about pregnancy, since oophorectomy is no longer performed adjuvantly and more women are bearing children in later years. Even the earlier literature suggested that about 7% of women who are fertile after mastectomy have one or more pregnancies, and 70% of these pregnancies were to be expected within the first 5 years.[10]

It has been generally observed that women who subsequently become pregnant survive very well, usually better than those with concurrent pregnancy, and often the same or slightly better than mastectomy patients with no subsequent pregnancy. Eight (67%) of White's[15] 12 patients who became pregnant lived at least 5 years, and 58% for 10 years. A similar finding was recorded by Rissanen,[74] whose 53 patients had 5- and 10-year survival rates of 77% and 69%, respectively. Fifty percent of patients in Cheek's series[75] survived 5 years, but only 29% of Applewhite and colleagues'[21] series survived 5 years. Holleb and Farrow[53] reported on 52 patients with an overall 5-year survival rate of 52%, whereas a 75% 5-year survival rate was reported by Cooper and Butterfield[76] in 32 patients. In the most recent analysis,[77] 41 Memorial Hospital patients who became pregnant after breast cancer treatment had an 80% 5-year survival rate. Sixteen had undergone first-trimester abortions, but this group did not have a survival rate different from that of patients undergoing a full-term delivery. Are these good results purely a function of selection? Is it only women with a good prognosis from the outset and no recurrence who live long enough to become pregnant? Medical personnel may not have warned good-prognosis patients as strenuously against pregnancy, and a personal belief in their favorable outlook may subconsciously have allowed women with a good prognosis to become pregnant.

The factor of a better prognosis is supported by the lower frequency of axillary lymph node metastases present in the group who later became pregnant when compared with other mastectomy populations. For example, in Holleb and Farrow's[53] large series, only 46% of patients who subsequently became pregnant had involved lymph nodes at the time of their mastectomy, compared, for example, with 72% of patients who had mastectomy while pregnant or postpartum.

The case-matching studies attempt to eliminate the obvious factor of pregnancy occurring only in those with a good prognosis. Ninety-six patients with subsequent pregnancy were matched by Peters with respect to both age and clinical stage.[61] The patients with subsequent pregnancy not only had a longer survival time than those without subsequent pregnancy but also had longer disease-free intervals when cases of recurrence were compared. Furthermore, when the factor of selection through early death was minimized by considering only those who became pregnant within 6 months after mastectomy, a respectable 54% were found to survive 5 years. In a more recent analysis, Cooper[76] matched each of 40 patients who subsequently became pregnant with two controls as determined by the clinical stage, age, status of lymph node involvement, and equal survival at least to the time of pregnancy. The patients with subsequent pregnancy still had a survival time superior to that of the controls.

Although these studies offer no evidence that pregnancy protects against breast cancer recurrence, they show no promotion of the disease. Theoretically, some of the multiple hormonal changes of pregnancy might be beneficial.[78] Urinary excretion of estriol is increased 1000 times during normal pregnancy, compared with 100-fold increase in estrone and estradiol. Estriol competes for estrogen binding sites and could displace estradiol from urine cytosol receptors. Estriol is an inhibitor of rat mammary carcinogenesis.[78]

As regards advice to the individual patient about pregnancy, most clinicians recommend at least a 2- to 3-year delay to allow aggressive disease to become manifest. After that time interval, the rate of breast cancer recurrence is smaller and more constant, year for year. If a pregnancy occurs even before 2 to 3 years, there is no evidence supporting routine termination. On the contrary, the 1981 Memorial Hospital study[77] on subsequent pregnancies could find no effect on survival, even when the patients who became pregnant within 2 years were compared with those who did so later.

REFERENCES

1. Wallack MK, Wolf JA Jr, Bedwinek J, et al: Gestational carcinoma of the female breast. Curr Probl Cancer 7:1–58, 1983
2. Moolgavkar SH, Day NE, Stevens RG: Two-stage model for carcinogenesis. Epidemiology of breast cancer in females. J Natl Cancer Inst 65:559–569, 1980
3. Donegan WL: Mastectomy in the primary management of invasive mammary carcinoma. In Hardy JD et al (eds): Advances in Surgery, Vol. 6, pp 1–101. Chicago, Year Book Medical Publishers, 1972
4. White TT: Carcinoma of the breast and pregnancy. Ann Surg 139:9–18, 1954
5. Peete CH, Honeycutt HC, Cherny WB: Cancer of the breast in pregnancy. NC Med J 27:514, 1966
6. Betson JR, Golden ML: Cancer and pregnancy. Am J Obstet Gynecol 81:718–728, 1961
7. Treves N, Holleb AI: A report of 549 cases of breast cancer in women 35 years of age or younger. Surg Gynecol Obstet 107:271–283, 1958
8. Horsley JS III, Alrich EM, Wright CB: Carcinoma of the breast in women 35 years of age or younger. Ann Surg 196:839–843, 1969
9. Hoeffken W, Lanyi M: Mammography. Philadelphia, WB Saunders, 1977

10. Donegan WL: Pregnancy and breast cancer. Obstet Gynecol 50:244–251, 1977
11. Byrd BF, Bayer DS, Robertson JC, et al: Treatment of breast tumors associated with pregnancy and lactation. Ann Surg 155:940–947, 1962
12. Majmudar B, Rosales-Quintana S: Infarction of breast fibroadenomas during pregnancy. JAMA 231:963–964, 1975
13. Rickert RR, Rajan S: Localized breast infarcts associated with pregnancy. Arch Pathol 97:159–161, 1974
14. Donegan WL: Mammary carcinoma and pregnancy. Major Probl Clin Surg 5:170–178, 1967
15. White TT: Carcinoma of the breast in the pregnant and the nursing patient. Am J Obstet Gynecol 69:1277–1286, 1955
16. Petrek JA: Pregnancy-associated (PA) breast cancer is not a different disease (Abstr). Submitted to The Society of Surgical Oncology, December 1, 1985
17. Zeigerman JH, Honigman FH, Crawford RW: Inflammatory mammary cancer during pregnancy and lactation. Obstet Gynecol 32:373–375, 1968
18. Westberg SV: Prognosis of breast cancer for pregnant and nursing women. Acta Obstet Gynecol Scand 25 (Suppl) 4:1, 1946
19. Haagensen CD: Carcinoma of the breast in pregnancy. In Haagensen CD: Diseases of the Breast, 2nd ed. Philadelphia, WB Saunders, 1971
20. Fleming U, Sheridan B, Atkinson L, et al: The effects of childbearing on carcinoma of the breast. Med J Aust 1:1252–1256, 1970
21. Applewhite RR, Smith LR, DiVincenti F: Carcinoma of the breast associated with pregnancy and lactation. Am Surg 39:101–104, 1973
22. Anderson JM: Mammary cancers and pregnancy. Br Med J 1:1124–1127, 1979
23. Hall EJ: Effects of radiation on the developing embryo. In Hall EJ: Radiobiology for the Radiologist, pp 231–239. New York, Harper and Row, 1973
24. Miller R, Mulvihill S: Small head size after atomic radiation. Teratology 14:355–357, 1976
25. Orr JW, Shingleton HM: Cancer in pregnancy. Curr Probl Cancer 8:1–50, 1983
26. Miller RW: Epidemiological conclusions from radiation toxicity studies. In Late Effects of Radiation. London, Taylor and Francis, 1970
27. Brent RL: The effects of ionizing radiation, microwaves, and ultrasound on the developing embryo: Clinical interpretations and applications of the data. Curr Probl Pediatr 14:61–87, 1984
28. Cloutier RJ, Smith SA, Watson EF: Dose to the fetus from radionuclides in the bladder. Health Phys 25:147–161, 1973
29. Harbert JC: Efficacy of bone and liver scanning in malignant disease. Facts and options. In Nuclear Medicine Annual. New York, Raven Press, 1982
30. National Council on Radiation Protection and Measurements Report #39: Basic Radiation Protection Criteria. Washington, DC, NCRP Productions, 1971
31. Roboz J, Gleicher N, Wu K, et al: Does doxorubicin cross the placenta? Lancet 2:1382–1383, 1979
32. Williamson RA, Karp LE: Azathioprene teratogenecity: Review of the literature and case report. Obstet Gynecol 58:247–250, 1981
33. Powell HR, Ekert H: Methotrexate-induced congenital malformations. Med J Aust 2:1076–1077, 1971
34. McLain CR Jr: Leukemia in pregnancy. Clin Obstet Gynecol 17:185–195, 1974
35. O'Dell RF: Leukemia and lymphoma complicating pregnancy. Clin Obstet Gynecol 22:859–870, 1979
36. Pizzuto J, Aviles A, Noreiga L, et al: Treatment of acute leukemia during pregnancy: Presentation of nine cases. Cancer Treat Rep 64:679–683, 1980
37. Alegre A, Chunchurreta R, Rodriguez-Alarcon J, et al: Successful pregnancy in acute promyelocytic leukemia. Cancer 49:152–153, 1982
38. Sanz MA, Rafecas FJ: Successful pregnancy during chemotherapy for acute promyelocytic leukemia. N Engl J Med 306:939, 1982
39. Schwartz PE, Vidone RA: Pregnancy following combination chemotherapy for a mixed germ cell tumor of the ovary. Gynecol Oncol 12:373–378, 1981
40. Rosenshein NB, Grumbine FC, Woodruff JD, et al: Pregnancy following chemotherapy for an ovarian immature embryonal teratoma. Gynecol Oncol 8:234–239, 1979
41. Sweet DL Jr, Kinzie J: Consequences of radiotherapy and antineoplastic therapy for the fetus. J Reprod Med 17:241–246, 1976
42. Barber HRK: Fetal and neonatal effects of cytotoxic agents. Obstet Gynecol 58:41S--47S, 1981
43. Nicholson HO: Cytotoxic drugs in pregnancy. J Obstet Gynaecol Br Emp 75:307–312, 1968
44. Stutzman L, Sokal JE: Use of anticancer drugs during pregnancy. Clin Obstet Gynecol 11:416–427, 1968
45. Potter JF, Schoeneman M: Metastases of maternal cancer to the placenta and fetus. Cancer 25:380–388, 1970
46. Smythe AR, Underwood PB, Kreutner A: Metastatic placental tumors. Report of three cases. Am J Obstet Gynecol 125:1149–1151, 1973
47. Fox H: Non-trophoblastic tumors of the placenta. In Fox H (ed): Pathology of the Placenta. pp 357–360. Philadelphia, WB Saunders, 1978
48. Pedersen H, Finster M: Anesthetic risks in the pregnant surgical patient. Anesthesiology 51:439–451, 1979
49. Nunn FJ: Faulty cell replication, abortion, congenital abnormalities. In Cottrell JE (ed). International Anesthesiology Clinics. Occupational Hazards to Operating Room and Recovery Room Personnel. Vol 19(4), pp 82–83. Boston, Little, Brown & Co, 1981
50. Haagensen CD, Stout AP: Carcinoma of the breast: Criteria of operability. Ann Surg 118:859–870, 1032–1051, 1943
51. Haagensen CD: The treatment and results in cancer of the breast at the Presbyterian Hospital, New York. Am J Roentgenol 62:328–334, 1949
52. Adair FE: Cancer of the breast. Surg Clin North Am 33:313, 1953
53. Holleb AI, Farrow JH: The relation of carcinoma of the breast and pregnancy in 283 patients. Surg Gynecol Obstet 115:65–71, 1962
54. Nugent P, O'Connell TX: Breast cancer and pregnancy. Arch Surg 120:1221–1224, 1985
55. King RM, Welch JS, Martin JK, et al: Carcinoma of the breast associated with pregnancy. Surg Gynecol Obstet 160:228–232, 1985
56. Bunker ML, Peters MV: Breast cancer associated with pregnancy or lactation. Am J Obstet Gynecol 85:312–321, 1963
57. Kilgore AR, Bloodgood JC: Tumors and tumor-like lesions of the breast in association with pregnancy. Arch Surg 18:2079–2098, 1929
58. Harrington SW: Carcinoma of the breast: Results of surgical treatment when the carcinoma occurred in course of pregnancy or lactation and when pregnancy occurred subsequent to operation. 1910–1933. Ann Surg 106:690–700, 1937
59. Montgomery TL: Detection and disposal of breast cancer in pregnancy. Am J Obstet Gynecol 81:926–933, 1961

60. Miller HK: Cancer of the breast during pregnancy and lactation. Am J Obstet Gynecol 83:607–611, 1962
61. Peters MV: The effect of pregnancy in breast cancer. In Forrest APM, Kunkler PB (eds): Prognostic Factors in Breast Cancer. pp 65–80. Baltimore, Williams & Wilkins, 1968
62. Mickal A, Torres JE, Mule JG: Carcinoma of breast in pregnancy and lactation. Am Surg 29:509–514, 1963
63. Rosemond GP: Carcinoma of the breast during pregnancy. Clin Obstet Gynecol 6:994–1001, 1963
64. DeVitt JE, Beattie WG, Stoddart TG: Carcinoma of the breast and pregnancy. Can J Surg 7:124–128, 1964
65. Holleb AI, Farrow JH: Breast cancer and pregnancy. Acta Unio Int Contra Cancrum 20:1480, 1964
66. Crosby CH, Barclay THC: Carcinoma of the breast: Surgical management of patients with special conditions. Cancer 28:1628–1636, 1971
67. Clark RM, Reid J: Carcinoma of the breast in pregnancy and lactation. Int J Radiat Oncol Biol Phys 4:693–698, 1978
68. Ribeiro GG, Palmer MK: Breast carcinoma associated with pregnancy: Clinicians' dilemma. Br Med J 2:1524–1527, 1977
69. Deemarsky LJ, Neishtadt EL: Breast cancer and pregnancy. Breast 7:17–21, 1980
70. Sakai F, Saez S: Existence of receptors bound to endogenous estradiol in breast cancers in premenopausal and postmenopausal women. Steroids 27:99–110, 1976
71. Sarrif WM, Durant JR: Evidence that estrogen-receptor-negative progesterone-receptor-positive breast and ovarian carcinoma contain estrogen receptor. Cancer 48:1215–1220, 1981
72. Katzenellenbogen JA, Johnson HJ Jr, Carlson KE, et al: Studies on the uterine, cytoplasmic estrogen binding protein. Thermal stability and ligand dissociation rate. An assay of empty and filled sites by exchange. Biochemistry 12:4092–4099, 1973
73. Garola RE, McGuire WL: An improved assay for nuclear estrogen receptor in experimental and human breast cancer. Cancer Res 37:3333–3337, 1977
74. Rissanen PM: Carcinoma of the breast during pregnancy and lactation. Br J Cancer 22:663–668, 1968
75. Cheek JH: Cancer of the breast in pregnancy and lactation. Am J Surg 126:729–731, 1973
76. Cooper DR, Butterfield J: Pregnancy subsequent to mastectomy for cancer of the breast. Ann Surg 171:429–433, 1970
77. Harvey JC, Rosen PP, Ashikari H, et al: The effect of pregnancy on the prognosis of carcinoma of the breast following radical mastectomy. Surg Gynecol Obstet 153:723–725, 1981
78. Lemon HM: Estriol and prevention of mammary carcinoma. Cancer Detect Prev 1:263–264, 1976

Occult Primary Tumor With Axillary Metastases

W. Bradford Patterson

On rare occasions, a breast cancer presents with enlarged axillary lymph nodes as the first sign of disease. Such patients, in whom a primary lesion is not apparent on physical examination or on a mammogram, pose a diagnostic and therapeutic dilemma: how far to pursue the search and how to treat the cancer that has almost certainly started elsewhere.

Until quite recently, the recommendations made by Halsted in 1907 have been the mainstay of treatment.[1] He described three patients who appeared first with axillary nodes and proved on subsequent follow-up to have breast cancer. Each was treated by radical mastectomy and included in his series. Subsequent authors have emphasized that when axillary nodes contain carcinoma, the ipsilateral breast will prove to be the source more often than not and that modern diagnostic aids such as electron microscopy, estrogen receptor determination, and mammography all are useful in making an accurate diagnosis. Mastectomy, with or without radiotherapy, has been most often recommended. This therapeutic plan needs to be more closely examined, in view of the evidence that local control of breast cancer can be achieved without immediate mastectomy. Breast-sparing approaches will be considered for more of the occult primaries in the future, although some local failures are predictable. How much impact the greatly improved techniques of mammography will have on exact diagnosis remains to be seen.

OCCURRENCE AND NATURAL HISTORY

In one of the few series that attempted to estimate the incidence of occult breast cancers, Owen reported finding 25 occult cases in 5451 patients with breast cancer. He calculated that, since two-thirds of the breast cancer patients seen at the Mayo Clinic in those years had axillary node involvement, 0.3% of breast cancers presented as occult primaries.[2] However, most series are reported from breast cancer clinics and centers, where diagnostic problems are often referred by community physicians and surgeons, and it is likely that the true incidence is somewhat less.

The age distribution of reported patients is similar to that of other patients with breast cancer. The reported range is 31 to 78 years and the average is 53. The predilection of breast cancer for the left side may be mimicked in the special situation when the primary tumor is occult, but the numbers are very small. An aspect of the natural history of greater interest is the length of time between diagnosis of cancer in an axillary node and the appearance of cancer in an untreated breast. Such data are anecdotal, since in most instances the breast has either been removed or irradiated. In Halsted's report of three patients, "a few months" to 2 1/2 years elapsed, but Haagensen reported one patient with an interval of 5 years and 4 months.[3]

AXILLARY ADENOPATHY AS A PRESENTING COMPLAINT

Transient node enlargement may occur with viral syndromes, infections in the arm or hand, and allergies. Persistent enlargement is more often due to cancer but, even when malignant, further progression may occur very slowly. Patients whose nodes proved malignant have given a history of enlargement for more than 4 years,[4] but most have been enlarged for a few weeks or months. Pierce studied 72 patients with enlarged axillary nodes in whom a biopsy was done. In 55, the node was not malignant. Of the remaining 17, malignant lymphoma was diagnosed in 10, metastatic adenocarcinoma in 5, squamous cell carcinoma in 1, and melanoma in 1.[5]

When malignant axillary nodes are the first sign of a breast cancer, the number of palpable nodes and the size of the mass may vary widely and probably depend on such variables as the patient's body habitus and regularity of medical care. Patients with a single node no larger than 0.9 cm have been reported as often as those with large fixed masses. In those patients who have an axillary lymph node dissection, which has usually been done as part of a radical or modified radical mastectomy, the number of additional involved nodes varies from none to more than 50. Among 142 patients reported with data concerning numbers of axillary nodes, 97 had additional involved nodes in the radical axillary dissection, whereas in 45 the only positive node was that initially palpable and excised to establish the diagnosis.[3,6–14]

The histology of axillary nodes identified as metastatic from occult breast cancers has been of interest to many authors. The most common microscopic finding has been infiltrating ductal carcinoma, but essentially all other variants—including medullary, comedocarcinoma, lobular, and papillary—have been regularly encountered. In a series of 27 cases reported from the Mayo Clinic in 1963, Owen and colleagues noted that 75% were comedocarcinomas and suggested that the relatively favorable prognosis in their series (9 of 18 living at 5 years and 6 of 12 living at 10 years) was related to this known favorable histology.[2] Later authors have not corroborated this pattern. For example, Patel and colleagues found that 21 of 29 patients had poorly differentiated adenocarcinoma.[12]

More than one investigator has raised the question of possible unique features in the cell type or histologic appearance of these as compared with other breast cancers. A recent report from the Memorial Sloan-Kettering Cancer Center states that the histology in two-thirds of their patients is characterized by a "diffuse infiltrate in the lymph node of large undifferentiated cells having clear to pink granular cytoplasm resulting in a distinctly apocrine look."[9] In 28 (65%) of 43 patients, this was the predominant pattern; in 7 (16%) a mixture of this pattern and the more common invasive ductal pattern was seen, and in 8 (18%) all sections showed a more usual histology. These observations should not be construed to mean that the "relatively undifferentiated cells with clear or granular pink cytoplasm" are unusual in breast cancer, but only that their appearance in two-thirds of a series is high. In this series, the occurrence of this pattern was similar in the lymph nodes and in the primary tumor.

A report from Duke University describes the use of electron microscopy to enhance the certainty with which breast cancer is implicated as the source of a malignant axillary node.[10] They report five cases in which initial histology (light microscopy) led to diagnoses of undifferentiated squamous carcinoma (1), lymphoma (1), melanoma (1), and undifferentiated carcinoma (2). With the aid of electron microscopy, all were shown to be highly consistent with breast cancer. To permit electron microscopic study, it is essential that tissue either be initially fixed in glutaraldehyde or at least that some thin-sliced tissue be kept in buffered formalin and not processed through paraffin embedding. Ultrastructural characteristics found in their five cases included differentiated features of adenocarcinomas, intracellular canaliculi, apical desmosomes, microvilli, and secretory vesicles. These authors and others stress the usefulness of estrogen and progesterone receptor determinations on the axillary nodal tissue. Results in the negative or borderline range are not helpful, but strongly positive receptor levels greatly aid in a diagnosis of breast cancer.

OCCULT CANCER IN THE BREAST

When a mastectomy has been performed on patients with occult breast cancer, careful sectioning of the breast tissue has disclosed a cancer in 55% to 100%.[2,3,6,8–10,12,15] The variation largely appears to be due to patient selection, and data suggest that in hospitals where a modified radical or radical mastectomy is routinely performed when adenocarcinoma is diagnosed in axillary nodes, 62% to 75% have a primary cancer identified in the specimen.[3,6,8,9]

Since by definition these breast cancers are occult, a careful search through any removed breast tissue is obligatory. Most commonly, thin sections of a few millimeters are cut by hand. In those cases in which no cancer can be found in the breast, it remains uncertain whether a very small primary lesion was overlooked or in fact was located elsewhere in the body.

In various reported series, the size of primary tumors has varied from 0.1 cm to 5.0 cm, with most in the 1- to 2-cm range.[3,6,8,10,14] Histologically, the primary cancers cover the same range of types reported above as being found in the axillary nodes.

Infrequently, noninvasive intraductal or lobular cancer is found. Rosen has reviewed a number of possible explanations for the finding of metastatic carcinoma in axillary nodes with only noninvasive carcinoma in the breast.[16] These include the following: (1) a focus of invasive cancer may be missed despite careful sectioning, (2) invasion may be occurring even though it is not detectable with light microscopy, (3) metastases may cross from the contralateral breast, (4) carcinoma from heterotopic breast tissue may be present in a lymph node, (5) invasive cancer may be present in breast tissue in the axillary fat and not examined, and (6) heterotopic glands in a lymph node may be misinterpreted as carcinoma.

We have recently seen a patient with an axillary mass that on excision proved to be adenocarcinoma consistent with a primary breast cancer, rather than an involved axillary node. On taking a history, the patient described a sizable axillary mass that had developed when she was nursing her one child 15 years previously, which "hung down from the under side of her arm like an egg." Clearly, she had ectopic breast tissue, the "axillary breast," a well-known occasional phenomenon.

WORK-UP AND STAGING

A pretreatment work-up of a patient with adenocarcinoma in axillary nodes and no obvious primary tumor is shown in Table 15-15. If lymphoma or sarcoma instead of carcinoma is diagnosed by the pathologist, the breast will be a much less likely primary site, and a somewhat different search should be made.

More careful attention to physical examination of the breast, as advocated by Halsted[1] and Haagensen,[3] might reduce even further the number of cases in which primary cancer is not found in the presence of enlarged axillary nodes. Halsted's advice to his audience in 1907 may strike some as preposterous, but experienced clinicians today may remember at least one instance in which his advice still seems appropriate.

> It well repays the experienced surgeon to spend perhaps an hour in the examination of certain breasts. The diagnosis has usually been exceedingly and unfortunately simple. But women are now presenting themselves more promptly for examination, realizing that a cure of breast cancer is not only possible, but, if operated upon early, quite probable. Hence the surgeon is seeing smaller and still smaller tumors, cancers which give not one of the cardinal signs. About as difficult a case as any, excepting, of course the adenoma in a transitional stage, is a tiny retromammary adenocarcinoma or a colloid carcinoma in a breast covered with one or two inches of fat. If in such a case there should be no shortening whatever of the trabeculae the diagnosis could hardly be made. The fat on pressure being elastic and the tumor so deep, the differential diagnosis from cyst might not be possible. But given even very slight shortening of the trabeculae from tumor to skin, this fact might be determinable by making both breasts take the widest possible excursions on the chest wall, under the skin. The faintest conceivable trace of a difference on the two sides, in a minor pectoral crease, for example, may suffice for the diagnosis.

Mammography is now being used routinely to examine the suspected breast. The percentage of positive mammograms found in the larger series reported during the past 25 years ranges from 12% to 55%.[6,12] Patel and colleagues[12] reported 8 of 17 mammograms positive, whereas Ashikari and colleagues,[6] who included all patients encountered from 1946 to 1975, found only 3 of 25 positive but do not state how many of the early patients in this series did not have this test. It is tempting to hope that more occult cancers with positive nodes will be found with the greatly improved x-ray techniques now in use, but it may just as well be true that the particular characteristics of occult breast cancers as reported by Haupt and Rosen (see above) do not produce a positive mammogram, since it is the dense stroma and the intraductal proliferation of cells with consequent degenerative calcium deposition that lead to a positive mammogram.

Table 15-15
Work-up of Patient With Cancer in Axillary Nodes Without a Known Primary Site

Diagnostic Procedure	*Special Considerations*
Physical examination	Pay particular attention to moles, thyroid, breasts, other nodes, genitalia, and prostate.
Laboratory studies	Complete blood count, liver function tests, and carcinoembryonic antigen.
Radiographic and nuclear studies	
Mammogram	Should be repeated on state-of-the-art equipment if available films are not optimal.
Chest film	Look for cancer of the lung or other metastases.
Bone scan	Can be deferred until after a working diagnosis of breast cancer is made.
Axillary node biopsy	
Routine pathology	Look for apocrine-like cells.[9] Mucicarmine stain can be helpful.
Electron microscopy	Intracellular canaliculi, apical desmosomes, microvilli, and secretory granules suggest adenocarcinoma.[10]
Receptor proteins	Estrogen and/or progesterone receptor elevation is consistent with breast cancer.

Is there advantage to a blind breast biopsy in the absence of any clue on physical examination or on a mammogram? A generous biopsy in the upper outer quadrant, or even a quadrantectomy, has been reported to demonstrate an occult cancer in all of three patients, where this approach was tested.[15] If a totally excised cancer is found, further treatment will still be required for the breast and nodes. If an incompletely excised cancer is found, re-excision or mastectomy should be done. A negative biopsy should not influence the decision about further treatment, since a cancer may still be present elsewhere in the breast. Thus, one cannot show that a policy of breast biopsy in these unusual cases will lead to better outcomes.

Numerous studies have demonstrated that there is little value in performing an extensive radiographic evaluation of these patients.[17,18,19] Experienced clinicians will focus on possible diagnoses for which there is effective therapy. Therefore, with the exception of a chest x-ray to identify occult lung cancer or other metastases, bilateral mammograms, and a bone scan to eliminate occult metastatic involvement prior to therapy, no other scans and x-rays are indicated in asymptomatic patients. Of course, a rare bit of pathology will be found on gastrointestinal x-rays and computerized tomography, but the probability of a payoff will be about the same if volunteers are brought in off the street for similar studies. This advice does not apply to the patient with enlarged axillary nodes who also has a 40-lb weight loss, digestive symptoms, and back pain, which may suggest a pancreatic or other gastrointestinal cancer.

TREATMENT AND OUTCOME

Since Halsted's original report in 1907, a radical mastectomy, initially conventional but recently "modified," has been the recommended treatment in the United States. Adjunctive radiotherapy was added in many of the earlier treatment reports. In two series, radiotherapy has been considered to be the principal modality of treatment, but in both of these series, surgical removal of the breast or some axillary nodes or both was often added before or afterward.[20,21]

Generally, aggressive local therapy has been restricted to patients in whom the histology of the axillary node biopsy specimen was consistent with breast cancer origin. Of 109 patients who were culled from various reports and for whom survival rates were given, 70, or 64%, were alive at 5 years.[2,3,6–8,15,20,21] The range in these series was from 50% to 89%. It is not possible to sift out the contributions of the various treatments, which included simple mastectomy, modified radical and Halsted radical mastectomy, biopsy excision of axillary nodes or radical axillary dissection, and pre- or postoperative or no radiotherapy. Reports from surgeons often failed to state whether radiotherapy was used routinely or selectively. If one selects from reported series only those patients who were followed for 5 years or more and who had an invasive cancer in the breast when treated by radical mastectomy, with or without radiotherapy, the overall survival rate is 23 out of 38, or 60.5% (Table 15-16).

A report on the use of radiotherapy in 11 patients by Vilcoq and colleagues indicates that 8 of the 11 patients with an axillary mass 3 cm or less in diameter had an "excisional biopsy" of the nodes prior to definitive radiotherapy.[21] Since many patients in all reported series had no positive nodes except those palpated, this "biopsy" may have removed all positive nodes in a number of his patients. In three patients with an axillary mass greater than 3 cm in diameter, two had axillary dissection after radiotherapy because of "persistent adenopathy that proved on pathologic examination to be involved by carcinoma." Therefore, Vilcoq's data demonstrate that breast preservation is possible but provides no conclusive information about the axilla. With radiation doses from 5000 to 6500 cGy given over 5 to 6 weeks, Vilcoq's patients had an excellent survival rate despite local recurrence in the breast in three patients (6, 11, and 14 years). He reported no pulmonary fibrosis but moderate fibrosis of the breast in two patients, along with "some" limitation of arm movement, and one patient with moderate arm edema. The limitation to the use of radiotherapy is that the occult primary tumor in the breast can neither be excised nor treated with supplementary radiation ("boosted"). If the occult primary lesion is larger than microscopic in size, it is likely to be undertreated by this approach.

Thus, despite wide variations in treatment of the breast and the lymph nodes, outcomes in this group of patients have certainly been as good as, and frequently better than, those in comparable patients whose primary breast cancer was not occult and whose axillary nodes were clinically and pathologically positive. The number of involved nodes in the axilla should be one of the best predictors of outcome in patients with occult primaries, as it is with other patients, but exact data have not yet been gathered. The initial biopsy on these patients has varied from a limited one to a thorough, extensive procedure. When later a formal axillary dissection was done, the number of recovered nodes and number involved by cancer were not systematically related to the original biopsy report, so the total number of involved axillary nodes can be assessed in only a few reports.

Table 15-16
*Five-Year Survival in Patients With Axillary Metastases**

Author	*Number of Patients* Treated	*Number of Patients* Surviving	
Owen et al[2]	5	3	
Haagensen[3]	9	8	
Fitts et al[8]	18	9	
Westbrook and Gallager[14]	6	3	
Total	38	23	60.5%

* Only those patients are included here who had a cancer demonstrated in the excised breast.

RECOMMENDATIONS FOR MANAGEMENT

Surgical management of the newly discovered axillary mass varies with the clinical presentation. Needle biopsy of the axillary mass is often easy but may not provide sufficient tissue for special studies and usually precludes hormone receptor analysis. If the axillary mass is small and easily reached, excision under local anesthesia is preferable, with the pathologist at hand to evaluate the specimen, assure that there is viable tissue for studies including receptor determination, and preserve tissue in glutaraldehyde for electron microscopy. Touch preparations to study cellular morphology may be useful if a lymphoma is suspected. If the axillary mass is large, a generous incisional biopsy is recommended. This should be done in such a manner as to permit an axillary resection at a later time. A radial incision will make it easier for subsequent mastectomy to encompass this scar, and is also compatible with breast preservation approaches (see Chapter 3). Immediate decisions about therapy based on frozen sections are contraindicated, since evaluation of the biopsy specimen is best performed on permanent sections.

Once the diagnosis of "probable" or "consistent with" breast cancer is made by the pathologist, the next step should be a bone scan, since a positive scan will lead the treatment away from further focus on the primary tumor and since the baseline bone scan will be almost inevitably wished for, if and when the patient develops symptoms during follow-up. In patients with breast cancer with positive nodes, from 0% to 32% have been reported to have a positive bone scan, and the mean is 7%.[22]

If the bone scan is negative, treatment of the breast and the axillary nodes is the next consideration. The arguments for several plans of management can be paraphrased as follows:

1. A mastectomy, following or with an axillary node dissection, is the treatment of choice because the breast will more often than not prove to contain a cancer when carefully sectioned. In the absence of proven systemic spread of breast cancer, a modified radical mastectomy is the accepted form of management to achieve local and regional control and is associated with a significant likelihood of long-term survival.
2. The breast need not be resected, since most of the primary cancers in the breast will be very small and irradiation can achieve local control. Axillary nodes likewise can be sterilized by irradiation, and, if there is persistent enlargement, later surgical removal is feasible. A theoretical drawback to this approach is that the occult cancer may be several centimeters in diameter, and even aggressive external beam irradiation has a significant failure rate in controlling such primary tumors, with or without a local boost.
3. Immediate treatment of the breast is not necessary. In a significant fraction of these patients, no primary tumor will be found in the breast, and a lesion may be located in other tissues. Since there are no persuasive data showing that immediate "prophylactic" treatment of the breast affects survival, close surveillance of the patient will permit immediate intervention where and when it is indicated.

The first and most traditional approach, removal of the breast, has a substantial chance of identifying the primary cancer so that the patient can be assured about its nature and that it has been removed. Breast reconstruction (Chapter 16) and adjuvant chemotherapy (Chapter 10) are additional considerations. Adjuvant radiotherapy has not been shown to change survival favorably and would seldom be recommended for these patients.

The third option, that of withholding all treatment of the breast until clinical or radiographic evidence of a primary tumor appears, cannot be recommended on the basis of any scientific rationale and will only appeal to those who are completely resigned to the "biologic predeterminism" concept of breast cancer biology. If one accepts the strong likelihood that an occult breast cancer is present and that this cancer, if untreated, will continue to seed metastases into the lymphatics and vascular system, a policy of watchful waiting appears to deny the patient any chance of benefiting from treatment.

Most patients find the loss of a breast easier to tolerate than uncertainty about a primary cancer that might be lurking in the breast. Mastectomy provides at least a 70% chance of identifying the malignant focus. Other patients will much prefer an approach that spares the breast, accepting the knowledge that the effectiveness of radiotherapy to the breast in this situation is less well documented. There is support for this approach in data from Vilcoq and colleagues[21] and Montague,[20] which suggest that survival rates are high with this form of breast-preserving treatment. The policy at the Dana-Farber Cancer Institute and the Joint Center for Radiation Therapy is to recommend mastectomy in these patients.

REFERENCES

1. Halsted W: The results of radical operations for the cure of carcinoma of the breast. Ann Surg 46(1):1–19, 1907
2. Owen HW, Dockerty MB, Gray HK: Occult carcinoma of the breast. Surg Gynecol Obstet 98:302–308, 1954
3. Haagensen CD: The diagnosis of breast carcinoma. In Haagensen CD: Diseases of the Breast. Philadelphia, WB Saunders, 1971
4. Klopp CT: Metastatic cancer of axillary lymph node without a demonstrable primary lesion. Ann Surg 131:437–439, 1950
5. Pierce EH, Gray HK, Dockerty MB: Surgical significance of isolated axillary adenopathy. Ann Surg 145:104–107, 1957
6. Ashikari R, Rosen PP, Urban JA, et al: Breast cancer presenting as an axillary mass. Ann Surg 183:415–417, 1976
7. Breslow A: Occult carcinoma of second breast following mastectomy. JAMA 226:1000–1001, 1973
8. Fitts WT, Steiner GC, Enterline HT: Prognosis of occult carcinoma of the breast. Am J Surg 106:460–463, 1963
9. Haupt HM, Rosen PP, Kinne DW: Breast carcinoma presenting with axillary lymph node metastases: An analysis of specific histopathologic features. Am J Surg Pathol 9(3):165–175, 1985
10. Iglehart JD, Ferguson BJ, Shingleton WW, et al: An ultrastructural analysis of breast carcinoma presenting as isolated axillary adenopathy. Ann Surg 196:8–13, 1982
11. Kaplan IW, Reinstine H: Occult carcinoma of the breast. Am Surg 20:575–582, 1954
12. Patel J, Nemoto T, Rosner D, et al: Axillary lymph node metastasis from an occult breast cancer. Cancer 47:2923–2927, 1981
13. Weinberger HA, Stetten D: Extensive secondary axillary lymph node carcinoma without clinical evidence of primary breast lesion. Surgery 29:217–222, 1951
14. Westbrook KC, Gallager HS: Breast carcinoma presenting as an axillary mass. Am J Surg 122:607–611, 1971
15. Feigenberg Z, Zer M, Dintsman M: Axillary metastases from an unknown primary source: A diagnostic and therapeutic approach. Isr J Med Sci 12:1153–1158, 1976
16. Rosen PP: Axillary lymph node metastases in patients with occult noninvasive breast carcinoma. Cancer 46:1298–1306, 1980
17. Neilan BA: Adenocarcinoma of unknown origin. CA 33:237–241, 1983
18. Nystrom JS, Weiner JM, Heffelfinger-Juttner J, et al: Metastatic and histologic presentations in unknown primary cancer. Semin Oncol 4:53–58, 1977

19. Ultmann JE, Phillips TL: Management of the patient with cancer of unknown primary site. In DeVita VT, Hellman S, Rosenberg SA (eds): Cancer: Principles and Practice of Oncology, pp 1518–1533. Philadelphia, JB Lippincott Co, 1982
20. Montague ED: Axillary metastases from unknown primary sites. In Fletcher G (ed): Textbook of Radiotherapy. Philadelphia, Lea & Febiger, 1980
21. Vilcoq JR, Calle R, Ferme F, et al: Conservative treatment of axillary adenopathy due to probable subclinical breast cancer. Arch Surg 117:1136–1138, 1982
22. Harbert JC: Efficacy of bone and liver scanning in malignant diseases: Facts and opinions. In Freeman LM, Weissmann HS (eds): Nuclear Medicine Annual 1982. New York, Raven Press, 1982

Lymphedema

Sumner A. Slavin Mark E. Weinstein

HISTORY

As breast cancer and its treatment have become the focus of intense medical scrutiny, lymphedema has attracted renewed attention. Current controversies relating to lymphedema can be traced historically to the time of Hippocrates,[1] when the earliest observations of "white blood" in nodes were recorded. Aristotle[2] correctly described the proper anatomical position of lymphatic ducts in relation to blood vessels and nerves, but it was Herophilus[3] (335 to 280 B.C.) who may have performed the first dissection of such structures. Cadaveric dissection languished during the Roman period of Galen[4] and remained an obscure source of medical information until the modern era of Vesalius. In 1622, Aselli[5] discovered lacteal vessels in a canine mesentery, perhaps abetting the first demonstration of human lymphatics by Pecquet[6] in 1651. There ensued a series of major advances in which lymphatics were identified in different anatomical regions by Bartholinus[7] and Rudbeck.[8] In 1692, Nuck[9] was the first to inject the lymphatic system using a mercury compound. Sappey[10] in 1874 duplicated this effort, producing a degree of anatomical detail that remains a standard for comparison in 1986. The physiology of the lymphatic system was elucidated by the investigations of Yoffee and Courtice[11] in the early 20th century. They were among the first to prove that serum proteins that had traversed capillary endothelium could be retrieved by the lymphatics for ultimate restoration to the circulation.

The history of the embryonic origin of the lymphatic system is primarily an outgrowth of research in the current century. Sabin[12] is credited with providing the definitive work in this area. She was able to prove that lymphatic endothelium and channels form primitive buds from rudimentary venous sacs. In 1911, she termed lymphatics "modified veins," correctly noting their relationship to the venous system at large.

Difficulties involved in the actual visualization of lymphatic channels *in vivo* prevented further physiological advances until 1933. In that year, Hudack and McMaster[13] injected patent blue dye intracutaneously, successfully staining lymphatic channels in living animals. The culmination of the arduous process of visualizing lymphatics occurred in 1952, when Kinmonth[14] of St. Thomas Hospital, London, performed the world's first lymphangiogram. The subsequent use of isotopes, which will be described in this chapter, represents another major advance in our efforts to study the lymphatic system.

CLASSIFICATION

Lymphedema is usually classified as either primary or secondary. Primary lymphedema, which is identified at birth, is characterized by lymphatics that can vary from aplastic to hypoplastic or hyperplastic. The consequences of defects in the lymphatic system may not become manifest until the second or third decade of life, when the term "lymphedema praecox" is applied, or later in life, when the term "lymphedema tarda" is used. Secondary lymphedema may be associated with neoplasia, infection, inflammation, radiation, surgery, or trauma.[15–20] In the context of breast cancer, however, secondary lymphedema implies an association with the primary breast cancer or its treatment. Therefore, it is possible to detect clinical lymphedema in the upper extremity of a patient whose breast cancer has metastasized extensively to local nodes in the absence of any treatment. Often, lymphedema has been associated with either surgical or radiation treatment directed toward eradication of the tumor.

ANATOMY AND PHYSIOLOGY

The lymphatics form a rich plexus or network of channels that traverse the human body in close contiguity with the vascular system.[21] Valveless lymphatics in the dermis communicate with a subcutaneous system of deeper lymph vessels endowed with numerous valves and three histologic layers: inner, middle, and outer. The inner lining consists of vascular endothelium, the middle layer is primarily muscular, and the outer is of elastic origin. These channels greatly outnumber veins and are generally distinguishable from them on the basis of their thinner, transparent walls. In terms of physiology, lymph is usually propelled by a number of mechanisms, of which contraction by surrounding skeletal muscle units is the most important. Some intrinsic contractility exists, but its contribution to lymphatic flow remains poorly substantiated or quantified.[22,23] Gravity can aid lymph transport when the position of a limb is altered to take advantage of this force. Numerically, a preponderant number of lymphatic channels are superficial to fascia and are scattered at different levels of the subcutaneous compartment. Below the deep fascia of the arm or leg, larger lymphatic channels are intimately associated with subfascial neurovascular structures. Muscle contains no lymphatics, but some vessels do occupy the inter- and intramuscular septal compartments.[21]

Ultimately, progressively larger lymphatic channels coalesce and join the confluence of the internal jugular and subclavian veins on each side. Surgeons interested in the operative management of lymphedema of the upper extremity are aware that the major lymphatic pathways accompany the radial and ulnar arteries. This anatomical fact facilitates intraoperative identification of lymphatics.

Pathophysiologically, lymph collects in the subcutaneous compartment of an extremity when the channels are obliterated or obstructed. It is not known precisely what percentage of available lymphatic channels must be nonfunctional to result in inefficient delivery of interstitial lymph to the vascular system. If obstructed, lymphatic channels can dilate from the normal range of 0.2 to 1.0 mm in diameter up to 2 to 3 mm. Such extreme dilation appears to cause valvular dysfunction and incompetency, resulting in leakage of plasma proteins through injured basement membrane. As a result of obstruction, intralymphatic pressure can rise from zero to a positive value.[24] Increased hydrostatic pressure within lymphatics allows egress of fluid and protein into the interstitial space, culminating in a swollen subcutaneous compartment. The resulting increase in tissue oncotic pressure can lead to further edema accumulation as some lymph channels collapse and others become obstructed.

SYMPTOMS AND PHYSICAL FINDINGS OF LYMPHEDEMA IN THE BREAST CANCER PATIENT

As subcutaneous fluid pressure increases, a number of gross changes become clinically detectable. Initially, the skin surface remains soft but there is a mild pitting edema. Persistent swelling and unremitting collection of tissue protein eventually produce fibrosis in the subcutaneous compartment. Such a process can be abetted by recurrent bacterial infections, which thrive in the fluid medium. This chain of events can accelerate, as recurrent bouts of cellulitis and lymphangitis occur. Cutaneous surfaces can become inflamed by bacterial infection; in time, there occurs a progressive thickening of the skin similar to the classic peau d'orange changes of breast cancer. Progressive fibrosis in the subcutaneous compartment of the extremity is clinically apparent; it is associated histologically with the deposition of thick sheets of white connective tissue. The normal suppleness of the soft tissue is lost as the limb becomes firm and tense. Such changes typically occur in the forearm before the upper arm becomes involved (Fig. 15-10).

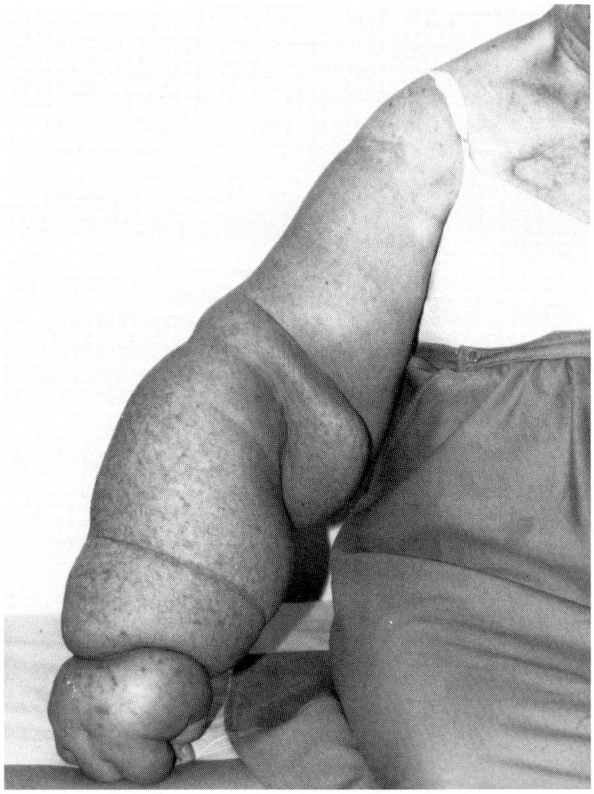

FIGURE 15-10. Severe postmastectomy lymphedema of upper extremity.

DIAGNOSIS

Severe lymphedema may be self-evident, but lesser degrees of swelling may require careful evaluation in order to detect it. After the quality of the soft tissue has been inspected, it is helpful to perform measurements of limb circumference. In the usual situation, the mid forearm and mid upper arm are measured using a bony landmark such as the olecranon for a standard reference point. Comparisons are made with a normal contralateral limb, but bilateral breast cancer may limit the value of this measurement. Circumferential measurements of the limb should be recorded prior to any major therapy such as breast surgery, axillary sampling, extensive lymphadenectomy, or radiation therapy. Volumetric measurements using water displacement techniques also assist in the quantification of lymphedema.[25]

Lymphangiography, an effective test for visualization and assessment of the lymphatic system, should not be routinely used in the evaluation of arm edema. Currently used Lipiodol contrast medium can exert toxic effects on the endothelial lining of lymphatics.[26] O'Brien showed that 17 of 53 patients with established lymphedema experienced a worsening of their condition following lymphangiography. During the 7-month follow-up period, ten patients' lymphedema measurements returned to prelymphangiographic levels; seven patients' measurements remained elevated.

LYMPHEDEMA FOLLOWING SURGERY

Dr. William Halsted made the earliest observations on the relationship between radical breast surgery and arm lymphedema. His observations of the relationship between poor wound healing, early and late postoperative infection, and trauma and the development of postoperative arm edema remain unchallenged.[15,16] In 1913, Halsted[15] presented his observations emphasizing the importance of primary wound healing without infection following radical mastectomy in the prevention and lessening of arm edema. To this end he recommended skin grafting of the large open area of tissue following removal of the breast. Skin grafting allowed for shortening of the length of skin flaps, decreased tissue necrosis and closure of the axillary dead space, improved arm motion, and lessened edema. Later, he observed that the combination of disruption of axillary lymphatics and infection led to the development of lymphedema.[16] However, disruption of the axillary lymphatics with occlusion of the axillary vein did not cause permanent swelling of the arm. The onset of lymphedema was extremely variable, ranging from months to years following surgery. Our current understanding of the pathogenesis of lymphedema reaffirms Halsted's original precepts.

In 1962, Britton and Nelson[27] reported their findings in 94 patients with lymphedema of the arm after radical mastectomy. None had local recurrence of their cancer. Seventy-seven percent of the patients had evidence of chronic infection of the arm. Two-thirds of the patients who developed lymphedema within 3 months of operation had postoperative wound complications, and 50% of those who developed lymphedema more than 3 months following surgery had delayed healing of their operative wound. Say and Donegan[17] conducted an analysis of 1551 patients with carcinoma of the breast treated between 1940 and 1965 and reported their results in 1974. They confirmed the findings of Halsted regarding the significant association between postoperative wound serum collection and skin flap necrosis and the subsequent development of lymphedema of the arm. Their overall incidence of arm edema following radical mastectomy without axillary radiation was 30.9%. This incidence should be compared with the incidences ranging from 3.4% to 62.5% reported in other studies of patients having axillary dissections without axillary radiation (Table 15-17).[17,18,28–35] Jolly and Viar[18] noted that the incidence of arm lymphedema following radical mastectomy increased from 15% to 28% when there was postoperative skin flap necrosis. Most likely, the wide variation in the reported incidence of lymphedema following axillary dissection has a twofold explanation: differences in the method of diagnosis and measurement of arm edema as well as differences in surgical technique and complication rate.

Since Halsted observed that the extent of axillary surgery was an important factor in the development of postoperative lymphedema, there have been few studies available comparing the incidence of arm edema after radical mastectomy versus after a limited axillary procedure. There is, however, a general trend toward a lower incidence of edema when limited axillary operations are performed without axillary radiation. Say and Donegan[17] found that patients treated by simple mastectomy had a 9.1% incidence of postoperative arm lymphedema compared with an incidence of 30.9% following radical mastectomy. Brismar and Ljungdahl[19] noted a 14% incidence of arm edema following radical mastectomy and a 6% incidence following modified radical mastectomy. Budd and colleagues[36] noted an incidence of arm edema of 3.4% following radical mastectomy and 2.6% after modified radical mastectomy. Simple mastectomy was not associated with any significant arm edema.

LYMPHEDEMA FOLLOWING RADIATION THERAPY

Radiation, in addition to surgery and wound complications, has been identified as a cause of edema of the arm. Say and Donegan[17] found the incidence of arm edema

Table 15-17
Incidence of Arm Edema Following Radical Mastectomy

Author	*Year*	*Number of Patients*	*Without Radiation (%)*	*With Radiation (%)*
Devenish & Jessop[28]	1940	90	8	—
Holman et al[29]	1944	100	31	50
MacDonald[30]	1948	40	62.5	—
Bell[31]	1949	568	3.4	5.8
Lobb & Harkins[32]	1949	51	40	81.8
Daland[33]	1950	90	20.7	69.2
Treves[34]	1952	84	8	—
Fitts[35]	1954	130	46	79
Say & Donegan[17]	1974	1323	30.9	37.5
Budd et al[36]	1978	89	3.4	—
Veronesi et al[42]	1981	349	6.6	—
Brismar & Ljungdahl[19]	1983	59	14	32

following radical mastectomy combined with axillary irradiation to be 42%, compared with 30.9% following radical mastectomy alone (see Table 15-17). Brismar and Ljungdahl[19] found that the incidence of arm edema increased from 14% to 32% under similar circumstances. In the latter study, however, those patients whose axillae were irradiated had more advanced axillary disease. It is difficult to isolate the effect of axillary irradiation because of the past tendency to irradiate the axillae of patients with axillary metastases (Table 15-17).[32,33,37]

Larson and associates[20] evaluated the incidence of edema of the arm among 475 women with early breast cancer treated between 1968 and 1980 at the Joint Center for Radiation Therapy. Among the patients who were treated with radiation to the axilla and who did not undergo any axillary surgery, there was only a 4% 6-year actuarial risk of arm edema. The use of limited axillary surgery followed by axillary irradiation did not result in a significantly increased incidence of arm edema. Those patients who underwent axillary irradiation following the removal of axillary lymph nodes without clearing of the axillary vein had a 6% risk of postradiation arm edema at 6 years. The combination of a full axillary dissection with clearing of the axillary vein followed by irradiation of the axilla, however, resulted in a 6-year actuarial risk of arm edema of 33%. An adequate number of control patients who had a full axillary dissection without axillary irradiation was not available in this series, nor was their follow-up of sufficient duration to evaluate the additional effect, if any, of irradiation to the development of arm edema. These results stress that the combination of full axillary dissection and axillary irradiation results in an unacceptably high risk of arm edema. Other investigators have found similar results.[38–42] This improved understanding of the relationship between the extent of axillary surgery and axillary irradiation in the development of lymphedema should allow surgeons and radiation therapists to better coordinate their diagnostic and therapeutic interventions.

CHEMOTHERAPY AND ARM EDEMA

The effect of chemotherapy on the development of arm edema following axillary surgery or irradiation is not known. Larson and co-workers[20] could demonstrate no effect of adjuvant chemotherapy on the incidence of postirradiation arm edema, whereas Danoff and associates[43] did note an increase. Larson and colleagues suggest that the discrepancy may be explained by differences in the number of chemotherapy cycles given.

LYMPHOSCINTIGRAPHY

The feasibility of using radionuclide scanning for evaluation of lymphatic anatomy and physiology was demonstrated in 1969.[44] Since then, it has become possible to inject technetium (^{99}Tc) sulfur colloid into the web space of a lymphedematous extremity to assess lymphatic function on the basis of the visualized lymphatic channels. In view of the recent recognition of the toxic hazard of Lipiodol contrast medium used in routine lymphangiography, lymphoscintigraphic evaluation techniques provide the only safe and accurate means for noninvasive investigation of the lymphatic system.

At the Dana Farber Cancer Institute, patients presenting with clinical evidence of lymphedema undergo by lymphoscintigraphy in order to assess lymphatic anatomy and function. A quantification of lymphatic flow and axillary nodal uptake of radionuclide tracer is possible. Kaplan and colleagues[45] showed that the mean percentage of axillary nodal uptake of tracer injected into the web space of the hand of a lymphedematous arm was significantly decreased compared with that of normal controls. Improved lymphatic flow with increased drainage was documented scintigraphically in lymphedematous arms after exercise and elevation.

The flare phenomenon appears to be a reliable lymphoscintigraphic sign of lymphedema.[46] The flare sign consists of a widening of the usual band of radiopharmaceutical activity in the area of existing lymphatic channels. Physiologically, the flare phenomenon indicates significant lymphatic obstruction with back-flow of radionuclide tracer through the walls of dilated, dysfunctional lymphatic channels. The migration of the tracer mimics the extravasation of plasma proteins through lymphatic walls and into the interstitial space, where accumulation occurs.

Using the initial examination as a baseline, objective assessment of lymphatic function at regular intervals is now possible. Increased resolution of the test indicates that lymphatic channels can be identified preoperatively and their location mapped (Fig. 15-11). Furthermore, the extent of collateralization and dilatation of existing lymphatic pathways can be determined with this study. Since much of the information provided by lymphoscintigraphy can be obtained by careful clinical examination, the most useful application of lymphoscintigraphy may be in the preoperative selection of candidates for microsurgical reconstruction and postoperative evaluation of the patency of microlymphaticovenous anastomoses.

NONOPERATIVE MANAGEMENT

A myriad of treatment regimens has been proposed for the management of lymphedema.[48,49] Current approaches emphasize conservative regimens during the early course of the disease, with surgery reserved for refractory cases. Unfortunately, there is evidence to suggest that such a program is illogical.[50,51] As severity of the lymphedema increases, certain microsurgical options may be precluded. A more thorough review of surgical options will be discussed in the next section, but it is important to recognize that severe, end-stage lymphedema is presently incurable and largely untreatable.

Nonoperative management has traditionally relied on bandaging and compression techniques in association with

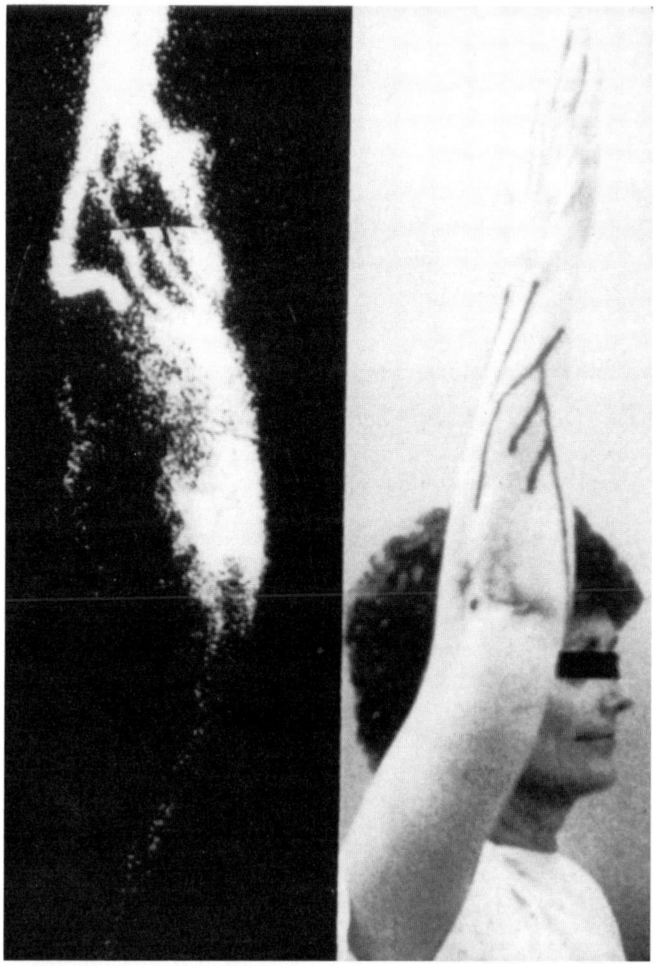

FIGURE 15-11. Lymphoscintigram with channels marked on the skin.

elevation of the affected extremity.[52] Fundamentally, external devices aid the patient by facilitating some degree of fluid mobilization from the congested subcutaneous compartment into the intravascular space. Patients note significant symptomatic relief as limb size is reduced and a more normal appearance of the extremity is restored. The increased pressure generated by the external pneumatic compression pump achieves a more rapid clearance of lymphedema fluid than do low-pressure stockings or garments.

Although intermittent external compression can reduce both limb girth and volume, the benefits are usually transient. A newer technique, known as sequential pneumatic compression,[53,54] uses a series of overlapping, pressurized cells exerting a distal to proximal compression cycle. Separate chambers inflate sequentially to milk fluid from one compartment to another. This system generates a peak pressure of 100 to 110 mm Hg in conjunction with a short cycle. It appears that lymphedema fluid can be mobilized by any compression device, including the familiar elastic compression garments, but more fluid is distributed in a proximal direction when sequential pumping is used. Simple elastic garments tend to distribute fluid both proximally and distally. In a prospective controlled trial, Richmand and co-workers[54] studied seven patients who had upper extremity lymphedema and who underwent 24 hours of treatment with the sequential compression device. They found a 28% decrease in the circumferential measurement of the limb at the mid forearm and a 45% decrease at the level of the wrist.

As lymphedema progresses, the increased tissue turgor and fibrosis become less responsive to compression devices. Nonoperative management for such patients emphasizes prolonged elevation, antibiotics, occasional diuretics, and strict hygiene of the limb. Despite the most compulsive efforts by the patient, it may be difficult or impossible to achieve sustained improvement. In such situations, patients may be candidates for surgical therapy, but no specific guidelines exist for appropriate timing of surgical intervention. Some authors recommend surgery for severe lymphedema, defined as a circumference of the lymphedematous limb 30% greater than that of the normal side.[55]

SURGICAL MANAGEMENT

The history of surgical approaches toward management of lymphedema reflects the frustrations inherent in treating this disorder. Generally, surgery is recommended when all nonoperative efforts have failed to relieve the relentless swelling and discomfort of a lymphedematous limb. Indications for surgery include impaired limb function, recurrent cellulitis and lymphangitis, a desire for improved cosmesis, and chronic pain and fatigue.[56] No procedure appears to provide a permanent cure, but some offer significant palliation.[57] There is no evidence that any surgical treatment for lymphedema can avert a lymphangiosarcoma, an extremely rare but feared and usually fatal complication of long-standing lymphedema.[58,59]

Historical reviews of the surgical management of lymphedema usually commence with Lisfranc, who attempted percutaneous drainage of edema fluid with needles in 1841.[60] Early in the 20th century, attempts were made to create artificial conduits from the superficial to deep lymphatic systems.[61,62] It was hoped that implantations of threads of nylon or silk or various types of rubber tubing might increase lymphatic drainage. Tissue bridges or bypasses using pedicled skin flaps have also been employed in an effort to restore flow across areas of obstruction such as the groin or axilla.[63,64] The best-known technique in this particular category is that of Goldsmith and colleagues,[65] who used an omental transposition flap sutured to the diseased limb. Long-term studies have failed to confirm the efficacy of such a technique; in particular, there is no evidence that lymphatic connections are established between the omentum and the recipient lymphedematous tissue.[66]

The most recent application of the tissue bridge concept was reported in 1983, when a latissimus dorsi myocutaneous flap was transposed across a diseased axilla in a patient suffering from postmastectomy lymphedema.[67] Of two patients in whom the technique was attempted, one had clinical improvement lasting for 3 years. Unfortunately, the authors did not provide evidence of enhanced lymphatic flow through the flap, nor did they state whether adjunctive measures were used to control lymphedema. Preliminary experimental evidence in rats suggests that rectus abdominus myocutaneous flaps transposed from the abdomen into the groin can relieve a lower extremity rendered lymphedematous by surgery and radiation.[68] The mechanism for improved lymphatic flow is conjectural at this time; however, new lymphatic connections between the diseased extremity and the pedicled myocutaneous flap appear on lymphoscintigraphy performed as early as 2 weeks after flap surgery. Whether such improved flow occurs as a result of regeneration of new lymphatics or as a result of anastomosis of existing injured lymphatics to healthy flap channels is presently unknown. It is hoped that, further research in this particular area will produce an answer that can be translated into clinical application.

Surgical efforts to achieve improved lymphatic flow from superficial to deep planes have emphasized excision of intervening tissue as a means to such an end. In 1912, Kondoleon[69] excised the fibrotic layer of deep fascia to facilitate flow to deep lymphatics. Sistrunk[70] elaborated on the same concept but recommended the additional excision of adjacent subcutaneous fat. Earlier, Charles[71] had reported on the radical excision of all diseased skin and subcutaneous tissues down to the deep fascial level, closing such an extensive wound with skin grafts. Homans,[72] in 1936, devised a procedure in which diseased tissue was removed from the lower extremity below the knee, and the wound was immediately reconstructed with skin flaps. Miller's modification of Homans' original procedure represented another important milestone when he extended the procedure above the knee level to an entire extremity.[62] Staged subcutaneous excision, as Miller's procedure became known, is currently considered one of the best palliative procedures for patients with severe lymphedema. This operation can achieve immediate, drastic reduction of limb volume during the course of a single or two-stage procedure. The technique suffers from a failure to deal with lymphedema on a physiological level; diseased tissue is removed, but the underlying pathophysiology may be unaffected. However, Miller noted increased clearance of radioactive human serum albumin in lymphedematous limbs after staged subcutaneous excision. In his series of 14 patients undergoing 29 excisions, 6 patients were observed for 4 to 6 years; all had normal functional use of the involved limb and good aesthetic appearance. The success of the procedure is limited, as further lymphedema fluid collection inexorably develops. Despite this fact, many patients are satisfied with the limb reduction provided by the procedure.

Microsurgical advances in the past 15 years have provided surgeons with a possible opportunity to treat lymphedema at a physiological level. Dr. Bernard O'Brien of Australia demonstrated the feasibility of such an approach in 1975, when he performed the first lymphovenous anastomoses in patients suffering from postmastectomy lymphedema.[55] Unfortunately, he combined his microsurgical approach with subcutaneous excision in adjacent areas of the same limb. This combination of excisional and microsurgical treatment resulted in a distinct reduction of limb volume but confused efforts to assess the relative merit of each technique. To date, there have been no prospective, controlled studies of the long-term patency results of microlymphaticovenous anastomosis. Puckett and colleagues reported discouraging results when lymphovenous anastomoses were conducted in dogs.[24] In their research model, 100% of the lymphaticovenous anastomoses created in experimentally induced lymphedematous limbs of dogs were occluded within 21 days after the microsurgery. These results suggest that the driving force of increased lymphatic pressure relative to the venous system may represent a self-defeating mechanism for sustained lymph flow. The author reasoned that subsequent decrements in intralymphatic pressure contribute to occlusion of the microvascular anastomosis and on that basis concluded that the connections may be hemodynamically unsustainable. The optimal pharmacologic agents for maintenance of microlymphaticovenous anastomoses have not yet been determined, and little if any data exist regarding any drug regimen or method of anticoagulation.

The current available data indicate that microlymphaticovenous anastomoses remain patent in approximately two-thirds of patients for periods of 12 to 15 months following the surgery.[47] From a theoretical point of view, the ability of a few such microvascular connections to act as effective, sustainable conduits of lymphatic flow has been seriously questioned. Yet, microlymphaticovenous surgery is appealing because it mimics the physiologic drainage of lymph into the venous system. Recent advances in lymphoscintigraphy permit the preoperative selection of patients based on scintigraphic mapping of available lymphatic channels. Current surgical management, whether it be excisional treatment or microlymphaticovenous anastomosis, is predicated on careful evaluation of preoperative lymphoscintigrams in any patient suffering from lymphedema. Most surgeons would agree that absence of visualization of functioning lymphatic channels on preoperative lymphoscintigraphy represents a potential indication for excisional surgery when the lymphedema is severe or disabling. If two or more lymphatic channels are visualized, microsurgery may be indicated. A recent study from China by Huang and co-workers[50] reported significant reductions in limb circumference and volume over a 24-month follow-up period when four or more microsurgical anastomoses were performed. The results improved proportionately with greater numbers of connections, with a maximum number of 11 microsurgical anastomoses performed.

Formerly, swelling of the upper extremity was accepted as an inevitable consequence of a myriad of factors: radical mastectomy, lymphadenectomy, radiation, and wound-healing complications. Modern concepts have relegated radical surgery to a lesser role, emphasizing instead the biology of breast cancer. As our understanding of the pathogenesis of lymphedema increases, fewer patients will suffer from this problem in the future. A critical review of the studies presented in this chapter indicates that the incidence of lymphedema can be reduced by scrupulous adherence to surgical techniques that avoid injury to lymphatic structures. Similarly, extensive axillary dissection combined with axillary irradiation should be modified to reflect our understanding of their injurious effects.

The extreme lack of data regarding the efficacy of surgical and nonsurgical management of established lymphedema underscores the need for more research in this area.

REFERENCES

1. Majno G: The Healing Hand. Cambridge, Harvard University Press, 1977
2. Bartels P: Das Lymphgefassystem. In Bardeleben K von (ed): Handbuch der Anatomie des Menschen, Vol 3, part 4. Jena, Gustav Fischer, 1909
3. Mayerson HS: On lymph and lymphatics. Circulation 28:839, 1963
4. Lyons MC, Towers B (eds): Galen on Anatomical Procedures (Translated by WHL Duckworth) Cambridge, Cambridge University Press, 1962
5. Aselli G: De lactibus sive lacteis venis, quarto vasorum mesarai corum genere novo invento. Milano JB, Biddellium, Mediolani, 622
6. Pecquet J: Experimenta nova anatomica quibus incognitum chyli receptaculum, et ab eo per thoracem in ramos usque subclavis vasa lacetea defergunter. Paris, 1651
7. Bartholinus T: Vasa lymphatica hafniae. Petrus hakius, 1653
8. Rudbeck O: Novo exercitatio anatomica, exhibens ductus hepaticos, aquoso et vasa glandularum serosa. Arosiae, exud e Lauringerus, 1653 (English translation in Bull Hist Med 11:304, 1942)
9. Nuck A: Adenographia curiosa et uteri foeminei anatome nova. Lugd B, 1692
10. Sappey PC: Anatomie, Physiologie, Pathologie des Vaisseaux Lymphatiques. Paris, Adrien Delahaye, 1874
11. Yoffee JM, Courtice FC: Lymphatics, Lymph and the Lymphomyeloid Complex. New York, Academic Press, 1970
12. Sabin FR: A critical study of the evidence presented in several recent articles on the development of the lymphatic system. Anat Rec 5:417, 1911
13. Hudack SS, McMaster PD: The lymphatic participation in human cutaneous phenomenon. J Exp Med 57:751, 1933
14. Kinmonth JB: Lymphangiography in man. Clin Sci 11:13, 1952
15. Halsted WS: Swelling of the arm after operations for cancer of the breast—elephantiasis chirurgica—its cause and prevention. Bull Johns Hopkins Hosp 32:309, 1921
16. Halsted WS: Developments in the skin-grafting operation for cancer of the breast. JAMA 60:416, 1913
17. Say CC, Donegan W: A biostatistical evaluation of complications from mastectomy. Surg Gynecol Obstet 138:370, 1974
18. Jolly P, Viar W: Reduction of morbidity after radical mastectomy. Am Surg 47:377, 1981
19. Brismar B, Ljungdahl I: Postoperative lymphoedema after treatment of breast cancer. Acta Chir Scand 149:687, 1983
20. Larson D, Weinstein M, Goldberg I, et al: Edema of the arm as a function of the extent of axillary surgery in patients with Stage I-II carcinoma of the breast treated with primary radiotherapy. Int J Radiat Oncol Biol Phys 12(9):1575, 1986
21. Haagensen CD: Diseases of the Breast, Chapters 2, 3, and 8, 2nd rev ed. Philadelphia, WB Saunders, 1971
22. Smith RO: Lymphatic contractility. J Exp Med 90:497, 1949
23. Wang GY, Zhong SZ: Experimental study of lymphatic contractility and its clinical importance. Ann Plast Surg 15:278, 1985
24. Puckett CL, Jacobs GR, Hurvitz JS, et al: Evaluation of lymphovenous anastomosis in obstructive lymphedema. Plast Reconstr Surg 66:116, 1980
25. Swedborg I: Voluminometric estimation of the degree of lymphedema. Scand J Rehabil Med 9:131, 1977
26. O'Brien B, Das SK, Franklin JD, et al: Effect of lymphangiography on lymphedema. Plast Reconstr Surg 68:922, 1981
27. Britton RC, Nelson PA: Causes and treatment of postmastectomy lymphedema of the arm. JAMA 180:95, 1962
28. Devenish EA, Jessop WHG: Nature and cause of swelling of the upper limb after radical mastectomy. Br J Surg 28:222, 1940
29. Holman C, McSwain B, Beal JM: Swelling of the upper extremity following radical mastectomy. Surgery 15:757, 1944
30. MacDonald I: Resection of axillary vein in radical mastectomy: Its relation to mechanism of lymphedema. Cancer 1:618, 1948
31. Bell HG: Cancer of the breast. Ann Surg 130:310, 1949
32. Lobb AW, Harkins HN: Postmastectomy swelling of the arm with a note on the effect of segmental resection of the axillary vein at the time of radical mastectomy. West J Surg 57:550, 1949
33. Daland EM: The incidence of swollen arms after radical mastectomy and suggestions for prevention. N Engl J Med 242:497, 1950
34. Treves N: Prophylaxis of postmastectomy lymphedema by the use of Gelfoam laminated rolls. Cancer 5:73, 1952
35. Fitts WT: Swelling of arm after radical mastectomy: Clinical study of its causes. Surgery 35:460–464, 1954
36. Budd DC, Cochran RC, Sturtz DL, et al: Surgical morbidity after mastectomy operations. Am J Surg 135:218, 1978
37. Smedal MI, Evans JA: The cause and treatment of edema of the arm following radical mastectomy. Surg Gynecol Obstet 111:29, 1960
38. Veronesi U, Valagussa P: Inefficacy of internal mammary node dissection in breast cancer surgery. Cancer 47:170, 1981
39. Vilcoq JR, Calle R, Stacey P, et al: The outcome of treatment by tumorectomy and radiotherapy of patients with operable breast cancer. Int J Radiat Oncol Biol Phys 7:1327, 1981
40. Wilkinson EJ, Hause L: Probability in lymph node sectioning. Cancer 33:1269, 1974
41. Zimmerman KW, Montague ED, Fletcher GH: Frequency, anatomical distribution and management of local recurrences after definitive therapy for breast cancer. Cancer 19:67, 1966
42. Veronesi U, Saccozzi R, Del Vecchio M, et al: Comparing radical mastectomy with quadrantectomy, axillary dissection and radiotherapy in patients with small cancers of the breast. N Engl J Med 305:6, 1981
43. Danoff BF, Goodman RL, Glick JH, et al: The effect of adjuvant chemotherapy on cosmesis and complications in patients with breast cancer treated by definitive irradiation. Int J Radiat Oncol Biol Phys 9:1625, 1983
44. Sacks GA, Sandler MP, Born ML, et al: Lymphoscintigraphy as an adjunctive procedure in the perioperative assessment of patients undergoing microlymphaticovenous anastamoses. Clin Nucl Med 8:309, 1983
45. Kaplan WD, Slavin SA, Marquisz JA, et al: Qualitative and

quantitative upper extremity radionuclide lymphoscintigraphy (abstr). Presented at the Soc Nucl Med meeting, St Louis, 1983
46. Jackson FI, Lentle BC: The scintilymphangiographic flare sign of lymphangitic obstruction. Clin Nucl Med 2:211, 1977
47. Slavin SA, Kaplan WD, Henderson IC: The important role of lymphoscintigraphy in the microsurgical management of lymphedema (in preparation)
48. Dale WA: The swollen limb. Curr Probl Surg, Sept 1973
49. Miller TA: Lymphedema. In Grabb WC, Smith JW (eds): Plastic Surgery, p 826. Boston, Little, Brown & Co, 1979
50. Huang GK, Hu RQ, Liu ZZ, et al: Microlymphaticovenous anastomosis in the treatment of lower limb obstructive edema: Analysis of 91 cases. Plast Reconstr Surg 76:671, 1985
51. Slavin SA: Microlymphaticovenous anastomosis in the treatment of lower limb obstructive edema: Analysis of 91 cases (discussion). Plast Reconstr Surg 76:684, 1985
52. Brush BE, Wylie JH, Benison BJ: Some devices for management of lymphedema of the extremities. Surg Clin North Am 39:1493, 1959
53. Zelikovski A, Melamed I, Kott I, et al: The "Lymphopress" — a new pneumatic device for the treatment of lymphedema: Clinical trial and results. Folia Angiol 28:165, 1980
54. Richmond DM, O'Donnell TF, Zelikovski A: Sequential pneumatic compression for lymphedema. A controlled trial. Arch Surg 120:1116, 1985
55. O'Brien B, Sykes PJ, Threlfall GN, et al: Microlymphaticovenous anastomosis for obstructive lymphoedema. Plast Reconstr Surg 60:197, 1977
56. Savage RC: The surgical management of lymphedema. Surg Gynecol Obstet 159:501, 1984
57. Miller TA: Surgical Management of lymphedema of the extremity. Plast Reconstr Surg 56:633, 1975
58. Stewart FW, Treves N: Lymphangiosarcoma in postmastectomy edema. Cancer 1:64, 1948
59. Martin MB, Kon ND, Kawamoto EH, et al: Postmastectomy angiosarcoma. Am Surg 50:541, 1984
60. Miller TA, Harper J, Longmire WP: The management of lymphedema by staged subcutaneous excision. Surg Gynecol Obstet 136:586, 1973
61. Handley WS: Lymphangioplasty: A new method for the relief of the brawny arm of breast cancer and for similar conditions of lymphatic oedema. Lancet 1:783, 1908
62. Miller TA: Surgical Management of lymphedema of the extremity. Plast Reconstr Surg 56:633, 1975
63. Smith JW, Conway H: Selection of appropriate surgical procedures in lymphedema; introduction of hinged pedicle. Plast Reconstr Surg 30:10, 1962
64. Hirshowitz B, Goldan S: A bihinged chest-arm flap for lymphedema of the upper limb. Plast Reconstr Surg 7:411, 1981
65. Goldsmith HS, De Los Santos R: Omental transposition in primary lymphoedema. Surg Gynecol Obstet 125:607, 1967
66. Danese CA, Papaioannou AN, Morales LE, et al: Surgical approaches to lymphatic blocks. Surgery 64:821, 1968
67. Medgyesi SA: Successful operation for lymphedema using a myocutaneous flap as a "wick". Br J Plast Surg 36:64, 1983
68. Kanter M, Slavin SA: An experimental model for chronic lymphedema in rats (submitted for publication)
69. Kondoleon E: Die operative Behandlung der elephantiastisher odeme. Zentralbl Chir 39:1022, 1912
70. Sistrunk WE: Elephantiasis treated by the Kondoleon operation. Surg Gynecol Obstet 26:388, 1918
71. Charles RH: A system of treatment, Vol. 3, p 504. London, J&A Churchill, Ltd, 1912
72. Homans J: Treatment of elephantiasis of legs; preliminary report. N Engl J Med 215:1099, 1936

Management of the Contralateral Breast

David W. Kinne

Bilateral breast carcinoma is not an uncommon clinical problem, and its occurrence is not surprising in this paired organ in which carcinoma of one side is frequently multifocal, highly curable, and detected in fairly young patients with long life expectancies.

The initial diagnostic consideration is to distinguish new primary cancers in the second breast from metastasis from the first side. Although different histologic types would establish the second side as a new primary, most breast cancers have similar microscopic appearances (ductal patterns). Robbins and Berg[1] addressed this problem in a series of bilateral breast cancers in 94 patients and outlined the following points:

1. Second primaries develop within breast parenchyma, whereas metastases to the breast tend to be in subcutaneous fat.
2. Metastases tend to be multiple and well-circumscribed, unlike the infiltrative stellate pattern characteristic of primaries.
3. Primary cancers are often associated with an *in situ* component, whereas metastases lack this feature. The presence of *in situ* disease establishes these tumors as primaries, but its absence does not indicate that these lesions are metastases.
4. Isolated metastases to the contralateral breast in the absence of recurrence at other sites is rare. A negative extent-of-disease evaluation increases the likelihood that contralateral tumors are primaries. The presence of distant metastases influences the approach to the second breast tumors, weighing against a potential curative approach even if these are second primaries.

An absolute distinction between these two is often difficult to establish. Many clinicians interpret second breast tumors as more likely to be new primaries if the interval after mastectomy is long.[2,3,] Leis[4] accepted the diagnosis of new primaries if nuclear differentiation was greater than in the first cancers or if the second lesions occurred more than 5 years after the first with no intervening evidence of metastases.

Bilateral primary breast cancers are categorized as synchronous (simultaneous) or metachronous (nonsimultaneous) according to whether they are diagnosed at the same time or the second side is detected at a later date, after the first side has been treated. This distinction is somewhat arbitrary because of variable growth patterns and the possible long preclinical phase of breast neoplasms. However, most reports document that metachronous bilateral primary breast cancer is the more common presentation. Leis and colleagues[5] summarized 22 articles published before 1965, with bilateral breast cancer reported in 1% to 20% of all breast cancer patients. Synchronous presentation occurred in 0.1% to 2.0% of all patients, whereas metachronous disease was reported in 1.0% to 12% of cases, with a median figure of 3.2%. This variation in metachronous disease presentation is a function of the length of follow-up.

In the first publication of bilateral breast cancer, Kilgore in 1921 estimated that 7% to 10% of women surviving the first cancer would develop contralateral breast cancer.[6] These figures remain valid today. Several reports have documented the incidence of bilateral breast cancer to be in this range.[7–11] The risk of developing cancer in the second breast is approximately five times greater than the normal risk of initial breast cancer in the general population.[1,12] Another way of expressing this risk, noted by Robbins and Berg,[1] is that almost 1% of patients who have undergone mastectomy for one breast cancer will develop a new primary cancer in the contralateral breast during each year of follow-up.

RISK FACTORS

Several factors have been implicated in increasing the risk of bilateral breast cancer. Age at presentation with the first cancer, success of treatment of that lesion, family history, multicentricity in the first breast, and certain histologic types are of importance.

Age

Robbins and Berg,[1] in a long-term study of Memorial Hospital patients treated by mastectomy, noted that patients developing their initial breast cancers before age 50 had a 10 to 14 times greater risk of developing contralateral breast cancers compared with the general population. For women over 70, the risk of bilateral breast cancer was two times that of the normal population. Prior and Waterhouse[13] gave the incidence of contralateral breast cancer in the Birmingham Regional Cancer Center (England) among nearly 22,000 patients whose primary breast cancer was treated between the years 1936 and 1964. This assessment represented more than 90,000 woman-years at risk. Three hundred and ninety-nine contralateral breast cancers developed, with 23% considered synchronous (defined as tumors diagnosed at the same time or within 1 month of the primary). When analyzed by a method including synchronous and metachronous second primaries, the overall risk of contralateral breast cancer was 3.0 times that of a first primary in the general population. The corresponding risks for three main age-groups (at the time of diagnosis of the first primary) were 5.6 for ages 15 to 44 years, 3.7 (45 to 59 years), and 1.8 (60 years and older). When synchronous tumors were excluded, the relative overall risk was 2.4 times that of the general population, and risks of 5.2, 3.0, and 1.0 for the three age ranges, respectively, were noted. These analyses documented that the level of risk of contralateral breast cancer was greatest in the young population, that it was negatively correlated with age, and that the relative risk remained constant over time.

A prospective study of patients presenting with a second primary breast cancer to Guy's Hospital from 1980 to 1982 was reported by Chaudary and colleagues.[14] The percentage of new simultaneous tumors detected clinically or by mammography was approximately 3%. The importance of mammography in detection is apparent in this series; with the routine mammographic screening of contralateral breasts in patients with unilateral disease, the rate of detection of simultaneous bilateral cancers increased fivefold over prior years. By placing more clinically unsuspected cancers in the simultaneous group, it might be assumed that a decrease in the rate of clinically nonsimultaneous cancers occurring in the early years of follow-up would occur. However, the detection rate of metachronous bilateral cancers in this series also increased, perhaps because of the more general use of mammography in the follow-up of women with unilateral disease.

There are three possible explanations for these findings. First, the incidence of breast cancer is increasing in the population (an unlikely occurrence). Second, mammography allows the detection and treatment of occult breast cancers that might never have become clinical problems to these patients. The third possibility is that earlier detection has been achieved in both the synchronous and the metachronous group and that with longer follow-up the rate of metachronous contralateral breast cancer development will diminish.

In this series, the patients developing their first cancers before the age of 40 had a risk of contralateral cancer that was three times that in women older than 40 at the development of their first lesion (Fig. 15-12). This higher risk could not be explained as an artifact of their better survival. As shown in Figure 15-13, there was no difference in the survival curves of patients who developed unilateral disease before age 40 compared with those who developed their disease at a later age. In fact, the mortality was slightly greater in the younger women. The authors concluded that a greater than average life expectancy, and thus exposure to a longer period of risk, could account only to a small extent for the increased risk of second cancers in the age-group under 40.

Some objections to these analyses remain. Two methodologic demands are required to establish reliable data on the risk run by breast cancer patients for developing contralateral primaries, namely lifelong complete follow-up of large cohorts to assess cumulative risk and reliable age-specific incidence figures in the population from which the unilateral cases are derived. The latter information, necessary to calculate relative risk in cohort studies, has been available in relatively few reports[1,12,13,15–17] and might be considered questionably valid in some of them.

These objections were answered in an epidemiologic investigation in Uppsala, Sweden, reported by Adami and colleagues.[18] In a well-defined geographic area, 1351 of 1423 women consecutively diagnosed as having primary breast cancer were compared with 1351 age-related women in a control group from the same area. This population-based study covered nearly one-third of the total

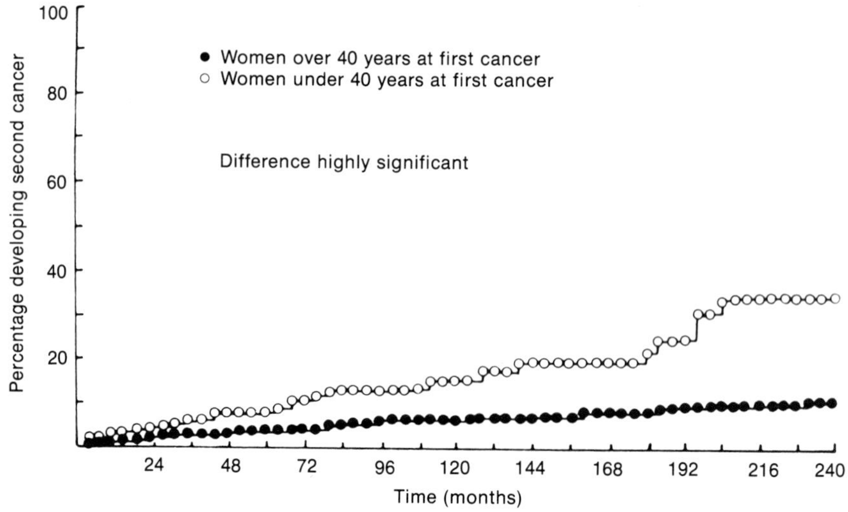

FIGURE 15-12. Occurrence of second cancers in relation to age at first cancer. (Chaudary MA, Millis RR, Hoskins EOL, et al: Bilateral primary breast cancer: A prospective study of disease incidence. Br J Surg 71:711, 1984)

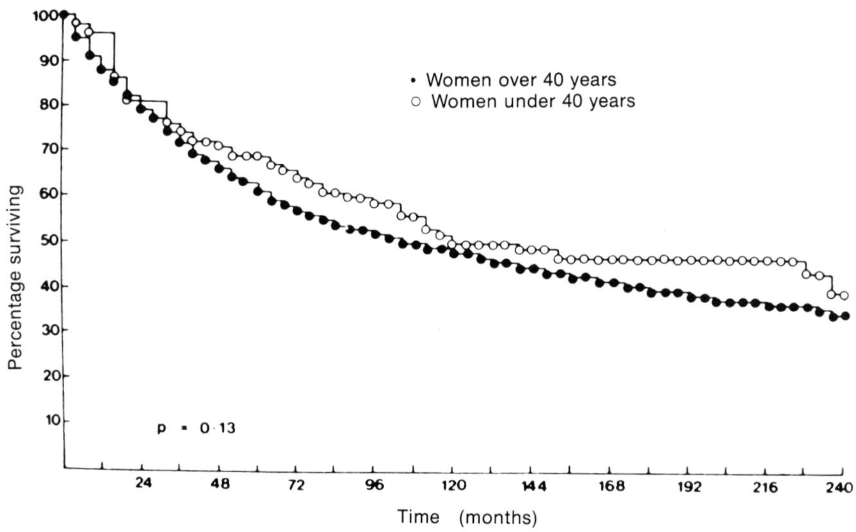

FIGURE 15-13. Survival in relation to age at diagnosis of breast cancer. (Chaudary MA, Millis RR, Hoskins EOL, et al: Bilateral primary breast cancer: A prospective study of disease incidence. Br J Surg 71:711, 1984)

Swedish population. Patients excluded from the 1423 initial group had either died, not responded, or incompletely answered the questionnaire. Thus, 95% of all initially reported cases were analyzed. All cases of breast cancer were confirmed by pathologic review by the same pathologist.

In the study group, simultaneous bilateral disease occurred in only one patient, whereas a history of previous cancer in the contralateral breast was reported by 65 patients. This prevalence was compared with that of 23 previous breast cancer cases in the control population. The relative risk of developing a second primary was 2.9% for the whole series and remained constant over several decades at a level determined by the age at first diagnosis. This risk was 9.9% before the age of 50 and 1.9% after that age. The cumulative risk of developing a second primary in this stable, well-defined population was 13.3% and 3.5% for women younger and older than 50 years, respectively, at first diagnosis. Also, there was not a steadily decreasing risk with increasing age over 50, as might be expected in view of the decreasing number of person-years at risk. Thus, bilateral breast cancer seemed to be characteristic of women younger than 50 years at first diagnosis.

Family History

Anderson[19,20] reported a high prevalence of bilateral breast cancer among the first-degree relatives of probands with bilateral primary breast cancer. If the probands' bilateral disease occurred premenopausally, first-degree relatives had a risk of bilateral breast cancer nine times higher than would be expected. The corresponding figure for postmenopausal females was four times higher than would be expected. In the Guy's Hospital series,[21] the prevalence of family history was established in 54 patients with bilateral primary breast cancer and 208 women with unilateral disease. Women with bilateral disease had a significantly greater prevalence of family history than patients with unilateral disease, and a greater proportion of first-degree relatives affected. Also, affected relatives of probands with bilateral cancer had a significantly higher prevalence of bilateral breast cancer compared with relatives of patients with unilateral disease.

Although it is agreed that familial breast cancer tends to occur early in life, in this study early occurrence was not necessarily a familial trait. In patients with bilateral breast cancer, no difference was noted in the mean age of onset of disease in those with a family history as compared with those without a family history. This was true for patients with unilateral cancers also. The implication is that the more powerful determining factor in bilateral breast cancer risk is the early age of onset of unilateral disease, compared with the impact of family history, although family history is an important factor.

Multicentricity

The definition of multicentric breast cancer varies, and the degree to which it is looked for in mastectomy specimens (i.e., the number and location of sections taken) accounts for the wide range of reported incidence. As reviewed by Lagios and colleagues[22] the frequency of multicentricity in the breast containing cancer has been stated to vary from 9% to 75%.

The association of multicentricity and bilaterality was explored by Lesser and colleagues[23] in a consecutive series of 1024 women with primary operable breast cancer treated at Memorial Hospital between October, 1976, and June, 1978. Multicentric carcinoma was defined as the presence of *in situ* or invasive carcinoma or both in a quadrant other than the one that harbored the original lesion. Two sections were taken per quadrant and pathologic review of all specimens was carried out by Rosen.

Multicentricity was present in 30% of specimens (16% *in situ* and 14% invasive carcinoma). The incidence was significantly higher in patients with larger primaries and in patients with pathologically involved axillary lymph nodes.

In this series, 501 women (57%) had had a previous mastectomy or a concurrent biopsy of the opposite breast. Among these women, the status of the opposite breast was significantly related to the frequency of multicentric disease. Patients with bilateral cancer, either previous or concurrent, had a higher frequency of multicentric disease in the ipsilateral breast than did patients whose opposite breast had atypia or benign lesions. The authors concluded that multicentricity and bilaterality are manifestations of similar factors involved in neoplastic transformation of breast epithelium leading to the development of breast cancer. These data confirmed the earlier findings of Robbins and Berg,[1] who noted that patients presenting with two or more grossly evident independent primary tumors in one breast had four times the average risk of developing contralateral breast cancers.

Pathology

Lobular carcinoma *in situ* (LCIS) was shown by Newman, in 1963, to carry a high rate of bilaterality.[24] Subsequently, many authors have described a bilateral rate of between 25% and 40%, detected by all diagnostic methods, including elective biopsy of the contralateral breast.[25–30]

Rosen showed the frequency of bilaterality to be related to the histologic type of primary carcinoma.[23] Patients with infiltrating duct carcinoma and LCIS in the primary side had a 57% higher rate of bilaterality (30 of 53 patients). Infiltrating lobular carcinoma or infiltrating duct carcinoma alone in the primary tumor carried bilateral rates of 28% and 22%, respectively. On the other hand, medullary carcinoma of the primary breast was associated with bilateral carcinoma in only 12%. Bilateral carcinoma was most common in patients with lower-grade invasive duct carcinomas, and there was a trend for contralateral carcinomas to be of the same histologic type as the ipsilateral tumors.

A search for factors that might be predictors of bilaterality was carried out by the National Surgical Adjuvant Breast Project (NSABP).[31] Thirty-eight pathologic factors and eight clinical factors were assessed; significant association with bilateral disease was found when the initial tumor measured more than 2 cm and was associated with invasive cancer or proliferative fibrocystic disease, nipple involvement, absent nodal sinus histiocytosis, LCIS, and invasive lobular or tubular carcinoma. In the 10 years of observation of patients in this study, 4.2% developed contralateral breast cancers (3.7% invasive), all of them metachronous. The second tumors measured only 1 cm less in diameter than the first, averaging 2.4 cm. Yet there was no significant difference in pathologic nodal status between the first and second cancers or that of patients with unilateral disease. Also, no difference in survival rate was noted between patients with bilateral or unilateral cancers.

Estrogen Receptors

Kiang and colleagues[32] reported 11 patients with simultaneous bilateral cancers; 8 of 11 had estrogen-receptor(ER)-positive tumors, 2 were negative on both sides, and 1 was asymmetric in receptor status. Six of 11 had similar histologic types on both sides. However, 5 of 7 metachronous cancers demonstrated different receptor status, with the primary side most often ER negative. Lesser and colleagues[23] noted that if the ipsilateral cancers were ER positive, bilaterality was significantly more likely than if the tumors of the first side were ER negative.

DETECTION

Three principal means of detecting contralateral breast cancer have been reported: close clinical follow-up, mammographic examinations at periodic intervals, and contralateral biopsy at the time the primary tumor is treated.

Clinical Follow-up

As noted in the report of Robbins and Berg,[1] the risk of developing contralateral breast cancer is less than 1% per year of follow-up in patients treated for unilateral breast cancer. This figure was confirmed in the summary article by Leis and colleagues[5] and also by the NSABP.[31] In a 30-year follow-up of patients treated from 1940 to 1943 with unilateral breast cancer, Adair and colleagues[33] described the actuarial 5-year risks of developing a second breast cancer (Table 15-18). A new clinical invasive cancer developed in 100 patients of the original 1458 patients in this series (6.9%), with half of these detected in the first 7 years of follow-up. Most patients died of breast cancer or other cancers in this long-term study, indicating the force of mortality of the first breast cancer or other illnesses in removing patients from the risk of contralateral disease.

Table 15-18
Actuarial 5-Year Risk of Developing Contralateral Breast Cancer

Years After First Breast Cancer	*Percentage*
0–4	3.8
5–9	3.1
10–14	2.9
15–19	3.8
20–24	2.4
25–29	1.6

(Adair F, Berg J, Joubert L, et al: Long-term follow-up of breast cancer patients: The 30 year report. Cancer 33:1145, 1974)

Mammography

In the Guy's Hospital series, the introduction of routine mammography increased the detection of simultaneous bilateral breast cancer fivefold over prior experience, to 2.4%.[14] An increase in detection of metachronous cancer was also noted. Other authors have reported similar findings,[34–37] and mammography of the contralateral breast at the time of initial diagnosis and at appropriate intervals afterward is accepted as standard practice today.

Contralateral Biopsy

Urban reported a 15% incidence of contralateral breast cancer in his series of patients surviving extended radical mastectomy for 10 years[38,39] and advocated contralateral breast biopsy to detect occult cancer at early stages. This procedure removed approximately 20% of breast tissue from the upper, outer quadrant, as well as the mirror image of the proven breast cancer. Sixteen percent of 159 contralateral biopsies showed carcinoma (11% simultaneous); however, 5 of 13 infiltrating carcinomas found were suspected clinically. In a later series, Urban listed 1204 patients, 80% of whom had contralateral biopsy. Patients excluded from this procedure were elderly or had advanced disease on the first side. As noted in Table 15-19, simultaneous bilateral carcinoma was detected in 12.5% of patients undergoing biopsy. Of 301 patients undergoing random biopsy (with no clinical or mammographic findings), 7.6% had carcinoma, with the majority noninfiltrating. Patients with minimal or positive findings had a higher percentage of infiltrating carcinoma found. Of note was that 75 patients had mammography, with 24 suggesting carcinoma in both breasts. Although many lesions missed were *in situ*, 24 of 40 patients with infiltrating carcinoma of the contralateral breast were missed by mammography. However, the quality of the mammograms was not evaluated. One would surmise that modern, high-quality films would detect more lesions.

Some authors have found a similar or higher incidence of contralateral breast cancer through biopsy,[41,42] and others have reported a lower yield.[43,44] In the Wanebo series,[42] 13 of 62 patients had contralateral cancer detected by biopsy; 11.3% had radiologically and clinically occult cancer.

PROGNOSIS

The survival rate of patients with bilateral breast cancer has been reported by many authors to be the same as for unilateral breast cancer, as long as the stage of the unilateral group is comparable to the more advanced of the two lesions in the bilateral series.[30,31,45–50] This relatively favorable course led some to suggest a possible immunologic stimulation by the first cancer, especially when *in situ*. Black and colleagues[51] showed that cancers subsequent to *in situ* cancers were often types exhibiting a more favorable prognosis.

Others have reported that patients with bilateral breast cancer have a poorer prognosis.[1,5,42,52–54] In a recent report by Fracchia and colleagues,[54] 403 patients with bilateral breast cancer were observed at least 10 years after treatment of the second side. Patients with simultaneous bilateral Stage I breast cancer had an overall recurrence rate of 29%, compared with a 16% recurrence rate for unilateral Stage I patients at 10 years. This subgroup suggested that bilateral breast carcinoma patients have a poorer outlook than patients with unilateral disease.

RECOMMENDATIONS

Two general approaches have been adopted for management of the second breast, depending on how one interprets the conflicting data presented in this chapter. One school believes that (1) patients with bilateral breast can-

Table 15-19
Contralateral Breast Cancer Detected by Biopsy 1964–1975 in 1204 Cases (80% Had Biopsy)

	Cancer			
Number of Biopsies	*Infiltrating*		*Noninfiltrating*	***Benign***
301 without signs	5		18	278
625 minimal signs	30		44	551
28 positive signs	20		2	6
954 total biopsies	55	119	64	835 (88 atypia)

12.5% simultaneous bilateral cancer in breasts biopsied (119/954); 10% simultaneous bilateral cancer in overall group (119/1204)

(Urban JA, Papachristou D, Taylor J: Bilateral breast cancer: Biopsy of the opposite breast. Cancer 40: 1968, 1977)

cer have a poorer prognosis than patients with unilateral disease, (2) contralateral biopsy is likely to detect a significant incidence of carcinoma, and (3) finding and treating contralateral disease, even lobular carcinoma *in situ* (LCIS) or lobular neoplasia (LN) improves the chances of cure. Members of this school advocate at least contralateral breast biopsy and treatment of the contralateral side, even when there is *in situ* duct or lobular carcinoma. In certain cases, prophylactic mastectomy has been advised. Leis[55] has advocated contralateral total mastectomy in young patients with early stage disease on the first side, significant family history, or when disease is multifocal or of the lobular type. Pathologic sectioning of these contralateral breasts revealed carcinoma in 17%, with one-half invasive. The 5-year survival rate from treatment was 96%. Accepting these figures, many argue that unnecessary mastectomies have been carried out in too many patients. Chaudary and colleagues[14] estimated that contralateral cancer would develop in 15 of 100 patients surviving 20 years and that prophylactic mastectomy would therefore benefit 15 and be needless in 85 patients. Close follow-up is their recommended approach.

A significant problem exists in patients who undergo breast preservation of the primary side with partial mastectomy, axillary dissection, and radiation therapy. To search for occult carcinoma in the contralateral breast, perhaps finding *in situ* disease, presents a therapeutic quandary. Would one advise mastectomy for *in situ* disease while the primary invasive tumor has been treated with a breast-preserving approach? This is unlikely—either bilateral primary irradiation or observation of the *in situ* side would seem preferable.

Subcutaneous mastectomy of the contralateral breast has been advocated by others,[56] with pathologic findings of atypical epithelial hyperplasia more often than in similar specimens from patients having no contralateral carcinoma. However, this operation does not remove all breast tissue,[57] and carcinoma has developed in residual tissue left behind after this procedure.[58] Subcutaneous mastectomy is not advised for prevention or treatment of breast carcinoma.

The other interpretation of available data is that (1) bilateral breast carcinoma does not carry a poorer prognosis than unilateral disease, (2) contralateral biopsy is unlikely to find disease of significance, and (3) treating the second side, especially when *in situ* disease is found, is unlikely to benefit patients. Unnecessary mastectomies will be performed, in this view. The risk of contralateral disease is recognized, so close monitoring of the contralateral breast by physical examination and mammography is advised.

The best approach is somewhere between these two, considering a patient's individual situation. Advocates of the first school should not be too concerned with the contralateral breast of elderly patients or those with advanced disease; finding and treating occult contralateral carcinoma would not benefit these groups. On the other hand, management of young patients with early stage disease and risk factors as noted by Leis[55] would likely benefit from more than a "watch and wait" policy. Consideration should be given to a contralateral biopsy, and discussion is advisable regarding prophylactic mastectomy, especially in subgroups who are extremely worried about the contralateral side or who seek reconstruction and will require a symmetry procedure for the other side.

REFERENCES

1. Robbins GF, Berg JW: Bilateral primary breast cancers. Cancer 17:1501–1527, 1964
2. Shellito JG, Bartlett WC: Bilateral carcinoma of the breast. Arch Surg 94:489–494, 1967
3. Egan RL: Bilateral breast carcinoma: Role of mammography. Cancer 38:931–938, 1976
4. Leis HP Jr: Selective, elective, prophylactic contralateral mastectomy. Cancer 28:956, 1971
5. Leis HP Jr, Mersheimer WL, Black MM, et al: The second breast. NY State J Med 65:2460–2468, 1965

6. Kilgore AR: The incidence of cancer in the second breast. JAMA 77:454, 1921
7. Pack GT: Bilateral mastectomy. Surgery 29:929, 1951
8. Hubbard TB Jr: Non-simultaneous bilateral carcinoma of the breast. Surgery 34:706, 1953
9. Trevor W: Bilateral breast cancer. NY State J Med 54:1937, 1954
10. McGill RA: Carcinoma of the breast. J Int Coll Surg 21:42, 1954
11. Fitts WT Jr, Patterson LT: The spread of mammary cancer. Surg Clin North Am 36:1539, 1955
12. Ryan AJ, Groswold MH, Allen EP, et al: Breast cancer in Connecticut 1935–1953. A study of 8396 proved cases. JAMA 167:298–307, 1958
13. Prior P, Waterhouse JAH: Incidence of bilateral tumors in a population-based series of breast cancer patients. Br J Cancer 37:620–634, 1978
14. Chaudary MA, Millis RR, Hoskins EOL, et al: Bilateral primary breast cancer: A prospective study of disease incidence. Br J Surg 71:711–714, 1984
15. Schottenfeld D, Berg J: Incidence of multiple primary cancer: IV. Cancers of the female breast and genital organs. J Natl Cancer Inst 46:161–170, 1971
16. Newell GR, Rawlings W, Krementz ET, et al: Multiple primary neoplasms in blacks compared to whites: III. Initial cancer of the female breast and uterus. J Natl Cancer Inst 53:369–373, 1974
17. Veronesi U, Rilke F, Salvadori B, et al: Bilateral cancer of the breast. In Severi L (ed): Multiple Primary Malignant Tumors. Perugia, Division of Cancer Research, 1974
18. Adami HO, Bergstrom R, Hansen J: Age at first primary as a determinant of the incidence of bilateral breast cancer. Cancer 55:643–647, 1985
19. Anderson DE: Some characteristics of familial breast cancer. Cancer 28:1500–1504, 1971
20. Anderson DE: Genetic study of breast cancer: Identification of a high risk group. Cancer 34:1090–1097, 1974
21. Chaudary MA, Millis RR, Bulbrook RD, et al: Family history and bilateral primary breast cancer. Breast Cancer Res Treat 5:201–205, 1985
22. Lagios MD, Westdahl PR, Rose MR: The concept and implications of multicentricity in breast carcinoma. Pathol Annu 16:83–102, 1981
23. Lesser ML, Rosen PP, Kinne DW: Multicentricity and bilaterality in invasive breast carcinoma. Surgery 91:234–240, 1982
24. Newman W: In situ lobular carcinoma of the breast: Report of 26 women with 32 cancers. Ann Surg 157:591, 1963
25. Urban JA: Biopsy of the "normal" breast in treating breast cancer. Surg Clin North Am 49:291, 1969(a)
26. McDivitt RW, Hutter RVP, Foote FW Jr, et al: In situ lobular carcinoma. JAMA 201:96, 1967
27. Peters TG, Donegan WL, Burg EA: Minimal breast cancer: A clinical appraisal. Ann Surg 186:704, 1977
28. Anderson JA: Lobular carcinoma in situ of the breast: An approach to rational treatment. Cancer 39:2597, 1977
29. Fisher ER, Fisher B: Lobular carcinoma of the breast: An overview. Ann Surg 185:377, 1977
30. Donegan WL, Perez-Mesa CM: Lobular carcinoma—an indication for elective biopsy of the second breast. Ann Surg 176:178, 1972
31. Fisher ER, Fisher B, Sass R, et al: Pathologic findings from the National Surgical Adjuvant Breast Project (Protocol No. 4). XI. Bilateral breast cancer. Cancer 54:3002–3011, 1984
32. Kiang DT, Kennedy BJ, Snover DC: Biological and histological characteristics of simultaneous bilateral breast cancer. Lancet 2:1105–1107, 1980
33. Adair F, Berg J, Joubert L, et al: Long term follow-up of breast cancer patients: The 30 year report. Cancer, 33:1145–1150, 1974
34. Egan RL: Bilateral breast carcinomas: Role of mammography. Cancer 38:931–938, 1976
35. Krause CA, Wagner DE: An evaluation of bilateral breast carcinoma: Simultaneous and sequential lesions. West J Med 24:187–190, 1976
36. Kesseler HJ, Grier WRN, Seidman I, et al: Bilateral primary breast cancer. JAMA 236:278–280, 1976
37. Egeli RA, Urban JA: Mammography in symptomatic women 50 years of age and under and those over 50. Cancer 43:872–882, 1979
38. Urban JA: Bilaterality of cancer of the breast. Biopsy of the opposite breast. Cancer 20:1867–1870, 1967
39. Urban JA: Bilateral breast cancer. Cancer 24:1310–1313, 1969
40. Urban JA, Papachristou D, Taylor J: Bilateral breast cancer: Biopsy of the opposite breast. Cancer 40:1968–1973, 1977
41. Pressman PI: Bilateral breast cancer: The contralateral breast biopsy. Breast 5(3):29–33, 1979
42. Wanebo HJ, Senofsky GM, Fechner RE, et al: Bilateral breast cancer: Risk reduction by contralateral biopsy. Ann Surg 201:667–677, 1985
43. Fenig J, Arlen M, Livingston SF, et al: The potential for carcinoma existing synchronously on a microscopic level within the second breast. Surg Gynecol Obstet 141:394–396, 1975
44. King RE, Terz JJ, Lawrence W Jr: Experience with opposite breast biopsy in patients with operable breast cancer. Cancer 37:43–45, 1976
45. Finney GC Jr, Finney GG, Montague AC, et al: Bilateral breast cancer, clinical and pathological review. Ann Surg 175:635–646, 1972
46. Khafagy MM, Schottenfeld D, Robbins GF: Prognosis of the second breast cancer—the role of previous exposure to the first primary. Cancer 35:596–599, 1975
47. Slack NH, Nemoto T, Fisher B: Experience with bilateral primary carcinoma of the breast. Surg Gynecol Obstet 136:433, 1973
48. Huff L: Bilateral carcinoma of the breast. Am J Surg 118:550, 1969
49. Wilson ND, Alberty RE: Bilateral carcinoma of the breast. Am J Surg 126:244, 1973
50. Haagensen CD: Diseases of the Breast, 2nd ed, pp 449–458. Philadelphia, WB Saunders, 1971
51. Black MM, Cutter SJ, Barclay THC: Post biopsy breast carcinoma: A natural experiment in cancer immunology. Cancer 29:61, 1972
52. DeVitt JE: Bilateral mammary cancer. Ann Surg 174:774–778, 1971
53. McCredie JA, Inch WR, Alderson M: Consecutive primary carcinomas of the breast. Cancer 35:1472–1477, 1975
54. Fracchia AA, Robinson D, Legaspi A, et al: Survival in bilateral breast cancer. Cancer 55:1414–1421, 1985
55. Leis HP Jr: Selective, elective prophylactic contralateral mastectomy. Cancer 28:956–961, 1971
56. McCarty KS Jr, Kesterson GHD, Wilkinson WE, et al: Histopathologic study of subcutaneous mastectomy specimens from patients with carcinoma of the contralateral breast. Surg Gynecol Obstet 147:682–688, 1978
57. Goldman LD, Goldwyn RM: Some anatomical considerations of subcutaneous mastectomy. Plast Reconstr Surg 51:501–505, 1973

58. Goodnight JE Jr, Quagliana JM, Morton DL: Failure of subcutaneous mastectomy to prevent the development of breast cancer. J Surg Oncol 26:198–201, 1984

Posttreatment Sarcomas

Jeanne A. Petrek

POSTMASTECTOMY LYMPHANGIOSARCOMA

Incidence

Development of lymphangiosarcoma in a lymphedematous upper extremity after mastectomy was first described in 1948 by Stewart and Treves,[1] reporting six cases at Memorial Hospital. In all six cases of the Stewart-Treves syndrome, the limb was swollen. Four of six patients had preoperative or postoperative radiotherapy, and one patient, though having no breast cancer, had undergone a radical mastectomy for a benign lesion. As of 1977, 206 cases had been reported in a review[2] of the literature. According to Shirger,[3] who studied 894 patients surviving 5 years or more after radical mastectomy, 0.45% will develop the syndrome. Another author[4] calculated 0.07% on finding seven patients in more than 9000 breast cancer patients.

Major series of lymphangiosarcoma from any site are reported from the Mayo Clinic (21 patients),[5] from the M. D. Anderson Hospital and Tumor Institute (22 patients),[6] and from Memorial Sloan-Kettering Cancer Center (44 patients).[7] Postmastectomy lymphangiosarcoma almost invariably occurs in the ipsilateral arm.[5] Only two cases of the malignancy arising in an irradiated chest wall after mastectomy (without apparent arm or chest lymphedema) have been recorded.[8,9] Besides the postmastectomy situations under discussion, lymphangiosarcoma can arise in other chronically lymphedematous limbs,[5,10] in benign vascular malformations[11] as well as in apparently normal skin of the head and neck,[12,13] and in the breast.[14] There have also been 13 case reports of postirradiation lymphangiosarcoma without lymphedema.[9] In 12 of these, the skin was still the site of origin.

Histology

The accepted diagnostic criteria require that angiosarcoma possess anastomosing spaces lined by atypical hyperchromatic endothelial cells. The branching pattern may be layered so that the vasoformative pattern is obscured.[15] Appropriate reticulin stains should identify the vasoendothelial walls of the neoplastic vessels and establish the endothelial relation of the tumor cells. Some cases of postmastectomy lymphangiosarcoma have not quite fulfilled these criteria but have been labeled only anaplastic or undifferentiated neoplasms.

There is considerable variation in the histologic appearance. In small superficial lesions, the tumor may be composed of cuboidal and spindle cells arranged around small capillary-like vessels. Sometimes sheets of neoplastic cells are seen, resembling Kaposi sarcoma. The cuboidal or oval cells can be arranged in cords or irregular clusters, which may have an epithelial appearance similar to breast cancer. Marked lymphangiectasia and proliferation of lymphatic vessels are also present. Electron microscopy has been used to investigate whether this is a lymphangiosarcoma or hemangiosarcoma.[16,17,18,19] At present, the ultrastructure analysis seems to favor hemangiosarcoma.[14]

Etiology

There are only occasional doubts about the independent nature of breast cancer-associated lymphangiosarcoma. That is, some[20,21] believe that many reported cases are metaplastic variants of the original breast carcinoma with an altered histologic picture as a result of the edema. Certainly, an autopsy rate of less than 20%[21] for the collected reported cases does not add confidence to defining this malignancy as a separate pathologic entity.

Nevertheless, there have been several cases of radical surgery for a *benign* breast tumor, with subsequent development of lymphangiosarcoma.[1] Although it is true that few cancers in the past have been critically assessed and compared with the original breast cancer with respect to their light microscopic, ultrastructural, and immunohistochemical characteristics, many recent publications have offered probing analyses.[10,14,23] The general consensus is one of a separate, independently arising malignancy.

Clinical Features

The first clinical sign of the Stewart-Treves syndrome is usually mistaken for an ecchymosis. Afterward, blue or bluish-red discrete nodules appear in the skin, and satellite nodules appear around the original lesions. These often coalesce, forming plaques that ooze serosanguineous fluid. Prior to ulceration, blebs or bullae containing hemorrhagic fluid may cap the tumor nodules. Some lesions undergo necrosis and form cystic cavities. The tumor usually spreads quickly to the forearm and chest wall, as well as circumferentially around the arm. The spread in the involved extremity is usually subcutaneous;[24] only rarely does it follow the intermuscular fascial planes to affect tissues deep inside the arm.[25]

Angiosarcoma has been recorded as early as 1 year[29,30] and as late as 49 years[28] after development of lymphedema, with the average at 8 to 10 years.[2] The oldest patient on record was 85 years,[26] and average age is in the mid-60s.[5,25,27] In three-fourths of patients with postmastectomy lymphangiosarcoma, the upper arm is the site of origin, usually the inner or medial side.

The tumor can resemble dermal metastases from the

original breast cancer or Kaposi sarcoma, melanoma, or pyogenic granuloma. Needless to say, accurate histologic determination is imperative because of the significant differences in treatments.

Prognosis and Treatment

More than half of patients die within 18 months of the diagnosis.[2] In a 1972 review of 162 published cases in the world literature, Woodward[5] found 11 patients who had survived more than 5 years. Seven were treated by amputation, two by wide excision, one with radiation therapy, and one with intra-arterial radioactive yttrium. The lungs are the most common site of metastases.[5,7] Skeletal metastases are frequently recorded, and rarer sites include the liver, gastrointestinal tract, peritoneum, thyroid, tonsils, and adrenals.

Although experience is limited, amputation offers the best chance of cure. In the Memorial Sloan-Kettering experience,[7] 24 of 40 patients were initially treated with surgery. Only 5 of 11 experienced recurrence after amputation, compared with all of 13 patients after wide resection. The median time to recurrence was 5 months. Of the six patients who were treated by amputation and who did not experience local recurrence, two subsequently developed distant metastases.

For the rare lesions arising in the forearm, disarticulation of the arm at the glenohumeral joint with a clear margin may be possible. For the more frequent origin in the upper arm, a forequarter (interscapulothoracic) amputation is the treatment of choice. However, many patients are not candidates for any curative surgical attempts, either because distant metastases are present or because the tumor has spread beyond surgical boundaries.

It is uncommon for amputation to yield good long-term cure rates. In the M. D. Anderson Hospital and Tumor Institute series,[6] 8 of 22 patients underwent forequarter amputation. Four of these cases remain free of disease after 6 months to 7 years of follow-up. The Mayo Clinic experience[5] recorded three of eight patients undergoing amputation as having long-term survival. An additional 16 cases reported from Memorial Sloan-Kettering[7] were treated with radiation therapy or chemotherapy. Although 12 of 31 courses of irradiation resulted in a response, only one case had a long-term response to radiation therapy, remaining free of disease 15 years after diagnosis. (A similar experience with radiation therapy was reported by Woodward and colleagues.[5])

Recently reported from M. D. Anderson[6] were 11 patients receiving a total of 19 trials of systemic chemotherapy, with a 42% response rate to various regimens including 5-fluorouracil; methotrexate; combinations of vincristine, actinomycin D, and cyclophosphamide; or a combination of Adriamycin and dacarbazine with or without vincristine. Responders survived a median of 26.5 months, compared with 4 months for nonresponders. Regional isolation-perfusion or infusion chemotherapy gave two complete responses and one partial response out of six patients treated. The Memorial Sloan-Kettering experience[7] with systemic chemotherapy showed only 6 responses out of 52 patient trials.

Lymphedema has been present in virtually every case, and though not truly causing the disease, lymphedema must be prevented to the fullest extent possible. This includes prompt and thorough treatment of cellulitis to prevent further lymphatic blockage, weight reduction for the obese, and adequate management of lymphedema by pressure gradient therapy and elastic support garments.

POSTIRRADIATION SARCOMAS

Incidence

Sarcomas are a rare but accepted complication of adjuvant radiotherapy after mastectomy for breast cancer. The first case was described in 1936.[31] Thirty-six cases have been reported in the English literature through 1985.[32]

Cahan and colleagues[33] (1948) at Memorial Hospital suggested the following criteria for a radiation-induced bone sarcoma: (1) localization within a previously irradiated area, (2) a clear histologic difference between the treated and the current lesion, (3) a relatively long latent interval, and (4) no bone abnormalities at the time of irradiation. Subsequent authors have also suggested histologic evidence of radiation damage.[34,35,36] Although the Cahan criteria were enumerated for bone sarcomas, they seem equally applicable to and have been used for postirradiation tumors at other sites.

Postirradiation sarcoma occurs in bone more frequently than in soft tissue. Presumably, this can be ascribed to the greater radiation absorption by bone, particularly when orthovoltage is used. The change from orthovoltage to supervoltage more than 20 years ago was expected to decrease postirradiation sarcomas because of lower energy attenuation in bone per roentgen with supervoltage irradiation.[37] However, by 1970, the first cases of sarcoma to appear after use of this modality were reported.[35] No one has yet reported a case developing after linear accelerator therapy.[37]

The rarity of postirradiation sarcomas, the long latency period, and the failure to recognize sarcomas (because of their clinical resemblance to local recurrence) make accurate estimates of both risk and incidence difficult. Nevertheless, the incidence of bone sarcomas in the normal population is 1 per 200,000.[38] Based on the postmastectomy irradiation statistics from the Massachusetts General Hospital, one author[35] estimates an incidence of one postirradiation sarcoma per 450 radiation-treated mastectomy patients alive at 10 years. This agrees with estimates proposed by the University of California Hospital[39] and is somewhat higher than those proposed by the Princess Margaret Hospital, which suggest that the occurrence rate is 1 per 2000 irradiated breast cancer patients surviving 5 years.[40]

Histology

Spontaneously acquired tumors cannot be distinguished histologically from radiation-induced tumors. Ultrastructural analysis, although it may be useful, has been noted in only a few cases.[41,42,43,44] Consequently, the diagnosis of radiation-induced tumor can only be inferred from a history of radiation exposure and with reference to criteria noted almost 40 years ago.[33] The most common tumors following irradiation for breast cancer have been osteosarcoma and fibrosarcoma. Chondrosarcoma,[45] mixed mesenchymal sarcoma,[42] malignant fibrous histiocytoma,[41,43] liposarcoma,[34] undifferentiated sarcoma,[42] and peripheral nerve sheath tumors[46] have also been reported. All sites of postirradiation bone sarcoma considered, 61.9% (104 cases) were osteogenic, 27.4% were fibrosarcomas, 8.9% were chondrosarcomas, and 1.8% were other types.[45] At Memorial Hospital, 5.5% of all osteogenic sarcomas treated were postirradiation.[47] The relative incidence of postirradiation to non–postirradiation fibrosarcoma was 6 to 214 and 4 to 204 at two different institutions.[36]

Sarcoma of the soft tissues and bones may initially be mistaken for postirradiation fibrosis and radiation osteitis.[34,35,48] This may be due to pathologic misdiagnosis or, more likely, to a superficial surgical biopsy. For example, multiple excisions were necessary to make the correct diagnosis in 5 of 11 reported patients with fibrosarcoma after irradiation for breast cancer.[49]

Etiology

A causal relationship seems to exist between x-ray therapy and sarcoma. However, osteogenic sarcoma of a rib following mastectomy has occurred in a patient who did not receive radiation therapy.[50] Certainly, a patient with one malignant tumor is statistically at risk from a second, unrelated neoplasm (the so-called "double primary" phenomenon).[35] Therefore, the term "postirradiation" (rather than "radiation-induced") better describes the sarcoma, insofar as it indicates only the chronology of events. Nevertheless, the incidence of postirradiation sarcoma, although low, is considerably higher than that of spontaneously occurring sarcomas, and almost all regard it as a definite entity.

The actual incidence of postirradiation sarcoma as a function of energy source and method of delivery is unknown. Too few of the previously reported cases provide sufficient data (kilovoltage, filters, fractionation, and field number/size/overlap) for such a determination. Such data are vital for estimation of the absorbed dose at the site of sarcoma induction. By combining several series,[39,51,52] one author[40] calculated the absorbed bone dose in cGy against the log% incidence of postirradiation sarcoma at any site among 5-year survivors. The findings showed a basically linear relationship of increased sarcoma risk with increased dose.

In their review of 262 cases of postirradiation bone sarcomas at any site, Yoshizawa and colleagues[53] noted that 1800 cGy was the lowest dose reported. Efforts to correlate the length of the latency period with the radiation dose have been unsuccessful. Specifically, higher doses do not seem to shorten the latency period. Even the age of the patient does not appreciably shorten the latency period. In sarcomas occurring after retinoblastoma irradiation (with young patients receiving large doses and sometimes repeated treatment courses), the latency period was still more than 10 years.[54] The latency periods for postirradiation bone sarcomas at all sites listed in papers from Memorial Hospital,[55] Roswell Park Cancer Institute,[56] and the Mayo Clinic[37] are 11, 12.5, and 14.3 years, respectively. Both shortening of the latency period and increased frequency of a second malignant neoplasm have been observed following chemotherapy and radiotherapy[57] and may indicate a deleterious consequence of multimodal treatment.

Clinical Features

Postirradiation sarcoma should be suspected when a patient presents with increasing pain or swelling in an irradiated area. Physical examination may reveal edema, tenderness, neurologic deficit, and perhaps a palpable mass. The skin overlying the irradiated area may show atrophy, fibrosis, telangiectasia, hyperpigmentation, dermatitis, and ulceration. Pain was present in 73% of patients and a mass was experienced by 78% in a study of 66 Memorial Hospital patients with postirradiation osteogenic sarcoma at all sites.[46] In two-thirds of these patients, the mass was 8 cm to 9 cm at the time of discovery. Progressive neurologic deficit attributable to postirradiation nerve sheath tumor was noted in six of eight patients in a recent Memorial Hospital series.[46]

As concerns postirradiation bone sarcomas at all sites, radiation osteitis was present in half of 43 recently reported cases.[58] Accompanying large soft tissue masses were found in virtually all patients and were readily apparent on plain films. Periosteal reaction was surprisingly uncommon. Aside from radiation osteitis, the radiographic features of postirradiation sarcomas are indistinguishable from those of spontaneous sarcomas. Computed tomography may be of use in delineating soft tissue sarcomas or the soft tissue component of bone sarcomas.

Needless to say, it is important to investigate pain, nerve deficit, or swelling and to perform a biopsy of the suspicious area. Early detection and proper treatment of postirradiation sarcoma are impeded if these clinical and radiographic findings are attributed merely to radiation fibrosis, osteonecrosis, or worse, to local recurrence.

Prognosis and Treatment

Few patients with radiation-induced sarcoma survive 5 years, compared with those with primary bone or soft tissue sarcoma. Sim and colleagues[59] at the Mayo Clinic, reporting 150 cases of postirradiation bone sarcoma, noted only 2 long-term survivors, the average survival being a little over 1 year. There were no survivors in the small Memorial Hospital series with postirradiation peripheral nerve sheath tumors.[46] With the recent series at Memorial Hospital[47] on postirradiation osteogenic sarcoma, the 5-year survival rate was 17%, median survival being 1 year. However, there were no survivors among trunk sarcomas.

The poorer outlook for breast cancer patients with postirradiation sarcomas may be due to delay when symptoms are thought secondary to the original disease or to radiation necrosis. In addition, the sarcoma is located in the less surgically accessible regions than the typical extremity sarcomas. Nevertheless, radical wide-margin removal, whether chest wall excision or forequarter amputation, is virtually the only recourse for these patients.

Ten patients have been reported with soft tissue fibrosarcoma occurring after radiation therapy for breast cancer.[49] Among the four patients who were reported in the English literature and who did not receive radical operative therapy, there was only a single 1-year survivor, whereas among the six treated surgically, all survived at least a year. Only one is a 5-year survivor. Recent technical improvements in chest wall reconstruction (musculocutaneous flaps, methylmethacrylate/mesh prosthesis, and so on) make it unnecessary for cancer surgeons to be reluctant about the size of the defect created in wide surgical incision.

As a rule, radiation-induced sarcomas cannot be treated by radiation therapy because of exceeding tissue tolerance. Chemotherapy may play a role, but recent reports are not optimistic. Kuten and colleagues[32] discussed six patients with soft tissue sarcoma after irradiation for breast cancer. Chemotherapy, consisting of the four-drug combination CYVADIC (cyclophosphamide, vincristine, Adriamycin, DTIC) was employed in six of seven patients. All died within 6 to 36 months from sarcoma diagnosis. Only two achieved partial remission, lasting 2 or 3 months. Using the CYVADIC regimen, Gottlieb and colleagues[60] reported 14% and 55% complete and overall response rates, respectively, in 136 patients with spontaneous soft tissue sarcomas. The poor response rate noted in the postirradiation group may be due to the fibrotic changes of previous irradiation, resulting in inadequate blood supply and thus reducing tissue concentration. It is therefore important to establish the correct diagnosis early to allow hopefully curative, complete, wide-margin surgical removal.

REFERENCES

1. Stewart FW, Treves N: Lymphangiosarcoma in postmastectomy lymphedema. Cancer 1:64–81, 1948
2. Sandsmark M: Angiosarcoma in post-mastectomy lymphoedema. J Chir Gynaecol 66:251–253, 1977
3. Schirger A: Postoperative lymphedema: Etiologic and diagnostic factors. Med Clin North Am 46:1045, 1962
4. Fitzpatrick PJ: Lymphangiosarcoma and breast cancer. Can J Surg 12:172–177, 1969
5. Woodward AH, Ivins JC, Soule EH: Lymphangiosarcoma arising in chronic lymphedematous extremities. Cancer 30:562–572, 1972
6. Yap B-S, Yap H-Y, McBride C, et al: Chemotherapy for postmastectomy lymphangiosarcoma. Cancer 47:853–856, 1981
7. Sordillo PP, Chapman R, Hajdu SI, et al: Lymphangiosarcoma. Cancer 48:1674–1679, 1981
8. Maddox JC, Evans HL: Angiosarcoma of skin and soft tissue. Cancer 48:1907–1921, 1981
9. Davies JD, Rees GJG, Mera SL: Angiosarcoma in irradiated post-mastectomy chest wall. Histopathology 7:947–956, 1983
10. Huey GR, Stehman FB, Roth LM, et al: Lymphangiosarcoma of the edematous thigh after radiation therapy for carcinoma of the vulva. Gynecol Oncol 20:394–401, 1985
11. Girard C, Johnson WC, Graham JH: Cutaneous angiosarcoma. Cancer 26:868–883, 1970
12. Rosai J, Sumner HW, Kostianovsky M, et al: Angiosarcoma of the skin. Hum Pathol 7:83–109, 1976
13. Hodkinson DJ, Soule EH, Woods JE: Cutaneous angiosarcoma of the head and neck. Cancer 44:1106–1113, 1979
14. Volmer J, Pickartz H, Jautzke G: Vascular tumours in the region of the breast. Virchow's Arch [A] 385:201–214, 1980
15. Stout AP: Haemangio-endothelioma: A tumour of blood vessels featuring vascular endothelial cells. Ann Surg 118:445–464, 1943
16. Silverberg SG, Kay S, Koss LG: Postmastectomy lymphangiosarcoma: Ultrastructural observations. Cancer 27:100–108, 1971
17. Dubin HV, Creehand EP, Headington JT: Lymphangiosarcoma and congenital lymphedema of the extremities. Arch Dermatol 110:608–614, 1974
18. Kermarec J, Varim J-P: Etude microscopique et ultrastructurale d'une tumeur de Stewart-Treves. Arch Anat Pathol 23:193–198, 1975
19. Winkler E: Das Stewart-Treves-Syndrom. Z Hautkr 50:593–600, 1975
20. Salm R: The nature of the so-called postmastectomy lymphagiosarcoma. J Pathol Bacteriol 85:445–456, 1963
21. Schafler K, McKenzie CG, Salm R: Postmastectomy lymphangiosarcoma: A reappraisal of the concept—a critical review and report of an illustrative case. Histopathology 3:131–152, 1979
22. McConnell E, Harris HR: Angiosarcoma in postmastectomy lymphoedema. Br J Surg 53:572–576, 1966
23. Miettinen M, Lehto V-P, Virtanen I: Postmastectomy angiosaracoma (Stewart-Treves syndrome): Light-microscopic, immunohistological, and ultrastructural characteristics of two cases. Am J Surg Pathol 7:329–339, 1983
24. Nelson WR, Morfit HM: Lymphangiosarcoma in the lymphedematous arm after radical mastectomy. Cancer 9:1189, 1956
25. Herrmann JB: Lymphangiosarcoma of the chronically edematous extremity. Surg Gynecol Obstet 121:1107–1115, 1965
26. Pantoja E, Beecher TS, Cross VF: Cutaneous lymphangiosarcoma of Stewart-Treves. Cutis 17:883–886, 1976
27. McSwain B, Whitehead W, Bennett L: Angiosarcoma: Report of three cases of postmastectomy lymphangiosarcoma and one of haemangiosarcoma. South Med J 66:102–106, 1973
28. Scott RB, Nydick I, Conway H: Lymphangiosarcoma arising in lymphedema. Am J Med 28:1008–1012, 1960
29. Birge RF, Peisen CJ, Thornton FR, et al: Angiosarcoma in

postmastectomy lymphedema. J Iowa Med Soc 47:491–495, 1957
30. Sternby NH, Gynning I, Hogeman KE: Postmastectomy angiosarcoma. Acta Chir Scand 121:420–432, 1961
31. Warren S, Sommer GN: Fibrosarcoma of the soft parts with special reference to recurrence and metastasis. Arch Surg 33:425–450, 1936
32. Kuten A, Sapir D, Cohen Y, et al: Postirradiation soft tissue sarcoma occurring in breast cancer patients: Report of seven cases and results of combination chemotherapy. J Surg Oncol 28:168–171, 1985
33. Cahan WG, Woodard HQ, Higginbotham N, et al: Sarcoma arising in irradiated bone. Report of eleven cases. Cancer 1:3–29, 1948
34. Arbari L, Warhol MJ: Pleomorphic liposarcoma following radiotherapy for breast carcinoma. Cancer 49:878–880, 1982
35. Hatfield PM, Schulz MD: Postirradiation sarcoma, including 5 cases after x-ray therapy of breast carcinoma. Radiology 96:593–602, 1970
36. Gane NFC, Lindup R, Strickland P, et al: Radiation-induced fibrosarcoma. Br J Cancer 44:705–711, 1970
37. Weatherby RP, Dahlin DC, Ivins JC: Postradiation sarcoma of bone. Review of 78 Mayo Clinic cases. Mayo Clin Proc 56:294–306, 1981
38. Took IM, Eisenberg H, Honeyman MS: Trends in cancer incidence and survival in Connecticut. Cancer 19:1573–1577, 1966
39. Philips TL, Sheline GE: Bone sarcomas following radiation therapy. Radiology 81:992–996, 1963
40. Tountas AA, Fornasier VL, Harwood AR, et al: Postirradiation sarcoma of bone. A perspective. Cancer 43:182–187, 1979
41. Hardy TJ, An T, Brown PW, et al: Postirradiation sarcoma (malignant fibrous histiocytoma) of axilla. Cancer 42:118–124, 1978
42. Travis EL, Kreuther A, Young T, et al: Unusual postirradiation sarcoma of chest wall. Cancer 38:2269–2273, 1976
43. Tsuneyoshi M, Enjoji M: Postirradiation sarcoma (malignant fibrous histiocytoma) following breast carcinoma. An ultrastructural study of a case. Cancer 45:1419–1423, 1979
44. Rennie JS, McLay A, Tanner NSB: Post-irradiation sarcoma of the lower lip. J Laryngol Otol 97:871–875, 1983
45. Fitzwater JE, Cabaud HE, Farr GH: Irradiation-induced chondrosarcoma. A case report. J Bone Joint Surg [Am]58:1037–1039, 1976
46. Foley KM, Woodruff JM, Ellis FT, et al: Radiation-induced malignant and atypical peripheral nerve sheath tumors. Ann Neurol 7:311–318, 1980
47. Huvos AG, Woodard HQ, Cahan WG, et al: Postradiation osteogenic sarcoma of bone and soft tissues. A clinicopathologic study of 66 patients. Cancer 55:1244–1255, 1985
48. Adam YG, Reif R: Radiation-induced fibrosarcoma following treatment for breast cancer. Surgery 81:421–425, 1977
49. O'Neill MB Jr, Cocke W, Mason D, et al: Radiation-induced soft-tissue fibrosarcoma: Surgical therapy and salvage. Ann Thorac Surg 33:624–628, 1981
50. Pendergrass EP: Adenocarcinoma of the right breast and osteogenic sarcoma of the right third rib in a patient who did not receive postoperative radiation. Cancer 22:644–649, 1968
51. Castro L, Choi SH, Sheehan FR: Radiation-induced bone sarcomas. Am J Roentgenol 100:924–930, 1967
52. Sagerman RH, Cassady JR, Tretter P, et al: Radiation-induced neoplasia following external beam therapy for children with retinoblastoma. Am J Roentgenol 105:529–535, 1969
53. Yoshizawa Y, Kusam T, Morimoto K: Search for the lowest irradiation dose from literatures on radiation-induced bone tumor. Nippon Acta Radiol 37:63–72, 1977
54. Soloway HB: Radiation-induced neoplasms following curative therapy for retinoblastoma. Cancer 19:1984–1988, 1966
55. Kim JH, Chu FC, Woodard HQ, et al: Radiation-induced soft-tissue and bone sarcoma. Radiology 129:501–508, 1978
56. Mindell ER, Shah NK, Webster JH: Postradiation sarcoma of bone and soft tissues. Orthop Clin North Am 8:821–834, 1977
57. Chabner BA: Editorial: Second neoplasm—a complication of cancer chemotherapy. N Engl J Med 297:213–215, 1977
58. Smith J: Radiation-induced sarcoma of bone: Clinical and radiographic findings in 43 patients irradiated for soft tissue neoplasms. Clin Radiol 33:205–221, 1982
59. Sim FH, Cupps RE, Dahlin DC, et al: Post-irradiation sarcoma of bone. J Bone Joint Surg [Am] 54:1479–1489, 1972
60. Gottlieb JA, Baker LH, O'Bryan RM, et al: Adriamycin used alone and in combination for soft tissue and bony sarcomas. Cancer Chemother Rep 6:271–282, 1975

Patient Rehabilitation and Support

16

Psychological Reactions to Breast Cancer and Its Treatment

Jimmie C. Holland Julia H. Rowland

Breast cancer has been the most widely studied cancer with respect to its psychological impact.[1] In part, this is because it is the most common cancer in women, affecting 1 of every 11; also, it is because this disease threatens an organ that is intimately associated with self-esteem, sexuality, and femininity, which are psychological issues of paramount concern to ill and healthy women alike. Although the threat imposed by a diagnosis of breast cancer does not distinguish it from that associated with other cancers, the fear of death that accompanies such a diagnosis is often heightened by the fact that many women can recall friends or relatives who died of breast cancer during an earlier period when fewer curative and supportive measures were available.

Breast cancer is a significant stress for any woman. Women vary widely, however, in their response to diagnosis and treatment.[2] It is important for physicians to understand both the normal emotional responses to the disease and the factors that contribute to them, as well as the range, nature, and types of abnormal responses they might encounter, including those characteristics that place certain women at high risk for poor adaptation. This section covers the following key issues: factors of social context, psychological and medical variables that contribute to the psychological response, and the usual responses of women to each phase of breast cancer (diagnosis, treatment, and rehabilitation). In addition, two special problems are reviewed: the impact of breast cancer upon female relatives, especially children, and the debate about whether personality contributes to breast cancer risk or length of survival.

FACTORS CONTRIBUTING TO PSYCHOLOGICAL RESPONSE

The accompanying display outlines the key factors that contribute to psychological response: the sociocultural context in which treatment options are offered, the psychological and psychosocial factors that the woman and her environment bring to the situation, and the medical factors or physical facts the woman must confront in terms of disease stage, treatment, response, and clinical course.

Sociocultural Context

Historical Background

Until the past decade, radical or modified radical mastectomy was the standard treatment for primary breast cancer in the United States. In earlier times, women were told at the time of diagnostic work-up that they had something "suspicious" in their breast. They gave permission for a biopsy under anesthesia and a mastectomy, which was done at the same time provided the results of frozen specimen analysis were positive. When the woman awakened in the Recovery Room, she discovered the outcome of the combined procedure. Mastectomy resulted in significant physical limitation owing to lymphedema of the affected arm and a deformed "washboard" chest wall. Early psychological studies performed at Memorial Hospital and elsewhere showed that, following radical mastectomy, women had significant postoperative depression, anxiety, poor self-esteem, and impaired physical and sexual function.[3–7] In addition to having to confront their major sur-

Factors Contributing to the Psychological Response of Women to Breast Cancer

Current Sociocultural Context, Treatment Options, and Decision-Making

- Changes in surgical management from a uniform approach
- Societal attitudes
  - Breast-conserving management; more acknowledged uncertainty
  - Public figures disclose having had breast cancer
  - Autobiographical accounts of treatment for breast cancer in popular press
- Women's movement concerns
- Ethical imperative for patient participation in treatment issues
- Legal imperative for knowledge of treatment options

Psychological and Psychosocial Factors

- Type and degree of disruption of life cycle tasks caused by breast cancer (e.g., marital, child-bearing)
- Psychological stability and ability to cope with stress
- Prior psychiatric history
- Availability of psychological and social support (partner, family, friends)

Medical Factors

- Stage of cancer at diagnosis
- Treatment(s) required: mastectomy, lumpectomy and radiation, adjuvant chemotherapy
- Availability of rehabilitation
  - Psychological (partner, support groups)
  - Physical (reconstruction)
- Psychological support provided by physicians and staff

gical defect, these women had few social or psychological supports beyond those available from their own family. The taboos associated with cancer in general and with the breast as a sexual organ dictated that the diagnosis of breast cancer be kept a secret, largely precluding discussion of it with others. As a consequence of a number of major changes in the primary treatment of breast cancer, largely brought about by greater public involvement in health care, a woman's experience with breast cancer today is very different.

In the early 1970s, a debate arose about the use of breast-conserving surgical procedures for the treatment of breast cancer; early data suggested that survival with this approach was comparable to that achieved with more radical surgery.[8] Controlled clinical trials conducted under the auspices of the National Surgical Adjuvant Breast Project (NSABP) and under the leadership of Bernard Fisher provided data supporting an approach to primary breast cancer treatment aimed at achieving maximal disease-free survival, optimal cosmetic results, and no compromise of the chances for cure.[9] Fisher pointed out that recognition of breast cancer as a systemic disease eroded the premise on which radical breast surgery had been based and which had previously led surgeons to attempt to remove "the last cancer cell."

In the past decade, the medical community has increasingly moved away from mastectomy as the uniform and standard treatment for primary breast cancer.[10,11] Newer approaches, although characterized by a greater degree of therapeutic uncertainty, have increasingly involved the use of breast-conserving procedures combined with irradiation. Comparable survival rates have been reported, although a thorough assessment of these new treatment approaches is necessarily limited by a shorter follow-up period. This uncertainty, the widely reported differences of opinion among breast cancer "experts" about optimal treatment, and the survival statistics, which are less than desirable with either treatment regimen, have been widely shared with the public, and with women in particular, through the popular press. "Consensus" meetings about breast cancer treatment, which have helped in establishing policy, have emphasized to women that no currently available procedure is likely to ensure 100% survival, a fact that previously was not widely discussed in public.

These changes in the approach to surgical management of primary breast cancer were paralleled by equally dramatic alterations in societal attitudes toward the disease during the 1970s. In 1974, Betty Ford and Happy Rockefeller publicly acknowledged having been treated for breast cancer. Mrs. Ford permitted disclosure of the fact that, because of malignant involvement of her axillary nodes, she received adjuvant chemotherapy. In the wake of these revelations, women began to inquire about the details of their mastectomy, specifically wanting to know their definitive diagnosis, the extent of disease spread, and whether they also had positive axillary nodes. Previously, women had often not been informed of these facts. At about the same time, several autobiographical accounts of individual women's confrontations with breast cancer were published, bringing the disease further into the public eye.[12,13]

These events occurred in the context of an increasingly active women's movement, which encouraged women's participation in decisions about medical care in general, and about breast cancer treatment in particular. Reach to Recovery, the first woman-to-woman support program, was an important self-help model that grew tremendously in the 1970s under the auspices of the American Cancer Society.[14] At the same time, societal support for a patient's right to participate in treatment decisions was growing, bringing with it an increased emphasis on ethical issues and patient autonomy. Laws were introduced to ensure this right. At least six states (California, Massachusetts, Wisconsin, New Jersey, New York, and Virginia) now require that women who are suspected of having breast cancer be given specific information. They must be informed about the option of having the biopsy and treatment done in two stages, as well as the option of having lumpectomy and irradiation as primary treatment.

These changes have resulted in a vastly altered sociocultural climate for women dealing with breast cancer. Table 16-1 summarizes the change in the focus of problems faced by women with breast cancer 15 to 20 years

Table 16-1
Changes in the Psychological Issues in Primary Breast Cancer Treament: Past and Present

15–20 Years Ago	*At Present*
Fears of breast cancer and mastectomy	Fears of breast cancer and choice of treatment options
One-stage biopsy/mastectomy under anesthesia	Laws that mandate a patient's knowledge of two-stage procedure, necessitating a decision between two treatment options
Little participation in treatment decision	Full participation in care and choices made by patient
Little discussion of survival/ prognosis	Full disclosure of survival/ prognosis
Full reassurance about future; Minimal follow-up	Limited reassurance about future; frequent and long-term observation

ago as compared to those issues that are the focus today. The emotional problems are different today, but equally compelling. Although fears about breast loss and threat to body image and sexual function have decreased with the introduction of breast-conserving treatment techniques, fears and anxieties about having made the right treatment choice and about the likelihood of survival have increased. A change that is integral to the initial emotional burden today is the patient's increased level of participation in primary treatment decisions.

Decision-Making Patterns

Today, women diagnosed with breast cancer will likely be aware of the plurality of views that exist concerning primary breast cancer treatment. Most will recognize that no "best" treatment exists, but rather that they have various options, and that their preference with respect to these options will be considered. Women now also have access to precise survival statistics for each mode of treatment, although consulting physicians may offer quite different interpretations of the data available from studies that compare mastectomy with lumpectomy and irradiation. Although the increased level of dialogue between physician and patient regarding diagnosis and care eases some of the stresses faced earlier by women, it also poses a new psychological burden, often at a time when anxiety is already great.

The steps through which a well-informed woman may go before primary breast cancer treatment is initiated highlight these new psychological problems (Fig. 16-1). Most women consult their gynecologist or a trusted and accessible physician when they find a breast lump (80% of which are found by women themselves). A mammogram may then be ordered and, depending upon its outcome, the woman may be advised of "suspicious" findings and referred to a surgeon. In some states, the law dictates that the surgeon must inform the woman of the difference between a one- and two-stage surgical procedure, reviewing with her the options of having a needle (outpatient) biopsy performed initially, with removal of the mass, if indicated, during a later, second procedure, versus having a diagnostic biopsy performed under general anesthesia with removal of the mass at the same time. In these states, the two treatment options of mastectomy or lumpectomy combined with irradiation must be presented as well. Some insurance carriers also mandate a second opinion prior to the performance of any elective surgical procedure. Although these policies provide a valuable impetus for women to obtain thorough medical evaluation and information, they also introduce yet another set of opinions.

After obtaining a second opinion or consulting several specialists, the woman may ask in desperation, "Which doctor should I trust?" "How do I know if I chose the right one?" "What if I pick the wrong treatment option?" "With which option can I be *sure* I am safe?" The woman must cope simultaneously with the need to keep her distressing emotions of anxiety and fear within tolerable limits while making the difficult decision about treatment for a disease which she knows may be fatal. To accomplish this, she must assimilate new medical information which, in itself, may produce more anxiety.

Valanis and Rumpler have provided a thoughtful review of the many issues faced by women in choosing among breast cancer treatment alternatives.[15] They note that a woman's previous experiences, her personal and demographic characteristics, as well as those of her social support network (family and friends) and her physician may influence her treatment selection. Findings by two researchers at Memorial Sloan-Kettering Cancer Center highlight the influence of two important factors—anxiety and the physician-patient relationship—on the decision-making process.

Scott studied three variables related to coping response in 85 women, aged 18 to 60 years, prior to and following breast biopsy.[16] The variables evaluated included state of anxiety, critical thinking ability, and information-processing capacity (concentration). Those who had negative biopsy results were tested again at 6 to 8 weeks. The key findings were that, prior to biopsy, anxiety levels were high, reasoning ability (critical thinking) was reduced, and the time required for processing information (roughly equated with ability to concentrate) increased. Six to eight weeks later, after recovery and after the negative results of the biopsy were known, the women's anxiety was reduced, and both reasoning and concentration had returned to normal. The group ($N=25$) with the highest pre-biopsy anxiety exhibited the greatest impairment in ability to reason. These findings suggest that anxiety and information overload may compromise decision-making at a critical period, making informed decisions difficult, even at best.[16]

An additional factor that must be considered in evaluating the decision-making process is the role of the phy-

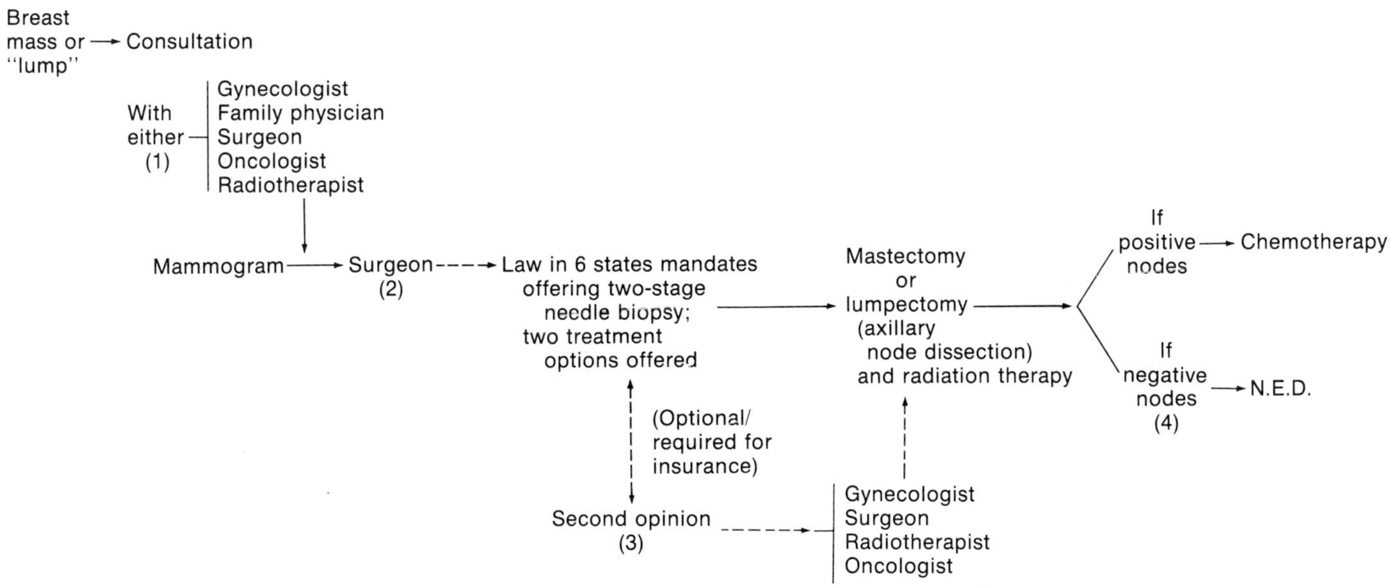

FIGURE 16-1. Steps in decision-making for treatment of patients with breast cancer.

sician-patient relationship. In a multicenter study of patients' perceptions of giving informed consent for chemotherapy, Penman and colleagues found that the information conveyed verbally by the physician played a principal role in their efforts to arrive at a decision about treatment, and that the written form contributed little.[17] Particularly pertinent to the present discussion was the fact that the primary reason cited for accepting the treatment outlined was "trust in the physician who discussed this treatment with me;" 86% said they relied strongly on the physician's recommendations. Current legal and ethical constraints that mandate the patient's independent choice may place a particularly heavy burden on some women who feel comfortable with decisions being made by others. In Penman's informed consent study, physicians estimated that one-third of their patients had assumed a passive or acquiescent stance in making a decision. Emphasis on informed decision-making also places a heavy responsibility on the physician to be cognizant of the individual patient's physical and psychological needs, and to tailor the discussion and recommendations accordingly.

The current climate which dictates a single approach to all women fails to take into account the fact that the reactions of women to the decision-making process vary widely. Ideally, information should be conveyed in different ways for each patient. At least four response types (presented below as extremes to highlight differences) may be delineated, each of which calls for an intervention or communication approach that is quite different.

Type 1: *"You decide for me, Doctor."* This is apt to be an older woman who has been accustomed to accepting the authority (and decisions) of physicians. She may be (or may choose to remain) less well informed about treatment options. She will cope best with a physician who outlines options, but who accepts a strong role in the decision. She will do poorly with the "come back in a week and let me know your decision" stance. Because she relates to a generation taught to expect the physician to recommend treatment, such a stance is interpreted as "the doctor doesn't know what to do" and is seen as frightening.

Type 2: *"I demand you do the——procedure."* This response is common among young women who are more medically sophisticated and who have consulted all available resources, obtained all relevant materials, and have already made a decision. These patients are often ready to assume an adversarial position if their requests are not heard or adopted. This response may be troublesome to the conscientious physician who may have to object to the patient's demand as inappropriate on sound medical grounds. Such a young woman needs to be treated as a full participant in the decision process, and may need to be given a careful outline of the relevant medical data, often supplemented upon request by written materials from authoritative sources, with which she can assure herself of the facts. Discussing the options, listening and responding to questions, and detailing the limits of the available options, based on data, will maximize the possibility that *both* the patient's and physician's points of view will be heard, and that a relationship of mutual respect will be established, allowing a true, shared decision to be reached.

Type 3: *"I can't decide."* This response is often seen in women who feel overwhelmed by the knowledge that they have a breast lump and are frightened by its threat to life; in such cases, the options are often too painful to consider. These women are often referred for psychiatric consultation. It is helpful for them to have the pressure temporarily removed and to be able to review the events and possible treatments in a setting where they feel secure in expressing concerns, recognizing that they must come to some closure. A useful procedure is to take them, step-by-step, through all the consequences and ramifications of each treatment option, asking at each juncture "How would you respond to that?" By this approach, with reduced anxiety, it usually becomes clear that certain aspects of one or the other treatment are more acceptable to the patient. These women may then return to their surgeon ready to proceed with therapy.

Type 4: *"Given the options, your recommendations, and my preferences, I choose. . . ."* This reaction suggests a mature patient who is anxious, but who is able to engage in a constructive interaction with the physician to arrive at a thoughtful decision. The exposition of relevant facts, with provision of pamphlets and discussion of all facets of the treatment and outcome, leads to a decision.

Clearly, the manner in which primary breast cancer treatment is determined leaves room for improvement. Some ways in which the current decision-making process could be improved are outlined below:

Information. Attention should be given to developing videotapes and written materials that extend the information provided by those currently available.

Breast Diagnostic Clinic. Major cancer centers, where many second opinions are given, could organize weekly clinic hours during which the participation of a surgeon, pathologist, and radiotherapist was assured. This multispecialty consultation could occur over a period of hours rather than the usual weeks, thus eliminating the attendant and prolonged lack of clear recommendations that currently occurs. The availability of a skilled counselor who is knowledgeable about breast cancer would ensure needed emotional support.

Nurse-Specialist in Breast Cancer. A nurse knowledgeable in breast cancer management who is sensitive to the psychological concerns of patients could provide an extremely valuable service in physicians' offices, expediting the discussion of options, listening to fears, assessing emotional stability in the decision-making process, supporting a doctor's recommendations, helping the patient to formulate questions, and correcting misinformation. The nurse could then convey information to the physician about the patient's psychological state, her ability to participate in the decision, and even her likely preferences, resulting in a more productive discussion between patient and physician. In a study done at Montefiore Hospital, we found that the nurse clinician who went to the patient's home before she underwent one-stage biopsy and mastectomy and who saw the patient during preoperative and postoperative visits, served as a powerful source of support. This support was as much a product of the continuity of care provided as the availability of a concerned advocate.[18]

Research. Studies of the decision-making process and the methods by which information about treatment options should be conveyed to ensure effective communication while remaining sensitive to the needs of different patients are needed. As legal and ethical constraints change medical practice in this area, it is imperative that we learn more about the decision process—in part, to influence legal authorities to develop laws that recognize individual differences and medical changes. Fisher points out that the mandate for a two-stage biopsy procedure, legislation which was originally intended to safeguard patients' options, may now be a hindrance.[19] He notes that biopsy procedures should increasingly include initial removal of the whole lump in order to ensure clean margins and an accurate pathologic evaluation. The current practice of obtaining multiple opinions, which are often sought after an inadequate or poorly performed initial biopsy done without anesthesia, may be a disservice to the woman and an impediment to optimal treatment.

On a reassuring note, it should be mentioned that research by Ashcroft and co-workers revealed that, given the choice of mastectomy or lumpectomy plus radiotherapy, women opting for either type of treatment had done well.[20] Levels of anxiety and depression for both groups were similar to those in other surgical patients. A one-year follow-up study failed to reveal any evidence of the profound anxiety and depression reported in other studies. The authors point out, however, that women choosing one treatment or the other may focus on different needs and concerns, an issue discussed later in this chapter section.

Psychological Factors

In an excellent review of the published studies on the psychosocial correlates of breast cancer and its treatment, Meyerowitz identified the psychosocial impact of breast cancer as falling into three broad areas: psychological discomfort (anxiety, depression, and anger), changes in life patterns (consequent to physical discomfort, marital/sexual disruption, or an altered activity level), and fears and concerns (mastectomy and death).[1] This psychological impact is modulated by variables within the woman, as well as her illness experience and her environment, all of which have been widely studied and which account for the remarkably wide range of responses to breast cancer. Using an outline of these variables to organize her review (see the accompanying display), Meyerowitz summarized the nature and direction of impact of these variables on premorbid and postmastectomy adjustment. A commonality of opinion and observation emerges despite the findings, which often lack a conceptual or historical framework. It is important to remember that most of the studies from the 1950s to the present have been done on women with breast cancer for whom mastectomy was the primary treatment, making it difficult to distinguish between the impact of mastectomy and that of breast cancer.

Summary of Variables Examined in the Psychological Literature on Breast Cancer and its Treatments*

Psychosocial Impact of Breast Cancer and its Treatment
- Psychological discomfort
  - Depression
  - Anxiety
  - Hostility
- Changes in life patterns
  - Physical discomfort
  - Marital/sexual upset
  - Reduced activity level
- Fears and concerns
  - Mastectomy/mutilation
  - Cancer/death

Variables That Influence Intensity and Duration of Psychosocial Impact
- Premorbid variables
  - Patient characteristics
    - Importance of physical appearance of the breast to patient
    - Age
    - Preoperative expectations
  - Environmental characteristics
    - Preoperative preparation by surgeon
    - Quality of marital/sexual relationship
- Postmastectomy variables
  - Coping styles of patients
    - Denial and related defenses (intensity and selectivity
    - Search for causes (self-blame and projection of blame)
  - Environmental variables
    - Time elapsed since surgery
    - Availability of support (physician/surgeon, spouse and family, other patients)
    - Additional medical treatments (radiotherapy and chemotherapy)

* (Meyerowitz B E: Psychosocial correlates of breast cancer and its treatments. Psychol Bull 87:127, 1980. Copyright 1980 by the American Psychological Association. Reprinted by permission of the author.)

We have regarded the key issues in psychological adaptation to breast cancer from three perspectives: the life stage at which it occurs; previous emotional stability, personality, and coping style; and the presence and availability of interpersonal supports. The point in the life cycle at which the breast cancer occurs and the social tasks that are threatened or interrupted are of prime importance. The threat to a sense of femininity and self-esteem occurs in all women, but it may be more pronounced in young women whose attractiveness and fertility are paramount, especially in those who are single and without a partner. In most instances, the meaning of the breast cancer is quite different for her than for the older woman who has a secure home and family, and for whom the risk to life may be predominant. However, the fact that breast cancer occurs frequently in older women who may be experiencing other losses, including the loss of a spouse, means that these individuals may also experience a difficult period of adaptation, having to adjust not only to losses in their social environment, but also to a threat to life. Preliminary reports by Fotopoulis of data from a multicenter study of the psychological aspects of breast cancer showed a high level of distress in older women.[21]

The second factor contributing to adaptation relates to the patient herself: her personality and coping patterns. Each woman has her own style of adapting to stress, shown to be a remarkably abiding quality. In a study by Gorzynski and colleagues of women evaluated before biopsy for breast cancer and 10 years later, coping styles and effectiveness in controlling emotional distress remained unchanged over time.[22] The coping strategies that have been found to be most effective in managing the stresses of breast cancer have been identified by Penman. Her research shows these strategies to be a cluster of behaviors, identifiable in the immediate postmastectomy period and characterized by a "tackling stance" to the problems raised by diagnosis and surgery.[23] Those women who use avoidance and capitulation, rather than "confrontive" coping strategies, are more emotionally distressed in the early rehabilitative stages following mastectomy than are women who deal more directly with the stress. Moreover, women who have a sense of control over events, actively taking a role in rehabilitation, have been found to do better than those with a helpless outlook. A pessimistic response usually reflects prior psychological patterns of poor coping with stressful events. Women who have had prior psychiatric illness are at higher risk for exacerbation of symptomatology and a more troubled response to breast cancer. Data from a large multicenter sample, compiled by Bloom and co-workers, showed that when women with a pre-existing psychiatric disorder were eliminated from a study of adaptation to breast cancer, there was an absence of serious psychopathological responses after mastectomy, despite the presence of higher levels of distress among patients with cancer than among those undergoing cholecystectomy or breast biopsy or those who constituted the healthy female control group.[24] Schain adds to the list of premorbid risk factors associated with poor adaptation a history of unsatisfactory or negative sexual experience, intense personal investment in the breasts, problems in body image, and difficulty discussing personal, especially sexual, problems.[25]

Adaptation may also be altered by the special meaning associated with breast cancer for a particular woman. Some women with a high investment in their bodies cannot even tolerate the idea of loss of or damage to a breast. Such women are at risk for delay in seeking consultation when a symptom occurs; they are also at risk for problems in adaptation following treatment. Today, women who are at increased genetic risk for breast cancer or those who have fibrocystic disease must deal with the anxiety aroused by regular breast self-examination, frequent physician visits, and repeated mammographic examinations. Some women may try to deny the risk, whereas others may become preoccupied with checking possible breast lumps, recalling their mother's, grandmother's, or sister's experience with breast cancer. When actual breast cancer develops, painful memories return under the stress of their own illness, causing significantly greater distress.

Adjustment also depends on the response of significant others—first and foremost, the response of spouse or partner, but also that of family and friends.[26–29] In their study of men's adjustment to breast cancer, Wellisch and co-workers found that, although they managed well overall, a subgroup remained distressed following their mate's mastectomy.[30] Adjustment appeared to be facilitated if the husband or partner was involved in the decision-making process, visited his spouse in the hospital, saw the scar early, and resumed sexual relations early. Support from other women, especially those who have been through mastectomy, has constituted the framework for such programs as Reach to Recovery, a highly effective form of group support. The efforts of this organization are becoming wider in scope today as a result of the addition to its services of peer visitors who can relate specifically to the woman who has had a mastectomy and reconstruction or lumpectomy and irradiation. The closer the visitor's experience is to that of the patient, the better her ability to provide an effective role model for coping and a source of practical and emotional support.

Some women have phobias about anesthesia or surgery, fearing the operating room, loss of control, or death during surgery. These individuals may have increased psychological difficulties and may require special management for successful treatment. A careful medical, family, and psychiatric history will reveal these and the other factors that may place a woman at high risk for emotional distress.

Medical Factors

Psychosocial adjustment also varies according to the stage of disease at diagnosis, the treatment required, and the likely prognosis and rehabilitative opportunities available. Central to all, however, is the relationship of the patient to a supportive surgeon or radiotherapist who is sensitive to concerns and monitors both emotional and physical well-being. The office or clinic nurse and hospital staff often become the patient's "second home," at times buffering and compensating for the absence of a more substantive physician-patient relationship. Recent work by Faulkner and Maguire has demonstrated that ward nurses can be trained to play an important role in monitoring the psychological problems of their breast patients.[31] Secretaries, as well as technicians, also contribute to the ambience of the medical care setting, and should be considered in any evaluation of psychosocial interventions and services.

Women's psychological responses to the stage and clinical course of their disease have been detailed elsewhere.[32] However, changes in the primary treatment and rehabilitative options currently available to women have led to concern about the impact of these newer approaches on women's adjustment. The extensive literature on the psychological aspects of breast cancer has been devoted almost exclusively to the patient's response to mastectomy. Only recently have studies begun to evaluate the effects on psychosocial morbidity of postmastectomy breast reconstruction or the use of lumpectomy and irradiation as primary treatment. In both cases, the fact that breast-sparing or reconstructive options exist appears to increase the morale of women in general. Some physicians and patients speculate that the awareness of these options also might reduce women's delay in seeking initial treatment, although this effect has yet to be clearly assessed. Because of the growing importance such procedures may have in the treatment of and response to breast cancer, they are discussed below in greater detail. Each new procedure raises special concerns for the women undergoing it; each must be evaluated and compared, with respect to its emotional and social sequelae, to the standard for care, mastectomy. Special issues related to adjustment to adjuvant chemotherapy and advanced disease will also be covered.

Reconstruction

An increasing number of women who are undergoing or who have already undergone mastectomy will consider breast reconstruction as a postsurgical treatment option. Interest in this procedure has grown as a result of several factors: the increasing use of tissue-sparing procedures which have resulted in more patients being better surgical candidates for reconstruction; rapid advances in the technologic aspects of the reconstructive surgery, leading to the development of procedures to correct defects from more radical surgeries, diminished complications, and the achievement of more optimal, "breastlike" outcomes; and the increasing demand by women for greater participation in their own health care. Although it is generally estimated that less than 10% of women undergoing mastectomy also undergo reconstruction, data collected by the American Society of Plastic and Reconstructive Surgeons suggest that this trend may be changing, especially for women treated a number of years ago. In a survey publicized in May of 1985, they reported that an estimated 98,000 reconstructions were performed by their 2600 member surgeons in 1984, in comparison to 20,000 such reconstructions recorded in 1981, just three years earlier.[33] Research conducted in 1980 by the National Cancer Institute on attitudes about breast cancer revealed that almost 40% of the women interviewed indicated that they would be interested in breast reconstruction if they underwent a mastectomy.[34] As Schain and colleagues noted in an excellent review, psychosocial issues in breast reconstruction fall into five major areas: information, economic factors, medical factors, intrapsychic factors or self-determined needs, and interpersonal factors, or other-determined needs.[35] Considerable progress has been made in women's exposure to information about breast reconstruction in contrast to an earlier period when there was a reluctance to provide women with appropriate information and to encourage their seeking out individuals who had undergone such surgery. A number of support groups sprang up around this latter issue (RENU, AWEAR). While the cost of these procedures has not diminished, coverage by health insurance carriers has increased, largely in response to pressure from health consumer and women's groups to reclassify the surgery as rehabilitative, not cosmetic. In addition, far fewer medical variables now preclude a woman from being a candidate for reconstruction.

The psychological variables associated with the decision to seek reconstruction or not and women's responses to reconstructive surgery were studied at Memorial Sloan-Kettering Cancer Center in a joint effort by the Psychiatry, Plastic and Reconstructive Surgery, and Breast Services.[36,37] The original research questions were:

Who seeks breast reconstruction and why?
What is the impact of this surgery on women's postmastectomy adaptation and functioning?
Are there any features of women's personality or surgical experience that mediate satisfaction with the outcome?
Are patients who seek this surgery different from those who do not?

One hundred and fifty women seeking postmastectomy reconstruction were evaluated according to a number of surgical and psychological parameters at the time of initial consultation. Eighty-three of the 117 women undergoing reconstruction were reassessed postoperatively. In addition, a comparison sample of 50 women who were not seeking reconstruction were also studied. The findings are summarized below.

Women seeking consultation for breast reconstruction ranged in age from 28 to 68 years (mean, 45.5) and tended to be middle or upper-middle class, white females who were married and Catholic. More than 60% were working full- or part-time. This profile is similar to that described by others doing research on reconstruction samples.[38,39] On the average, the women coming for consultation were 34 months postmastectomy, although intervals since mastectomy ranged from 1 month to 20 years. Seventy-three percent of the patients had undergone modified radical mastectomy; less than 25% had received adjuvant chemotherapy or radiotherapy. The plastic surgeons considered 85% of the women to be good to excellent candidates for reconstructive surgery.

On interview and self-report, these women, as a group, appeared to be psychologically well-adjusted and functioning well. Although they harbored some emotional pain related to cancer and the mastectomy, they were generally well informed about the nature of the surgery and approached reconstruction with realistic expectations of its potential benefits for them, both personally and physically. The reasons most frequently cited for seeking surgery were to be rid of the prosthesis, to "feel whole again," and to re-establish breast symmetry, thus diminishing self-consciousness about appearance. These motives have been echoed in other samples studied.[40,41]

The study's results largely underscored the positive effects of breast reconstruction. With few exceptions, the net effect of the surgery was to increase both observed and stated satisfaction with levels of psychological, social, and sexual function. Eighty-three percent of the women stated that they were happy or absolutely delighted with the overall results, and most found that the results of reconstructive surgery met or surpassed their expectations.

Response to reconstruction was found to be independent of a woman's age, social class, or her surgeon's estimate of the success of outcome. However, women who pursued this surgery primarily to please others or with the expectation of improving sexual and social relations were at risk for disappointment. Time from surgery also appeared to modify their response. Although satisfaction with overall results increased with the length of the interval since mastectomy, as the interval since completion of the reconstruction increased, so did the likelihood of a more critical response, both to the physical aspects of the surgery as well as to its net effect. Finally, it was concluded that a woman's ability to obtain clear and complete information about the surgery preoperatively, especially with respect to all surgery proposed for the remaining breast to achieve symmetry, and to have the opportunity postoperatively to express dissatisfaction or explore fears and concerns about results, were also potentially important mediators of later satisfaction.

The data derived from the study of the women in the reconstruction group was also compared to that for the group of 50 women who were not seeking breast reconstruction. This latter group was drawn from a pool of patients returning for routine mastectomy follow-up to one of Memorial Hospital's breast surgeons, and was roughly matched with the reconstruction sample in terms of age, time since mastectomy, and type of mastectomy. Results indicated that women seeking reconstruction resembled their nonreconstructed peers in many aspects. Comparison of these two groups revealed no differences in satisfaction with or ability to resume daily activities postmastectomy, levels of self-esteem, feelings of attractiveness, sexual functioning, or self-reported psychological symptoms. Nonreconstructed patients reported greater comfort with external prosthesis use, had less knowledge about reconstruction, and attached greater importance to their breasts. There was also a suggestion that women in the reconstruction group felt that their husband or sexual partner more frequently avoided touching or looking at the mastectomy site than did the husbands or partners of the nonreconstructed group.

Additional comparisons between women who sought consultation and eventually underwent reconstruction and those who sought consultation but later refused surgery for nonmedical reasons revealed some interesting differences. Those who refused surgery for nonmedical reasons tended to be older and of a lower socioeconomic status, and more often were single. They appeared to have experienced greater psychosocial dysfunction as a result of their mastectomy, were at greater risk for psychiatric symptoms, and were more likely to have seen a therapist for emotional problems. Finally, they tended to have undergone more radical treatment for their breast cancer and, therefore, were poorer candidates for plastic surgery. The differences in psychosocial and physical status between these groups indicate that women who are at increased risk for emotional or surgical disappointment following reconstructive procedures may select themselves out at the time of consultation.

Concerns that women seeking reconstructive procedures do so out of neurotic or psychotic needs were not supported by our or other investigators' research.[40,41] Most women sought surgery for personal reasons. Importance of "personal" versus "public" body image was a consistent theme echoed by patients in Daniel's study.[42] After undergoing reconstruction, many women found themselves less preoccupied with their health and the fact that they had had cancer; they no longer had the constant reminder of the physical defect. Teimourian and Adham found increased sexual activity in women postreconstruction,[43] and work by Gerard suggested that reconstructed patients achieved more sexual responsivity than did their mastectomy peers.[44] Goin and Goin reported that, in postclimacteric women, the request for breast reconstruction may serve as a catalyst for more adequate adjustment to the mid-life crises that are often complicated by a diagnosis of cancer.[45]

The key concerns of women about reconstruction include the cost of the surgery; the safety of the techniques used, both with respect to the potential for complications and the risk of masking or promoting recurrent disease; and the cosmetic results achievable. Surgeons differ in their approach to this latter concern. Some prefer to use written materials only, others show pictures of reconstructed breasts, whereas many use a combination of these approaches and may, at times, refer a woman to a previously reconstructed patient for more details. In our own research and that of others,[35,46] several additional issues seemed to be of importance in counseling women who were considering or undergoing these procedures. These factors included the need for discussion of all facets of the surgical steps (including the number and length of hospitalizations); a thorough review of plans for symmetry procedures, if needed; and consideration of the timing of the procedure. The psychological impact of the timing of reconstruction has been the focus of additional studies.

IMMEDIATE VERSUS DELAYED RECONSTRUCTION. Although debate about the medical efficacy and outcome of immediate versus delayed reconstruction persists, the psychological literature has begun to indicate that early reconstruction may prevent some of the trauma associated with loss and disfigurement experienced by women undergoing mastectomy. Recent research with women undergoing immediate reconstruction has shown not only high levels of patient satisfaction with surgical results, but also significantly less psychosocial morbidity among these women than among those who undergo mastectomy alone.[47–50] The patients undergoing immediate reconstruction were less depressed and suffered less impairment of their sense of femininity, self-esteem, and sexual attractiveness than their peers who delayed or did not seek reconstruction. These studies also suggest that immediate reconstruction does not interfere with the necessary mourning process associated with the threat to life and breast loss.

In a single study by Stevens and associates, women undergoing immediate reconstruction exhibited less psychiatric and psychosocial impairment in the early postreconstruction period (within 6 months) than did women undergoing delayed surgery.[49] However, a number of patients in the delayed group had more extensive disease initially, and were not followed longitudinally, as was the group undergoing immediate reconstruction. In preliminary analyses of a larger, randomized, comparative trial of patients undergoing immediate versus delayed reconstruction, Schain and colleagues noted that initial differences in adjustment may be minimal, and are likely to disappear over time.[50]

The survey conducted by the American Society of Plastic and Reconstructive Surgeons revealed that 34% of the breast reconstructions performed by member surgeons in 1984 were done at the same time as, or within a few days of, mastectomy.[33] As more women request these procedures, additional research will be needed to determine who will benefit from immediate reconstruction and who will be better served by having a waiting period between cancer surgery and reconstructive procedures.

Lumpectomy and Irradiation

The use of alternatives to mastectomy has increased as a function of a number of changes in the treatment of breast cancer: the increased role of outpatient biopsies, a clearer understanding of the biology of the disease, and the encouraging therapeutic results of breast-conserving approaches to management. Data that show survival rates in women treated by breast-conserving procedures to be equal to that in women undergoing more radical procedures have begun to have an impact on practice in all communities, although differences in interpretation of survival data still exist among physicians. The impetus to adopt less radical approaches has also been spurred on by women's own requests for less mutilating treatment and their increasingly active role in decision-making. Combined lumpectomy and irradiation, because it is a cosmetic alternative to mastectomy, has grown in importance, not only as a means of providing equivalent survival, but also because it provides equivalent or improved psychosocial function. For this reason, it has been the focus of a number of recent comparative studies.

Steinberg reviewed six "first-generation" studies in which the adaptation of women undergoing lumpectomy and irradiation versus those undergoing mastectomy was compared.[51] In general, the studies showed that women who undergo breast-sparing surgery are less self-conscious, have a better body image, manifest better overall adjustment, and report greater satisfaction with sexual ac-

Table 16-2
Controlled Studies of Psychological Response to Mastectomy (M) versus Lumpectomy and Radiation Therapy (L-RT) *

Study	*No. Subjects* *L-RT*	*M*	*Satisfaction With Body Image*	*Marital Adjustment*	*Satisfaction With Sexual Function*	*Psychological Adjustment*	*Fear of Recurrence*
Sanger and Reznikoff, 1981[52]	20	20 (Modified)	L-RT group–more positive feelings	Equal		Equal	
Schain et al., 1983[53]	18	20 (Modified)	L-RT group–less negative feelings	Equal	Equal	Equal	Equal (M = 80%; L-RT = 83%)
Steinberg, Juliano, and Wise, 1985[54]	21	46 (Modified)	L-RT group–more positive feelings	Equal	L-RT group report that husbands/ partners are more sexual	Equal in terms of depression and anxiety; L-RT group better in general	Equal
Bartelink, Van Dam, and Van Dongen, 1985[55]	114	58 (Modified)	L-RT group–less self-conscious		L-RT group–less sexually inhibited		M–greater
Taylor et al., 1985[56]	26	31 (Simple/ Modified) 9 (Radical)	L-RT group–fewer concerns about disfigurement	Equal	L-RT group having sex more frequently, more affectionate husbands/ partners	L-RT group–best global adjustment	
Haes and Welvaart, 1985[57]	21	18 (Radical)	L-RT group–less negative feelings	Equal	Equal	Equal	Equal (older patients less fearful)
Wellisch, 1986[58]	22	30 (Modified)	L-RT group–more positive feelings	Equal	L-RT group–higher libido	Equal	Equal

* (Modified from Steinberg M: Psychological aspects of lumpectomy-radiation treatment for early breast cancer. In Syllabus for Early Breast Cancer: The Psychologic Perspective, a conference sponsored by Long Island Jewish Medical Center and Memorial Sloan-Kettering Cancer Center, New York, New York, October 11, 1985.)

tivity than do those undergoing mastectomy. The results of these studies, together with those of two others, are presented in Table 16-2 and are discussed briefly below.[52–58] Despite the small numbers of patients represented in each, data from these research studies suggest that women undergoing lumpectomy and irradiation have, as a group, adapted well.

The study reported by Schain and co-workers is of particular interest in that the women interviewed had all agreed to be randomized between the two procedures.[53] Data showed more positive feelings about body image in the lumpectomy-irradiation group, but little difference with respect to other parameters of mental well-being, psychological symptoms, or fears of recurrence. Bartelink's study reported an increased incidence of fear of recurrence among women undergoing mastectomy, but all of the patients in his study had undergone radical mastectomy.[55] Observations from our clinical practice indicate elevated fears of recurrence among patients undergoing combined lumpectomy-irradiation. However, the prevalence of such fears may, in part, reflect the fact that women who have had lumpectomy-irradiation in the first years of the procedure's common use, have frequently done so over the admonitions of skeptical surgeons who have advised them that they might be saving the breast but putting their lives in jeopardy. As Steinberg notes, these women chose an unpopular, poorly accepted treatment, and were thus likely to differ from women electing mastectomy, the more traditional and established treatment.[51] The decision to undergo lumpectomy-irradiation may also depend on women's attitudes about cancer. The thought of leaving any tumor cells in the breast is intolerable for some women who believe that mastectomy offers them greater assurance that the cancer has been removed.

Research by Ashcroft and colleagues[20] and Margolis and Goodman[59] suggests that personality characteristics also influence a woman's preference for treatment. Both sets of researchers found that women selecting lumpectomy and irradiation were more concerned about insult to their body image and were more dependent upon their breasts for self-esteem than were women choosing mastectomy. Patients selecting lumpectomy and irradiation also strongly believed that they would have difficulty adjusting emotionally to the effects of a mastectomy. In contrast, patients choosing mastectomy more often perceived the affected breast as foreign, and wanted to have it removed; they were also more fearful of irradiation. For some women, excision and irradiation will not yield the best cosmetic result, particularly in light of recent technologic advances in plastic and reconstructive breast surgery.

The disadvantages of lumpectomy-irradiation include the increased demands placed on patients by the treatment. Although initial hospitalization is shortened by allowing women to be discharged from the hospital with the drainage pump in place, returning later for its removal, daily radiation therapy extends the total treatment period to more than 2 months. For some women, this time represents a small burden if they can manage to keep the breast; others may prefer the single procedure and subsequent reconstruction over a longer period of being a "patient." In all cases, discussion of safety, side effects, cosmesis, personal needs, and professional views must be reviewed prior to final decision-making. Clearly, one side benefit of irradiation is the opportunity to derive additional support from the physician as a result of frequent visits and contact with the radiotherapy staff.

A greater psychological burden is placed on women who are told that positive nodes were found at surgery and that chemotherapy must be added to their treatment regimen. Treatment for these patients is lengthened significantly. Some women in this group describe their early weeks of treatment as being characterized by "one piece of bad news after another."

Adjuvant Chemotherapy

The news that adjuvant chemotherapy is required demands adjustment, not only to yet another treatment modality, but also to the heightened threat to survival signified by the spread of disease to the axillary nodes. Anticipation of chemotherapy may be difficult. Women's fears of the potential adverse sequelae often arise from their knowledge of other chemotherapeutic regimens. They should be told about the drugs that will be used and the side effects of each, with special emphasis placed on the fact that alopecia is not permanent. At this point, counseling for reactive anxiety and depression may be helpful in reducing later distress. Despite these fears, few women refuse treatment, and most comply with their regimen. Taylor and co-workers found a compliance rate of 92% in women receiving an adjuvant regimen of Adriamycin, cyclophosphamide, methotrexate, and 5-fluorouracil.[60] However, their data do support the bad image that chemotherapy has in the public's mind, as evidenced by the fact that a number of women were initially resistant to accepting chemotherapeutic treatment.

The nausea and vomiting associated with chemotherapy are generally well tolerated if antiemetic drugs are used. Use of behavioral interventions may provide a means of regaining a sense of self-control and reducing anxiety. Anticipatory nausea and vomiting are particularly susceptible to control by this means.

A troublesome side effect of chemotherapy that can have psychological consequences is weight gain. The cause of such weight changes remains unclear. A recent study revealed that 50% of patients gained more than 10 pounds.[61] No difference was found in these patients in terms of treatment regimens (cyclophosphamide, methotrexate, and 5-fluorouracil versus cyclophosphamide, methotrexate, 5-fluorouracil, vincristine, and prednisone), estrogen receptor status, age, or menopausal status, although a decrease in activity level was found in those who experienced weight gain. The added insult to self-esteem posed by significant weight gain suggests that more attention should be paid to this problem.

A recent consensus meeting on breast cancer reviewed whether adjuvant therapy was effective and for whom, since in 50% of all women with early breast cancer disease has spread to the lymph nodes.[62] There was support for the use of chemotherapy in premenopausal women with positive nodes. In addition, it was recommended that postmenopausal women with involved lymph nodes and tumors containing estrogen receptors receive tamoxifen, which has virtually no side effects. These changes in management approaches alter the treatment experience for older women. However, the need to encourage women to participate in clinical trials persists since treatment for breast cancer is still far from being as effective as it should be.

Psychological preparation for chemotherapy is essential, and should incorporate patient educational materials, nursing input, and an outline of disease and treatment-related expectations provided by the physician. It is important to anticipate and plan for emotional reactions to ending treatment when, as with radiotherapy, fears of recurrence peak.[63] Our clinical experience suggests that many women experience severe reactive anxiety and depression at this time, perhaps because of their greater awareness of relative survival statistics.

Advanced Disease

Supportive care for patients with advanced breast cancer is aimed at palliative management and control of symptoms. Different metastatic sites, especially those involving bone, lung, or brain, present special supportive problems. Bone pain must be controlled. Hypercalcemia causes mental changes that must be monitored. The use of groups has been found to be an effective means of providing psychological support. The work of Spiegel and co-workers demonstrated an improved ability to communicate with family and to deal with illness and fatal outcome among those women participating in a support group with other patients with advanced breast cancer.[64] Advanced care is best provided at home with support from the family and, if needed, a homemaker, although a hospice setting with home care components may also serve the needs of these patients. Central to the success of a supportive program is a sense of continuity of care with physicians and staff and continued support of family and friends.

Psychiatric consultation should be considered when a patient's distress is not responsive to the usual supportive measures. Depressive symptoms may reach great proportions, and although suicide is unusual, suicidal ideation is common. A management approach that combines psychological support with psychopharmacologic use of antidepressants is often helpful. Amitriptyline is beneficial for its antidepressant, analgesic, and sedative properties when given at bedtime in doses of 50 to 75 mg. Anxiety may be high and very distressing, especially in the presence of hypoxia or prolonged pain. Anxiolytic drugs, particularly, diazepam and alprazolam, are also helpful for control of symptoms during daytime hours. It is best to administer these drugs initially at regular intervals to achieve control, thereafter tapering the dose or administering the drug as needed. In general, if given control of their dose initially, women will take too little of a drug to be effective. Agitated behavior associated with an irreversible metabolic encephalopathy may require control by administration of haloperidol in small doses.

SPECIAL ISSUES

Experiencing the diagnosis and treatment of breast cancer in a friend or family member can arouse intense feelings of threat and helplessness. Female relatives in particular may find themselves worrying about their altered risk status; all involved, however, may wonder whether there is something they can do to reduce risk of cancer in themselves or alter the course of it in their loved one. Although not always openly raised, these are issues that may have important ramifications for management that clinicians may need to monitor and discuss. Each is discussed separately below.

Children of Women With Breast Cancer

For all female first-degree relatives, breast cancer in a sister, mother, or daughter is known to mean a heightened risk for all, particularly if the disease has occurred premenopausally. The increased need to monitor these survivors closely for breast cancer is becoming more widely appreciated. The traumatic effect on children, both sons and daughters, is great when the mother develops breast cancer. Behavioral disorders, conflicts with parents, and regressive and acting out behaviors in children have been seen to increase during a parental illness.[65–67] Lichtman and colleagues noted that in 78 patients with breast cancer, deterioration of the mother-child relationship was evident in 12%.[68] Problems were more likely to arise in those situations in which the mother had a poor prognosis, extensive surgery, poor psychological adjustment, and to a lesser extent, difficulty adjusting to chemotherapy or irradiation. A prior history of parent-child conflicts also placed the relationship at risk during the mother's illness. Mothers' relationships with their daughters were significantly more stressed than their relationships with their sons. Daughters were more likely than sons to show signs of fearfulness, withdrawal, and hostility, emanating perhaps from their fear of developing disease and the greater demands placed on the daughters. These findings parallel those reported by Litman[67] and Wellisch,[65] who noted that mothers rely more often on daughters than sons during illness, and that adolescent daughters may be particularly vulnerable to disruption in their lives. Support and intervention among daughters may be particularly important. These studies and experiences suggest that supportive measures should include careful evaluation and discussion of hereditary risk, an explanation of recommended breast examination practices, and whenever possible, alleviation of additional burdens. The monitoring of all children, especially when the mother's breast cancer is advanced, is important.

Psychological Factors in Breast Cancer Risk and Survival

Breast cancer has been the most widely studied malignant disease not only because of its psychological impact, but also because the breast is the cancer site that has been explored most extensively for possible psychological factors associated with risk and survival. As with the debate about breast cancer treatment, the role of emotions in breast cancer risk and progression has received much attention in the news media. The impact of such press has not been studied directly, but in dealing with their illness, many women have expressed concern that they "brought the disease on themselves" or that they are afraid that their attitude is bad, and that they may be making the cancer worse. Others have sought out a psychiatrist, asking for a "mental check-up" prior to beginning treatment.

In a study of what women considered to be the cause of their breast cancer, Taylor and associates found that 41% of their well-educated sample thought that they were responsible for the development of the disease, and that stress was a major factor in its development.[69] The belief that they are responsible for their illness and its outcome has become an added psychological burden for many women; indeed, it is a hazard for those who, based on these beliefs, seek psychological therapy as primary treatment for their breast cancer, never starting or discontinuing conventional treatment. Thus, it is important that oncologists and clinicians know the status of research on possible psychosocial risk factors in order to answer their patients' questions on the subject, provide clarification and reassurance, and strengthen the patient-physician relationship that is vital to their patients' optimal care. The following is a brief review of the related research intended for the clinician. For a more extensive critique of the biobehavioral issues in cancer, the reader is referred to the publications of Fox[70,71] who has offered a continuing critique of this area of study.

Data relating stress and illness have come both from animal and human studies. Briefly, a series of studies by Riley showed that cage conditions of crowding, noise, and manipulation caused elevated corticosterone levels which, in turn, caused involution of the thymus and enhanced mammary tumor growth.[72,73] However, studies of other models of stress and tumor types have shown protective effects as well as no effects on carcinogenesis.[74] Miller has offered some hypotheses to explain the discrepancy in results related to type of stress, timing (i.e., precarcinogenic versus postcarcinogenic exposure), type of tumor, and outcome measures used, but it is clear that in animal models, stress can have both protective and deleterious effects.[75]

Another model from animal studies has been introduced by Sklar and Anisman.[76] These researchers found that tumor growth in mice implanted with P815 mastocytoma tumor cells was greatest in those mice that were yoked in a paradigm in which they received inescapable shock.[76] Exposure to the "learned helplessness" model was associated with norepinephrene depletion and suppressed lymphocytic stimulation to phytohemagglutinin (PHA) and Concanavilin A (Con A).[77] The animal studies by Ader have also been provocative, showing that the immune response could be conditioned to an aversive stimulus.[78] These data and evidence of regulatory links between the brain, the immune system, and the endocrine system have accounted for a challenging new area of immune research that is being pursued actively.[79] Although stress has an effect on immune function, the relationship between stress and carcinogenesis remains unclear. However, there has been a tendency to extrapolate these exciting data prematurely to individual human patients with cancer.

The role of personality factors in breast cancer carcinogenesis has also been examined. Studies in this area have focused on the impact of personality on behavior that may affect exposure to carcinogens or optimal health practices and the impact of emotions on changes within the body on the humoral or cellular level. Most of the human psychosomatic medical studies of women with breast cancer were done in the 1950s using an approach in which premorbid personality patterns were deduced from anecdotal reports of women in whom breast cancer had already developed.[70] These personal histories, typified by repression, denial, and inhibition of emotions—especially anger—could not differentiate prior personality from response to disease. A controlled prospective study that would confirm a personality type associated with risk for breast cancer has not been done. One study in progress is designed to assess women who are at high risk for breast cancer, prospectively studying their genetic and biologic state, as well as their response to life events.[80] Similarly, a study of a large cohort of healthy women is beginning in which women will be followed prospectively over a period of 5 years for all known environmental and biologic risk factors. As part of this longitudinal follow-up, psychological state, social supports, and stressful events will also be assessed.[81] It is hoped that these efforts will help clarify the impact of psychosocial variables on cancer risk. It may be that a psychological state or event could act as a promoter in the presence of an initiator factor, particularly if the external or internal stressor occurs during a period when breast tissue is most vulnerable to abnormal change. A personality type that is prone to breast cancer has not yet been adequately substantiated, however.

An increasing number of recent studies have examined psychological factors in breast cancer that might influence survival. Pettingale and co-workers have carried out a series of studies in England suggesting that recurrence-free survival was greater in women who showed either denial or a "fighting spirit," as compared to those who exhibited stoic acceptance or feelings of helplessness or hopelessness.[82] Data from a study of 20 of these survivors examined 10 years later showed that these traits remained predictive of survival, even when controlled for eight other prognostic factors.

Derogatis and colleagues found a positive correlation between survival and expression of negative emotions in a group of women studied from the time that chemotherapy for metastatic disease was initiated.[83] Long-term survivors (those who survived for more than 1 year) showed more negative emotions and more symptoms of anxiety, depression, and hostility than those surviving for less than 1 year. Levy and co-workers reported findings for a cohort of women studied at the time of mastectomy.[84] Those patients with a greater number of positive axillary nodes showed "better" psychological adjustment (measured by fewer expressions of distress) and lower natural killer cell activity than patients with few or no positive nodes. This careful study of the correlates of immune and psychological function represents a new level of sophistication within such studies of breast cancer, studies that had previously suffered from small sample sizes and methodologic flaws.

Gorzynski and co-workers[22] conducted a follow-up study of 10-year survivors of breast cancer who had been studied for psychological state and cortisol production at the time of biopsy by Katz and colleagues.[85] The women were found to have similar psychological coping responses and cortisol production as they had had 10 years earlier, suggesting that these represent stable traits. Mean cortisol production was higher in the group with breast cancer than in the group with benign biopsy results, both initially and 10 years later. Women who were alive at 10 years were compared to those who had died in the interim with respect to their prebiopsy characteristics. Psychological state was not significantly different; however, the mean weight of those who had died was significantly higher than that of the survivors.[86] These data support those of Donegan and co-workers, who reported a strong correlation between lower weight and longer survival, a relationship found to be second in significance to nodal status.[87] It may be that studies showing personality differences are actually measuring the association of personality with some behavioral variable, such as diet or weight. As increasing attention is being directed to dietary factors—especially fat intake, which may correlate with greater caloric intake and obesity—and their role in risk and survival, these cofactors will need to be examined further.

These studies are provocative and suggest new directions for research. The "fighting spirit" described by Pettingale and associates[82] in women with breast cancer has received increasing interest as a psychological construct in adaptation. Validated scales are needed to test this construct, as it is currently being measured differently from one study to another. "Fighting" cancer has such a universal appeal, at both a personal and societal level, that one must be cautious in evaluating the studies.

Marshall and Funch examined survival in 352 women with breast cancer who completed crude social stress and social involvement measures at the time of diagnosis between 1958 and 1960.[88] Records for 283 who had died were available for review. Using regression analysis, they found that the stage of disease at diagnosis was the most powerful predictor of length of survival, accounting for 15% to 20% of the variance. However, 9% of the variance in survival in the younger group could be explained by social variables; this was not true in the older group. Social stress was consistently found to have an adverse effect, and involvement with others was positively related to length of survival. Although the authors suggest that the significance of their findings is limited because of the crude measures used, their data are interesting in light of the large study of over 6000 elderly persons conducted by Berkman and Syme.[89] In the latter study, the researchers found that longevity was associated with social support. Although the number of subjects studied was not sufficient to gauge impact on cancer alone, early mortality from a range of diseases occurred more frequently in those who earlier had reported themselves to be isolated and lacking in social support.

In a recent study using some of the variables isolated in earlier research, Cassileth and colleagues tested the ability of seven social and psychological factors reported to be associated with longevity to predict survival: social ties, life satisfaction, job satisfaction, use of psychotropic drugs, subjective view of adult health, hopelessness/helplessness, and perception of adjustment required to cope with the diagnosis.[90] Two groups of patients were followed—those with irreversible cancer ($n = 204$) who were followed until death, and those with Stage II breast cancer or melanoma ($n = 155$) who were followed until disease recurrence. None of the factors delineated, either individually or in combination, was found to influence survival or time to recurrence for either advanced or early stages of disease. Recently, Holland and co-workers attempted to replicate the Derogatis study in the Cancer and Leukemia Group B using the SCL-90 psychological symptom self-report scale. Their study, done at the time of initiation of adjuvant chemotherapy in 360 women with Stage II breast cancer, did not show any psychological differences between the 106 patients who had recurrences or died and those who survived.[91]

There remains a need for further research that uses a prospective, multi-tier design to identify possible predictors that could then be tested in a larger model. Psychological factors play an important role as they affect ability and willingness to obtain and comply with available treatment. Dietary patterns may also be important. In addition, psychological and social variables contribute to qualify of life, if not directly to survival time. Whether there are psychosocial factors, however, that influence the biology of breast cancer, in terms of either risk or survival is not clear. Fox has suggested that psychological factors, if they do play a role, may be salutary or detrimental, but that they likely constitute a small part of the variance in relation to the other known factors that relate to disease.[71]

Advice to patients should reflect the preliminary nature of the data. In addition, women with breast cancer should be encouraged to recognize the fact that the available data do not support their fears that they caused the breast cancer to develop. "Fighting spirit" and active participation are desirable, but a period of distress associated with illness is not, according to available data, likely to cause tumor progression as some women currently believe. Women who have a need for greater participation (and a sense of control) in their care that may be served by alternative treatment methods should be encouraged to employ these methods, provided they do not interfere with conventional therapy and have no deleterious effect.

Women should be encouraged to participate in clinical trials of breast cancer treatment when they are available. The mortality from this disease is still too high, and much is to be learned about treatment and about the interaction of psychological and biologic variables. It can be pointed out that the large multicenter studies compare the best present treatment with one that may be better. Women who agree to enter these trials are assured of care by physicians who constitute the cutting edge of science as it is applied to clinical trials. Participation in such studies also serves the altruistic goal of helping to reduce the toll that this disease takes on all women. Answers will only be found in large prospective studies in which the range of variables, well-defined and controlled, may be assessed.

SUMMARY

In summary, breast cancer remains the most common tumor in women; it has a unique and, at times, a complex psychological impact, but one to which psychologically healthy women respond well without developing serious psychological symptoms. Current modes of primary treatment using breast-conserving procedures are reducing the negative impact on women's self-image and body image. However, current ethical and legal constraints relating to treatment options have added significantly to decision-making dilemmas and to fears of recurrence, which, by virtue of the detailed information given about survival statistics, may persist for an indefinite period. Reconstruction has had a significant benefit in terms of quality of life in women who undergo mastectomy.

Special attention must be directed to the psychological well-being of first-degree relatives of women with breast cancer, especially their daughters. Large prospective studies of the biologic and psychological aspects of breast cancer are needed to understand the possible role of psychosocial factors in risk and outcome of breast cancer. At present, the influence of these factors appears to figure prominently in issues of quality of life, although positive attitudes and "fighting spirit" are associated with responses and behaviors that are likely to enhance survival.

REFERENCES

1. Meyerowitz BE: Psychosocial correlates of breast cancer and its treatment. Psychol Bull 87:108, 1980
2. Holland JC, Mastrovito R: Psychologic adaptation to breast cancer. Cancer 46:1045, 1980
3. Bard M, Sutherland AM: Psychological impact of cancer and its treatment. IV. Adaptation to radical mastectomy. Cancer 8:656, 1955
4. Schottenfeld D, Robbins GF: Quality of survival among patients who have had radical mastectomy. Cancer 26:650, 1970
5. Craig TJ, Comstock GW, Geiser PB: The quality of survival in breast cancer: A case-control comparison. Cancer 33:1451, 1974
6. Maguire GP, Lee EG, Bevington DJ, et al: Psychiatric problems in the first year after mastectomy. Br Med J 1:963, 1978
7. Lee E, Maguire GP: Emotional distress in patients attending a breast clinic. Br J Surg 62(2):162, 1975
8. Crile G: Management of breast cancer: Limited mastectomy. JAMA 230:95, 1974
9. Fisher B, Barboni P: Breast cancer. In Holland JF, Frei E III (eds): Cancer Medicine, 2nd ed, pp 2025–2056. Philadelphia, Lea & Febiger, 1982
10. Veronesi U, Saccozzi R, Del Vecchio M, et al: Comparing radical mastectomy with quadrantectomy, axillary dissection and radiotherapy in patients with small cancers of the breast. N Engl J Med 305:6, 1981
11. Harris JR, Levene MB, Hellman S: Results of treating stages I and II carcinoma of the breast with primary radiation therapy. Cancer Treat Rep 62:985, 1978
12. Rollin B: First You Cry. Philadelphia, JB Lippincott, 1976
13. Kushner R: Breast Cancer: A Personal History and Investigative Report. New York, Harcourt, Brace & Jovanovich, 1975
14. Markel WM: The American Cancer Society's program for the rehabilitation of the breast cancer patient. Cancer 28:1676, 1971
15. Valanis BG, Rumpler CH: Helping women to choose breast cancer treatment alternatives. Cancer Nurs 8(3):167, 1985
16. Scott DW: Anxiety, critical thinking and information processing during and after breast biopsy. Nurs Res 32:24, 1983
17. Penman DT, Holland JC, Bahna GF, et al: Informed consent for investigational chemotherapy: Patients' and physicians' perceptions. J Clin Oncol 2:849, 1984
18. Wieder S, Schwartzfeld J, Fromewick J, et al: Psychosocial support program for patients with breast cancer at Montefiore Hospital: Team effort. Qual Rev Bull 4:10, 1978
19. Fisher B: Choice of surgery in early breast cancer. Presented at The Conference on Early Breast Cancer: The Psychological Perspective, Long Island Jewish Medical Center and Memorial Sloan-Kettering Cancer Center, New York, New York, October 11, 1985
20. Ashcroft JJ, Leinster SJ, Slade PD: Breast cancer—patient choice of treatment: Preliminary communication. J R Soc Med 78:43, 1985
21. Fotopoulis S, Cook MR: Psychological aspects of breast cancer: Age. Presented at the American Psychological Association Meetings, Montreal, Quebec, Canada, September, 1980
22. Gorzynski JG, Holland J, Katz JL, et al: Stability of ego defenses and endocrine responses in women prior to breast biopsy and ten years later. Psychosom Med 42(3):323, 1980
23. Penman DT: Coping Strategies in Adaptation to Mastectomy, Doctoral dissertation, Yeshiva University, New York, 1979
24. Bloom J, Cook M, Holland J, et al: (for Psychological Adjustment to Breast Cancer Cooperative, NCI): A prospective comparison study of women's psychological response to mastectomy. Proc Am Soc Clin Oncol 3:73, 1984
25. Schain WS: Breast cancer surgeries and psychosexual sequelae: Implications for remediation. Semin Oncol Nurs 1:200, 1985
26. Bloom JR: Social support, accommodation to stress and adjustment to breast cancer. Soc Sci Med 16:1329, 1982
27. Funch DP, Mettlin C: The role of support in relation to recovery from breast surgery. Soc Sci Med 16:91, 1982
28. Peters-Golden H: Breast cancer: Varied perceptions of social support in the illness experience. Soc Sci Med 16:483, 1982
29. Wortman CB: Social support and the cancer patient. Cancer 53:2339, 1984
30. Wellisch DK, Jamison KR, Pasnau RO: Psychosocial aspects of mastectomy: II. The man's perspective. Am J Psychiatry 135:543, 1978
31. Faulkner A, Maguire P: Teaching ward nurses to monitor cancer patients. Clin Oncol 10:383, 1984
32. Holland JC: The clinical course of breast cancer: A psychological perspective. Front Radiat Ther Oncol 11:133, 1976
33. American Society of Plastic and Reconstructive Surgeons, Inc: Breast reconstructions quadruple. News Release, May 16, 1985
34. National Survey on Breast Cancer: A Measure of Progress in Public Understanding. Washington, DC, National Cancer Institute, Department of Health and Human Services, 1980
35. Schain WS, Jacobs E, Wellisch DK: Psychosocial issues in breast reconstruction: Intrapsychic, interpersonal, and practical concerns. Clin Plast Surg 11:237, 1984
36. Jacobs E, Holland J, Rowland JH, et al: Who seeks breast reconstruction? A controlled psychological comparison. (abstr). Psychosom Med 45:80, 1983
37. Rowland JH, Holland JC, Jacobs ER, et al: Psychological response to breast reconstruction. Paper presented at the 137th Annual Meeting of the American Psychiatric Association, Los Angeles, CA, May 11, 1984
38. Clifford E, Clifford M, Georgiade NG: Breast reconstruction following mastectomy: II. Marital characteristics of patients seeking the procedure. Ann Plast Surg 5(5):344, 1980
39. Clifford E, Clifford M, Georgiade NG: Breast reconstruction following mastectomy: I. Social characteristics of patients seeking the procedure. Ann Plast Surg 5(5):341, 1980
40. Goin JM, Goin MK: Breast reconstruction after mastectomy. In Changing the Body, Psychological Effects of Plastic Surgery, pp 163–189. Baltimore, Williams & Wilkins, 1981
41. Clifford E: The reconstruction experience: The search for restitution. In Georgiade NG (ed): Breast Reconstruction Following Mastectomy, pp 22–34. London, CV Mosby, 1979
42. Daniel E: Breast Reconstruction Postmastectomy: A psychosocial Study, Doctoral dissertion, University of California, San Francisco, 1984 Dissertation Abstr Int 46(5):1741B, 1985
43. Teimourian B, Adham M: Survey of patients' responses to breast reconstruction. Ann Plast Surg, 9:321, 1982
44. Gerard D: Sexual functioning after mastectomy: Life vs. lab. J Sex Marital Ther 8:305, 1982
45. Goin MK, Goin JM: Midlife reactions to mastectomy and sub-

sequent breast reconstruction. Arch Gen Psychiatry 38:225, 1981
46. Winder AE, Winder BD: Patient counseling: Clarifying a woman's choice for breast reconstruction. Patient Educ Counseling 7:65, 1985
47. Dean C, Chetty U, Forrest APM: Effects of immediate breast reconstruction on psychosocial morbidity after mastectomy. Lancet i:459, 1983
48. Noone RB, Frazier TG, Hayward CZ, et al: Patient acceptance of immediate reconstruction following mastectomy. Plast Recon Surg 69:632–640, 1982
49. Stevens LA, McGrath MH, Druss RG, et al: The psychological impact of immediate breast reconstruction for women with early breast cancer. Plastic Reconstr Surg 73:619, 1984
50. Schain WS, Wellisch DK, Pasnau RO, et al: The sooner the better: A study of psychological factors in women undergoing immediate versus delayed breast reconstruction. Am J Psychiatry 142:40, 1985
51. Steinberg MD: Psychological aspects of lumpectomy-radiation treatment for early breast cancer. In Syllabus for Early Breast Cancer: The Psychological Perspective, a conference sponsored by Long Island Jewish Medical Center and Memorial Sloan-Kettering Cancer Center, New York, New York, October 11, 1985
52. Sanger CK, Reznikoff M: A comparison of the psychological effects of breast-saving procedures with the modified radical mastectomy. Cancer 48:2341, 1981
53. Schain W, Edwards BK, Gorrell CR, et al: Psychosocial and physical outcomes of primary breast cancer therapy: Mastectomy vs. excisional biopsy and irradiation. Breast Cancer Res Treat 3:377, 1983
54. Steinberg MD, Juliano MA, Wise L: Psychological outcome of lumpectomy versus mastectomy in the treatment of breast cancer. Am J Psychiatry 142:34, 1985
55. Bartelink H, Van Dam F, van Dongen J: Psychological effects of breast-conserving therapy in comparison with radical mastectomy. Radiat Oncol Biol Phys 11:381, 1985
56. Taylor SE, Lichtman RR, Wood JV, et al: Illness-related and treatment-related factors in psychological adjustment to breast cancer. Cancer 55:2506, 1985
57. Haes JCJM, Welvaart K: Quality of life after breast cancer surgery. J Surg Oncol 28:123, 1985
58. Wellisch DK: Unpublished data, personal communication, 1986
59. Margolis GJ, Goodman RL: Psychological factors in women choosing radiation therapy for breast cancer. Psychosomatics 25:464, 1984
60. Taylor SE, Lichtman RR, Wood JV: Compliance with chemotherapy among breast cancer patients. Health Psychol 3:553, 1984
61. Huntington M: Weight gain in patients receiving adjuvant chemotherapy for carcinoma of the breast. Cancer 56:472, 1985
62. Kolata G: Breast cancer consensus. Science 229:1378, 1985
63. Holland JC, Rowland J, Lebovits A, et al: Reactions to cancer treatment. Assessment of emotional response to adjuvant radiotherapy as a guide to planned interventions. Psychiatr Clin North Am 2:347, 1979
64. Spiegel D, Bloom JR, Yalom I: Group support for patients with metastatic cancer. Arch Gen Psychiatry 38:527, 1981
65. Wellisch DK: Adolescent acting out when a parent has cancer. Int J Family Ther 1:230, 1979
66. Buckley IG: Listen to the Children: A study of the Impact on the Mental Health of Children of a Parent's Catastrophic Illness. New York, Cancer Care, 1977
67. Litman TJ: The family as the basic unit in health and medical care: A social behavioral overview. Soc Sci Med 8:495, 1974
68. Lichtman RR, Taylor SE, Wood JV, et al: Relations with children after breast cancer: The mother-daughter relationship at risk. J Psychosoc Oncol 2:1, 1984
69. Taylor SE, Lichtman RR, Wood JV: Attributions, beliefs about control, and adjustment to breast cancer. J Pers Soc Psychol 46:489, 1984
70. Fox BH: Premorbid psychological factors as related to cancer incidence. J Behav Med 1:45, 1978
71. Fox BH: Current theory of psychogenic effects on cancer incidence and prognosis. J Psychosoc Oncol 1:17, 1983
72. Riley V: Mouse mammary tumors: Alteration of incidence as an apparent function of stress. Science 189:465, 1975
73. Riley V: Psychoneuroendocrine influences on immunocompetence and neoplasia. Science 212:1100, 1981
74. Newberry BH: Effects of presumably stressful stimulation on the development of animal tumors: Some issues. In Weiss SM, Herd JA, Fox BH (eds): Perspectives on Behavioral Medicine, pp 329–350. New York, Academic Press, 1981
75. Miller N: Effects of emotional stress on immune function. Pavlov J Biol Sci 20:47, 1985
76. Sklar L, Anisman H: Stress and coping factors influence tumor growth. Science 205:513, 1979
77. Laudenslager M, Ryan S, Drugan R, et al: Coping and immunosuppression: Inescapable but not escapable shock suppresses lymphocytic proliferation. Science 221:568, 1983
78. Ader R (ed): Psychoneuroimmunology. New York, Academic Press, 1981
79. Jemmott JB, Locke SE: Psychosocial factors, immunologic mediation and human susceptibility to infectious diseases: How much do we know? Psychol Bull 95:78, 1984
80. Tross S, Rowland J, Dermatis H, et al: Prospective psychologic study of women at high risk of breast cancer. Personal communication, 1985
81. Tross S, Strax P, Rowland J, et al: Prospective study of healthy women for risk of breast cancer. Personal communication, 1985
82. Pettingale KW, Morris T, Greer S, et al: Mental attitudes to cancer: An additional prognostic factor. Lancet I:750, 1985
83. Derogatis LR, Abeloff MD, Melisaratos N: Psychological coping mechanisms and survival time in metastatic breast cancer. JAMA 242:1504, 1979
84. Levy SM, Herberman RB, Maluish AM, et al: Prognostic risk assessment in primary breast cancer by behavioral and immunological parameters. Health Psychol 4:99, 1985
85. Katz JL, Ackman P, Rothwax Y, et al: Psychoendocrine aspects of cancer of the breast. Psychosom Med 32:1, 1970
86. Zumoff B, Gorzynski JG, Katz JL, et al: Nonobesity at the time of mastectomy is highly predictive of 10-year disease-free survival in women with breast cancer. Anticancer Res 2:59, 1982
87. Donegan WL, Hartz AJ, Rimm AA: The association of body weight with recurrent cancer of the breast. Cancer 41:1590, 1978
88. Marshall JR, Funch DP: Social environment and breast cancer: A cohort analysis of patient survival. Cancer 52:1546, 1983
89. Berkman LF, Syme LS: Social networks, host resistance and mortality: A nine year followup study of Alameda County residents. Am J Epidemiol 109:186, 1979
90. Cassileth BR, Lusk EJ, Miller DS, et al: Psychosocial correlates of survival in advanced malignant disease. N Engl J Med 312:1551, 1985
91. Holland JC, Korzun AH, Tross S, et al: Psychosocial factors and disease-free survival in Stage II breast carcinoma (abstr). Proc Am Soc Clin Oncol 5:237, 1986

Educational and Support Groups for Breast Cancer Patients and Their Families

Grace H. Christ
Mary Ellen Bowles Laurie J. Bauman

Studies conducted in the past 15 years have documented the psychological and social stresses associated with breast cancer treated by mastectomy and, more recently, by lumpectomy and irradiation. A range of psychosocial interventions have proved to be helpful in mitigating these stresses.[1–10] Some of these interventions are addressed in other sections of this chapter. This section will emphasize group interventions that have been used to help patients cope with these adaptive challenges. The groups that are described here include postsurgical rehabilitation groups, self-help groups, family groups, psychoeducational groups for continuing care, and groups for patients with metastatic and terminal illness.

Patients treated by mastectomy have been found to experience depression, anxiety, and a reduced interest in sex[6,11–13] as well as concern about how to cover the mastectomy site or camouflage the prosthesis.[14–16] Recent studies suggest that patients who receive a lumpectomy and irradiation may experience less disruption of their body image, sexual functioning, and overall adjustment. However, they do not seem to differ from patients treated by mastectomy in the frequency of separation and divorce, social changes, or overt emotional symptoms.[17–22] A more comprehensive understanding of the psychosocial consequences of treatment with lumpectomy and irradiation is developing.

Many of the group interventions used with patients treated by mastectomy also appear to be beneficial for patients treated by lumpectomy. However, these interventions require modifications to accommodate differences in treatment and in the personal concerns related to those differences. Further development of interventions tailored to the specific needs of women treated with lumpectomy and irradiation will be developed as the treatment process and the needs of these patients become better understood.

The purpose of most of the groups described here is to enhance the coping ability of patients confronted with predictable stress, rather than to prevent psychological breakdown or to treat those at high risk of social or psychological morbidity. More intensive interventions are required with patients who have pre-existing emotional problems, other high-risk characteristics, or prolonged and persistent emotional reactions.

Although patients often experience emotional disequilibrium in response to a diagnosis of breast cancer, few request counseling, supportive interventions, or psychiatric consultation. Despite the fact that patients are often overwhelmed by their reactions, most are unable to request support for a number of reasons. Some are psychologically immobilized and cannot exert the emotional energy needed to get help. Others view a request for support as an inability to cope, a loss of autonomy, or a sign of mental illness. Furthermore, most patients are unaware that counseling may help assuage the existential terror evoked by a diagnosis of cancer or alleviate grief over the loss of a breast. The dilemma is that, later, these same patients will resent not receiving enough psychosocial help or support. For these reasons, patients are most likely to use services to mitigate their normal distress if those services are universally prescribed and easily available. The breast surgery rehabilitation (BSR) group at Memorial Sloan-Kettering Cancer Center in New York City is an example of such a service.

BREAST SURGERY REHABILITATION GROUP

Ninety-eight percent of the patients who have participated in the BSR group at Memorial Sloan-Kettering Cancer Center over the past 15 years have rated the group as being helpful.[9] Early studies found that participation in the group reduced the time required for physical and emotional adjustment and shortened the hospital stay. Physicians routinely refer patients who have had a mastectomy or a lumpectomy with axillary node dissection to the BSR group; more than 90% of patients who undergo breast surgery at Memorial Hospital participate in the group. The fact that physicians refer their patients to the group accounts for the unusually good rate of attendance. The physicians review ahead of time all of the information that patients will receive in the BSR group to ensure that it is consistent with their education of their patients. Typical questions that physicians ask about patient groups arose at the inception of the BSR program. "Won't it increase patients' anxieties if they compare notes and find differences in surgeons' procedures?" "Won't the patients who are more upset make the calmer ones more anxious?" "Will the patients' discussions make them ask us more questions and make patient care more time-consuming?" The physicians' skepticism was reduced by ongoing discussions between group leaders and surgeons and by the positive responses of patients to the group. Although the program did not eliminate the tendency for patients to ask their physicians repetitive questions, the physicians found that many of the patients' questions were answered in the group and that, in most instances, the patients' anxieties were reduced. Patients talk with one another and compare notes in any case, but doing so in a group with experienced professionals present more readily corrects any misinformation and misconceptions.

Group Structure

The BSR group meets daily for 90 minutes and is led by a physical therapist, a nurse, and a social worker who use a psychoeducational model. Physical therapy exercises and self-care information focus the patients' attention on the physical changes that often trigger emotional reactions and thoughts about what these changes will mean in their lives.

The size of the group ranges from 9 to 15 patients per session, and each patient attends two to four sessions before she is discharged.

The first 45 minutes of each group session is led by the physical therapist, who explains the difference between incisional and referred sensations, outlines techniques for preventing lymphedema in the affected arm, and teaches a series of exercises for restoring the full range of motion.

Twice a week, the nurse uses the second 45 minutes to discuss self-care information. Using an anatomical drawing of the chest, the nurse reviews the surgical procedures for mastectomy and lumpectomy-axillary node dissection. Hand and arm precautions are reviewed, an explanation of the purpose of the Reliavac and the proper method for caring for the wound after discharge from the hospital is offered, the need for self-examination of the other breast is emphasized, a gradual return to normal activities is recommended, and preliminary information about breast prostheses is provided. Three times a week, a social worker and a volunteer (a former patient) spend the second 45 minutes discussing emotional rehabilitation. Because professionals often wonder how such discussions can be of help to patients immediately after surgery, the subject will be elaborated on here.

Group Discussions

One goal of the BSR group is to help patients to identify the psychological and social rehabilitative tasks confronting them as a result of diagnosis and treatment and to begin to plan how they will accomplish those tasks. We have found that the group provides patients with an opportunity to anticipate problems and to rehearse solutions, which, in turn, increases their feelings of mastery and control.

Another goal of the group is to desensitize patients to the horror they felt about the very idea of having cancer—a potentially life-threatening disease. One volunteer explained how this had happened for her: "There, I said it! In the group was the first time I could say 'I had cancer.' I used to think this was the worst thing that could happen to a woman. But the other day, my daughter asked me, 'How is it for you, Mom?' I said, 'It's O.K.' "

The most important goal, however, is to mitigate the profound feelings of isolation and loneliness that cancer evokes. Patients say they feel that the other group members empathize with them. Also, they often begin to accomplish their own psychological tasks by assisting others in their first steps toward recovery.

Confronting the diagnosis of cancer—a potentially life-threatening, disfiguring, and painful disease—is one of the patient's most difficult tasks. Talking about it in the group helps participants to realize that their fear is a universal one; this places the fear in a different context. The subject often arises when the patient-volunteer is introduced. "This is Mrs. Smith, a Reach to Recovery volunteer, which means she has had a mastectomy. It's been 15 years since she was sitting where you are." Typically, patients respond with statements such as "That's a relief. It's good to see someone alive." When the issue of fear of death is raised, a patient recalls: "Well, my mother had breast cancer when she was my age. I'll never forget how she suffered. I don't know how I'll ever put it out of my mind." Another patients says: "Well, I think that's everybody's fear—that the cancer will come back. I try to be positive and live each day, but the worry is there." Then the patient-volunteer offers her perspective: "I know what you mean. When I had my mastectomy 15 years ago, the doctor said 'Go home, and don't worry.' I went home and started to worry. I thought, he knows he took the cancer out of my breast, but how about the rest of me? I had some bad moments. Every ache and pain, even ones I had before the surgery, made me think the cancer had come back."

Hearing that the volunteer was also frightened does not remove the patient's fear, but it does help her view her own fear as a normal reaction that will diminish with time. She places her own anguished confrontation with mortality into the context of universal human experience. "Well, everybody has to die. I could be hit by a car. At least with this, I have a chance." "If you have to have cancer, the breast is the best place to have it. At least it's not a vital organ." "It could have been much worse. Oh God, when you see the children with cancer. That's what really gets you. I'm just grateful it's me and not my children."

The group provides a safe place to begin acknowledging fear and grief—emotions that some patients avoid for fear they may be overwhelmed or may overwhelm others who are close to them. For those who might feel ashamed because they are not meeting their own standards of courage in facing the crisis, it can be reassuring to know that others who seem to be coping well have their own fears and low moments. "Go ahead, cry. It helps. I've cried plenty myself." "Of course I'm scared that they didn't get it all. I think everyone is afraid that it will come back. I try to be positive and live each day, but the worry is there." The group member who initially may be unable to put her experience in any context but one of personal terror and anguish hears that others are finding a way to reframe their experience and live with it. "Well, I think that when I get back to work and I'm busy, it will be easier. That's what saved me when my husband died." The confrontation with mortality can become an impetus to enjoy life more. "You know, I've been doing for others. I think that now I'm going to be little more selfish and do things I want to do."

Becoming reconciled to the loss of a breast may also be facilitated by participation in the group. "I don't think I'll ever be able to look." "I've looked; it's not so bad." "My husband says it won't make any difference. I think I'll always wonder if he really means it, or if he is just saying it to make me feel good." "Well, I wasn't any Miss America to begin with and my husband loved me. I don't think this will make much difference." "Last night, my husband and I looked together. He cried—not for himself, for me." "I don't feel bad about losing the breast. I wanted to live, and if that's the price, I'll pay it." The Reach to Recovery volunteer shares her experience: "Our sex life is better than it ever was because we realize what we almost lost."

Other common issues addressed in the group include anticipating the reactions of friends, work colleagues, and children; learning practical ways to deal with physical limitations; preparing for chemotherapy; and dealing with individual concerns. The group leader is responsible for ensuring that the critical issues are discussed and that the topics addressed are relevant to most patients. The social worker handles highly individual reactions or complex personal problems outside the group or refers the patient to another mental health professional.

The group leader is responsible not only for keeping patients from trivializing their emotions but also for maintaining a positive focus on coping. The discussion is intended to label the issues the patients are facing, not to produce despair. "Yes, it is frightening that there isn't a 100% guarantee of cure. How do you think you are going to help yourself live with that fear?" The volunteer may be able to help patients with this issue, too. "I was in the shower one day. I felt like screaming and running. Then I realized that I was the problem. I had to cope, or I might as well go ahead and die. It wasn't easy, but now I feel better about myself than I did before I had the mastectomy."

Finally, respecting individual coping styles is vitally important. The volunteer is trained to share her own experience but not to give advice to others regarding how they must react.

Because the numbers of patients being treated by lumpectomy and irradiation are not large enough yet to establish a separate group, they participate in the group with patients who have been treated with mastectomy. Although much of the physical therapy and nursing information and group discussion is relevant to the patients who have undergone lumpectomy and irradiation, these patients are always eager to talk with a patient who has undergone their particular treatment, and they would prefer their own group if that were possible.

Sometimes, patients who have had lumpectomy and irradiation feel guilty about their strong emotional reactions. "How can I be so upset if I didn't lose a breast?" Although they may be less traumatized initially because they do not have to deal with amputation, the diagnosis of a life-threatening illness must not be trivialized. For this reason, a patient volunteer program for patients who have undergone lumpectomy has been developed at Memorial Sloan-Kettering Cancer Center. Such programs are now included as part of most Reach to Recovery programs throughout the country. The beginning of radiotherapy treatment seems to be a critical time for these patients, but educational and support groups have proved to be useful throughout the course of radiotherapy.

SELF-HELP GROUPS

The number of self-help groups for people with a chronic illness, such as cancer, has grown astronomically. Gussow and Tracey reported that there is a self-help group for every major disease listed by the World Health Organization.[23] All of these groups share the philosophy that people who have experienced a crisis or a threatening situation have a unique contribution to make to others who also are undergoing the same experience.

Several mechanisms have been suggested to explain the appeal of self-help groups. First, because they have been through it themselves, "veterans" of a crisis can provide insight and understanding to those who are now coping with that crisis—i.e., these veterans have what Borkman called "experiential knowledge."[24] In fact, Katz said that sharing a central problem is what defines membership in a self-help group.[25] It is this shared status that explains the oft-quoted statement that "only another woman with a mastectomy can really understand my feelings."

A second possible mechanism through which group members experience benefits is the destigmatizing and normalizing effects that groups seem to have.[24] Another way self-help works is through the helper-therapy principle,[26] which suggests that the "helper" may benefit more than the recipient does because the helper's sense of interpersonal competence is increased by her role as adviser, what she learns from the women she helps, the social approval she receives for helping others, and the reinforcement of her own success in coping. Because members of self-help groups are both care givers and care receivers, all of them can benefit. Another way that self-help groups may provide benefits is through the modeling of successful recovery—a role that veteran patients, such as Reach to Recovery volunteers, consciously adopt to encourage successful adaptation to the illness.

Reach to Recovery

The first group to provide systematic assistance to women with breast cancer was Reach to Recovery, a self-help organization composed of former mastectomy patients. The Reach to Recovery program is the largest and best known self-help service for women with breast cancer. Since 1969, it has been a rehabilitation program of the American Cancer Society (ACS), and visits to patients have grown to approximately 65,000 per year in the United States alone.[27] Volunteers must have had their own mastectomy at least 1 year before and are screened and trained by their local ACS unit. They visit newly diagnosed women in the hospital (or occasionally at home) a few days after the patient's surgery. In most cities, the patient's physician must give written permission before a volunteer is called. When the ACS office receives a request from the hospital, it obtains patient data, such as age, marital status, and stage of illness so that the volunteer who makes the visit will share as many characteristics with the patient as possible. This similarity is important because the meaning of the diagnosis of breast cancer and the loss of a breast is different for younger and older women and for married and single ones.

The volunteer usually begins the visit by describing

the Reach to Recovery program and identifying herself as a cancer survivor who has had a mastectomy. She brings with her a standard kit containing a temporary prosthesis, a ball, a rope, and a booklet that illustrates exercises designed to help patients retain the full range of arm motion. The volunteer demonstrates the exercises and how to use the ball and rope. The rapport that is established through this shared activity facilitates achievement of the other purpose of the visit—to encourage the patient to talk about her fears and concerns. Currently, Reach to Recovery is beginning to train volunteers who have been treated by lumpectomy and irradiation as well. Educational materials also are being developed for lumpectomy patients.

Few studies on the efficacy of self-help groups have been done,[7,28] and until recently, no studies evaluating the effects of the Reach to Recovery program had been conducted. However, in a study of 652 patients with breast cancer, Rogers and co-workers found that 90% of patients who had seen a volunteer perceived the program as helpful.[29,30] The main reason the visits were beneficial was that the volunteer herself had had a mastectomy. More than three-quarters of the patients agreed that "just seeing someone who had recovered helped me feel I could, too," and two-thirds agreed that the volunteer "could understand my feelings because she could remember feeling the same way." In addition, a majority of the women said that they felt less isolated and alone and that their morale was better after the volunteer's visit.

Few respondents criticized the program. Thirty percent said that the volunteer had not taught them anything new, 15% said that they could not confide in the volunteer because she was "too different" (e.g., in age or marital status), 11% maintained that the visit had occurred too soon after their surgery, and 7% said that the volunteer had talked too much about herself.

Overall, 59% reported that the visit had been very helpful, 30% described the visit as somewhat helpful, 7% said that it had been of no consequence, and 4% said that it had not been helpful at all. Patients consistently rated the visit as helpful regardless of their age, marital status, stage of illness, social stratum, or employment. Furthermore, the presence or absence of support from their family, friends, physician, or other health professionals also did not influence the patients' ratings about the helpfulness of the visit. Even the patients who talked informally with a friend, family member, neighbor, or colleague who had had a mastectomy rated the visit as helpful.

When Rogers and her colleagues evaluated the possible benefits of the Reach to Recovery program in areas such as depressive symptoms, fear about recurrence, concern about disfigurement, and length of time required to return to normal activities, they were unable to demonstrate significant effects.[31] However, a nonsignificant trend was found among those who had seen a volunteer. They tended to return to their usual activities about 1 week sooner than did those who had not seen a volunteer. Overall, the data clearly indicate that the bond of common experience enables Reach to Recovery volunteers to provide a unique kind of understanding and to act as a role model of successful recovery.

The Reach to Recovery program is not the only hospital visitation program for patients with breast cancer. In some hospitals, health care professionals recruit their own patients to become visitors, usually because the professionals prefer to retain some control over who visits their patients and what information and exercises the patients receive. The BSR program at Memorial Sloan-Kettering provides additional training for Reach to Recovery volunteers to enable them to participate effectively in the group. Furthermore, because of Betty Ford's and Happy Rockefeller's battles against breast cancer, more women share their diagnosis with friends and relatives. Rogers and her colleagues reported that fully 80% of the patients they interviewed had talked informally with someone who had had a mastectomy (a relative, co-worker, neighbor, friend, or friend of a friend).[29-31]

Self-Help Groups for Survivors

Many community groups have formed to help patients with breast cancer to return to a normal life and to help them cope with the disease and its treatment. Some groups, such as the "I Can Cope" program that the ACS offers nationwide, are open to patients with all kinds of cancer. Others, such as the YMCA's "Encore" program, have limited their membership to patients with breast cancer. Still others have limited their membership to patients with breast cancer who have undergone a specific treatment—for example, those who were treated by mastectomy and are coping with the loss of a breast, those who are receiving adjuvant chemotherapy, or those who were treated with a lumpectomy and irradiation. What these groups have in common is the emphasis on survivorship—the needs of those who are at the stage of illness where their future health is ambiguous. Groups that limit their membership usually focus on specific issues relating to the treatment of breast cancer or to particularly troubling aspects of the illness.

Some of the groups are organized and run by mental health professionals; others are organized and controlled by patients. Some groups sponsor intense, short-term sessions that are held for several months, then are disbanded; others have ongoing programs that involve the same members and that are closed to newcomers. Still others are open to new members at all times. In all cases, the underlying mechanisms of the groups are the same: all of them help members help one another by sharing their problems, being role models of successful recovery, and destigmatizing the illness.

The BSR group program at Memorial Sloan-Kettering has been used in a modified form in cancer centers and hospitals that have enough patients to make the program cost-effective.[32] In hospitals that have fewer patients, professionals use the content of the BSR program in their individual contacts with patients in smaller groups, relying more on self-help groups such as Reach to Recovery for other patient experiences. Furthermore, the information generated in the BSR group about the postoperative experience has been disseminated to professionals from health care institutions and agencies throughout the United States.

FAMILY ISSUES AND GROUP INTERVENTIONS

Concerns of Patients' Partners and Children

The process of hospitalization is a period of extreme stress for families as well as patients. Family members, too, want information and guidance about treatment, how to respond best to the patient, and how to understand and cope with their own reactions. For this reason, the rehabilitation team on the Breast Service at Memorial Sloan-Kettering Cancer Center conducts weekly group sessions for families of inpatients to address their concerns and to provide them with an opportunity to meet with others facing the same experience. Common concerns of family members are discussed below.

The psychological, social, and emotional consequences of breast cancer and its treatment have been studied extensively in patients, but the concerns of patients' husbands or partners have received little attention.[2] Wellisch and co-workers documented some of the concerns of the husbands of mastectomy patients, particularly their fear that their wives would die, their frequent episodes of depression, and their concern about intimacy and sexuality.[33] They concluded, however, that men generally cope well with their partner's disease and usually are sympathetic to their wife's distress.

Gotay studied the concerns of patients with breast cancer and their spouses and found that men tended to be more concerned about their wives' possible death than were their wives.[34] The men also described the problems they had in coping with their wives' emotional distress, especially with extremes of optimism and despair. It also has been reported that men fear they may fail to respond to their wives sexually, hurt her during sex, or react badly to the scar. They also fear that their wife may reject them or may no longer respond to them sexually.[35]

Witkin described some of the common myths men believe about mastectomy and how they can best help their wives to cope with it.[10] Some men believed that the best strategy was to act as though nothing had happened; others believed that their wives would change in some fundamental way because of the diagnosis and mastectomy. Many believed that they should be strong for their wives and thus not discuss their own fears or concerns. Many men postponed making sexual overtures in the belief that their wives would not be interested in sex.

These myths often interfered with open communication and intimacy between spouses. Although the men's actions were well intentioned, their wives often misinterpreted the behavior as rejection or withdrawal.[33] In some instances, the men were in a double-bind whereby any action they took was perceived as wrong.[4] For example, when one husband attempted to reassure his wife about her good prognosis, she accused him of lying. When he stopped trying to reassure her, she accused him of withholding bad news. When another husband made sexual overtures, his wife rejected him as being insensitive; when he stopped making overtures, she accused him of rejecting her.

Although such double-bind situations are not uncommon, they do not seem to be characteristic of couples who are coping with mastectomy. Most authors believe that marriages that suffer as a result of a mastectomy were tenuous before the surgery.[36,37] A survey conducted in 1984 reported that 81% of men said that if their wife had a mastectomy, they would respond with compassion and support;[35] according to clinical observation, most husbands actually do react this way when breast cancer is diagnosed. Little research is available to confirm these clinical impressions, but unpublished data from research conducted in New York State and involving 652 patients with breast cancer provide some evidence to support them.[29,38] Sixty-eight percent of these patients said that they had not experienced marital problems because of the mastectomy, 16% reported "a few" problems, 13% said that they had had "some" problems, and only 3% reported having "many" problems. Fifty percent of the women reported that the mastectomy had strengthened the marriage, 47% said that the marriage had not changed, and 3% reported that the surgery had weakened their relationship with their spouse. Almost all women (94%) who had been sexually active before the surgery were sexually active afterward; 24% had initiated sexual activity by the end of the first week after surgery, and 60% had done so by the fourth week after surgery. Seventy-eight percent of patients reported that their sex life had not changed, 7% said it had improved, and 14% said it was less satisfying than before.

Divorce was extremely rare in this sample of patients. After an average of 12 months following discharge from the hospital, only 10 women said that their husband was no longer living with them. More than 50% of those couples had decided to separate or divorce before the diagnosis of cancer. The data from this study seem to support earlier reports that most patients with breast cancer do not experience serious long-term problems with their marriages, their relationships with their husbands, or their sex lives because of the diagnosis of breast cancer or a mastectomy. Nevertheless, most patients with breast cancer and their partners are concerned about sexual functioning, and counseling programs for couples and groups of couples have been initiated to address this issue.[10]

Children also are vulnerable to the stresses resulting from the diagnosis of breast cancer. Lichtman and colleagues, in their study of 78 patients with breast cancer and their perceptions of changes in the relationships of these patients with their children, identified some of these stresses.[39] Although the majority of mother-child relationships remained strong or grew stronger after diagnosis and treatment of breast cancer, 12% of those relationships had deteriorated to some degree. Problems with children were more likely to occur if the patient's prognosis was poor, her surgery was extensive, her psychological adjustment was poor, or if she had serious difficulty with radiation therapy or chemotherapy.

Women's relationships with their daughters were at

significantly greater risk than were their relationships with their sons. Lichtman and colleagues believed that the fear of inheriting breast cancer and the mother's demands for support were the major factors contributing to problems with adolescent and postadolescent daughters.

Groups for Patients' Families

Families of newly diagnosed patients need information about cancer and its treatment, about how to respond best to the patient, and about how to understand and cope with their own reactions. At Memorial Sloan-Kettering Cancer Center, this information is given to family members individually and in weekly family group meetings for relatives and friends of current inpatients.

During family group meetings, participants receive a condensed version of the information about physical therapy and personal care given to patients in the BSR group. They also learn about some of the common patient reactions at this time. For example, patients usually perceive the diagnosis as a gut-wrenching blow rather than an intellectual abstraction. Cancer causes a loss of trust in one's body; thus, it is normal for patients to regard every ache and pain as a sign of recurrent cancer for a period of time. Most patients with newly diagnosed breast cancer feel well, and usually, it is a small, painless lump that necessitates surgery. Thus, the treatment causes pain; it does not alleviate pain or correct a functional deficit.

Experiencing symptoms of grief is normal for both patients and family members at diagnosis. Feelings of unreality (e.g., "Is this really happening? Maybe it's a mistake") may persist for some time. As the reality of the diagnosis takes hold, sadness and anger usually become the dominant emotions; these feelings may persist for some time. We emphasize to families that these feelings are normal for anyone who experiences a loss.

Patients tend to respond to this crisis in the same way that they responded to previous life stresses, but family members may anticipate the following common patterns. Generally, patients are relieved when the surgery is completed. They may have had fantasies about dying during surgery and are relieved to be alive and able to get out of bed. Some feel euphoric after surgery. They see other patients coping with the same surgery and may feel that the worst is over and that the surgery was not as bad as they had expected. After several days, they become more aware of the reality of their situation and, in many cases, feel depressed. They may fluctuate between laughter and tears. It is normal to experience such abrupt mood shifts.

Family members ask the following kinds of questions: "Actually, she seems pretty good—better than before the surgery. But how long will it be until she gets home?" "Should I treat her the way I usually do?" "Is it good to talk about it?" "How will I know if she is recovering normally?" "How long will it take for her to get back to her old self?"

Although patients recover physically from a mastectomy or lumpectomy relatively quickly, and most people are greatly relieved to return to normal, families must be reminded that the emotional healing will proceed at a slower pace. Many patients do not experience the full impact of the diagnosis and surgery until they return home. They want to be viewed as normal, but they continue to feel the pain of the losses they have sustained, sometimes believing that everyone around them is oblivious to their ongoing struggle to live with the fear of recurrence and metastases.

Family members also are encouraged to recognize the disruption in their own lives that has been caused by the cancer and to accept the fact that they may resent it. This may be difficult because they feel closer to the patient as a result of the threat of losing her and therefore feel guilty about their negative feelings and personal worries.

Because the diagnosis of cancer evokes fear in the family, as well as in the patient, family members may be anxious about their own health and may be more worried than usual about aches and pains. A patient often feels irrationally guilty for having "brought this on" her family, and family members may be angry at her. Group leaders treat these worries as normal reactions; however, they may suggest that the group member have a physical check-up for reassurance. This suggestion may be particularly helpful for the patient's first-degree female relatives, who are statistically at higher risk once their mother, sister, grandmother, or aunt has been diagnosed as having breast cancer. These women often benefit from being checked by a breast specialist or being followed in a specialized clinic for high-risk women.

The question of what to tell young children about the diagnosis and treatment is often raised in the family group. Both clinical experience and research studies support the idea that children cope better with the known than the unknown. Thus, families are usually advised to tell their children about the surgery. It may be easier to hear the word cancer from their parents than to overhear it from neighbors or other adults. Children often wonder whether cancer is contagious, whether they caused it somehow, and whether their mother will get better again. Parents are encouraged to explore their children's understanding of the situation, clarify their misconceptions, and reassure them that the patient will recover and continue to care for them.

Another question that parents frequently ask about children is whether the patient should show them her incision. The group leader discusses this as an individual matter that depends on the nature of the parent-child interaction about nudity before the surgery. Some women believe they should show the wound to their children, but prefer to wait until the wound has healed. Others inform the children about it by drawing a simple figure and outlining the location of the incision.

In summary, families often are as profoundly affected by the diagnosis of breast cancer as is the patient herself. They also need information and the opportunity to explore their thoughts and reactions. The family group is one method of lessening their feelings of isolation and enlisting them as knowledgeable partners in the rehabilitation process.

GROUPS FOR CONTINUING CARE

The groups described previously address the needs of patients who have been newly diagnosed and treated for breast cancer. However, in coping with the many stresses that occur after they are discharged from the hospital, patients often have ongoing needs for information and assistance. Groups can be a cost-effective means of providing this service to patients. The three types of groups described in this section are appropriate at later points in the disease process, and address specific issues related to post-hospital care, adjuvant therapy, and metastatic illness.

Follow-up Groups

Clinical experience and research suggest that the months after hospitalization are an extremely difficult period for patients with breast cancer and that during this period, they have ongoing needs for information and emotional support.[13] At Memorial Sloan-Kettering Cancer Center, all patients with breast cancer have the opportunity to attend a workshop 3 months after they are discharged from the hospital. The format of the workshop includes a review of information presented during the inpatient group sessions, opportunities to ask questions, information about nutrition and breast reconstruction, and small-group discussions on selected topics. A social worker coordinates the program, and other team members (physician, nurse, physical therapist, nutritionist, and psychiatrist) discuss topics related to their specialty.

Patients learn that they share common concerns and that the strange postsurgical sensations they are experiencing are normal. They typically ask questions such as the following: "Why do I still feel numbness in my arm?" "Should I continue the exercises?" "Is it true that I can't ever have a manicure?" "Why did I have a bone scan?" Although patients have already received the answers to many of these questions, they need to reinforce and validate their understanding and clarify their misconceptions. They also need to feel supported in their responses to family, friends, and others who may question their treatment and may suggest alternative therapies.

Nutrition is an important topic for patients at this time. During the workshops, they receive basic facts about the benefits of a low-fat, high-fiber, well-balanced diet. The importance of sufficient calcium and iron is stressed, but megavitamin doses are discouraged. Their questions often reflect an intense desire to find an anticancer diet: "What do you think about vitamin E?" "Should I give up coffee?" "Will a macrobiotic diet prevent the cancer from coming back?" Although patients may feel anxious and frustrated when they find that no anticancer diet exists, they learn that these feelings are normal and that they must learn how to manage them.

Breast reconstruction is another topic of great interest to patients treated with mastectomy. During the workshop, a nurse reviews reconstructive surgery, explaining implantation of the prosthesis, symmetry procedures, and construction of the areola and nipple. Patients ask questions about whether the implant is safe, whether it interferes with the ability to detect a recurrence, whether there is sensation in the nipple, and whether pain is associated with the operation.

Patients then receive information about the psychological issues involved in a decision for or against reconstruction. Although research studies document a high degree of satisfaction among women who undergo breast reconstruction, a patient must not make her decision until she has had a consultation with the breast surgeon and the plastic surgeon. Group members learn that women choose breast reconstruction for several reasons: it obviates the need for a prosthesis, it allows them to wear strapless clothes or go back to wearing bikinis, and it removes the constant reminder of cancer. However, the most important predictor of whether a woman will be satisfied with reconstruction is a good understanding between her and the plastic surgeon about what results can be expected. Middle-aged or older women often feel that it is inappropriate to have breast reconstruction; thus, it should be made clear to them that women of all ages are candidates for the procedure.

The final part of the workshop is devoted to emotional rehabilitation. Mental health professionals lead small-group discussions on topics such as coping with chemotherapy, managing fears about recurrence, adjusting to the loss of a breast, sexual functioning after surgery, and stress-reduction techniques.

Approximately one-third of the patients invited to these follow-up workshops attend, and those who do attend are extremely positive about them. Some refer to the workshop as a "reunion" with their inpatient experience. They document on our evaluation form that continued provision of information, normalization of their experience, and contact with the health care team and other patients increase their sense of control and mastery. In the future, we plan to study the characteristics of women who attend these workshops and compare them with those who do not.

Groups for Patients Receiving Adjuvant Chemotherapy

Patients anxiously await the final pathology report. When lymph node involvement is documented and adjuvant chemotherapy is recommended, patients face another crisis. They may feel as threatened as they did at the original diagnosis; they interpret this recommendation to mean that their prognosis is less favorable and assume that the side effects of chemotherapy will be devastating. At this time, patients ask questions such as the following "Will I be vomiting all the time?" "Will I lose my hair?" "Will I be able to go to work?" "Will I have to go into the hospital for chemotherapy?" "Does it work?" "Is it worth it?"

Patients need reassurance that they are not being treated with chemotherapy because of documented cancer but because they are at increased statistical risk of metastases. At Memorial Sloan-Kettering Cancer Center, a social worker coordinates monthly groups for patients who are undergoing adjuvant chemotherapy and their families. Each meeting focuses on one topic of interest to patients: for example, diet and chemotherapy, an introduction to medical terminology, how to communicate with your physician, the side effects of adjuvant chemotherapy, or stress-reduction techniques. In these groups, professionals provide authoritative information; however, the input of volunteers who have completed adjuvant therapy successfully and share their experiences may be extremely helpful. "No, I didn't lose my hair." "I wasn't hungry at dinner time after I had my chemotherapy, so I used to have a light supper, go to bed early, and be fine the next morning." "Yes, I did lose my hair. I got a wig, which really wasn't so bad, and the minute the chemotherapy was over, my hair started to grow back. Actually, it came back curly." "I was a basket case when I heard I needed chemotherapy. I thought it meant I had cancer throughout my body. But I'm still here eight years later."

The adjuvant chemotherapy group identifies the usual physical and psychological reactions that patients experience. Through statements such as the following, patients indicate that this information is reassuring: "I was so scared. But as soon as I started chemotherapy, I felt less frightened. I could see how I was reacting. Even though I felt queasy, as long as I knew it was normal it wasn't so bad." Individual problems that require more intensive follow-up counseling or referral also are identified in the group.

Groups for Patients with Metastatic Disease

The interval between the time metastasis is detected and the time the patient dies may be a prolonged period during which multiple chemotherapy regimens are used. These regimens have an uncertain outcome and often are as debilitating and painful as the symptoms of the metastasis. Because the precise nature of the disease and its progressive course are not always fully understood, patients feel confused, fearful, angry, and depressed. This experience is probably described best in *Hanging in There,* a book written by Natalie Spingarn, a patient who has lived with metastatic disease for more than 10 years.[40]

The conclusions of Spiegel and associates about the effectiveness of weekly support groups for women with metastatic cancer coincide with our clinical experience and that of others.[7] In a 1-year, randomized, prospective study, they found that patients who participated in this program had significantly lower mood-disturbance scores on the Profile of Mood State scale, had fewer maladaptive coping responses, and were less fearful than the control group. The group helped members improve their communication with physicians, explore difficult family relationships, and discuss issues such as life and death and how to have as rich a life as possible in the face of a terminal illness. These are the usual issues that emerge in groups for women with metastatic illness. Women who choose to participate in these groups usually regard them as valuable and believe that the quality of their lives improves as a result of their participation. However, these groups are the most difficult ones for the group leader because of the issues addressed and because a number of members are likely to die during the course of the group sessions. Therefore, skilled group leaders are not always readily available.

CONCLUSIONS

This section has discussed only a few of the types of groups that are tailored to address the specific problems of patients with breast cancer. Loneliness and fear often confront the woman with breast cancer, thus creating a greater need for contact than her family and friends may be able to provide. Psychological support obtained in a group may offer this additional help.

Family members, too, are profoundly affected by the disease and its treatment, and they often suffer from the loneliness caused by hiding feelings they believe would overwhelm the patient. This "putting up a brave front" results in mutual withdrawal and diminishes the quality of their relationship with the patient.

The groups described here fulfill several functions. They enable the patient to maintain contact with people who are as interested in treatment issues as she is, they ensure the accuracy of the information the patient and family receive and help to clarify their misperceptions, they help the patient continue with scientifically developed treatment rather than turning in desperation to alternative therapies, and they allow the patient to deal with her emotional reactions in a way that enables her to continue living with dignity and meaning.

REFERENCES

1. Bloom JR: Social support, accommodation to stress and adjustment to breast cancer. Soc Sci Med 16:1329, 1982
2. Christensen DN: Postmastectomy couple counseling: An outcome study of a structured treatment protocol. J Sex Marital Ther 9:266, 1983
3. Euster S: Rehabilitation after mastectomy: The group process. Soc Work Health Care 43:251, 1979
4. Gates CC: Husbands of mastectomy patients. Patient Counseling Health Ed 2:38, 1980
5. Joiner JG, Fisher JZ: Postmastectomy counseling. In Howell E, Hayes M (eds): Women and Mental Health. New York, Basic Books, 1981
6. Schain WS: Sexual problems of patients with cancer. In DeVita VT, Hellman S, Rosenberg S (eds): Cancer: Principles and Practice of Oncology. Philadelphia, JB Lippincott, 1982
7. Spiegel D, Bloom JR, Yalom I: Group support for patients with metastatic cancer. Arch Gen Psychiatry 38:527, 1981
8. Wellisch DK: Implementation of psychosocial services in managing emotional stress. Cancer 53:828, 1984
9. Winich L, Robbins G: Physical and psychological readjustment after mastectomy. Cancer 39:478, 1977

10. Witkin MH: Psychosexual myths and realities of mastectomy. Med Aspects Hum Sexuality 67, 13:67, 1979
11. Abt V, McGurrin MC, Heitz AA: The impact of mastectomy on sexual self-image and behavior. Sex Ed Ther 4(2):45, 1978
12. Maguire GP, Lee EG, Bevington RF, et al: Psychiatric problems in the first year after mastectomy. Br Med J 1:963, 1978
13. Morris T, Greer HS, White P: Psychological and social adjustment to mastectomy: A two-year follow-up study. Cancer 40:2381, 1977
14. Jamison KR, Wellisch DK, Pasnau RO: Psychosocial aspects of mastectomy: I. The woman's perspective. Am J Psychiatry 135:432, 1978
15. Silberfarb PM, Maurer LH, Crouthamel CS: Psychosocial aspects of neoplastic disease. I. Functional status of breast cancer patients during three different treatment regimens. Am J Psychiatry 137:450, 1980
16. Thomas SG: Breast cancer: The psychosocial issues. Cancer Nurs 1:53, 1978
17. Ashcroft JJ, Leinster SJ, Slade PO: Breast cancer—Patient choice of treatment: Preliminary communication. J R Soc Med 78:43, 1985
18. Bartelink H, Van Dam F, Van Dongen J: Psychological effects of breast-conserving therapy in comparison with radical mastectomy. Radiat Oncol Biol Physics 11:381, 1985
19. Sanger CK, Reymikoff M: A comparison of the psychological effects of breast-saving procedures with the modified radical mastectomy. Cancer 48:2341, 1981
20. Schain W, Edwards BK, Gorell CR, et al: Psychosocial and physical outcome of primary breast cancer therapy: Mastectomy vs. excisional biopsy and irradiation. Breast Cancer Res Treat 3:377, 1983
21. Steinberg MD, Juliano MA, Wise L: Psychological outcome of lumpectomy versus mastectomy in the treatment of breast cancer. Am J Psychiatry 142:34, 1985
22. Taylor SE, Lichtman RR, Wood J, et al: Illness-related and treatment-related factors in psychological adjustment to breast cancer. Cancer 55:2506, 1985
23. Gussow Z, Tracey GS: The role of self-help clubs in adaptation to chronic illness and disability. Soc Sci Med 10:407, 1976
24. Borkman T: A cross-national comparison of stutterers' self-help organizations. N Z Speech Ther J 29:6, 1974
25. Katz AH: Self-help organizations and volunteer participation in social welfare. Soc Work 15:51, 1970
26. Riessman F: The "helper" therapy principle. Soc Work 10:27, 1965
27. Sabo D: The male role and mastectomy: Support groups and men's adjustments. J Psychosoc Oncol 4(1/2):1986
28. Killilea M: Mutual help organizations: Interpretations in the literature. In Caplan G, Killilea M (ed): Support Systems and Mutual Help. New York, Grune & Stratton, 1976
29. Rogers TF, Metzger LM, Bauman LJ: The effects of lay groups on recovery and functioning. Grant No. CA 22219, National Cancer Institute, 1979
30. Rogers T, Bauman L, Metzger L: Effects of peer support: Reach to Recovery and the cancer patient. In Engstrom PF, Anderson PN, Mortenson LE (eds): Advances in Cancer Control: Epidemiology and Research. New York, Alan R. Liss, 1984
31. Rogers T, Bauman L, Metzger L: An assessment of the Reach to Recovery program. CA 35::116, 1985
32. Sachs SH, Davis JM, Reynolds SA, et al: Postmastectomy rehabilitation in a community hospital. J Fam Pract 11:395, 1980
33. Wellisch D, Jamison K, Pasnau R: Psychosocial aspects of mastectomy: The man's perspective. Am J Psychiatry 135:543, 1978
34. Gotay CC: The experience of cancer during early and advanced stages: The views of patients and their mates. Soc Sci Med 18:605, 1984
35. Breast Cancer Digest, 2nd ed. Bethesda, MD, National Cancer Institute, 1984
36. Bard M, Sutherland AM: Psychological impact of cancer and its treatment. Cancer 8:656, 1955
37. Downie PA: Rehabilitation of the patient after mastectomy. Nurs Mirror 140:58, 1975
38. Metzger LM, Rogers RF, Bauman LJ: Effects of age and marital status on emotional distress after a mastectomy. J Psychosoc Oncol 1:17, 1983
39. Lichtman RR, Taylor SE, Wood JU, et al: Relations with children after breast cancer: The mother-daughter relationship at risk. J Psychosoc Oncol 2:1, 1984
40. Spingarn ND: Hanging in There: Living Well on Borrowed Time. New York, Stein & Day, 1982

Patient Rehabilitation: Nursing

Susan McKenney Keohan

Nurses interact with women in every phase of the breast cancer process: screening and detection, diagnosis, primary treatment, adjuvant therapy, first recurrences, secondary treatment, and palliative care. Through their care, these women are provided with a means to receive information, explore concerns and needs, discern treatment alternatives in the midst of crisis, and establish and reinforce a therapeutic relationship that promotes positive coping and comfort within each patient's unique physical, psychosocial, and spiritual capacity.[1–3] Probably the nurse's most significant contribution is to play the role of patient advocate. To maximize optimal rehabilitation, the nurse must be knowledgeable in breast self-examination (BSE) as a secondary preventive measure, in counseling of women premastectomy and postmastectomy, in providing anticipatory guidance in dealing with surgery, in choosing a temporary and permanent prosthesis, and in teaching postmastectomy exercises and interventions to prevent lymphedema. In addition, nurses should be able to answer questions about the alternatives in breast reconstruction, the indications and side effects of primary radiotherapy and chemotherapy, and the effects of breast cancer treatments on a woman's sexual identity.

THE ROLE OF THE NURSE IN SECONDARY PREVENTION OF BREAST CANCER

When the American Cancer Society (ACS) surveyed women in 1983, 96% reported that they knew about breast examinations.[4] The frequency with which they reported practicing BSE is reviewed in Table 16-3.[11] One contention, however, is that a consistent BSE technique has not been reported. Studies show that being taught BSE either by a nurse or physician may result in improved proficiency in self-examination.[9,11–13] Nurses are often able to spend more time than other health professionals exploring patients' concerns in a nonthreatening fashion, explaining

Table 16-3
Frequency with which Breast Self-Examination (BSE) Is Practiced

Study	No. of Participants	Type*	Percentage of Women Who Practice BSE				
			Ever	This Year	1–2 Times/Yr	3–11 Times/Yr	Every Month
NCI(5)	1580	A	83	77	13	24	40
ACS(4)	752	A	80	69	19	23	27
Huguley and Brown(6)	2092	B		67	13	19	34
Feldman et al.(7)	996	B		67	26	22	19
Foster and Costanza(8)	1004	B				28	23
Senie et al.(9)	1216	B	71			40	29
Celantano and Holtzman(10)	308	A		76			35

*A, women without breast cancer; B, women with breast cancer.
(Modified. with permission, from Morra ME; Breast self-examination today: An overview of its use and its value. Semin Oncol Nurs 1:171, 1985)

Table 16-4
Number of Biopsies Recommended and Performed and Number of Cancers Detected on Physical Examination: Data From the Cincinnati Breast Cancer Detection Project Only (as of 6-1-78)

Type of Clinician	No. of Patients Examined	No. of Biopsies Recommended	No. of Biopsies Performed	% of Biopsies Performed Per Biopsies Recommended	No. of Biopsies Documenting Cancer
Surgeon	6609	530	239	45%	18
Nurses	25,587	1075	352	33%	28
Physicians other than surgeons	8007	458	239	52%	29
Total	40,203	2063	830		75

(Modified, with permission, from Moskowitz M: Clinical examination of the breasts by nonphysicians. Cancer 44:313, 1979)

BSE techniques and establishing a relationship that will reinforce and encourage a woman to examine her breast. Because of this, nurses are in a good position to teach a more thorough method of examination, and to build awareness, discuss risks, and refute myths about BSE and the development of breast cancer. Recent studies report that nurses in expanded roles are as successful as physicians in examining breasts and detecting suspicious lesions.[14–18] In the West London Breast Cancer Screening Study, 999 women were examined independently by a nurse and a physician.[19] Although the nurses and physicians referred the same number of patients (89) for further evaluation and possible biopsy, only 43 of the patients were thought to have a suspicious mass by both the nurse and the physician. There were 8 cancers in the 89 patients referred for further evaluation by clinic doctors and 6 cancers among the 89 referred by nurses. The physicians missed one cancer and the nurses failed to find three.

In a comparative study sponsored by the National Cancer Institute (NCI) and the ACS, 40,203 women were examined by nurses, surgeons, and other physicians over a four-year period as part of the Cincinnati Breast Cancer Detection Network.[17] The data in Table 16-4 indicate that, in a screening situation, nurse practitioners are at least comparable to surgeons and nonsurgical physicians in detecting breast lesions. About one third of the patients referred by nurses for consideration of biopsy, and 8% of these biopsies were positive. These results were not strikingly different from those of the surgeons and general physicians; 45% of the patients referred by surgeons and 52% of the patients referred by other physicians had biopsies, and a cancer was diagnosed in 7.5% and 12% of these biopsies respectively.

There remains considerable controversy about the optimal method of BSE. The ACS has promoted a standard format that diagrams an optimal method of performing breast examinations; however, there is some preliminary evidence to suggest that this may not be adequate in teaching and reinforcing the practice of BSE. Hence, new breast examination programs have been developed in an attempt to be more comprehensive in teaching women the technique of BSE.

The Finland Mammacare Program (1975) uses nurses as the key persons responsible for teaching and reinforcing BSE.[20] They have used reminder calendars to individualize and promote monthly examinations and have reported an increase in the monthly practice of BSE from 20% (preparticipation) to 70%.

The Breast Examination Training (BET) Center in California is a program that has been modeled after the Mammacare program.[21] This program is run by nurses who provide individual education, support, and guidance, on a one-to-one basis, for women interested in BSE and screening. The nurses incorporate the use of simulated breast models with private practice sessions that permit immediate feedback on technique. The success of such programs remains undocumented, as there are few randomized or controlled studies that compare programs that do and do not use practice models. Some preliminary evidence suggests that the use of such models may increase a woman's confidence level and ability to detect lesions;[21] however, this remains to be confirmed. In addition, programs that incorporate simulated breast models are very expensive, both for the person being trained and the agency utilizing them, and they are training-intensive for the nurses involved. Thus, they may actually be less cost-effective to use than screening programs.

The Breast Evaluation Center at the Dana Farber Cancer Institute has designed a nursing approach to teaching BSE. The goal of the program is to teach a thorough and realistic approach to BSE in a uniquely personalized fashion. This program does not use training models. A woman is taught to understand the specific characteristics of her own breasts, and is encouraged only to detect changes within them during monthly examinations. Initially, a woman's knowledge of BSE, the particular technique she uses, and her confidence level during practice are assessed, along with any factors that may inhibit BSE practice. Each patient's perception of personal risk is also explored. After identifying the patient's readiness and motivation to learn, a teaching session incorporates common facts about breast cancer, normal developmental anatomy and physiology, basic definitions used by health care providers, BSE guidelines, and the rationale for early detection. Then, specific instructions for each woman are given with respect to timing and frequency of examinations, and written materials from the ACS and NCI are provided.

The nurse clinician describes and demonstrates each step of BSE. Inspection includes examining breast contour for changes, both with the arms positioned overhead in an interlocked position and on the hips. The chest muscles are flexed with each maneuver. Identifying and documenting each woman's own unique breast characteristics provides a baseline to which she can compare her breast characteristics during examinations. Signs that patients are taught to observe and report include skin changes of redness, swelling, pitting, or peau d'orange; nipple inversion or eversion from a previously normal position; spontaneous nipple discharge, or any obvious dimpling, bulging, or puckering.

Breast palpation is typically not something most women do correctly without instruction. The two most common mistakes include incorrect pressure and covering the chest wall and axilla incompletely. The nurse first shows the patient how to palpate tissue, using the pads of three fingers and moving them in a circular fashion on the knuckles of the woman's hand. This demonstrates technique, as well as correct pressure. The patient is then asked to demonstrate palpation on the nurse's hand. The goal of this practice is to help the woman focus on technique. Palpation of the breast is done while lying down, placing the hand of the side being examined behind the head. Using the pads of three fingers on the opposite hand, the breast is systematically palpated in a spindle fashion, progressing in approximately 1-inch sections that extend along the sternum, clavicle, axilla, and inframammary ridge.

While conducting a breast examination in a patient, every attempt is made to provide a careful description of the woman's breast for her. Common anatomical areas that are often misconstrued as lumps or problems are described. These areas include the ribs along the medial aspect of the chest wall along the sternum, as well as physiologic nodularities in the upper and outer breast quadrants and the inframammary ridge. In addition, any unique breast characteristics are described in considerable detail, including regions prone to recurrent cysts, a fibroadenoma, previous biopsy scarring, radiation induration, high-risk areas for *in situ* cancer, mastectomy scars, and sites of breast reconstruction. The literature on teaching BSE does not address these specific issues. Although women are encouraged to practice BSE, they commonly report that they have no baseline with which to compare, nor do they know what they should be feeling, nor have they ever been told what is normal for them. Demonstration of the breast examination technique by the patient allows for feedback and reinforcement by the nurse and her surgeon.

NURSING CARE OF THE MASTECTOMY PATIENT

The modified radical mastectomy is currently the most widely used surgical procedure for treatment of malignant tumors of the breast. A major component of nursing care for women undergoing mastectomy is to provide emotional support and to explore psychosocial concerns. This aspect of care is covered in depth in the first section of this chapter.

The goals of rehabilitation for a woman undergoing mastectomy include "physical restoration of the use and function of the shoulder and arm; emotional support focusing on the psychological responses to the cancer diagnosis and loss of the breast; adjustment and resumption of preoperative social and sexual activities; occupational/vocational efforts to aid in regaining preoperative function; prevention of complications, such as frozen shoulder, infection, and lymphedema; and cosmetic rehabilitation through a prosthesis or breast reconstruction."[22,23]

The preoperative period has been identified as a time of considerable anxiety during which the critical thinking and information processing abilities of patients with breast cancer are compromised.[24] Providing anticipatory guidance, identifying specific teaching needs, and exploring concerns regarding various aspects of mastectomy and rehabilitation are especially difficult during this time, and it is often helpful for the nurse to involve family members or significant others in accomplishing these goals. Also, it is important to let the patient know that, although the length of hospitalization varies from surgeon to surgeon, the average expected hospital stay is between 3 days and 1 week. Explaining the underlying rationales for the use of antibiotics, pain medication, intravenous (IV) lines, drainage tubes, and dressings may also help the woman understand the normal expected course of recovery. A discussion of the temporary limitations of the shoulder and the need for arm exercises, as well as probable sensation changes, is also important if the woman is to adjust optimally postoperatively.

Teaching and demonstrating postmastectomy hand and arm exercises is an important nursing intervention that may prevent or reduce lymphedema in the affected arm and promote optimal postoperative range of motion in the shoulder. Exercises may begin immediately after or within 1 week of surgery at the discretion of the attending surgeon. Each exercise should initially be repeated three to four times, after which the patient should progress to 10 repetitions over a period of time. A description of these postmastectomy exercises follows.[25]

Hand and Wall Climbing—Stand in a comfortable position facing a wall with toes as close to the wall as possible. Place the hands against the wall at about shoulder level, with the elbows bent. Work hands up the wall parallel to each other until the arms are fully extended, then work them back down to shoulder level again.

Pulley Motion—This exercise may be completed by tossing a rope over a rod in the home. Using a see-saw motion with the arms stretched sideways, slide the rope up and down over the rod, extending the arms without bending at the waist.

Elbow Pull-in—Standing straight and comfortably, extend the arms sideways to shoulder level. In rhythm, bend the elbows, clasping the fingers at the back of the neck, pull elbows in toward each other until they touch, and then return to former position. Unclasp the fingers and extend the arms sideways at shoulder level, returning to the initial position.

Paddleswing—From a standing, straight position, bend forward from the waist, allowing the arms to hang. Without bending the elbows, and in rhythm, swing the right arm back while bringing the left arm forward. Then, allow both arms to hang forward in the initial position.

The Pendulum Swing—Starting from a comfortable standing position, bend forward from the waist, allowing the arms to hang. Swing both arms together, from one shoulder to the other, without bending the elbows and while keeping the arms parallel. Then, return arms to the hanging position.

Forehead Touch—Standing straight at arms' length distant from a wall, place hands against the wall at shoulder level and parallel to each other. Slowly bend the elbows, leaning forward until the forehead touches the wall. Then, straighten the elbows slowly, pushing the body away from the wall.

Lymphedema

Lymphedema is the most frequent long-term side effect of mastectomy and axillary dissection, and is characterized by a difference in measurement between extremities of greater than or equal to 1 cm to 1.5 cm. Mild edema ranges from 1 cm to less than 3 cm, moderate lymphedema from 3 cm to 5 cm, and severe lymphedema is classified as a difference of greater than 5 cm or 6 cm.[26,27] This is discussed in detail in Chapter 15. Assessment of lymphedema begins immediately postoperatively and is accomplished by measuring each of the arms 6 cm above and below the olecranon process.

Primary intervention in preventing lymphedema requires that the patient have information regarding potential risks, complications, and how to perform hand and arm exercises postmastectomy.[28,29] Hand and arm care precautions, listed in the accompanying display, are self-explanatory. In addition to providing this information, surgeons often have patients elevate the affected arm for periods of 20 minutes four times daily beginning 24 to 48 hours postoperatively.

Secondary nursing interventions for lymphedema focus on instructing and encouraging the patient to monitor herself for signs and symptoms of tightness, swelling, impaired movements, and cellulitis.[28] During follow-up visits, the nurse is able to assess the patient for lymphedema and, if it is present, may instruct the patient to elevate her affected arm three to four times daily for approximately 20 minutes. Tertiary interventions are instituted when excessive or prolonged problems with lymphedema occur. Such problems are manifested by structural problems, muscle weakness, and impaired circulation. In such cases, the nurse's role would be to reinforce previous intervention, as well as to assess activities of daily living and pain control. Antibiotics may also be administered for recurrent episodes of cellulitis.

Hand and Arm Care Measures

Avoid vaccinations, injections, drawing of blood in the affected arm.
Avoid occupational injuries.
Avoid infections and burns.
Avoid constricting clothing, jewelry, or arm bags.
Avoid lifting heavy objects.
Avoid shaving with a razor or using deodorant.
Avoid harsh chemicals.
Avoid measuring blood pressure in the affected arm.

Breast Prostheses

If a woman chooses to undergo mastectomy as her primary therapy and does not opt for immediate breast reconstruction, she will need to learn about the use of temporary and permanent prostheses. Reach to Recovery volunteers have been invaluable in providing peer support, as well as necessary information about these devices. The volunteers usually provide the woman with her first temporary prosthesis, a simple piece of cotton fluff that may be placed in the bra to provide breast contour form without aggravating the surgical site. A permanent prosthesis is generally not fitted until adequate postoperative healing has taken place, usually within a few weeks. The nurse may offer practical advice by providing current information on how to go about choosing a permanent prosthesis. It is recommended that women see experienced fitters who are aware of all the available breast forms. Table 16-5 lists the most common prostheses, along with their individual characteristics, advantages, and disadvantages. Patients should be encouraged to act as a responsible consumer and to avoid selecting the first prosthesis they see until they have had an opportunity to try all of the different styles for comfort. Prostheses may be found in most lingerie departments of major stores, in medical supply houses, or in surgical appliance stores. Generally, most of the prostheses require that you either use a good support bra or a mastectomy bra, which has a pocket specially designed to accommodate the prosthesis. Whichever bra is chosen, it is important that the prosthesis feel secure against the chest wall so that slipping or discomfort may be avoided.

Breast Reconstruction

Women today are faced with many treatment alternatives in the management of their breast cancer. Breast reconstruction is an option which, until recently, was never considered until after a woman had had her mastectomy; in many cases, it may not have been discussed at all. The usual reasons women contemplate breast reconstruction are a desire for physical restitution, enhancement of their self-esteem, decreased dependency on their external pros-

Table 16-5
Prostheses

Brands/Types of Prostheses	*Main Characteristics*	*Major Advantages/Disadvantages*
Amoena brands	Silicone gel with a smooth, shiny covering and side wings	Made for left and right breasts; secures to chest wall and bra forms; has air vents that ensure ventilation; has a concave back which decreases skin friction; must be warmed before placement
Comfort 2000	Similar to the Amoena brand, but has a flat back; worn in a bra with a specially designed pocket	May cause scar irritation
Cameo natural breast Prosthesis	Made of organic material called Kunsleakahout, which is also used for creating artificial veins and skin; is worn directly on the skin; has 3 small air holes for ventilation; has nipple on form	Not filled with liquid or silicone so there is no danger of leaking or skrinking; hygienic and odorless; chlorine- and salt-waterproof; made in left and right breast forms; warms quickly and remains at room temperature.
Nearlyme	Has side tapers that fill in the hollow under the arm and top tapers to that help fit the form closer to the chest wall (especially important for those who have undergone a radical mastectomy); must be worn in bra and may need to use a breast form cover for comfort; made of nonsticky polyurethane filled with silicone; no nipple on form	Designs for both radical and modified radical mastectomies are available; has left and right breast forms; may be worn in chlorinated or salt water or in sauna.
Cherish II	Soft, mobile silicone gel encased in a smooth silicone elastomer skin; has a base seam to ensure dimensional stability; no need for a breast form cover in most cases; has nipple on breast form	One breast form only; has graduated weights
Trulife	Has foam and liquid breast forms; has nipple on form; must be worn with cotton covers for comfort; oil-filled prosthesis has sponge back	No seams to irritate skin; has only one breast form; oil-filled form is the least expensive, but it does not last as long as the form model
Carefree	Silicone gel prosthesis with a silastic rubber skin; available in pink or brown	Does not breath well; less pre-formed; one breast form available
Custom Breast Prosthetics	Customized prosthesis using a preopeative impression; made with silicone	Costs $600

thesis, more natural feeling in clothing, and the renewal of sexual enjoyment.[30] However, women may often feel very guilty for considering reconstruction.

In order to counsel effectively a woman who is undergoing or contemplating breast reconstruction, the nurse should emphasize that the decision to undergo such a procedure is her decision alone, not one forced upon her. The patient must also understand that the reconstructed breast will differ from her pre-mastectomy breast in many ways. In addition, the nurse must be knowledgeable about the psychological needs of women who have had a mastectomy and the psychosexual sequelae of mastectomy and reconstruction. Encouraging women to seek second opinions on breast reconstruction requires a knowledge of the community resources available, referrals to plastic surgeons, a knowledge of the costs and insurance coverage involved (Table 16-6). It is also important that the nurse have a basic knowledge of breast cancer, as most women have many fears and anxieties about the reconstruction masking a possible recurrence. An in depth discussion of reconstructive techniques is provided in the section that follows.

Postoperative nursing care of the reconstructed patient involves care of the operative wound, which may range from simple, dry, dressing changes and care of a drain to major postoperative care measures for abdominal surgery. Women should be instructed to wear a good support bra without underwires, preferably one that fastens in the front. Patients are generally instructed to avoid excessive exposure to the sun, stretching or heavy lifting that might injure the incision, and excessive pressure on the chest wall during sexual activities for approximately 6 weeks until healing has occurred. The woman should be encouraged to return to her normal activities of daily living and to continue practicing BSE. Women who have had simple implants may be taught how to do breast massage in order to assist in the expansion of the new breast mound and to diminish capsule formation. This usually begins 2 to 3 days postoperatively, but the exact timing is determined by the individual plastic surgeon. Generally, the woman is instructed to use the palm of her hand to gently press the breast mound on each side for a count of five, moving in a forward-to-back and an upward-to-downward motion. This is then repeated on each side five times for 10 to 15 minutes daily. Patients are encouraged to continue this exercise for approximately 1 year following surgery. Women who have undergone a myocutaneous flap procedure should be informed that it may take weeks to months before the breast assumes a natural shape. Sensation changes—both hyperesthesia and hypoesthesia—often occur, and completion of the procedure may take more than one operation.

The nipple and areola complex is generally reconstructed after the breast mound has settled or the tissue flap has healed and edema has decreased. Women should understand that the nipple and areola will look and feel different from their original complex. Generally, the differences appreciated are color changes; specifically, the areola may be slightly lighter than that of the opposite breast. Because tanning or exposure of the reconstructed tissues to the sun is generally discouraged, a more natural look may be achieved using organic hennas that will not compromise the tissue.

NURSING IMPLICATIONS OF PRIMARY RADIOTHERAPY

Nursing interventions in the care of patients undergoing radiotherapy include education of the patient with regard to the treatment and its side effects, skin care during treatment, and radiation safety precautions. Patient education is directed at providing women with accurate and detailed information that covers the rationale for treatment, the procedures involved in planning the treatment course, the various methods of delivering radiation therapy, and the potential risks and side effects of the procedure.

Prior to initiating radiotherapy, a second surgical procedure may be performed to achieve a wider excision and axillary dissection. The use of a drain or Hemovac for the first 24 hours is indicated to reduce the likelihood of

Table 16-6
Resources Related to Breast Reconstruction

Source	*Basic Characteristics*
American Society of Plastic and Reconstructive Surgeons Chicago, IL (312) 856-1834	Provides 24-hour patient referral service for certified plastic surgeons specializing in breast cancer reconstruction
Reconstruction Education for National Understanding (RENU) Philadelphia, PA: (215) 635-1499 Cleveland, OH: (216) 356-2683 Washington, DC: (202) 483-2600	Similar to the ACS program, Reach to Recovery; provides a trained volunteer to discuss reconstruction issues with patients
Cancer Information Service (CIS) 1-800-4 CANCER	May provide information on local resources available on breast reconstruction

hematoma or seroma. A sterile dressing is usually all that is needed. Patients should be informed that any sign of redness, purulent drainage, pain, or fever is to be reported. However, scar tissue formation and induration are to be expected, and will resolve over time. Periodic twinges of pain or a pulling sensation should be explained as expected outcomes and are not necessarily signs of recurrence or spread. Since, like modified radical mastectomy, this treatment involves axillary dissection, the same arm precautions and exercises are recommended.

The planning or simulation period is a time when radiotherapists design the radiation treatment, and internal mammary nodes are located and ports are calculated. It is important to inform patients that markings or tattoos are made on the skin as alignment points, and that lead shields are specifically designed for the protection of other organs.

The treatment phase of radiotherapy takes approximately 5 to 6 weeks, with the patient typically receiving 180 to 200 cGy per day 5 days per week.[31] The treatment plan may also include booster doses, delivered to the primary tumor site either by a concentrated, external beam of irradiation using high-energy photons from a linear accelerator or by an interstitial implant of radioactive iridium-192 at the site of the tumor in the breast.[32] Common side effects include fatigue, breast edema, skin reaction, hyperpigmentation, and asymmetrical fibrosis. Less commonly, rib fractures, pneumonitis, arm edema, myositis, and pain may occur.[31]

The cause of fatigue secondary to radiation therapy is not clearly understood. Recommending that the patient follow a diet high in protein and carbohydrates and balance exercise and rest periods may help to modify the stress of radiation therapy. Skin reactions are the most common and most variable of the side effects of primary radiotherapy. If they occur, they generally develop within the last few weeks of treatment. Those who are most susceptible to reactions are women who have undergone prior chemotherapy. A common reaction is desquamation, or peeling of the skin. This may develop weeks after radiation therapy has been completed; itching is the predominant sensation reported. Hypopigmentation or hyperpigmentation may also occur, with color changing over a period of months. Wet desquamation, which produces effects similar to a second degree burn, is a more severe reaction involving sloughing of the tissue layers. This occurs much less commonly now that newer techniques for delivering primary radiotherapy have been developed.

Teaching good skin care to women undergoing breast irradiation is important, as it may reduce overall discomfort and promote optimal skin integrity. Women are advised to keep their skin clean and dry, using tepid water and mild soap for cleansing. Soaps, such as Ivory or Neutrogena, are acceptable for use. The skin should be patted dry, never rubbed. Patients should be instructed to avoid using perfumes, cosmetics, creams, lotions, or deodorants on the treated area, as they are irritants and may potentiate burns. Instead, unscented hydrophilic lotions, such as Lubriderm, Aquafore, Eucerin, or lanolin, may be used to soothe dry, irritated skin. Radiation therapy nurses have recommended using Aveeno oatmeal bar or cornstarch to relieve itching. Women should avoid wearing tight, constricting clothing during treatment as it may aggravate already tender skin. Exposure to excessive temperatures and ultraviolet sunlight, as well as heating pads and salt or chlorinated water, should also be avoided.

The nursing care of patients receiving radiation implants is focused on providing emotional support during isolation periods and maintaining safety precautions for staff personnel, other patients, and visitors. There is actually very little technical care necessary once the implant is inserted. A dry, sterile dressing is changed on a p.r.n. basis, mild analgesics are administered for local discomfort, and vital signs are monitored. The implant is also checked for signs of dislodging. An explanation of all protective isolation measures is important if the patient is to cope with the anxiety of being alone and undergoing treatment that has the potential for being dangerous to others.

Protective measures include limiting time spent with visitors to 30 minutes per day at distances of one foot and time spent with staff to 30 minutes per shift. Private rooms that are labeled well with precautionary signs are used. Lead shields are utilized around the patients while direct care is being given. Bed linens are kept in patients' rooms until after the iridium seeds have been removed.[32]

THE PSYCHOSEXUAL SEQUELAE OF BREAST CANCER

Sexuality is a major variable in a patient's physiological and psychological adaptation to breast cancer treatment. The meaning of breasts to women in society,[33,34] and the anxiety fostered by changes in body image and self-concept as a result of mastectomy have been well documented.[23]

A sexual assessment requires nurses to first identify their own feelings and biases about discussions of sexuality. Taking responsibility for such discussions and interventions requires nurses to become knowledgeable about male and female sexuality and the resources available for referrals, as well as to be proficient in taking a careful sexual history and in limited counseling techniques. Gaining the trust of a patient provides the basis for a therapeutic relationship. Clinicians should employ a philosophy that reinforces self-worth, is nonjudgmental, and conveys affirmation and normalcy if communication is to be facilitated.

The assessment is begun by identifying the age, developmental level, socioeconomic status, educational level, and ethnic background of the couple. MacElveen-Hoehn has reviewed strategies that may help clinicians initiate discussions in a nonthreatening manner.[35] She suggests the following approaches:

Talk with couples whenever possible.
Begin with the least sensitive question; i.e., "I'd like to

hear what each of you perceives as the strengths and assets of your relationship."

Proceed from general discussions to more specific ones; i.e., "Radiation therapy affects body systems in different ways. Have you noticed any changes in your sex life?"

Ask "when" or "how often" instead of "do you."

Use the third person to introduce a question.

Prepare questions with a statement that validates a range of normalcy.

Refer to how commonly an experience occurs.

Move from past to present.

Once the assessment is completed, any problems identified should be explored in much the same way that a history of present illness is for a medical problem. This further evaluation might include eliciting a description of the problem from the couple, and determining the problem's onset and frequency, as well as any variables governing its occurrence or its nature. The couple should be asked to describe their perceptions of the problem, as well as interventions they might have attempted. The clinician should also ask the couple how he or she might provide help—for instance, by supplying information or making therapeutic plans or referrals.[36]

The P-LI-SS-IT model of sexual counseling is frequently used in intervention.[36] The acronym stands for permission, limited information, specific suggestions, and intensive therapy. *Permission,* identified as the first level, involves a general discussion of the impact of cancer treatment on sexuality. Permission implies conveyed acceptance of lifestyle. Couples are encouraged to take risks and experiment with different things. Books and pamphlets that address aspects of sexuality should be made available. The nurse must be able to answer questions, provide follow-up, or to make referrals.

Limited information implies giving couples specific information to address specific concerns of sexuality and misconceptions related to current treatment (e.g., initiating sexual relations after mastectomy or protecting the mastectomy site or the reconstructed breast from physical trauma associated with different positions).

Specific suggestions refers to instances in which the couple and clinician contract to develop and work on a prescribed program. A program may be developed to foster better communication skills between partners, or to promote greater sensitivity with regard to physical intimacy, exploring new methods, sexual expression, or symptom management.

Intensive therapy requires referral to a specialist in sex therapy. Couples requiring this level of counseling are those with long-standing sexual difficulties or severe psychological distress.

NURSING MANAGEMENT OF CHEMOTHERAPY

The nursing management of women receiving chemotherapy has two major points of focus. One is providing the patient and family with verbal and written information about specific chemotherapeutic regimens, their therapeutic goals, potential risks, and toxicities, along with proposed interventions designed to maintain self-care and to promote safe participation in therapy and optimal living. The second focus of care relates to the intravenous administration of chemotherapy, protocols for safe handling, aseptic technique, guidelines for administration, and management of extravasation.

It is beyond the scope of this section to discuss all aspects of the nursing management of patients receiving chemotherapy. Therefore, the reader is referred to Table 16-7 for review of the most common side effects, presenting signs and symptoms, and interventions involved.[37–40]

Nausea and vomiting are two of the most comon and most distressing symptoms resulting from chemotherapy that affect a woman's overall adjustment to treatment and quality of life. Management with antiemetics has been approached in the past on a trial and error basis. There is evidence to suggest that the nursing management of nausea and vomiting, using progressive muscle relaxation and guided imagery, may effectively alleviate these symptoms.[41–43] The advantages of a behavioral program in managing these symptoms are that it provides the woman with a sense of control over her life, it is virtually devoid of side effects, it is cost-effective and relatively easy to learn, and it may be used in either the clinical or home setting. In order to teach relaxation techniques to women, clinicians must first evaluate the patient's motivation and readiness to learn. Four key elements that have been identified by Benson as being essential for the achievement of relaxation are a quiet environment, decreased muscle tonus, a mental device, and a passive attitude.[44]

The side effect of alopecia is probably one of the most devastating consequences of chemotherapy. This assault on body image may be comparable to that of the mastectomy itself. It is important for nurses to explore the potential impact of alopecia prior to initiating chemotherapy. The most helpful approach is to remind the patient that her hair will grow back after the treatment is finished. Providing referrals to local hair salons that supply wigs and that have personnel who work with patients receiving chemotherapy is a valuable nursing intervention. The effectiveness of inducing scalp hypothermia with cold caps in order to prevent hair loss is questionable,[45,46] but if a patient who has been fully informed of its level of efficacy wishes to try this approach, she should be allowed to do so.

Weight gain during the course of adjuvant chemotherapy has also been reported by several researchers,[47–50] although its exact etiology is still unknown. Foltz, in 1985, studied the variables of activity, depression, dietary intake, serum estradiol levels, and metabolic rate as possible influencing factors.[47] Her study suggested that only reductions in estradiol levels were significantly related to weight gain. However, a functional association was not clearly identified. Studies investigating weight gain in women with breast cancer receiving adjuvant chemotherapy have some limitations, including small sample size and a lack of on-

Table 16-7
Nursing Management of Chemotherapy

Side Effect/Toxicity	*Signs/Symptoms*	*Intervention*
Nausea and Vomiting		
Complex reflex mediated in the vomiting center of the medulla	Range from queasiness to intractable nausea and vomiting	Administer antiemetics 30 minutes prior to administration of chemotherapy. phenothiazines sedatives antihistamines dexamethasone
May be anticipatory; psychological component associated with negative stimulus conditioning		
Involves a chemotherapy trigger zone, which is a small area located at the base of the fourth ventricle bilaterally		Modify diet; cold foods and clear liquids are preferable; instruct patient to eat meals 3–4 hrs before receiving chemotherapy and then lightly for the rest of the day; recommend avoidance of sweet, fatty, or warm foods.
		Provide distraction or use visual imagery and relaxation techniques.
Cardiac Toxicity		
Dose-dependent with use of Adriamycin	EKG changes, tachycardia, extrasystoles, ST-T wave changes (12%–30% of patients) apparent within 1 week of drug administration	Limit cumulative drug dose to < 450 mg/m^2
Incidence of cardiomyopathy is 0.5% if patient receives a total dose of <550 mg/m^2; incidence increases to 30% with doses ≥600 mg/m^2.	Rhythm changes are transient and reversible.	
	Congestive heart failure that is chronic if permanent cardiomyopathy results	Treat congestive heart failure with diuretics, digoxin, other cardiotonic drugs.
Bladder Toxicity		
Hemorrhagic/chemical cystitis from excretion of cyclophosphamide metabolites in bladder.	Burning or pain on urination, urgency, frequency, dysuria, hematuria	Encourage fluid intake (2–3 liters for 48 hours following IV hydration); with oral cyclophosphamide, encourage intake of 1–3 liters of fluid per day.
Occurs in 5%–10% of patients		Recommend frequent voiding.
		Monitor creatinine values if patient has renal disease

going control groups of women with breast cancer who have not received chemotherapy.

REFERENCES

1. McNally JC, Stair JC, Somerville ET: Guidelines for Cancer Nursing Practice. New York, Grune & Stratton, 1985
2. Delisa JA, Miller RM, Melnick RR, et al: Rehabilitation of the cancer patient. In Devita VT, Hellman S, Rosenberg S (eds): Cancer: Principles and Practices of Oncology, pp 1738–1743. Philadelphia, JB Lippincott, 1982
3. Donovan MI, Girton SE: Cancer Care Nursing. Norwalk, Connecticut, Appleton-Century-Crofts, 1984
4. American Cancer Society: 1983 Survey of Public Awareness and Use of Cancer Detection Tests, pp 17–25. New York, Gallup Omnibus, 1983.
5. National Cancer Institute: Breast Cancer: A Measure of Progress in Public Understanding. Technical Report, no. 81-2291, pp 158–161. Bethesda, MD, National Institutes of Health Publication, 1980
6. Huguley CM, Brown RL: The value of BSE. Cancer 47:989, 1981
7. Feldman JG, Carter AC, Nicastri AD, et al: Breast self-examination, relationship to stage of breast cancer at diagnosis. Cancer 47:2740, 1981
8. Foster RS, Costanza MC: Breast self-examination practices and breast cancer survival. Cancer 53:999, 1984
9. Senie RT, Rosen PP, Lesser ML, et al: Breast self-examination and medical examination related to breast cancer stage. Am J Public Health 71:583, 1981

Table 16-7
(Continued)

Side Effect/Toxicity	*Signs/Symptoms*	*Intervention*
Myelosuppression Dose-limiting; nadir occurs within 7–14 days; recovery by day 21–28 occurs with all chemotherapeutic agents	Anemia—tachycardia, dizziness, headache, dyspnea, pallor, fatigue	Consider RBC infusion if the hematocrit is < 25% or if there is active bleeding.
	Thrombocytopenia—increased bruising, petechiae, nosebleeds, hematuria, retinal hemorrhage	Advise patient to maintain adequate nutrition and to balance rest and exercise periods.
	Leukopenia—granulocyte count decreased to $1000/mm^3$, resulting in an increased risk of infection; is the most frequent cause of death in patients with cancer; clinical signs and symptoms less evident in neutropenic patients	Monitor patient for subtle symptoms of infection (dyspnea, temperature > 100.8°F, pain, burning on urination).
		Use agents or medications that might alter platelet function with caution.
		Maintain integrity of skin and mucous membranes.
		Minimize performance of invasive procedures.
Alopecia Dependent on sensitivity of the hair follicles	Sudden or slow hair loss	Prepare patient for psychological impact and body image change by fitting for wig.
Adriamycin may cause of 90%–100% loss within 14–21 days.		Advise patient of the availability of hypothermal scalp techniques; explain that the procedure produces variable results without guaranteed benefit. (Cool caps are worn 30 minutes before and for 30 minutes after chemotherapy.)
Cyclophosphamide + methotrexate are associated with moderate sensitivity.		
Hair will grow back after drug is discontinued.		
Extravasation Vesicants: Adriamycin, vinblastine	Minor skin irritation, vein discoloration, necrosis of skin and underlying tendons and neurovascular structures	Attempt to prevent extravasation by following appropriate protocol established by each hospital for administration of chemotherapy. Some protocols recommend avoiding use of the veins in the hand, wrist, or antecubital region, using the large veins in the forearm instead.
Damage to tissue surrounding vein		When using a free-running IV line, administer IV vesicant at a rate of 1 mg/1 ml/1 min.
Renal Toxicity Methotrexate nephrotoxicity is secondary to precipitation of the drug in the renal tubules and is related to high doses.	Elevated creatinine levels	Maintain hydration.
		Monitor BUN, serum creatinine levels.
Rare when CMF protocol is used*		Measure creatinine clearance.
		Order serum uric acid and electrolyte studies.

Table 16-7
(Continued)

Side Effect/Toxicity	*Signs/Symptoms*	*Intervention*
Anorexia		
May be caused by nausea, vomiting, diarrhea stomatitis, chemotherapy Depression Cyclophosphamide may cause hypogeusia (decreased taste activity).	Inability to eat food and resultant weight loss	Recommend a program of mouth care before each meal. Serve small, attractive meals; cold foods are better tolerated. Administer zinc sulfate tablets, 25 mg QID, PO to combat metallic taste. Institute program for management of anxiety and depression.
Stomatitis		
Ulcerative lesions in the mouth and oropharynx; oral inflammation Potential source of infection during immunosuppression Usually occurs 7–14 days after drug administration Exfoliation of oral epithelium Adriamycin may cause xerostomia (a decrease in saliva production and an increase in saliva viscosity). Gram-negative organisms are the most likely infective agents. Fungus—Candida albicans Herpes simplex virus	Mild erythema and edema of mucocutaneous junction; dryness of the mouth; burning sensation on the lips; hemorrhagic ulcerations secondary to trauma, pressure, dentures, dry or hard foods, or toothbrush use; glossal edema or infection; superficial inflammation that may cause white, fluctuant patches; herpetic lesions	Promote good oral hygiene before and during chemotherapy. Examine oral cavity daily. Perform oral care before and after meals. Gargle, swish or spit out either: hydrogen peroxide and saline or water (ratio of 1:2 or 1:4) baking soda and water, 1 tsp in 500 ml (Avoid lemon and glycerine as they are too drying.) Maintain hydration. Recommend bland, soft foods and protein and vitamin supplements, as well as the avoidance of hot, spicy foods. Keep lips moist with Chapstick, Vaseline, or vitamin E preparations. Administer pain medication for discomfort. Topical anesthetics dyclonine, 1% lidocaine (Viscous), 15 ml per dose lidocaine (Viscous, 2%) Bendadryl elixir (12.5 ml/5 ml) and Kaopectate Orabase Administer Nystatin (for thrush) after oral rinsing every 6 hr. Administer antibiotic suspensions as ordered.

Table 16-7
(Continued)

Side Effect/Toxicity	*Signs/Symptoms*	*Intervention*
Cutaneous Manifestations		
Methotrexate is the chemotherapeutic agent that is most commonly involved, followed by fluorouracil and Adriamycin. Dermatologic reactions from chemotherapy usually resolve without serious complications.	Transient maculopapular erythema occuring 1–3 days after drug administration, hyperpigmentation, photosensitivity, hyperkeratosis, acne-like reaction, pruritus, radiation recall (sunburn reaction to previously irradiated breasts), nail banding	Advise use of a sunblock (#15). Recommend avoiding direct exposure to the sun while receiving chemotherapy.
Hepatotoxicity		
Methotrexate administered over a long period of time may cause liver damage. Pre-existing liver disease increases patient's risk.	Hepatic fibrosis, jaundice, elevated liver enzymes	Monitor liver function tests prior to administration of chemotherapy.
Sexual and Reproductive Toxicity		
Temporary or permanent sterility Possible teratogenic or mutagenic changes	Menstrual dysfunction, amenorrhea, irregular vaginal bleeding, hot flashes, weight gain, sleep disturbances, vaginal tissue atrophy, diminished libido, inability to conceive	Provide sexual counseling prior to chemotherapy. Continue counseling on birth control. Discuss use of lubricants, such as KY jelly. Discuss vaginal estrogen creams, the use of which is very controversial in premenopausal women. Administer clonidine, 1mg TID, for hot flashes.

* CMF, Cyclophosphamide, methotrexate, and 5-fluorouracil.

10. Celantano DD, Holtzman D: Breast self-examination competency: An analysis of self-reported practice and associated characteristics. Am J Public Health 73:1321, 1983
11. Morra ME: Breast self-examination today: An overview of its use and its value. Semin Oncol Nurs 1:170, 1985
12. Calnan MW, Chamberlain J, Moss S: Compliance with a class teaching breast self-examination. J Epidemiol Community Health 37:264, 1983
13. Holtzman D, Celentano D: The practice and efficacy of breast self-examination: A critical review. Am J Public Health 73:1324, 1983
14. Hall DC, Adams CK, Stein GH, et al: Improved detection of human breast lesions following experimental training. Cancer 46:408, 1980
15. Kaku K, Gilbert FI, Sachs RR: Comparison of health appraisals by nurses and physicians. Public Health Rep 85:1042, 1970
16. George MG, Sellwood RA, Asbury D, et al: Role of non-medical staff in screening for breast cancer. Br Med J 19:147, 1980
17. Moskowitz M: Clinical examination of the breasts by nonphysicians. Cancer 44:311, 1979
18. Richards DB, Holcombe JK: The nurse's role in screening and cancer detection. Semin Oncol 7:56, 1980
19. Chamberlain J, Rogers P, Price JL, et al: Validity of clinical examination and mammography as screening tests for breast cancer. Lancet 2:1026, 1975
20. Howard J: Breast self-examination: Issues for research. Proceedings of Working Group Meeting, Health Promotion and Sciences Branch, Division of Cancer Prevention and Control, National Cancer Institute, Bethesda, Maryland, 1982
21. Pennypacker HS, Goldstein MK, Stein GH: A precise method of manual breast self-examination. In Murphy LM (ed): Progress in Cancer Control IV. Research in the Cancer Center, pp 304–311. New York, Alan R. Liss, 1983
22. Kroehl SA: Nursing care of the patient undergoing mastectomy. In Pfeiffer CH, Mulliken JB (ed): Caring for the Patient with Breast Cancer, pp 53–58. Reston, Virginia: Reston Publishing/Prentice-Hall, 1984
23. Mast M: Primary care of the mastectomy patient. Nurse Practitioner 2:27, 1984
24. Scott DW: Anxiety, critical thinking and information processing during and after breast biopsy. Nurs Res 32:24, 1983
25. American Cancer Society: Reach to Recovery: Exercises After Mastectomy. New York, American Cancer Society, 1956
26. Knobf MK: Primary breast cancer: Physical consequences and rehabilitation. Oncol Nurs 1:214, 1985

27. Markowski J, Wilcox JP, Helm PA: Lymphedema incidence after specific postmastectomy therapy. Arch Phys Med Rehabil 62:444, 1981
28. Getz DH: Primary, secondary and tertiary nursing interventions of lymphedema. Cancer Nurs 6:177, 1985
29. Rudolph BJ: Lymphedema following a radical mastectomy. Oncol Nurs Forum 6:13, 1979
30. Mulliken JB: Reconstruction of the breast following mastectomy. In Pfeiffer CH, Mulliken JB (eds): Caring for the Patient with Breast Cancer. Reston, Virginia, Reston Publishing, 1984
31. Harris JR, Hellman S: Primary radiation therapy for early breast cancer. Cancer 51:2547, 1983
32. Hassey KM: Radiation therapy for breast cancer: A historic review. Semin Oncol Nurs 1:181, 1985
33. Schain WS, Wellisch DK, Pasnau RO, et al: The sooner the better: A study of psychological factors of women undergoing immediate versus delayed reconstruction. Am J Psychiatry 142:40, 1985
34. Schain WS: Breast cancer surgeries and psychosexual sequelae: Implications for remediation. Semin Oncol Nurs 1:200, 1985
35. MacElveen P: Sexual assessment and counseling. Semin Oncol Nurs 1:70, 1974
36. Annon JS: The Behavioral Treatment of Sexual Problems. Honolulu, Mercantile Printing, 1974
37. Brager BL, Yasko J: Care of the Client Receiving Chemotherapy. Reston, Virginia, Reston Publishing, 1984
38. Flaherty AM: Symptom management: Nausea and vomiting. Cancer Nurs 8:36, 1985
39. See-Lasley K, Ignoffe R: Manual of Oncology. St. Louis, CV Mosby, 1981
40. Yasko JM: Guidelines for Cancer Care: Symptom Management. Reston, Virginia, Reston Publishing, 1983
41. Cobb SC: Teaching relaxation techniques to cancer patients. Cancer Nurs 4:157, 1984
42. Contanck PH: Relaxation training for control of nausea and vomiting in patients receiving chemotherapy. Cancer Nurs 8:277, 1983
43. Frank JM: The effects of music therapy and guided visual imagery on chemotherapy-induced nausea and vomiting. Oncol Nurs Forum 12:47, 1985
44. Benson H: The Relaxation Response. New York, Morrow, 1977
45. Hunt JM, Anderson JE, Smith IE: Scalp hypothermia to prevent Adriamycin-induced hair loss. Cancer Nurs 2:25, 1982
46. Dean JC, Salmon SE, Griffith KS: Medical intelligence: Prevention of doxorubicin-induced hair loss with scalp hypothermia. N Engl J Med 301:1427, 1979
47. Foltz AT: Weight gain among stage II breast cancer patients: A study of five factors. Oncol Nurs Forum 12:21, 1985
48. Heasman KZ, Sutherland HJ, Campbell JA, et al: Weight gain during adjuvant chemotherapy for breast cancer. Breast Cancer Res Treat 5:195, 1985
49. Subramarian VP, Raich PC, Walker BK: Weight gain in breast cancer patients undergoing chemotherapy. Breast Cancer Res Treat 1:170, 1981
50. Knobf MK, Mullen JC, Xistris D, et al: Weight gain in women with breast cancer receiving adjuvant chemotherapy. Oncol Nurs Form 10:28, 1983

Breast Reconstruction After Mastectomy

John Bostwick III

When a woman develops cancer of the breast, the focus of management is to provide optimal treatment of the tumor, both locally and systemically. Because of the importance of the breast as a symbol of femininity, as well as the fear of deformity from the local treatment of the breast cancer, the emotional sequelae of the treatment must be addressed when the initial treatment plan is developed. The concerns of women about the physical deformity of mastectomy and its psychological impact have encouraged breast management teams to pursue less deforming local treatment while providing acceptable local control of the tumor. The modified radical mastectomy and breast reconstruction, as well as conservative surgery and radiation therapy, have evolved to meet the desires of patients for local treatment with minimal permanent residual physical deformity. Breast and chest wall reconstruction are operative interventions that enhance the function, appearance, and psychological well-being of women who have a deformity after the local treatment of breast cancer.[1]

Breast reconstruction evolved when women were unwilling to accept the permanent deformity resulting from mastectomy. Breast reconstruction is best integrated into the initial treatment plan for and management of the patient with breast cancer. Because of the complexity of the management of breast cancer today, teamwork among the specialties is necessary. The breast management team involved in the diagnosis and management of patients with breast cancer now includes a reconstructive surgeon. When the possibility of breast reconstruction is mentioned as a part of the comprehensive plan for the management of a woman with breast cancer, she can make a more informed decision for her treatment.

The deformity that results from the local treatment of breast cancer is a constant reminder to the woman that she has breast cancer, and it is a symbol of her diminished femininity.[2] A breast deformity in a woman who has chosen conservative treatment for her breast cancer is especially devastating because of the high priority she assigns to her body image, as evidenced by her selection of conservative treatment over a more deforming procedure. When a woman develops a deformity after conservative treatment, such as significant asymmetry or a fibrotic breast, or if a mastectomy is required because of persistence or recurrence of local cancer, breast reconstruction may be especially useful in lessening her sense of deformity.[3] These feelings of deformity and the psychological impact of the breast deformity not only affect the woman's emotional status, but also her social adjustment and her relations with her family and friends.

The goal of breast reconstruction is to alleviate the breast and chest wall deformity and to provide attractive and symmetrical breasts that meet the woman's expectations while still adhering to sound oncologic principles and management. Breast reconstruction must be incorporated into the comprehensive management of the woman with breast cancer. Because the woman is the final arbiter of her attractiveness, it is important for the breast reconstructive surgeon to clearly define her expectations before the plan for the breast reconstruction is developed. There are many techniques for breast reconstruction. The simplest technique that meets the patient's expectations while providing a lasting, attractive, breast reconstruction is usually the one that is selected. A number of decisions must be made when breast reconstruction is planned. For example, the timing of the reconstructive surgery must be coordinated with the adjunctive management of the patient. The management of the opposite breast is also important, and the oncologic, aesthetic, and psychological issues that affect the care of the woman's opposite breast must be considered. Some women would rather undergo a more extensive operation on the missing breast in order to avoid an operation and the resulting scar on the attractive opposite breast. Other women desire an aesthetic correction of their opposite breast, such as augmentation mammaplasty, reduction mammaplasty, or mastopexy. The goal of breast reconstruction in these cases, then, is to match the corrected opposite breast.

The breast reconstruction must also be incorporated into the overall plan for the patient's management, and this requires close interspecialty consultation. The woman should participate in the decisions about her management; however, it must be remembered that the primary goal of her care is to provide the best management possible of the breast cancer. The timing and technique of the breast reconstruction must take into consideration the overall management of the patient. For example, an elective breast reconstruction is usually delayed until the completion of adjunctive chemotherapy or radiation therapy. The techniques of breast reconstruction must not compromise the follow-up of the local treatment. Breast reconstruction should neither adversely modify the course of the breast cancer nor hide a local recurrence. Silicone breast implants for breast reconstruction are usually placed behind the musculofascial layer of the mastectomy field so that proper follow-up and monitoring are possible, and so that there is minimal risk that a recurrence will be hidden.[4]

The patient's clinical status is also a determinant in the selection of breast reconstruction. For the patient with Stage I breast cancer, the breast reconstruction may be done immediately at the time of the modified radical mastectomy, although most breast reconstructions are delayed a few months or until local and adjunctive therapy is completed.[5] When there is systemic disease, the advisability and timing of the breast reconstruction must be determined carefully, with input from all of the members of the breast management team. Breast cancer is considered to be a chronic disease, and because of the possibility of excellent long-term control of systemic disease, some women with metastases have experienced an enhancement of the quality of their life with breast reconstruction. The breast management team should be sensitive to the overall quality of life of their patients.

TIMING AND TYPES OF BREAST RECONSTRUCTION

A broad range of techniques of breast reconstruction has been developed to address each specific area of the mastectomy deformity, as well as to provide a breast reconstruction that is symmetrical to the opposite breast. The expectations of the patient must be taken into consideration when planning the breast reconstruction, as must the type of deformity and any oncologic or aesthetic considerations. The mastectomy deformity may range from a mild asymmetry after lumpectomy to an irradiated ulcer containing locally recurrent tumor after an extended radical mastectomy.

Techniques of breast reconstruction are available for this broad range of deformities. For simple deformities, a modification of an aesthetic surgical procedure, such as a breast implant, may be satisfactory (Fig. 16-2). Final symmetry of the breast reconstruction with the opposite breast is important, and the appearance of the opposite breast influences the type of breast reconstruction selected. For large, irradiated mastectomy defects with ulceration, additional resection of the chest wall may be necessary before the deformity is reconstructed. In such cases, distant flaps are either pedicled into the area with their own blood supply intact or are transferred to the chest area and reconnected by microvascular technique.

Breast reconstruction may be done immediately, at the time of the local surgical treatment of the breast cancer, or it may be delayed until a later time. The option for immediate breast reconstruction should be considered when the initial treatment plan is formulated by the members of the breast management team (Fig. 16-3). The desires and wishes of the patient are incorporated into this plan.[6] The availability of immediate breast reconstruction may influence some patients' selection of the type of local treatment of the breast cancer. Immediate breast reconstruction permits the patient to have a modified radical mastectomy without having to face the spectre of the mastectomy deformity.[7] Immediate breast reconstruction requires careful patient selection and planning by the breast management team. A few years ago, it was thought that a woman should live with the mastectomy deformity for a time so that she could appreciate the breast reconstruction. It has now been shown that this is not necessary. Moreover, immediate breast reconstruction may lessen the psychological trauma of the breast cancer experience when modified radical mastectomy is selected as the local treatment.

Breast reconstruction using either available tissue and a silicone breast implant or the tissue expander is the most frequently selected technique for immediate reconstruction. The general surgeon and the reconstructive surgeon consult before the operation to plan the incision, as well as the sequence and specifics of the operation. After the general surgeon has performed the mastectomy and the specimen has been examined by the pathologist, breast reconstruction is begun. The musculofascial layer is elevated from the chest wall to create a cover for the silicone

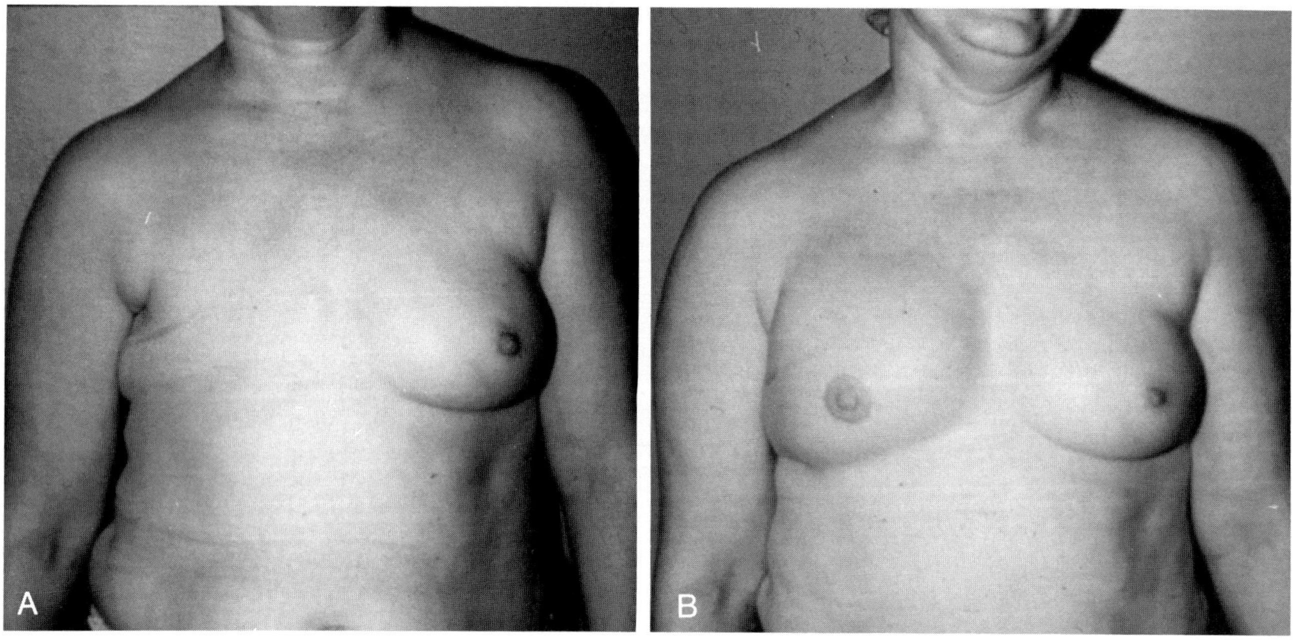

FIGURE 16-2. *(A)* A 38-year-old woman 2 years after undergoing a modified radical mastectomy for Stage I breast cancer. *(B)* The same woman 1 year after breast reconstruction with a silicone breast implant placed beneath the musculofascial layer and the skin.

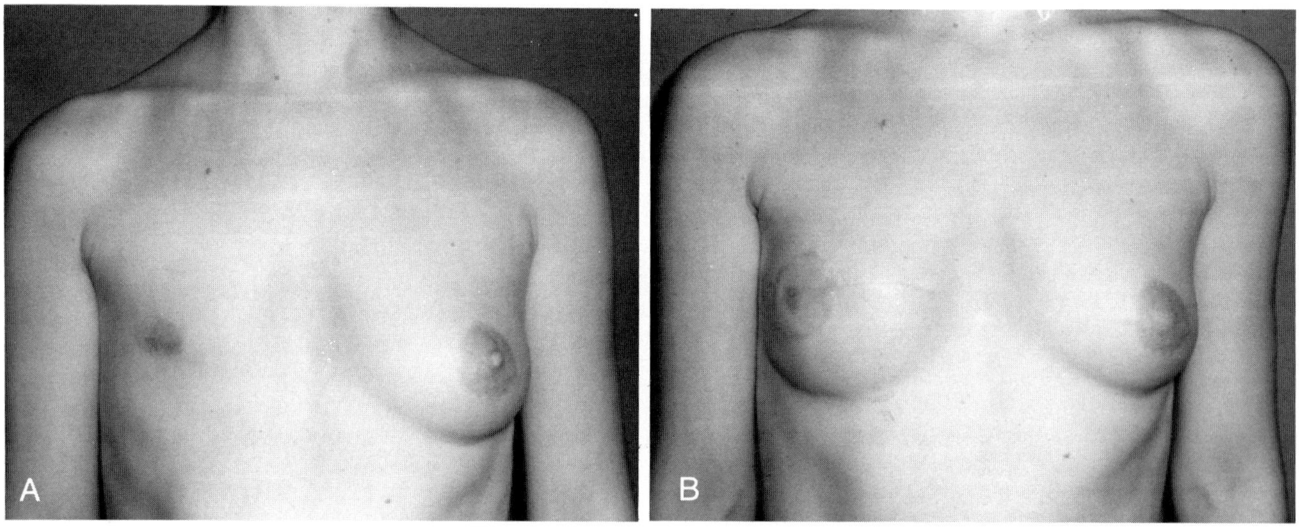

FIGURE 16-3. *(A)* This 28-year-old woman had breast agenesis following breast irradiation for a hemangioma at 2 years of age. A biopsy confirmed infiltrating ductal carcinoma of the right breast. *(B)* One year after undergoing a right modified radical mastectomy with immediate breast reconstruction using a silicone breast implant placed beneath the musculofascial layer and skin. The nipple-areolar complex was reconstructed using an upper inner thigh graft. (Bostwick J, Stevenson TR, Nahai F, et al: Radiation to the breast: Complications amenable to surgical treatment. Ann Surg 200:550, 1984.)

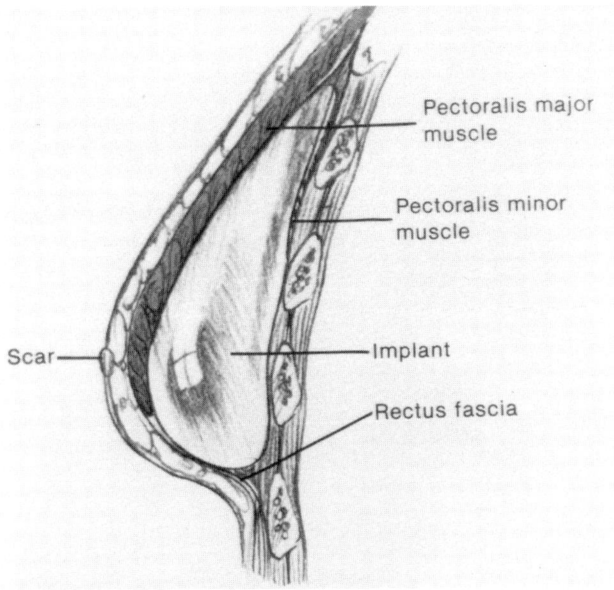

FIGURE 16-4. The silicone breast implant is placed under the musculofascial layer of the chest wall. This technique provides good coverage for the silicone breast implant, and the implant remains soft and retains a natural shape. (Bostwick J: Aesthetic and Reconstructive Breast Surgery, p 361. St. Louis, CV Mosby, 1983.)

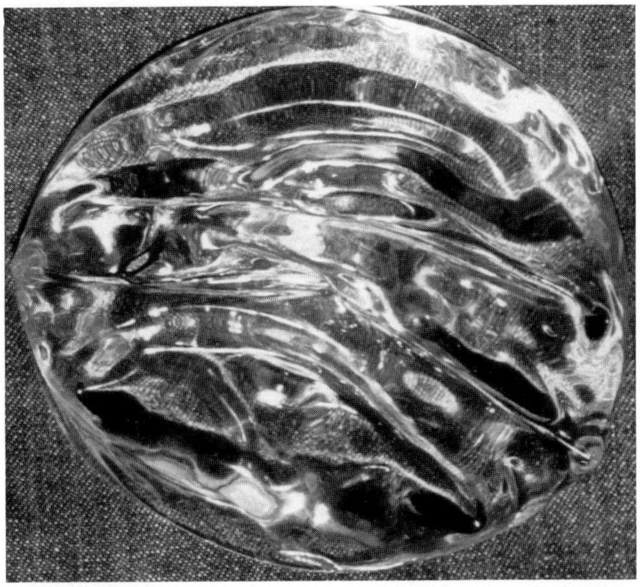

FIGURE 16-5. The silicone breast implant is an envelope of silicone sheeting that contains a silicone gel which is the consistency of breast tissue.

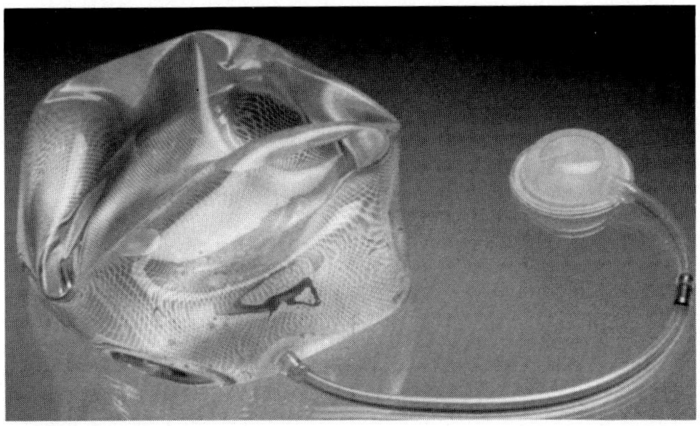

FIGURE 16-6. The tissue expander is an envelope of silicone sheeting connected to a fill valve. After the device is positioned under the musculofascial layer and the wound has healed, it is inflated with saline solution during outpatient visits.

breast implant (Fig. 16-4).[8,9] When this "pocket" is of satisfactory dimensions to accommodate a silicone breast implant, an implant is positioned for optimal symmetry (Fig. 16-5). When the quality of the mastectomy flaps is questionable, or if the breast must be reconstructed to a size larger than can be achieved safely with a silicone breast implant, a tissue expander is used (Fig. 16-6). The tissue expander is then inflated slowly over a period of a few weeks during the postoperative period until a satisfactory size is obtained. The tissue expander may then be replaced by a permanent silicone breast implant. Flaps, such as the latissimus dorsi or the rectus abdominis musculocutaneous flap, may also be used at the time of immediate breast reconstruction; however, these procedures represent major operations and are usually not the primary techniques of choice.

Breast reconstruction is usually delayed until after local surgical treatment of the breast cancer. This allows the patient and the members of the breast management team to focus on the treatment of the breast cancer. Breast reconstruction is also usually delayed until 2 to 3 months after adjunctive treatment. By waiting 6 to 9 months, the patient has time to recover from the initial treatment, to make a definitive decision concerning breast reconstruction, and to consider the management of her opposite breast. She may also select a reconstructive surgeon during this period, discussing and evaluating the type of breast reconstruction that would be most likely to meet her expectations.

Both immediate and delayed breast reconstructions are done in two or three stages. It is important for the patient to know that the breast reconstruction is not complete after the first operation. During the first operation, the breast mound is reconstructed and the chest wall contour is restored. Correction of the opposite breast is done whenever necessary, either during the first operation or, when immediate breast reconstruction is done, at the time of the second operation. During the second operation, the nipple-areolar complex is reconstructed and any other corrections necessary for symmetry are performed. When the tissue expander technique is used, an additional operation is required to replace the tissue expander with a permanent silicone breast implant.

Complications of immediate breast reconstruction

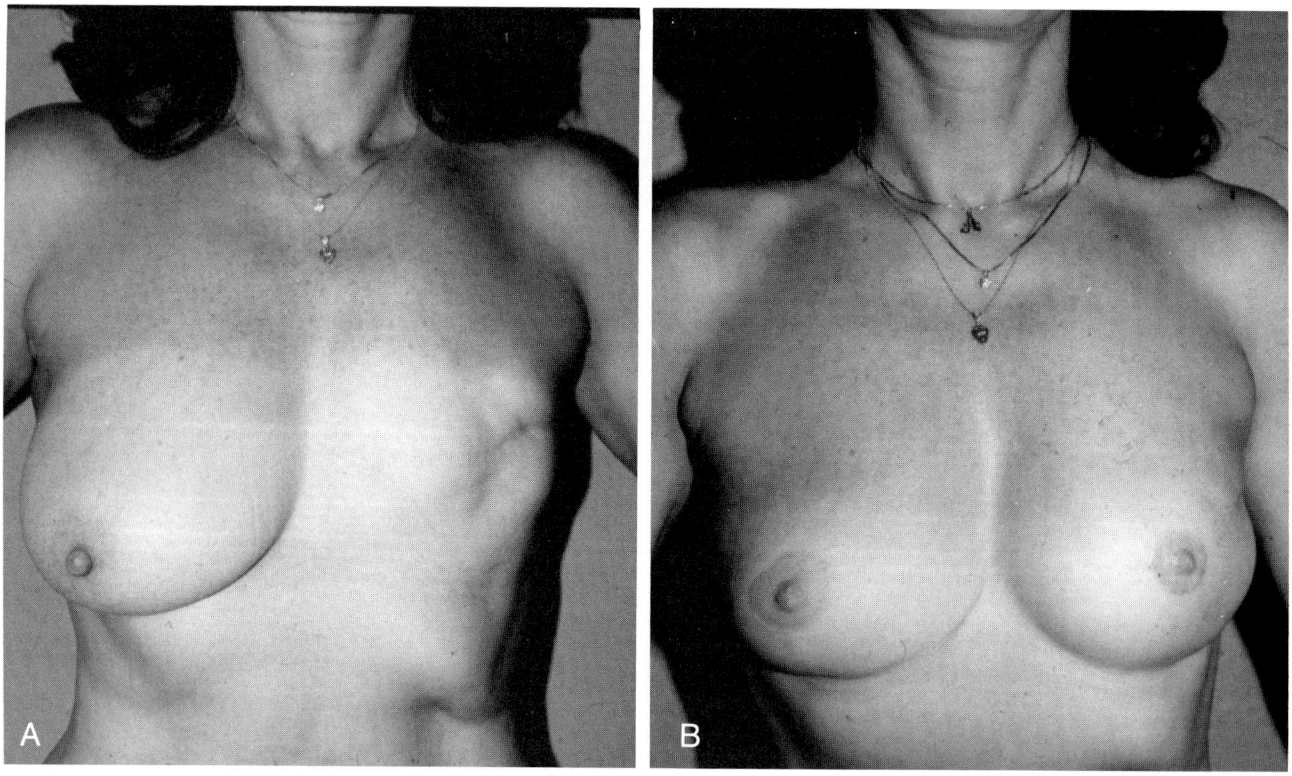

FIGURE 16-7. *(A)* This 35-year-old woman had a total mastectomy 14 years before her breast reconstruction. *(B)* The left breast was reconstructed with a silicone breast implant beneath the musculofascial layer. A reduction mammaplasty of the right breast was done to achieve symmetry. The nipple-areolar complex was reconstructed 3 months later. (Bostwick J: Aesthetic and Reconstructive Breast Surgery, p 366. St Louis, CV Mosby, 1983.)

may be related to either psychological or technical factors. When the patient has unrealistic expectations of the results of the breast reconstruction, she may be unhappy with the initial outcome. During preoperative discussions, it is important to stress that the initial result is not the final appearance and that it will take additional operations to achieve attractive and symmetrical breast reconstruction. Other complications are usually related to problems with the skin flaps. If they are thin and undergo some necrosis in the postoperative period, there is the possibility of exposure of the silicone breast implant. When this occurs, the silicone breast implant usually must be removed temporarily and the wound allowed to heal. The reconstruction may then resume as a delayed breast reconstruction.

METHODS OF BREAST RECONSTRUCTION

Use of Available Tissue and Silicone Breast Implants

The reconstructive technique that involves the use of available tissue and placement of a silicone breast implant is performed following total mastectomy in patients in whom the creation of a breast mound will provide symmetry with the other breast.[10,11] A silicone breast implant is placed under the total mastectomy site, beneath the musculofascial layer of the chest wall. It is usually placed through the mastectomy scar, obviating the need for any additional scars on the reconstructed breast. The silicone breast implant is chosen for its symmetry with the opposite breast. The tight tissues of the mastectomy site are gradually stretched by the silicone breast implant, so the final result is not achieved until several months after the implant placement. After a few months, reconstruction of the nipple-areolar complex is done; at the same time, any modification of the silicone breast implant that is necessary for maximal symmetry may be accomplished (Fig. 16-7).

A modification of this technique involves the use of an upper abdominal advancement flap.[12,13] The tissue of the upper abdomen below the proposed breast reconstruction is elevated and moved upward on the chest wall to provide additional tissue for the lower portion of the breast reconstruction. It is necessary to make a scar in the inframammary crease in order to attach the upper abdominal flap in its new position.

The technique of breast reconstruction that utilizes the silicone breast implant is suitable for achieving symmetry with opposite breasts that are not large and do not have significant ptosis. The most common complication of

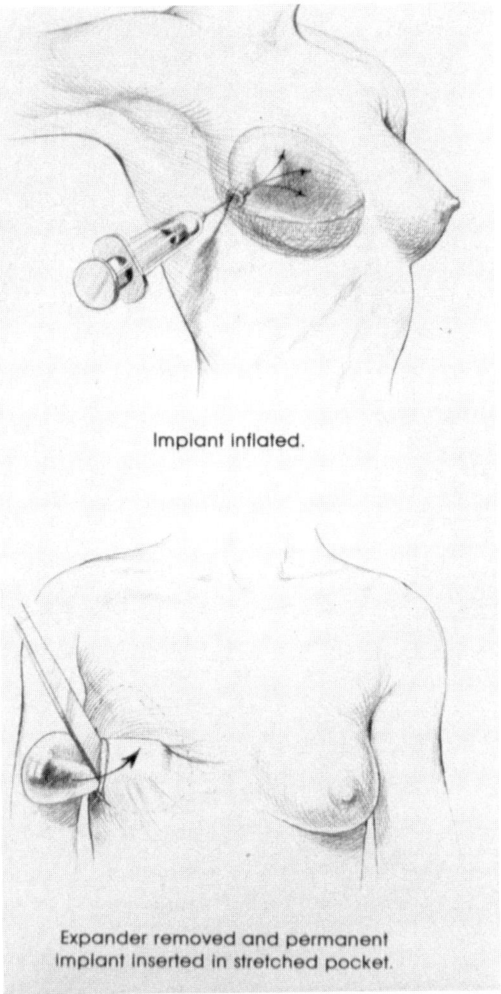

FIGURE 16-8. The tissue expander is placed in the proper position for breast reconstruction. It is then inflated during the postoperative period to provide the proper size breast. The tissue expander is later replaced by a permanent silicone breast implant. (Berger K, Bostwick J: A Woman's Decision: Breast Care, Treatment and Reconstruction, p 98. St Louis, CV Mosby, 1984.)

this technique is the development of a fibrous capsule around the silicone breast implant. This results in firmness of the reconstructed breast. The capsular contracture may distort the breast reconstruction, leading to eventual asymmetry. This asymmetry may require an additional operation to revise or change the silicone breast implant, or the silicone breast implant may be exchanged for autogenous tissue from an abdominal flap.

Use of Available Tissue and a Tissue Expander

A tissue expander is used when the local tissues that remain after total mastectomy are deficient or are too tight for a silicone breast implant.[14,15] The tissue expander is placed beneath the musculofascial layer and is gradually inflated during the postoperative period by injecting saline solution through a subcutaneous valve connected to the tissue expander (Fig. 16-8). After the local tissues have been expanded satisfactorily, the tissue expander is exchanged for a permanent silicone breast implant. This technique of breast reconstruction allows the use of available tissue and obviates the need for more complex reconstructions that involve distant flaps and additional scars (Fig. 16-9). The tissue expander technique is suitable for patients with ptosis, and also permits reconstruction of large breasts.

The possible complications of breast reconstruction using a tissue expander are the same as those associated with breast reconstruction using available tissue.[16] In addition, the complications specific to the use of the expander device include valve failure and the introduction of bacteria at the time of expansion, which may lead to secondary infection.

Use of a Latissimus Dorsi Musculocutaneous Flap

The latissimus dorsi musculocutaneous flap supplements the tissue of the chest wall in postmastectomy reconstructions by transposing latissimus dorsi muscle or skin to the mastectomy area (Fig. 16-10). The latissimus dorsi flap is elevated on the thoracodorsal pedicle in the axilla; the blood supply remains intact while the flap is moved to the area of the breast reconstruction.[17,18] The latissimus dorsi flap provides fill for the infraclavicular area and allows reconstruction of the anterior axillary fold after a radical mastectomy. When the mastectomy site is tight, the flap may also be used to replace missing skin (Fig. 16-11). The latissimus dorsi musculocutaneous flap places a donor scar across the back or along the side of the chest. Replacement of missing tissue with a flap is essential after a radical mastectomy (Fig. 16-12). Patients in whom mastectomy has resulted in tight or grafted skin and those with radiation changes of the skin also often require a flap for satisfactory breast reconstruction.

Use of the latissimus dorsi musculocutaneous flap is also helpful when matching an opposite breast that is full and relatively large or ptotic.[19,20] The latissimus dorsi skin is placed onto the reconstructed breast laterally and inferiorly in order to supplement the reconstructed breast (Fig. 16-13). A silicone breast implant is then placed beneath the flap to give the proper size to the reconstructed breast.

The latissimus dorsi musculocutaneous flap is one of the most reliable and safest flaps to use in reconstructive surgery. Its use is associated with a low incidence of necrosis of the flap. Other possible complications include capsular contracture around the silicone breast implant and insufficient reconstruction in cases in which more tissue is needed than is supplied by the flap. In addition, infections and hematoma are unusual but possible complications of this complex flap surgery.

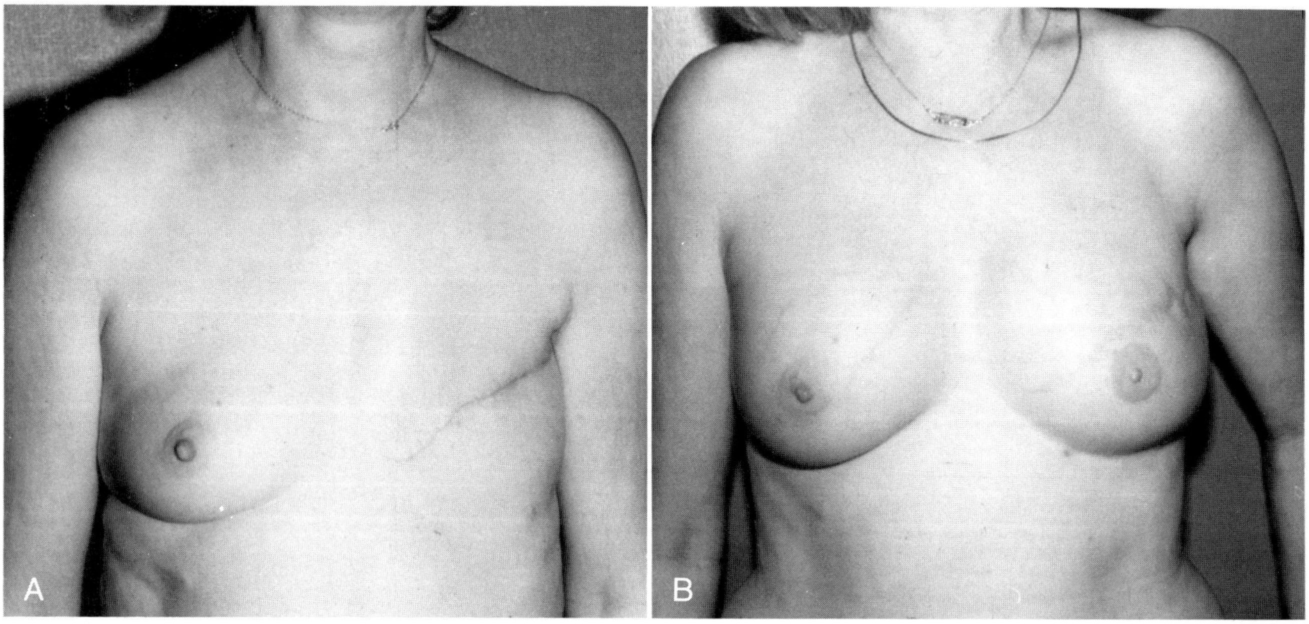

FIGURE 16-9. *(A)* A 45-year-old woman 3 months after a left modified radical mastectomy. *(B)* The same woman 2 years after tissue expansion of the left breast area and an augmentation of the right breast with a silicone breast implant placed beneath the musculofascial layer. (Berger K, Bostwick J: A Woman's Decision: Breast Care, Treatment and Reconstruction, p 100. St Louis, CV Mosby, 1984.)

Use of Abdominal Flaps

The lower transverse rectus abdominis musculocutaneous (TRAM) flap may be used for breast reconstruction when the patient needs additional tissue, has an excess of tissue in the lower abdomen, or does not want breast reconstruction with a silicone breast implant.[21,22] An ellipse of lower abdominal skin and fat (Fig. 16-14) is moved to the chest area and pedicled as a musculocutaneous flap on the upper rectus abdominis muscle (Fig. 16-15). The blood supply to the flap is derived from the musculocutaneous perforators coursing into it from the rectus abdominis muscle fascia in the periumbilical area. Patients with compromised microcirculation, such as those who are heavy cigarette smokers or who have diabetes mellitus, may not have sufficient blood supply to nourish the flap.

This is a very complex operation that requires an experienced surgeon and a healthy patient who is willing to undergo a major operation in order to achieve a soft and natural-feeling breast reconstruction using abdominal fat.[23] In the properly selected patient, this reconstructive procedure may be accomplished using the excess lower abdominal tissue and without the use of a silicone breast implant (Fig. 16-16). As a result of the operation, the abdominal donor area is flatter and more attractive because the lower excess has been removed and transferred to reconstruct the new breast.

This technique is useful when a major tissue deficit results from the mastectomy. It is especially helpful when the opposite breast is full and somewhat ptotic. In the properly selected patient, there is enough skin and fat to match the opposite breast. For women who have had a radical mastectomy and who have a significant infraclavicular defect, the TRAM flap may provide the best opportunity for achieving breast symmetry.

The potential complications of the TRAM flap method of breast reconstruction are more numerous than those associated with less complex methods of breast reconstruction. The patient must have excellent microcirculation to preserve the viability of the tissue. When the amount of tissue required is relatively great, the TRAM flap may be moved to the breast area on two pedicles of rectus abdominis muscle. Fat necrosis may develop if a relative decrease in blood flow to the fat of the flap occurs. This may result in a thickening in the fat of the reconstructed breast, which may mimic a tumor. It is sometimes necessary to biopsy these areas. The abdominal wall may also be weakened by the transfer of the rectus abdominis muscles to the chest area. A secure abdominal closure supplemented with Prolene mesh provides a strong abdominal wall that will not stretch with time or with vigorous physical activity.

Free Flap Breast Reconstruction

Free flap reconstructive techniques involve the transfer of composite tissue from a distant area. In this procedure,

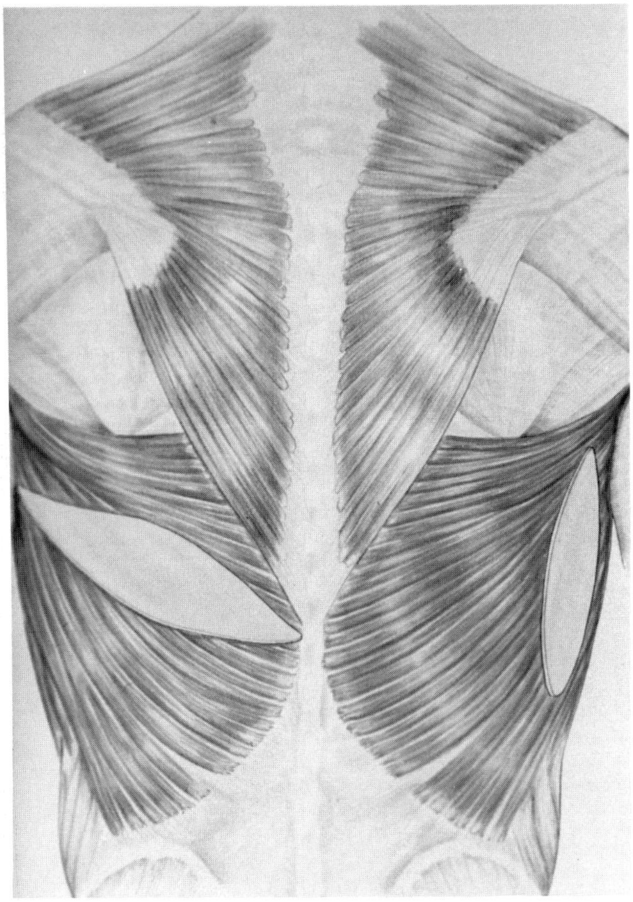

FIGURE 16-10. Skin islands from the back may be transferred along with the underlying latissimus dorsi muscle. (Contemporary Surgery, Vol. 27, No. 1. Redondo Beach, California, Bobit Publishing Co., July, 1985.)

the gluteus maximus musculocutaneous flap from the buttocks is anastomosed into the internal mammary vessels in the area of the breast reconstruction.[24] This technique requires a high level of technical expertise because the tissue transfer is done with microvascular technique. The advantages of this method are that abundant tissue is available and that the donor scar is practically out of sight, being easily hidden beneath clothing.

The surgeon plans the precise amount and type of buttocks tissue needed for the breast reconstruction, including both skin and fat. This tissue, along with the underlying gluteus maximus muscle and its pedicle, is elevated and then divided. The flap is then transferred to the breast area. The internal mammary artery is then dissected deep to the fourth and fifth medial costal cartilages. These vessels are then attached to the pedicle vessels coursing into the flap. When there is not a recipient vein of sufficient size, vein grafts or the use of a pedicled vein from the neck may be necessary.

The most frequent concern when tissue is removed and reattached with microvascular technique is survival of the tissue with adequate blood supply. A potential complication of this technique is failure of the flap. Other possible complications include hematomas or infection of the donor site for the reconstructed breast.

SELECTION OF A BREAST RECONSTRUCTION METHOD

The type of breast reconstruction chosen to achieve the expectations of the patient is determined after consultation with the reconstructive surgeon. In planning a reconstructive approach, the surgeon should consider all pertinent information available from the other members of the breast management team. The stage of the disease and the recommendations of the general surgeon and oncologists are both considered in formulating a plan for the breast reconstruction.

Final symmetry after breast reconstruction is a major consideration. Determinants of the management of the opposite breast include its appearance and oncologic status. When the opposite breast is to be changed, a technique of breast reconstruction that will allow optimal matching of the corrected breasts is selected. The patient's attitude concerning the use of a silicone breast implant may determine whether the techniques that use the patient's own tissues, such as the TRAM flap or the gluteus maximus musculocutaneous flap, are used. If the opposite breast is full and attractive and there has been a significant amount of tissue removed from the upper part of the chest, a flap technique is usually the best method for providing natural fill to this area.

The simplest and least involved technique of breast reconstruction that will achieve symmetry and attractive breasts is usually selected. When sufficient tissue is available, a silicone breast implant is placed beneath the available tissues at the site of the mastectomy. The tissue expander technique is used when there is a relative deficiency of tissue at the mastectomy site, and when the patient does not want to undergo a distant flap procedure because of the additional scars, complexity, and morbidity associated with such a technique. The use of the tissue expander also requires additional office visits for filling and expansion of the device, as well as a subsequent operation to replace it with a permanent silicone breast implant.

When the patient has undergone a radical mastectomy, additional tissue is needed to fill in the infraclavicular region, as well as to recreate the anterior axillary fold. The latissimus dorsi musculocutaneous flap or the TRAM flap technique is usually selected for these patients. The latissimus dorsi musculocutaneous flap method is usually selected when the tissue requirements are not too great, or when there is some concern about the potential safety of the TRAM flap technique. The latter method provides the largest amount of autogenous tissue for reconstruction of the breast after radical mastectomy. When the breast reconstruction is planned with a silicone breast implant but the skin is deficient either in volume or thickness, the latissimus dorsi musculocutaneous flap is useful for sup-

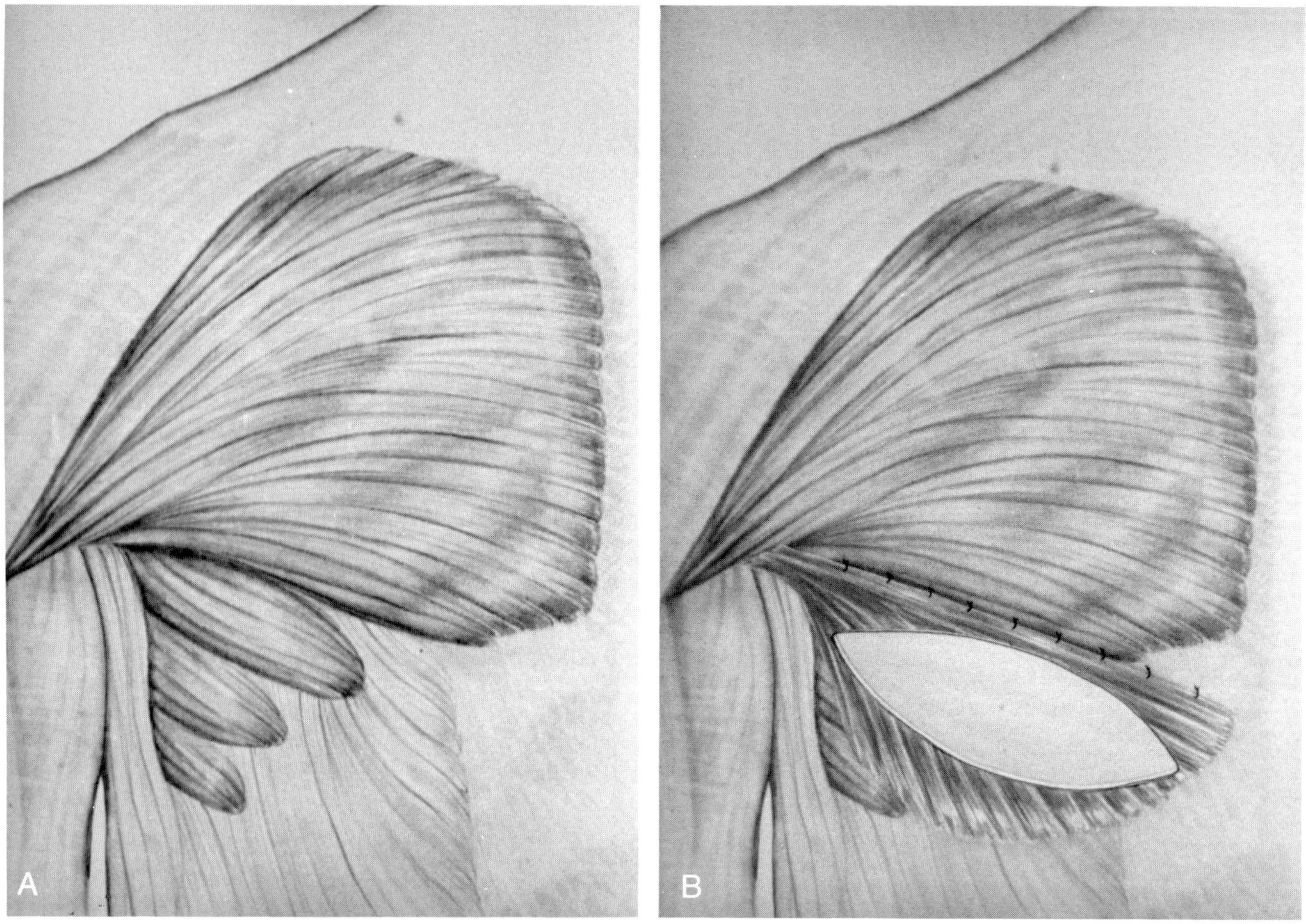

FIGURE 16-11. *(A)* A mastectomy defect on the chest wall. *(B)* The latissimus dorsi flap is transferred to the mastectomy site to supplement missing or tight skin and to provide muscle coverage of the silicone breast implant. (Contemporary Surgery, Vol. 27, No. 1, p 19. Redondo Beach, California, Bobit Publishing Co., July, 1985.)

plementing the tissue and for providing adequate coverage of the silicone breast implant.

The TRAM flap technique is selected when the patient has an abundance of lower abdominal tissue and desires a breast reconstruction with this tissue without the use of a silicone breast implant. These women must be healthy, have good microcirculation, and must understand the magnitude of this operation. This method has the advantages of avoiding the silicone breast implant and providing a satisfactory breast reconstruction with minimal long-term problems.

A gluteus maximus musculocutaneous flap may be transferred from the buttocks region to the breast area and attached by microvascular technique. This method of breast reconstruction is selected when autogenous tissue is required, when the abdominal site is not suitable for the TRAM flap type of breast reconstruction, or when the patient desires reconstruction without the use of a silicone breast implant. It may also be selected when the other breast cannot be matched with a silicone breast implant. This method requires that the surgeon be experienced in microvascular techniques and that the patient be healthy with good microcirculation. In this procedure, the gluteus maximus musculocutaneous flap is transferred to the breast area and the gluteal vessels are anastomosed to the internal mammary vessels after a window has been created in the medial lower costal cartilages.

IRRADIATION AND RECONSTRUCTIVE SURGERY

The management of complications from radiation therapy, especially radiation ulcers or radionecrosis involving bone, involves removal of the irradiated tissue and reconstruction with tissue that has its own blood supply (Figs. 16-17 and 16-18). Treatment of the wound requires excision of the ulcer and the surrounding irradiated tissues and closure with a musculocutaneous flap.[25,26] The latis-

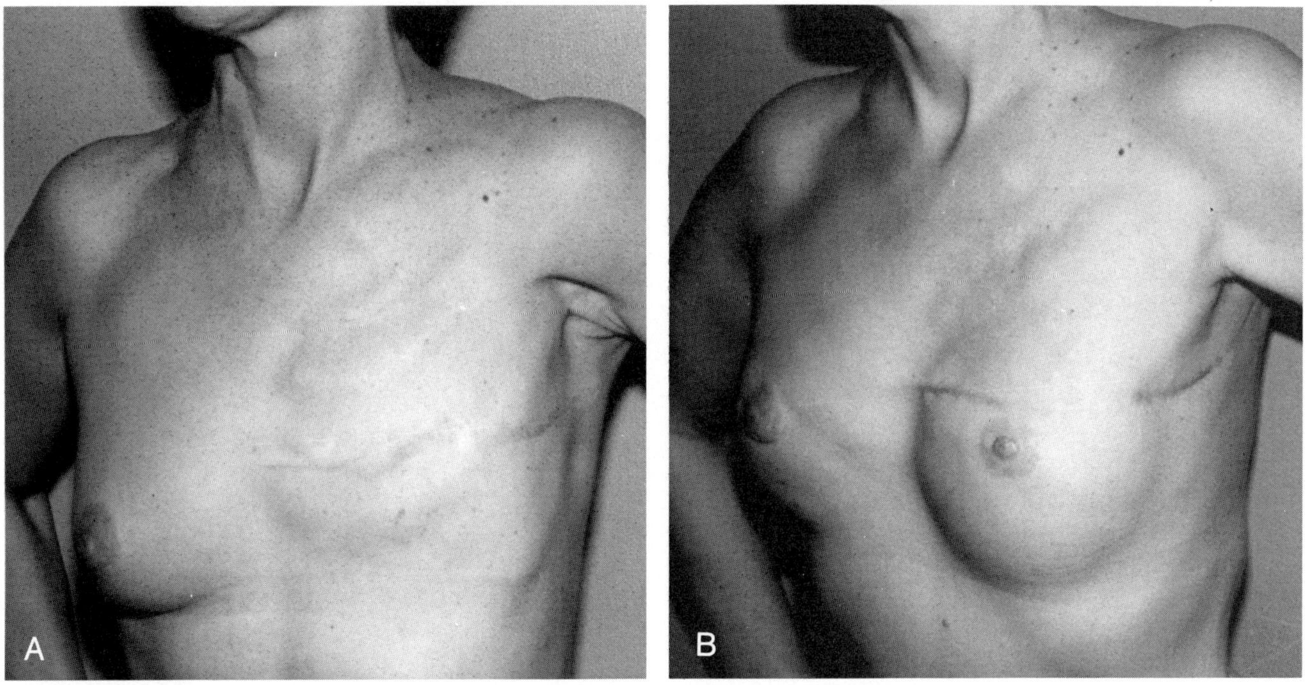

FIGURE 16-12. *(A)* A 48-year-old woman 10 years after undergoing a left radical mastectomy. *(B)* The same woman 1 year after breast reconstruction using a latissimus dorsi musculocutaneous flap and a silicone breast implant. A prophylactic total mastectomy with immediate breast reconstruction was performed in the opposite breast.

simus dorsi musculocutaneous or rectus abdominis musculocutaneous flap is useful in these clinical situations. These large musculocutaneous flaps provide sufficient tissue to fill the wounds, and a breast reconstruction may be accomplished with the additional tissue. When recurrent breast cancer is not present, the chest wall resection is conservative. The outer cortex of the ribs may be removed, thus preserving the stability of the chest wall.

The latissimus dorsi musculocutaneous flap technique is selected when the radiation ulcer is in the upper part of the chest area, or when the defect is less than 10 cm in diameter. This flap is used even if the axilla has been irradiated, and is indicated if both of the internal thoracic vessels that supply the rectus abdominis musculocutaneous flap have been irradiated. The area of radiation injury is excised, and a latissimus dorsi musculocutaneous flap is taken from the back in such a way that, when it is pedicled on the thoracodorsal vessels to the anterior chest to fill the defect, the skin will replace the missing skin, and the latissimus dorsi muscle will bring additional blood supply to a relatively avascular area. When the area of the wound is greater than the amount of back skin that can be transposed, the muscle of the latissimus dorsi is transposed and covered with a split-thickness skin graft.

If the area of the radiation injury is large, or if the patient is also interested in a simultaneous breast reconstruction, a TRAM flap from the abdomen may provide sufficient tissue. In this technique, a large flap is designed to cover the excised chest wall defect. Additional tissue is then designed to provide cover and fill for the reconstructed breast. The flap is pedicled to the chest area on the superior epigastric vessels contained in the rectus abdominis muscle. In patients who have undergone mediastinal irradiation, it is usually safest for the pedicle to be based on the contralateral internal thoracic and superior epigastric vessels. The use of two vascular pedicles with the bilateral TRAM flap increases the blood supply to the flap and provides better assurance that the flap will survive.

When the latissimus dorsi musculocutaneous flap or the TRAM flap is not suitable, the greater omentum is another source of tissue for filling chest wall defects after radiation necrosis.[27] The greater omentum is pedicled to the chest wall after a laparotomy. The omental flap is then developed on the gastroepiploic vessels. The greater omentum is then pedicled to the chest area and placed into the defect, and a split-thickness skin graft is applied for optimal wound healing.

The use of microvascular techniques is sometimes necessary for the treatment of patients with radiation injuries. A free flap is indicated when the flaps of choice are not available, and when the wound is life-threatening. The opposite latissimus dorsi musculocutaneous flap may be moved to the chest area. Because of the radiation damage to the vessels of the chest area, vessels in the neck are usually selected for the site of the anastomosis.[28]

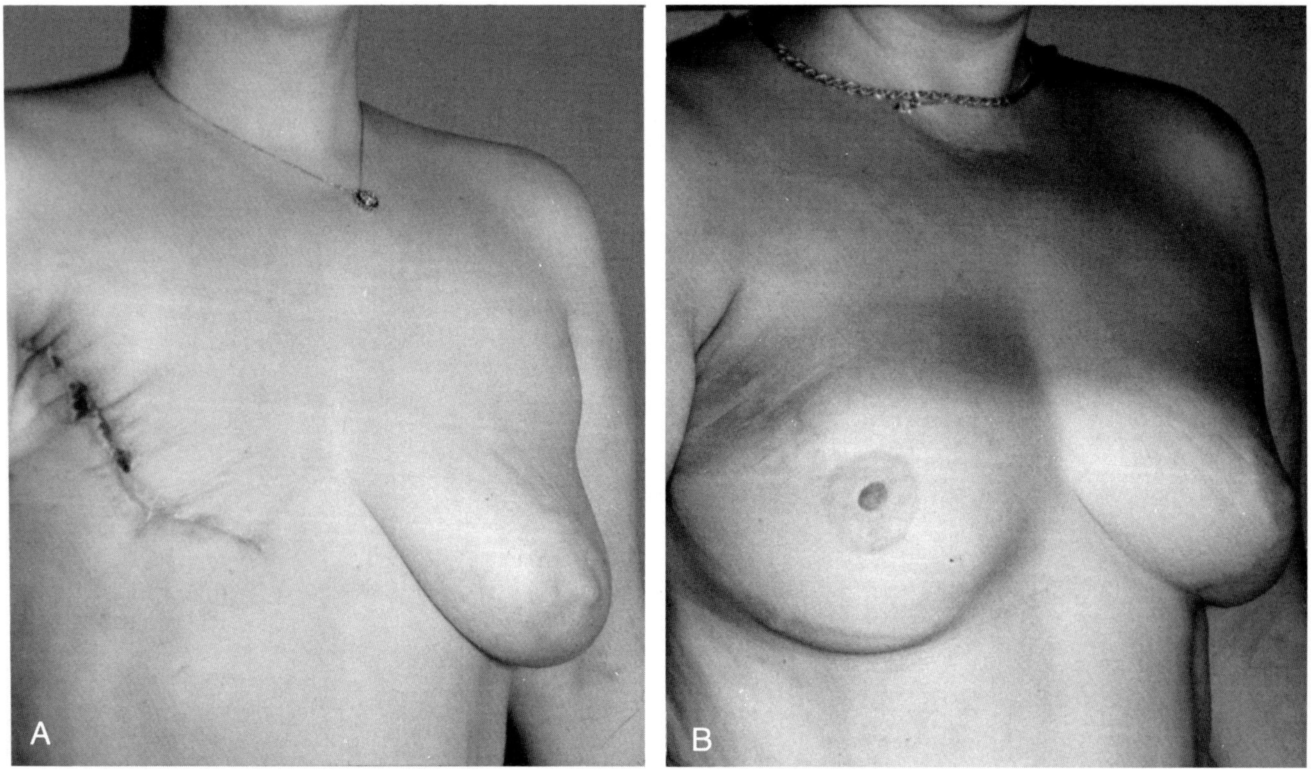

FIGURE 16-13. *(A)* A 48-year-old woman following a modified radical mastectomy. *(B)* The same patient after a breast reconstruction with a latissimus dorsi musculocutaneous flap from the back and a silicone breast implant. A reduction mammaplasty was done on the opposite breast. The nipple-areolar complex was reconstructed 3 months after the breast reconstruction. (Contemporary Surgery, Vol. 27, No. 1, p 19. Redondo Beach, California, Bobit Publishing Co., July, 1985.)

Complications after breast reconstruction for radiation-associated problems are related to the adequacy of the removal of the involved tissue and the quality and appropriate volume of the reconstructive tissues provided. When infected and irradiated tissue persists, the symptoms of infection, pain, and ulceration will continue. When there is recurrence of the breast tumor, the resection should be done widely, with frozen section control, to ensure the complete removal of the tumor. Other possible complications of such reconstructions are related to problems with the flaps. The risk of necrosis of these flaps is always present; however, the latissimus dorsi musculocutaneous flap and the TRAM flap have been associated with few problems when used for such reconstructions.

MANAGEMENT OF THE OPPOSITE BREAST

Oncologic, reconstructive, and aesthetic considerations of the opposite breast must all be considered when developing a plan for breast reconstruction. The opposite breast is the key to the symmetry and final result of the breast reconstruction. Since it must be matched to obtain symmetry, the appearance of the opposite breast determines the selection of the specific technique of breast reconstruction. Because patients with breast cancer have an increased risk for development of a second primary breast cancer, the oncologic management of the opposite breast may include careful monitoring with breast self-examinations, monitoring by a physician, breast imaging, or consideration of a prophylactic mastectomy.

The psychological and aesthetic considerations related to the opposite breast also influence the type of breast reconstruction chosen. When the opposite breast is attractive and the woman does not want it operated on or changed, the goal of the breast reconstruction is to match the opposite breast. This usually requires a flap technique of breast reconstruction. Most women with an attractive opposite breast would rather have a scar on their back, lower abdomen, or buttocks than a scar on the remaining breast.

When the opposite breast is hypoplastic and lacks significant projection, a silicone breast implant may not provide satisfactory breast symmetry. In these women, an augmentation mammaplasty with a silicone breast implant of the opposite breast may provide the best chances for symmetry while enhancing the overall breast form.[29] An operation, such as an augmentation mammaplasty, on the

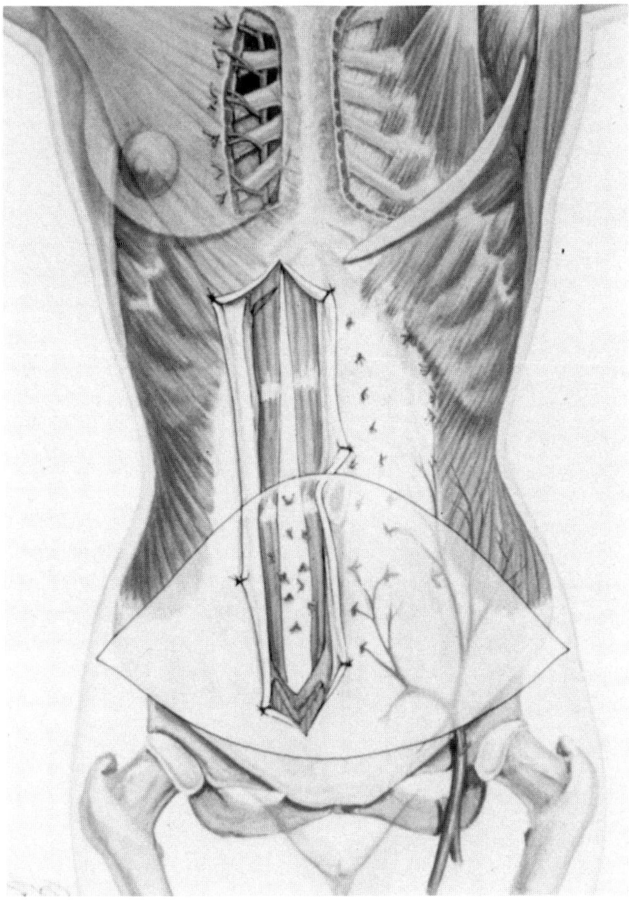

FIGURE 16-14. The lower transverse rectus abdominis musculocutaneous (TRAM) flap is designed as an ellipse over the lower abdominal excess. (Contemporary Surgery, Vol. 27, No. 1, p 20. Redondo Beach, California, Bobit Publishing Co., July, 1985.)

opposite breast also provides an opportunity for a biopsy if this is indicated by high-risk factors. The silicone breast implant is placed in the submusculofascial position behind the breast tissue. This permits monitoring of the opposite breast without interference with the silicone breast implant. Breast self-examination, breast imaging, and even a breast biopsy or total mastectomy may be performed in these patients because the silicone breast implant is behind the tissues under consideration. When breast ptosis is associated with breast hypoplasia, a symmetrical breast reconstruction usually requires a submusculofascial silicone breast implant and a mastopexy. These procedures are done to elevate the nipple-areolar complex and to remove the excess skin that lies vertically beneath the nipple-areolar complex and horizontally in the inframammary crease. The removal of the excess skin and elevation of the nipple-areolar complex may be accomplished without interfering with the breast parenchyma and without creating scars on the breast that might make oncologic monitoring more difficult.

It is difficult to obtain symmetry in patients with a large, heavy, and ptotic opposite breast without reducing this breast at the time of breast reconstruction.[30] The chances of symmetry are increased by modifying both breasts during the same operation. The patient's expectations concerning the size and contour of the opposite breast must be considered during the planning of such breast reconstructions. When the opposite breast is large and the patient does not want it modified, a TRAM flap may provide enough skin and fat to match the reconstructed breast. However, the usual strategy is to plan a reduction of the opposite breast and a breast reconstruction to match the reduced breast. Sometimes, it is necessary to use a flap for breast reconstruction in order to ensure that the expected size is achieved.

Breast reduction is accomplished by removing breast tissue from the areas of greatest tissue excess, usually the lower and lateral aspects of the breast. The excess skin is removed through both a verticle ellipse located below the nipple-areolar complex and a horizontal ellipse at the inframammary crease. This results in an inverted "T" incision and scar. The nipple-areolar complex is then moved upward to its new position, either by a pedicle on the retained breast parenchyma or, when the distance of transposition is great, by a skin graft technique. Some breast scars may result from a reduction mammaplasty. The reconstructive breast surgeon, the patient, and other members of the breast management team should become familiar with the characteristics of the reduced breast; if a change develops, breast imaging and a breast biopsy may be indicated.

A family history of breast cancer in a first-degree maternal relative (a mother or sister) is a major risk factor for the development of breast cancer.[31] Also, when breast cancer occurs, especially in premenopausal women, the risk of developing cancer in the opposite breast is increased significantly. Breast cancer in one breast doubles the chances of cancer developing in the opposite breast. Younger women also have a greater risk of developing a breast cancer in the opposite breast. There are specific pathologic markers for an increased relative risk of developing breast cancer, some of which are multifocal areas of carcinoma, lobular carcinoma *in situ,* pathologic changes of epithelial hyperplasia and atypia, and multiple areas of *in situ* intraductal carcinoma.[32,33] Fibrocystic disease is not associated with an increased risk, although there are certain pathologic changes associated with fibrocystic disease that correlate with an increased relative risk.

Prophylactic mastectomy is an operation that is performed before the actual development of breast cancer to reduce the risk and worry of developing breast cancer by removing a high percentage of breast tissue. A total mastectomy is preferred over subcutaneous mastectomy because 95% to 98% of the breast tissue can be removed, and the tissue that remains is just under the skin and thus can be monitored easily for the development of breast cancer. The nipple-areola skin may be left in position or removed and replaced as a skin graft. The total mastectomy may be extended to remove a sample of the Level I axillary

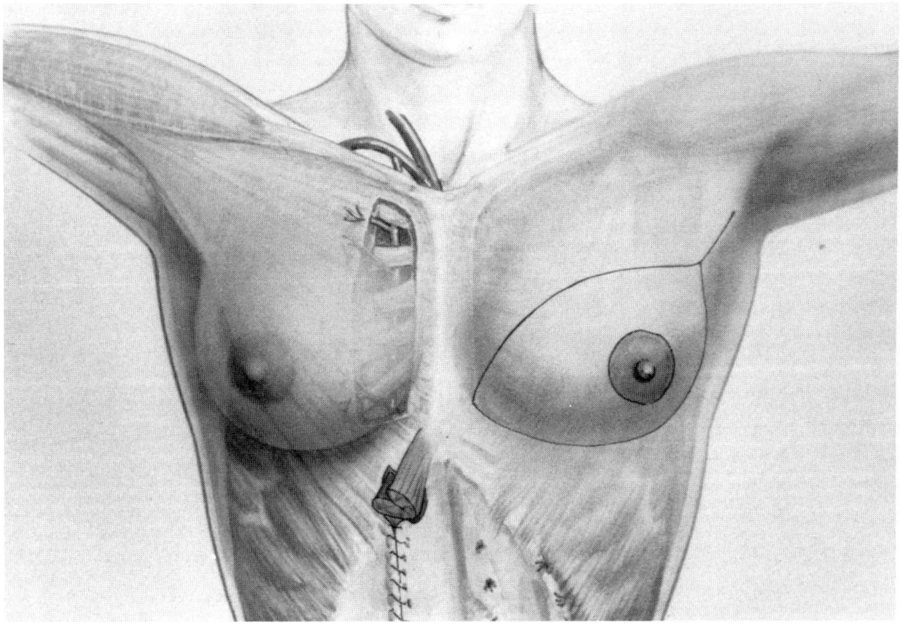

FIGURE 16-15. Breast reconstruction is accomplished using lower abdominal excess tissue and without the need for a silicone breast implant. (Contemporary Surgery, Vol. 27, No. 1, p 20. Redondo Beach, California, Bobit Publishing Co., July, 1985.)

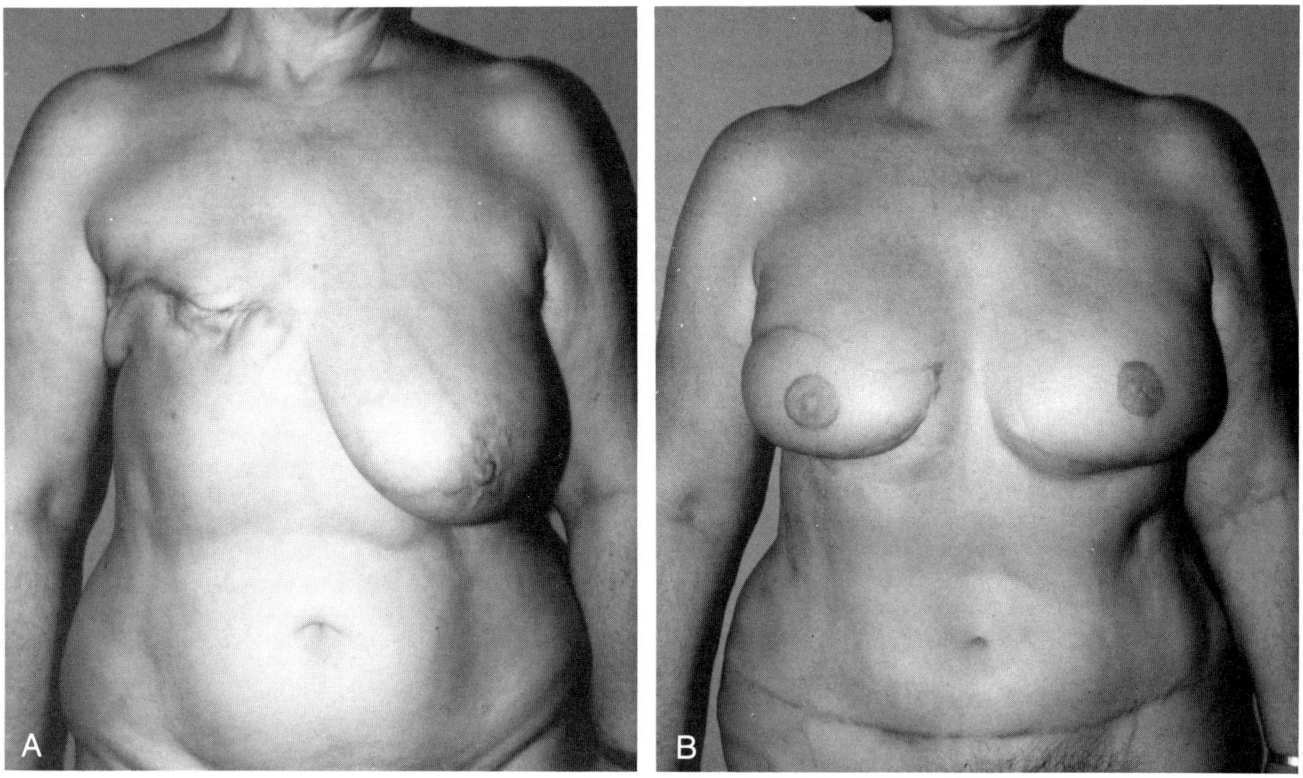

FIGURE 16-16. *(A)* A 52-year-old woman 6 months after undergoing a modified radical mastectomy. *(B)* The same patient 9 months after undergoing a left total mastectomy and bilateral breast reconstruction using bilateral lower TRAM flaps.

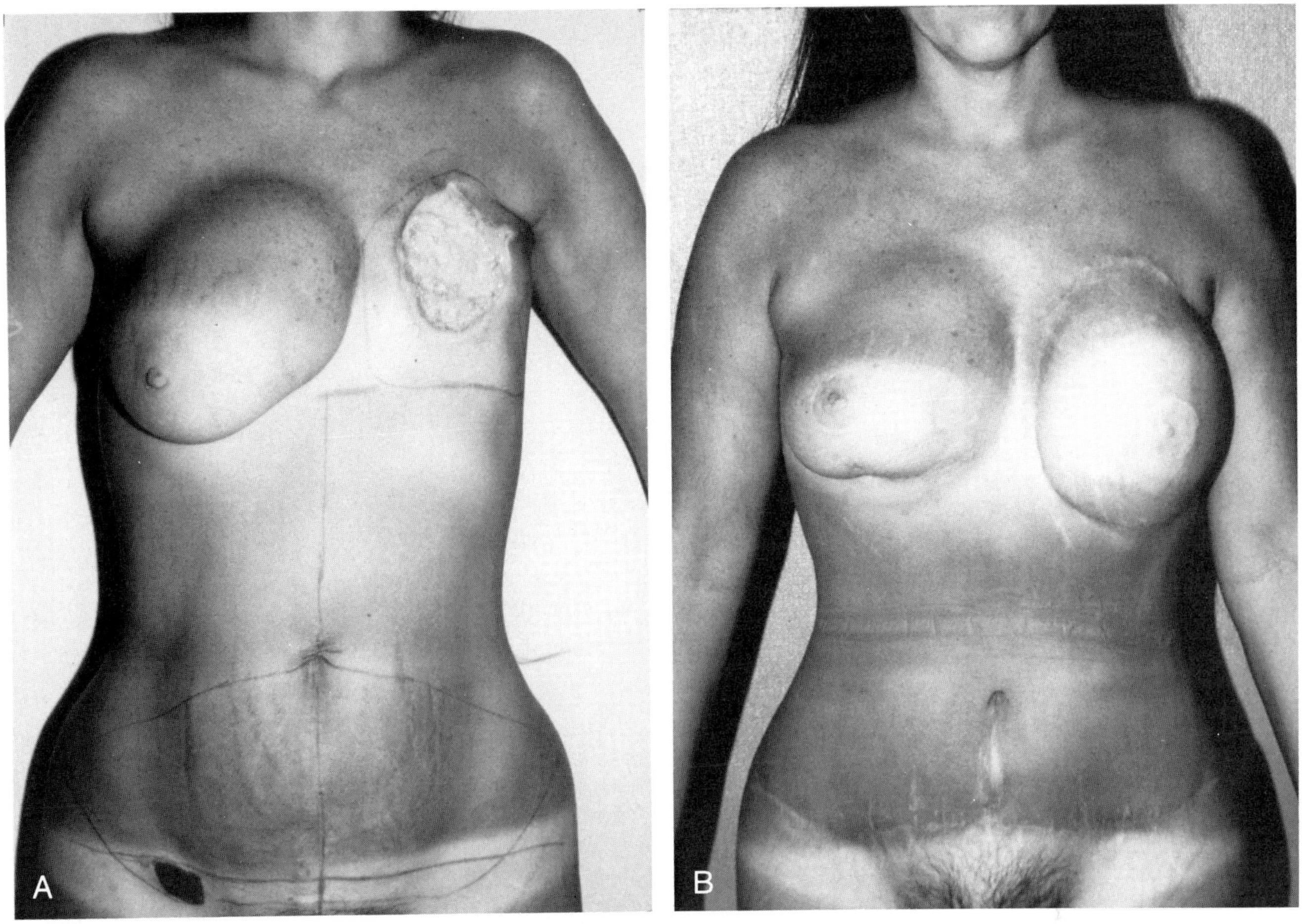

FIGURE 16-17. *(A)* A 31-year-old woman with radiation necrosis of the breast after lumpectomy–radiation treatment. Breast cancer was found at the time of augmentation mammaplasty, and the patient refused a mastectomy. *(B)* The same patient 2 years after undergoing bilateral breast reconstruction using lower TRAM flaps. She also underwent a revision of the right breast to improve symmetry. (Ishii CH, Bostwick J, et al: Double-pedicle transverse rectus abdominis musculocutaneous flap for unilateral breast and chest wall reconstruction. Plast Reconstr Surg 76:905, 1985.)

lymph nodes when there is an especially high risk of early invasive breast cancer. If an invasive breast cancer is found, no additional surgery is needed for local treatment. This option of prophylactic mastectomy has become more attractive for women at high risk since the development of effective methods of immediate breast reconstruction.

In patients in whom a prophylactic mastectomy is done at the time of breast reconstruction, the opposite breast that is at increased risk for breast cancer may be either hypoplastic, ptotic, or hypertrophic. The adjustment of the opposite breast in these women requires an aesthetic correction, a prophylactic mastectomy, and a breast reconstruction. This is one of the most complex corrections in breast reconstruction. The reconstructive surgeon understands the specific findings after the breast reconstruction and should participate in the patient's follow-up to interpret specific masses thought to be local recurrence.

Prophylactic mastectomy is an operation that is subject to a number of complications. These complications include all those associated with total mastectomy and immediate breast reconstruction, in addition to the potential problems associated with breast reconstruction using a silicone breast implant. In addition to the possible complications of infection and hematoma, breast and nipple-areola skin may be lost. When the silicone breast implant is not completely covered by the musculofascial layer, exposure of the silicone breast implant may occur, necessitating removal of the implant in most cases. Prophylactic mastectomy and immediate breast reconstruction remain controversial procedures, but represent options for the woman who is very worried about the development of breast cancer.

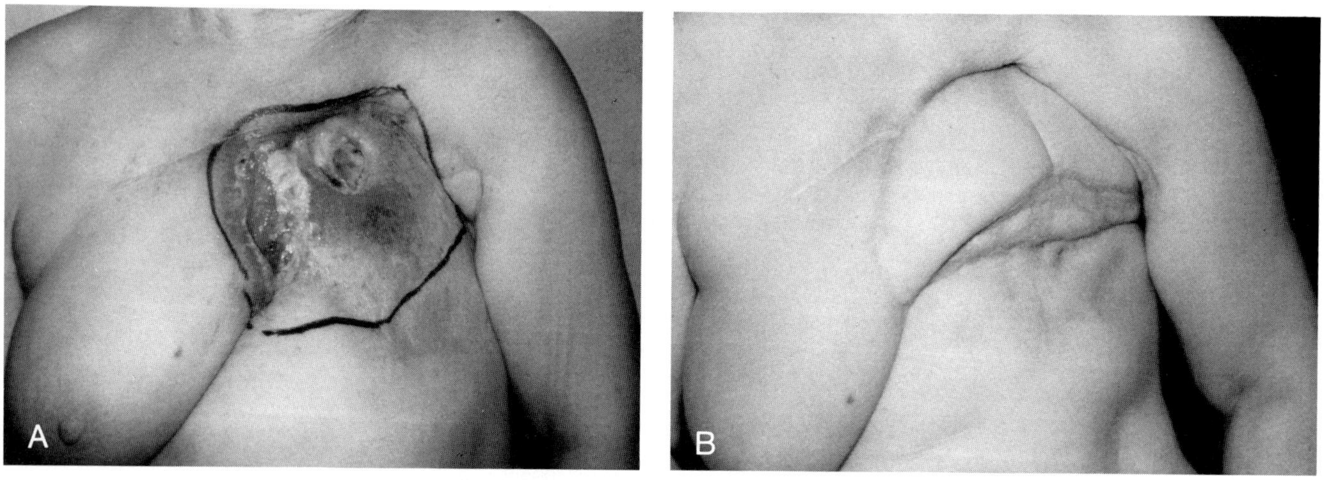

FIGURE 16-18. *(A)* This 72-year-old woman developed osteoradionecrosis of the chest wall after radiation therapy for a local recurrence of breast cancer. Initially, she received adjuvant radiation therapy after the radical mastectomy. *(B)* The same patient 9 months after resection of the ulcer and breast reconstruction with a latissimus dorsi musculocutaneous flap. (Bostwick J, Stevenson TR, Nahai F, et al: Radiation to the breast: Complications amenable to surgical treatment. Ann Surg 200:547, 1984.)

RECONSTRUCTION OF THE NIPPLE-AREOLAR COMPLEX

Nipple-areolar reconstruction is done after symmetry of the reconstructed breasts has been achieved. It is the last phase of breast reconstruction. The goal is to reconstruct a nipple-areolar complex that is symmetrically positioned and is similar in size and appearance to the opposite nipple-areolar complex.[34] In bilateral reconstructions, both nipple-areolar complexes should be positioned properly on attractive, reconstructed breasts. Nipple-areolar reconstruction is usually not done at the time of breast reconstruction because if the breast shape changes, asymmetry or malposition of the nipple-areola complex may develop. Delayed nipple-areolar reconstruction allows the patient to participate in the planning of its position, size, and appearance, which may coincidentally improve the chances that the reconstruction will meet the expectations of the patient. Reconstruction of the nipple-areolar complex is done for the sake of appearance only, as there is no sensation other than the minimal sensation that is present on postmastectomy skin flaps.

Tissue for nipple-areolar reconstructions should match the opposite nipple-areolar complex in color, texture, and overall appearance. Tissue from the opposite nipple-areolar complex, obtained at the time of reduction mammaplasty of the opposite breast, is particularly well suited as a donor site. The pigmented skin of the upper inner thigh crease is also a good choice for donor skin. This donor site is closed as a line in the upper inner thigh crease. The lower half or end of the opposite nipple is often selected as donor tissue because of the excellent symmetry that can be achieved. In bilateral reconstructions in which the opposite nipple is not available, or when the opposite nipple is small, the earlobe or local flaps of the chest skin may be used for nipple reconstruction.

REFERENCES

1. Bostwick J: Aesthetic and Reconstructive Breast Surgery. St. Louis, CV Mosby, 1983
2. Goin JM, Goin MK: Changing the Body: Psychological Effects of Plastic Surgery. Baltimore, Williams & Wilkins, 1981
3. Pearl RM, Wisnicki J: Breast reconstruction following lumpectomy and irradiation. Plast Reconstr Surg 76:83, 1985
4. Gruber RP, et al: Breast reconstruction following mastectomy: A comparison of submuscular and subcutaneous techniques. Plast Reconstr Surg 67:312, 1981
5. Noone RB, et al: Patient acceptance of immediate reconstruction following mastectomy. Plast Reconstr Surg 69:632, 1982
6. Georgiade GS, Riefkohl R, Cox E, et al: Long-term clinical outcome of immediate reconstruction after mastectomy. Plast Reconstr Surg 76:415, 1985
7. Little JW, Golembe EV, Fisher JB: The "living bra" in immediate and delayed reconstruction of the breast following mastectomy for malignant and non-malignant disease. Plast Reconstr Surg 68:392, 1981
8. McCraw JB, Bostwick J, Horton CE: Methods of soft tissue coverage of the mastectomy defect. Clin Plast Surg 6:57, 1979
9. Woods JE, Irons GB, Arnold PG: The case for submuscular implantation of prostheses in reconstructive surgery. Ann Plast Surg 5:115, 1980
10. Snyderman RK, Guthrie RH: Reconstruction of the female breast following radical mastectomy. Plast Reconstr Surg 47:565, 1971

11. Dowden RV, Dinner MI: Breast reconstruction without skin flaps. Clin Plast Surg 11:265, 1984
12. Lewis JR: Use of a sliding flap from the abdomen to provide cover in breast reconstructions. Plast Reconstr Surg 64:491, 1979
13. Ryan JJ: A lower thoracic advancement flap in breast reconstruction after mastectomy. Plast Reconstr Surg 70:153, 1982
14. Radovan C: Tissue expansion in soft-tissue reconstruction. Plast Reconstr Surg 74:482, 1984
15. Argenta LC: Reconstruction of the breast by tissue expansion. Clin Plast Surg 11:247, 1984
16. Manders EK: Soft-tissue expansion: Concepts and complications. Plast Reconstr Surg 74:493, 1984
17. Schneider WJ, Hill HL, Brown RG: Latissimus dorsi myocutaneous flap for breast reconstruction. Br J Plast Surg 30:277, 1977
18. Bostwick J, Vasconez LO, Jurkiewicz MJ: Breast reconstruction after a radical mastectomy. Plast Reconstr Surg 61:682, 1978
19. Biggs TM, Cronin ED: Technical aspects of the latissimus dorsi flap in breast reconstruction. Ann Plast Surg 6:381, 1981
20. Maxwell GP: Latissimus dorsi breast reconstruction: An aesthetic assessment. Clin Plast Surg 8(2):373, 1981
21. Hartrampf CR, Scheflan M, Black PW: Breast reconstruction following mastectomy with a transverse abdominal island flap. Anatomical and clinical observations. Plast Reconstr Surg 69:216, 1982
22. Dinner MI, Dowden RV, Scheflan M: Refinements in the use of the transverse abdominal island flap for postmastectomy reconstruction. Ann Plast Surg 11:362, 1983
23. Elliott LF, Hartrampf CR: Tailoring of the new breast using the transverse abdominal island flap. Plast Reconstr Surg 72:887, 1983
24. Shaw WW: Breast reconstruction by superior gluteal microvascular free flaps without silicone implants. Plast Reconstr Surg 72:490, 1983
25. Bostwick J, Stevenson TR, Nahai F, et al: Radiation to the breast: Complications amenable to surgical treatment. Ann Surg 200:543, 1984
26. Ferguson DJ, Sutton HG, Dawson PJ: Late effects of adjuvant radiotherapy for breast cancer. Cancer 54:2319, 1984
27. Jurkiewicz MJ, Arnold PG: The omentum: An account of its use in the reconstruction of the chest wall. Ann Surg 185:548, 1977
28. Serafin D, Georgiade NG, Given KS: Transfer of free flaps to provide well-vascularized, free cover for breast reconstructions after radical mastectomy. Plast Reconstr Surg 62:527, 1978
29. Truppman ES, Ellenby JD: A 13-year evaluation of subpectoral augmentation mammaplasty. In Owsley JQ Jr, Peterson RA (eds): Symposium on Aesthetic Surgery of the Breast, pp 341–343. St. Louis, CV Mosby, 1978
30. Courtiss EH, Goldwyn RM: Breast sensation before and after plastic surgery. Plast Reconstr Surg 58:1, 1976
31. Anderson DE, Badzioch MD: Bilaterality in familial breast cancer patients. Cancer 56:2092, 1985
32. Jarrett JR, Cutler RG, Teal DF: Subcutaneous mastectomy in small, large, or ptotic breasts with immediate submuscular placement of the implants. Plast Reconstr Surg 62:702, 1978
33. Woods JE, Irons GB, and Arnold PG: The case for submuscular implantation of prostheses in reconstructive breast surgery. Ann Plast Surg 5:115, 1980
34. Gruber RP: Nipple-areola reconstruction: A review of techniques. Clin Plast Surg 6:71, 1979

Diagnosis and Treatment of Pain in Breast Cancer

Mark Stillman Kathleen M. Foley

Pain is a common symptom in patients with breast cancer, reported by 52% of patients with metastatic breast cancer in active therapy and by as many as 75% to 80% of patients with far-advanced disease.[1] The clinical assessment of pain in such patients requires a specific expertise and is based on an understanding of the nature of pain and its underlying pathophysiology. Of particular importance is the recognition that its presence does not imply recurrent or persistent disease. There are a series of common specific pain syndromes in patients with breast cancer and often several causes of pain in a single patient.[1,2] A detailed diagnostic evaluation helps to assure the appropriate use of available therapeutic procedures.

COMMON PAIN SYNDROMES IN BREAST CANCER

There are certain general principles that should be followed in the full assessment of the patient with pain, and these have been previously reviewed.[3] Equally important, the type of pain (acute versus chronic) and the pathophysiological mechanisms (somatic, visceral, or deafferentation) need to be identified. Breast cancer patients have both acute and chronic pain. This classification is based on an increased understanding of pain mechanisms and recognition that the central modulation for acute pain may be different from that of chronic pain.[4] Different types of pain may require different management approaches, and patients may vary in their responses to treatment. Acute pain is relatively easy to recognize and is more amenable to many of the therapeutic procedures available. For example, in the patient with breast cancer and bone metastases, the use of radiation therapy will dramatically relieve the acute pain syndrome. In patients with chronic pain—for example, the patient with tumor infiltration of the brachial plexus and deafferentation pain—the persistent pain usually has failed to respond to those modalities directed at the cause of the pain. In these patients, pain usually has led to significant changes in personality, lifestyle, and functional ability. Such patients need a treatment approach that encompasses not only treatment of the cause of the pain but also treatment of the complications that have arisen in the patient's functional status, social life, and personality.

Breast cancer is often associated with several physiological types of pain. Somatic and visceral pain result from activation and sensitization of nociceptors and mechanoreceptors by mechanical (tumor compression or infiltration) or chemical (metastases in bone) stimuli. Acute, intermittent, or continuous pain results. Most therapeutic approaches are partially effective in controlling this kind of pain.[5] In contrast, deafferentation pain is pain that results from nerve injury after nerve section or from chronic tumor infiltration or compression. There is partial damage of axons and nerve membranes, which become extremely sensitive to any mechanical or chemical stimuli. Chronic, unremitting pain results, and it is poorly controlled by the majority of therapeutic approaches. Experimental studies indicate that pain from deafferentation leads to central neuronal hyperactivity in the spinal cord and possibly in the thalamus.[6] These different physiological mechanisms account, in part, for the differences in response of various types of cancer pain to analgesic, neurosurgical, and anesthetic approaches. For example, drug therapy and neurosurgical procedures are often effective in managing pain from brachial plexopathy in its early acute stage, but once deafferentation has occurred, the success of such procedures diminishes rapidly. Pain in the patient with breast cancer is also influenced by the patient's stage of disease. A useful classification for deciding therapeutic approaches in patients with acute or chronic pain is listed below and has been developed to allow the physician to further understand the multidimensional components of pain, specifically psychological distress and pain significance.

1. Patients with acute cancer-related pain
   a. Occurring at the time of diagnosis (e.g., bone metastases)
   b. Resulting from cancer therapy (surgery, chemotherapy, or radiation)
2. Patients with chronic cancer-related pain
   a. Associated with tumor progression (e.g., brachial plexopathy)
   b. Associated with cancer therapy (e.g., postmastectomy syndrome following surgery)
3. Patients with preexisting chronic pain and cancer-related pain (e.g., patients with chronic low back pain and bone metastases)
4. Patients with a history of drug addiction and cancer-related pain
   a. Actively involved in illicit drug use
   b. In methadone maintenance programs
   c. With a history of drug abuse
5. Dying patients with cancer-related pain

Lastly, a classification of common pain syndromes has been developed and includes three major categories.[1] The first and most common cause of pain in breast cancer patients is that associated with direct tumor involvement. Metastatic bone disease, nerve compression, and infiltration and involvement of the hollow viscus are the most common causes of pain in this group (see the accompanying display). The second group of pain syndromes is associated with cancer therapy. This group accounts for 20% of pain patients in an inpatient population and includes those with pain that occurs in the course of or as a result of surgery, chemotherapy, or radiation therapy. In patients with breast cancer, this group represents a significant number because these patients have initial successful antitumor therapy and live long enough for these complications to be noted. The third category of pain syndromes includes those unrelated to the cancer or the cancer therapy. From 3% to 10% of patients who present with a history of breast cancer and a new onset of pain can be placed in this category.

Common Pain Syndromes in Patients With Breast Cancer

Pain Syndromes Associated with Direct Tumor Infiltration

Tumor Infiltration of Bone

1. Metastases to the base of the skull
   a. Jugular foramen syndrome
   b. Orbital syndrome
   c. Parasellar syndrome
   d. Middle fossa syndrome
2. Metastases to vertebral bodies
   a. Odontoid metastases fractures
   b. C7-T1 vertebral metastases
   c. Lumbar metastases L1
   d. Sacral metastases

Tumor Infiltration of Nerve, Plexus, Root, Meninges, and Spinal Cord

1. Tumor infiltration of peripheral nerve
2. Tumor infiltration of the brachial plexus
3. Tumor infiltration of the lumbar pléxus
4. Leptomeningeal metastases
5. Epidural spinal cord compression

Tumor Infiltration of Hollow Viscus

Pain Syndromes Associated with Cancer Therapy

Postsurgical Pain Syndromes

1. Peripheral neuropathy
2. Steroid pseudorheumatism
3. Aseptic necrosis of bone
4. Postherpetic neuralgia

Postradiation Therapy Pain Syndromes

1. Radiation fibrosis of the brachial plexus
2. Radiation myelopathy
3. Irradiation-induced peripheral nerve tumors
4. Radiation necrosis of bone

Pain Syndromes Associated with Direct Tumor Infiltration

Tumor Infiltration of Bone

Invasion of bone by metastatic tumor is the most common cause of pain in patients with breast cancer. Both the periosteum and all the structures of joints except the articular cartilage are pain-sensitive structures, whereas the cortex and bone marrow are considered to be pain-insensitive bone structures. The vascular supply to bone has its own nerve fiber network, but the role of such nerves in the generation of pain remains unstudied. Current hypotheses for the origin of bone pain relate to the role of prostaglandins in the metastatic process. Drugs that inhibit prostaglandin synthesis inhibit pain and, in some instances, tumor growth in both clinical and experimental studies.[7,8] From the clinical point of view, metastatic breast tumor involvement of bone produces pain in one of two ways: (1) by the direct involvement of the bone and activation of the nociceptors locally or (2) by compression of adjacent nerves, soft tissue, or vascular structures. Specific pain syndromes involving bone are briefly considered here:

METASTASES TO THE BASE OF THE SKULL. Greenberg has reported a series of syndromes associated with metastases to the base of the skull.[9] All share two common features: (1) Pain is the earliest complaint, often preceding neurologic signs and symptoms by several weeks or months, and (2) documentation on plain x-ray films is often difficult, and tomography and CT scanning are often required. CT scans appear to be superior to all other radiologic diagnostic studies in evaluating tumor involvement in this region. Seventeen of the 43 patients reported in this series had breast cancer. The metastases at the base of the skull usually appeared at the same time as other bony metastases from breast cancer, and at the time of diagnosis, 29 of the 43 had metastases elsewhere in the body, 19 to other bones. The median time from primary diagnosis to onset of neurologic signs ranged from 0 to 192 months, with a median time of 66 months for patients with breast cancer.

JUGULAR FORAMEN SYNDROME. Occipital pain referred to the vertex of the head and ipsilateral shoulder and arm is the early presenting symptom. The pain is often exacerbated by head movement and associated with local tenderness over the occipital condyle. The patient's signs and symptoms vary with the cranial nerve involved and can include hoarseness, dysarthria, dysphagia, neck and shoulder weakness, and ptosis. The neurologic examination can help to localize the lesion by determining the function of cranial nerves IX, X, XI, and XII, since involvement of all four of these nerves suggests jugular foramen and hypoglossal canal involvement with secondary nerve dysfunction. The presence of a Horner's syndrome suggests sympathetic involvement extracranially but in close proximity to the jugular foramen.

ORBITAL SYNDROME. Pain in the supraorbital area is the earliest sign, followed by blurred binocular vision leading to diplopia and eventually proptosis and external ophthalmoplegia. Sensory loss in the opthalmic division of the fifth nerve is often common.

PARASELLAR SYNDROME. Parasellar or cavernous sinus metastases present with unilateral frontal headache and ocular paresis without proptosis. Oculomotor and abducens paresis are the most common cranial nerve manifestations, and papilledema is also observed.

MIDDLE FOSSA SYNDROME. Pain, numbness, and paresthesias in the distribution of the second and third divisions of the trigeminal nerve are the presenting complaints. Dull aching pain or acute lancinating pain and headache were the characteristic pain complaints. This was the most common pain syndrome due to breast cancer.

METASTASES TO VERTEBRAL BODIES. These syndromes share two common features: (1) Pain is an early symptom preceding neurologic signs and symptoms, and (2) if the nature of the pain is not accurately diagnosed, irreversible neurologic deficits including paraplegia and quadriplegia may occur. Eighty-five percent of patients with epidural spinal cord compression had vertebral body metastases in a recent series, and 10% of patients with epidural spinal cord compression had pain as their only complaint in the absence of any neurologic findings.[10] Some typical pain syndromes are described below.

ODONTOID FRACTURES. Disease in this region can result from pathologic fracture and secondary subluxation, with resulting spinal cord or brain stem compression. Fractures of the odontoid process are most often secondary to destruction of the atlas and represent an important group of vertebral metastases from breast cancer.[11] Of 18 patients with odontoid fracture treated at Memorial Sloan-Kettering Cancer Center (MSKCC), the clinical features consisted of severe neck pain and neck stiffness in 17 patients, with signs of cord compression noted in only 4 patients. The pain is characteristically noted to radiate over the posterior aspect of the skull to the vertex, exacerbated by neck movement and particularly by neck flexion. Neurologic signs include progressive sensory and motor findings beginning in the upper extremities with associated autonomic dysfunction, but pain is the earliest symptom. Neck manipulation in these patients is dangerous, and tomography is necessary to confirm the diagnosis. Early diagnosis of tumor in the vertebral body before subluxation or fracture occurs is important, because therapy directed at the control of tumor growth (e.g., radiation therapy) should be instituted before misalignment becomes evident.

C7–T1 VERTEBRAL METASTASES. This is a common site for metastatic disease originating from the breast. The pain is usually localized to the adjacent paraspinal area and is characterized by a constant, dull, aching pain radiating bilaterally to both shoulders. There may be tenderness to percussion over the spinous process at this level. With nerve root compression, radicular pain in the C7, C8, T1 distribution most commonly occurs unilaterally in the posterior arm, elbow, and ulnar aspect of the hand. The neurologic symptoms include paresthesias and numbness in the fourth and fifth fingers, with progressive hand weakness and triceps weakness. The presence of a Horner's syndrome suggests paravertebral sympathetic involvement. Metastatic bone disease at this level results from either hematogenous spread to bone or more commonly from tumor originating in the brachial plexus or paravertebral space and spreading along the nerves to the contiguous vertebral body and epidural space. Plain x-rays of the cervical and thoracic spine do not provide adequate visualization of the C7–T1 area because of overlapping cardiac and bony structures. CT scan is the diagnostic procedure of choice to define the presence of metastatic disease.[12] In patients with bilateral radicular symptoms or signs of spinal cord dysfunction, myelography should be performed to rule out an associated epidural spinal cord compression.

LUMBAR METASTASES—L1. Dull, aching midback pain exacerbated by lying or sitting and relieved by standing is the most usual presenting complaint. The pain is exacerbated by movement and is particularly significant when the patient goes from the recumbent to the standing position. The pain is often referred bilaterally to the sacroiliac regions or radicular to the superior iliac crests unilaterally or bilaterally. Lack of knowledge of these referred points for L1 disease often confuses the diagnostic work-up.

SACRAL METASTASES. Aching pain beginning insidiously in the lower back or coccygeal region and exacerbated by lying or sitting and relieved by walking is the common clinical complaint for tumor infiltration of the sacrum. Increasing pain with neurologic signs and symptoms of perianal sensory loss, bowel and bladder dysfunction, and impotence help to localize the site of the disease. Certain patients may complain of specific tenderness over the sciatic notch and radicular symptoms in the sciatic nerve distribution associated with nerve compression from local bony changes in the sacrum. The diagnostic evaluation should include the CT scan, which is the most useful diagnostic procedure. In certain instances the barium enema, intravenous pyelogram, or lymphangiogram may help in identifying the presence of presacral tumors.

Tumor Infiltration of Nerve, Plexus, Root, Meninges, and Spinal Cord

The pain syndromes in this group occur either by direct tumor infiltration of nerve, by progressive compression of nerve structures, or by sudden compression by metastatic fractures of bone adjacent to nerves or nerve roots. The neuropathology of these lesions has not been correlated with the nature of pain, but on the basis of neurophysiological evidence it has been suggested that persistent mechanical and noxious stimulation of nociceptors combined with the partial damage of axons and nerve membranes may account for the types of pain encountered in this group of syndromes.

TUMOR INFILTRATION OF PERIPHERAL NERVE. Constant burning pain with hyperesthesia and dysesthesia in the area of sensory loss is the usual clinical presentation. The most common cause of infiltration of the peripheral nerve is tumors that invade the paravertebral or retroperitoneal space. The pain is commonly radicular and unilateral, and a careful sensory examination can often delineate the site of nerve compression. The most common example of infiltration of peripheral nerve is metastatic tumor involvement of rib, producing intercostal nerve entrapment. The diagnosis of these syndromes can be made clinically, with confirmation by CT scanning to document the anatomical region of nerve compression.

TUMOR INFILTRATION OF THE BRACHIAL PLEXUS. Pain is the earliest and most consistent symptom, and its differential diagnosis has been discussed in Chapter 14.

TUMOR INFILTRATION OF THE LUMBAR PLEXUS. In a study of the natural history of lumbosacral plexopathy in cancer patients,[13] breast cancer was the tumor diagnosis in 15% of patients (9 of 85). Pain is the presenting complaint in 91% of patients, with weakness occurring in 60% and numbness in 42%. The pain is of two types: (1) local pain in the sacrum or sacroiliac joint, lower back, or groin and (2) radicular pain in either the lateral, posterior, or anterior leg. CT scanning is the most useful diagnostic study to define soft tissue masses or bone abnormalities in the lumbosacral and pelvic regions. Specific studies like intravenous pyelography may give additional information necessary to suggest the presence of tumor in adjacent lymph tissue. The differential diagnosis includes lumbar neuritis, postsurgical lumbar plexopathy, radiation fibrosis, and lumbar disk disease. Each of these entities has a characteristic neurologic presentation and should be differentiated from tumor infiltration of the lumbar plexus.

LEPTOMENINGEAL METASTASES. Pain occurs in 40% of these patients and is of two types: (1) headache with or without neck stiffness and (2) back pain commonly localized in the lower back and buttock area. The pain results from traction on or infiltration of nerves and meninges. The clinical spectrum of this disorder is discussed in Chapter 14.

EPIDURAL SPINAL CORD COMPRESSION. Pain is the presenting symptom in 95% of patients and in 85% of patients is associated with vertebral body metastasis. (See Chapter 14 for further discussion.)

Pain Syndromes Associated With Cancer Therapy

In cancer therapy, clinical pain syndromes may occur in the course of or subsequent to treatment of cancer patients undergoing the common treatment modalities of surgery, chemotherapy, or radiation therapy. These syndromes are of two types. First are those that occur acutely (within weeks) from the introduction of the specific therapy, such as immediate postoperative pain syndromes, the mucositis of chemotherapy, and the radiation-induced esophagitis. These syndromes are readily recognized, and the associated pain is a self-limited illness. The second type, comprising those that occur several weeks to months and, in certain instances, years later, presents a clinical problem: Is the pain a complication of therapy or recurrent disease? The incidence of pain syndromes associated with cancer therapy is not known, but they represent an important aspect of the differential diagnosis of the pain complaint for both the patient and physician. They include the syndromes discussed below.

Postsurgical Pain Syndromes

POSTMASTECTOMY PAIN SYNDROME. Four percent to 10% of women having any surgical procedure on the breast, from lumpectomy to radical mastectomy, develop this syndrome.[14,15] The pain can occur immediately or up to several months following surgery and is characterized as a tight, constricting, burning pain in the posterior arm, axilla, and anterior chest wall. There is often a trigger area in the axilla which on palpation recreates the pain. The pain is exacerbated by movement, and patients often maintain their arms in a flexed position close to the chest wall. This posture leads to the development of a frozen shoulder and secondary pain, with disuse atrophy of the arm and shoulder muscles from the immobilization. The pain results from interruption of the intercostal brachial nerve, a sensory cutaneous branch of T1–T2, and subsequent formation of a traumatic neuroma at the end of the severed nerve. Neuroanatomical studies reveal that there is a wide variation in the size and distribution of this nerve, which may account for the varied clinical appearance of the pain syndrome. The syndrome can be clearly distinguished from tumor infiltration of the brachial plexus. Treatment with physical therapy to prevent shoulder immobilization, local rubbing of the area, nerve blocks of the trigger point with local anesthetics, and small doses of amitriptyline are approaches that have had some limited success. Breast reconstruction does not improve the pain or the sensation of tightness in the anterior chest wall.

PHANTOM BREAST PAIN. Following mastectomy, phantom breast sensations have been reported, but phantom pain is rarely if ever noted. Phantom sensations occur in almost all patients but are rarely reported to physicians. The sensations slowly dissipate over months and are associated with the breast telescoping in size.[16]

Postchemotherapy Pain Syndromes

This group includes a series of pain problems that occur in cancer patients receiving chemotherapy. The major features of these entities are briefly described below.

PERIPHERAL NEUROPATHY. The painful dysesthesias following treatment with the vinca alkaloid drugs occur as part of a symmetrical polyneuropathy characterized as a burning pain exacerbated by superficial stimuli. The syndrome is self-limited, usually lasting from 4 to 6 weeks, with resolution of the pain associated with partial return of nerve function. Amitriptyline has been of particular use in the management of this group of pain syndromes.[17]

STEROID PSEUDORHEUMATISM. This entity can follow both rapid and slow withdrawal of steroid medication from patients who have been taking these drugs for either short or long periods of time.[18] The syndrome consists of prominent diffuse myalgias and arthralgias, with muscle and joint tenderness on palpation but without objective inflammatory signs. A sense of generalized malaise and fatigue is common. The signs and symptoms revert with reinstitution of the steroid medication. This pain syndrome is common in breast cancer patients who are being pulsed with steroids as part of their chemotherapy regimen. It is not unusual to see marked exacerbation of pain from bone metastases or epidural cord compression in the setting of steroid withdrawal.

ASEPTIC NECROSIS OF BONE. Aseptic necrosis of the humeral and, much more commonly of the femoral head is a known complication of cancer therapy, and particularly of chronic steroid therapy.[19] Pain in the shoulder or knee is the common presenting complaint, and changes that are visible on x-ray examination occur several weeks or months after the onset of pain. Limitation of joint movements with progressive inability to use the arm or hip functionally is the natural history of this illness. The bone scan is the most useful diagnostic procedure and is usually positive before changes appear in plain films. The appropriate treatment is replacement of the diseased area, which leads to dramatic resolution of the pain complaint.

POSTHERPETIC NEURALGIA. This is a well-described clinical entity characterized by pain that persists after the cutaneous eruptions from herpes zoster infection have cleared. In patients with cancer, herpes zoster infection commonly occurs in an area of tumor pathology or in a port of previous radiation therapy. The true incidence of postherpetic neuralgia in patients with cancer is unknown but appears to be more common in patients who develop the infection after the age of 50. There are generally three types of pain: (1) continuous burning pain in the area of sensory loss, (2) painful dysesthesias, and (3) intermittent shocklike pain. The management of patients with postherpetic neuralgia has recently been reviewed,[20] and the current approach includes the use of mild analgesics, amitriptyline in low doses, and carbamazepine (Tegretol) for management of the intermittent shocklike pain. Although the site of the postherpetic neuralgia pain does not necessarily correspond to the site of previous tumor in patients, the presence of the pain can often obscure underlying pathologic conditions. Again, careful attention to the patient's complaint and to the motor and sensory examination is imperative. If the sensory loss is more extensive than the scarring or if the motor findings are out of the distribution of the nerves involved, further work-up of the patient may be necessary to rule out some other cause such as metastatic disease in bone, paraspinal space, or epidural space.

Postradiation Therapy Pain Syndromes

RADIATION FIBROSIS OF THE BRACHIAL PLEXUS. Pain occurs in 35% of patients presenting with this entity but is characterized by a dull, heavy, burning pain in the hand. The clinical findings have been discussed in the section on brachial plexopathy (Chapter 14).

RADIATION MYELOPATHY. Pain is an early symptom in 15% of patients with this entity.[21] The pain may be localized to the area of spinal cord damage or may be referred, with dysesthesias below the level of injury. Clinically the neurologic symptoms and signs are those of a Brown-Sequard syndrome characterized by an ipsilateral motor paresis with a contralateral sensory loss at a cervicothoracic level. The syndrome progresses to a complete transverse myelopathy. Careful plain x-ray films of the spine and myelography should be undertaken and commonly show normal anatomy. Occasionally, widening of the cord at the injured area may be noted. The differential diagnoses include intramedullary tumor, epidural spinal cord compression, arteriovenous malformation, or a transverse myelitis, but the clinical history, taken with the neurologic findings, can usually make the diagnosis. Management of the pain with carbamazepine (Tegretol) may be of some value, but there are no good therapies available for managing this group of patients.

RADIATION-INDUCED PERIPHERAL NERVE TUMORS. A painful enlarging mass in an area of previous irradiation suggests this entity. Two of the nine patients in the series who developed irradiation-induced peripheral nerve tumors had had previous radiation therapy to the brachial plexus regions 6 to 10 years earlier as part of their primary breast cancer therapy.[22] This particular group of patients points up the need to assess the patient who has recurrent pain and who presents in an atypical fashion or late in the course of an illness. Such patients require needle biopsy or surgical exploration to define the nature of the tumor.

RADIATION NECROSIS OF BONE. Pain that presents in an irradiated site years following radiation therapy needs reassessment to rule out recurrent tumor, but radiation necrosis occurs with a typical radiographic picture. In breast cancer patients, radiation necrosis of the clavicle or rib is the most common type, and bone resection often ameliorates the local bone pain.

Pain Syndromes Unassociated With Cancer or Cancer Therapy

Common pain syndromes that occur in the general population and that are unassociated with cancer or cancer therapy include pain from cervical and lumbar osteoarthritis, osteoporosis, and collapsed vertebral bodies.

MANAGEMENT OF PAIN ASSOCIATED WITH BREAST CANCER

Therapeutic Approaches

The management of pain associated with breast cancer requires an understanding of pain pathophysiology, analgesic pharmacology, and the knowledge of new and established neurosurgical and anesthetic techniques.

The goals of therapy vary with the patient and the clinical setting. For patients undergoing diagnostic evaluation or therapeutic intervention, pain control should allow them to undergo the necessary procedures while at the same time allowing them to function. For terminal patients with metastatic disease, alternatively, an effective pain regimen will allow them to function at a reasonable level with a minimal amount of pain. The tailoring of such a regimen frequently requires the talents of a multidisciplinary team composed of a nurse, social worker, oncologist, neurologist, psychiatrist or psychologist, anesthesiologist, clinical pharmacologist, and neurosurgeon.[1]

Conventional Drug Therapy

The medical management of cancer pain has been the recent topic of several extensive reviews.[3,23–26] Because the pain syndromes associated with breast cancer are frequent and varied and many times are due to multifocal involvement, medical therapy deserves particular emphasis.

As discussed, the first step in the management of pain is the identification of the source and an attempt to eliminate the offending cause with surgery, chemotherapy, or radiation therapy.[27,28] For patients on active antitumor therapy and for those in whom the primary modalities have failed, therapy aimed at symptom control is crucial. Analgesic drug therapy is the first-line approach, with behavioral, anesthetic, and neurosurgical approaches reserved for selected cases.

The analgesic drugs belong to three different categories based on their putative mechanisms of action: (1) the non-narcotic analgesics such as acetaminophen, and the nonsteroidal anti-inflammatory drugs (NSAIDs), which act on peripheral nociceptors; (2) the opiate agonists, mixed agonist-antagonist drugs, and partial agonists that activate opiate receptors in the central and peripheral nervous systems; and (3) the adjuvant analgesic drugs that potentiate the opiates and produce analgesia in certain pain states. The effective use of these categories of drugs requires an appreciation of their clinical pharmacologic characteristics and the recognition that the choice of a drug or combination of drugs must be individualized in each case.

NON-NARCOTIC ANALGESICS AND NSAIDs. These drugs, with aspirin as the prototype, function as a first-line approach in the management of cancer pain and are the drugs of choice for mild to moderate pain. A heterogeneous group, this class of drugs has analgesic potency similar to aspirin, though many of the drugs differ in their anti-inflammatory and antipyretic properties. The mechanism of their analgesic action is through reduction of nociceptor stimulation by inhibition of prostaglandin synthesis. The NSAIDs, in particular, may play an important part in the management of bone metastasis-related pain, in which prostaglandins are believed to have a role.[8]

Table 16-8
Oral and Parenteral Narcotic Analgesics for Severe Pain

	Route	*Equianalgesic Dose (mg)**	*Duration (Hours)*	*Plasma Half-life (Hours)*	*Comments*
Narcotic Agonists					
Morphine	I M P O	10 60	4–6 4–7	2–3.5	Standard for comparison; also available in slow-release tablets.
Codeine	I M P O	130 200+	4–6 4–6	3	Biotransformed to morphine; useful as initial narcotic analgesic.
Oxycodone	I M P O	15 30	3–5	—	Short-acting; available alone or as 5-mg dose in combination with aspirin and acetaminophen.
Levorphanol (Levodromoran)	I M P O	2 4	4–6 4–7	12–16	Good oral potency, requires careful titration in initial dosing because of drug accumulation.
Hydromorphone (Dilaudid)	I M P O	1.5 7.5	4–5 4–6	2–3	Available in high-potency injectable form (10 mg/ml) for cachectic patient and in rectal suppositories; more soluble than morphine.
Meperidine (Demerol)	I M P O	75 300+	4–5 4–6	3–4 Normeperidine 12–16	Contraindicated in patients with renal disease, accumulation of active toxic metabolite normeperidine, produces CNS excitation.
Methadone (Dolophine)	I M P O	10 20		15–30	Good oral potency, requires careful titration in initial dosing to avoid drug accumulation.
Mixed Agonist-Antagonists					
Pentazocine (Talwin)	I M P O	60 180+	4–6 4–7	2–3	Limited use in cancer pain; psychotomimetic effects with dose escalation; available only in combination with naloxone, aspirin, or acetaminophen; may precipitate withdrawal in physically dependent.
Nalbuphine (Nubain)	I M P O	10 —	4–6	5	Not available orally; less psychotomimetic effects than pentazocine, may precipitate withdrawal in physically dependent patients.
Butorphanol (Stadol)	I M P O	2 —	4–6	2.5–3.5	Not available orally; produces psychotomimetic effects; may precipitate withdrawal in physically dependent patients.
Partial Agonists					
Buprenorphine (Temgesic)	I M S L	0.4 0.8	4–6 5–6	?	Not available in United States; no psychotomimetic effects; may precipitate withdrawal in tolerant patients.

* Based on single dose studies in which an I M dose of each drug listed was compared with morphine to establish relative potency. Oral doses are those recommended when changing from parenteral to oral routes. For patients without prior narcotic exposure, the recommended oral starting doses are 30 mg morphine, 5 mg methadone, 2 mg levorphanol, 4 mg hydromorphone.

Unlike opiates, these agents have a ceiling effect, a dose above which no further analgesic benefit will be accrued. Likewise, they do not produce tolerance, but gastrointestinal and hematologic side effects limit their usefulness in the cancer population.

OPIATE AGONISTS, MIXED AGONIST-ANTAGONISTS, AND PARTIAL AGONISTS. Morphine is the standard opiate agonist and produces analgesia by binding specific opioid receptors in the central and peripheral nervous systems. The other drugs in this category, like morphine, are used in the management of moderate to severe pain (Table 16-8). There is no "best" drug, and choice of an analgesic is empiric. The mixed agonist-antagonist opiates have potent analgesic properties but also possess the ability to block opiate receptors when given in large doses. As a rule, these drugs have a limited role in cancer patients because of the psychotomimetic side effects that appear with larger doses. The exception to this is buprenorphine, which is presently only available for parenteral use.[29]

Several properties of the opiate drugs should be considered if they are used chronically. The first is the development of tolerance, a state in which larger or more frequent doses of opiates are needed to maintain analgesic effect. This is to be distinguished from physical dependence, which in turn must be separated from psychological dependence or addiction. Physical dependence refers to the tendency of opiate drugs to induce symptoms and signs of a withdrawal (nausea, vomiting, abdominal cramps, diaphoresis, diarrhea) if they are suddenly discontinued or if an opiate antagonist (e.g., naloxone) or agonist-antagonist is administered to the patient. This state of physical dependence is the expected result of long-term use of opiates and must be anticipated when any change or discontinuation of medication is planned. In contrast, psychological dependence or addiction is not an expected behavioral characteristic in the cancer population.[30] A form of sociopathic behavior, addiction is characterized by drug-craving behavior and obsessive attempts to obtain and use the opiate analgesic. Current knowledge suggests that certain psychological and socioeconomic factors other than chronic drug use are responsible for its development.[31]

In the practical use of opiates, a working knowledge of equianalgesic drug doses will prevent undermedication when switching from one opiate analgesic to another and from one route of administration to another (i.e., from the parenteral route to oral). Studies have shown that cross-tolerance among the opiate analgesics is incomplete, thus providing the physician with a convenient method of prolonging effective analgesia in the population with chronic cancer pain.[32,33] As a starting dose, one-half the calculated equianalgesic dose of the new drug is prescribed, and the dose can be titrated upward as indicated.

Another frequently overlooked point is the clearcut distinction among some opiates between the duration of analgesic action and the plasma half-life. The shorter-acting opiate drugs such as morphine or hydromorphone have the advantage of causing less sedation with chronic dosing but have to be given more frequently in order to maintain analgesic efficacy. Methadone has a plasma half-life of 15 to 30 hours, and levorphanol has a half-life of 12 to 16 hours, but both produce analgesia for only 4 to 6 hours in clinical studies.[34,35] Therefore, with repetitive dosing, oversedation and respiratory depression may occur.[36] For effective analgesia with drugs of long plasma half-lives, an as-needed regimen rather than fixed-interval dosing should therefore be employed. When the patient's pain has stabilized, a fixed-interval dosing schedule will allow the patient to have continuous pain relief.

The use of non-narcotic and adjuvant drugs in combination with opiates provides additive analgesia. The additions of aspirin, acetaminophen,[32] ibuprofen,[37] an antihistamine such as hydroxyzine,[38] or an amphetamine[39] have all been reported to provide increased analgesia. Diazepam, chlorpromazine, and cocaine do not provide additive analgesia, and there is little evidence favoring "cocktail" formulas over individually tailored combinations of drugs.[40–42]

The side effects and potential complications of opiate analgesics deserve mention in any discussion of their use. Anticipated side effects include sedation, respiratory depression, nausea, vomiting, and constipation. Sedation varies with the drug and dose and is particularly common with repetitive administration. Management includes the reduction of dosage, changing the dosage interval, or switching to an opiate with a shorter half-life. The addition of amphetamine is effective in counteracting sedation as well as augmenting analgesia.[39] Respiratory depression is a serious complication, but tolerance to this effect develops with chronic use. When respiratory depression occurs in a cancer patient chronically receiving opiates, it can be rapidly reversed by the specific opiate antagonist, naloxone. In order to prevent severe withdrawal reactions, 0.4 mg of naloxone should be diluted in 10 mg of saline and slowly infused intravenously. Repeated administrations may be necessary, including an intravenous drip. In patients receiving meperedine, naloxone may precipitate seizures by lowering the seizure threshold.

Nausea and vomiting due to opiate activation of the medullary chemoreceptor zone may occur with all the opiates but are not predictable side effects. Tolerance to these side effects may also develop, but the use of antiemetics and antiemetic histamines is often necessary when the patient is first started on a drug regimen.

Constipation, on the other hand, is a predictable side effect due to opiate effects at multiple sites of the gastrointestinal tract and its neuromusculature. Several prophylactic regimens have been recommended, but the choice of any one must be empiric as there are no controlled studies.[43]

Finally, myoclonus and seizures may complicate the long-term use of opiates. These signs of central nervous system hyperirritability have been encountered most commonly with meperidine. Normeperedine, an active hepatic metabolite of meperidine, is excreted by the kidneys, and accumulation from repeated chronic dosing or renal insufficiency may cause myoclonus or generalized seizures.[44]

Alternate Methods of Drug Administration

Alternate methods and routes of drug delivery have been employed to avoid the inconveniences and inadequacies of conventional opiate administration (e.g., poor oral bioavailability, the discomfort of intermittent parenteral administration, and peak-trough phenomena). Slow-release forms of oral morphine are now available and provide more continuous gastrointestinal absorption, thereby minimizing peak and trough side effects. Unlike immediate-release morphine, the dosage interval for oral slow-release morphine preparations is every 8 to 12 hours. The sublingual route of administration has the benefit of bypassing the first-pass effect of the liver, and a sublingual preparation of the partial agonist buprenorphine will soon be available in the United States.[29]

Continuous intravenous and subcutaneous infusions provide constant plasma levels of opiate and preclude the need for and discomfort of repeated intravenous, intramuscular, or subcutaneous injections. Morphine, hydromorphone, meperedine, methadone, and levorphanol all have been used, and guidelines have been developed for their use.[45]

Epidural and Intrathecal Opiate Administration

Epidural and intrathecal opiate administration provides significant analgesia through the activation of opiate receptors in the spinal cord.[46–48] The advantage of this method of opiate administration is selective suppression of ascending spinothalamic pathways without additional sensory or motor blockade. With small doses of opiate, there is minimal distribution to the supraspinal opiate receptors responsible for mediating the intolerable side effects that accompany systemically administered drugs (sedation, respiratory depression, constipation, myoclonus). Both continuous administration and intermittent bolus administration of opiates have been studied and found to be effective in cancer patients with pain. Unfortunately, the cross-tolerance induced by systemically administered drugs and the rapid development of tolerance with spinal administration of drugs in cancer patients influence the usefulness of this procedure.[47] There is controversy over the optimal timing for employing these approaches, and comparative trials with oral opiate administration are lacking.

Adjuvant Analgesic Drugs

Adjuvant analgesic drugs, with few exceptions, do not possess major analgesic properties in and of themselves but are used to enhance the analgesic effects of other drugs and to counteract side effects. Aside from methotrimeprazine, a potent phenothiazine analgesic, these drugs rarely function as independent analgesics. They include anticonvulsants, antidepressants, and neuroleptics.

The anticonvulsants carbamazepine and phenytoin have well-established roles in the treatment of neuropathic pain and trigeminal neuralgia. Their mechanism of action is supposedly the suppression of unrestrained neuronal firing. In cancer pain, their specific roles involve the management of lancinating neuralgic pain associated with tumor infiltration or surgical nerve injury (plexopathy, stump pain). Doses start at 100 mg per day and approach the dosages used for seizure management.

Of the phenothiazine drugs, only methotrimeprazine possesses analgesic qualities, and 15 mg intravenously is equivalent to 10 mg of intramuscular morphine. This drug is particularly useful as a short-term opiate-sparing analgesic in circumstances in which opiates are undesirable or ineffective—for example, in bowel obstruction or after gastrointestinal surgery. In addition to its analgesic properties, it also has antiemetic and sedative properties.

The tricyclic antidepressants have a proven record as analgesics in the management of patients with migraines, postherpetic neuralgia, and diabetic neuropathy.[17,20,49] The serotonergic antidepressants such as amitriptyline have been found useful in doses lower than those used for depression. Controlled studies in the population with cancer pain are necessary to further define their role.

Corticosteroids possess anti-inflammatory, antitumor, and mood-altering effects and play a useful role in patients with cancer pain.[50–52] In particular, the ability of steroids to produce euphoria, improved appetite, and a sense of well-being has been praised as beneficial in terminally ill cancer patients and is associated with prolonged survival time and reduced narcotic requirements in some studies. In certain cases, such as epidural spinal cord compression[10] and lumbosacral and brachial plexopathies, steroids have demonstrated analgesic efficacy.

Of particular relevance to patients with breast cancer and pain are the reports of the successful use of L-dopa in the management of metastatic bone pain.[53,54] In one study,[53] 10 of 30 patients with breast cancer metastatic to bone responded to a 48-hour course of L-dopa and showed objective signs of tumor regression (normalization of bone scans and bone films). In three patients, a positive response to L-dopa predicted a beneficial response to surgical pituitary ablation, and a total of nine patients demonstrated the suppression of prolactin levels to less than one-half of baseline while taking L-dopa. The significance of pituitary and, more specifically, prolactin suppression in mediating analgesia in breast cancer is controversial and has not been confirmed in neurosurgical series when analgesia following hypophysectomy was independent of endocrine function (see below).[55]

Anesthetic Approaches to Pain

These approaches require specific expertise, and certain guidelines apply to their use (Tables 16-9 and 16-10). Historically these procedures have been employed late in the course of a patient's illness because patients prefer to defer these procedures until they complete their anticancer therapy. Also, when informed about the potential risks of neurologic impairment associated with the procedures, many patients are unwilling to accept such a risk for pain control alone. Some of these procedures are briefly considered in the paragraphs that follow.

TRIGGER POINT INJECTIONS. Myofascial trigger points represent painful, hyperirritable areas of muscle or fascia and can be relieved by local injections of either short-acting local anesthetic or saline.

PERIPHERAL NERVE BLOCKS. This technique is most useful for the control of pain associated with tumor infiltration of the chest wall as in locally recurrent breast cancer. Successful injection of a local anesthetic blocks nerve conduction, and a permanent nerve block can be achieved with the injection of a neurolytic agent such as absolute alcohol or phenol. These agents cause nerve demyelination and secondary axonal degeneration. This technique is usually limited to the chest or abdominal wall, where the disruption of both sensory and motor function will not be disabling.

Table 16-9
Types of Anesthetic Procedures Commonly Used for Cancer Pain

Type of Procedure	*Most Common Indications*
Nerve block	
Peripheral	Pain in discrete dermatomes in chest and abdomen
Epidural	Unilateral lumbar or sacral pain Midline perineal pain Bilateral lumbosacral pain
Intrathecal	Midline perineal pain Bilateral lumbosacral pain
Autonomic Stellate ganglion	Reflex sympathetic dystrophy (e.g., frozen shoulder) Arm pain
Lumbar sympathetic	Reflex sympathetic dystrophy Lumbrosacral plexopathy Vascular insufficiency of the lower extremity
Celiac plexus	Midabdominal pain
Continuous epidural infusion with local anesthetics	Unilateral and bilateral lumbosacral pain Midline perineal pain
Chemical hypophysectomy	Diffuse bone pain
Inhalation therapy	Generalized pain Incident pain
Trigger-point injection	Focal muscle pain

(Foley KM: The treatment of cancer pain. N Engl J Med 313:84–95, 1985)

Table 16-10
Neuroablative, Neurostimulatory, and Neuropharmacologic Procedures for Relief of Pain from Cancer

Site	*Procedure*		
	Neuroablative	*Neurostimulatory*	*Pharmacologic*
Peripheral nerve	Neurectomy	Transcutaneous and percutaneous electrical nerve stimulation	Local anesthetics
Nerve root	Rhizotomy		Local anesthetics Neurolytic agents
Spinal cord	Dorsal-root entry-zone lesions Cordotomy Myelotomy	Dorsal-column stimulation	Epidural and intrathecal local anesthetics and opiates
Brain stem	Mesencephalic tractotomy	Periaqueductal stimulation	Intraventricular opiates
Thalamus	Thalamotomy	Thalamic stimulation	
Cortex	Cingulumotomy Frontal lobotomy		
Pituitary	Transsphenoidal hypophysectomy		Chemical hypophysectomy

(Foley KM: The treatment of cancer pain. N Engl J Med 313:84–95, 1985)

AUTONOMIC NERVE BLOCKS. Autonomic nerve blocks involve the injection of a local anesthetic or neurolytic agent into the stellate ganglion for brachial plexus and other arm pain, the celiac plexus for midabdominal pain, and the lumbar sympathetic chain for lumbosacral plexus pain. In patients with brachial plexopathy, local anesthetic infiltration followed by neurolytic infiltration of the stellate ganglion on the involved side may provide temporary relief. However, inconsistent results and the frequent distortion of the anatomy due to local disease recurrence limit the usefulness of this procedure.[56]

EPIDURAL AND INTRATHECAL NERVE BLOCKS. Epidural and intrathecal nerve blocks play a significant role in the management of specific pain syndromes, and both local anesthetic and neurolytic solutions have been used.[57,58] For lumbosacral plexus or spine pain, intermittent or continuous epidural infusion of local anesthetic is useful, providing analgesia with relative sparing of motor and autonomic function. Side effects are minimal, and the risk of infection is low, especially if the device is internalized. The benefit of this approach is in its opiate-sparing potential, allowing for a reduction or a "holiday" from systemic opiates and enabling the partial reversal of established opiate tolerance.

Permanent intrathecal or epidural nerve blocks with phenol or alcohol are used to manage patients with advanced disease. This chemical rhizotomy can be used for localized pain in the abdomen and thorax and has been useful in midline perineal pain as well.[56] The neurolytic agent is introduced into the thecal sac or epidural space, where it contacts afferents emanating from (and efferent traveling to) areas of nociception and destroys the nerve fibers. Ideally, by positioning the patient and controlling the concentration of the agent, dorsal sensory roots can be preferentially affected. Unfortunately this is not always the case, and motor and autonomic involvement are frequent complications. For this reason, this ablative technique is reserved for patients who (1) have failed all modes of medical pain and tumor control, (2) are poor candidates for surgical neuroablative procedures, (3) cannot tolerate aggressive opiate therapy, (4) have had successful diagnostic epidural or intrathecal blocks with local anesthetics, and (5) have no epidural block shown on myelography.

Lastly, nitrous oxide, when administered with oxygen through a non-rebreathing mask, has analgesic properties. When it is added to systemic opiates, relief of anxiety and pain is augmented without additional sedation in the patient with far-advanced disease.[59]

Neurosurgical Approaches to Pain

The neurosurgical management of cancer pain includes a series of neuroablative and neurostimulatory procedures.[2,60–63] Neuroablative procedures involve the creation of surgical or radio-frequency lesions along the ascending pain pathways, and neurostimulatory procedures require the stereotactic placement of stimulatory electrodes in pathways or areas that modulate or inhibit the ascending neospinothalamic pathways.

The common neuroablative procedures are listed in Table 16-10.

DORSAL RHIZOTOMY. This procedure has most commonly been used to manage brachial plexopathy pain. It involves the truncation of sensory roots, sparing the motor roots and resulting in complete anesthesia in a restricted area. It requires a laminectomy, and, because multiple nerve roots must be cut, the patient is left with a complete sensory deficit, rendering the limb functionless. A more selective approach entailing microsurgical section of anterolateral fibers as they enter the spinal cord is said to result in less proprioceptive loss, but detailed experience is lacking.[64]

DORSAL ROOT ENTRY ZONE LESIONS (DREZ). DREZ lesions are a more recent procedure involving the stereotactic thermocoagulation of the dorsal root entry zone as well as the dorsal roots. There has been particular interest in using DREZ lesions to treat the pain associated with malignant brachial plexopathies and traumatic avulsion of the brachial plexus. Limited data suggest the usefulness of this procedure.[65]

ANTEROLATERAL CORDOTOMY. The anterolateral cordotomy is a procedure that surgically interrupts the neospinothalamic tract in the cervical or thoracic cord, and it can be performed either by an open surgical approach or by a percutaneous stereotactic procedure. The procedure is most useful for pain in the lower thoracic and lumbosacral dermatomes and is particularly useful in patients with localized unilateral disease.[66] High cervical cordotomy has been of only limited value in patients with brachial plexopathy, because the level of pain relief often falls following the cordotomy. Midline pain syndromes, such as those in lumbosacral spine disease or localized pelvic disease, require bilateral cordotomies. The procedure is associated with certain risks, particularly when high cervical cordotomies or bilateral cordotomies are performed. With cervical cordotomies, there is a risk of phrenic nerve paralysis in addition to the risks that accompany the sectioning of the spinal cord—hemiparesis, ataxia, or urinary tract dysfunction. Unfortunately, within 6 months of a cordotomy, up to 50% of patients who initially achieved relief develop new pain either on the mirror side or in a previously unrecognized site. In patients living longer than 18 months, the development of a postcordotomy dysesthetic deafferentation syndrome may occur.

MIDLINE MYELOTOMY. Midline myelotomy or commissural myelotomy is a procedure that has stimulated new interest in the management of midline or bilateral cancer pain. After a T9 to L1 laminectomy, the spinal cord is split through the ventral sulcus, sparing the anterior spinal artery, using either a myelotome or a carbon dioxide laser.[67–69] This procedure reportedly does not disturb sphincter or motor function but may cause cutaneous dysesthesias in as many as 30% of patients.

Neurostimulatory Procedures

Neurostimulatory procedures include transcutaneous nerve stimulation (TENS), dorsal column and direct nerve stimulation, brain stem periventricular stimulation, and thalamic stimulation.

TENS. TENS has its theoretical basis in the gate theory of pain.[70] Both low- and high-intensity stimulation are applied to peripheral nerves in order to activate large-diameter fiber afferent nerves and facilitate inhibition of nociceptive afferents as they enter the dorsal horn. As many as 40% of cancer patients may respond to TENS, particularly if the pain is acute,[71] but the transient benefit reduces the usefulness of this procedure.

DORSAL COLUMN STIMULATION. Similar techniques are used in stimulating the cervical and thoracic spinal cord. In one series, about 50% of patients achieved some relief from cancer pain. Recently the enthusiasm for the technique has waned.[72]

BRAIN STEM AND THALAMIC STIMULATION. A limited number of studies have demonstrated beneficial effects of this technique in patients with bilateral or midline pain syndromes.[73] These early studies have used chronic depth electrodes placed under local anesthesia. Fifty percent of patients have achieved pain relief, at least temporarily, but more patients need to be studied in a randomized fashion.

Chemical and Transsphenoidal Hypophysectomy

As mentioned in the discussion of the effect of L-dopa on bone pain, there is evidence that neuroendocrine ablative procedures may provide at least palliative benefit in patients with breast cancer metastatic to bone. Both chemical hypophysectomy (suprasellar injection of alcohol) and transsphenoidal hypophysectomy have been associated with palliation of pain in 35% to 75% of patients.[74,75] In one study, transfrontal hypophysectomy in six patients with epidural spinal cord compression from breast cancer resulted in pain relief in four patients and evidence of tumor regression.[76] The mechanism for production of analgesia is uncertain. It may be related to disruption of the hypothalamic-thalamic endorphinergic pain pathways. Despite earlier evidence in studies with L-dopa suggesting that pituitary hormonal suppression mediated analgesic effects,[53] there are little data to support this contention in patients who have undergone transsphenoidal hypophysectomy.[55]

SUMMARY AND CONCLUSIONS

From the above description of the pain syndromes associated with breast cancer and the available methods of analgesia, the initial approach to the management of a patient's pain should be an attempt to control the causative factors. When this fails, an individually tailored analgesic regimen should be constructed with the assistance and expertise of a variety of pain specialists. The rational use of systemic opiates and nonopiate analgesics form the first line of treatment and are supplemented by various anesthetic and neurosurgical procedures.

REFERENCES

1. Foley KM: Pain syndromes in patients with cancer. In Bonica JJ, Ventafridda V, Fink RB, Jones LE, et al (eds): Advances in Pain Research and Therapy, Vol. 2, pp 59–75. New York, Raven Press, 1979
2. Twycross RG, Fairfield S: Pain in far-advanced cancer. Pain 14:303–310, 1982
3. Foley KM: The treatment of cancer pain. N Engl J Med 313:84–95, 1985
4. Basbaum AI, Fields HL: Endogeneous pain control mechanisms: Review and hypothesis. Ann Neurol 4:451–462, 1978
5. Payne R, Foley KM: Advances in the management of cancer pain. Cancer Treat Rep 68:173–183, 1984
6. Tasker RR, Tsuda T, Hawrylyshyn P: Clinical neurophysiological investigation of deafferentation pain. In Bonica JJ, Lindblom U, Iggo A (eds): Advances in Pain Research and Therapy, Vol. 5, pp 713–738. New York, Raven Press, 1981
7. Brodie GN: Indomethacin and bone pain. Lancet 2:1160, 1974
8. Galasko CSB: Mechanisms of bone destruction in the development of skeletal metastases. Nature 263:507–510, 1976
9. Greenberg JS, Deck MDF, Vikram B, et al: Metastasis to the base of the skull: Clinical findings in 43 patients. Neurology 31:530–537, 1981
10. Gilbert RW, Kim J-H, Posner JB: Epidural spinal cord compression from metastatic tumor: Diagnosis and treatment. Ann Neurol 3:40–51, 1978
11. Sundaresan N, Galicich JH, Lane J: Treatment of odontoid fractures in cancer patients. J Neurosurg 54:187–192, 1981
12. Cascino FL, Kori S, Krol G, et al: CT of the brachial plexus in patients with cancer. Neurology 33:1553–1557, 1983
13. Jaeckle KA, Young DF, Foley KM: The natural history of lumbosacral plexopathy. Neurology 35:8–15, 1985
14. Granike I, Ashikari R, Foley KM: The postmastectomy pain syndrome. Proc American Society of Clinical Oncology 3:122, 1983
15. Temple WJ, Ketcham AS: Preservation of the intercostobrachial nerve during axillary dissection for breast cancer. Am J Surg 150:585–588, 1985
16. Staps T, Hooyenhout J, Wobbes T: Phantom breast sensation following mastectomy. Cancer 56:2898–2901, 1985
17. Watson CP, Evan RJ, Reed K, et al: Amitriptyline vs. placebo in postherpetic neuralgia. Neurology 32:671–673, 1984
18. Rotstein J, Good RA: Steroid pseudorheumatism. Arch Intern Med 99:545–555, 1957
19. Fisher DE, Bickel WH: Corticosteroid-induced avascular necrosis: A clinical study of seventy-seven patients. J Bone Joint Surg 53:859–873, 1971
20. Portenoy RK, Duma C, Foley KM: Acute herpetic and postherpetic neuralgia: Review of clinical features and current therapy. Ann Neurol (in press) 1986
21. Palmer JJ: Radiation myelopathy. Brain 95:109–122, 1972
22. Foley KM, Woodruff TM, Ellis FT, et al: Radiation-induced malignant and atypical peripheral nerve sheath tumors. Ann Neurol 7:311–318, 1980

23. Foley KM, Sundaresan N: Management of cancer pain. In DeVita VT, Hellman S, Rosenberg SA (eds): Cancer: Principles and Practice of Oncology, pp 1940–1961. Philadelphia, JB Lippincott, 1985
24. Foley KM: Analgesic management of bone pain. In Weiss L, Hilbert HA (eds): Bone Metastases, pp 348–368. Boston, GK Hall Medical Publishers, 1981
25. Beaver WT: Management of cancer pain with parenteral medication. JAMA 244:2653–2657, 1980
26. Foley KM: The practical use of narcotic analgesics. In Reidenberg MM (ed): The Medical Clinics of North America, pp 1091–1104. Philadelphia, WB Saunders Co, 1982
27. Bonadonna E, Molinari R: Role and limits of anticancer drugs in the treatment of advanced cancer pain. In Bonica JJ, Ventafridda V (eds): Advances in Pain Research and Therapy, Vol. 2, pp 81–88. New York, Raven Press, 1979
28. Trodella L, Ausili-Cefaro G, Turrizianian A, et al: Pain in osseous metastases: Results of radiotherapy. Pain 18:387–396, 1984
29. Robbie DS: A trial of sublingual buprenorphine in cancer pain. Br J Clin Pharmacol 7:315S–385S, 1979
30. Porter J, Jick H: Addiction rare in patients treated with narcotics. N Engl J Med 302:123, 1980
31. Newman RG: The need to redefine "addiction." N Engl J Med 308:1096–1098, 1983
32. Houde RW, Wallenstein SL, Beaver WT: Evaluation of analgesics in patients with cancer pain. In Lasagna L (ed): International Encyclopedia of Pharmacology and Therapeutics, pp 59–97. New York, Pergamon Press, 1966
33. Inturrisi CE, Foley KM: Narcotic analgesics in the management of pain. In Kuhar M, Pasternak G (eds): Analgesics: Neurochemical, Behavioral and Clinical Perspectives, pp 257–287. New York, Raven Press, 1984
34. Inturrisi CE, Verebely K: Disposition of methadone in man after a single oral dose. Clin Pharmacol Ther 13:923–930, 1972
35. Dixon R, Crews T, Mohasci C, Inturrisis CE, Foley KM: Levorphanol: Radioimmunoassay and plasma concentration profiles in dog and man. Res Commun Chem Pathol Pharmacol 29:535–547, 1980
36. Symonds P: Methadone and the elderly. Br Med J 1:512, 1977
37. Ferrer-Brechner T, Ganz P: Combination therapy with ibuprofen and methadone for chronic cancer pain. Am J Med 77:78–83, 1983
38. Beaver WT, Feise G: Comparison of analgesic effects of morphine sulfate, hydroxyzine and their combination in patients with postoperative pain. In Bonica JJ, Albe-Fessard D (eds): Advances in Pain Research and Therapy, Vol. 1, pp 553–557. New York, Raven Press, 1976
39. Forrest WH, Brown BW, Brown CR, et al: Dextroamphetamine with morphine for the treatment of postoperative pain. N Engl J Med 296:712–715, 1977
40. Singh PN, Sharma P, Gupta PK, et al: Chemical evaluation of diazepam for relief of postoperative pain. Br J Anaesth 53:831–835, 1981
41. Dundee JW, Moore J: The myth of phenothiazine potentiation. Anaesthesia 16:95–96, 1961
42. Kaiko RF, Kanner R, Foley KM, et al: Morphine and cocaine in patients with cancer pain. Proc 4th World Congress on Pain, 1984
43. Maguire LC, Yan JL, Miller E: Prevention of narcotic-induced constipation. N Engl J Med 305:1651, 1981
44. Kaiko RF, Foley KM, Grabinski P, et al: Central nervous system excitatory effects of meperidine in cancer patients. Ann Neurol 13:180–185, 1983
45. Campbell CF, Mason JB, Weiler JM: Continuous subcutaneous infusion of morphine for the pain of terminal malignancy. Ann Intern Med 98:51–52, 1983
46. Cousins MJ, Mather LE: Intrathecal and epidural administration of opioids. Anesthesiology 61:276–310, 1984
47. Greenberg H, Taren J, Ensminger WD, et al: Benefit from and tolerance to continuous intrathecal infusion of morphine for intractable cancer pain. J Neurosurg 57:300–364, 1982
48. Max MB, Inturrisi CE, Grabinski P, et al: Epidural opiates: Plasma and cerebrospinal fluid (CSF) pharmakokinetics of morphine, methadone, and beta-endorphin. Pain (Suppl 2): Third World Congress on Pain, IASP, S122, 1981
49. Walsh TD: Antidepressants in chronic pain. Clin Neuropharmacol 6:271–295, 1983
50. Schell HW: The risk of adrenal corticosteroid therapy in far advanced cancer. Am J Med Sci 252:641–644, 1966
51. Schell HW: Adrenal corticosteroid therapy in far advanced cancer. Geriatrics 27:131–141, 1972
52. Twycross RG, Ventfridda V (eds): The continuing care of terminal cancer patients. Oxford, Pergamon Press, 1980
53. Minton JP: The response of breast cancer patients with bone pain to L-dopa. Cancer 33:358–363, 1974
54. Tolis GJ: L-dopa for pain of bone metastases. N Engl J Med 292:1353–1354, 1975
55. LaRossa JT, Strong MS, Melby JC: Endocrinologically incomplete transethmoidal trans-sphenoidal hypophysectomy with relief of bone pain in breast cancer. N Engl J Med 298:1332–1335, 1978
56. Swerdlow M: Role of nerve blocks in pain involving the chest and brachial plexus. In Bonica JJ, Ventafridda V (eds): Advances in Pain Research and Therapy, Vol. 2, pp 567–576. New York, Raven Press, 1979
57. Moore DC: Role of nerve blocks with neurolytic solutions in visceral and perineal pain. In Bonica JJ, Ventafridda V (eds): Advances in Pain Research and Therapy, Vol. 2, pp 593–605. New York, Raven Press, 1979
58. Brechner VL, Ferrer-Brechner T, Allen GD: Anesthetic measures in the management of pain associated with malignancy. Semin Oncol 4:99–108, 1977
59. Fosburg MT, Crone RK: Nitrous oxide analgesia for refractory pain in the terminally ill. JAMA 250:511–513, 1983
60. Nathan PW: Pain in cancer: Comparison of results of cordotomy and chemical rhizotomy. In Fusek I, King I (eds): Present Limits of Neurosurgery, pp 513–516. Amsterdam, Excerpta Medica, 1972
61. Nathan PW: Results of antero-lateral cordotomy for pain in cancer. J Neurol Neurosurg Psychiatry 26:353–362, 1963
62. Friedberg S: Neurosurgical treatment of pain caused by cancer. Med Clin North Am 59:481–485, 1975
63. White JC, Sweet WH: Pain and the Neurosurgeon. Springfield, IL, Charles C Thomas, 1969
64. Sindou M, Fischer G, Mansuy L: Posterior spinal rhizotomy and selective posterior rhizotomy. Prog Neurol Surg 7:201–250, 1976
65. Nashold BS, Ostdahl RH: Dorsal root entry zone lesions for pain relief. J Neurosurg 512:59–69, 1979
66. Kanner RM, Foley KM, Galicich J: Patient selection for cordotomy in patients with cancer. Neurology 31:45, 1981
67. King RB: Anterior commissural myelotomy for intractable pain. J Neurosurg 47:7–11, 1977
68. Cook AW, Kawakami Y: Commissural myelotomy. J Neurosurg 47:1–6, 1977
69. Fink RA: Neurosurgical treatment of non-malignant intractable rectal pain: Microsurgical commissural rhizotomy with the Larkin dioxide laser. Neurosurgery 14:64–65, 1984

70. Melzack R, Wall PD: Pain mechanisms: A new theory. Science 150:971–979, 1965
71. Ventafridda V, Sganzerla EP, Fochi C, et al: Transcutaneous nerve stimulation in cancer pain. In Bonica JJ (ed): Advances in Cancer Pain, pp 509–515. New York, Raven Press, 1979
72. Loeser JD: Dorsal column and peripheral nerve stimulation for relief of cancer pain. In Bonica JJ, Ventafridda V (eds): Advances in Pain Research and Therapy, Vol. 2, pp 499–507. New York, Raven Press, 1979
73. Meyerson BA: Central nervous system stimulation for cancer pain: Possible methods of manipulating the physiology of pain control. In Bonica JJ, Ventafridda V (eds): Advances in Pain Research and Therapy, Vol. 4, pp 149–164. New York, Raven Press, 1982
74. Moricca G: Chemical hypophysectomy for cancer pain. In Bonica JJ (ed): Advances in Neurology, Vol. 4, pp 707–714. New York, Raven Press, 1974
75. Miles J, Lipton S: Mode of action by which pituitary alcohol injection relieves pain. In Bonica JJ (ed): Advances in Pain Research and Therapy, Vol. 1, pp 867–869. New York, Raven Press, 1976
76. Sengupta RP, Lassman LP: Hypophysectomy for severe spinal cord complications from breast carcinoma. Paraplegia 12:111–117, 1974

Interpreting Clinical Data

17

Rebecca Gelman Marvin Zelen

In 1924, Major Greenwood[1] (of life-table fame) published an article in the *Lancet* entitled "Is the statistical method of any value in medical research?" He mentioned the contention of some researchers that "there is, properly speaking, no special method or art of medical statistics; plain good sense is all that is required" and countered this contention with some examples of "terrible results of common sense." Greenwood's position was that "there is a kind of statistical tact, which is rather more than simple good sense; some are born with it; . . . the rest of us have to acquire it." He also noted that relations between statisticians and physicians had improved over time: "Twenty years ago, there was some tendency to treat the statistician or biometrician as a pariah, and he acquired the virtues and vices of a minority, a certain courage and a certain trick of overemphasis—they always characterize a fighting minority. Now, statistics and statisticians are perfectly respectable; there may even be a risk of putting the claims of the statistical expert too high."

Since Major Greenwood's time, there has been a remarkable evolution in the development of methodology motivated by problems arising in the planning, execution, and analysis of clinical trials. This development represents a joint effort by both statisticians and clinical investigators. It has flourished because of the widespread recognition of the need to objectively evaluate the effects of therapy rather than depend on individual subjective assessments. The variability in prognosis associated with the natural history of breast cancer and the need to have long-term follow-up make the application of objective methods of evaluation particularly important with regard to assessing the benefits of therapy.

Although as statisticians we are loath to admit that it is possible to "put the claims of statistics too high," the widespread acceptance of modern statistical methods by medical investigators has sometimes resulted in an overemphasis of some statistical concepts. A particularly notorious example is the ubiquitous acceptance by medical journal editors of the need to have "$p < 0.05$" as a requirement for acceptance of articles.

This chapter is an attempt to provide examples of "statistical tact." There are three principal situations in clinical trials in which one has a chance to demonstrate such tact: designing a study, analyzing a study, and evaluating the medical literature. The first two situations are described in the two main sections of this chapter. To some extent, evaluating the medical literature involves evaluating how well the authors designed and analyzed their studies. So it is hoped that consumers of medical literature will develop statistical tact by reading both of the sections presented here.

DESIGN OF STUDIES

This section discusses some of the more controversial issues in study design for breast cancer trials: randomization, eligibility criteria, stratification, sample size, and response definitions.

Randomization

Randomization is a process by which treatments are assigned to patients so that each patient registered for a trial has the same opportunity of being assigned to any of the treatments under investigation. The implementation of this equal opportunity is a chance mechanism based on the laws of probability. The simplest situation is a clinical trial investigating two treatments in which the assignment of a treatment to an individual patient is made so that there is an equal probability (one in two) of receiving either of the two treatments. Conceptually, this is equivalent to tossing a fair coin to decide the assignment. In practice, the assignment is carried out by using a table of random numbers. (Random-number tables consist of an array of digits in which each digit has an equal probability (one in ten) of appearing in any row or column.) For the case of two treatments, the assignment could be made by choosing odd versus even numbers for the randomization. One essential feature is that at the time of registration neither the physician nor the patient knows which treatment will be assigned. (Hence allocating treatments according to the patient's name, hospital number, day first seen, or according to a randomization schedule to which the physician has access does not result in a randomized trial, since in each case it is possible for the physician to know the treatment assignment before entering the patient in the study.) In more complicated clinical trial designs, the randomization may be blocked or stratified or both. Blocking ensures exact balance in the numbers of patients assigned to each treatment after predetermined numbers of patients have been entered in a trial. For example, one could have a scheme that, after each set of ten patients is entered, results in five of these new patients being assigned to treatment A and five to B. Stratification ensures balance of treatment assignments within important patient subgroups. Both blocking and stratification can be carried out with a predetermined schedule or dynamically at each randomization (taking into account how much imbalance would be caused by each possible treatment assignment).[2]

There are three main purposes of randomization: to balance on average all known and unknown prognostic factors, to provide a basis for statistical inference (i.e., significance tests), and to eliminate conscious and unconscious bias.[3] The phrase "on average" is sometimes misunderstood, to the extent that "when it is shown that there are appreciable differences between groups or one or more baseline characteristics" some investigators "conclude that the randomization has failed in its purpose and that standard analyses are no longer relevant."[3] In fact, some imbalance among prognostic factors not used for stratification is expected in a randomized trial. For example, in a randomized study with 14 prognostic variables, there is a 50% chance that at least one of the prognostic variables will be imbalanced across treatments enough so that a naive computation of the significance level of the imbalance would yield $p < 0.05$. In the extreme, the probability is less than 0.05 that a nonstratified randomized trial with 58 prognostic factors will have no "statistically significant" prognostic factor imbalance. To balance prognostic factors on average means that there will be balance among treatments with respect to all factors over a hypothetically infinite number of trials studying the same issue.

The second important property provides "a scale of variability on which an observed difference (in treatment outcomes) may be assessed in order to judge whether it is a larger one than a random allocation would normally produce"[3] between two equally effective treatments. "It is thus the process of randomization that generates the significance test, and this process is independent of prognostic factors, known or unknown,"[4] balanced or not.

The third reason for randomization is to control bias. The term "bias" here refers to any factor other than treatment that might influence outcome. Various categorizations of biases eliminated by randomization have been listed by many authors.[4–8] As R.A. Fisher stated in 1925,[8] randomization "relieves the experimenter from the anxiety of considering and estimating the magnitude of the innumerable causes by which his data may be disturbed." Such causes include the following:

Selection bias, either patient (e.g., patients destined to have shorter survival time tend to select a treatment requiring fewer visits to the cancer center) or physician (e.g., physicians tend to put patients who will have poor compliance on regimens with less toxicity).

Eligibility bias (e.g., patients are excluded from the analysis of several regimens for different reasons).

Diagnostic bias, sometimes called "stage creep" (as diagnostic and staging tests get better, each stage except the worst loses some bad prognostic patients and each stage except possibly the first gains some good prognostic patients; hence, survival appears to improve within each stage although overall survival may stay the same).

Bias due to changes in definitions over time (e.g., response, severe toxicity) or of the people doing the evaluation (e.g., the well-known July 1 effect related to change in hospital staff).

Bias due to differences in follow-up, either extent of follow-up (e.g., for some statistical tests censored observations cannot count "against" a treatment; therefore, a group with short follow-up may appear to have better survival rates than a group with long follow-up, even though both groups will have the same survival curves when all data are available) or frequency of follow-up (patients who have more frequent blood counts will, as a group, have lower nadir counts than patients who have less frequent blood counts).

Bias due to changes in ancillary therapy or supportive care (including such things as propensity to hospitalize, availability of different antibiotics, pain relief protocols).

Bias due to regression to the mean (e.g., metastatic patients tend to be put on a new treatment when their disease is rapidly growing or when they have new or worsening symptoms; the normal fluctuations of tumor growth rates or symptoms within a single patient guarantee that some patients will improve simply because the bad symptoms were a transient phenomenon).

The three goals of randomization can never be completely met using nonrandomized designs. This does not mean that there is no place in breast cancer research for nonrandomized or even uncontrolled trials. As Gehan and Freireich[9] point out, "the primary purpose of many clinical trials is not evaluation of relative effectiveness, so that a control group is not needed." For this reason, phase I drug trials, early phase II drug trials, and early studies of new surgical or radiotherapy techniques are usually nonrandomized. The purpose of such studies is to allow physicians to gain enough expertise in the new treatments to permit a fair comparison with established treatments in a future phase III trial and to document that the new treatments show enough promise to justify a phase III trial. Because such uncontrolled trials are subject to all the biases listed above, they should be interpreted with care. In Moertel and Reitemeier's report[10] of 20 phase II trials of the use of 5-fluorouracil (5-FU) in advanced bowel cancer, the percentage of responders ranged from 8% to 85%, with the 6 largest trials (40 to 150 patients) having response percentages ranging from 11% to 55%.

Although uncontrolled phase II studies may be very unreliable, there is some reason to encourage the use of more of such studies before a randomized comparative trial is done. It has been estimated[11] that in the current research environment, more than half of the clinical trials reported as positive in the literature (i.e., showing a significant difference with $p < 0.05$) are actually false-positives. That is, if the a priori probability that a clinical trial will result in a significant advance is 5% and if only trials large enough to have a false-negative rate of 10% are undertaken (and most trials reported in the literature are smaller than this), then there will be equal numbers of true-positive and false-positive trials reported. One way to increase the proportion of true-positive studies is to do much bigger randomized studies. However, another way is "to carry out pilot studies before launching a definitive study. If the pilot studies are encouraging, then proceed with a large comparative study."[11] One problem with this approach is that the more encouraging the pilot studies, the less likely are physicians to be willing to randomize patients on a subsequent comparative study. Hence, Chalmers and colleagues[12] have argued that even pilot studies should be randomized. Our view is that pilot studies in breast cancer treatment should be carried out with the clear objective of developing programs that can be used in randomized comparative trials as soon as feasibility issues are resolved by the phase II data. All nonrandomized studies of breast cancer treatment must be viewed cautiously, and in almost all cases effectiveness should be tested in randomized comparative trials.

On the other hand, there are situations in which randomization is clearly impossible for ethical reasons. Most people would agree that randomization would not be appropriate in studying the effects of malnutrition on patients with primary breast cancer. However, for almost any other study there will be a wide range of opinion on the ethics of randomization. One problem is that it is very difficult to be completely neutral about which of two treatments one would "bet on" as being the best even in the absence of relevant human data. This has led the authors of an introductory statistics textbook[13] to state, "We feel that it is more forthright to admit that the physician who puts a patient in a (randomized) clinical experiment is surely subjecting the patient to the chance of getting a therapy that, in the physician's best judgment at the moment, is not the best treatment for that patient." The key phrase is, "in the physician's best judgment at the moment." How often are these best judgments, made in advance of a randomized trial, correct? Since a new treatment would not be studied unless there was some hope of its being better for some outcome than standard treatment, this is almost equivalent in some situations to asking how often a new treatment is more beneficial than a standard. Using reports in medical journals (in English) during the period of 1964 to 1972, Gilbert and colleagues studied surgical trials comparing an innovative therapy with a standard therapy.[14] Among 36 comparisons (Table 17-1), they found that "while some innovations turned out to be highly preferred, in almost as many comparisons the standard was highly preferred" and that "averaged across these studies, the patient in the control group does about as well as the patient in the experimental group." Therefore, even if investigators are not "perfectly unsure" which of two treatments is better, it may be ethical for them to randomize by virtue of knowing that such "hunches" or "theoretical reasoning" or "conclusions from pilot studies" are incorrect almost as often as they are correct.

Even when a randomized trial is ethical, there may be economic reasons for deciding to do a different type of study. Consider the case of a standard regimen that has been used on thousands of patients and has been associated with a response rate of p (based on data from all these patients, not based on a small subset of them). Then some would argue that the response rate to this standard can be considered known (i.e., having no random error). In this case, a prospective study on a new therapy that is compared with a historical control requires only one-quarter of the number of patients needed for a randomized trial comparing the new treatment versus standard.[9] The problem is that without randomization it is usually impossible to verify that the patients on trial are "just like" historical controls. There is one exception: when the outcome on the standard treatment is homogeneous. Response is homogeneous when 0% (or 100%) of the patients respond; survival time is homogeneous when all of

Table 17-1
Comparisons of Innovations (I) With Standards (S) for 36 Randomized Clinical Trials

	Primary	*Secondary*	*Total*
$I \gg S$	1	4	5
$I > S$	5	2	7
$I = S$	2	2	4
$S = I$	7	3	10
$S > I$	3	3	6
$S \gg I$	1	3	4
Comparisons	19	17	36
Papers	18	14	32

$\gg$ Highly preferred
$>$ Preferred
= Equivalent
I = S means equivalence, but I a success; S = I means equivalence, but I a disappointment.
(Gilbert JP, McPeck B, Mosteller F: Progress in surgery and anesthesia: Benefits and risks of innovative therapy. In Bunker JP, Barnes BA, Mosteller F (eds): Costs, Risks, and Benefits of Surgery, pp 124–169. New York, Oxford Press, 1977)

the patients die at the same time (e.g., 293 days after diagnosis). Survival time homogeneity seems to be found only among some particular strains of small rodents, but response homogeneity is occasionally found in certain subgroups of breast cancer patients (e.g., metastatic patients with performance status 4 and nonfunctioning livers seldom respond to anything). It would not take many responses of such patients, treated in a nonrandomized way with a new therapy, to convince all clinicians of the benefit of using the new therapy.

However, most of the studies with historical controls reported in the medical literature do not deal with homogeneous patient subgroups. Although the frequency of such reports appears to be decreasing,[15] some will probably continue to be published for a long time. Several authors[9,16] have listed conditions under which nonrandomized studies can be reliable. In general, articles using nonrandomized controls should describe attempts to minimize biases and should estimate the effects of possible bias; the believability of results is in direct proportion to how many biases seem to be small. For example, studies with literature controls or "data base" controls[17] are usually far less reliable than studies using one arm of a recent prior trial done by the same investigators as a control, because the former are more subject to selection, eligibility, diagnostic, definitional, follow-up frequency, and ancillary therapy biases. However, even the best historically controlled study can be misleading. Pocock[18] examined 19 instances in which a clinical trials group used the same treatment in two consecutive trials. "If historical comparisons of this type are without bias, one would not expect any notable difference in survival for two groups receiving the same treatment. In fact, the 19 changes in death rate ranged from -46% to $+24\%$, and in four instances the difference was statistically significant (each $p < 0.02$)." Similar examples exist in the breast cancer literature. Changing one of the treatments in an Eastern Cooperative Oncology Group (ECOG) randomized trial of metastatic breast cancer resulted in significant changes in the response rate, response duration, time to failure, and survival time of patients given the treatment that *remained* the same; these changes were significant even when adjusted (in statistical models) for the possible effects of institution and 35 prognostic factors.[19] Similar unexplainable differences exist in the survival experience of adjuvant chemotherapy breast cancer patients treated with L-phenylalanine mustard (L-PAM) on two successive National Surgical Adjuvant Breast and Bowel Project protocols.[20,21] The reliability of historical controls is challenged even more directly when the results of historically controlled trials show significant differences[22] that are not verified by the results of randomized trials.[23,24]

Eligibility and Stratification

Eligibility criteria in clinical trials have both ethical and statistical rationales. Ethical eligibility criteria exclude from study patients in whom the risk-benefit ratio of the trial is highly unfavorable, either for toxicity reasons (e.g., excluding pregnant women and women with impaired renal or hepatic function from drug trials) or for efficacy reasons; that is, excluding patients who a priori have a very small chance of benefitting from the trial treatment, either because they have a very bad prognosis (e.g., patients confined to bed) or a very good prognosis (e.g., patients with *in situ* cancer) or disease unaffected by the modalities being tested (e.g., patients with brain metastases only in drug trials and patients with estrogen-receptor (ER)-negative tumors in oophorectomy trials). In addition, patients unable to give informed consent for psychological reasons are usually excluded from cancer trials.

There are several statistical considerations that affect eligibility criteria. First, patients who are unevaluable for the main outcome variable might be excluded (e.g., patients with no clinical evidence of disease on a response study or breast cancer patients with prior lung cancer on a study of survival). Second, there might be eligibility criteria with the main purpose of avoiding length bias problems (e.g., excluding from randomization patients who are more than 2 months postdiagnosis; see Chapter 5 for a discussion of length biasing). Third, eligibility criteria are used to increase the homogeneity of the study population (e.g., restricting a study of adjuvant therapy to Stage II premenopausal ER-negative patients). There are two statistical advantages of homogeneity: The more homogeneous the patients are with respect to outcome variables, the smaller is the number of patients required to answer the main question of the trial; and the more homogeneous patients are with respect to the hypothesized effect of the two treatments of the trial, the more reasonable it is to ignore patient characteristic–treatment interactions in the planning of sample size and analysis. For example, if it is hypothesized that treatment differences are likely to be bigger among premenopausal than among postmenopausal patients on a specific trial and if both premenopausal and postmenopausal patients are eligible, then the accrual goal for that trial should be set high enough to allow either a test for menopause-treatment interaction or else separate estimates of treatment difference for premenopausal and postmenopausal patients. In either case, many more patients are needed than would be required in a trial restricted to premenopausal patients. Of course, study results can only be generalized to patients similar to those eligible for the study. So a trial that enrolls only premenopausal patients provides no information about results in postmenopausal patients, whereas a trial unrestricted with respect to menopause provides at least some information on both menopause groups.

Sometimes investigators are not concerned about interactions of treatment and patient characteristics but are worried that an imbalance with respect to a particularly important patient characteristic could bias treatment comparisons. For example, primary breast cancer patients with fewer pathologically positive nodes tend to live longer than patients with a greater number of positive nodes. If a randomized trial of adjuvant chemotherapy (against control) resulted in the treatment with apparently shorter survival time having been assigned to patients with substantially more positive nodes, a simple statistical comparison of the two groups would be suspect. Perhaps the treatment with the poorer survival time is comparable to the other treatment, and the apparently shorter survival time associated with it was due to the worse prognosis of patients randomized to that regimen. The statistical comparison of the treatment groups could be adjusted for the prognostic factor imbalance by using a statistical model, but this has the following three drawbacks:

1. The assumptions used by the model may be incorrect and hence inferences drawn from the model may be incorrect.
2. In the absence of a prognostic factor imbalance, the simple statistical comparison between groups is more understandable and more easily verified and hence more likely to influence clinicians than a comparison using a complicated statistical model.
3. Even if the model assumptions are correct, there will be some loss of statistical power (efficiency) using a model (i.e., the use of a model is equivalent to making simple comparisons among groups with smaller sample sizes).

As mentioned above, randomization balances prognostic factors on average but does *not* guarantee that the trial will be balanced with respect to any particular prognostic factor. The more patients who are randomized, the less likely are large imbalances with respect to any particular prognostic factor, but this is cold comfort to an investigator who finds at the end of the accrual period that his trial has been unlucky enough to result in a large imbalance. Also, even in large clinical trials, if interim analyses could result in changes in study design (e.g., stopping the trial), then it is desirable that important prognostic factors be balanced at the times of interim analyses, when the sample size might be rather small.

There are two ways of ensuring balance of particular prognostic factors in a randomized trial. The first and more commonly used method has historically been called stratified randomization.[25] In this method, randomization is done separately within each possible patient prognostic group, and hence imbalances within a subgroup are not very likely, particularly if randomization is blocked. For example, if it is desirable to stratify a metastatic breast cancer trial on the basis of dominant metastatic site (visceral, osseous, or soft) and performance status (completely ambulatory versus partially nonambulatory), then randomization can be done separately within each of the six possible prognostic groups (visceral and ambulatory, visceral and nonambulatory, osseous and ambulatory, osseous and nonambulatory, soft and ambulatory, soft and nonambulatory). From the point of view of the randomization scheme, it is as if six independent randomized trials are being done concurrently. This approach has the advantage of taking care of possible interactions of prognostic factors by balancing treatments in subgroups with each possible combination of patient characteristics. However, as the number of prognostic factors increases, so does the number of subgroups, and it is not unusual for a proposed protocol to contain more possible subgroups than patients in the accrual goal (e.g., five prognostic factors with two, two, three, three, and four levels results in $2 \times 2 \times 3 \times 3 \times 4 = 144$ subgroups to randomize). As Simon has pointed out, "if there is extensive stratification, numerous strata will contain very few patients. Consequently, balance with regard to the most important factor or factors may be seriously impaired by the inclusion of factors of secondary importance. Even the total numbers of patients assigned to each of the treatments may be very unequal. Extensive overstratification becomes equivalent to randomization with no stratification at all."[26]

One way to accommodate more stratification factors is to balance each individual prognostic factor but not to try to balance all possible combinations. This method has several names: "dynamic randomization," "minimization," and "dynamic stratification." First, one has to find out which treatment assignment would result in least imbalance. This is done by calculating two sums, as described by Pocock:[27]

> The method is best described with the aid of an example. Consider the situation reached in the advanced breast cancer trial after 80 patients have already entered and the next patient is ready to receive treatment assignment. Table 17-2 shows the numbers of patients on each of the two treatments, A and B, according to each of the four patient factors. Thus, each one of the 80 patients appears four times in this table, once for each factor. Suppose the next patient is ambulatory, age <50, has disease-free interval ≥2 years and visceral metastasis (as indicated by the arrows in Table 17-2). Then for each treatment one adds together the number of patients in the corresponding four rows of the table.
>
> Thus, for A this sum = 30 + 18 + 9 + 19 = 76
> while for B this sum = 31 + 17 + 8 + 21 = 77

Table 17-2
Treatment Assignments by the Four Patient Factors for 80 Patients in an Advanced Breast Cancer Trial

Factor	*Level*	*Number on Each Treatment* A	B	*Next Patient*
Performance status	Ambulatory	30	31	←
	Nonambulatory	10	9	
Age	< 50	18	17	←
	≥ 50	22	23	
Disease-free interval	< 2 years	31	32	
	≥ 2 years	9	8	←
Dominant metastatic lesion	Visceral	19	21	←
	Osseous	8	7	
	Soft tissue	13	12	

Table 17-3
Priority List for Stratification Factors in Breast Cancer Clinical Trials (Highest Priority at Top of List)

Category	*Examples*
Factors not used for eligibility criteria but that are used as eligibility criteria by most other investigators	Pathologic nodal status (0 vs. 1 or more positive nodes) in an adjuvant trial
Factors for which there is an a priori reason to believe a treatment interaction exists but this trial will not accrue sufficient numbers of patients to have good statistical power in testing the interaction	Estrogen receptor status (positive vs. negative vs. indeterminate) in a metastatic trial of hormonotherapy vs. chemotherapy
Factors used as strata by most other investigators	Performance status in metastatic breast cancer trial; menopause in adjuvant trial
Factors that are (when tested) almost always shown to be highly significant in models for outcome variables	Number of organs with metastases in metastatic trial

In its simplest form, minimization requires one to give the treatment with the smallest such sum of marginal totals to the next patient. In this case, the 81st patient is therefore assigned to treatment A. If the sums for A and B were equal, then one would use simple randomization to assign the treatment. Other methods of minimization use unbalanced randomization (rather than direct assignment) when one treatment assignment would result in less unbalance than another[28,29,30] or use simple randomization unless the resultant imbalance in any single prognostic factor exceeds some prespecified amount.[25]

However, even these methods break down when the number of stratifying factors gets very large. Sometimes curtailing the number of strata becomes simple when investigators realize what stratification *does not* do: It does not ensure that enough patients are entered in each subgroup to have sufficient data to estimate treatment effects within subgroups; it does not make tests of interaction of treatment and patient characteristics more powerful; and it does not limit the variables that can be used in statistical modeling. Not all prognostic characteristics should be stratified. Some factors should be eligibility criteria, some should be stratification factors, and some could be effectively balanced using statistical models (which is sometimes called "post hoc stratification"). What category to assign any particular prognostic characteristic in a specific study is a matter of controversy; some authors even argue that stratification is more bother than it is worth and should never be used.[31,32]

Table 17-3 lists general categories of prognostic characteristics in a priority list for strata variables. Several categories involve assessing what other current trials use as strata or eligibility criteria on the theory that one important function of stratification is to convince other clinicians that the trial results are believable. Table 17-4 gives the results of a survey of randomized breast cancer trials published in the *New England Journal of Medicine*, the *Journal of Clinical Oncology, Breast Cancer Treatment and Research, Cancer*, the *European Journal of Cancer*, the *British Journal of Cancer*, and *Lancet* between October of 1984 and September of 1985. Attention was restricted to randomized trials, because nonrandomized trials do not have stratification factors. No attempt was made to survey the many articles evaluating the value of "new" prognostic factors, for two reasons: There have been very few reports of prospective trials confirming the results of these studies (probably because of a lack of interest in confirmatory studies rather than because such variables are not prognostic), and many such articles do not evaluate the new variables in statistical models that use all the commonly available prognostic factors.

Among the ten metastatic trials, eight used some multivariate models. The most common eligibility variables were prior chemotherapy (seven trials *either* required that all patients have prior chemotherapy *or* required that no patients have prior chemotherapy), presence of measurable or evaluable disease, performance status better than 4 (i.e., patients could not be 100% bedridden), time since last therapy (usually specified as at least 4 weeks), and no prior treatment with the drugs used on the protocol. The most common stratification factors (performance status 0 to 1 versus 2 to 3, dominant metastatic site, and ER status) were also the variables most often found significant in multivariate models, but it is not clear what is cause and what is effect. That is, it was not always possible to tell what variables were tried in multivariate models, and investigators are more likely to use their strata variables than other variables.

Of the 12 adjuvant therapy trials, only two reported multivariate models. However, six other articles reported results separately within two or more patient subgroups. The variables used to define these subgroups are shown in the last column of Table 17-4. Nine of the trials had eligibility criteria that would exclude patients with a lumpectomy (this figure includes the NSABP trial of total mastectomy versus radical mastectomy). Half of the trials were limited to only premenopausal or only postmenopausal patients, and three trials were stratified by age 50, which could be considered a pseudovariable for menopause. All but two trials used pathologically positive nodes as an eligibility criterion, a stratification factor, or in reporting results, or they found it significant in models (these are

Table 17-4
Commonly Used Eligibility and Strata Variables in 1985

	10 Metastatic Breast Trials (References 34–41)					*12 Adjuvant Breast Trials (References 33, 42–48)*			
Characteristics and Levels	*Trials Using it for Eligibility*	*Trials Using it for Stratification*	*Trials Where it was Significant in Response Models*	*Trials Where it was Significant in Time to Failure Models*	*Trials Where it was Significant in Survival Models*	*Trials Using it for Eligibility*	*Trials Using it for Stratification*	*Trials Where it was Significant in Survival Models*	*Trials Reporting Separate Results by Treatment by Levels of Characteristics*
Age									
≤ 65–75 (upper limit)	3					5			
60		1	1	1					
50			2	1	1		3		2
< 35						1			1
in years								1	
Menopause	3					6			3
Performance status									
≤ 3	6								
0,1 vs. 2,3		5	2	3	3	1			
Estrogen receptor status		4	3	2	3		1	2	2
Progesterone receptor status								2	1
Measurable/evaluable disease	7				1				
Number of metastatic sites		1	2		2				
Dominant metastatic site*		5	2	2	4				
Skin metastases			1						
Bone metastases				1					
			1						
Disease-free interval			1	2	2				
Time since recurrence				1	1				
Time since last therapy	5								
Prior chemotherapy									
Yes/No	7								
Drugs of this protocol	5	1							
Prior hormonotherapy									
Yes/No	1	1	1	1					
Response			2	1	1				
Tumor size									
< 5 cm						3		1	
< 4 cm						1			
< 2 cm							2		1
in mm								1	
Nodal status									
Clinically positive						2			
Pathologically positive						4	2	2	3
Path 1-3 vs. 4+						1	4		5
Path 4–6, 4–8, or 4–10								2	3
Pathologic grade								1	1
Surgery (Mx vs. lumpectomy)						9			
Number of nodes examined								1	
Tumor location									4
Obesity								1	
Institution		6					4		

* Dominant metastatic site = Visceral vs. Others; sometimes Others are divided into Osseous and Soft.

not mutually exclusive categories); and all but four trials did the same with one to three versus four or more pathologically positive nodes. Tumor size was used for eligibility or stratification in half the trials.

Of course, it could be argued that the trials represented in Table 17-2 are "old." Although they were published within the past year, several were started a decade ago. A better guide to current strata variables would be a survey of currently accruing clinical trials. Pocock and Lagakos did such a survey of 15 clinical trials groups in 1982.[49] They found that European groups had fewer stratification factors (0 to 2) and hence fewer patient subgroups (1 to 4) than U.S. groups (2 to 5 stratification factors, 4 to 50 patient subgroups). Table 17-5 lists the stratification factors used by the ten active adjuvant therapy breast trials. Although they did not tally eligibility factors, they noted that "one can see some consistency in the choice of factors, number of positive nodes and menopausal status being fairly standard. Some of the trials were without these patient factors because they were restricted to node-negative or premenopausal patients."[49]

Sample Size

There is no single answer to the question, "How many patients are needed in this trial?" Before one can begin to formulate accrual guidelines, one needs to determine the main purpose of the trial, the principal outcome measure, and the main method of statistical analysis. A trial in which the main goal is to show that one treatment is better than another will require far fewer patients than a trial in which the main goal is to show that two treatments are equally effective. The measure of patient outcome chosen to document treatment effect will also have a large effect on sample size. Outcomes that will be measured on all patients (e.g., time to failure in a study of metastatic breast cancer in which all patients are considered evaluable for this outcome) require a smaller total sample size than outcomes that will be measured on only some patients (e.g., duration of response, which is only measured in responders). For the same relative effect of treatments, outcome variables that have many different possible values (e.g., survival in days) require smaller sample sizes than outcomes that have only a few possible values (e.g., survival of at least 5 years, which has only the value "yes" or "no"). Also, the magnitude of treatment differences is likely to vary among outcome variables, and smaller differences require larger trials. For example, Table 17-6 lists the relative treatment effects on five outcome measures in a Ludwig adjuvant breast cancer trial of observation versus CMFpT.[50] The treatment difference in disease-free interval (measured by odds ratio) was more than 2½ times as great as the treatment difference in overall survival. Even a single outcome variable may be analyzed by several statistical methods. The analysis method chosen can make a differ-

Table 17-5
Commonly Used Strata Variables

Center	*Stratification Factors*
1	None
2	None
3	Stages I or II Pre- or postmenopausal
4	Positive nodes (+ or −) Radiotherapy (+ or −)
5	Number of + nodes Pre- or postmenopausal
6	Simple or radical mastectomy Pre- or postmenopausal
7	Number of + nodes (1−3 or 4+) Pre- or postmenopausal Estrogen receptor (+ or −)
8	Number of + nodes (0−3 or 4+) Tumor size (<3 or ≥3 cm) Pre- or postmenopausal Unfavorable signs (+ or −)
9	Number of + nodes (1−3 or 4+) Estrogen receptor (+ or −)
10	Number of + nodes (1−3 or 4+) Pre- or postmenopausal Tumor size (<2, 2–5 or >5 cm) Radiotherapy (+ or −) Estrogen receptor (+ or −)

Pocock SJ, Lagakos SW: Practical experience of randomization in cancer trials: An international survey. Br J Cancer 46:368–375, 1982)

Table 17-6
Treatment Effect Differences as Evaluated by Five Different Outcome Measures: 4-Year Kaplan-Meier Rate, Ludwig III

End-point Measure	Observation n=156	CMFp+T n=154	Odds Ratio CMFpT/OBS
Disease-free interval	32%	66%	4.1
Disease-free survival	31%	61%	3.5
Systemic disease-free survival rate	41%	62	2.3
Survival (breast cancer deaths only)	69%	81%	1.9
Overall survival	67%	76%	1.6

(Goldhirsh A, Gelber R for the Ludwig Breast Cancer Study Group: Adjuvant treatment for early breast cancer: The Ludwig breast cancer studies. National Cancer Inst Monogr 1:55–70, 1986

Table 17-7
Sample Size Calculations

Category of Outcome Variable	Examples	Type of Test and Reference for Sample Size and Form of Information
Binary (two-valued)	Response percent, proportion surviving 5 years, complete response rate, percent with severe or worse toxicity, percent with disease-free interval over 2 years	Chi-squared, 55, tables and formulas Binomial, 56, graphs Fisher's Exact, 57, tables and formulas
Categorical (three to seven ordered values)	Type of response (CR, PR, NC, PD), degree of toxicity (none, mild, moderate, severe, life-threatening)	Wilcoxon, 63, formulas
Continuous (many-valued)	Time to response, duration of response, time to failure (progression or relapse, whichever comes first), time from failure to death, survival, disease-free interval, disease-free survival, systemic disease-free survival, time from recurrence to death	F-test, 58, formulas F-test, 60, tables F-test, 62, computer program F-test, 61, graphs Logrank test, 59, formulas Logrank test, 64, tables

ence in required sample sizes, but it is not usually easy to generalize those circumstances in which a particular method will be associated with a smaller required trial size than other methods. Fortunately, the influence of different analysis methods on sample size is generally smaller than the effect of choice of outcome measures.

Table 17-7 shows some outcome measures common in breast cancer clinical trials together with references for methods of calculating sample size. Because uncontrolled or nonrandomized studies have more complicated (and often nonstandardized) statistical considerations, only methods for calculating sample sizes of randomized controlled trials are included here. Some of the articles referenced have tables of sample sizes, some give formulas, and some include computer program listings. In all cases, the calculation of sample size requires the trial planner to specify the following three quantities:

1. *The relevant treatment effect.* Either the smallest treatment difference it is clinically important to detect (for trials trying to show treatment differences) *or* the largest difference that is clinically unimportant (for trials trying to show treatment equivalence). How the difference is expressed depends on both the outcome measure chosen and the statistical test to be used. For instance, if the outcome measure is response percent and the statistical method is the chi-square test, then the difference might be specified as "a 20% difference in response—for example, from 50% to 70%." If the outcome measure is survival and the statistical method is the F-test (based on the assumption of exponentially distributed survival times), then the difference might be specified as "a 20% increase in median survival—for example, from 5 years to 6 years." It is important that the difference specified be both clinically relevant (Would this much of an improvement be important to the patient?) and scientifically realistic (Based on past studies of these and other treatments, is it reasonable to expect these treatments to differ this much in effect?). For instance, a 40% increase in response rate (e.g., from 50% to 90%) in a trial of two combination chemotherapies for metastatic breast cancer would be highly unusual, so such a large difference would probably not

be realistic. Similarly, a doubling of median survival time in a trial of adjuvant hormonotherapy among a group of primary breast cancer patients who in the past have had a 10-year median survival would also be unrealistic.

2. *The false-positive error rate.* The false-positive error rate is the probability that the statistical test will show a significant treatment effect when there is no real treatment difference. (It is sometimes referred to as the type I error rate or the significance level and is often denoted by α.) If the nonequivalence of treatments A and B is only possible if B is better than A, then a one-sided error rate is used (e.g., when A is placebo and B is a treatment without any possible detrimental effect). Otherwise, a two-sided error rate is used. Generally, a two-sided calculation should be done unless a significant result in one direction (e.g., A better than B) would be ignored.

3. *The false-negative error rate.* The false-negative error rate is the probability that the statistical test will fail to show a significant treatment effect when the true treatment results are as different as specified by item 1 above. (The false-negative rate is sometimes called the type II error rate and is often denoted by β.) The power or sensitivity of the trial refers to the true-positive rate (the probability of finding a statistically significant result if there is a real difference between treatments). Power is equal to $1-\beta$.

The sample size is related to all three of the above quantities. If sample size is held constant, then one can lower the false-positive error rate only by either raising the false-negative error rate or by increasing the treatment difference that is to be detected. Alternatively, keeping sample size constant, an increase in the false-positive error rate will raise the power of detecting smaller treatment differences. Increasing the sample size is the only way to decrease one of the three quantities (the false-positive rate or the false-negative rate or the magnitude of the difference the trial will be able to detect) without causing an increase in at least one of the other quantities.

In trials that are designed to find a treatment difference, the false-positive rate is usually chosen to be 1% or 5% and the false-negative rate is usually chosen to be 5%, 10%, 20%, or sometimes even 30%. In trials that are designed to show treatment equivalence, the false-positive rate is often larger (10% to 20%) and the false-negative rate is usually chosen to be 5% or 10%.

Many methods of calculating sample size also require the trial planner to assume something about the expected outcome on at least one of the treatments. For example, it may be necessary to estimate the percent response one would expect on the standard treatment or the median survival of control patients. It is a good idea to see what difference (if any) in needed sample size occurs for various estimates of expected outcome. It is important to note that sample size requirement for time outcomes (e.g., survival time) are based on the number of observed events (e.g., deaths). So if the trial is to be analyzed before all patients have had an event observed (e.g., before all have died), then some estimate must be made of what percentage of the patients will have an event observed before the analysis is done. In this respect, there is a trade-off between total number of patients needed and the length of follow-up, since increasing either will increase the number of deaths.

The same formulas that are used to estimate the necessary accrual (based on desired power) before a trial is started can be used to calculate the power or type II error probability (based on actual accrual) when a trial is reported in the literature. This is especially important in trials in which the observed treatment differences were not found to be significant. In such a case, one of two explanations may be true: Either the treatment effects truly do not differ, or it may be that the treatment effects truly differ but not enough patients were accrued to have a good chance of detecting the difference. If the type II error probability is low, this would be evidence in favor of the first alternative; if the type II error probability is high, one would have to worry about the second alternative.

There have been several surveys of the medical literature that show that most trials do not have enough patients to have a good chance of detecting even large differences in treatment outcome. Freiman and colleagues[51] reviewed 71 "negative" trials (not restricted to cancer studies) in major medical journals and found 50 of the trials had at least a 10% risk of missing a 50% therapeutic improvement. Zelen[52] surveyed articles on randomized trials appearing in *Cancer* between 1977 and 1979 and found the median trial size to be 50 per treatment (range 10 to 400; 70% less than 100 patients per treatment; 15% between 100 and 200 patients per treatment). Mosteller and colleagues[53] reviewed cancer trials referenced in the book *Randomized Trials in Cancer: A Critical Review by Sites.*[54] They found 108 randomized breast cancer trials, 93 reported in articles and 15 reported in abstracts. The distribution of sample sizes was similar to that found by Zelen: median size 45 per treatment, range 5 to 750; 82% less than 100 patients per treatment, 12% between 100 and 200 patients per treatment. In the small survey conducted to obtain commonly used strata variables (see Table 17-4), the median accrual for randomized trials in metastatic breast cancer was 57 per treatment (range 21 to 110); the median accrual for randomized adjuvant trials was 190 per treatment (range 36 to 614). These surveys probably overestimate the median size of clinical trials because small "negative" trials do not always get published. In order to put these surveys in perspective, Table 17-8 uses the methods given in references 55 and 62 to calculate what differences would have an 80% chance of being detected as significant in trials with 25, 50, 100, 200, 400, and 600 patients per treatment. To calculate these numbers, it was assumed that the false-positive error probability (two-sided) was 0.05 and the false-negative error probability was 0.20. The response example assumes that a chi-square test will be used and that the lower response

Table 17-8
Differences That Could Be Detected in Tests with a False-Positive Error Probability of 0.05 (Two-Sided) and False-Negative Error Probability of 0.20

		Survival Examples:[60] *Lower Median = 10 years, Accrual Period = 2 Years; Ratio of Medians:*	
Number of Patients per Treatment	*Response Example:*[53] *Lower Rate = 50%; Difference in Rates:*	*Additional Follow-up = 3 Years*	*Additional Follow-up = 8 Years*
25	41%	18.00	4.40
50	29%	4.40	2.61
100	20%	2.60	1.92
200	14%	1.90	1.58
400	10%	1.57	1.37
600	8%	1.44	1.29

percent is 50%. A difference in response rates of 41% would correspond to the higher response percent, being 91% = 50% + 41%, which is too big a difference to be scientifically reasonable. A difference in response percents of 20% (e.g., 50% versus 70%) is usually considered a clinically important difference in metastatic breast cancer trials. It would take 100 patients per treatment to have a power of 80% to detect such a difference, yet most published trials accrue only half this many patients. The survival example assumes that an F-test of exponential death rates is used and that the worse treatment is associated with a median survival of 10 years and that accrual takes 2 years. It is also assumed that there is either 3 years or 8 years of additional follow-up after accrual ends (for a 5-year or 10-year study, respectively). A ratio of medians of 18.0 corresponds to a median survival of 180 years on the better treatment, clearly an absurd "improvement." Not until the sample size reaches 400 or so does the detectable difference (to a median of 15.7 or 13.7 years for 3 and 8 years of follow-up) become reasonable. There are many who would argue that even 600 patients per treatment are not enough, since a 2-year improvement in median survival time (ratio of 1.20) would be of great clinical importance.

The desire to see if adjuvant therapy has been associated with small increases in survival time has led to several overviews of breast cancer trials, in which data from several centers are combined.[65,66] The methodology of such overviews is briefly discussed below. It should be pointed out that overviews are no substitute for large clinical trials. By their nature, overviews can only answer the most general questions about outcome variables with a universal definition (e.g., is chemotherapy of all types combined associated with longer survival). To decide which particular chemotherapies are most beneficial or to evaluate their effects on relapse-free survival requires large clinical trials.

Defining an Outcome Variable: Response

Defining outcome variables *before* starting a study is as important as deciding eligibility criteria *before* any patient is entered. In both cases, it appears to be humanly impossible to come up with unbiased rules after the results of the study are known. Since few outcome variables have caused as much discussion as response and since the definition of response affects the definitions of response duration and time to treatment failure, we shall concentrate on that outcome variable in this section.

The justification often given for measuring response at all is twofold: (1) It is an outcome measure available early in the trial and is correlated with survival and (2) it is one way of assessing palliation. Neither of these two justifications is supported by much data. One article compares the use of response as a marker for survival time to using height as a marker for weight in evaluating a diet program.[67] The common practice of comparing the survival time of responders versus nonresponders is incorrect because of the bias resulting from the requirement that responders survive long enough for the response to be observed.[67,68] Often the definition of response is such that a response cannot be observed less than 2 or 3 months after treatment starts; there is no such minimum survival time required for nonresponders. If it were true that higher response rates caused longer survival, then treatments that differ greatly in response rates should differ greatly in survival time. This certainly does not happen in breast cancer. In one study[68] involving two sequential trials conducted by the same cooperative group on premenopausal women with metastatic breast cancer, one treatment had a response rate of 21% (5% complete); the other had a response rate of 71% (28% complete). The crude analysis of survival of response showed that for both treatments, responders appeared to live longer than nonresponders. However, the overall survival time on the two treatments

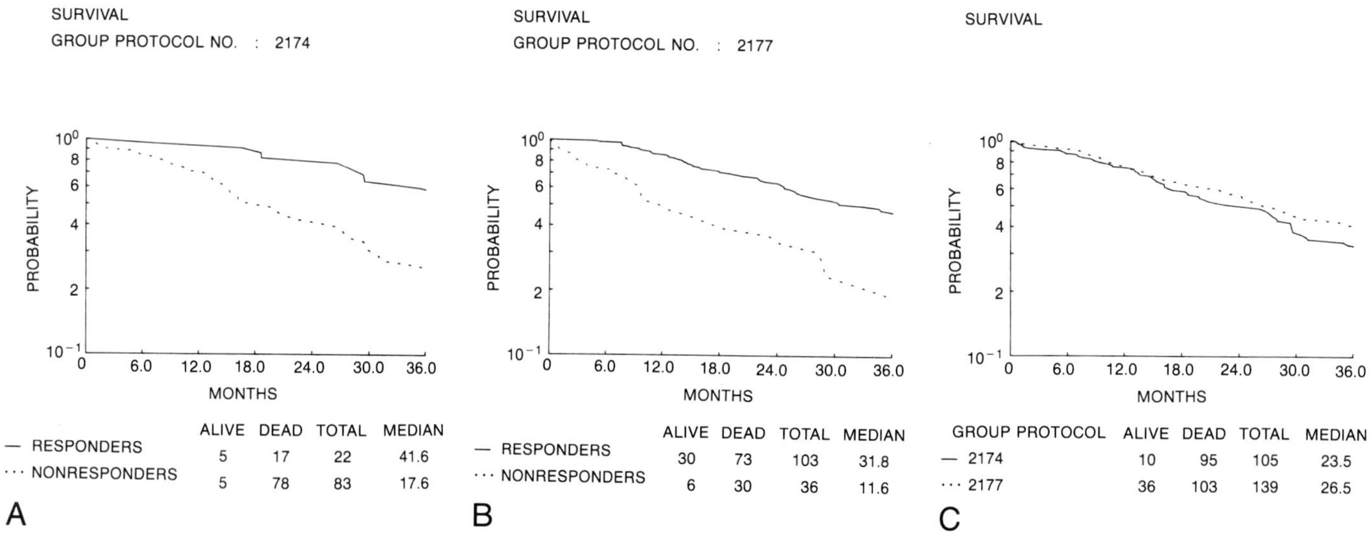

FIGURE 17-1. Illustration of fallacy of comparing survival time of responders to that of nonresponders. *(A)* Survival by response for study EST 2174. *(B)* Survival by response for study EST 2177. *(C)* Survival by study EST 2174 and 2177.

was identical (Fig. 17-1). Even when appropriate statistical techniques are used to eliminate the bias in comparing responders to nonresponders,[67,69] within a single study there is no way to tell if response "causes" longer survival. For at least some patients, response simply acts as a marker for favorable pretreatment characteristics, either known or unknown. It is not unusual to find in a randomized trial that the treatment associated with a higher response rate is also associated with a shorter duration of response.[70] This is precisely what would be expected if response does not benefit the patients at all but is positively correlated with good prognostic factors. In such a situation, one treatment (say, A) identifies more patients with the "response marker"; of necessity, these extra patients have a slightly worse prognosis than those also identified as "responders" by treatment B, so duration of response for the whole group of responders on A is "pulled down" by these patients with a worse prognosis. This is the same idea as the "stage creep" mentioned previously. Some medical journals now refuse to publish survival curves for responders versus nonresponders,[71] but they continue to appear in many other journals.[72] Cross-study comparisons of response rates and survival time have sometimes shown studies with higher response rates to have longer survival times,[73] but they have sometimes shown the opposite.[67] All such analyses suffer from the multiple biases inherent in historical control studies. It may be easier to document that response is associated with palliation;[74] oddly enough, very few researchers have attempted to study this.

However, as a recent article[75] points out, "until better methods of assessing palliation become available we believe that some measure of change in tumor size will continue to be viewed as an acceptable endpoint." It is obviously to everyone's advantage to standardize this measure, and several groups have tried to do so for breast cancer trials (National Cancer Institute [NCI],[76] Union Internationale Contre le Cancer [UICC],[77] British Breast Group[78]) or for solid tumors in general (World Health Organization [WHO],[79] ECOG[80]). Tables 17-9 to 17-12 are an abstract of the NCI guidelines, which seem to be the most popular in the United States. The UICC guidelines differ from these in the following ways:

Organ response is not defined (only lesion response and patient response are defined).

A patient partial response requires "≥50% decrease in measurable lesions . . . and objective improvement in evaluable, but nonmeasurable lesions. No new lesions. It is not necessary for every lesion to have regressed to qualify for partial response, but no lesion should have progressed .... If nonmeasurable but evaluable lesions represent the bulk of disease and these clearly do not respond, even though measurable lesions have improved, then this is considered 'no change,' not 'objective regression.' "

Progression is defined as new lesions or "a 25% or more increase in the sum of products of the diameters of each lesion measured, except that if an increase of less than 25% makes additional treatment necessary, this is also regarded as progression."

There is no stated minimum duration of response; the NCI definition requires at least two measurements 4 weeks apart to be classified as response before a patient can be called a responder.

The phrase "of each individual lesion, or those selected for study" seems to imply that the investigator is free to decide *not* to measure some lesions; the NCI guidelines require at least all measurable lesions to be used in deciding if a patient has a partial response, and all evaluable lesions must be used (in addition to all measurable ones) in deciding on complete response and progression.

Table 17-9
Methods of Tumor Measurement of Individual Organ Site Involvement

1. Measurable, Bidimensional

a. Surface area approximation will be used by multiplying the longest diameter by the greatest perpendicular diameter.
b. If multiple lesions are available for a single organ site, the sum of the products will be determined and used as the "total parameter pool" for objective response determination of that site.
c. Ruler or caliper will be used for measurements (not estimates or finger-breadths).
d. Record in metric system.

2. Measurable, Unidimensional

a. In those lesions in which unidimensional measurements only are possible, these measurements will be made by ruler and recorded in the metric system.
b. In measurable liver enlargement, the sum of the linear measurements below the right costal margin (RCM) in the nipple line, xiphoid and left costal margin (LCM) in the nipple line will be used.

3. Evaluable

a. Whenever possible, photographs will be taken before therapy and during therapy to document estimated response.
b. Scans of liver or brain may be used to estimate the extent of the involvement and the response.

4. Unevaluable

a. Pretreatment and serial measurements (hepatic or bone enzymes, scans) will be made but cannot be used as the sole measure for objective response.
b. Scans (bone, neoplasm scans with "tumor-seeking" agents) will be used to document presence or absence of tumor in the specific organ but will not be used to measure disease.

Mammography measurements are specifically mentioned as a way to document breast response; they are not mentioned in the NCI guidelines. In one study of 35 patients with advanced primary breast cancer, response judged by physical examination differed from response judged by mammography in 12 (34%) of the cases.[81]

Pleura metastases and ascites—pleura nodules are mentioned and presumably count as measurable disease, whereas the NCI does not count pleura metastases as measurable and requires evaluable pleural effusions and ascites to have positive cytologic findings and to be uninfluenced by diuretics.

Bone metastases—the UICC allows bone scans to be used in documenting response, although stating, "it should be noted that other processes can produce increased uptake in bone scans and that both progression and regression of lesions may be reflected by an increase in uptake"; the NCI guidelines do not allow bone scans to be the "sole measure for objective response" for bone metastases. (The literature on the relative value of bone scans and bone x-rays seems divided.[82,83])

Mediastinal nodes—the UICC does not require a pre-involvement x-ray; the NCI does for measurable (rather than evaluable) disease.

Lymphedema—counted as measurable disease by the UICC but as unevaluable by NCI.

Skin ulcers—the UICC states, "neither the development nor healing of skin ulcers should be taken as sole evidence of change"; the NCI does not specifically mention skin ulcers.

Table 17-10
Possible Classification of Organs

Organ	*Bidimensional*	*Unidimensional*	*Evaluable*	*Unevaluable*
Skin and subcutaneous	X	X	X	
Peripheral lymph nodes*	X	X		
Other lymph nodes*	X	X	X	
Lung	X	X	X	
Pleural effusion			If positive cytology X	No cytology or diuretics X
Mediastinum*	Meas. on CT or x-rays X	If pre-involvement x-ray X	No pre-involvement x-ray X	
Bone			X	Scan or enzyme only X
Liver		X	X	Chemistries only X
Intra-abdominal mass	X	X	X	
Primary/contralateral breast	X	X	X	
Central nervous system			X	

*All count as nodal "organ"

Table 17-11
Definitions of Response by Organ Site Involvement

Complete Response

Complete disappearance of all clinically detectable malignant disease for at least 4 weeks. A patient who has radiographic evidence of bone metastases prior to therapy has to have normalization of radiographs or complete sclerotic healing of lytic metastases in association with a normal bone scan.

Partial Response

Greater than or equal to 50% decrease in tumor area for at least 4 weeks without increase in size of any area of known malignant disease of >25% or appearance of new areas of malignant disease.

1. Measurable, bidimensional. Greater than or equal to 50% decrease in tumor area (multiplication of longest diameter by the greatest perpendicular diameter) or a 50% decrease in the sum of the products of the perpendicular diameters of multiple lesions in the same organ site for at least 4 weeks.
2. Measurable, unidimensional. Greater than or equal to 30% decrease in linear tumor measurement for at least 4 weeks.
   a. Mediastinal and hilar width response may be determined by this formula:

      A = On-study width
      B = Normal width (pre-involvement x-ray)
      C = Width after treatment

      $$\text{P.R. if } \frac{(A-B) - (C-B)}{(A-B)} \geq 0.3$$

   b. Palpable masses that can be measured in only one dimension may be evaluated for response by using this formula:

      A = On-study measurement
      B = Measurement after treatment

      $$\text{P.R. if } \frac{A - B}{A} \geq 0.3$$

   c. A partial response of malignant hepatomegaly has occurred if the sum of the liver measurements below the costal margin(s) decreased by ≥ 30%.
3. Nonmeasurable, evaluable: Definite improvement in evaluable malignant disease estimated to be in excess of 50%.
   a. Serial evaluations of chest x-rays (i.e., confluent multinodular and lymphangitic metastases, malignant pleural effusions) and physical measurements (i.e., abdominal girth) should be documented in the records and by photograph when practical.
   b. The response should last for at least 4 weeks.
   c. A partial response of bone metastases occurs if there is a partial decrease in the size of lesions, blastic transformation of lytic lesions, or decreased density of blastic lesions, lasting for at least 4 weeks.

Stable

No significant change in measurable or evaluable disease for at least 4 weeks (≥8 weeks for bone metastases).

1. No increase in size of any known malignant disease.
2. No disappearance of new areas of malignant disease.
3. This designation includes decrease in malignant disease of <50% or increase in malignant disease of <25% in any site.
4. No deterioration in ECOG performance status of ≥1 level related to malignant disease.

Progression

Significant increase in size of lesions present at the start of therapy or after a response or appearance of new metastatic lesions not previously identified.

1,2. Measurable, bidimensional and unidimensional:
   a. Greater than or equal to 25% increase in the area of any malignant lesions >2 cm^2 or in the sum of the products of the individual lesions in a given organ site (comparison of products of the longest diameter by the greatest perpendicular diameter).
   b. Greater than or equal to 50% increase in the size of the product of diameters if only one lesion is available for measurement and was ≤2 cm^2 in size at the initiation of therapy.
   c. Greater than or equal to 25% increase in the sum of the liver measurements below the costal margins and xyphoid.
   d. Appearance of new malignant lesions.

3. Nonmeasurable, evaluable:
   a. Definite increase in the area of malignant lesion estimated to be greater than 25%.
   b. Appearance of new malignant lesions.
   c. Increase in size or number of bone metastases (occurrence of compression or pathologic fractures do not represent progression).
4. Nonmeasurable, nonevaluable: Definite evidence of new clinically detectable (physical or radiographic) malignant disease.

Table 17-12
Evaluation of Patient's Total Response

Organ Site Evaluation

1. Record responses as complete (CR), partial (PR), stable (S), progression (P), or NED under appropriate methods of evaluation.
2. If more than one type of evaluation method exists for a given organ site, each must be recorded separately.
3. If there is more than one measurable lesion per organ site, an organ site PR occurs if there is a greater than 50% decrease in the sum of the products of the perpendicular diameters of all measurable lesions.
4. In patients with measurable disease, the worst response will prevail in determining response by organ site.
5. Stabilization of evaluable disease will not detract from a PR of measurable disease by organ site but will reduce a CR to a PR.
6. Progression in any classification of measurability or evaluability in an organ site shall prevail as the response for that organ site.

Overall Objective Patient Response

1. If progression occurs in any organ site, the overall response will be progression.
2. If *all* organ sites are a CR, then overall response is CR.
3. If in the totals of responses by organ site there are equal or greater numbers of CR plus PR than stabilizations, then the overall response is PR.
4. Stabilization of evaluable organ site does not detract from CRs or PRs in measurable organ sites, but the patient's overall response should be a PR, not CR.

The WHO guidelines are much briefer; ignoring omissions, the main difference with the NCI guidelines seems to be in the definition of partial response as "a 50% decrease in the sum of the products of the perpendicular diameters of the multiple lesions."

Other definitions of partial response have been used in the past; in reading the older literature, it is important to note that most of these definitions would result in *higher* response rates than the current NCI definition of at least a 50% decrease in tumor area in at least 50% of the involved organs with measurable lesions. At one time it was common to measure only "indicator"[84] or easily measured lesions and to ignore other metastatic sites in calculating response. Soft tissue (skin, nodes, breast) lesions and discrete lung nodules were often chosen. Since these lesions have often been found to be more sensitive to chemotherapy than bone or other visceral disease,[85] the use of indicator lesions results in a higher calculated response rate (and higher calculated complete response rate) than if all lesions are used to determine response. Using a 25% decrease instead of a 50% decrease in the partial response definition will obviously result in a higher response rate; for the same reason, defining progression to be at least a 50% increase[86] instead of at least a 25% increase will result in fewer patients being called progressors and give most patients a longer time in which to demonstrate a response. Similarly, if baseline measurements are used to calculate a progression instead of the minimum measurements observed, there will be fewer progressors and progressions will occur later than using the NCI guidelines. In a study of 116 breast cancer patients evaluated for response according to the 1971 criteria of four cooperative cancer groups, it was found that about 15% of the patients (a third of the partial responders) had a partial response based on an observed response in less than half of their sites of disease; these patients would not be deemed responders by the NCI criteria.[87] A study of chemotherapy trials of non-breast cancers (metastatic colorectal cancer, non-small cell cancer of the lung, and squamous cell cancer of the head and neck) surveyed the authors of 62 articles appearing in three cancer journals between January of 1980 and December of 1983.[88] It was found that 28 of the trials reported (45%) required only one measurement to satisfy the definition of response. One would assume this to be a less stringent requirement than requiring measurements at two separate times to satisfy the response definition; however, there was a nonsignificant tendency for trials requiring only one measurement to have a lower response rate. Defining a partial response to be *either* a 50% decrease in the sum of products of diameters of all lesions *or* a complete response in 10% of the lesions measured also results in a higher response rate than the NCI criteria.[87] It is conceivable that someone could have defined a patient partial response as a partial response in *all* organs with disease or at least a 50% decrease in the size of *all* lesions, and this definition would result in a *lower* response rate than the current NCI guidelines; however, we do not know of any report that actually used this definition. So it seems safe to assume that articles not using the NCI (or UICC or WHO) guidelines to determine response will have higher response rates reported than if they used the NCI guidelines.

The use of clearly defined response guidelines in the planning of a trial does *not* guarantee that these guidelines are followed. In re-evaluating response from data records of 401 patients treated on a 1961 protocol,[89] Rimm found that three physicians agreed with each other only 67% of the time and each agreed with the protocol definitions about 67% of the time. He states, "It is apparent from these data that the existence of a set of precise criteria does not guarantee that it will be applied to the data as originally proposed. Consequently, the problem of evaluating results is not, as many expect, resolved simply by establishing a protocol." Sears and Olson reviewed 385 responses of advanced breast cancer and agreed with the original physician in 79%.[90] Slack found the agreement of three physicians with themselves, when reviewing tumor measurements recorded on data forms, was only slightly better than agreement with each other.[91]

In addition to error in following response guidelines, there is clearly a great deal of error in measuring tumors. Studies of simulated tumor nodules[75,92,93] have shown that the probability of falsely declaring a partial response based on a single measurement in addition to the "baseline" when the simulated tumor is the *same* size, when both measurements are done by the *same* physician, and when the definition of response is a 50% decrease in area of the lesion, varies from 0.3% to 8% (for nodules larger than 3 cm in diameter). For two different physicians, the corresponding percentages of false partial responses are 3% to 8% for large (>3 cm) lesions and perhaps as high as 13% for nodules smaller than 3 cm in diameter. Since the definition of progression involves a change of 25%, measurement error has an even bigger effect on determining progression: As many as 13% to 19% of simulated lesions that were the *same* size were declared progressions by a single investigator as a result of measurement error; 26% to 30% of lesions of the same size were declared progressions based on the measurements of two different investigators. Although smaller simulated nodules are associated with more measurement error than larger nodules in all three reports, the same may not be true of enlarged neck nodes[75] and may[94] or may not[75] be true of lung metastases measured on x-rays. In one study[75] of 15 patients with hepatomegaly measured by eight physicians, partial response would have been (erroneously) declared 9% of the time when two different physicians measured the same patient (and a 50% decrease in sum of linear measurements was used to define response). In another study based on 32 patients with hepatomegaly, there was far less measurement error between physicians when liver-spleen scans were used to document response than when physical examination was used.[95] Finally, from autopsy studies[96] we know that many sites of metastases are undetected clinically before death; some of these must be counted as errors in response determination.

Several aspects of the response definitions have been shown to lower the number of false partial responses:

summing up the areas of more than one lesion,[75] requiring two sequential measurements at least 4 weeks apart to be in response,[75] and the fact that the natural history of most lesions is to become larger as time from diagnosis increases.[75,93] None of these extra safeguards are available for the determination of progression: Only one measurement in one lesion is enough to document progression. In addition, there is more measurement error in progression than response. We suggest that, for consistency with past studies, the NCI definition of progression should continue to be used for calculations of response rate and duration of response on protocols but that investigators should not necessarily change treatment whenever this minimal progression definition is met.

Another source of variation in response rates concerns the definition of "unevaluable" response and how unevaluable responses are handled in calculating the response rate. In a 1979 review[97] of 35 reports on metastatic breast cancer, it was noted that 39% of the reports either defined partial response to be something less than a 50% decrease in lesion size or excluded unevaluable patients from the calculation of response rate. A 1975 survey[98] of 30 articles on all forms of cancer found 40% of articles excluded at least one unevaluable patient from the response rate calculation. Altogether, 12% of the 12,000 patients in uncontrolled studies and 5% of the 5,000 patients in controlled studies were excluded. The most common reasons given for nonevaluability were "protocol failure" (51% of the patients excluded from controlled studies) and early death (33% of the patients excluded from controlled studies). In a comparison of the 1971 response definitions for metastatic breast cancer of four cooperative groups, it was found that they each omitted 13% to 14% of the eligible patients from calculation of response rate because of nonevaluability; omitting such patients raised the calculated response rates by 6% to 7% (since the patient group evaluated had about a 50% response rate). It would be helpful if all investigators agreed on how to deal with unevaluable patients in calculating response rates. Since most reasons for nonevaluability (early death, excessive toxicity, refusal of the patient to stay in the study) seem by definition to preclude the possibility that the patient could have benefitted from the therapy, it would seem to be less misleading to classify such patients as "nonresponders" and use them in the denominator of the response fraction.

Two other aspects of protocol design indirectly affect calculation of response: follow-up schedules and time elapsed since hormonotherapy. Although many studies have been done on the optimal scheduling of follow-up examinations in adjuvant therapy patients,[99–103] not much research seems to have been done on metastatic follow-up. If the response criteria require two measurements at least a month apart to be decreased, then a protocol that specifies that chest x-rays should be done once a month will document more responses in patients with lung metastases than a protocol that specifies that chest x-rays should be done once every 3 to 6 months. Perhaps the proposed application of diagnosis-related-group calculation of medical costs for outpatients will encourage investigators in the United States to agree on follow-up schedules. Another area that could use standardization is the eligibility criteria with regard to the interval between prior hormonotherapy and registration on a protocol. Response to ablative surgery is not immediate, so allowing nonprogressing patients to enter a treatment trial within a month or two of oophorectomy will result in a higher response rate on that trial than in a study that requires patients with prior oophorectomy to demonstrate progression before entry. Similarly, withdrawal responses have been documented when either estrogens[104] or other hormones[105] are stopped, so it seems reasonable to require sufficient time to elapse after terminating hormone treatment before starting a new treatment.

ANALYSIS OF RESULTS

This section describes some of the basic ideas that are useful for the analysis of clinical trial data. This material is not intended to be a substitute for a statistics text but is designed to reduce some of the confusion that often accompanies the application of statistical methods to clinical data.

Analysis of Categorical Data

Measurements on patients in clinical trials often can take only one of two values. Examples are response (yes or no), severe toxicity (yes or no), refusing treatment (yes or no), living at least 5 years (yes or no). Other outcomes can take one of four or five different values (e.g., complete, partial, stable, progression for response; none, mild, moderate, severe, life-threatening for toxicity). Both types of outcomes are examples of categorical data. This section will discuss only binary (two-valued) outcomes, but the methods can be extended to outcomes that can take a few more values.

For example, in a trial evaluating objective tumor response at 12 weeks following bilateral oophorectomy for premenopausal patients with advanced breast cancer, 21 complete and partial responses were observed for 95 patients, giving an observed response rate of 22%.[106] It would not be surprising if another group of independent investigators reported a different observed proportion of success for the same procedure and the same patient population used in the example above. Both clinical trials would yield estimates of the same theoretical success rate. Statistical inference refers to the logic and reasoning of using estimates (based on data) and relating them to theoretical probabilities. This is illustrated in Figure 17-2. The result observed in the sample (of 95 patients entered on protocol) is a 22% response. It is important to distinguish this observed result from the population characteristic being estimated (the response rate at 12 weeks to oophorectomy if the entire population of premenopausal women with metastatic breast cancer were castrated). The

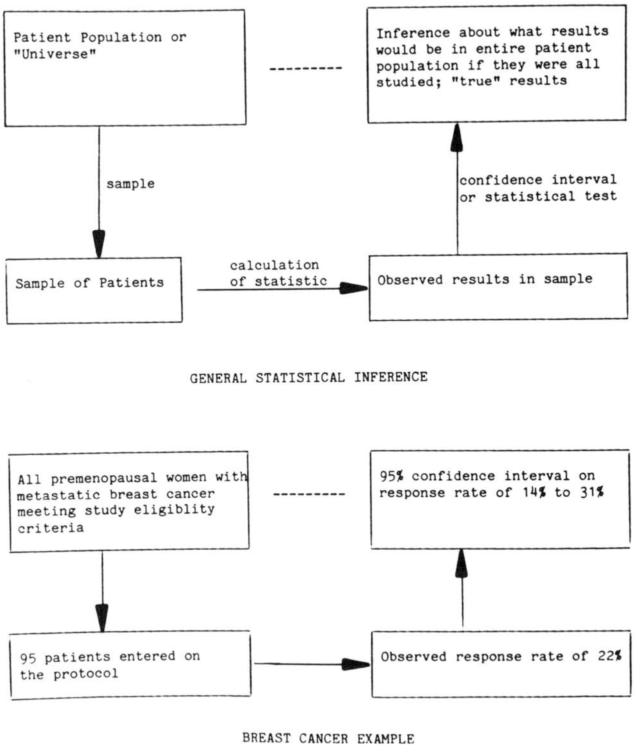

FIGURE 17-2. The process of inference.

observed result is an estimate of the population result and is subject to fluctuations due to sampling variability. One role of statistical methods is to quantify the uncertainty of results due to sampling. Statistical methods enable one to measure variation. This in turn enables one to judge how closely experimental outcomes would agree if the same study were independently replicated. Thus, one can predict in advance the agreement of different institutions on different trials carrying out the same study on the same patient population. As a result, one can provide a standard for objectively deciding when the outcome of two or more treatment groups differs by more than chance.

Confidence Limits

Placing confidence limits on an estimate is a statistical technique that enables one to infer how close the observed proportion is to the theoretical probability. In general, the greater the sample size, the closer the observed proportion will be to the theoretical probability. Often one can quote an uncertainty associated with an observed response rate that denotes limits within which the theoretical probability is likely to be.

In order to judge how far the observed or estimated proportion is from the theoretical success probability, one can calculate a confidence interval for the theoretical probability. Figure 17-3 can be used to calculate 95% confidence intervals as follows: The bowed lines correspond to sample size, the horizontal scales correspond to the observed proportion, and the vertical scales correspond to the theoretical probabilities representing the limits of the 95% confidence interval. For our example, the observed response rate is 21/95 = 22%. To use Figure 17-3, we first find 0.22 on the lower horizontal scale. Looking up the vertical 0.22 line, the lower confidence limit is found on the left vertical scale where the bowed line for 100 patients meets the 0.22 line, and the upper confidence limit is found where the upper 100 patient bow meets the 0.22 line. These limits are 14% and 31%, respectively. (The bowed lines corresponding to n = 100 are used as a convenient approximation to the real sample size of n = 95.)

The interpretation of the range of the interval 14% to 31% is that the observed rate may have been generated by any of the theoretical probabilities within this interval. That is, the observed oophorectomy response rate of 22% is consistent with theoretical rates that are as low as 14% and as high as 31%. The confidence interval is simply a declarative statement, giving the plausible values of the theoretical success probability that could have produced the observed result. In truth, the confidence interval either contains the true success probability or does not—that is, it is correct or incorrect. The 95% figure associated with the confidence interval states the proportion of times these confidence statements are likely to be correct. It is as if we are talking to a person who does not tell the truth all of the time but only 95% of the time. We do not know whether any individual conversation is correct. Because, however, 95% of the statements are correct, we would tend to believe everything the person says. The 95% is called a confidence coefficient. This magnitude is arbitrary, and one can choose different confidence coefficients. However, the confidence coefficient of 95% is widely used.

If the graph in Figure 17-3 is not readily available, approximate 95% confidence intervals can be calculated by taking the estimate ± 2 × standard error of the mean (SEM). The SEM is a measure of sampling variability inherent in an observed response rate, and it is usually estimated by

$$\text{SEM} = \sqrt{p(1-p)/n},$$

where p is the observed proportion of patients responding and n is the number of patients observed. For values of the observed proportion between 20% and 80%, using 2 × SEM provides reasonable approximations for the 95% confidence interval. For the example of the oophorectomy study, the approximate limits (14%, 30%) are almost the same as those obtained from Figure 17-3. A conservative way of calculating the 95% confidence limit is to use the value $\sqrt{1/n}$ as the half-width of the confidence interval. Hence, for our example, n = 95 and $\sqrt{1/95} = 0.10$. Therefore, a conservative 95% confidence limit is 22% ± 10%. This gives 12% and 32% as the confidence limits.

All three calculations of the confidence interval assume that the patients entered in the trial are typical of all

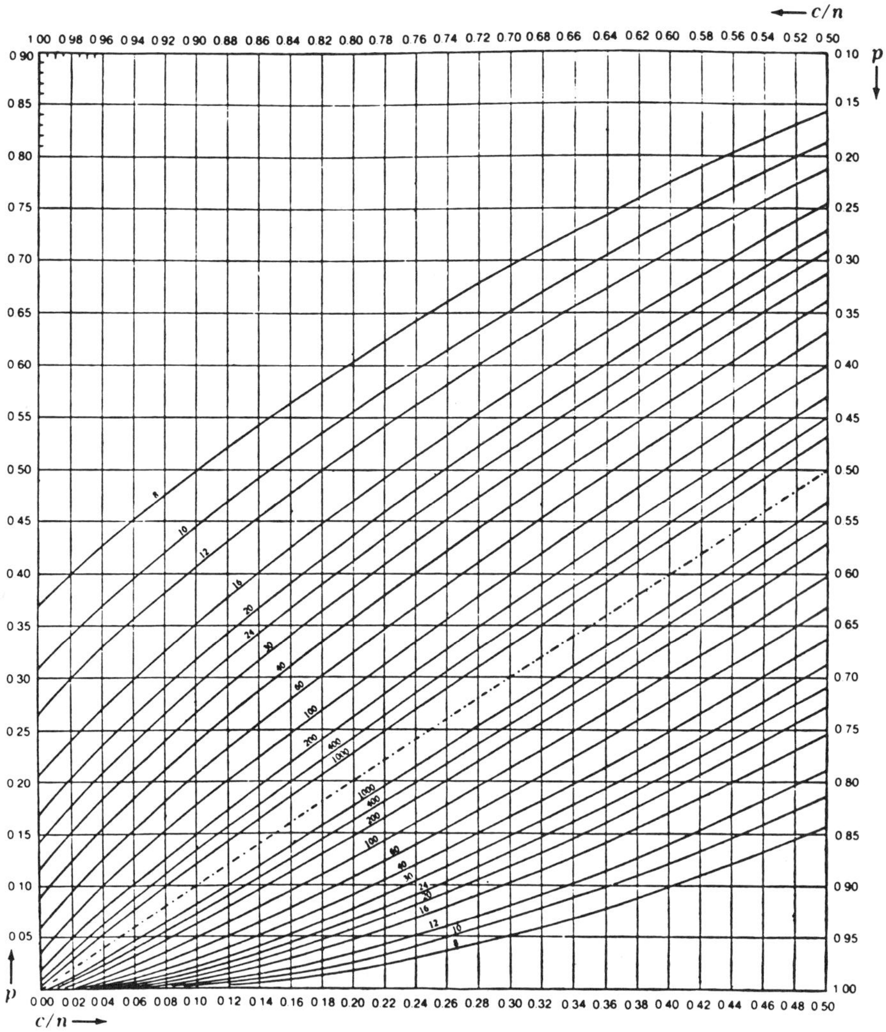

FIGURE 17-3. Chart providing confidence limits for P in binomial sampling, given a sample fraction c/n. Confidence coefficient: $1 - 2\alpha = 0.95$. The numbers printed along the curves indicate the sample size n. If for a given value of the abscissa c/n, P_A and P_B are the ordinates read from (or interpolated between) the appropriate lower and upper curves, then $\Pr\{P_A \leq P \leq P_B\} \geq 1 - 2\alpha$. (Biometrika Tables for Statisticians, Vol. 1, 3rd ed. London, Biometrika, 1976. Reprinted by permission of the Biometrika Trustees.)

patients who meet the eligibility criteria of the protocol. That this assumption may not be exactly correct is shown by a recent article documenting physician bias in selecting patients for a sarcoma trial.[107] Patients and their physicians were asked to participate in a randomized trial comparing Adriamycin versus no treatment. Some patients did actually enter the trial, whereas others declined. Many of the patients who were not entered in the trial received no further treatment. Hence, one had two groups of patients receiving no treatment—one group who were randomized and the other who received it as the treatment of choice by their physician. At the end of 30 months, the randomized treatment group had a 68% survival rate compared with a 29% rate for the other no-treatment group. Obviously both physician and patient selection factors were important in choosing the no-treatment option as the treatment of choice. Hence, when applying the confidence interval methodology to clinical data, one has to keep in mind the role of possible selection factors that may make the statistical calculation irrelevant.

Comparing Response Rates Using a Statistical Test of Significance

Using a statistical test of significance to compare response rates is also a common problem. For example, suppose that 13 patients are randomized and 4 of 6 respond on treatment A (67%) compared with 1 of 7 on treatment B (14%). These results are often presented in a 2×2 contingency table, as shown in Table 17-13. The goal of the statistical analysis problem is to objectively decide whether the theoretical response probabilities are different for the two groups or whether the observed results could be due only to random variation when the treatments have the same theoretical response probabilities.

The logic for judging the evidence proceeds as follows: We assume that the theoretical success probabilities of both A and B are equal. Under this assumption, the probability of each possible outcome of the trial with fixed marginal totals (i.e., five successes, eight failures, seven patients on treatment B, and six patients on treatment A) is computed. Trial outcomes can be enumerated explicitly by looking at "a," the number of successes on treatment A, because, with fixed marginal totals, setting a value for "a" determines the remaining table entries. If the observed result (a=4) is to be judged as evidence in favor of treatment A, then any stronger result (i.e., a=5) should also be judged as favoring A. Furthermore, the same reasoning would apply to treatment B, if the results had been reversed (i.e., a=0, c=5). Thus, by adding together the probabilities of all possible outcomes that represent evidence against equality of treatment effects, we obtain a probability that is called a p value or significance level. This probability assumes that the theoretical success probabilities are the same for both treatments. The entire process is called significance testing. The operational interpretation of a test of significance is that if the p value is less than a small probability, either we have observed a result that would rarely occur or else the assumption of equality of treatment effects is incorrect. Because rare events occur infrequently (by definition), we would tend to place more credence in the second explanation and declare that the treatments are significantly different. It is commonly accepted that p values less than 0.05 are sufficiently small to "declare" that the treatments show a statistically significant difference, although it is perfectly reasonable to use some other small values (e.g., 0.01 or 0.005). The chosen probability is called the significance level of the test. The choice of a significance level depends on the consequences of a false-positive conclusion in a given situation. Because different people have different opinions on what is "really unlikely," many investigators report the actual probability levels (e.g., $p = 0.027$, $p = 0.06$) rather than lumping them into two categories (<0.05 or ≥ 0.05). It is important to note that the p value is not the probability that the treatments are equal; rather, it is the chance of obtaining the observed result or one more extreme if we assume that the effects of the treatments are equal.

The particular calculation described above (as applied to Table 17-13) is known as Fisher's exact test.[108,109] The p value for the example is 0.10. Each possible table is associated with the probability

$$\frac{m!n!s!f!}{a!b!c!d!T!}$$

where $i! = i(i-1)(i-2) \ldots (1)$, so, for example, $6! = 6\times5\times4\times3\times2\times1 = 720$. Although this method provides exact p values, a computer or specialized statistical tables are generally required to carry out the calculations for large samples. Because most scientists do not have easy access to these, the p value is often calculated using an approximation called the chi-square test.

One version of the chi-square statistic is calculated by using the formula

$$\begin{aligned}\chi^2 &= (a-sm/T)^2/\{sfmn/(T-1)T^2\}\\ &= (aT-sm)^2(T-1)/(sfmn).\end{aligned}$$

The approximate p value (two-sided) is the area under a chi-square distribution (1 degree of freedom) to the right of the value of χ^2. Values of χ^2 and corresponding two-sided p values are shown in Table 17-14. Values of χ^2 greater than 3.84 provide statistically significant evidence of a treatment difference (at the $p = 0.05$ level of significance). The approximate p value obtained for the example in Table 17-14 is 0.17.

Analysis of Survival Data

Many of the outcome measures mentioned previously can be expressed as the time between two events—for example, survival (time from randomization or diagnosis or birth to death), duration of response (time from first documentation of partial response to documentation of relapse), disease-free interval (time from primary treatment to first metastases or recurrence). The essential statistical feature of these outcome measures is that the date of the first event is known for all patients in the group but that the date of the second event may be unknown for some patients. For example, literature reports on survival of primary breast cancer patients almost always include data on some patients who had not yet died by the time of the publication. If a patient diagnosed in 1978 was still alive when a survival analysis was done in 1984, the patient is said to be "censored for survival" with a "censored time of 6 years." We know that the patient survived at least 6 years, but we do not know how much longer the patient will live. The usual elementary methods of plotting histograms, calculating means and medians, and comparing two groups (e.g., with the Student t test or the original Wilcoxon test) all assume that the outcome measure is completely known for all patients; hence these methods cannot be used when some patients have censored times. The following sections discuss the analyses of censored data. Many of the examples use survival as the end point, but the methods are the same no matter what time variable is being studied.

Actuarial Curves

Five-year survival percents have often been used to describe the prognosis of cancer patients[110] or to compare different treatments.[111] The advantage of the 5-year survival percent is that it is a single number and hence is easy to remember. The disadvantage is that it does not provide very much information about the survival experience of a group of patients. Physicians soon noticed that different diseases could have the same 5-year survival but be associated with very different short-term (or long-term) prognoses.[112] Since there was no reason to concentrate on 5 years rather than some other time period, investigators began to list 2-year and 10-year survival percents as well as 5-year values. Eventually, tables of survival percents for many time periods were replaced by plots of survival curves, with the time indicated on the horizontal axis (going from 0 to some maximum time) and the percent

Table 17-13
2×2 Contingency Table

	Success	*Failure*	*Total*	*Success Rate*
Treatment A	a=4	b=2	m=6	67%
Treatment B	c=1	d=6	n=7	14%
TOTAL	s=5	f=8	T=13	—

(survival probability) represented on the vertical axis (going from 0% to 100%). Because a curve has an infinite number of points and any study has only a finite number of patients, survival plots use either step functions (Fig. 17-4) or straight lines to connect points corresponding to distinct death times (for ungrouped data) or yearly survival percents (for grouped data).

If no patients are censored, then the T-year survival percent can be simply calculated as the number of patients who survive at least T years divided by the total number of patients. If some patients have censored survival times, then the calculation is more complicated. Table 17-15 shows survival data for premenopausal patients with metastatic breast cancer assigned to combination chemotherapy in an ECOG study.[113] The trial accrued patients from 1978 to 1983, and the analysis was done in 1985. Ten patients entered in 1978; one was still alive at the time of analysis and so is censored in the interval 6 to 7 years. Four patients entered in 1983; two were still alive at the time of analysis and so are censored in the 1 to 2-year interval. Table 17-16 shows the same data summarized by interval. All 95 patients are used to estimate the 1-year survival percent as 1 − 26/95 = 0.73 = 73%. In the life table or actuarial method,[114,115] patients who are censored are assumed to be just like uncensored patients; for example, their survival times are censored simply because they have not yet been on trial long enough to die.[116] Patients who are censored within an interval are also assumed to have been followed for half the interval (in the example, half a year). Hence the number of patients entering an interval minus half the number censored during that interval is used as the number of patient years at risk (69 − 1/2×2 = 68 for the second interval in the example). Hence, of the people who survive at least 1 year, 1 − 22/68 = 0.68 = 68% survive 2 years. Since 73% survive 1 year and 68% of the 1-year survivors survive 2 years, the 2-year survival percent is 0.73 × 0.68 = 0.50 = 50%. This actuarial method is used for large data sets when the individual survival times are grouped—for example, a tumor registry that records survival only to the closest year. Clinical trial reports more commonly use a modification of the life table proposed by Kaplan and Meier.[117] In this method, the survival percent is calculated at each individual death time rather than at yearly intervals (see Fig. 17-4).

Even when the assumption is reasonable that censored patients are just like uncensored ones, some phy-

Table 17-14
Table of Chi-Square, One Degree of Freedom, Two-Sided p Values

χ^2	*p Value*
1.07	0.300
1.64	0.200
2.07	0.150
2.71	0.100
3.17	0.075
3.84	0.050
5.02	0.025
6.63	0.010
7.83	0.005
10.83	0.001

sicians mistrust actuarial calculations,[118] referring to them as "projections"[119] and contrasting them with "absolute" or "real" survival percents. It is important to note that the actuarial method is the only way to use all the data to obtain an unbiased estimate of the T-year survival percent. In the example of Table 17-16, if one simply ignored the fact that 12 patients were censored in the first four intervals, the 4-year survival percent would be calculated as 1 − 69/95 = 27%. This estimate is too high because it is equivalent to assuming that all 12 patients censored before 4 years would survive at least 4 years. If one dropped all censored patients from the calculations, the 4-year survival percent would be computed as 1 − 69/83 = 17%. This estimate is too low because it is equivalent to assuming that we know only that the 12 patients censored before 4 years survived at least 0 days, when in fact we know that all of them survived at least a year and 5 survived at least 3 years.

One could obtain an unbiased estimate of the 4-year survival percent by using data from only those patients entered early enough to make 4-year follow-up possible. In the example, if only patients entered into the trial in 1978, 1979, and 1980 are used, one obtains an estimate of the 4-year survival percent of 1 − 47/61 = 23%, very close to the life table estimate of 24% based on all 95 patients. However, as in the analysis of binomial data, we need more than an estimate of the 4-year survival percent. We need to know the uncertainty of that estimate. The estimate based on the 61 patients entered before 1981 is more

Table 17-15
Survival of Premenopausal Metastatic Breast Cancer Patients Treated with Combination Chemotherapy

Year of Entry Into Trial	*Interval*	*Number Alive at Start of Interval*	*Number Dying During Interval*	*Number Withdrawn Alive = Number Censored During Interval = Number Still Alive on Date of Analysis*
1978	0–1	10	4	0
	1–2	6	1	0
	2–3	5	2	0
	3–4	3	1	0
	4–5	2	1	0
	5–6	1	0	0
	6–7	1	0	1
1979	0–1	25	5	0
	1–2	20	5	0
	2–3	15	5	0
	3–4	10	3	0
	4–5	7	3	0
	5–6	4	1	0
1980	0–1	26	8	0
	1–2	18	8	0
	2–3	10	5	0
	3–4	5	0	0
	4–5	5	2	3
1981	0–1	11	2	0
	1–2	9	3	0
	2–3	6	1	0
	3–4	5	0	5
1982	0–1	19	7	0
	1–2	12	3	0
	2–3	9	4	5
1983	0–1	4	0	0
	1–2	4	2	2

variable than the estimate based on all 95 patients. That is, if all premenopausal patients with metastatic breast cancer similar to the patients in this study were treated with the drug regimen of this study, their 4-year survival percent would probably not be exactly 24%. If we had data on only those patients entered before 1981, we would have a 95% confidence interval of 12% to 34% for the true 4-year survival percent. (This confidence interval was calculated using the normal or SEM approximation to a binomial confidence interval, described previously.) If all the data in Table 17-16 are used in the estimate, then the 95% confidence interval would be 15% to 31% (using Greenwood's formula[120] for the variance). Thus, the 95% confidence interval is narrower when actuarial methods are used.

There are situations in which the actuarial method would be inappropriate or misleading. The essential feature of such situations is that censoring and survival times are statistically dependent—that is, the mechanism causing patients to have censored survival times is for at least some patients related to their true survival time. Two examples of situations where the actuarial method is inappropriate are described below:

1. *A clinical trial in which some patients are lost to follow-up because they or their physicians withdraw them from study for reasons related to therapy or disease status.*

Sometimes sicker patients (those who have had serious toxicity or whose disease is more extensive or who are progressing) are more likely to drop out of a clinical trial than healthier patients; sometimes healthier patients are more likely to be lost (because they move to another city or resume working and miss clinic appointments); sometimes there is a combination of both. Because ascertaining whether a patient who is lost to follow-up is alive or dead is relatively easy (using the National Death Registry or state death certificate offices), this type of dependent censoring may not be a problem in survival analysis. However, it can be a serious problem for end points such as duration of response or disease-free interval. It is sometimes reasonable to count patients who

Table 17-16
Summary of Table C1 Life-Table Calculations

i = *Interval*	n_i = *Number Alive at Start of Interval*	d_i = *Number Dying During Interval*	c_i = *Number Censored During Interval*	*Patient Years at Risk* $n_{i^*} = n_i - c_i/2$	$p_i = 1 - d_i/n_i^*$	1-Year Survival Percent = $S_i = S_{i-1} \times P_i$	KM
0–1	95	26	0	95.0	0.73	0.73	0.73
1–2	69	22	2	68.0	0.68	0.50	0.52
2–3	45	17	5	42.5	0.60	0.30	0.33
3–4	23	4	5	20.5	0.80	0.24	0.24
4–5	14	6	3	12.5	0.52	0.12	0.14
5–6	5	1	3	3.5	0.71	0.09	0.11
6–7	1	0	1	0.5	1.00	0.09	—

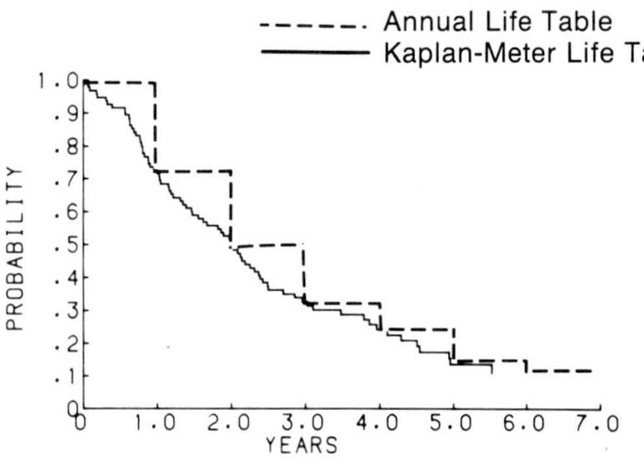

FIGURE 17-4. Actuarial survival curves.

are lost because they are sicker as "relapses" or "recurrences" rather than as censored observations. For instance, many investigators use disease-free survival time (time to recurrence *or* death) as an outcome measure rather than disease-free interval (time to recurrence with patients who die before recurrence counted as censored observations). Another way of handling this problem (for either patients who drop out because they are too sick or patients who drop out because they are too healthy) is to make some assumptions about the shape of the survival curve and/or about a specific mathematical form for the relationship between survival and censoring. That these assumptions can make a practical difference and that the usual actuarial curve can be very misleading is shown in Figure 17-5. These data are from a lung cancer clinical trial with 61 patients, 33 of whom had died and 28 of whom were still alive at the time of analysis or who were lost to follow-up because they developed metastases.[122] The top curve is the usual Kaplan-Meier actuarial estimate; the two straight-line curves are estimates based on different assumptions about the relationship between censoring and survival, and the fourth curve is the estimate obtained when all 61 survival times were available. Clearly,, the Kaplan-Meier estimate and the higher straight-line curve are not good estimates of the survival experience of this group.

2. *A set of data in which there are several causes of death (or failure) and patients who die of causes of secondary interest are recorded as censored observations for the cause of primary interest.*

This problem can arise in a survival analysis when deaths not attributable to cancer are counted as censored; in an analysis of time to local recurrence when distant recurrences or deaths are counted as censored, or in an analysis of duration of response in bone metastases when progressions in other sites are counted as censored. These problems differ from those listed above because no amount of patience and diligent record keeping would enable the investigator to obtain an uncensored data set—for example, some patients will die before local failure and hence time to local failure will never be observed for them. Also, patients with poor prognosis will, as a group, tend to have earlier local failure and will also, as a group, tend to die earlier, so one cannot assume that censoring (possibly due to death) and time to local failure are unrelated. Use of simple actuarial methods in such cases can lead to anomalies, with one group appearing to have a longer time to one type of failure than another group only because it has more of a second type of failure (which is counted as censored). This may have happened in a recent breast cancer trial.[124] Negative-node patients, not given chemotherapy, had an actuarial curve of time to breast failure that appeared to be worse than the corresponding curve for positive-node patients who were given chemotherapy. A far higher percentage of positive-node patients than negative-node patients had died, and patients dying before local recurrence were considered censored for time to local failure. The classification of death without local recurrence as a censored observation could have led to a misleading actuarial curve. Similar problems have occurred in studying other types of cancer—for example, in classifying children with central nervous system failure as censored for time to bone marrow failure.[125] One way around this

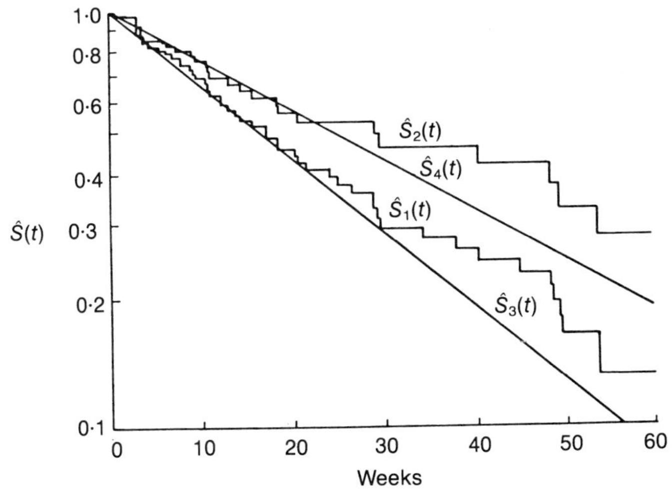

FIGURE 17-5. Semilog graphs of four estimates calculated from data: $\hat{S}_1(t)$, empirical estimate calculated from complete data; $\hat{S}_2(t)$, constant-sum (Kaplan–Meier, 1958) estimate calculated from censored data; $\hat{S}_3(t)$, cone-model estimate calculated from censored data; $\hat{S}_4(t)$, constant-sum exponential estimate calculated from censored data. (Lagakos SW, Williams JS: Models for censored survival analysis: A cone class of variable sum models. Biometrika 65:181-189, 1978. Reprinted by permission of the Biometrika Trustees.)

problem is to analyze time to first unfavorable event—for example, time to death from any cause, time to first recurrence counting death as a recurrence, or time to failure in any site. With such definitions, censoring may be restricted to patients who have not yet been followed long enough to observe an unfavorable event, and hence actuarial methods would be appropriate. Although in many cases such "compound" end points are not of primary interest, they may be adequate for comparisons since big changes in time to any single "simple" end point would be reflected in similar changes in time to the compound end point. When such compound end points are unacceptable, specific assumptions about the relationship between types of failure may allow actuarial-type estimates to be computed.[126,127]

Comparing the Survival Time of Two Groups of Patients

Deciding whether one of two treatments is associated with better survival time would not necessarily be easy even if the two true survival curves were known exactly (e.g., from divine revelation rather than from estimates based on data). One problem in doing such a comparison is shown in Figure 17-6*A*. Treatment A is associated with higher mortality early in the follow-up period and lower mortality later in the follow-up period. When there are two different *integers,* it is always possible for a group of people to come to a consensus on which number is larger; when there are two different *curves* it may be impossible for a group of people to agree on which is "better."

Figure 17-6*B* shows a more subtle problem in comparing two survival curves. Here treatment B is associated with a higher percentage of patients being alive at each follow-up time. However, at any time more than 5 years from the start of the study, patients on treatment B actually have a higher mortality rate than those on treatment A. (When a survival curve is plotted with a log scale for the vertical axis, the slope of the curve at time T is proportional to the mortality rate at time T.) If the survival curves of only those patients who survived at least 5 years are plotted, so that the number of patients alive at 5 years becomes "100%," then the curves in Figure 17-6*C* result. Most investigators would choose treatment B as "better overall" but might hesitate to use it on a patient who has such good risk factors that the patient is expected to survive at least 5 years on either treatment.

The problem of comparing two curves becomes more difficult when the curves are estimated from data. Hence they are not known exactly but have random (sampling) variation. Because the estimate of the late survival curve (the survival near the end of the follow-up period) is based on fewer patients than the estimate of the early survival curve, the estimate of the late part of the curve is always less reliable than the estimate of the early part of the curve; a data set with many censored values exacerbates this problem.

Sometimes survival curves appear to differ early in the follow-up period and then seem to "come together," as in Figure 17-7*A*. Sometimes the opposite happens—that is, the curves are very similar at first and only differ later in the follow-up period, as in Figure 17-7*B*. Not all statistical tests are equally effective (powerful) in these two situations; that is, a test that is very likely to produce a significant result in comparing the two curves of Figure 17-7*A* might be very unlikely to produce a significant result in comparing the two curves of figure 17-7*B*. Before a clinical trial starts to accrue patients, the trial planner needs to decide which type of survival difference (early or late) is of most interest and should choose the most appropriate test statistic for detecting such a difference. It would be misleading to try several statistical tests and report only the most significant.

Two of the most commonly used tests of differences in survival curves are the logrank test (slight variations are known as the proportional hazards test, the Mantel-Haenszel test, the generalized Savage test, or the exponential order scores test[127–130]) and the generalized Wilcoxon test (slight variations are known as the Gehan modification of the Wilcoxon test, the Gilbert modification of the Wilcoxon test, and the Breslow test.[131–134]) The generalized Wilcoxon test is more sensitive to differences in survival distributions that occur earlier in time, and the logrank test is more sensitive to differences that occur later in time. As Fleming and colleagues[135] and Lagakos[136] point out, both statistics can be expressed as the weighted sum of statistics from a series of 2×2 contingency tables.

Consider an example with survival curves obtained

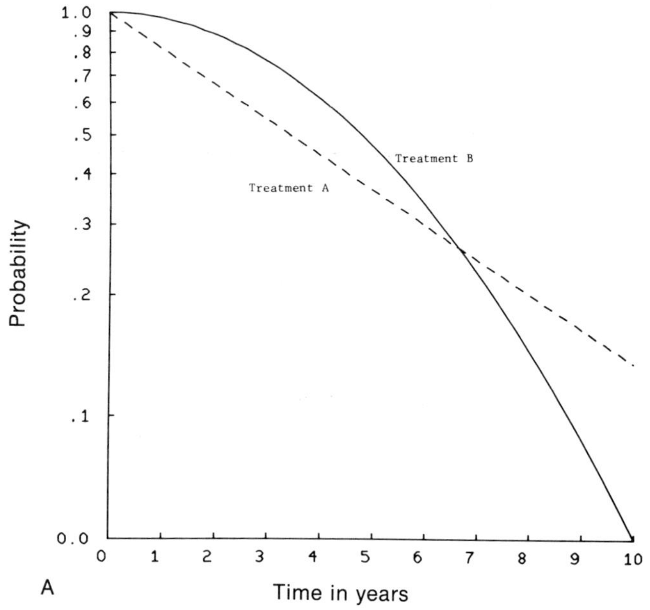

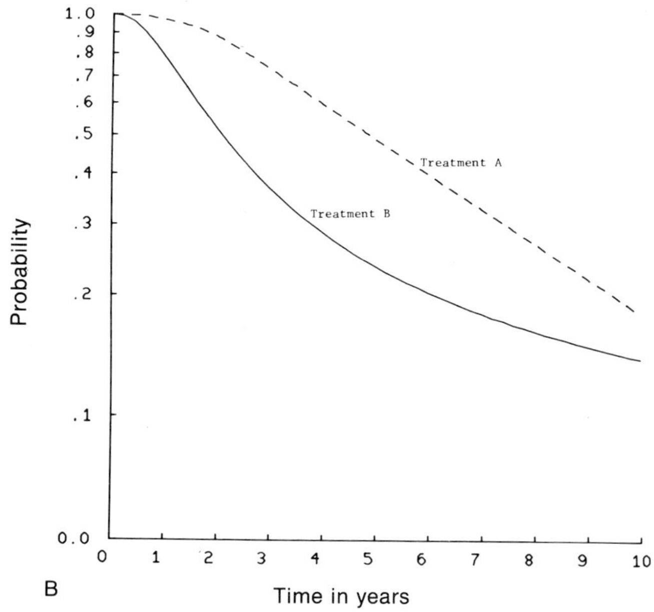

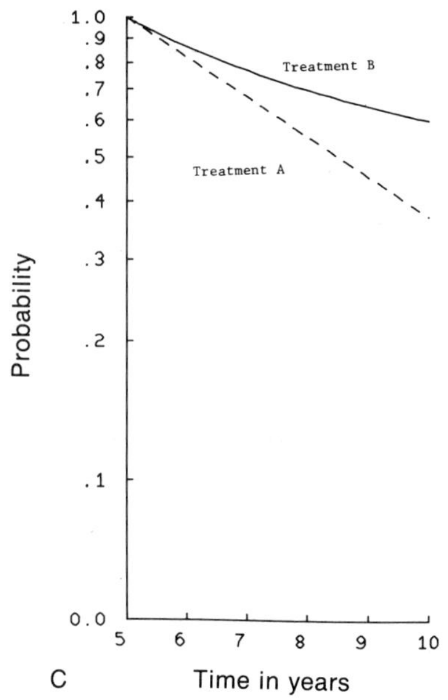

FIGURE 17-6. Two problems in comparing survival curves. *(A)* Crossing survival curves. *(B)* Crossing hazard rates. *(C)* Same survival curves as in *B,* but plots start 5 years after randomization.

from two groups of patients. We designate the groups as A and B. Assume there are M patients treated with A and N treated with B, and that there are J distinct death times, labeled $t_1 < t_2 < \ldots < t_J$. The data can be summarized by forming a 2×2 contingency table corresponding to each death time t_j:

Treatment	*Number of Deaths at Time t_j*	*Number Alive at Time t_j*	*Total Alive Just Before Time t_j*
A	a_j	b_j	m_j
B	c_j	d_j	n_j
Total	s_j	f_j	T_j

If we just consider a single table (the one at time t_j), then conditional on the marginal totals s_j, f_j, m_j, and n_j, the expected value for a_j under the null hypothesis assumption of no difference between treatments is

$$E_j = s_j m_j / T_j$$

and the conditional variance is

$$V_j = \frac{m_j n_j s_j f_j}{(T_j - 1)T_j^2}$$

(If n_j *or* m_j is 0, then we set $E_j = 0$ and $V_j = 0$, because if

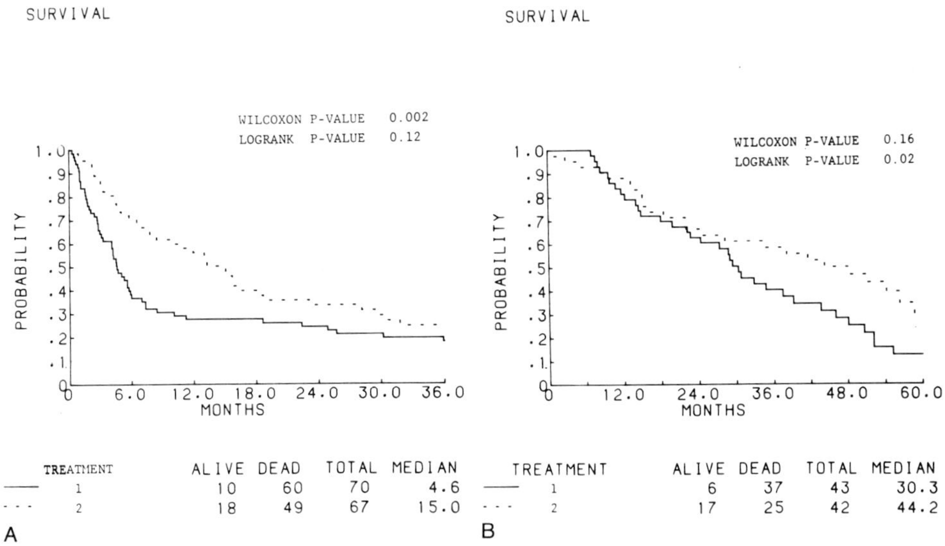

FIGURE 17-7. Illustration of different results from logrank and modified Wilcoxon tests. *(A)* Early difference in survival curves. *(B)* Late difference in survival curves.

only one treatment has patients followed for t_j years, we cannot estimate the difference between survival curves at t_j.) These are the same as the expected value and variance for the chi-square test of differences in proportions. However, now there are J 2×2 tables instead of just one. How should we add up all the E_j and V_j values? Should 2×2 tables with small number of total patients (T_j) be given the same weight as 2×2 tables with large numbers of total patients? One way to answer these questions is to choose some numbers $w_1, w_2, \ldots, w_j$ to use as "weights" and to form the statistic

$$Q = \frac{[\Sigma_j w_j(a_j - E_j)]^2}{\Sigma_j w_j^2 V_j}.$$

It turns out that under the assumption that the null hypothesis is true (i.e., under the assumption that the survival curves do not differ), the statistic Q has a chi-square distribution with one degree of freedom. Hence, the significance level can be found by comparing Q to the values in Table 17-14.

If $w_j = T_j$ (total number of patients alive at the jth death), then Q is the Gehan modification of the Wilcoxon test statistic. If one combines both treatment groups into one and calculates the Kaplan-Meier survival curve, the survival probabilities associated with a death (failure) can be used as the weights in Q—that is, if P_j is the survival probability associated with the jth failure, then $w_j = P_j$. This is another modification of the Wilcoxon test (Breslow, Peto, Prentice). Note that as time increases, both T_j and P_j become smaller. So the Wilcoxon modifications put most weight on early differences and hence are more sensitive to early differences than late.

If $w_j = 1$ for all j, then Q is the Mantel form of the logrank statistic. In this case Q could be simplified as

$$Q = \frac{(O - E)^2}{V}$$

where $0 = \Sigma n_j$ is the number of deaths observed on treatment B, $E = \Sigma E_j$ is the number of deaths expected on treatment B, and $V = \Sigma V_j$. The logrank statistic as introduced by Peto and Peto is

$$Q = \frac{(O - E)^2}{1/EA + 1/EB}$$

where EA and EB are the expected number of deaths on each treatment. The logrank statistic gives the same weight to all tables, even though differences that occur later in the follow-up affect far fewer patients (because fewer are still alive at that point) than differences that occur earlier in the follow-up. Hence the logrank test is more sensitive to late differences than to early ones.

As an example, the significance levels of the generalized Wilcoxon and the logrank test were calculated for the data represented in figure 17-7. For the early difference data set (Fig. 17-7*A*), the generalized Wilcoxon statistic has a value of 10.13 for a significance level of 0.0015, whereas the log-rank statistic has a value of 2.45 for a significance level of 0.12. In contrast, the logrank statistic is more significant in the late difference example (value 5.67, significance level 0.017, compared with the generalized Wilcoxon value 1.97 and significance level 0.16; Fig. 17-7*B*).

We point out that the generalized Wilcoxon and logrank tests will give incorrect significance levels if the censoring and survival times are statistically dependent—that is, if the mechanism causing patients to have censored survival times is for at least some patients related to their true survival time. In a randomized trial, a necessary (but not sufficient) condition for independent censoring is identical follow-up and data collection schedules for both regimens. Simply planning identical data collection schedules is not always enough, as demonstrated by a multi-institutional study of a 6-month induction regimen versus a 16-month induction regimen used to treat metastatic breast cancer.[137] The outcome variable of interest was time to failure rather than survival. Although follow-up data were supposed to be submitted every 6 months, delinquent institutions would often wait until the end of the induction period to mail in data unless the patient failed earlier. This resulted in dependent censoring, with the proportion of patients affected by the dependent censoring being higher in the 16-month induction group (because they had a longer induction period). The logrank test calculated from the available data had a nonsignificant result for a year after accrual ended and then became significant; over the same period of time (from the date accrual ended until a year later), estimates of median time to failure from the Kaplan-Meier curve went from 4.0 to 5.7 months for the 6-month regimen and from 4.7 to 10.2 months for the 16-month regimen. If censoring had been independent of survival, the logrank test would have had a significant result on the date accrual ended and the estimates of median survival at that time would have been 5.6 and 10.4 months.

Dependent censoring can sometimes result in an erroneous decision that two treatments are different. For example, in a study of brain cancer in which data were mailed to a central office once every 6 months, there was at one point a telephone survey of toxicity on one of the study drugs (based on an NCI alert about the drug).[138] The phone interviewers not only recorded toxicity but also noted the death date of the patient or the last date the patient was seen in the clinic. Since frequency of clinic visits was affected by toxicity and since serious toxicity was not completely unrelated to survival time, this survey inadvertently induced dependent censoring for the survival outcome. For about 6 months after the phone survey, the logrank test showed the treatment for which information was obtained in the survey to be associated with significantly worse survival. The treatments never afterward differed significantly in survival times. Had censoring been independent of survival time in all treatments, the logrank test would not have had a significant result at any time.

Use of Multiple Regression Models

Multiple regression models are one group of methods for quantitating the effect of several prognostic variables simultaneously on an outcome measure. The word "effect" does not imply causation, but only association. For example, a regression model based on data of the inhabitants of a town with age as an outcome measure and length of first name and height as "prognostic" variables might show both of the latter variables to have a "significant effect" on age. However, this finding would probably have been induced by time changes in the popularity of certain names and the fact that children tend to be shorter and younger than adults. In no way does the model imply that tallness and brevity of first name cause longevity.

Statistical models can be put to three different uses: prediction, explanation, and post hoc adjustment. Prediction models can help an investigator use data from past studies to predict results in future studies, taking into account possible changes in patient mix. For instance, suppose a study found the response rate of metastatic patients to CMF to be 50% among a group of patients, 50% of whom were premenopausal, 70% of whom had visceral dominant disease, 20% of whom had osseous dominant disease, 50% of whom were completely ambulatory, 50% of whom were partially nonambulatory, and so on. If the article reporting on the study includes a well-defined model of response, then a reader would be able to predict that this regimen might have a 65% response rate in his own metastatic breast clinic, which he knows to be composed of 60% premenopausal patients, 50% visceral dominant patients, 40% osseous dominant patients, 70% completely ambulatory patients, 30% partially nonambulatory patients, and so on. However, a statistical model alone would not enable the reader to use such an article to predict the response rate of totally nonambulatory patients, since the original study did not have any of this type of patient. Also, most medical journal reports of statistical models are not detailed enough to allow this sort of adjusted prediction. Another use of prediction models is in deciding what patient characteristics to use for stratification (or eligibility) in future studies. Fortunately, most literature reports of models do clearly state which characteristics were found to be most prognostic.

Explanation models are used to suggest biologic hypotheses. For example, suppose a model of survival of Stage II breast cancer patients treated with a particular chemotherapy that controlled for various pathologic variables found age to be far more prognostic than menopausal status or hormone receptor status. This could lead to an investigation of drug metabolism at different ages. A similar model that found menopausal status and hormone receptor status to be far more prognostic than age might lead to an investigation of the endocrine effects of the chemotherapy. In either case, the model is used to generate rather than test hypotheses.

Post hoc adjustment models are used in randomized trials to enable a more precise treatment comparison. The simple treatment comparison unadjusted for any patient characteristics would be an unbiased test of treatment effects, but accounting for the variability associated with prognostic factors would increase the sensitivity of the comparisons. If a randomized trial resulted in a large imbalance in an important prognostic factor, it would be important to examine treatment comparisons with and without post hoc adjustment. In nonrandomized studies, post hoc adjustment has a different purpose: to eliminate some of the bias resulting from a lack of balance of known prognostic factors. In such studies, the simple treatment comparison is never unbiased unless patients are completely homogeneous.

There are some post hoc adjustment models available for handling a few prognostic factors that are conceptually simpler than regression models. The most commonly used are called stratified tests. In a stratified test, each prognostic variable must be divided into a few groups, just as it would be for purposes of stratification (e.g., age categorized as less than 50 years, 50 to 60, and more than 60 rather than being used as age in years). The test statistic for comparing treatments is computed within each possible subgroup. Hence, a test using two categories for menopause and three for nodal status would require the calculation of $6 = 2 \times 3$ subgroup statistics. Then the subgroup statistics are combined to obtain an overall test of treatment effect. The variables used to form subgroups for a stratified test need not have been used for stratified randomization. There are stratified versions of all the tests mentioned in the two previous sections on data analysis.[139–142] The advantages of stratified tests over regression models are that it is very easy to tell which subgroup contributes most (or least) to an overall significant treatment difference and that only one extra assumption (over and above those needed for the unstratified test) is necessary. The extra assumption takes the form that the appropriate measure of treatment difference is approximately constant over subgroups. For instance, in using menopausal status (pre or post) and number of positive nodes (either one to three or more than four) in a stratified logrank test of the effect of chemotherapy and control on survival, one must assume that the ratio of hazards (i.e., the mortality rate on chemotherapy divided by the mortality rate on control) is about the same in each of the four subgroups (although the control mortality rate may differ in the four subgroups).

The main disadvantage of stratified tests over regression models is that they become unwieldy with more than a few prognostic variables. Also, there is no way to handle a variable with many values (e.g., age or number of positive nodes) without grouping it into categories. The groupings used may be arbitrary (e.g., age <50, 50 to 60, >60 years), but the results of the model depend heavily on the groupings used. In addition, one loses precision (compared with a simple treatment comparison) if there are any subgroups in which all patients in the subgroup were given the same treatment. In the case of survival analysis, precision is lost if there are any subgroups where all deaths were among patients on one treatment. This greatly limits the number of prognostic factors that can be used in stratified tests.

Regression models have an assumption similar to the constant-difference assumption of stratified tests: the linearity assumption. In each regression model, it is assumed that the outcome variable (or a specific function of it) can be expressed as a function of a linear combination of the effects of the prognostic factors plus an error term. The simplest regression model is linear regression (sometimes called "ordinary least-squares regression"), in which the functions involved are "multiply by 1." If Y is the outcome measure and Z is the treatment variable (coded 1 for one treatment and 0 for the other) and if there are four prognostic factors labeled X_1, X_2, X_3, X_4, then the simple linear model assumes

$$Y = \alpha + \beta Z + \gamma_1 X_1 + \gamma_2 X_2 + \gamma_3 X_3 + \gamma_4 X_4 + f$$

where f is an error term with a gaussian distribution (also called a normal distribution or a bell-shaped distribution). The Greek letters (called coefficients) represent the magnitude of effects. The purpose of the model is to estimate the terms represented by Greek letters. As in the stratified test, this model implies that the difference in treatment effects is assumed to be constant over subgroups (and equal to β). However, it also implies that the difference in outcome between levels of any prognostic factor (e.g., the difference between patients with one positive node and two positive nodes) is the same in all subgroups (e.g., is the same among patients on treatment 0 who are premenopausal and have T1 lesions and are ER negative as it is among patients on treatment 1 who are postmenopausal and have T2 lesions and are ER negative, to name only two subgroups).

In addition to the linearity assumption, regression models assume that the patients in a study constitute a random sample from a much larger target population and that the treatment outcomes within each subgroup follow the distributions presumed by the model.[143] Significance tests and confidence intervals formed from regression models depend directly on this distributional assumption for their validity, not on randomization. This is why nonrandomized studies are usually analyzed by means of these models. It is very important to check that the model assumptions are approximately correct before putting much trust in conclusions based on models. Unfortunately, adequate testing of distributional assumptions usually takes far more patients than are available in either randomized or nonrandomized studies. A few generalities are possible, however. Simple linear regression on survival or binary outcomes is almost never appropriate because the outcome variables by definition cannot follow a gaussian (normal, or bell-shaped) distribution. Response is a two-valued outcome (yes or no) or an ordered categorical outcome (e.g., complete, partial, stable, progression), and neither two spikes nor four spikes can ever be considered bell-shaped (see the frequency diagrams in Figs. 17-8*A* and 17-8*B*). Even if one did not have to worry about censored times, survival would not be bell-shaped because it is always positive (only coding errors live negative years) and because the survival experience of most human groups (whether or not they have cancer) is not symmetric. For example, the median survival time of a group of patients with newly diagnosed metastases from breast cancer all followed to death could be 24 months. Since by definition all survival times are positive, 0 patients died at 0.00 months (although 0.03 is a possible survival time if someone died the day of diagnosis of metastases). So if survival were symmetrically distributed, one would expect all patients to have died by 48 months. But this seldom happens in breast cancer studies; in a study with a median survival time of 24 months, it would not be surprising to find 20% to 30% of the patients still alive at 48 months. In other words, breast cancer survival time tends to have a longer (right-hand) tail than would be expected from a symmetrical distribution. (Some less frequently used regression models such as the log-normal for survival data and the empirical logit for response data[144] partially overcome the above problems of simple regression.)

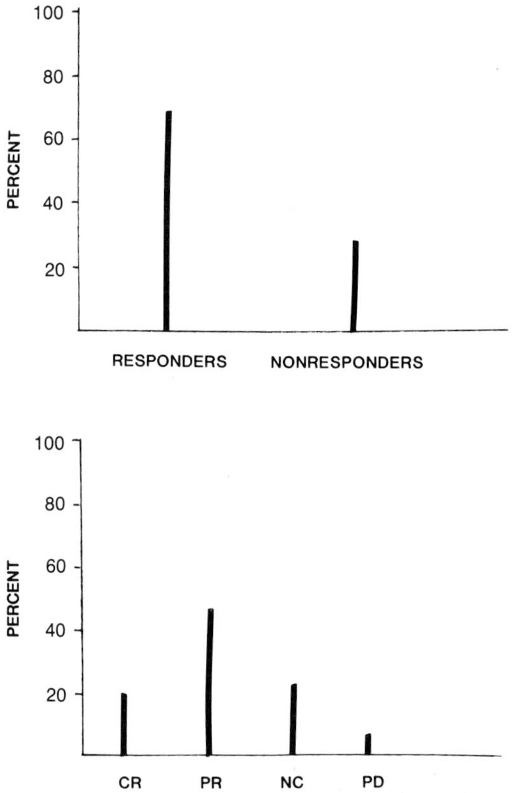

FIGURE 17-8. Histograms of response.

Some cancer survival data may be adequately described by the exponential probability law. Models assuming exponential survival were among the first used in cancer research (Fig. 17-9).[145] The exponential distribution is a member of a family of probability distributions called the Weibull distributions. General Weibull models other than the exponential have been used on breast cancer trials.[146,147] The use of the general Weibull model may be particularly appropriate when the tail of the distribution seems larger than expected from an exponential model. Determining which model most accurately fits the data is difficult. The problem is that many models differ most in the tails (the later part of survival follow-up), which is precisely the part of the curve based on the fewest patients and is subject to the most censoring. So it is often difficult to choose between a Weibull and the exponential model.

The proportional hazards model of Cox[148] is based on a different type of assumption. Instead of assuming a particular mathematical form for the survival curves, it is assumed that there is an underlying unknown survival distribution and that the effect of a value or a prognostic factor (e.g., premenopausal) is to multiply the instantaneous risk of death by a specific constant. The instantaneous risk of death associated with the underlying survival function may not be constant over time, but each multiplicative term associated with a prognostic factor is assumed to be constant over time. Figure 17-10 shows two survival curves with proportional hazards. Since they are plotted with a log scale for the vertical axis, the slopes of the curves at any time point are proportional to their associated death rates. The slope of the lower curve is always 30% larger than the slope of the higher curve. This assumption of proportional hazards applies to every prognostic factor (and to treatment) within every subgroup formed by a specified value assigned to all the other prognostic factors. So it is not an easy assumption to check, although there have been some articles on overall tests of proportionality over time.[149]

A different approach is used to analyze categorical data, particularly outcome variables with only two values, although the method can be extended to an outcome with several values. When the actual outcome has only two possible values (e.g., it is coded 0 for nonresponders and 1 for responders) there is not much use in trying to predict the outcome in individual patients using a linear function. Figure 17-11*A* illustrates this problem for one prognostic factor. The best-fitting line through a set of points at 0 and 1 does not fit any of them very well. So instead of using an individual patient's response as the outcome variable in a model, we use the probability of response among a group of patients with the same characteristics. Probabilities are numbers between 0 and 1. One could consider using a linear model for fitting probability of response, as in figure 17-11*B*. One problem with this approach is that the best-fitting line may well predict probabilities less than 0 or more than 1 for some values of the prognostic factor (e.g., ages less than 35 or more than 70 years in Fig. 17-11*B*). So such data are usually modeled by functions that only take on values between 0 and 1. One such function is the logistic (sometimes called logit analysis).[144] Instead of a linear function to predict probability of response,

$$\Pr(\text{response}) = \alpha + \beta Z + \gamma_1 X_1 + \gamma_2 X_2 + \gamma_3 X_3 + \gamma_4 X_4,$$

the logistic model uses the function

$$\Pr(\text{response}) = \frac{e^{\alpha + \beta Z + \gamma_1 X_1 + \gamma_2 X_2 + \gamma_3 X_3 + \gamma_4 X_4}}{1 + e^{\alpha + \beta Z + \gamma_1 X_1 + \gamma_2 X_2 + \gamma_3 X_3 + \gamma_4 X_4}}$$

where e is the base for natural logarithms. This looks complicated, but since Pr(nonresponse) = 1 − Pr(response) and since, in the logistic model,

$$\Pr(\text{nonresponse}) = \frac{1}{1 + e^{\alpha + \beta Z + \gamma_1 X_1 + \gamma_2 X_2 + \gamma_3 X_3 + \gamma_4 X_4}},$$

then

$$\ln\left[\frac{\Pr(\text{response})}{\Pr(\text{nonresponse})}\right]$$

$$= \ln\,[\text{odds of response}]$$

$$= \alpha + \beta Z + \gamma_1 X_1 + \gamma_2 X_2 + \gamma_3 X_3 + \gamma_4 X_4,$$

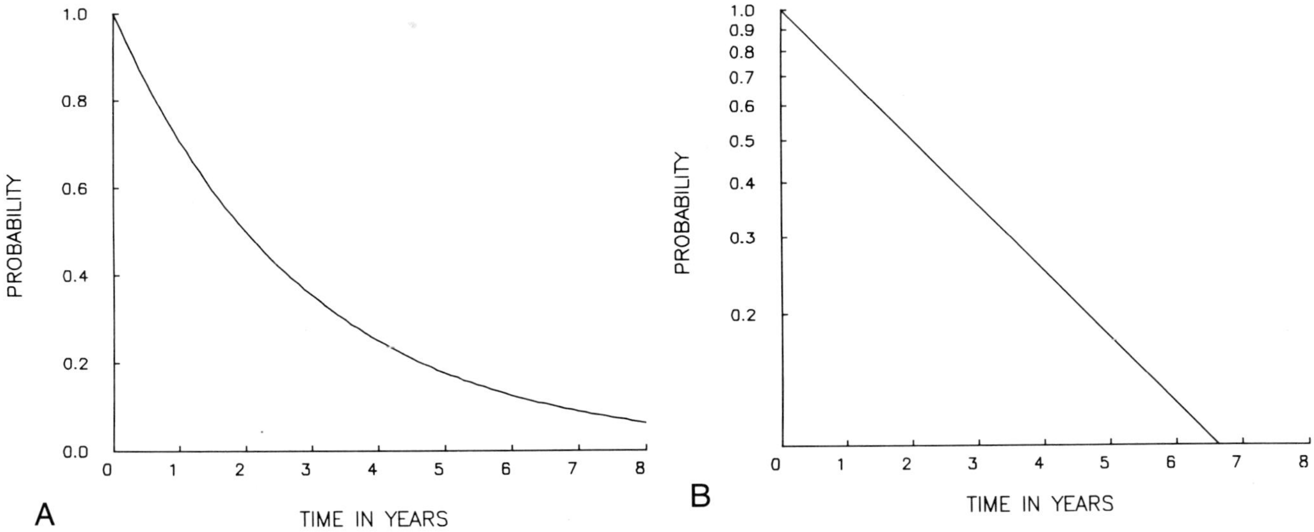

FIGURE 17-9. Exponential survival curve. *(A)* Linear scale for probability axis. *(B)* Log scale for probability axis.

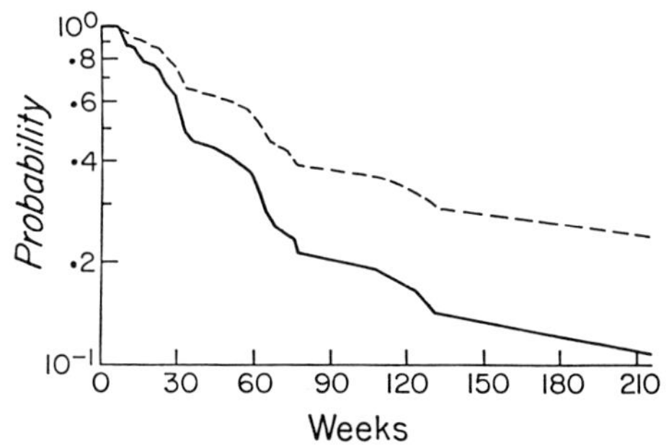

TREATMENT	ALIVE	DEAD	TOTAL	MEDIAN
——— PAM	7	35	42	32.3
- - - CMF	7	35	42	62.6

FIGURE 17-10. Illustration of the proportional hazards assumption.

where ln stands for natural logarithm. In cancer clinical trials, the logistic model is the most common one used for binary outcomes, but any function that takes on values between 0 and 1 could be used, and in fact the probit model (which is based on a different function) is more common than the logistic model for animal carcinogenicity studies.[150] Of course, there are situations in which the logistic and probit models would give different answers. The two models differ most for extreme high or low values for the prognostic factor (i.e., for probabilities of response close to 0 or 1). So to have a good idea of whether the logistic or probit model fits the data better, one would have to have many patients in subgroups that have very low (but not zero) or very high (but less than 1) probabilities of response. (To even obtain an estimate of 1% for the chance of response requires at least 100 patients in a poor-prognosis subgroup, so most trials do not come close to being large enough to allow an accurate choice between the probit and logistic models.) Even in small trials, however, one can choose a few characteristics that seem to be highly prognostic in the model, group them into a few levels, and see how well the logistic model estimates response in the subgroup thus formed.[151]

One sometimes sees a similar sort of checking of survival models. The curve predicted by the model is compared with the actuarial survival curve for some subgroups.[147] It is important to note that this sort of checking of model predictors (whether for survival or binary outcomes) against the data the model was based on is only meant to provide a rough guide to whether model assumptions are strongly violated in one data set. Such checking *cannot* verify that the model is good for prediction. The only way to do that is to obtain a totally different data set (e.g., run another trial) and see how well a model fitted to the old data predicts the new data. Since few investigators have the luxury of repeating a clinical trial, this prediction checking is usually accomplished by dividing the patient group in half. One group is used for model development and the other group is used to assess the predictive accuracy of the model[151] (although very few investigators seem to bother with any sort of prediction checking). There are also other methods of cross-validation using many small subgroups instead of one large one as the test sample.[152,153]

Investigators who do cross-validation are sometimes shocked when a model that seems to fit the development data set very well does a horrible job of predicting outcome in the test group. Part of the explanation is in the great variation of both cancer patients and treatment. We really do not know all the important prognostic factors, and most models account for only a very small amount of the natural variation among cancer patients. However, part of the explanation is purely statistical and involves overfitting and collinearity. Overfitting refers to using too many prognostic factors in the model. Although one major ad-

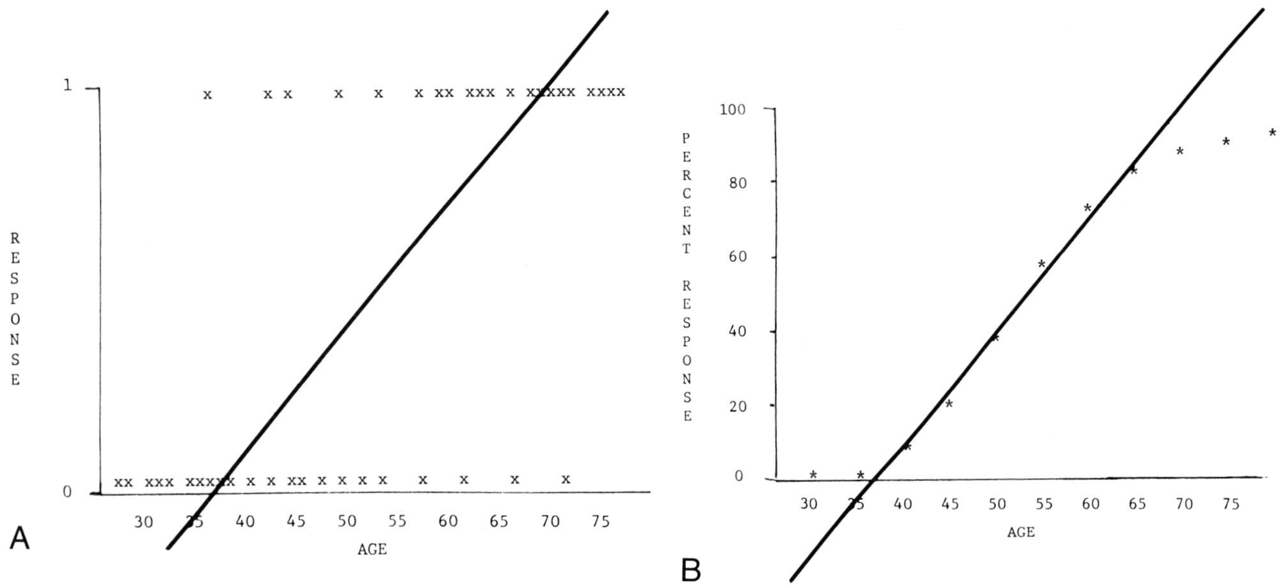

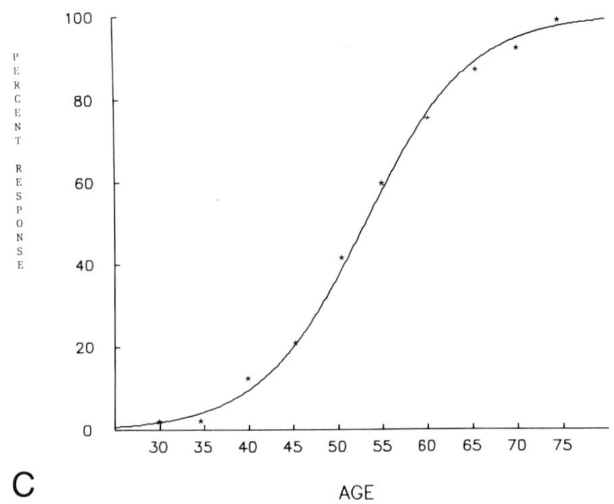

FIGURE 17-11. Reason for using logistic regression for binary data. *(A)* Best-fitting straight line relating response to age. *(B)* Best-fitting straight line relating proportion responding to age. *(C)* Best-fitting logistic curve relating proportion responding to age.

vantage of regression models over stratified tests is that the former can handle more patient characteristics, there is still a limit. For example, if one had complete survival data on 50 patients and one used 49 variables in a model, the model would perfectly fit the survival times of those 50 patients, even if all 49 "prognostic factors" were fabricated by being assigned a value of 1 if a coin toss resulted in heads and 0 otherwise. However, since the prognostic factors are only random numbers, the model based on them would have *no* predictive accuracy on any other data set. A rough rule of thumb is that one should not try to fit a regression model "when there are fewer than ten times as many events in the training sample as there are" prognostic factors.[151] In survival analysis, an event is death; in response analysis with an overall response percent over 50%, an event is nonresponse; in response analysis with an overall response percent under 50%, an event is response. So a proportional hazards model developed on a data set with 80 patients of whom 20 have died could only really handle two possible prognostic factors, and even that would be a problem if the two factors were collinear. Exact collinearity refers to a situation in which two or more prognostic factors are linearly related,[155] for example,

$$X_2 = 32 + 9/5\ X_3$$

where X_2 is temperature in Fahrenheit and X_3 is temperature in Celsius. One could not use both X_2 and X_3 as prognostic factors in the same model. Such exact collinearity seldom occurs in clinical trials. Approximate collinearity is a problem whenever two (or more) patient characteristics are highly correlated—for example, age under 50 years and menopausal status, or more than three organs with metastases and visceral dominant metastases. If two prognostic factors are highly correlated among patients who have an event in the development data set, then the significance levels associated with those factors will be unreliable and the estimates of coefficients for those factors when both are in the model will be random. So the only way to explore whether menopause or age is most correlated with survival is to obtain a data set with many young postmenopausal and old premenopausal women (less collinearity).

Statistical Methods of Combining Data from Different Studies

It is not unusual for a clinical question in breast cancer research to be associated with several separate but very similar randomized trials. Often each of the trials involved has an accrual that is too small to have a reasonable chance of detecting clinically important treatment differences. (See the section above entitled "Sample Size.") In addition, the results of the separate trials are not identical and can be contradictory. Hence medical journals include many breast cancer literature reviews that attempt to draw overall conclusions from the wealth of published reports.

Some of these reviews[156–159] use statistical methodology to combine data. The statistical methods used differ primarily in how much homogeneity of studies is assumed. Conceptually, the simplest way of combining data from several randomized trials using the same two treatments (call them A and B) and the same definition for some outcome variable would be to combine all data on patients treated with A, to combine all data on patients treated with B, and then to compare these two large groups using one of the statistical tests described above in the sections entitled "Analysis of Categorical Data" and "Analysis of Survival Data." Let us call this "combined group analysis" just to have a name for it. This method assumes complete homogeneity between trials. Such an analysis would be unbiased and would be more sensitive to small differences than the analysis of one of the studies of A versus B. However, since the trials undoubtedly differ at least a little in patient mix, treatment outcome, or length of follow-up, the sensitivity of the analysis could be improved by treating the individual trials as strata and doing one of the stratified tests alluded to in the beginning of this section. Stjernsward[156] used a stratified chi-square test on 5-year survival percents to evaluate the benefit of adjuvant radiotherapy. More recently, Peto[158] in an yet unpublished analysis used a stratified logrank test to evaluate (separately) adjuvant chemotherapy and adjuvant hormonotherapy.

A simpler and cruder way of combining studies involves combining results rather than patient data. Suppose there are five trials comparing A with B and that in all five, a survival analysis shows A better than B (although not necessarily significantly better). Under the null hypothesis that A and B are associated with the same survival, the probability that five out of five trials would favor A is $(0.5)^5 = 0.03125$. So this is evidence that A is associated with longer survival than B. In general, if there are a total of n trials and A appears to be better in k of them, the p value associated with this distribution of trial results is

$$(0.5)^n \sum_{i=k}^{n} \frac{n!}{i!(n-i)!}$$

where $i! = i(i-1)(i-2)\ldots(2)(1)$ and $0! = 1$. This method is called the sign test and has been used by Stjernsward and Day[157] in combining evidence from trials of adjuvant radiotherapy. Its advantages are that it is simple to calculate and the data needed for its calculation are always available in published reports of clinical trials. Its disadvantage is that all trials are equally weighted (i.e., a trial of 5 patients counts the same as a trial of 5000). In either a stratified test or the combined group analysis, the result of each trial is weighted proportionally to the number of events (e.g., death or response) in the trial. Hence the stratified tests and the combined group tests are more sensitive to small differences than the sign test.

The combined group analysis works best when the outcomes on treatment A are very similar in all the trials and the outcomes on treatment B are very similar in all the trials. If the outcomes (or distributions of prognostic characteristics) vary much from trial to trial, it would be better to use a stratified test (or the sign test), since such tests are not based on the assumption of homogeneity of treatment A outcomes and of treatment B outcomes. Instead, stratified tests and the sign test assume that some appropriate measure of treatment difference is approximately the same for all trials. Although homogeneity of differences is a more reasonable assumption than homogeneity of outcomes within treatment groups, it has often been criticized.[160,161,162] There is a group of models, called random effects models, which allow one to test whether the treatment differences are more heterogeneous than could be expected from the sizes of the trials and, if so, to account for this "extra" variation in a stratified test. Himel and colleagues[159] used such a model in analyzing published reports of adjuvant chemotherapy.

There is one other type of heterogeneity to worry about in combining data from many studies when the outcome variable used is the time until an event—for example, survival time. Even if one is willing to assume homogeneity over trials of differences, one may not be willing to assume homogeneity over time of differences. That is, the difference between A and B may not be constant over time. For example, in the first year following randomization, A may be twice as good as B as measured by the odds ratio of death; in the second year A may be only 80% better, in the third year 40% better, and in the fourth year two treatments may be associated with the same risk of death. There is some evidence[163] that survival time and time to recurrence differences between adjuvant chemotherapy (or hormonotherapy) and control are not constant over time. If this is true, then combining data from trials with different lengths of follow-up could be a problem. If a statistic that puts proportionally more weight on the tail of the survival curve were used (e.g., the logrank test), then the trials followed for the longest time would be given much more weight than the other trials. It may be that the trials followed longest are not typical of the studies being combined. If so, the results of the combined analysis might change drastically when more follow-up is obtained on recently started trials. A related problem is that a test for homogeneity of differences over trials is limited by the amount of follow-up available on each trial.

Even if the trials seem very similar for the first 3 years of follow-up, there is no way to test if they will be similar for the next 3 years unless all have at least 6 years of follow-up. For this reason, it would be better to find the trial with the minimum follow-up and only combine data up to that time. Unfortunately, literature reports often do not include enough detail to allow calculation of the observed difference at an earlier time.

It seems clear that reviews combining data from many trials on breast cancer will continue to be written. It also seems clear that investigators will continue to argue about whether the particular trials combined are similar enough with regard to treatment, patient characteristics, follow-up schedules, and outcomes to make a combined analysis at all reliable. It would certainly be easier to draw conclusions from a few well-run large trials than from many small ones. We hope that in the future more mechanisms for cooperation in clinical research will be developed.

REFERENCES

1. Greenwood M: Is the statistical method of any value in medical research? Lancet 2:153–158, 1924
2. Zelen M: The randomization and stratification of patients to clinical trials. J Chron Dis 27:365–375, 1974
3. Meier P: Statistical Analysis of Clinical Trials. In Shapiro SH, Lewis JA (eds): Clinical Trials, p 168. New York, Marcel Dekker, 1983
4. Byar DP, Simon RM, Friedewald WT, et al: Randomized clinical trials: Perspectives on some recent ideas. N Engl J Med 295:74–80, 1976
5. Pocock SJ: Clinical Trials, pp 50–65. New York, John Wiley & Sons, 1983
6. Friedman LM, Furberg CD, DeMets DL: Fundamentals of Clinical Trials, pp 28–36. Boston, John Wright & Sons, 1982
7. Bailar JC III, Brown BW, DeCosse JJ, et al: Issues in the design of clinical trials. In Miké V, Stanley KE (eds): Statistics in Medical Research, pp 189–218. New York, John Wiley & Sons, 1982
8. Gelber RD, Zelen M: Planning and reporting of clinical trials. In Calabresi P, Scheir PS, Rosenberg SA (eds): Medical Oncology, pp 406–425. New York, Macmillan, 1985
9. Gehan EA, Freireich EJ: Nonrandomized controls in cancer clinical trials. N Engl J Med 190:198–203, 1974
10. Moertel CG, Reitemeier RJ: Advanced Gastrointestinal Cancer: Clinical Management and Chemotherapy. New York, Paul E Hoeber, 1969
11. Zelen M: Strategy and alternate randomized designs in cancer clinical trials. Cancer Treat Rep 66:1095–1100, 1982
12. Chalmers TC, Block JB, Lee S: Controlled studies in clinical cancer research. N Engl J Med 287:75–78, 1972
13. Brown BW, Hollander M: Statistics, A Biomedical Introduction, p 138. New York, John Wiley & Sons, 1977
14. Gilbert JP, McPeck B, Mosteller F: Progress in surgery and anesthesia: Benefits and risks of innovative therapy. In Bunker JP, Barnes BA, Mosteller F (eds): Costs, Risks, and Benefits of Surgery, pp 124–169. New York, Oxford Press, 1977
15. Chalmers TC, Shroeder B: Controls in "Journal" articles. N Engl J Med 301:1293, 1979
16. Pocock SJ: The combination of randomized and historical controls in clinical trials. J Chron Dis 29:175–188, 1976
17. Moon TE, Jones SE, Tong T, et al: Development of a natural history data base of breast cancer studies. In Salmon SF, Jones SE (eds): Adjuvant Therapy of Cancer IV, pp 227–234. New York, Grune & Stratton, 1984
18. Pocock SJ: Letter: Randomized clinical trials. Br Med J 1:1661, 1977
19. Tormey D, Gelman R, Falkson G: Prospective evaluation of rotating chemotherapy in advanced breast cancer. Am J Clin Oncol 6:1–18, 1983
20. Fisher B, Redmond C: Studies of the NSABP. In Salmon SE, Jones SE (eds): Adjuvant Therapy of Cancer, pp 67–81. New York, Elsevier-Dutton Holland, 1977
21. Fisher B, Redmond C, Fisher ER: A summary of findings from NSABP trials of adjuvant therapy. In Salmon SE, Jones SE (eds): Adjuvant Therapy of Cancer IV, pp 185–194. New York, Grune & Stratton, 1984
22. Gutterman JU, Cardenas JO, Blumenschein GR, et al: Chemoimmunotherapy of disseminated breast cancer—prolongation of remission and survival. Br Med J 2:1222–1225, 1976
23. Muss HB, Richards F, Cooper MR, et al: Chemotherapy vs. chemoimmunotherapy with methanol extraction residue of bacillus Calmette-Guerin in advanced breast cancer: A randomized trial by the Piedmont Oncology Association. Cancer 47:2295–2301, 1981
24. Malick GR, Blumenschein SS, Legha GN, et al: A randomized trial of high dose 5-fluorouracil, doxorubicin, and cyclophosphamide vs. conventional FAC regimen in metastatic breast cancer. Proc Am Soc Clin Oncol (abstract C303) 1:1982
25. Zelen M: The randomization and stratification of patients to clinical trials. J Chron Dis 27:365–375, 1974
26. Simon R: Design and conduct of clinical trials. In DeVita VT Jr, Hellman S, Rosenberg SA (eds): Cancer: Principles and Practice of Oncology, Vol. 1, p 334. Philadelphia, JB Lippincott Co, 1985
27. Pocock SJ: Clinical Trials, pp 84–85. New York, John Wiley & Sons, 1983
28. White SJ, Freedman LS: Allocation of patients to treatment groups in a controlled clinical study. Br J Cancer 37:849–857, 1978
29. Pocock SJ, Simon R: Sequential treatment assignment with balancing for prognostic factors in the controlled clinical trial. Biometrics 31:103–115, 1975
30. Begg CB, Iglewicz BB: A treatment allocation procedure for clinical trials. Biometrics 36:81–90, 1980
31. Peto, R, Pike MD, Armitage P, et al: Design and analysis of randomized clinical trials requiring prolonged observation of each patient. I. Introduction and design. Br J Cancer 34:585–612
32. Randomized clinical trials (leader). Br Med J 1:1238–1239, 1977
33. Ludwig Breast Cancer Study Group: Chemotherapy with or without oophorectomy in high risk premenopausal patients with operable breast cancer. J Clin Oncol 3:1059–1067, 1985
34. Jain KK, Caspar ES, Geller NC, et al: A prospective randomized comparison of epirubicin and doxorubicin in patients with advanced breast cancer. J Clin Oncol 3:818–826, 1985
35. Cummings FJ, Gelman R, Horton J: Comparison of CAF versus CMFP in metastatic breast cancer: Analysis of prognostic factors. J Clin Oncol 3:932–940, 1985
36. Wils JA, Bron H, VanLange L, et al: A randomized trial of combined versus alternating therapy with cytostatic drugs and high dose medroxyprogesterone acetate in advanced breast cancer. Cancer 56:1325–1331, 1985
37. Mann GB, Hortobagyi GN, Buzdar AU, et al: A comparative

study of PALA, PALA plus 5-FU, and 5-FU in advanced breast cancer. Cancer 56:1320–1324, 1985
38. Zekan PJ, Muss HB, Capizzi RL, et al: High dose cyclophosphamide and 5-fluorouracil versus vincristine, doxorubicin, and cyclophosphamide in advanced carcinoma of the breast. Cancer 54:2338–2343, 1984
39. Krook JE, Ingle JN, Green SJ, et al: Randomized clinical trial of cyclophosphamide, 5-FU, and prednisone with or without tamoxifen in postmenopausal women with advanced breast cancer. Cancer Treat Rep 69:355–361, 1985
40. Falkson G, Gelman RS, Tormey DC: Mitomycin and tamoxifen versus mitolactol, doxorubicin, and tamoxifen in patients with previously treated breast cancer. Cancer Treat Rep 69:755–760, 1985
41. Mouridsen HT, Rose C, Engelsman E, et al: Combined cytotoxic and endocrine therapy in postmenopausal patients with advanced breast cancer: A randomized study of CMF vs. CMF plus tamoxifen. Eur J Cancer Clin Oncol 21:291–299, 1985
42. Taylor G IV, Kalish LA, Olson JE: Adjuvant CMFP versus CMFP plus tamoxifen versus observation alone in postmenopausal, node-positive breast cancer patients: Three-year results of an ECOG study. J Clin Oncol 3:145–154, 1985
43. Klefstrom P, Halsti P, Grohn P, et al: Levamisole in the treatment of Stage II breast cancer. Cancer 55:2753–2757, 1985
44. Meier P, Ferguson DJ, Karrison T: A controlled trial of extended radical mastectomy. Cancer 55:880–891, 1985
45. Bonadonna G, Valagussa P, Rossi A, et al: Ten year experience with CMF-based adjuvant chemotherapy in resectable breast cancer. Breast Cancer Res Treat 5:95–115, 1985
46. Fisher B, Bauer M, Margolese R, et al: Five-year results of a randomized clinical trial comparing total mastectomy and segmental mastectomy with or without radiation in the treatment of breast cancer. N Engl J Med 312:665–673, 1985
47. Fisher B, Redmond C, Fisher ER, et al: Ten year results of a randomized clinical trial comparing radical mastectomy and total mastectomy with or without radiation. N Engl J Med 312:674–681, 1985
48. Ribeiro G, Swindel R: The Christie Hospital tamoxifen (Nolvadex) adjuvant trial for operable breast carcinoma—7 year results. Eur J Cancer Clin Oncol 21:897–900, 1985
49. Pocock SJ, Lagakos SW: Practical experience of randomization in cancer trials: An international survey. Br J Cancer 46:368–375, 1982
50. Goldhirsh A, Gelber R for the Ludwig Breast Cancer Study Group: Adjuvant treatment for early breast cancer: The Ludwig breast cancer studies. Cancer Treat Rep Natl Cancer Inst Monogr 1:55–70, 1986
51. Freiman JA, Chalmers TC, Smith H, et al: The importance of beta, the type II error, and sample size in the design and interpretation of the randomized controlled trial. N Engl J Med 290:690–694, 1978
52. Zelen M, Grehan E, Glidewell O: Biostatistics. In Hoogstraten B(ed): Cancer Research: The Impact of the Cooperative Groups, pp 291–312. New York, Mason Publishing, 1980
53. Mosteller F, Gelbert JP, McPeek B: Reporting standards and research strategies for controlled trials. Controlled Clin Trials 1:37–50, 1980
54. Staquet MJ (ed): Randomized Trials in Cancer: A Critical Review by Sites. New York, Raven Press, 1978
55. Fleiss JL: Statistical Methods for Rates and Proportions, pp 38–48, 260–280. New York, John Wiley & Sons, 1981
56. Feigl P: A graphical aid for determining sample size when comparing two independent proportions. Biometrics 34:111–122, 1978
57. Casagrande JT, Pike MC, Smith PG: The power function of the exact test for comparing two binomial distributions. Appl Stat 27:176–180, 1978
58. George SL, Desu MM: Planning the size and duration of a clinical trial studying time to some critical event. J Chron Dis 27:15–24, 1974
59. Peto R, Pike MC, Armitage P, et al: Design and analysis of clinical trials requiring prolonged observation of each patient. Br J Cancer. Part I 34:585–612, 1976; Part II 35:1–39, 1977
60. Lesser ML, Cento SJ: Tables of power for the F-test for comparing two exponential survival distributions. J Chron Dis 34:533–544, 1981
61. Schoenfeld DA, Richter JR: Nomograms for calculating the number of patients needed for a clinical trial with survival as an endpoint. Biometrics 38:163–170, 1982
62. Bernstein D, Lagakos SW: Sample size and power determination for stratified clinical trials. J Stat Comput Simul 8:65–73, 1978
63. Lehmann EL: Nonparametrics: Statistical Methods Based on Ranks, pp 69–75. San Francisco, Holden-Day, 1975
64. Freedman LS: Tables of the number of patients required in clinical trials using the logrank test. Stat Med 1:121–129, 1982
65. Peto R: Presentation to NCI sponsored consensus conference on adjuvant breast cancer treatment, Bethesda, Maryland. September, 1985
66. Himel HN, Liberati A, Gelber RD, et al: Adjuvant chemotherapy for breast cancer: A pooled estimate based on results from published randomized control trials. JAMA 256:1148–1159, 1986
67. Schneiderman MA, Krant MJ: What shall we measure on whom: Why? Cancer Chemother Rep 50:107–112, 1966
68. Anderson JR, Cain KC, Gelber RD: Analysis of survival by tumor response. J Clin Oncol 1:710–719, 1983
69. Mantel N, Byar DP: Evaluation of response time data involving transient states: An illustration using heart transplant data. J Am Stat Assoc 69:81–86, 1974
70. Vogel CL, East DR, Lafonte J, et al: Alternating cytoreductive and cycle active chemotherapy in patients with poor risk patterns of metastatic breast cancer. Proc Am Soc Clin Oncol 22:409, 1980
71. Wittes R: Discussion: Cancer Treat Rep 69:1145–1146, 1985
72. Kiang DT, Gay J, Goldman A, et al: A randomized trial of chemotherapy and hormonotherapy in advanced breast cancer. N Engl J Med 313:1241–1246, 1985
73. Tonkin K, Tritchler D, Tannock I: Criteria of tumor response used in clinical trials of chemotherapy. J Clin Oncol 3:870–875, 1985
74. Baum M, Priestman T, West RR, et al: A comparison of subjective responses in a trial comparing endocrine with cytotoxic treatment in advanced carcinoma of the breast. In Mouridsen HT, Palshoff T (eds): Breast Cancer—Experimental and Clinical Aspects, pp 223–226. Oxford, Pergamon Press, 1980
75. Warr D, McKinney S, Tannock I: Influence of measurement error on assessment of response to anticancer chemotherapy: Proposal for new criteria of tumor response. J Clin Oncol 2:1040–1046, 1984
76. Hoogstraten B, Irewin L, Ahmann D, et al: Breast Cancer: Suggested Protocol Guidelines for Combination Chemotherapy Trials, DHEW Publication No. (NIH) 77-1192. Bethesda, MD, 1977
77. Hayward JL, Carbone PP, Heuson JC, et al: Assessment of

response to therapy in advanced breast cancer. Cancer 39:1289–1294, 1977

78. British Breast Group: Assessment of response to treatment in advanced breast cancer. Lancet 1:38–39, 1974
79. Miller AB, Hoogstratten B, Staquet M, et al: Reporting results of cancer treatment. Cancer 47:207–214, 1981
80. Oken MM, Creech RH, Tormey DC, et al: Toxicity and response criteria of the Eastern Cooperative Oncology Group. Am J Clin Oncol 5:649–655, 1982
81. Coccini G, DiBlasio B, Alberti G, et al: Problems in evaluating response of primary breast cancer to systemic therapy. Breast Cancer Res Treat 4:309–313, 1984
82. Bitran JD, Bekerman C, Desser RK: The predictive value of serial bone scans in assessing response to chemotherapy in advanced breast cancer. Cancer 45:1562–1568, 1980
83. Citrin DL, Hougen C, Zweibel W, et al: The use of serial bone scans in assessing response of bone metastases to systemic therapy. Cancer 47:680–685, 1981
84. Lavin PT: An alternative model for the evaluation of antitumor activity. Cancer Clin Trials 4:451–457, 1981
85. Smalley RV, Bartolucci AA: Variations in responsiveness and survival of clinical subsets of patients with metastatic breast cancer or two chemotherapy combinations. In Mouridsen HT, Palshoff T (eds): Breast Cancer—Experimental and Clinical Aspects, pp 223–226. Elmsford, NY, Pergamon Press, 1980
86. Kusma J: Some problems in evaluating tumor responses in the clinical drug evaluation program. Cancer Chemother Rep 50:113–118, 1966
87. Davis HL, Multhauf P, Klotz J: Comparison of cooperative group evaluation criteria for multiple-drug therapy for breast cancer. Cancer Treat Rep 64:507–517, 1980
88. Tonkin K, Tritchler D, Tannock I: Criteria of tumor response used in clinical trials of chemotherapy. J Clin Oncol 3:870–875, 1985
89. Rimm AA: Electronic computers for evaluation of clinical data. I. Man versus machine. Cancer Chemother Rep 50:141–149, 1966
90. Sears ME, Olson KB: Extramural review of clinical response of breast cancer to cytotoxic chemotherapy. Cancer 46:2928–2929, 1980
91. Slack NH: Electronic computers for evaluation of clinical data. II. Man versus man. Cancer Chemother Rep 50:150–163, 1966
92. Lavin PT, Flowerdew G: Studies in variation associated with the measurement of solid tumors. Cancer 46:1286–1290, 1980
93. Moertel CG, Hanley JA: The effect of measuring error on the results of therapeutic trials in advanced cancer. Cancer 38:388–394, 1976
94. Gurland J, Johnson R: How reliable are tumor measurements? JAMA 194:125–130, 1965
95. Blendis LM, McNeilly WJ, Sheppard L, et al: Observer variation in the clinical and radiological assessment of hepatosplenomegaly. Br Med J 1:727–730, 1970
96. Hagemeister FB, Buzdar AU, Luna MA, et al: Causes of death in breast cancer. Cancer 46:162–167, 1980
97. Hoogstraten B: Reporting treatment results in solid tumors. In Buyse ME, Staquet MJ, Sylvester RJ (eds): Cancer Clinical Trials, p 144. Oxford, Oxford University Press, 1984
98. Block JB, Schneiderman M, Chalmers TC, et al: Nonevaluable patients in cancer research. Cancer 36:1169–1173, 1975
99. Arnstein NB, Harbert JC, Byrne PJ: Efficacy of bone and liver scanning in breast cancer patients treated with adjuvant chemotherapy. Cancer 54:2243–2247, 1984
100. Scanlon EF, Oviedo MA, Cunningham MP, et al: Preoperative and follow-up procedures on patients with breast cancer. Cancer 46:977–979, 1980
101. Wickerham L, Fisher B, Cronin W, et al: The efficacy of bone scanning in the follow-up of patients with operable breast cancer. Breast Cancer Res Treat 4:303–307, 1984
102. McNeil BJ, Hanley J: Analysis of serial radionuclide bone images in osteosarcoma and breast carcinoma. Radiology 135:171–176, 1980
103. Pandya KJ, McFadden ET, Kalish LA, et al: Frequency and patterns of early disease recurrence and method of detection in operable breast cancer with pathologically positive axillary lymph nodes on Eastern Cooperative Oncology Group adjuvant studies: A preliminary report. Cancer Treat Symp 2:117–122, 1983
104. Nesto RW, Cady B, Oberfield RA, et al: Rebound response after estrogen therapy for metastatic breast cancer. Cancer 38:1834–1937, 1976
105. Kaufman RJ, Escher GC: Rebound regression in advanced mammary carcinoma. Surg Gynecol Obstet 113:635–640, 1961
106. Rossof AH, Creech RH: Randomized evaluation of combination chemotherapy versus observation following oophorectomy for metastatic breast cancer (abstr C-349). Proc Am Assoc Cancer Res and Clin Oncol 22: 1980
107. Antman K, Amato D, Wood W, et al: Selection bias in clinical trials. J Clin Oncol 3:1142–1147, 1985
108. Fisher RA: Statistical Methods for Research Workers. Edinburgh, Oliver & Boyd, 1934
109. Fleiss JL: Statistical Methods for Rates and Proportions, pp 24–26. New York, John Wiley & Sons, 1981
110. Harrington SW: Survival rates of radical mastectomy for unilateral and bilateral carcinoma of the breast. Surgery 154–166, 1945
111. Axtell LM, Cutler SJ, Myers MH (eds): End Results in Cancer—Report No. 4 (DHEW Publication No. NIH 73-272). Washington, DC, U.S. Government Printing Office, 1972
112. Fletcher RH, Fletcher SW, Wagner EH: Clinical Epidemiology: The Essentials, p 114. Baltimore, Williams & Wilkins, 1982
113. Falkson G, Gelman RS, Tormey DC, et al: The ECOG experience with Cyclophosphamide, Adriamycin, and 5-Fluorouracil (CAF) in patients with metastatic breast cancer. (Cancer) Cancer 56:219–224, 1985
114. Berkson J, Gage RP: Calculation of survival rates for cancer. Mayo Clin Proc 25:270–286, 1950
115. Cutler SJ, Ederer F: Maximum utilization of the life table method in analyzing survival. J Chronic Dis 8:699–712, 1958
116. Breslow N, Crowley J: A large sample study of the life table and product limit estimates under random censorship. Ann Stat 2:437–453, 1974
117. Kaplan EL, Meier P: Nonparametric estimation from incomplete observations. J Am Stat Assoc 53:457–481, 1958
118. Wanebo HJ: Letter: Treatment of breast cancer. N Engl J Med 3113:116, 1985
119. Fisher B, Redmond C: Reply to letters: Treatment of breast cancer. N Engl J Med 313:117–118, 1985
120. Greenwood M: The natural duration of cancer. Reports on Public Health and Medical Subjects. London, 33 Her Majesty's Stationery Office, 1926
121. Miller RG: Survival Analysis, pp 44–45, 50–52. New York, John Wiley & Sons, 1981
122. Lagakos SW, Williams JS: Models for censored survival analysis: A cone class of variable sum models. Biometrika 65:181–189, 1978
123. David HA, Moeschberger MC: The Theory of Competing Risks. London, Griffen, 1978
124. Fisher B, Bauer M, Margolese R, et al: Five-year results of a

randomized trial comparing total mastectomy and segmental mastectomy with or without radiation in the treatment of breast cancer. N Engl J Med 312:665–673, 1985

125. Peto J: Calculation and interpretation of survival curves. In Buyse MC, Staquet MJ, Sylvester RJ (eds): Cancer Clinical Trials: Methods and Practice, pp 361–380. Oxford, Oxford University Press, 1984
126. Prentice RL, Kalbfleisch JD, Peterson AV, et al: The analysis of failure times in the presence of competing risks. Biometrics 34:541–554, 1978
127. Peto R, Peto J: Asymptotically efficient rank test procedures. J R Stat Soc [A] 135:185–206, 1972
128. Savage IR: Contributions to the theory of rank order statistics. Ann Math Stat 27:590–615, 1956
129. Mantel N: Evaluation of survival data and two new rank order statistics arising in its consideration. Cancer Chemother Rep 50:163–170, 1966
130. Gelber RD, Zelen M: Planning and reporting of clinical trials. In Calabresi P, Schein PS, Rosenberg SA (eds): Medical Oncology, pp 406–425. New York, Macmillan, 1985
131. Gehan EA: A generalized Wilcoxon test for comparing arbitrarily singly-censored data. Biometrika 52:203–223, 1965
132. Elandt-Johnson RC, Johnson NL: Survival Models and Data Analysis, pp 225–264. New York, John Wiley & Sons, 1980
133. Breslow N: A generalized Kruskal-Wallis test for comparing k samples subject to unequal patterns of censorship. Biometrika 57:579–594, 1970
134. Tarone RE: On the distribution of the maximum of the logrank statistic and modified Wilcoxon statistic. Biometrics 37:79–96, 1981
135. Fleming TR, Green SJ, Harrington DP: Performing serial testing of treatment effects. In Baum M, Kay R, Scheurlen H (eds): Clinical Trials in Early Breast Cancer: Second Heidelberg Symposium, pp 469–484. Basel, Birkhaeuser Verlag, 1982
136. Lagakos SW: Inference in survival analysis: Nonparametric tests to compare survival distributions. In Miké V, Stanley KE (eds): Statistics in Medical Research: Methods and Issues with Applications in Cancer Research, pp 340–364. New York, John Wiley & Sons, 1982
137. Gelman R: Effects of reporting lags on interim inferences from clinical trials. In Baum M, Kay R, Scheurlen H (eds): Clinical Trials in Early Breast Cancer: Second Heidelberg Symposium, pp 175–186. Basel, Birkhaeuser Verlag, 1982
138. Hanley J, Gelman R: Effects of reporting lags on interim inferences from clinical trials (abstr): Proc Soc Clin Trials 1:142, 1980
139. Cox DR: Analysis of Binary Data, pp 58–71. London, Methuen & Co, 1970
140. Zelen M: The analysis of several 2 × 2 contingency tables. Biometrika 58:129–137, 1971
141. Mantel N, Haenszel W: Statistical aspects of the analysis of data from retrospective studies of disease. J Natl Cancer Inst 22:719–748, 1959
142. Kalbfleish JD, Prentice RL: The Statistical Analysis of Failure Time Data, pp 18–19. New York, John Wiley & Sons, 1980
143. Koch GG, Gillings DB, Stokes ME: Biostatistical implications of design, sampling, and measurement to health science data analysis. Annu Rev Public Health 1:163–225, 1980
144. Cox DR: Analysis of Binary Data, pp 14–26, 30–42. London, Methuen, 1970
145. Feigl P, Zelen M: Estimation of exponential survival probabilities with concomitant information. Biometrics 21:826–838, 1965
146. Fischer B, Redmond C, Brown A, et al: Influence of tumor estrogen and progesterone receptor levels on the response to tamoxifen and chemotherapy in primary breast cancer. J Clin Oncol 1:227–241, 1983
147. Byar DP: Analysis of suurvival data: Cox and Weibull models with covariates. In Miké V, Stanley KE (eds): Statistics in Medical Research, pp 365–401. New York, John Wiley & Sons, 1982
148. Cox DR: Regression models and life tables. J R Stat Soc [B] 34:187–220, 1972
149. Schoenfeld D: Partial residuals for the proportional hazards regression model. Biometrika 69:239–241, 1982
150. Finney DJ: Statistical Methods in Biological Assays. London, Griffen, 1964
151. Tsiatis AA: A note on the goodness-of-fit test for the logistic regression model. Biometrika 67:250–251, 1981
152. Harrel FE, Lee KL, Matcher DB, et al: Regression models for prognostic prediction: Advantages, problems, and suggested solutions. Cancer Treat Rep 69:1071–1077, 1985
153. Geisser S: The predictive sample reuse method with application. J Am Stat Assoc 70:320–328, 1975
154. Simon R: Use of regression models: Statistical aspects. In Buyse ME, Staquet MJ, Sylvester RJ (eds): Cancer Clinical Trials: Methods and Practice, pp 444–466. Oxford, Oxford University Press, 1984
155. Weisberg S: Applied Linear Regression, pp 174–182. New York, John Wiley & Sons, 1980
156. Stjernsward J: Decreased survival related to irradiation postoperatively in early operable breast cancer. Lancet 1:1285–1286, 1974
157. Stjernsward J, Day N: Rebuttal of two articles by Dr. Levitt et al. Cancer 40:381, 1977
158. Peto R: Presentation to NCI sponsored consensus conference on adjuvant breast cancer treatment. Bethesda, Maryland, September, 1985
159. Himel HN, Liberati A, Gelber RD, et al: Adjuvant chemotherapy for breast cancer: A pooled estimate based on results from published randomized control trials. JAMA 256:1148–1159, 1986
160. Levitt SH, McHugh RB: Letter: Early breast cancer and postoperative irradiation. Lancet 1:1258–1259, 1975
161. Levitt SH, McHugh RB, Song CW: Radiotherapy in the postoperative treatment of operable cancer of the breast. II. Cancer 39:933–940, 1976
162. Levitt SH, McHugh RB: Reply to rebuttal letter by Drs. Stjernward and Day. Cancer 40:382, 1977
163. Zelen M, Gelman R: The assessment of adjuvant trials in breast cancer. NCI Monographs, August, 1986

Index

Page numbers followed by *f* indicate a figure; *t* following a page number indicates tabular material.